Comprehensive Applied Basic Sciences

CABS

for MDS Students

Second Edition

As per DCI Syllabus:
New MDS Course Regulations, 2017

Questions–Answers

Presented in **Question–Answer** Form for Quick and Easy Review of Basic Subjects

The Book Covers

Human Anatomy, Embryology and Histology

Dental Anatomy and Dental Histology

Physiology

Biochemistry

Microbiology

Pathology

Pharmacology

Biostatistics and Research Methodology

Dental Materials

Genetics and Miscellaneous

Comprehensive Applied Basic Sciences

for MDS Students

CABS

Second Edition

As per DCI Syllabus:
New MDS Course Regulations, 2017

Questions–Answers

Suresh K Sachdeva MDS

Professor
Department of Oral Medicine and Radiology
Surendera Dental College and Research Institute
Sri Ganganagar, Rajasthan

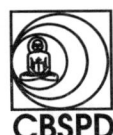

CBSPD

CBS Publishers & Distributors Pvt Ltd

New Delhi • Bengaluru • Chennai • Kochi • Kolkata • Mumbai

Hyderabad • Jharkhand • Nagpur • Patna • Pune • Uttarakhand

Comprehensive
Applied Basic Sciences
for MDS Students

CABS

Second Edition

Questions–Answers

ISBN: 978-81-94708-23-0

Second Edition: 2021
Reprint: 2022, 2023, **2024**
First Edition: 2016
Reprint: 2019, 2020

Published by **Satish Kumar Jain** and produced by **Varun Jain** for
CBS Publishers & Distributors Pvt Ltd
4819/XI Prahlad Street, 24 Ansari Road, Daryaganj, New Delhi 110 002, India
Ph: 011-23289259, 23266861   Website: www.cbspd.com
                                     e-mail: delhi@cbspd.com

Corporate Office: 204 FIE, Industrial Area, Patparganj, Delhi 110 092, India
Ph: 011-4934 4934   Fax: 011-4934 4935   e-mail: publishing@cbspd.com;
                                               publicity@cbspd.com

Branches

- **Bengaluru:** Seema House 2975, 17th Cross, KR Road, Banasankari 2nd Stage, Bengaluru 560 070, Karnataka, India
  Ph: +91-80-26771678/79   Fax: +91-80-26771680   e-mail: bangalore@cbspd.com
- **Chennai:** 7, Subbaraya Street, Shenoy Nagar, Chennai 600 030, Tamil Nadu, India
  Ph: +91-44-26680620, 26681266   Fax: +91-44-42032115   e-mail: chennai@cbspd.com
- **Kochi:** 42/1325, 1326, Power House Road, Opp KSEB, Power House, Ernakulum Kochi 682 018, Kerala, India
  Ph: +91-484-4059061-65,67   Fax: +91-484-4059065   e-mail: kochi@cbspd.com
- **Kolkata:** 147, Hind Ceramics Compound, 1st Floor, Nilgunj Road, Belghoria, Kolkata-700056, West Bengal, India
  Ph: +033-25633055, 033-25633056   e-mail: kolkata@cbspd.com
- **Lucknow:** Basement, Khushnuma Complex, 7 Meerabai Marg (Behind Jawahar Bhawan),Lucknow-226001, UP, India
  Ph: +91-522-4000032   e-mail: tiwari.lucknow@cbspd.com
- **Mumbai:** PWD Shed, Gala no 25/26, Ramchandra Bhatt Marg, Next to JJ Hospital Gate no. 2, Opp. Union Bank of India Noorbaug,
  Mumbai-400009, Maharashtra, India
  Ph: 022-66661880/89   e-mail: mumbai@cbspd.com

Representatives

- Hyderabad   0-9885175004   • Jharkhand   0-9811541605   • Nagpur   0-9421945513
- Patna   0-9334159340   • Pune   0-9923910676   • Uttarakhand 0-9716462459

Printed at: Mudrak, Noida, UP, India

to

my parents, wife and daughter

for their love and patience

and

all the students for making this ordinary book as "Extraordinary"

Foreword

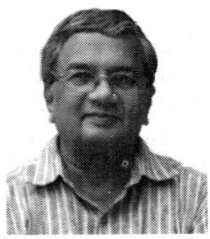

I am delighted to write the Foreword to the Second Edition of *Comprehensive Applied Basic Sciences* popularly known as **CABS for MDS students**, authored by Dr Suresh K Sachdeva.

Dr Sachdeva has carefully updated the art and science of basic science in the Second Edition using the same multidisciplinary approach that has been the hallmark of success of its First Edition. The fact that this book has reached its Second Edition is the best sign that you are holding in your hands a very successful book, and probably one of the dental bestsellers published in recent times. Up to now, it has been used by thousands of students and I am sure that it will continue to be read and cherished in the new edition as well.

For the Second Edition, Dr Sachdeva has partially restructured the book, substantially revised it, and updated the text wherever it was necessary, as per **DCI syllabus: New MDS Course Regulations, 2017.**

Furthermore, the author has dramatically increased the number of diagrams/illustrations, which are essential for understanding the subject of applied basic sciences. It will provide a helpful study material to MDS students and help them review the subject for examinations.

In summary, it is my distinct pleasure and honor to most enthusiastically endorse the new edition of an established book. Dr Sachdeva deserves the full appreciation for this compilation and providing the MDS students with such an attractive, comprehensive, up-to-date and useful book of applied basic science.

It is my hope and expectation that this book will provide an effective learning experience and referenced resource for MDS students and other potential readers.

H. R. Umarji

Prof (Dr) Hemant R Umarji
Former Head
Department of Oral Medicine and Radiology
Government Dental College and Hospital
Mumbai, Maharashtra
India

Foreword

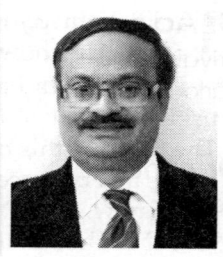

It gives me a great pleasure and sense of satisfaction in writing Foreword to the Second Edition of *Comprehensive Applied Basic Sciences (CABS), for MDS Students* authored by my junior colleague, Dr Suresh K Sachdeva. I have seen him as a young hardworking student, preparing for postgraduate entrance metamorphosing into a teacher of his capabilities. The newer guidelines set by the Dental Council of India prescribe basic sciences exam at the end of first year. Writing a theory book for the postgraduates is a herculean task that too in an examination point of view. The author has put a great effort to bring all the basic sciences under one umbrella and presented it as a compendium common to all the branches. Our present theory examination system, assess the results of a year-long study of entire basic sciences by a single question paper. The student sometimes finds it challenging to revise all the textbooks in the last phase of preparation. I do not hesitate to recommend that this a precious book in such a situation. The author has taken appropriate care to uniformly and reliably cover the entire basic sciences, but yet comprehensive. The subject is presented in a lucid manner in the form of question and answer type. The questions were drawn from previous year examination papers of various health universities. This gives an insight for the student what needs to be stressed during exam preparation. I have no doubt that dental postgraduates preparing for theory examinations will benefit from a careful study of this book. Careful thought and intelligent use of a sound knowledge of basic facts and principles will usually be more rewarding in the long run than plain memorizing. I wish him the very best in this and all his other professional endeavors.

Dr S Gowri Sankar
Professor
Department of Orthodontics
Narayana Dental College
Nellore, Andhra Pradesh
India

Contributors

Dr Aditi Mishra BDS
Private Practitioner
Faridabad, Haryana, India

Dr Ashok Galav MDS
Reader
Department of Oral Medicine and Radiology
Azamgarh Dental College
Azamgarh, UP, India

Dr Deepak Sharma MDS
Assistant Professor
Department of Periodontics
HP Government Dental College and Hospital
Shimla, Himachal Pradesh, India

Dr Manoj Vengal MDS
Professor
Department of Oral Medicine and Radiology
KMCT Dental College
Calicut, Kerala, India

Dr Poulomi Bhakta MDS
Senior Lecturer
Department of Oral Medicine and Radiology
Daswani Dental College and Research Centre
Kota, Rajasthan, India

Dr K Aravinda MDS
Professor and Head
Department of Oral Medicine and Radiology
Swami Devi Dyal Hospital and Dental College
Barwala, Haryana, India

Dr K Sridevi MDS
Professor and Head
Department of Oral Medicine and Radiology
Lenora Institute of Dental Sciences
Rajahmundry, Andhra Pradesh, India

Dr Sugandha Arya MDS
Reader
Department of Oral Medicine and Radiology
Vyas Dental College and Hospital
Jodhpur, Rajasthan, India

Preface to the Second Edition

"Your Own Work is More Inspirational Than Anything"

It is my pleasure to release the Second Edition of *Comprehensive Applied Basic Sciences (CABS) for MDS Students* within a few years of its First Edition with reprints in between as the book was well-accepted by students. This overwhelming success and all-round acceptance of the first edition was very encouraging and quite stimulating but at the same time put a huge responsibility and expectation to do better in the new edition. In preparing this edition, I pursued this goal with profound enthusiasm and passionate zeal with a wholly transformed appearance and updated contents in the Second Edition.

New Features: It is designed as per DCI syllabus according to New MDS Course Regulations, 2017 for MDS students (Applied Basic Sciences) with more illustrations, more diagrams and flowcharts. I have extensively done corrections in this edition as per the feedback received from students for previous edition. I have added many new materials with recent classifications, text details, new question papers (1999–2020) from major health universities Pan-India and insufficient topics are upgraded. The basic essence is maintained as all questions are provided with crisp, most refined and "to the point" answers to make it more interesting. "Suggested Reading" section contains more number of references from journals/textbook for students who want to read the subject/topics in depth.

How to Use this Book: Before starting this book, students are advised to go through the latest syllabus for Part I given at the beginning, as all the basic science subjects are not in the syllabus of all the specialties. Moreover, within the subjects, a few questions are speciality specific that can also be skipped by other speciality students. So, students preparing for Part I need to use this book in a smart, specific and precise manner, to get the best out of this edition. While this book has been compiled for postgraduate students, I am confident that it will serve as a useful reference for students preparing for NEET-MDS Exams, undergraduates and practitioners. I sincerely welcome all suggestions and constructive criticisms towards improving this book in subsequent editions at *cabsformds@rediffmail.com*

September, 2020

Suresh K Sachdeva

Preface to the First Edition

I have written *Comprehensive Applied Basic Sciences (CABS) for MDS Students* not as an author but as a student. When I was doing my postgraduation, every student used to read multiple books, seminars, articles for the applied basic science paper, which consumed a lot of precious time and create unnecessary stress during exam time. If we do preparations as per the previous year's question papers, some difficult and twisted questions make the situation worse. This lead a strong feeling in me to write a comprehensive book for the applied basic sciences which contains all the subjects as solved question–answers, from all over India. I have tried my best to bring out a book which can invoke interest in students in this subject. The basic aim of writing this book is to make the students familiar with the usually asked questions and to give a clear picture of an answer to be written in a particular question.

This book holds the potential of filling the gap that has been felt by dental postgraduate students for years. This book provides the readers a comprehensive and concise overview of the basic science subjects with ten chapters, each having the previous years' questions with answers from almost all the universities of India, arranged as per the syllabus prescribed by Dental Council of India.

The questions are answered as short notes, long questions with "to the point" answers. Also the variants of a question asked in different universities have also been added. Moreover, the answers are selected from the standard textbooks which are usually used by students, to avoid any confusion. And where the answers have been taken from the articles, proper citation of the reference has been given.

This book is written to bring out a concise, easily understandable resource for students to learn and guide them to write well structured answers in their examinations.

I hope that the book will fulfill the need of the students by giving them relevant guidance during their preparation for examination. I am confident that the readers will be greatly benefited by my effort.

I have tried my best to cover all the aspect of applied basic sciences as per the DCI syllabus in my book. As no one is perfect, I humbly accept my limitations regarding shortcomings in the book and I sincerely welcome the constructive suggestions from the readers of this book at cabsformds@rediffmail.com

April, 2016

Suresh K Sachdeva

Acknowledgments

I thank Almighty for the grand success of first edition of CABS for MDS students, which inspired me to work on Second Edition with more enthusiasm and zeal.

My family and friends deserve my heartfelt acknowledgement for their unconditional support.

I appreciate the support and guidance received from the Prof (Dr) Vishal Dang Sir, Past President, Indian Academy of Oral Medicine and Radiology, New Delhi, and Prof (Dr) Sreenivasan V, Principal, BVP Dental College, Navi Mumbai, Maharashtra, India, during the testing time of my professional career.

I would like to extend my special thanks and sincere regards to Prof (Dr) Hemant R Umarji sir and Prof (Dr) S Gowri Sankar sir for kind enough to me in writing the foreword to this book.

I would always be grateful to my teachers at Department of Oral Medicine and Radiology, Tamil Nadu Government Dental College and Hospital, Chennai and DAV (C) Dental College and Hospital, Yamunanagar.

The revision work was indeed a mammoth task to accomplish and would not have been possible without active cooperation from friends and colleagues, who provided valuable feedback of the first edition. I am thankful to Dr Shekhar Kapoor (CDC, Ludhiana), Dr Manas Gupta (Bhopal), Dr Pritesh Ruparelia (Ahmedabad), Dr Sanjay Dutta (GDC, Guwahati), Dr (Major) Ravi Athawale, Dr Purnendu Rout (KIDS, Bhubaneswar), Dr Avinash L Kashid (Ambajogai), Dr Abhishek Sinha (Lucknow), Dr Saurabh Srivastava (Lucknow), Dr Hemant Sawhney (Greater Noida), Dr Bhuvan Jyoti (Ranchi), Dr Ranjeeta Mehta (Rishikesh), Dr Lavina Taneja, Dr K Sashikumar Singh (RIMS, Imphal), Dr Mohsin Muzaffar Tak (GDC, Srinagar), Dr Varun Chopra (Chandigarh), Dr Ravleen Nagi (Panchkula), Dr P Redwin (Kanyakumari), Dr Bhaumik Joshi (Ahmedabad), Dr Ashish Kakkar (Sirsa) for provided me Question Papers from Pan-India on prompt basis.

Last but not the least; I am greatly indebted to Mr Satish Kumar Jain (CMD), Mr YN Arjuna (Senior Vice-President) for continuing faith in me in publishing second edition on time. I also need to say thanks to the entire staff of CBS Publishers & Distributors for patiently answering all my queries and beautifully doing the book work.

September, 2020   Suresh K Sachdeva

Contents

SYLLABUS FOR MDS IN VARIOUS SPECIALTIES

The syllabus for MDS course includes both Applied Basic Sciences and subjects of concerned specialty. The syllabus in Applied Basic Sciences shall vary according to the particular specialty; similarly the candidates shall also acquire adequate knowledge in other subjects related to their respective specialty.

Scheme of Examination: Part I: Basic Science Paper: 100 Marks (10×10). At the end of First year MDS.

1. PROSTHODONTICS AND CROWN AND BRIDGE

APPLIED ANATOMY OF HEAD AND NECK

General Human Anatomy: Gross Anatomy, anatomy of Head and Neck in detail: Cranial and facial bones, TMJ and function, muscles of mastication and facial expression, muscles of neck and back including muscles of deglutition and tongue, arterial supply and venous drainage of the head and neck, anatomy of the para nasal sinuses in relation to the Vth cranial nerve. General considerations of the structure and function of the brain, brief considerations of V, VII, XI, XII, cranial nerves and autonomic nervous system of the head and neck. The salivary glands, pharynx, larynx, trachea, esophagus, functional anatomy of masticatory muscles, deglutition, speech, respiration, and circulation, teeth eruption, morphology, occlusion and function. Anatomy of TMJ, its movements and myofacial pain dysfunction syndrome.

Embryology: Development of the face, tongue, jaws, TMJ, paranasal sinuses, pharynx, larynx, trachea, esophagus, salivary glands, development of oral and para oral tissues including detailed aspects of tooth formation.

Growth and Development: Facial form and facial growth and development overview of dentofacial growth process and physiology from fetal period to maturity and old age, general physical growth, functional and anatomical aspects of the head, changes in craniofacial skeletal development, relationship between development of the dentition and facial growth.

Dental Anatomy: Anatomy of primary and secondary dentition, concept of occlusion, mechanism of articulation, and masticatory function. Detailed structural and functional study of the oral and para oral tissues, normal occlusion, development of occlusion in deciduous mixed and permanent dentitions, root length, root configuration and tooth-numbering systems.

Histology: Histology of enamel, dentin, cementum, periodontal ligament and alveolar bone, pulpal anatomy, histology and biological consideration. Salivary glands and histology of epithelial tissues including glands. Histology of general and specific connective tissue including bone, salivary glands, histology of skin, oral mucosa, respiratory mucosa, connective tissue, bone, cartilage, cellular elements of blood vessels, blood, lymphatics, nerves, muscles, tongue and tooth.

Cell biology: Brief study of the structure and function of the mammalian cell Components of the cell and functions of various types of cells and their consequences with tissue injury.

APPLIED PHYSIOLOGY AND NUTRITION

Introduction, mastication, deglutition, digestion and assimilation, homeostasis, fluid and electrolyte balance, blood composition, volume, function, blood groups and hemorrhage, blood transfusion, circulation, heart, pulse, blood pressure, capillary and lymphatic circulation. Shock, respiration, control, anoxia, hypoxia, asphyxia, artificial respiration. Endocrine glands in particular reference to pituitary, parathyroid and thyroid glands and sex hormones. Role of calcium and Vit D in growth and development of teeth, bone and jaws. Role of Vit A, C and B complex in oral mucosal and periodontal health. Physiology and function of the masticatory system. Speech mechanism, mastication, swallowing and deglutition mechanism, salivary glands and saliva.

Endocrines: General principles of endocrine activity and disorders relating to pituitary, thyroid, pancreas, parathyroid, adrenals, gonads, including pregnancy and lactation. Physiology of saliva, urine formation, normal and abnormal constituents, physiology of pain, sympathetic and parasympathetic nervous system, neuromuscular coordination of the stomatognathic system.

Applied Nutrition

General principles, balanced diet, effect of dietary deficiencies and starvation, diet, digestion, absorption, transportation and utilization and diet for elderly patients.

Applied Biochemistry

General principles governing the various biological activities of the body, such as osmotic pressure, electrolytic dissociation, oxidation-reduction carbohydrates, proteins, liquids and their metabolism; Enzymes, vitamins, and minerals; Hormones; Blood; Metabolism of inorganic elements; Detoxification in the body and antimetabolites.

APPLIED PHARMACOLOGY AND THERAPEUTICS

Dosage and mode of administration of drugs. Action and fate of drugs in the body, drug addiction, tolerance and hypersensitive reactions; Drugs acting on the central nervous system, general anesthetics hypnotics, analeptics and tranquilizers. Local anesthetics; Chemotherapeutics and antibiotics; Antitubercular and antisyphilitic drugs; Analgesics and antipyretics; Antiseptics; Styptics; Sialogogue and antisialogogues; Haematinics; Cortisones; ACTH; Insulin and other antidiabetic vitamins: A, D, B-complex group C, K, etc. Chemotherapy and radiotherapy; Drug regime for antibiotic prophylaxis and infectious endocarditis and drug therapy following dental surgical treatments like placement of implants, pre- and periprosthetic surgery.

APPLIED PATHOLOGY

Inflammation, repair and degeneration; Necrosis and gangrene; Circulatory disturbances; Ischemia, hyperemia, chronic venous congestion, edema, thrombosis, embolism and infarction. Infection and infective granulomas; Allergy and hypersensitive reactions; Neoplasms; Classification of tumors; Carcinogenesis; Characteristics of benign and malignant tumors; Spread of tumors. Applied histopathology and clinical pathology.

APPLIED MICROBIOLOGY

Immunity, knowledge of organisms commonly associated with diseases of the oral cavity (morphology cultural characteristics, etc.) of Strepto, Staphylo; Clostridia group of organisms, spirochetes, organisms of tuberculosis, leprosy, diphtheria, actinomycosis and moniliasis, etc. Virology; Cross infection control, sterilization and hospital waste management.

a. **Applied Oral Pathology:** Developmental disturbances of oral and para oral structures, Regressive changes of teeth; Bacterial, viral and mycotic infections of the oral cavity. Dental caries, diseases of pulp and periapical tissues; Physical and chemical injuries of the oral cavity, oral manifestations of metabolic and endocrine disturbances; Diseases of the blood and blood forming organism in relation to the oral cavity; Periodontal diseases; Diseases of the skin, nerves and muscles in relation to the oral cavity.

b. **Laboratory Determinations:** Blood groups, blood matching, RBC and WBC count, bleeding and clotting time, PT, PTT and INR smears and cultures—urine analysis and culture. Interpretation of RBS, glycosylated Hb, GTT.

Biostatistics: Characteristics and limitations of statistics, planning of statistical experiments, sampling, collection, classification and presentation of data (tables, graphs, pictograms, etc.) and Analysis of data, parametric and nonparametric tests.

Introduction to Biostatistics

Scope and need for statistical application to biological data. Definition of selected terms—scale of measurements related to statistics, methods of collecting data, presentation of the statistical diagrams and graphs. Frequency curves, mean, mode of median; Standard deviation and co-efficient of variation, Correlation-Co-efficient and its significance, Binominal distributions normal distribution and Poisson's distribution, Tests of significance.

RESEARCH METHODOLOGY

Understanding and evaluating dental research, scientific method and the behavior of scientists, understanding to logic-inductive logic-analogy, models, authority, hypothesis and causation. Measurement and Errors of measurement, presentation of results, Reliability, Sensitivity and specificity diagnosis tests and measurements, Research Strategies, Observation, Correlation, Experimentation and Experimental design. Logic of statistical in(ter)ferences, balance judgments, judgment under uncertainty, clinical vs. scientific judgment, problems with clinical judgment, forming scientific judgments, the problem of contradictory evidence, citation analysis as a Means of literature evaluation, influencing judgment: Protocol writing for experimental, observational studies, survey including hypothesis, PICO statement, aim objectives, sample size justification, use of control/placebo, standardization techniques, bias and its elimination, blinding, evaluation, inclusion and exclusion criteria.

APPLIED RADIOLOGY

Introduction, radiation, background of radiation, sources, radiation biology, somatic damage, genetic damage, protection from primary and secondary radiation, Principles of X-ray production, Applied principles of radiotherapy and after care.

ROENTGENOGRAPHIC TECHNIQUES

Intra oral, extra oral roentgenography, Methods of localization digital radiology and ultrasounds. Normal anatomical landmarks of teeth and jaws in radiograms, temporomandibular joint radiograms, neck radiograms. Use of CT and CBCT in prosthodontics.

APPLIED MEDICINE

Systemic diseases and (its) their influence on general health and oral and dental health. Medical emergencies like syncope, hyperventilation, angina, seizure, asthma and allergy/anaphylaxis in the dental offices-Prevention, preparation, medicolegal consideration, unconsciousness, respiratory distress, altered consciousness, seizures, drug related emergencies, chest pain, cardiac arrest, premedication, prophylaxis and management of ambulatory patients, resuscitation, applied psychiatry, child, adult and senior citizens.

APPLIED SURGERY AND ANESTHESIA

General principles of surgery, wound healing, incision wound care, hospital care, control of hemorrhage, electrolyte balance. Common bandages, sutures, splints, shifting of critically ill patients, prophylactic therapy, bone surgeries, grafts, etc, surgical techniques, nursing assistance, anesthetic assistance. Principles in speech therapy, surgical and radiological craniofacial oncology, applied surgical ENT and ophthalmology.

APPLIED PLASTIC SURGERY

Applied understanding and assistance in programs of plastic surgery for prosthodontics therapy.

APPLIED DENTAL MATERIALS

Students should have understanding of all materials used for treatment of craniofacial disorders: Clinical, treatment, and laboratory materials, associated materials, technical considerations, shelf life, storage, manipulations, sterilization, and waste management. Students shall acquire knowledge of testing biological, mechanical and other physical properties of all materials used for the clinical and laboratory procedures in prosthodontics therapy.

2. PERIODONTOLOGY

APPLIED BASIC SCIENCES APPLIED ANATOMY

Development of the Peridontium, Micro and Macro structural anatomy and biology of the periodontal tissues, Age changes in the periodontal tissues, Anatomy of the Peridontium (macroscopic and microscopic anatomy, Blood supply of the Periodontium, Lymphatic system of the Periodontium, Nerves of the Periodontium), Temporomandibular joint, Maxillae and Mandible, Tongue, oropharynx, Muscles of mastication/Face, Blood Supply and Nerve Supply of Head and Neck and Lymphatics, Spaces of Head and Neck.

PHYSIOLOGY

Blood; Respiratory system—knowledge of the respiratory diseases which are a cause of periodontal diseases (periodontal Medicine); Cardiovascular system (Blood pressure, Normal ECG, Shock), Endocrinology-hormonal influences on Peridontium, Gastrointestinal system (Salivary secretion-composition, function and regulation, Reproductive physiology, Hormones—Actions and regulations, role in periodontal disease, Family planning methods), Nervous system (Pain pathways; Taste-Taste buds; primary taste sensation and pathways for sensation), Hemostasis.

BIOCHEMISTRY

Basics of carbohydrates, lipids, proteins, vitamins, enzymes and minerals; Diet and nutrition and Peridontium; Biochemical tests and their significance; Calcium and phosphorus.

PATHOLOGY

Cell structure and metabolism, Inflammation and repair, necrosis and degeneration, Immunity and hypersensitivity, Circulatory disturbances-edema, hemorrhage, shock, thrombosis, embolism, infarction and hypertension, Disturbances of nutrition, Diabetes mellitus, Cellular growth and differentiation, regulation, Lab investigations, Blood

MICROBIOLOGY

General bacteriology (Identification of bacteria, Culture media and methods, Sterilization and disinfection), Immunology and Infection, Systemic bacteriology with special emphasis on oral microbiology-staphylococci, genus actinomyces and other filamentous bacteria and actinobacillus actinomycetumcomitans, Virology (General properties of viruses, Herpes, Hepatitis, virus, HIV virus), Mycology (Candidiasis), Applied microbiology, Diagnostic microbiology and immunology, hospital infections and management.

PHARMACOLOGY

General pharmacology (Definitions-Pharmacokinetics with clinical applications, routes of administration including local drug delivery in Periodontics, Adverse drug reactions and drug interactions), Detailed pharmacology of Analgesics-opiod and nonopiod, Local anesthetics, Haematinics and coagulants, Anticoagulants, Vit D and Calcium preparations, Antidiabetics drugs, Steroids, Antibiotics, Antihypertensive, Immunosuppressive drugs and their effects on oral tissues, Antiepileptic drugs Brief pharmacology, dental use and adverse effects of General anesthetics, Antipsychotics, Antidepressants, Anxiolytic drugs, Sedatives, Antiepileptics, Antihypertensives, Antianginal drugs, Diuretics, Hormones, Pre-anesthetic medications, Drugs used in Bronchial asthma, cough, Drug therapy of Emergencies, Seizures, Anaphylaxis, Bleeding, Shock, Diabetic Ketoacidosis, Acute addisonian crisis Dental Pharmacology: Antiseptics, Astringents, Sialogogues, Disclosing agents, Antiplaque agents, Fluoride pharmacology.

BIOSTATISTICS

Introduction, definition and branches of biostatistics, Collection of data, sampling, types, bias and errors, Compiling data-graphs and charts, Measures of central tendency (mean, median and mode), standard deviation and variability, Tests of significance (chi square test, t-test and z-test), Null hypothesis.

3. ORAL AND MAXILLOFACIAL SURGERY

Applied Anatomy

1. Surgical anatomy of the scalp, temple and face
2. Anatomy of the triangles of neck and deep structures of the neck
3. Cranial and facial bones and its surrounding soft tissues with its applied aspects in maxillofacial injuries.

4. Muscles of head and neck; chest, lower and upper extremities (in consideration to grafts/flaps)
5. Arterial supply, venous drainage and lymphatics of head and neck
6. Congenital abnormalities of the head and neck
7. Surgical anatomy of the cranial nerves
8. Anatomy of the tongue and its applied aspects
9. Surgical anatomy of the temporal and infratemporal regions
10. Anatomy and its applied aspects of salivary glands, pharynx, thyroid and parathyroid gland, larynx, trachea, esophagus
11. Tooth eruption, morphology, and occlusion
12. Surgical anatomy of the nose
13. The structure and function of the brain including surgical anatomy of intra cranial venous sinuses
14. Autonomous nervous system of head and neck
15. Functional anatomy of mastication, deglutition, speech, respiration and circulation
16. Development of face, paranasal sinuses and associated structures and their anomalies
17. TMJ: Surgical anatomy and function. Physiology of nerve conduction, pain pathway, sympathetic and parasympathetic nervous system, hypothalamus and mechanism of controlling body temperature.

Physiology

1. **Nervous system:** Physiology of nerve conduction, pain pathway, sympathetic and parasympathetic nervous system, hypothalamus and mechanism of controlling body temperature
2. **Blood:** Composition, Haemostasis, various blood dyscrasias and management of patients with the same, Hemorrhage and its control, Capillary and lymphatic circulation, Blood grouping, transfusing procedures.
3. **Digestive system:** Saliva—composition and functions of saliva, Mastication, deglutition, digestion, assimilation, Urine formation, normal and abnormal constituents.
4. **Respiration:** Control of ventilation, anoxia, asphyxia, artificial respiration, Hypoxia—types and management.
5. **Cardiovascular System:** Cardiac cycle, Shock, Heart sounds, Blood pressure, Hypertension.
6. **Endocrinology:** General endocrinal activity and disorder relating to thyroid gland, Parathyroid gland, adrenal gland, pituitary gland, pancreas and gonads, Metabolism of calcium.
7. **Nutrition:** General principles of a balanced diet, effect of dietary deficiency, protein energy malnutrition, Kwashiorkor, Marasmus. Fluid and Electrolytic balance in maintaining haemostasis and significance in minor and major surgical procedures.

Biochemistry

General principles governing the various biological activities of the body, such as osmotic pressure, electrolytes, dissociation, oxidation, reduction etc. General composition of the body, Intermediary metabolism, Carbohydrates, proteins, lipids, and their metabolism. Nucleoproteins, nucleic acid and nucleotides and their metabolism, Enzymes, vitamins and minerals, Hormones, Body and other fluids. Metabolism of inorganic elements, Detoxification in the body, Antimetabolites.

Pathology

1. **Inflammation:** Repair and regeneration, necrosis and gangrene, Role of component system in acute inflammation, Role of arachidonic acid and its metabolites in acute inflammation, Growth factors in acute inflammation, Role of molecular events in cell growth and intercellular signaling cell surface receptors, Role of NSAIDs in inflammation, Cellular changes in radiation injury and its manifestation.
2. **Haemostasis:** Role of endothelium in thrombogenesis, Arterial and venous thrombi, Disseminated Intravascular coagulation
3. **Shock:** Pathogenesis of hemorrhagic, neurogenic, septic, cardiogenic shock, Circulatory disturbances, ischemia, hyperemia, venous congestion, edema, infarction
4. **Chromosomal abnormalities:** Marfans Syndrome; Ehlers-Danlos Syndrome; Fragile X- Syndrome

5. **Hypersensitivity:** Anaphylaxis, type 2 hypersensitivity, type 3 hypersensitivity and cell mediated reaction and its clinical importance, systemic lupus erythematosus, Infection and infective granulomas.
6. **Neoplasia:** Classification of tumors, Carcinogenesis and carcinogens- chemical, viral and microbial, Grading and staging of cancers, tumor Angiogenesis, Paraneoplastic syndrome, spread of tumors, Characteristics of benign and malignant tumors
7. **Others:** Sex linked agammaglobulinemia, AIDS, Management of immune deficiency patients requiring surgical procedures, Di George Syndrome, Ghons complex, post primary pulmonary tuberculosis—pathology and pathogenesis.

Oral Pathology

Developmental disturbances of oral and paraoral structures; Regressive changes of teeth. Bacterial, viral and mycotic infections of oral cavity. Dental caries, diseases of pulp and periapical tissues; Physical and chemical injuries of the oral cavity. Oral manifestations of metabolic and endocrinal disturbances. Diseases of jawbones and TMJ. Diseases of blood and blood forming organs in relation to oral cavity. Cysts of the oral cavity; Salivary gland diseases. Role of laboratory investigations in oral surgery.

Microbiology

Immunity, Knowledge of organisms commonly associated with diseases of oral cavity. Morphology cultural characteristics of strepto, staphylo, pneumo, gono, meningo, clostridium group of organisms, spirochetes, organisms of TB, leprosy, diphtheria, actinomycosis and moniliasis. Hepatitis B and its prophylaxis. Culture and sensitivity test, Laboratory determinations. Blood groups, blood matching, RBC and WBC count, Bleeding and clotting time etc, smears and cultures. Urine analysis and cultures.

Applied Pharmacology and Therapeutics

1. Definition of terminologies used
2. Dosage and mode of administration of drugs
3. Action and fate of drugs in the body
4. Drug addiction, tolerance and hypersensitivity reactions
5. Drugs acting on the CNS
6. General and local anesthetics, hypnotics, analeptics, and tranquilizers
7. Chemo therapeutics and antibiotics
8. Analgesics and antipyretics, Antitubercular and antisyphilitic drugs, Antiseptics, Sialogogue and antisialogogues
9. Haematinics, Antidiabetic, Vitamins A, B-complex, C, D, E, K

4. CONSERVATIVE DENTISTRY AND ENDODONTICS

Applied Anatomy of Head and Neck

Development of face, paranasal sinuses and the associated structures and their anomalies; cranial and facial bones; TMJ anatomy and function; Arterial and venous drainage of head and neck; Muscles of face and neck including muscles of mastication and deglutition; brief consideration of structures and function of brain. Brief consideration of all cranial nerves and autonomic nervous system of head and neck. Salivary glands; Functional anatomy of mastication, deglutition and speech. Detailed anatomy of deciduous and permanent teeth, general consideration in physiology of permanent dentition, form, function, alignment, contact, occlusion; Internal anatomy of permanent teeth and its significance, Applied histology-histology of skin, oral mucosa, connective tissue, bone, cartilage, blood vessels, lymphatics, nerves, muscles, tongue.

Anatomy and Development of Teeth

Enamel-development and composition, physical characteristics, chemical properties, structure, Age changes-clinical structure. Dentin-development, physical and chemical properties, structure type of dentin, innervations, age and functional changes and clinical considerations. Pulp-development, histological structures, innervations, functions, regressive changes, clinical considerations, Dentin and pulp complex. Cementum-composition, cementogenesis, structure, function, clinical considerations. Knowledge of internal anatomy of permanent teeth, anatomy of root apex and its implications in endodontic treatment. Periodontal ligament-development, structure, function and clinical considerations. Salivary glands-structure, function, clinical considerations.

Applied Physiology

- Mastication, deglutition, digestion and assimilation, fluid and electrolyte balance.
- Blood composition, volume, function, blood groups, haemostasis, coagulation, blood transfusion, circulation, heart, pulse, blood pressure, shock, respiration-control, anoxia, hypoxia, asphyxia, artificial respiration, and endocrinology-general principles of endocrine activity and disorders relating to pituitary, thyroid, parathyroid, adrenals including pregnancy and lactation.
- Physiology of saliva-composition, function, clinical significance.
- Clinical significance of vitamins, diet and nutrition-balanced diet.
- Physiology of pain, sympathetic and Para sympathetic nervous system, pain pathways, physiology of pulpal pain, Odontogenic and non Odontogenic pain, pain disorders-typical and atypical.
- Biochemistry such as osmotic pressure, electrolytic dissociation, oxidation, reduction, etc. Carbohydrates, proteins, lipids and their metabolism, nucleoproteins, nucleic acid and their metabolism. Enzymes, vitamins and minerals, metabolism of inorganic elements, detoxification in the body, anti metabolites, chemistry of blood lymph and urine.

Pathology

Inflammation, repair, degeneration, necrosis and gangrene, Circulatory disturbances-ischemia, hyperemia, edema, thrombosis, embolism, infarction, allergy and hypersensitivity reaction, Neoplasms-classifications of tumors, characteristics of benign and malignant tumors, spread of tumors, Blood dyscrasias. Developmental disturbances of oral and Para oral structures, dental caries, regressive changes of teeth, pulp, periapical pathology, pulp reaction to dental caries and dental procedures, Bacterial, viral, mycotic infections of the oral cavity.

Microbiology

- Pathways of pulpal infection, oral flora and micro-organisms associated with endodontic diseases, pathogenesis, host defense, bacterial virulence factors, healing, theory of focal infections, microbes relevance to dentistry–strepto, staphylococci, lactobacilli, corynebacterium, actinomycetes, clostridium, neisseria, vibrio, bacteriods, fusobacteria, spirochetes, mycobacterium, virus and fungi.
- Cross infection, infection control, infection control procedure, sterilization and disinfection.
- Immunology—antigen–antibody reaction, allergy, hypersensitivity and anaphylaxis, auto immunity, grafts, viral hepatitis, HIV infections and aids. Identification and isolation of microorganisms from infected root canals. Culture medium and culturing technique (Aerobic and anaerobic interpretation and antibiotic sensitivity test).

Pharmacology

- Dosage and route of administration of drugs, actions and fate of drug in body, drug addiction, tolerance of hypersensitivity reactions.
- Local anesthesia—agents and chemistry, pharmacological actions, fate and metabolism of anaesthetic, ideal properties, techniques and complications.
- General anesthesia—premedications, neuromuscular blocking agents, induction agents, inhalation anesthesia, and agents used assessment of anesthetic problems in medically compromised patients.
- Anaesthetic emergencies
- Antihistamines, corticosteroids, chemotherapeutic and antibiotics, drug resistance, haemostasis, and haemostatic agents, anticoagulants, sympathomimetic drugs, vitamins and minerals (A, B, C, D, E, K, iron), anti-sialogogue, immunosuppressant, drug interactions, antiseptics, disinfectants, antiviral agents, drugs acting on CNS.

Biostatistics

Introduction, Basic concepts, Sampling, Health information systems-collection, compilation, presentation of data. Elementary statistical methods-presentation of statistical data, Statistical averages-measures of central tendency, measures of dispersion, Normal distribution. Tests of significance-parametric and non-parametric tests (Fisher extract test, Sign test, Median test, Mann-Whitney test, Kruskal-Wallis one way analysis, Friedmann two-way analysis, ANOVA, Regression analysis), Correlation and regression, Use of computers.

Research Methodology

Essential features of a protocol for research in humans, Experimental and non-experimental study designs, Ethical considerations of research.

Applied Dental Materials

Physical and mechanical properties of dental materials, biocompatibility. Impression materials, detailed study of various restorative materials, restorative resin and recent advances in composite resins, bonding-recent developments, tarnish and corrosion, dental amalgam, direct filling gold, casting alloys, inlay wax, die materials, investments, casting procedures, defects, dental cements for restoration and pulp protection (luting, liners, bases) cavity varnishes. Dental ceramics-recent advances, finishing and polishing materials. Dental burs-design and mechanics of cutting-other modalities of tooth preparation. Methods of testing biocompatibility of materials used.

5. ORTHODONTICS AND DENTOFACIAL ORTHOPEDICS

Applied Anatomy

a. Prenatal growth of head: Stages of embryonic development, origin of head, origin of face, origin of teeth.
b. Postnatal growth of head: Bones of skull, the oral cavity, development of chin, the hyoid bone, general growth of head, growth of the face.
c. Bone growth: Origin of bone, composition of bone, units of bone structure, schedule of Ossification, mechanical properties of bone, roentgen graphic appearance of bone
d. Assessment of growth and development: Growth prediction, growth spurts, the concept of normality and growth increments of growth, differential growth, gradient of growth, methods of gathering growth data. Theories of growth and recent advances, factors affecting physical growth.
e. Muscles of mastication: Development of muscles, muscle change during growth, muscle function and facial development, muscle function and malocclusion
f. Development of dentition and occlusion: Dental development periods, order of tooth eruption, chronology of permanent tooth formation, periods of occlusal development, pattern of occlusion.
g. Assessment of skeletal age.

Physiology

Endocrinology and its disorders: Growth hormone, thyroid hormone, parathyroid hormone, ACTH. Calcium and its metabolism. Nutrition-metabolism and their disorders: Proteins, carbohydrates, fats, vitamins and minerals. Muscle physiology. Craniofacial Biology: Adhesion molecules and mechanism of adhesion. Bleeding disorders in orthodontics: Hemophilia.

Dental Materials

a. Gypsum products: Dental plaster, dental stone and their properties, setting reaction, etc.
b. Impression materials: Impression materials in general and particularly of alginate impression material.
c. Acrylics: Chemistry, composition physical properties
d. Composites: Composition types, properties, setting reaction
e. Banding and bonding cements.
f. Wrought metal alloys: Deformation, strain hardening, annealing, recovery, recrystallization, grain growth, properties of metal alloys
g. Orthodontic arch wires, Elastics: Latex and non-latex elastics.

h. Applied physics, Bioengineering and metallurgy, Specification and tests methods used for materials used in Orthodontics, Survey of all contemporary literature and recent advances in above mentioned materials.

Genetics: Cell structure, DNA, RNA, protein synthesis, cell division. Chromosomal abnormalities. Principles of orofacial genetics. Genetics in malocclusion. Molecular basis of genetics. Studies related to malocclusion. Recent advances in genetics related to malocclusion. Genetic counseling. Bioethics and relationship to Orthodontic management of patients.

Physical Anthropology: Evolutionary development of dentition, Evolutionary development of jaws.

Pathology: Inflammation, Necrosis

Biostatistics: Statistical principles. Data Collection, Method of presentation. Method of Summarizing. Methods of analysis, different tests/errors. Sampling and Sampling technique. Experimental models, design and interpretation. Development of skills for preparing clear concise and cogent scientific abstracts and publication

Applied Research Methodology in Orthodontics: Experimental design. Animal experimental protocol. Principles in the development, execution and interpretation of methodologies in Orthodontics. Critical Scientific appraisal of literature.

Applied Pharmacology: Definitions and terminologies used-Dosage and mode of administration of drugs. Action and fate of drugs in the body, Drug addiction, tolerance and hypersensitive reactions, Drugs acting on the central nervous system, general anesthetics hypnotics, analeptics and tranquilizers. Local anesthetics, Chemotherapeutics and antibiotics. Vitamins: A, D, B-complex group, C and K, etc.

6. ORAL AND MAXILLOFACIAL PATHOLOGY AND ORAL MICROBIOLOGY

1. **Biostatistics and Research Methodology:** Basic principles of biostatistics and study as applied to dentistry and research. Collection/organization of data/measurement scales/presentation of data and analysis. Measures of central tendency, Measures of variability. Sampling and planning of health survey. Probability, normal distribution and indicative statistics. Estimating population values. Tests of significance (parametric/non-parametric qualitative methods). Analysis of variance, Association, correlation and regression

2. **Applied Gross Anatomy of head and neck, histology and genetics:** Temporomandibular joint. Trigeminal nerve and facial nerve. Muscles of mastication, Tongue, Salivary glands, Nerve supply, blood supply, lymphatic drainage and venous drainage of oro-dental tissues. Development of face, palate, mandible, maxilla, tongue and applied aspects of the same. Development of teeth and dental tissues and developmental defects of oral and maxilla-facial region and abnormalities of teeth. Maxillary sinus. Jaw muscles and facial muscles. Introduction to genetics. Modes of inheritance. Chromosomal anomalies of oral tissues and single gene disorders

3. **Physiology (General and Oral):** Saliva, Pain, Mastication, Taste, Deglutition, Wound healing, Vitamins (influence on growth, development and structure of oral soft and hard tissues and paraoral tissues), Calcium metabolism, Theories of mineralization, Tooth eruption and shedding, Blood and its constituents, Hormones (influence on growth, development and structure of oral soft and hard tissues and paraoral tissues)

4. **Cell Biology:** Cell structure and function (ultra structural and molecular aspects).Intercellular junctions. Cell cycle and division. Cell cycle regulators. Cell–cell and cell-extracellular matrix interactions. Detailed molecular aspects of DNA,RNA and intracellular organelles, transcription and translation and molecular biology techniques

5. **General Histology:** Light and electron microscopy considerations of epithelial tissues and glands, bone. Light and electron microscopy considerations of hemopoetic system, lymphatic system, muscle, neural tissue, endocrinal system (thyroid, pituitary, parathyroid)

6. **Biochemistry:** Chemistry of carbohydrates, lipids and proteins. Methods of identification and purification. Metabolism of carbohydrates, lipids and proteins. Biological oxidation. Various techniques-cell fractionation and ultra filtration, centrifugation, electrophoresis, spectrophotometry and radioactive techniques.

7. **General Pathology:** Inflammation and chemical mediator, Thrombosis, Embolism, Necrosis, Repair, Degeneration, Shock, Hemorrhage, Pathogenic mechanisms at molecular level, Blood dyscrasias. Carcinogenesis and Neoplasia

8. **General Microbiology:** Definitions of various types of infections. Routes of infection and spread. Sterilization, disinfection and antiseptics. Bacterial genetics. Physiology, growth of micro-organisms

9. **Basic Immunology:** Basic principles of immunity, antigen and antibody reaction. Cell mediated and humoral immunity. Immunology of hypersensitivity. Immunological basis of auto immune phenomena. Immunodeficiency with relevance to opportunistic infections. Basic principles of transplantation and tumor immunity.

10. **Systemic Microbiology/Applied Microbiology:** Morphology, classification, pathogenicity, mode of transmission, methods of prevention, collection and transport of specimen for laboratory diagnosis, staining methods, common culture media, interpretation of laboratory reports and antibiotic sensitivity tests. Staphylococci, Streptococci, *Corynebacterium diphtheriae*, Mycobacterium, Clostridia, bacteroids and fusobacteria, Actinomycetales, Spirochetes, General structure, broad classification of viruses, pathogenesis, pathology of viral infections, Herpesvirus, Hepatitis virus, HIV, General properties of fungi, Superficial, subcutaneous, deep opportunistic infections, General principles of fungal infections, method of collection of samples, diagnosis and examination of fungi.

11. **Oral biology (Oral and Dental Histology):** Study of morphology of permanent and deciduous teeth. Structure and function of oral, dental and paraoral tissues including their ultra structure, molecular and biochemical aspects

12. **Basic Histo-Techniques and Microscopy:** Routine hematological tests and clinical significance of the same. Biopsy procedures for oral lesions. Tissue processing. Microtome and principles of microtomy. Various stains used in histopathology and their applications. Microscope, principles and theories of microscopy. Light microscopy and various other types including electron microscopy. Fixation and fixatives. Ground sections and decalcified sections. Cytological smears

7. PUBLIC HEALTH DENTISTRY

Applied Anatomy and Histology

a. **Applied Anatomy in relation to:** Development of face, Bronchial arches, Muscles of facial expression, Muscles of mastication, TMJ, Salivary gland, Tongue, Hard and soft palate, Infratemporal fossa, Paranasal air sinuses, Pharynx and larynx, Cranial and spinal nerves-with emphasis on trigeminal, facial, glossopharyngeal and hypoglossal nerve, Osteology of maxilla and mandible, Blood supply, venous and lymphatic drainage of head and neck, Lymph nodes of head and neck, Structure and relations of alveolar process and edentulous mouth, Genetics—fundamentals.

b. **Oral Histology:** Development of dentition, Innervations of dentin and pulp, Peridontium—development, histology, blood supply, nerve supply and lymphatic drainage, Oral mucous membrane, Pulp-periodontal complex.

Applied Physiology and Biochemistry

Cell, Mastication and deglutition, Food and nutrition, Metabolism of carbohydrates, proteins and fats, Vitamins and minerals, Saliva and Oral health, Fluid and electrolyte balance, Pain pathway and mechanism—types, properties, Blood composition and functions, clotting mechanism and erythropoiesis, Blood groups and transfusions, Pulse and blood pressure, Dynamics of blood flow, Cardiovascular homeostasis—heart sounds, Respiratory system: Normal physiology and variations in health and diseases, Asphyxia and artificial respiration, Endocrinology: thyroid, parathyroid, adrenals, pituitary, sex hormones and pregnancy, Endocrine regulation of blood sugar.

Applied Pathology

Pathogenic mechanism of molecular level, Cellular changes following injury, Inflammation and chemical mediators, Edema, thrombosis and embolism, Hemorrhage and shock, Neoplasia and metastasis, Blood disorders, Histopathology and pathogenesis of dental caries, periodontal disease, oral mucosal lesions, and malignancies, HIV, Propagation of dental infection.

Microbiology

Microbial flora of oral cavity, Bacteriology of dental caries and periodontal disease, Methods of sterilization, Infection control, dental office/camps, Virology of HIV, herpes, hepatitis, Parasitological, Basic immunology-basic concepts of immune system in human body: Cellular and humoral immunity, Antigen and antibody system, Hypersensitivity, Autoimmune diseases.

Oral Pathology

Detailed description of diseases affecting the oral mucosa, teeth, supporting tissues and jaws.

Physical and Social Anthropology

Introduction and definition, Appreciation of the biological basis of health and disease, Evolution of human race, various studies of different races by anthropological methods

Applied Pharmacology

Definition, scope and relations to other branches of medicine, mode of action, bioassay, standardization, pharmacodynamic, pharmacokinetics. Chemotherapy of bacterial infections and viral infections-sulphonamides and antibiotics. Local anesthesia Analgesics and anti-inflammatory drugs. Hypnotics, tranquilizers and antipyretics. Important hormones-ACTH, cortisone, insulin and oral antidiabetic. Drug addiction and tolerance. Important pharmacological agents in connection with autonomic nervous system-adrenaline, Noradrenaline, atropine. Brief mention of antihypertensive drugs. Emergency drugs in dental practice. Vitamins and Hemopoietic drugs. Effect of drugs on oral health.

Research Methodology and Biostatistics

Health Informatics—basic understanding of computers and its components, operating software (Windows), Microsoft office, preparation of teaching materials like slides, project, multimedia knowledge. Operative skills in analyzing the data.

Research Methodology—definitions, types of research, designing written protocol for research, objectivity in methodology, quantification, records and analysis.

Biostatistics—introduction, applications, uses and limitations of biostatistics in Public Health dentistry, collection of data, presentation of data, measures of central tendency, measures of dispersion, methods of summarizing, parametric and non parametric tests of significance, correlation and regression, multivariate analysis, sampling and sampling techniques–types, errors, bias, trial and calibration

8. PEDIATRIC AND PREVENTIVE DENTISTRY

Applied Anatomy of Head and Neck

Anatomy of the scalp, temple and face, triangles of neck and deep structures of the neck, Cranial and facial bones and its surrounding soft tissues with its applied aspects, Muscles of head and neck, Arterial supply, venous drainage and lymphatics of head and neck, Congenital abnormalities of the head and neck, Anatomy of the cranial nerves, tongue and its applied aspects, salivary glands, pharynx, thyroid and parathyroid gland, larynx, trachea, esophagus, Autonomous nervous system of head and neck, Functional anatomy of mastication, deglutition, speech, respiration and circulation, TMJ: anatomy and function.

Applied Physiology

Introduction, Mastication, deglutition, digestion and assimilation, Homeostasis, fluid and electrolyte balance. Blood composition, volume, function, blood groups and hemorrhage, Blood transfusion, circulation, Heart, Pulse, Blood pressure, Normal ECG capillary and lymphatic circulation, shock, respiration, control, anoxia, hypoxia, asphyxia, artificial respiration. Endocrine glands in particular reference to pituitary, parathyroid and thyroid glands and sex hormones. Role of calcium and Vit. D in growth and development of teeth, bone and jaws. Role of Vit. A, C and B complex in oral mucosal and periodontal health. Physiology and function of the masticatory system. Speech mechanism, swallowing and deglutition mechanism, salivary glands and Saliva.

Applied Pathology

Inflammation and chemical mediators, Thrombosis, Embolism, Necrosis, Repair, Degeneration, Shock, Hemorrhage, Blood dyscrasias, Pathogenesis of Dental Caries, Periodontal diseases, tumors, oral mucosal lesions, etc. in children.

Applied Microbiology

Microbiology and Immunology as related to Oral Diseases in Children: Basic concepts, immune system in human body, Auto Immune diseases and Immunology of Dental caries.

Applied Nutrition and Dietics: General principles, balanced diet, effect of dietary deficiencies and starvation, protein energy, malnutrition, Kwashiorkor, Marasmus. Fluid and Electrolytic balance in maintaining haemostasis. Diet, digestion, absorption, transportation and utilization

Genetics: Introduction to genetics, Cell structure, DNA, RNA, protein synthesis, cell division. Modes of inheritance. Chromosomal anomalies of oral tissues and single gene disorders

Growth and Development: Prenatal and Postnatal development of cranium, face, jaws, teeth and supporting structures. Chronology of dental development and development of occlusion. Dimensional changes in dental arches. Cephalometric evaluation of growth.

9. ORAL MEDICINE AND RADIOLOGY

Applied Anatomy

1. **Gross anatomy of the face:** Muscles of Facial Expression and Muscles of Mastication. Facial nerve, Facial artery, Facial vein, Parotid gland and its relations, Submandibular salivary gland and its relations
2. **Neck region:** Triangles of the neck with special reference to Carotid, Digastric triangles and midline structures, Facial spaces, Carotid system of arteries, Vertebral Artery, and Subclavian arteries, Jugular system: Internal jugular, External jugular, Lymphatic drainage, Cervical plane, Muscles derived from Pharyngeal arches, Infratemporal fossa in detail and temporomandibular joint, Endocrine glands Pituitary, Thyroid, Parathyroid. Exocrine glands: Parathyroid, Parotid, Thyroid. Sympathetic chain, Cranial nerves-V, VII, IX, XI, and XII.
3. **Oral Cavity:** Vestibule and oral cavity proper, tongue and teeth, Palate-soft and hard.
4. **Nasal Cavity:** Nasal septum, Lateral wall of nasal cavity, Paranasal air sinuses
5. **Pharynx.**
6. **Gross salient features** of brain and spinal cord with references to attachment of cranial nerves to the brainstem Detailed study of the cranial nerve nuclei of V, VII, IX, X, XI, XII
7. **Osteology:** Comparative study of fetal and adult skull, Mandible: Development, ossification, age changes and evaluation of mandible in detail.

Embryology

Development of face, palate, nasal septum and nasal cavity, paranasal air sinuses. Pharyngeal apparatus in detail including the floor of the primitive pharynx. Development of tooth in detail and the age changes. Development of salivary glands. Congenital anomalies of face must be dealt in detail.

Histology

Study of epithelium of oral cavity and the respiratory tract. Connective tissue, Muscular tissue, Nervous tissue, Blood vessels, Cartilage, Bone and tooth, Tongue, Salivary glands, Tonsil, thymus, lymph nodes.

Physiology

1. General Physiology: Cell, Body Fluid Compartments, Classification, Composition, Cellular transport, RMP and action potential
2. Muscle Nerve Physiology: Structure of a neuron and properties of nerve fibers, Structure of muscle fibers and properties of muscle fibers, Neuromuscular transmission, Mechanism of muscle contraction
3. Blood: RBC and Hb, WBC-Structure and functions, Platelets-functions and applied aspects, Plasma proteins, Blood Coagulation with applied aspects, Blood groups, Lymph and applied aspects
4. Respiratory System: Air passages, composition of air, dead space, mechanics of respiration with pressure and volume changes. Lung volumes and capacities and applied aspects. Oxygen and carbon dioxide transport. Neural regulation of respiration. Chemical regulation of respiration. Hypoxia, effects of increased barometric pressure and decreased barometric pressure.
5. Cardio-Vascular System: Cardiac Cycle, Regulation of heart rate/Stroke volume/cardiac output/blood flow, Regulation of blood pressure, Shock, hypertension, cardiac failure.
6. Excretory System: Renal function tests
7. Gastrointestinal tract: Composition, functions and regulation of: Saliva, Gastric juice, Pancreatic juice, Bile and intestinal juice, Mastication and deglutition
8. Endocrine System: Hormones—classification and mechanism of action, Hypothalamic and pituitary hormones, Thyroid hormones, Parathyroid hormones and calcium homeostasis, Pancreatic hormones, Adrenal hormones.
9. Central Nervous System: Ascending tract with special references to pain pathway
10. Special Senses: Gustation and Olfaction

Biochemistry

1. Carbohydrates: Disaccharides specifically maltose, lactose, sucrose, Digestion of starch/absorption of glucose, Metabolism of glucose, specifically glycolysis, TCA cycle, gluconeogenesis, Blood sugar regulation, Glycogen storage regulation, Glycogen storage diseases, Galactosemia and fructosemia
2. Lipids: Fatty acids-Essential/nonessential, Metabolism of fatty acids-oxidation, ketone body formation, utilization ketosis, Outline of cholesterol metabolism- synthesis and products formed from cholesterol
3. Protein: Amino acids-essential/nonessential, complete/incomplete proteins, Transamination/Deamination (Definition with examples), Urea cycle, Tyrosine-Hormones synthesized from tyrosine, Inborn errors of amino acid metabolism, methionine and transmethylation
4. Nucleic Acids: Purines/Pyrimidines, Purine analogs in medicine, DNA/RNA–Outline of structure, Transcription/translation, Steps of protein synthesis, Inhibitors of protein synthesis, Regulation of gene function
5. Minerals: Calcium/Phosphorus metabolism specifically regulation of serum calcium levels, Iron metabolism, Iodine metabolism, Trace elements in nutrition
6. Energy Metabolism: Basal metabolic rate, Specific dynamic action (SDA) of foods.
7. Vitamins: Mainly these vitamins and their metabolic role-vitamin A, Vitamin C, Vitamin D, Thiamin, Riboflavin, Niacin, Pyridoxine

Pathology

1. Inflammation: Repair and regeneration, necrosis and gangrene, Role of complement system in acute inflammation, Role of arachidonic acid and its metabolites in acute inflammation, Growth factors in acute inflammation, Role of molecular events in cell growth and intercellular signaling cell surface receptors, Role of NSAIDs in inflammation, Cellular changes in radiation injury and its manifestations
2. Homeostasis: Role of Endothelium in thrombo genesis, Arterial and venous thrombi, Disseminated Intravascular Coagulation, Shock: Pathogenesis of hemorrhagic, neurogenic, septic, cardiogenic shock, circulatory disturbances, ischemic hyperemia, venous congestion, edema, infarction
3. Chromosomal Abnormalities: Marfan's syndrome. Ehlers-Danlos Syndrome, Fragile X Syndrome
4. Hypersensitivity: Anaphylaxis, Type II Hypersensitivity, Type III Hypersensitivity, Cell mediated Reaction and its clinical importance, Systemic Lupus Erythematosus, Infection and infective granulomas
5. Neoplasia: Classification of Tumors, Carcinogenesis and Carcinogens – Chemical, Viral and Microbial, Grading and Staging of Cancer, tumor Angiogenesis, Paraneoplastic Syndrome, Spread of tumors, Characteristics of benign and malignant tumors
6. Others: Sex linked agammaglobulinemia, AIDS, Management of Immune deficiency patients requiring surgical procedures, DiGeorge's Syndrome, Ghon's complex, post primary pulmonary tuberculosis-pathology and pathogenesis

Pharmacology

1. Definition of terminologies used
2. Dosage and mode of administration of drugs
3. Action and fate of drugs in the body
4. Drugs acting on CNS
5. Drug addiction, tolerance and hypersensitive reactions
6. General and local anesthetics, hypnotics, antiepileptic and tranquilizers
7. Chemotherapeutics and antibiotics
8. Analgesics and anti-pyretic
9. Anti-tubercular and anti-syphilitic drugs
10. Antiseptics, Sialogogue, and anti-Sialogogue
11. Haematinics
12. Antidiabetics
13. Vitamins: A, B complex, C, D, E and K
14. Steroids

LIST OF INDIAN UNIVERSITIES INCLUDED (1990–2020)

1. All India Institute of Medical Sciences-Centre for Dental Education and Research.(AIIMS-CDER), New Delhi
2. Baba Farid University of Health Science (BFUHS), Faridkot
3. Bangalore University
4. Bombay University
5. Dr. N.T.R University of Health Sciences (NTR Uni.), Vijayawada
6. Dr. Ram Manohar Lohia Avadh University, Ayodhya (DRMLA Uni.)
7. Gujarat University, Ahmedabad
8. Guwahati University/Srimanta Sankaradeva University of Health Sciences.
9. Hemvati Nandan Bahuguna Garhwal University, Uttarakhand. (HNBG, Uni.), Srinagar
10. Himachal Pardesh University (HP Uni.), Shimla
11. Kerala University of Health Science (KUHS), Thrissur
12. Madhya Pradesh Medical Science University (MDMS Uni.), Jabalpur
13. Maharashtra University of Health Science (MUHS), Nashik
14. Nagpur University.
15. Pandit Deendayal Upadhyay Memorial Health Science and Ayush University of Chattisgarh (AHSUC Uni.), Raipur
16. Rajasthan University of Health Sciences (RUHS), Jaipur
17. Rajiv Gandhi University of Health Sciences (RGUHS), Bengaluru
18. Tamil Nadu Dr. M.G.R. Medical University (TNMGR), Chennai
19. University of Delhi (UOD)
20. University of Health Sciences, Rohtak (UHSR)
21. University of Kashmir (UOK)
22. Babu Banarasi Das University, Lucknow (BBD Uni.)
23. Bharati Vidyapeeth Deemed University, Pune (BVP Uni.)
24. DYP Uni., Navi Mumbai
25. KLE Deemed University, Belgaum
26. Manipal Academy of Higher Education (MAHE).
27. NITTE Uni. Mangaluru.
28. Pacific University (PAHER), Udaipur.
29. Sharda University, Greater Noida, Uttar Pradesh
30. Sumandeep Vidyapeeth University, Vadodara, Gujarat
31. Yenepoya University, Mangalore
32. Kaloji Narayana Rao University of Health Sciences, Warangal, Telangana (KNRUHS)
33. People's University, Bhopal

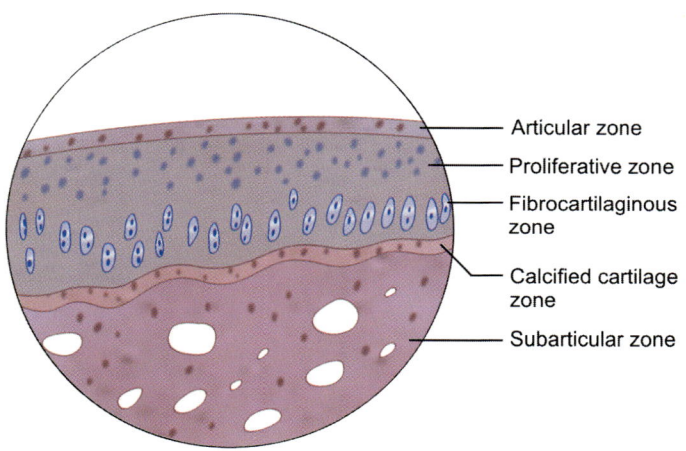

Fig. P-1: : Histology of articular surfaces of temporomandibular joint (TMJ)

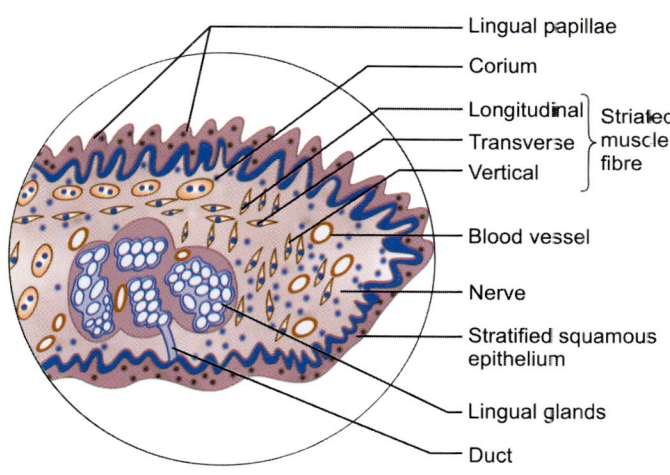

Fig. P-2: Histology of tongue

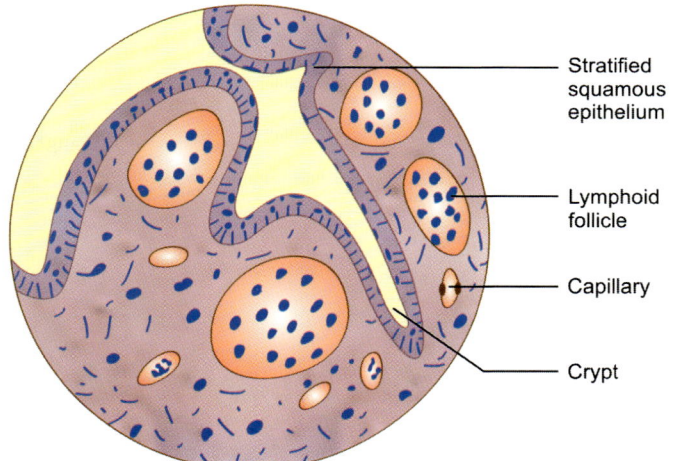

Fig. P-3: Histology of palatine tonsil

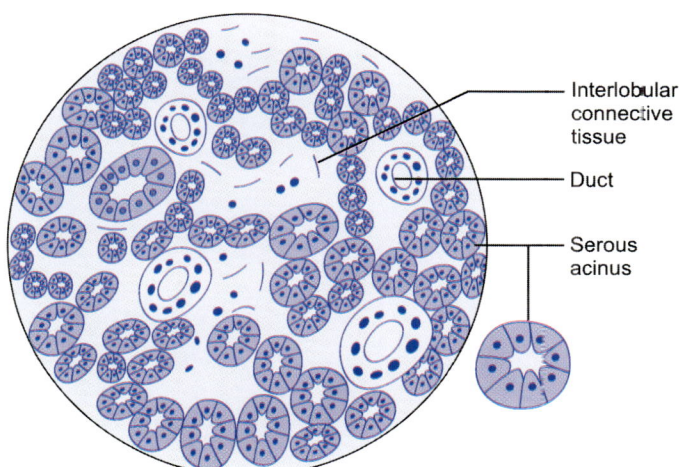

Fig. P-4a: Histology of parotid gland

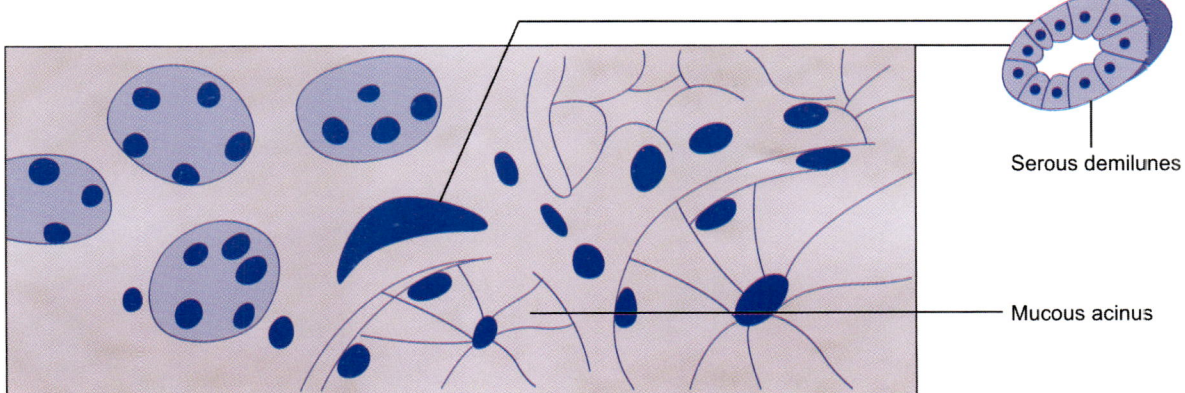

Fig. P-4b: Histology of submandibular gland

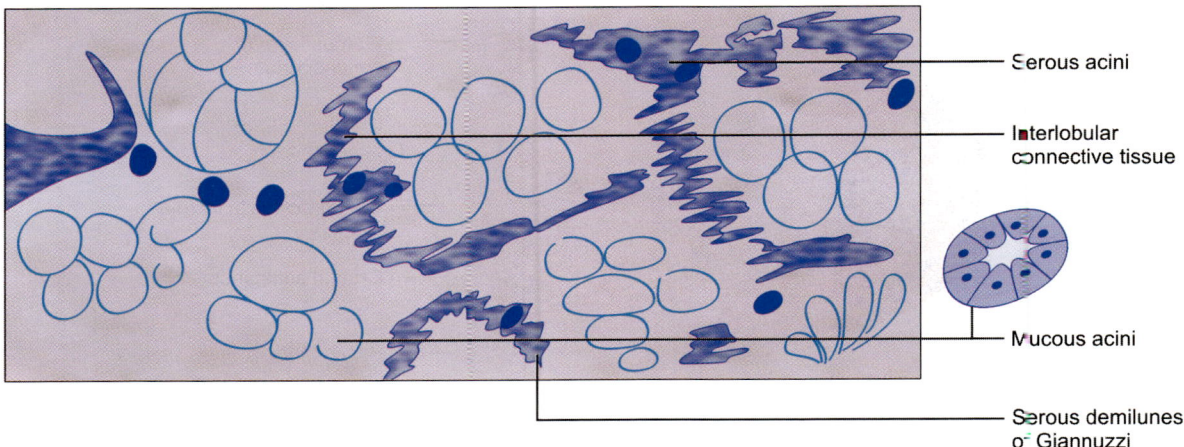

Serous acini

Interlobular connective tissue

Mucous acini

Serous demilunes of Giannuzzi

Fig. P-4c: Histology of sublingual gland

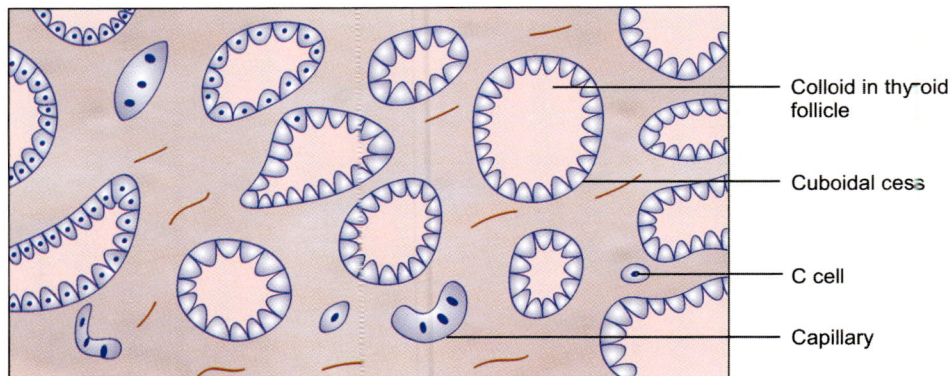

Colloid in thyroid follicle

Cuboidal cells

C cell

Capillary

Fig. P-5: Histology of thyroid gland

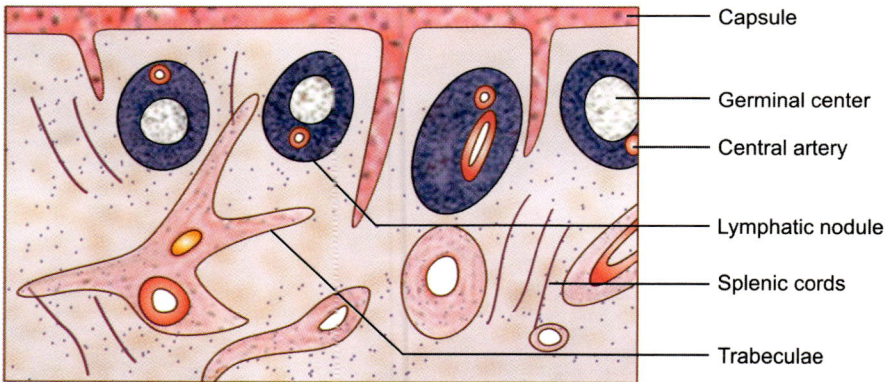

Capsule

Germinal center

Central artery

Lymphatic nodule

Splenic cords

Trabeculae

Fig. P-6: Histology of spleen

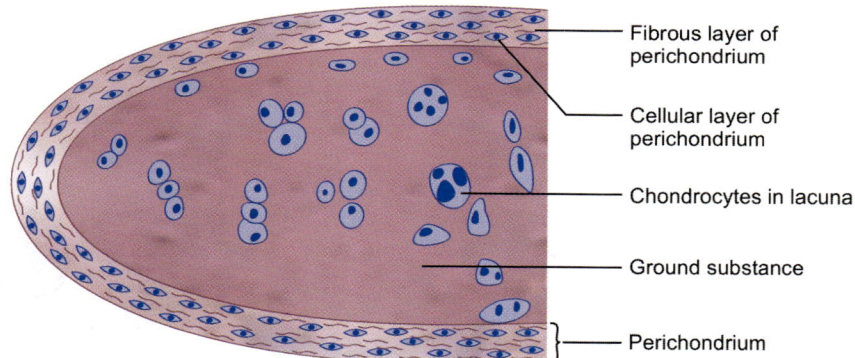

Fibrous layer of perichondrium

Cellular layer of perichondrium

Chondrocytes in lacuna

Ground substance

Perichondrium

Fig. P-7a: Histology of hyaline cartilage

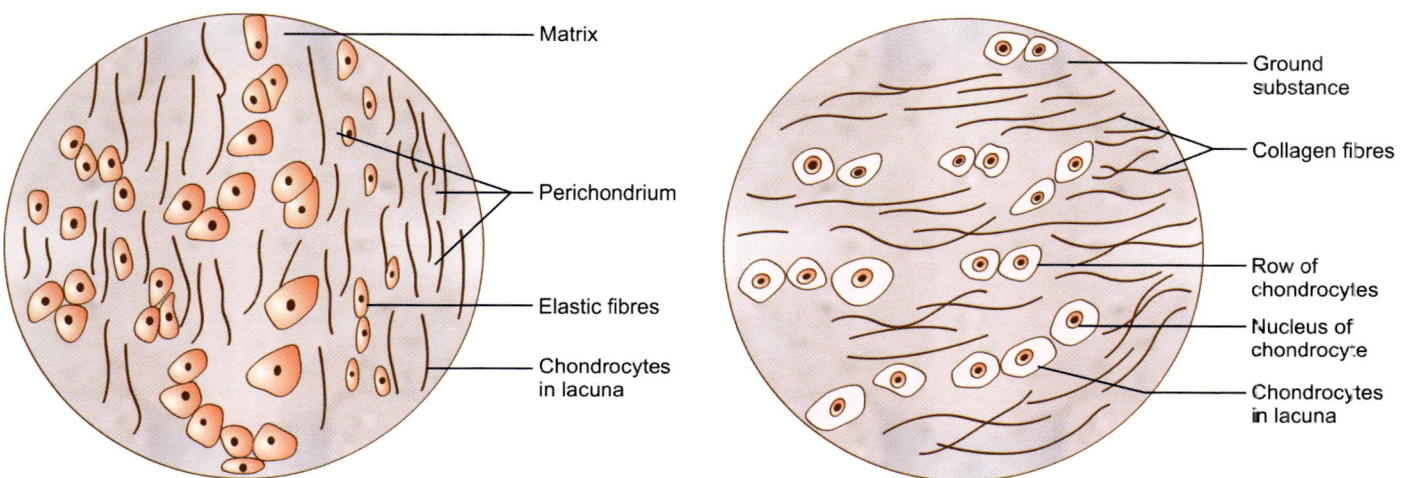

Matrix

Perichondrium

Elastic fibres

Chondrocytes in lacuna

Fig. P-7b: Histology of elastic cartilage

Ground substance

Collagen fibres

Row of chondrocytes

Nucleus of chondrocyte

Chondrocytes in lacuna

Fig. P-7c: Histology of fibrocartilage

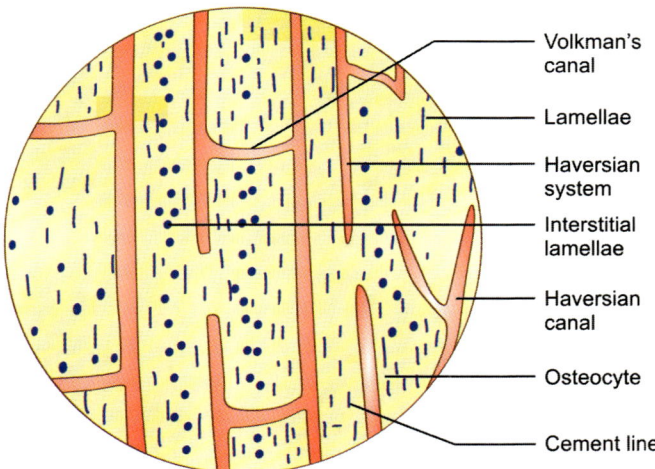

Volkman's canal

Lamellae

Haversian system

Interstitial lamellae

Haversian canal

Osteocyte

Cement line

Fig. P-8a: Histology of compact bone

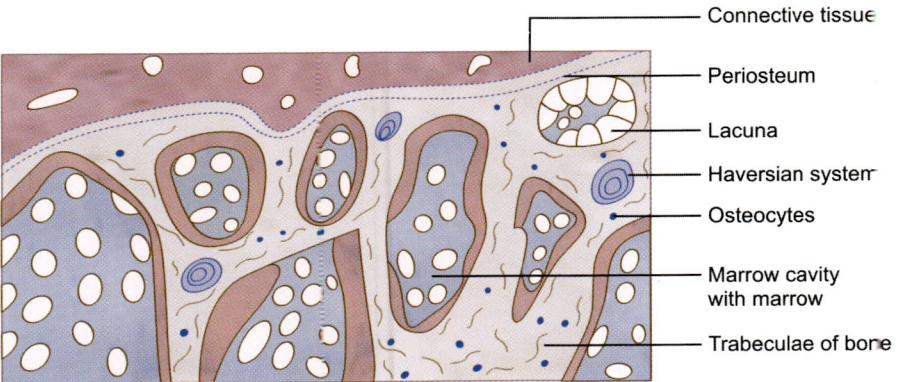

Connective tissue
Periosteum
Lacuna
Haversian system
Osteocytes
Marrow cavity with marrow
Trabeculae of bone

Fig. P-8b: Histology of cancellous bone

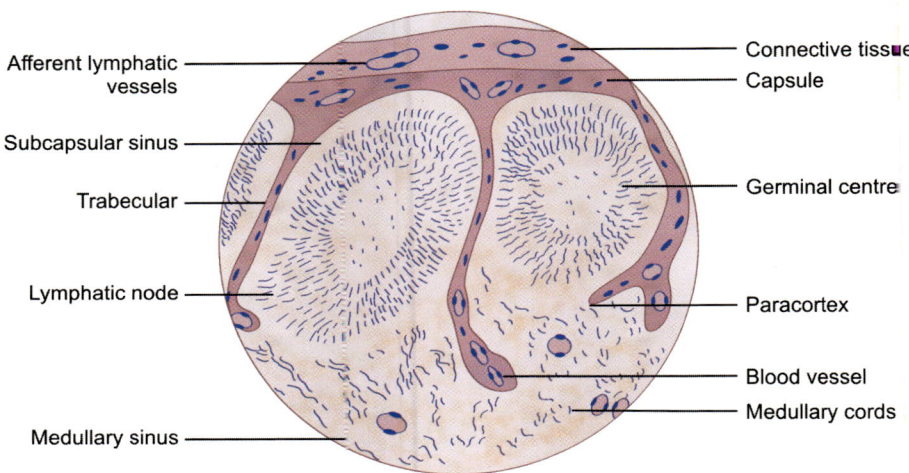

Afferent lymphatic vessels
Subcapsular sinus
Trabecular
Lymphatic node
Medullary sinus

Connective tissue
Capsule
Germinal centre
Paracortex
Blood vessel
Medullary cords

Fig. P-9: Histology of lymph nodes

Anatomy, Embryology and Histology

1. OSTEOLOGY

Q. 1. Discuss the development of mandible in detail. Write about age changes in mandible. Write a note on its clinical considerations.

(BFUHS, Nov. 2007; TNMGR, Sept. 2010; RUHS, May 2015; UOK, May 2015; MUHS, June 2016; HNBG Uni., May 2017; HP Uni., April 2019)

Ans. The mandible is the largest and the strongest bone of the face. It has following parts (Fig. 1.1a).

Body of mandible: The body is horseshoe shaped. It lodges teeth. Each half of the body has outer or external surface and inner or internal surface and upper (alveolar) and lower border (*base*) with muscle attachments.

Ramus: The ramus is quadrilateral in shape and has two surfaces (medial and lateral), four borders (upper, lower, anterior and posterior) and two processes: *Condyloid*—Latin *knuckle-like* and *coronoid*—Greek *crow's beak*. Ramus forms the posterior end of body and provides attachment to muscles of mastication.

Development of mandible: The development of mandible is described as (Fig. 1.1b):

a. **Development of body:** Most of the body is formed intramembranous in the mesenchyme of the deeper part of 1st branchial arch around 6th week of intra-uterine life (IUL) by one centre of ossification at the bifurcation of mental and incisive nerves. The ossification spreads medially below incisive nerve; ventrally around the mental nerve to form the *mental foramen* and upwards between the mental nerve and *Meckel's cartilage*. Anteriorly, the ossification takes place towards the midline to meet opposite side. Posteriorly, the bony trough containing nerve is formed (*mandibular canal*), till future lingula.

b. **Development of ramus:** Development takes place by rapid ossification posteriorly into mesenchyme of 1st branchial arch away from Meckel's cartilage marked by mandibular foramen.

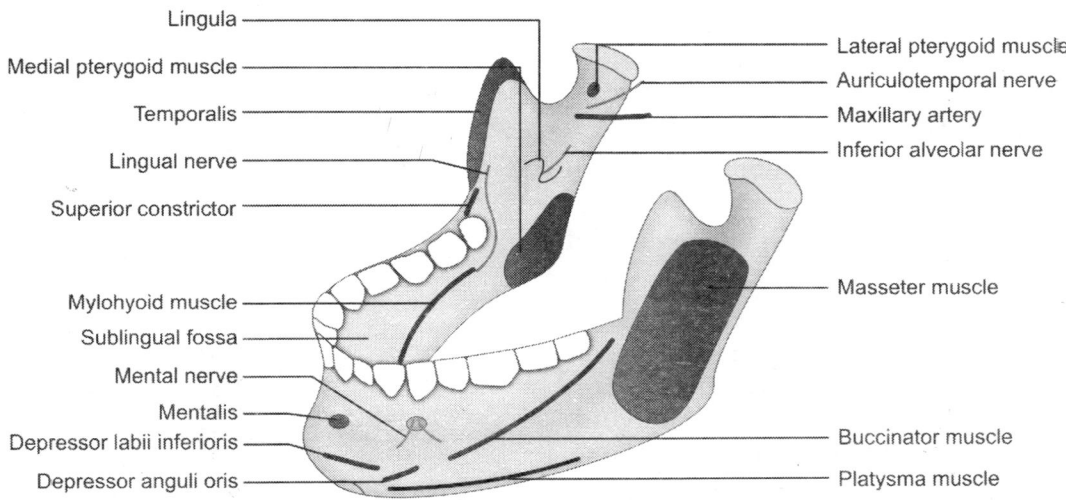

Lingula	Lateral pterygoid muscle
Medial pterygoid muscle	Auriculotemporal nerve
Temporalis	Maxillary artery
Lingual nerve	Inferior alveolar nerve
Superior constrictor	
Mylohyoid muscle	Masseter muscle
Sublingual fossa	
Mental nerve	
Mentalis	
Depressor labii inferioris	Buccinator muscle
Depressor anguli oris	Platysma muscle

Fig. 1.1a: Structure of mandible with muscle attachments

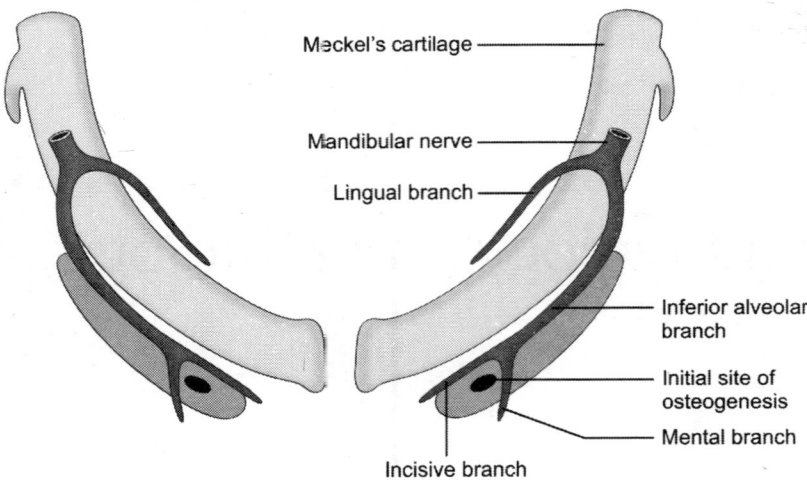

Fig. 1.1b: Development of mandible and role of Meckel's cartilage

Condylar cartilage (14th week of IUL) gives rise to condylar head and neck and posterior half of ramus. Coronoid cartilage (4th–6th week of IUL) gives rise to coronoid process and anterior half of ramus.

The symphyseal cartilage (2 in number) appears in the connective tissue between 2nd ends of Meckel's cartilage and gets obliterated within 1st year after birth.

c. **Development of alveolar process:** It starts when mandible begins to grow on each side of deciduous tooth germ during the early bell stage forming bony trough around the tooth germs, with bony septa between tooth germs.

Blood Supply

a. **Ramus:** Periosteal vessels from inferior alveolar artery (IAA).
b. **Body of the mandible:** Endosteal vessels from perimandibular branch of maxillary artery, facial artery, external carotid artery (ECA), and superficial temporal artery (STA).
c. **Mandibular teeth:** Dental branch from IAA.

Lymphatics: Submandibular and submental lymph nodes.

Nerves: Inferior alveolar nerve (IAN) and associated branches (br.)

Muscles (Fig. 1.1a)

Muscles origin: Mentalis, orbicularis oris, depressor labii inferioris, depressor anguli oris, buccinator, digastric anterior belly, mylohyoid, geniohyoid, genioglossus, superior pharyngeal constrictor.

Muscles insertion: Platysma, masseter, medial pterygoid, inferior head of the lateral pterygoid, temporalis.

Age changes (Fig. 1.1c)   *(Sumandeep Uni., April 2015)*
1. *In infants:*
    a. The body of bone is mere shell, containing the socket with deciduous teeth
    b. Condyloid process is almost in line with body.
    c. Coronoid process is of larger in size and projects above the level of condyle. Mandibular canal is of large size and runs near the lower border of mandible. Mental foramen opens below the socket of 1st deciduous molar tooth. The mandibular angle is obtuse (175°).
2. *In children:*
    a. The body becomes longer in its whole length. The two halves of the mandible fuse at the symphysis during the first year of life.
    b. The mandibular canal is situated just above the level of mylohyoid line.

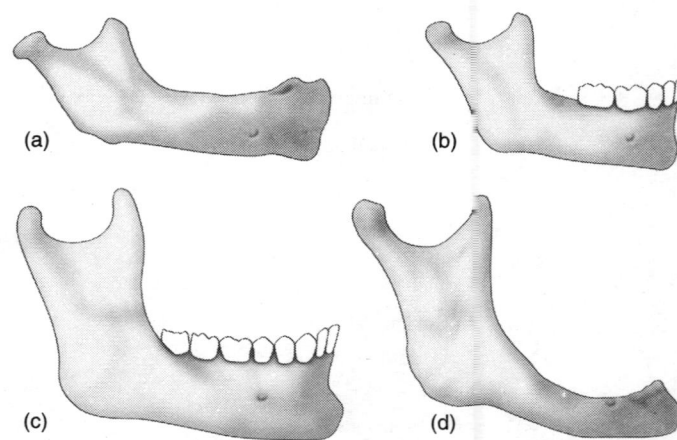

Fig. 1.1c: Age changes in mandible: (a) At birth, (b) childhood, (c) adulthood and (d) old age

c. Mental foramen opens below the sockets for deciduous molar teeth near lower border. The foramen and canal gradually shift upwards.

d. The coronoid process is large and projects upwards above the level of condyle.

e. The mandibular angle becomes less obtuse. It is 140° or more because the head is in line with the body.

3. *In adults:*

a. The body is almost equal divided between the alveolar and sub-alveolar parts.

b. The mandibular canal runs parallel with mylohyoid line.

c. The mental foramen opens midway between the upper and lower borders.

d. The angle reduces to about 110° or 120° because the ramus becomes almost vertical.

4. *In old age:*

a. The body becomes greatly reduced in size.

b. Because of loss of teeth, the alveolar process is absorbed, so that the height of body is markedly reduced.

c. The mental foramen and the mandibular canal are close to the alveolar border.

d. The angle again becomes obtuse about 140° because the ramus is oblique.

Applied Anatomy   *(Sumandeep Uni., April 2015; NTR Uni., May 2019)*

1. The mandible is commonly fractured at the canine socket where it is weak, followed by fracture of the mandible at angle and neck of mandible.

2. Involvement of the inferior alveolar nerve in the callus may cause neuralgic pain. If the nerve is paralyzed, the areas supplied by these nerves become insensitive.

3. Developmental disturbances include agnathia, micrognathia, facial hemihypertrophy, hemiatrophy, abnormalities of dental arch relation, developmental cysts like median mandibular cyst and alveolar cyst of newborn.

4. Dislocation of the mandible is most frequently in the posterior direction.

5. As mandible progressively changes over an individual's life, it is routinely used to determine the age of the deceased in forensic medicine.

Q. 2. Discuss in detail about the maxilla. Write about age changes in maxilla.   *(BFUHS, Nov. 2007; UOK, May 2015)*

Q. Describe the development of maxilla.
(Sumandeep Uni., June 2016; HP Uni., April 2019)

Ans. Maxilla is the second largest bone of the face. One maxilla is present on the either side of the midline and both together form the upper jaw. The body of maxilla is pyramidal in shape, with its base directed medially at the nasal surface, and the apex directed laterally at the zygomatic process. It has four surfaces and encloses a large cavity, the maxillary sinus. The surfaces are given below.

I. Anterior or Facial Surface (Fig.1.2a)

1. Anterior surface is directed forwards and laterally and forms part of *norma frontalis*.

2. Above the incisor teeth, there is a slight depression, *incisive fossa*, which gives origin to *depressor septi*. Incisivus arises from the alveolar margin below the fossa and the *nasalis* superolateral to the fossa along the nasal notch.

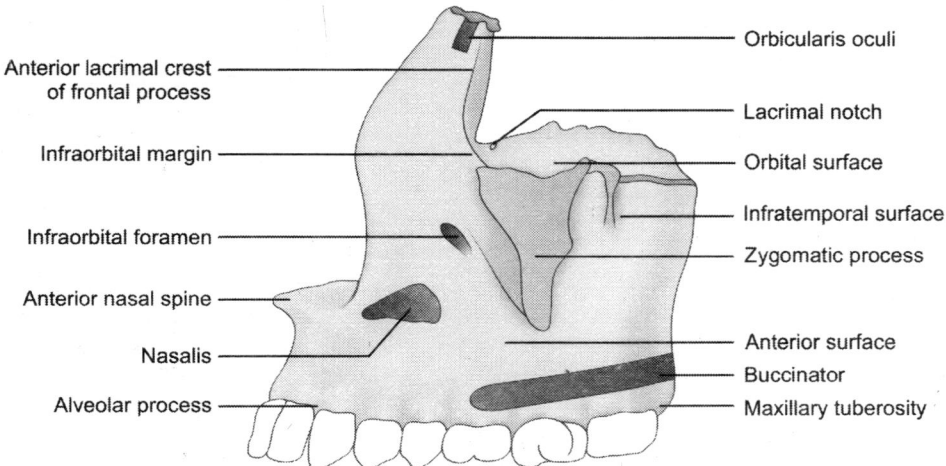

Fig. 1.2a: Lateral surface of maxilla with muscle attachments

3. Lateral to canine eminence, there is a larger and deeper depression, *canine fossa*, which gives origin to *levator anguli oris*.
4. Above the canine fossa, there is *infraorbital foramen*, which transmits infraorbital nerve and vessels.
5. *Levator labii superioris* arises between the infra-orbital margin and infraorbital foramen.
6. Medially, the anterior surface ends in a deeply concave border, *nasal notch*, which terminates below as projection, *anterior nasal spine*. Anterior surface bordering the nasal notch gives origin to nasalis and depressor septi.

II. Posterior or Infratemporal Surface

1. Posterior surface is convex, directed backwards and laterally and forms the anterior wall of *infratemporal fossa*.
2. It is separated from anterior surface by the zygomatic process and a rounded, vertical ridge (*Jugal crest*) at the level of first molar tooth going up to the zygomatic process.
3. In the centre, there are two or three alveolar canals (foramina) for posterior superior alveolar nerve and vessels.
4. Posteroinferiorly (behind the 3rd molar), there is a rounded eminence, *maxillary tuberosity*, which articulates superomedially with pyramidal process of palatine bone, and gives origin laterally to the superficial head of medial pterygoid muscle.
5. Above the maxillary tuberosity, the smooth surface forms anterior wall of pterygopalatine fossa, and is grooved by maxillary nerve. This continues upwards into orbital surface as *infraorbital groove*.

III. Superior or Orbital Surface

1. Superior surface is smooth, triangular and slightly concave, and forms the greater part of the floor of orbit, with an anterior, posterior and medial border.
2. Anterior border forms a part of infraorbital margin. Medially, it is continuous with the lacrimal crest of the frontal process.
3. Posterior border is smooth and rounded; it forms most of the anterior margin of inferior orbital fissure. In the middle, it is notched by the infraorbital groove that runs anteriorly and passes into the bone as the infraorbital canal.
4. Medial border presents anteriorly *lacrimal notch* which is converted into *nasolacrimal canal* by descending process of lacrimal bone. Behind the notch, border articulates antero posteriorly with lacrimal, labyrinth (orbital plate) of ethmoid, and the orbital process of palatine bone respectively.
5. The surface presents infraorbital groove leading forwards to infraorbital canal which opens on the anterior surface as infraorbital foramen. The groove, canal and foramen transmit the infraorbital nerve and vessels. Near the midpoint, the canal gives off laterally a branch, the canalis sinuous, for the passage of anterior superior alveolar nerve and vessels.
6. Inferior oblique muscle of eyeball arises from a depression just lateral to lacrimal notch at the anteromedial angle of the surface.

IV. Medial or Nasal Surface (Fig. 1.2b)

1. Medial surface forms base of body of maxilla and is a part of the lateral wall of nasal cavity.
2. Posterosuperiorly, it displays a large irregular opening of the maxillary sinus, *maxillary hiatus*.

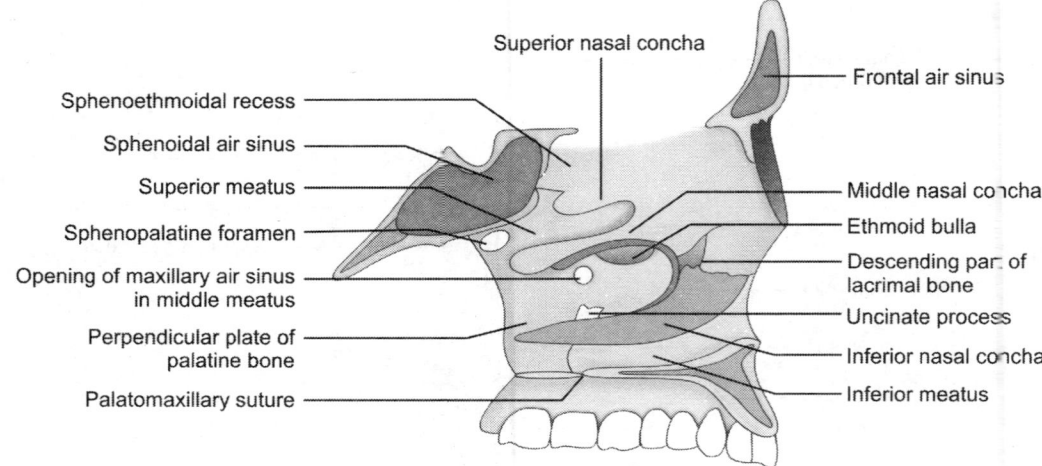

Fig. 1.2b: Medial surface of maxilla with muscle attachments

3. Above the hiatus, there are parts of air sinuses which are completed by the ethmoid and lacrimal bones.
4. Below the hiatus, the smooth concave surface forms a part of inferior meatus of nose.
5. Behind the hiatus, the surface articulates with perpendicular plate of palatine bone, enclosing the greater palatine canal which runs downwards and forwards, and transmits greater palatine vessels and the anterior, middle and posterior palatine nerves.
6. In front of the hiatus, there is nasolacrimal groove, which is converted into the nasolacrimal canal by articulation with the descending process of lacrimal bone and the lacrimal process of inferior nasal concha. The canal transmits nasolacrimal duct to the inferior meatus of nose.
7. More anteriorly, an oblique ridge forms the conchal crest for articulation with the inferior nasal concha.

Blood supply: Branches of maxillary artery.

Nerves: Maxillary nerve (V2) and its branches.

Development of maxilla: All parts of the maxilla undergo intramembranous ossification through two ossification centers. In the 7th week of IUL, there is differentiation between the maxilla and premaxilla (or incisive bone). In the third month, both parts fuse around the area of the alveolar process after which the premaxilla becomes anterior part of the maxilla. The maxillary sinuses are relatively small and become larger during development of maxilla and other skull bones.

Age Changes

1. *At birth*
   a. The transverse and anteroposterior diameters are more than the vertical diameter.
   b. Frontal process is well marked.
   c. Body consists of a little more than the alveolar process, the tooth sockets reaching to the floor of orbit.
   d. Maxillary sinus is a mere furrow on the lateral wall of nose.
2. *In the adults:* Vertical diameter is greatest due to development of the alveolar process and increase in the size of the sinus.
3. *In the old:* The bone reverts to infantile condition. Its height is reduced as a result of absorption of the alveolar process.

Applied Clinical Aspect

1. Periodontal disease is a common cause for bone resorption within the alveolar process.

2. Alveolar ridge resorption can also take place after extraction.
3. Maxillary fracture, most commonly the Le Fort fractures are classified into three types:
   a. Le Fort I fracture: Detachment of the alveolar process from the maxilla in a rectangular form.
   b. Le Fort II fracture: Pyramidal in shape, involving the alveolar process, midface and nasal bones.
   c. Le Fort III fracture: Separation of the viscerocranium from the neurocranium. The entire maxilla and nasal bones detach from the skull.

Q. 3. Write a short note on hyoid bone.
(*TNMGR, Sept. 2009; KUHS, Jan. 2014*)

Ans. The hyoid (Greek: *U-shaped*) bone is U-shaped. It develops from second and third branchial arches. It is situated in the anterior midline of the neck between the chin and the thyroid cartilage. At rest, it lies at the level of the third cervical vertebra behind and the base of the mandible in front. It is kept suspended in position by muscles and ligament. The hyoid bone provides attachment to the floor of the mouth and to the tongue above, to the larynx below, and to the epiglottis and pharynx behind. The bone consists of the central part, called the *body*, and of two pairs of *cornua*, greater and lesser.

Body: It has anterior and posterior surfaces, and upper and lower borders. The anterior surface is convex and is directed forwards and upwards. It is often divided by a median ridge into two lateral halves. Posterior surface is concave and is directed backwards and downwards. Posterior surface is separated from epiglottis by thyrohyoid membrane. In early life, body is connected with greater cornu by cartilage, but later they become united by bone.

Greater cornua: These are flattened from above downwards. Each cornua tapers posteriorly, but ends in a tubercle. It has **two surfaces**—upper and lower, **two borders**—medial and lateral and a tubercle.

Lesser cornua: These are small conical pieces of bone which project upwards from the junction of the body and greater cornua. The lesser cornua are connected to the body by fibrous tissue. Occasionally, they are connected to the greater cornua by synovial joints which usually persist throughout life, but may get ankylosed.

Attachments on Hyoid Bone (Fig. 1.3)

1. *Anterior surface of the body*: Insertion to geniohyoid and mylohyoid muscles, origin to hyoglossus.

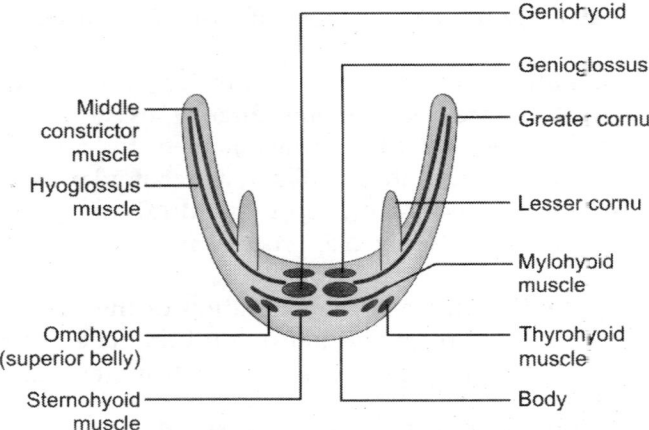

Fig. 1.3: Hyoid bone with muscle attachment

2. *Upper border of the body:* Insertion to the lower fibers of the genioglossi and attachment to the thyrohyoid membrane.

3. *Lower border of the body:* Attachment to the pretracheal fascia. In front of the fascia, the sternohyoid is inserted medially and the omohyoid laterally. Below the omohyoid, there is the linear attachment of the thyrohyoid, extending back to the lower border of the greater cornua.

4. *Medial border of the greater cornua:* Attachment to the thyrohyoid membrane, stylohyoid muscle and digastric pulley.

5. *Lateral border of the greater cornua:* Insertion to the thyrohyoid muscle anteriorly. The investing fascia is attached throughout its length.

6. *Lesser cornua:* Provide attachment to the stylohyoid ligament at its tip. The middle constrictor muscle arises from its posterolateral aspect extending onto the greater cornua.

Applied Clinical Anatomy

1. The primary role of the hyoid bone is to provide stability to adjacent structures through attached muscles.
2. Hyoid serves as a surgical landmark for approaching thyroglossal cysts and base of tongue.
3. Hyoid plays an integral role in the movement of the upper airways.

2. FACE, SCALP AND TEMPLE

Q. 1. Write a note on scalp. *(Gujarat Uni., Oct. 2004; HP Uni., April 2019)*

Ans. The soft tissue covering the cranial vault forms the scalp. The scalp is made of five layers (Fig. 2.1a).

1. **Skin** is thick and hairy, adherent to the epicranial aponeurosis through the dense superficial fascia.
2. **Subcutaneous or superficial fascia (dense connective tissue)** more fibrous and dense in the centre than at the periphery of the head. It binds the skin to the subjacent aponeurosis and provides proper medium for passage of vessels and nerves to the skin.
3. **Epicranial aponeurosis or galea aponeurotica** freely movable on the pericranium along with the overlying and adherent skin and fascia. Anteriorly, it receives insertion of frontalis; posteriorly it receives insertion of occipitalis and is attached to external occipital protuberance and nuchal lines. On each side, it is attached to superior temporal lines and extends down to zygomatic arch.

   First three layers of scalp are called *'surgical layers of the scalp'* or *'scalp proper'*.
4. **Loose areolar tissue:** extends anteriorly into the eyelids because the frontalis muscles have no bony attachment; posteriorly to the highest and superior

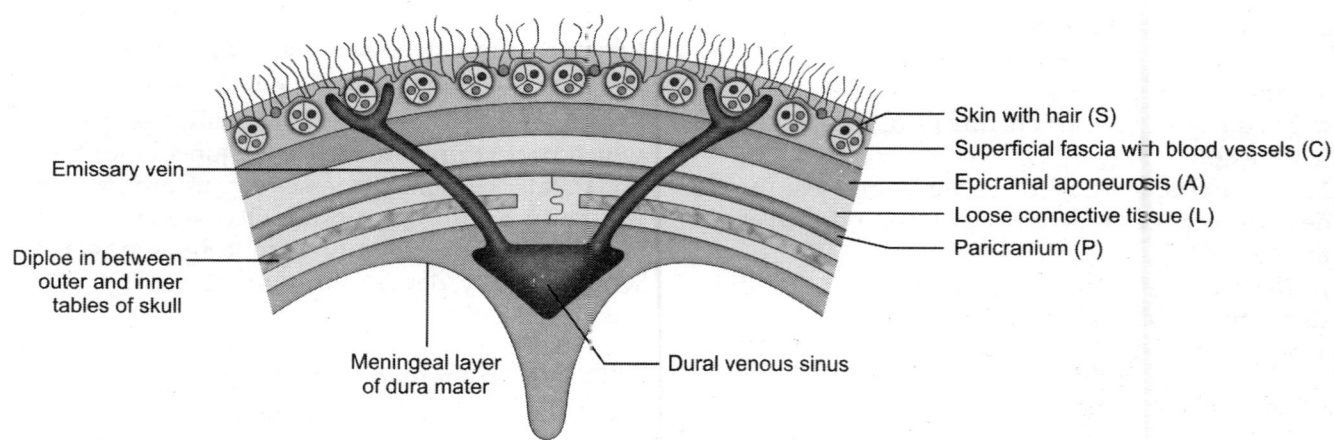

Fig. 2.1a: Layers of SCALP

nuchal line and on each side to the superior temporal lines. It gives passage to emissary veins, connecting extracranial veins to intracranial venous sinuses.

5. **Pericranium** loosely attached to the surface of the bones, but is firmly adherent to their suture where the sutural ligaments bind the pericranium to the endocranium.

Development

- Neural tube and crest forms the nervous system.
- External ectoderm forms epidermis which gives rise to skin of scalp.
- Mesoderm gives rise to connective tissue and subsequent layers of scalp.

Arterial Supply (Fig. 2.1b)

a. *In front of auricle (anterior)*: Supratrochlear, supraorbital, superficial temporal arteries.
b. *Behind the auricle (posterior)*: Posterior auricle, occipital arteries.

Venous Supply

a. Superficial scalp:
  1. Anterior part: Supratrochlear and supraorbital v.
  2. Posterior part: Superficial temporal, occipital and posterior auricular v.
b. Deep scalp: Pterygoid venous plexus.

Lymphatic

Anterior part: Parotid/preauricular lymph nodes.
Posterior part: Occipital and postauricular (mastoid) lymph nodes.

Nerve Supply (Fig. 2.1b)

Anterior: Supratrochlear and supraorbital nerve.

Lateral: Zygomaticotemporal nerve and auriculotemporal nerve.
Posterior: Lesser spinal nerve (cervical plexus) and greater spinal nerve (dorsal rami of the cervical spinal nerve (C2).
Muscle: Occipitofrontalis muscle.

Applied Anatomy

1. Wounds of the scalp gape when epicranial aponeurosis is divided transversely.
2. Scalp is common site for sebaceous cysts, because of plenty of sebaceous glands.
3. Scalp wounds bleed profusely, because once injured, vessels are prevented from retracting by fibrous fascia.
4. Subcutaneous hemorrhages are less extensive and inflammations cause small swelling with severe pain due to dense fascia.
5. Collection of fluid deep to pericranium is known as *cephalhematoma*.
6. The loose areolar tissue layer is known as *dangerous area of the scalp* as the emissary veins from here transmit infection from the scalp to the cranial venous sinuses.
7. Collection of blood in loose connective tissue layer causes generalized swelling of scalp, with no brain compression so known as *safety layer*. This blood may extend to root of nose and eyelids causing *black eye* as frontalis muscle has no bony attachment.
8. Subgaleal hematoma (SGH) is collection of blood between the tense tissue of the galea aponeurotica and the pericranium.
9. Giant cell arteritis: Vasculitis due to granulomatous inflammation of the superficial temporal artery and

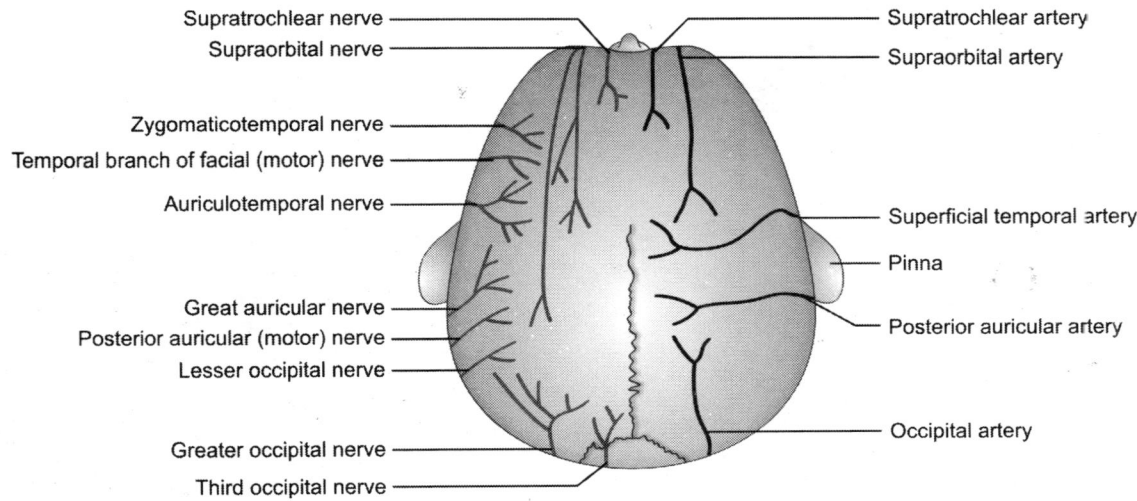

Fig. 2.1b: Arterial (R) and nerve supply (L) of scalp

symptoms include pain in the temple region, headache, flu-like symptoms, and jaw claudication.

Q. 2. Write a note on danger area of face.
(RGUHS, May 2007; UHSR, April 2014)

Ans. Danger area of face comprises upper lip, lower part of nose and adjacent area. It is a triangular area with apex opposite the medial angle of eye and nose and base formed by upper lip (Fig. 2.2). This area has been so named because boils, infections of the nose and injuries around the nose, especially those that become infected can readily spread to cavernous sinus resulting in cavernous sinus thrombosis (CST). CST is generally a fulminate process with high rates of morbidity and mortality.

Anatomical considerations: Anterior facial vein begins at the side of root of nose through the union of supraorbital and frontal veins. The vein drains upper lip, septum of nose and adjacent areas. The anterior facial vein communicates with the cavernous sinus through the ophthalmic veins. It also communicates with cavernous sinus via deep facial vein which connects the pterygoid plexus with anterior facial vein. Anterior facial vein has no valves and it makes possible bidirectional blood flow in the vein. Dangerous area of face is lacking in deep fascia, which acts as barrier to the spread of inflammation and the infective processes. The highly anastomotic and valve less venous system allows retrograde spread of infection to the cavernous sinus via the superior and inferior ophthalmic veins. Squeezing the pimples in the area of upper lip or side of nose or even the cheeks may cause infection which may be carried to the cavernous sinus leading to its

thrombosis, so the cheek area may be included in the dangerous area.

Q. 3. Write a note on muscles of facial expression.
(TNMGR, Sept. 2008; BFUHS, May 2011; UHSR, April 2009; Sumandeep Uni. April 2014; MUHS, June 2016; RGUHS, June 2018; NTR Uni. Oct. 2019)

Q. Write a short note on blood and nerve supply of the face.
(TNMGR, March 2010)

Ans. The facial muscles are striated muscles that attach to the bones of skull to perform important functions for daily life including mastication and facial expressions.

Embryologically, they develop from mesoderm of second branchial arch, therefore supplied by facial nerve.

Morphologically, they represent remnants of *panniculus carnosus* (a subcutaneous muscle sheet seen in some animals). All of them are inserted into the skin.

Topographically, the muscles are grouped under the following six heads (Fig. 2.3a).

A. Muscles of the Scalp
Occipitofrontalis

B. Muscles of the Auricle (Vestigial Muscles)
1. Auricularis anterior
2. Auricularis posterior
3. Auricularis superior

C. Muscles of the Eyelids
1. Orbicularis oculi
2. Corrugator (Latin—*to wrinkle*) supercilii
3. Levator palpebrae superioris (an extraocular muscle, supplied by the third cranial nerve)

D. Muscles of the Nose
1. Procerus
2. Compressor naris
3. Dilator naris
4. Depressor septi

E. Muscles around the Mouth
1. Orbicularis oris
2. Levator labii superioris alaeque nasi
3. Zygomaticus major
4. Levator labii superioris
5. Levator anguli oris
6. Zygomaticus minor
7. Depressor anguli oris
8. Depressor labii inferioris
9. Mentalis (Latin—*chin*)
10. Risorius (Latin—*laughter*)
11. Buccinators (Latin—*cheek*)

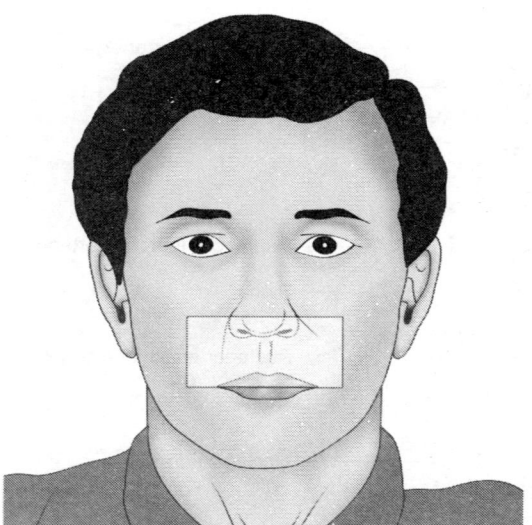

Fig. 2.2: Danger area of face

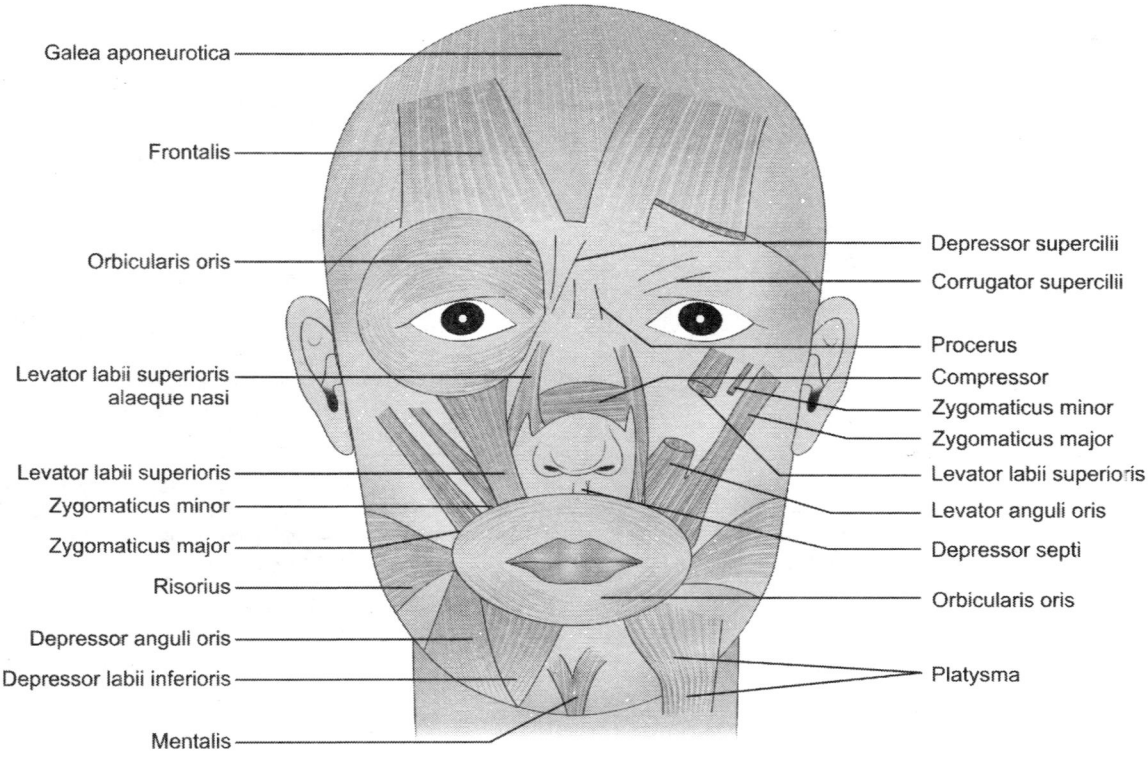

Fig. 2.3a: Muscles of facial expression

F. Muscles of the Neck

Platysma (Greek—*broad*)

Functionally, most of the muscles may be regarded primarily as regulators of three opening situated on the face, namely the palpebral fissures, the nostrils and the oral fissures. Each opening has a single sphincter and a variable number of dilators. Sphincters are naturally circular and the dilators radial in their arrangement.

Blood Supply (Fig. 2.3b)

- Lower and upper lips and mouth: Inferior and superior labial artery.
- Maxillary region: Maxillary artery.
- Muscles located inferior to the mandible: Submental artery.
- Forehead region: Superficial temporal artery.

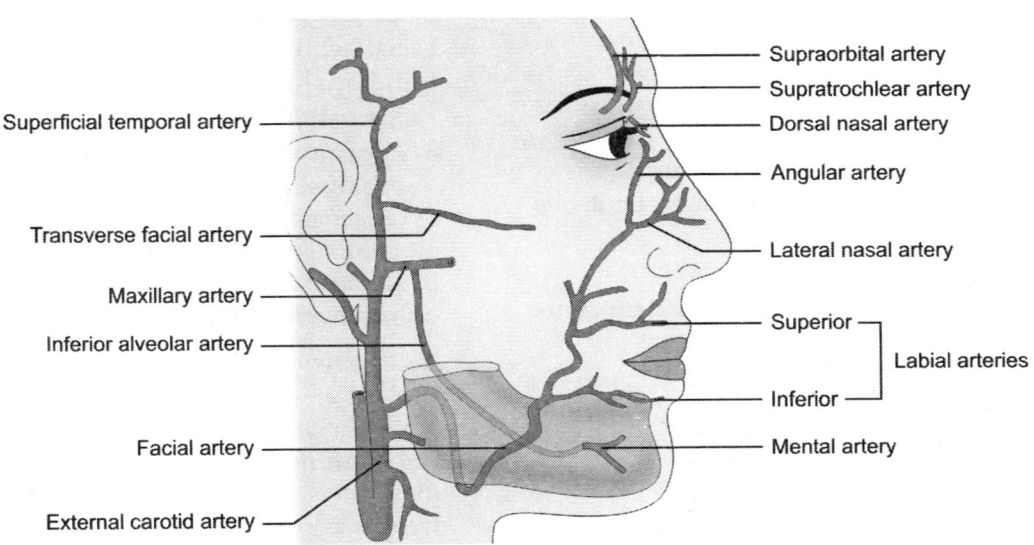

Fig. 2.3b: Arterial supply of face

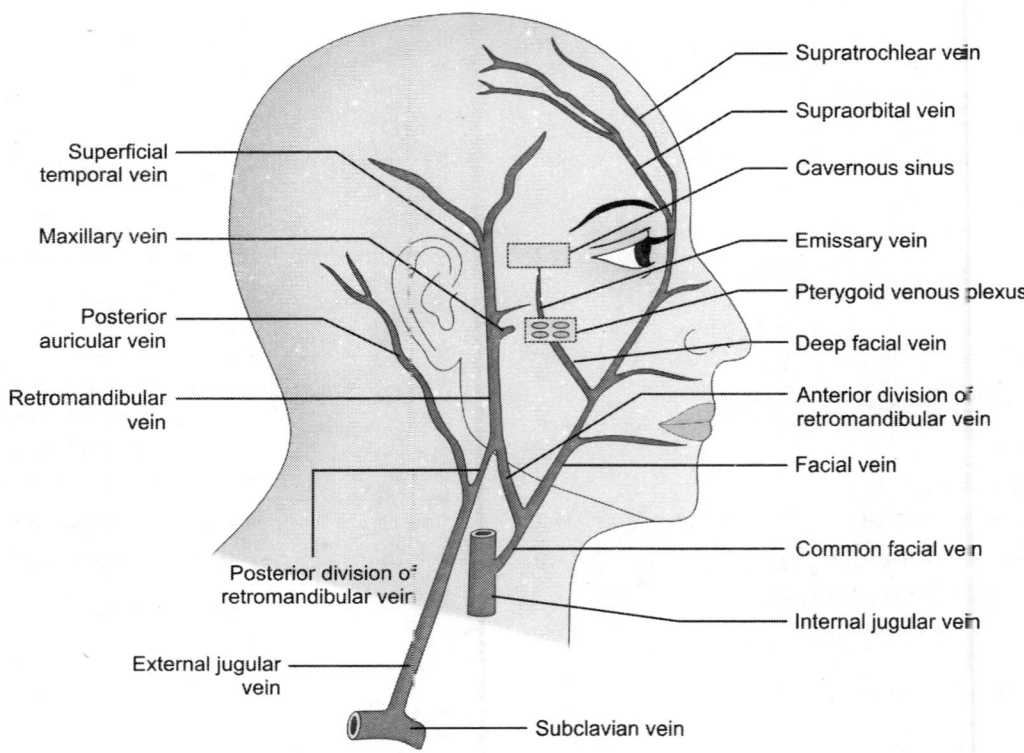

Fig. 2.3c: Venous supply of face and scalp

Venous supply (Fig. 2.3c): Supratrochlear + Supraorbital vein → angular vein → facial vein → internal jugular vein (IJV).

Lymphatics: Submental, submandibular, preauricular, and parotid.

Nerves

1. **Motor:** Facial nerve and mandibular nerve
2. **Sensory:** Trigeminal nerve (CN V)
   - Ophthalmic branch (V1): Forehead region.
   - Maxillary branch (V2): Maxilla region.
   - Mandibular branch (V3): Mandible region.
3. Cervical spinal nerves.

A few common facial expressions and the muscles producing them are given below.

1. *Smiling and laughing*: Zygomaticus major
2. *Sadness*: Levator labii superioris and levator anguli oris
3. *Grief*: Depressor anguli oris
4. *Anger*: Dilator naris and depressor septi
5. *Frowning/dislike*: Corrugator supercilii and procerus
6. *Horror, terror and fright*: Platysma
7. *Surprise*: Frontalis
8. *Doubt*: Mentalis
9. *Grinning*: Risorius
10. *Contempt*: Zygomaticus minor
11. *Closing the mouth*: Orbicularis oris
12. *Whistling*: Buccinators and orbicularis oris.

Applied Clinical Anatomy

1. Myotonia: Failure of muscle relaxation after cessation of voluntary contraction.
2. Myasthenia gravis.
3. The position and anatomy of face make it particularly vulnerable to trauma. Cosmetic results are better when minimal tension (i.e. parallel to natural skin tension lines) is placed on wound edges at the time of repair.
4. Facial hemiatrophy.
5. Facial hemi hypertrophy.
6. Hemifacial microsomia.
7. Facial paralysis:
   a. Supranuclear/upper motor neuron type of paralysis. Only lower part of opposite side of face is paralyzed, upper part is spared due to its bilateral representation in the cerebral cortex
   b. Nuclear: All signs of Bell's palsy except deafness.
   c. Infranuclear lesion also known as Bell's palsy:

Bell's palsy: Unilateral face appears to droop, while the other side of the face is normal in both appearance and function. It is the most common acute mononeuropathy and the most common diagnosis associated with facial nerve paresis (i.e. weakness) or paralysis (i.e. complete motor loss). The 2013 clinical practice guideline committee made the following recommendations for the management.

- Bell's palsy is a diagnosis of exclusion.
- Start oral steroids within 72 hours of symptom onset in patients 16 years and older.
- Clinicians should not prescribe oral antiviral treatment alone for patients with new-onset BP.
- Eye protection for patients presenting with difficulty or inability to close the eyelid.

8. Trigeminal neuralgia.
9. **Modiolus:** It is a fibro-muscular mass formed by the convergence of various muscles towards a focus just lateral to the buccal angle. They are divided into two group:
    a. Cruciate modiolar muscles: Zygomaticus major, levator anguli oris, depressor anguli oris, platysma pars modiolaris.
    b. Transverse muscles: Buccinator, risorius, orbicularis oris, incisivus superior and inferior.

The contraction of modiolus presses corner of mouth against the premolars so that the occlusal table is closed in front. Food is crushed by premolars and molars and it does not escape at the corner of mouth.

Prosthetic significance:

a. Border molding: The functional movements are made during border molding procedure by holding the modiolus with thumb and index finger. It helps in establishing height of occlusal plane of occlusal rim.
b. Corners of mouth are marked on the occlusal rims to provide dentist with anterior landmarks for height of first premolars.
c. The convergence of the muscles of facial expression into modiolus makes it a muscular knot of considerable strength with a wide versatility of movement up, down, forward and back.
d. It is in a strategic position to unseat mandibular dentures and sometimes maxillary dentures as well.

Q. 4. Discuss the course and branches of external carotid artery. Also discuss the applied anatomy of ECA. (TNMGR, Oct. 2003; Sept. 2008; RUHS, June 2017)

Ans. External carotid artery (ECA) lies anterior to internal carotid artery (ICA) and is the chief artery of supply to structures in the front of the neck and in the face. ECA develops from 3rd aortic arch during 4th–5th week of IUL.

Course and Relation

1. ECA begins in the carotid triangle at the level of upper border of thyroid cartilage, opposite 3rd and 4th cervical vertebrae. It runs upwards and slightly backwards and laterally and terminates behind the neck of mandible by dividing into maxillary and superficial temporal arteries.
2. It has a slightly curved course, so that it is anteromedial to ICA in its lower part and anterolateral in its upper part.
3. In carotid triangle, it lies under the cover of anterior border of sternocleidomastoid. The artery is crossed superficially by cervical branch of facial nerve, hypoglossal nerve, and facial, lingual and superior thyroid veins. Deep to the artery, there are: wall of pharynx; superior laryngeal nerve and ascending pharyngeal artery.
4. Above carotid triangle, it lies deep in the substance of parotid gland. Within the gland, it is related superficially to retromandibular vein and facial nerve. Deep to the artery, there are: ICA; Styloglossus, stylopharyngeus, 9th nerve, pharyngeal branch of 10th, and styloid process; superior laryngeal nerve and superior cervical sympathetic ganglion.

Branches (Fig. 2.4a)

Anterior: a. Superior thyroid, b. Lingual, c. Facial.

Posterior: a. Occipital, b. Posterior auricular.

Medial: Ascending pharyngeal.

Terminal: a. Maxillary, b. Superficial temporal.

Superior thyroid artery: Superior thyroid artery arises from ECA just below the level of greater cornua of hyoid bone. It runs downwards and forwards parallel and just superficial to external laryngeal nerve. It passes deep to the three long infrahyoid muscles to reach the upper pole of the lateral lobe of thyroid gland. The artery and external laryngeal nerve are close to each other higher up, but diverge slightly near the gland. To avoid injury to the nerve, the superior thyroid artery is ligated as near the gland as possible.

Branches: i. Terminal branch to thyroid gland, ii. Superior laryngeal artery, iii. Sternocleidomastoid branch, iv. Cricothyroid branch.

Lingual artery (TNMGR, Oct. 2003): The lingual artery arises from ECA opposite the tip of greater cornua of hyoid bone. Its course is divided into three parts by hyoglossus muscle. **First part** lies in the carotid triangle. It forms a characteristic upward loop which is crossed by the hypoglossal nerve. The lingual loop permits free movements of hyoid bone. **Second part** lies deep to hyoglossus along upper border of hyoid bone. It is superficial to middle constrictor of pharynx. **Third part** is called the *arteria profunda linguae* (**Ranine artery**), or

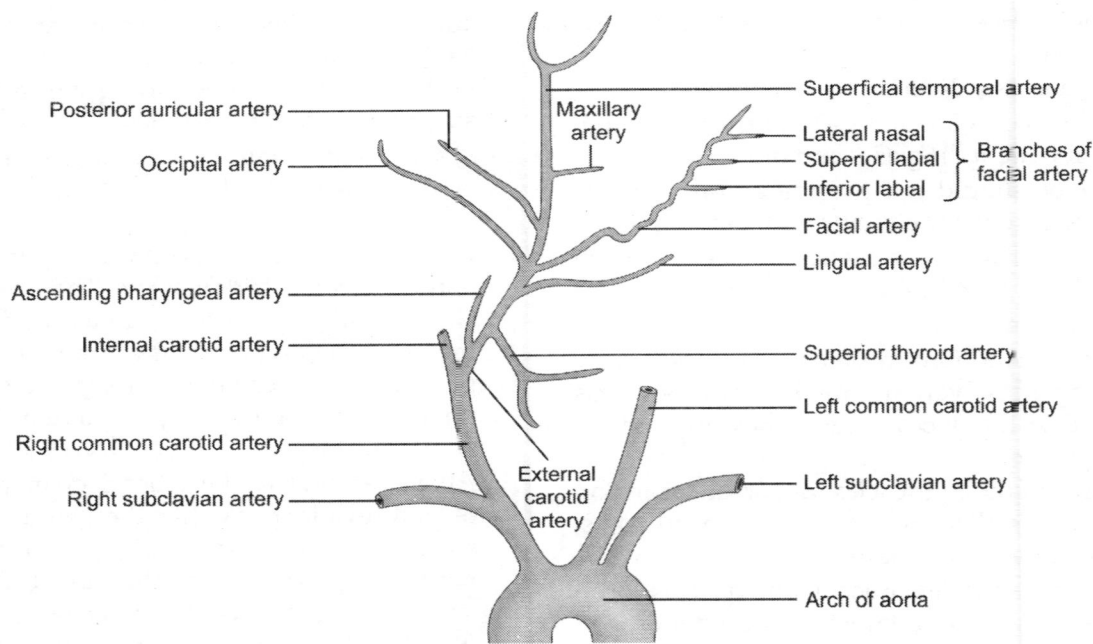

Fig. 2.4a: External carotid artery and its branches

deep lingual artery. It runs upwards along the anterior border of the hyoglossus, and then horizontally forwards on the undersurface of tongue as fourth part. In its vertical course, it lies between the genioglossus medially and the inferior longitudinal muscle of the tongue laterally. The horizontal part of the artery is accompanied by the lingual nerve. During surgical removal of the tongue, the first part of the artery is ligated before it gives any branch to the tongue or to the tonsil (Fig. 2.4b).

Facial artery *(RGUHS, May 2011; KUHS, July 2012)*: The facial artery arises from ECA just above the tip of greater cornua of hyoid bone. It runs upwards first in the neck as **cervical part** and then on the face as **facial part**. The course of the artery in both places is tortuous. The tortuosity in the neck allows free movements of the pharynx during deglutition. On the face, it allows free movements of the mandible, lips and the cheek during mastication and during various facial expressions.

1. **Cervical part:** It runs upwards on the superior constrictor of pharynx deep to posterior belly of digastrics with stylohyoid and to the ramus of the mandible. It grooves posterior border of the submandibular gland. Then the artery makes an

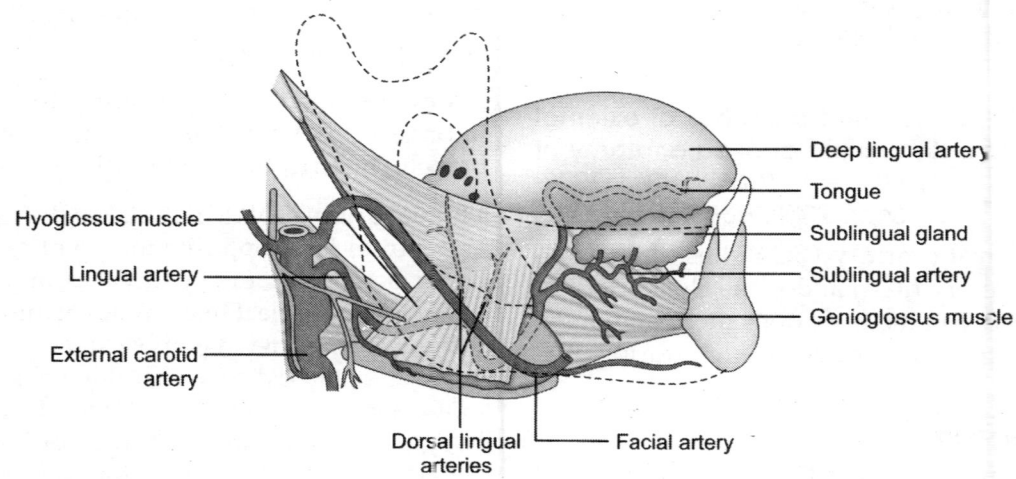

Fig. 2.4b: Lingual artery and its branches

S-bend, first winding down over submandibular gland and then up over the base of mandible.

Branches: i. Ascending palatine, ii. Tonsillar, iii. Submental, iv. Glandular branches for submandibular gland and lymph nodes.

2. **Facial part:** It enters the face at anteroinferior angle of masseter muscle (here it is called anesthetist's artery), runs upwards close to angle of mouth, side of nose till medial angle of eye.

Branches: i. Inferior labial, ii. Superior labial, iii. Lateral nasal, iv. Angular artery (terminal segment)

Surgical considerations

1. The facial artery has a role in reconstructive procedures of the face as it acts vascular supply for various flaps including local flaps, regional flaps, or free flaps, e.g. submental, platysma muscle, nasolabial, buccinator myomucosal, and facial artery musculo-mucosal flaps.

2. External approaches to mandible fracture repair can require ligation of the facial artery. If bleeding from the facial artery occurs, direct pressure should be applied to the angle of mandible over the vessel until the vessel is identified and bleeding controlled.

Occipital artery: It arises from the posterior aspect of ECA, opposite the origin of facial artery. It is crossed at its origin by hypoglossal nerve. In the carotid triangle, the artery gives two **sternocleidomastoid branches.** The upper branch accompanies the accessory nerve and the lower branch arises near the origin of the occipital artery.

Posterior auricular artery: It arises from the posterior aspect of ECA, just above the posterior belly of digastrics. It runs upwards and backwards deep to parotid gland but superficial to the styloid process. It crosses base of the mastoid process and ascends behind the auricle. It supplies back of the auricle, skin over mastoid process and over the back of the scalp. It is cut in incisions for the mastoid operations. Its **stylomastoid branch** enters the stylomastoid foramen and supplies middle ear, mastoid antrum and air cells, semicircular canals and facial nerve.

Ascending pharyngeal artery: This is a small branch that arises from the medial side of ECA, close to its lower end. It runs vertically upwards between the side wall of the pharynx and the tonsil, medial wall of the middle ear and the auditory tube. It sends meningeal branches into the cranial cavity through foramen lacerum, jugular foramen and hypoglossal canal.

Maxillary artery: This is larger terminal branch of ECA. It begins behind the neck of mandible under cover of

the parotid gland. It runs forwards deep to the neck of the mandible below the auriculotemporal nerve and enters the infratemporal fossa.

Superficial temporal artery: It is the smaller terminal branch of ECA, begins behind the neck of the mandible under cover of the parotid gland. It runs vertically upwards, crossing the root of zygoma, divides into anterior and posterior branches which supply the temple and scalp. The anterior branch anastomoses with the supraorbital and supratrochlear branches of the ophthalmic artery. In addition, it gives off a transverse facial artery and a middle temporal artery which runs on the temporal fossa deep to the temporalis muscle.

Applied Clinical Anatomy

1. **Carotid artery disease:** Atherosclerosis leading to blockages of vessel due to the build-up of fatty deposits (plaques).

2. **Aneurysm:** Damage to ECA leading to ballooning of a portion of the artery, or complete rupture.

3. Pulse of the facial artery is palpable at the anteroinferior angle of the masseter muscle against the bony surface of the mandible.

Q. 5. Write a note on maxillary artery.
(TNMGR, Sept. 2002; MAHE, April 2013)

Ans. Maxillary artery is larger terminal branch of ECA, given off behind the neck of the mandible. It has a wide territory of distribution and supplies:

a. External and middle ears and auditory tube.
b. Duramater.
c. Upper and lower jaws and teeth.
d. Muscles of the temporal and infratemporal regions.
e. Nose and paranasal air sinuses.
f. Palate.
g. Root of the pharynx.

Course and relations: Three parts (Fig. 2.5):

1. **First (mandibular) part:** Runs horizontally forwards, first between the neck of the mandible and sphenomandibular ligament, below the auriculotemporal nerve and then along the lower border of lateral pterygoid.

2. **Second (pterygoid) part:** Runs upwards and forwards superficial to the lower head of the lateral pterygoid.

3. **Third (pterygopalatine) part:** Passes between the two heads of the lateral pterygoid and through the pterygomaxillary fissure, to enter the pterygopalatine fossa.

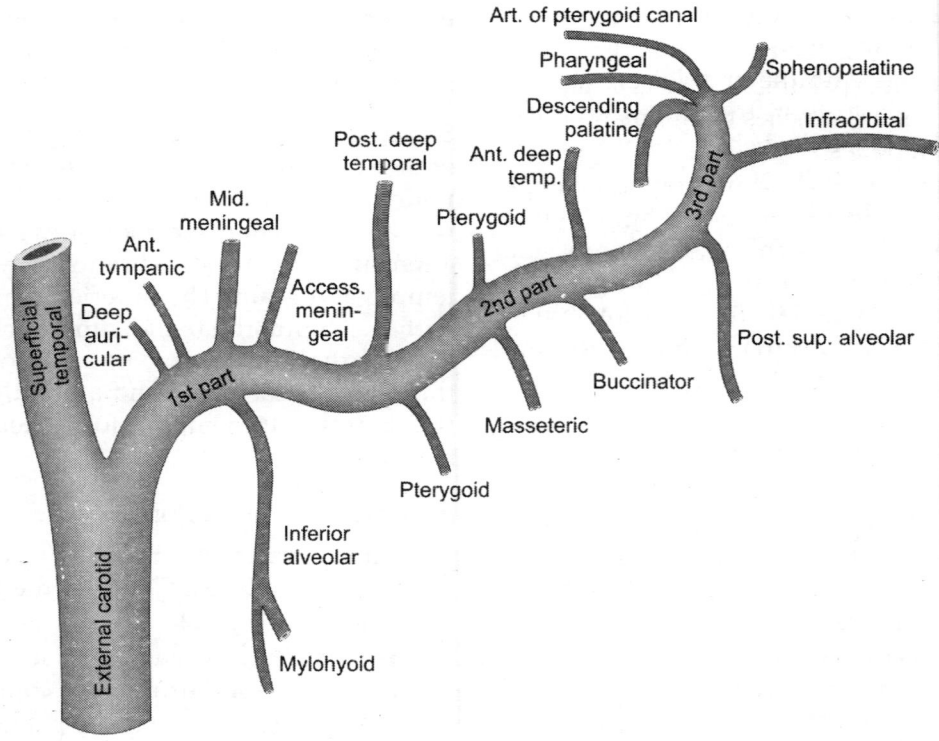

Fig. 2.5: Maxillary artery and its branches

Branches of first part (DAMAI)

1. **Deep auricular artery:** External acoustic meatus, outer surface of tympanic membrane and temporomandibular joint (TMJ).
2. **Anterior tympanic branch:** Middle ear, medial surface of tympanic membrane.
3. **Middle meningeal artery:** Bone, meninges, 5th, 7th nerves, middle ear and tensor tympani.
4. **Accessory meningeal artery:** Meninges and structures in the infratemporal fossa.
5. **Inferior alveolar artery:** Tongue, mylohyoid muscle, mandible, roots of mandibular teeth and chin

Branches of second part

1. **Masseteric:** Masseter muscle.
2. **Deep temporal (anterior and posterior):** Temporalis muscle.
3. **Pterygoid:** Lateral and medial pterygoid muscle.
4. **Buccal:** Buccinator muscle.

Branches of third part

1. **Posterior superior alveolar artery:** Maxillary molar and premolar teeth; gums and maxillary air sinus.
2. **Infraorbital artery:** Orbital branches—orbit; Middle superior alveolar branch—premolar teeth; Anterior superior alveolar branches—incisor and canine teeth. Also branches to lacrimal sac, the nose and the upper lip.
3. **Greater palatine artery:** Soft palate, tonsil, palatine glands and mucosa; upper gums.
4. **Pharyngeal branch:** Roof of nose and pharynx; auditory tube; sphenoidal sinus.
5. **Artery of the pterygoid canal:** Auditory tube; upper pharynx and middle ear.
6. **Sphenopalatine artery (artery of 'epistaxis'):** Lateral and medial walls of nose and paranasal sinuses.

Applied Clinical Anatomy

1. Epidural hematomas (EDH) forms due to trauma to middle meningeal artery (MMA) at the pterion (region where frontal, parietal, temporal and sphenoid bone meet on side of temple). The patient initially experiences a brief loss of consciousness following a *"lucid interval"* where the patient can function, again to become unconscious with increased mortality.
2. Sphenopalatine artery is a common cause of posterior epistaxis.

Q. 6. Write a short note on facial vein.

Ans. The common facial vein is formed by joining of facial vein and anterior branch of retromandibular vein.

Origin and course: Facial vein pierces the deep investing fascia of the neck just below the border of the mandible where it unites with the anterior branch of the retromandibular vein to form the common facial vein, which empties into IJV. It lies behind the maxillary artery and follows a less tortuous course. It runs obliquely downward and backward, beneath the zygomaticus and zygomatic head of the quadratus labii superioris, descends along the anterior border and then on the superficial surface of the masseter, crosses over the body of the mandible, to unite with posterior facial vein to form the common facial vein, The common facial vein crosses the external carotid artery and enters the IJV vein below the hyoid bone.

Tributaries: Submental, tonsillar, external palatine, submandibular, pharyngeal, and superior thyroid vein.

Q. 7. Write a short note on pterygoid venous plexus.
(Bangalore Uni., Jan. 1992)

Ans. It is the plexus of veins present around and within the lateral pterygoid muscle. It is the main venous component associated with the infratemporal fossa. The pterygoid plexus joins the maxillary vein as it passes posterior to the mandible. The maxillary vein joins the superficial temporal vein to form the retromandibular vein that lies within the parotid gland. It is formed by following veins:

1. Sphenopalatine vein.
2. Deep temporal vein.
3. Pterygoid vein.
4. Masseteric vein.
5. Buccal vein.
6. Alveolar veins.
7. Greater palatine vein.
8. Middle meningeal veins.
9. Branches from ophthalmic vein.

It drains into the following veins:
1. Facial vein via deep facial vein
2. Cavernous sinus via veins passing through foramen ovale and foramen lacerum.

Applied Clinical Anatomy

The pterygoid plexus is in connection with cavernous sinus through small emissary veins which do not contain venous valves, which can allow infections within the dental area to travel to the cavernous sinus, causing thrombosis.

3. TEMPOROMANDIBULAR JOINT AND MUSCLES OF MASTICATION

Q. 1. Write a short note on evolution of temporomandibular joint.
(Gujarat Uni., April 2019; TNMGR, Oct. 2019)

Ans. Evolution of TMJ: The earliest type of vertebrae, the *Agnatha* had the opening of their mouth on the ventral side anterior to the vertebral axis leading from the oropharyngeal channel to gut proper. The slits that opened to the outside served for both respiration and food filtration. These moved simultaneously in cooperation with a mouth through a series of cartilages called gill arches with bend known as the *synarthrosis* (primary jaw joint).

Amphibia: The amphibia has a single joint for the double jaws between nasal and frontal bone. The jaws of these creatures were used just for protection. In some mammals, direct tooth to tooth contact is necessary for sharpening of teeth which is absent in pelycosauria, a mammal-like reptile which may be considered as ancestors of all later mammals like reptiles. Their teeth are all of a simple blade-like form. The primary notable modification from the amphibian structure was the disappearance of the otic notch that supported the tympanum of the primitive ear.

Reptilia: They have loss of bony components within the pelycosauria. The dentary bone has a limited extension distal to the tooth row, while the postdentary bones are well developed and comprise the posterior third of the jaw. In the mammalian architectural theme, the mandible forms the lower jaw and articulates with the skull. It also forms the lateral walls of the upper food way, which is roofed above by a palate. The viscerocranium provides roof and walls to them. Upper food airway and the neurocrania house the brain. The mammalian skull has two characteristics—the carnivores and the herbivores. The herbivores form the pelycosauria did not show many evolutionary changes whereas the carnivores and the insectivorous showed.

Austrolopithecus: African skull is least differentiated. It has some characteristics features:
- The jaw protrudes sharply.
- Upper jaw has outstanding canine buttresses. It has a slender zygomatic arch when compared with *Austrolopithecus boisei* skull. It has massive zygomatic buttresses, and the jaws are retruded.

Muscular elements are specialization of the lateral pterygoid muscle with decrease in the bulk of temporalis muscle. The contraction of the lateral pterygoid muscle permitted modification of condylar movement.

Q. 2. Discuss the development of temporomandibular joint. (BFUHS, May 2007; AHSUC, May 2017)

Ans. In 8–9th week of IUL, Meckel's cartilage provides the skeletal support for the development of the mandible and extends from the midline backwards and dorsally. The articulation of malleus and incus functions as the primary TMJ.

At, 10th week of IUL: Two distinct regions of mesenchymal condensation appear between condylar cartilage and developing temporal bone, i.e. temporal blastema and condylar blastema. At the same time lateral pterygoid muscle attaches to condyle.

12th week of IUL: Two slit-like joint cavities and an intervening disc appear.

1st cleft appears immediately above condylar blastema becomes inferior joint cavity. The condylar blastema then differentiates into condylar cartilage.

2nd cleft appears in relation to the temporal ossification that becomes the superior joint cavity and primitive articular disk is formed. The mesenchyme around the joint begins to form the fibrous joint capsule. The developing superior head of the lateral pterygoid muscle attaches to the anterior portion of the fetal disk. The disk also continues posteriorly through the petrotympanic fissure and attaches to the malleus of the middle ear.

16th week of IUL: Malleus and incus begin transformation into middle ear bones and disappearance of primary joint starts.

18–20th week of IUL: Secondary joint becomes functional and Meckel's cartilage loses its function and disappears.

Mandibular fossa is flat at birth and there is no articular eminence, this becomes prominent only following the eruption of the deciduous dentition.

Q. 3. Describe in detail the anatomy of the temporomandibular joint?
(BFUHS, May 2011; MUHS, April 2012; UHSR, April 2013; CDER-AIIMS, May 2014; HP Uni., June 2016; AHSUC, July 2016; MPMS Uni., July 2017; TNMGR, Oct. 2018, 2019)

Q. Write a short note on articular disc of temporomandibular joint. (TNMGR, April 1998; March 2002; Sept. 2002)

Q. Describe the temporomandibular joint, its relations, movements, age changes and disorders of the TMJ.
(RGUHS, Nov. 2011; KUHS, Jan. 2014; MUHS, Sumandeep Uni., April 2014)

Q. Briefly describe development, anatomy and histological characteristics of TMJ. (BFUHS, May 2009; HP Uni., May 2017; April 2019)

Q. Give classification of joints. Describe the temporomandibular joint and discuss how it differs from other joints? (MUHS, November 2014)

Ans. A **joint/arthrosis** is a junction between two or more bones or cartilages.

Classification of joints

A. **Structural classification**
1. **Fibrous joint (immovable joint):** i. Sutures (e.g. Skull), ii. Syndesmosis (e.g. inter-osseous), iii. Gomphosis (e.g. joint between tooth root and socket).
2. **Cartilaginous joints (limited movement):** i. Primary cartilaginous joint or synchondrosis (e.g. hyaline cartilage at ends of long bones), ii. Secondary cartilaginous joints or symphysis (e.g. symphysis menti).
3. **Synovial joints:** Permits free movements between two bones surrounded by capsule enclosing joint cavity filled with synovial fluid. Types are:
   a. Based on complexity: i. Simple, ii. Complex, iii. Compound
   b. Based on degree of freedom: i. Uniaxial, ii. Biaxial, iii. Multiaxial
   c. Based on shape of the articulating surfaces: i. Planer joint, ii. Ginglymoid (hinge) joint, iii. Condylar or bicondylar joint, iv. Sellar or saddle joint, v. Spheroidal (ball and socket) joint, vi. Ellipsoid joints, vii. Pivot or trochoid joints.

B. **Functional classification** (according to the degree of mobility)
1. Synarthrosis (immovable), like fibrous joints.
2. Amphiarthrosis (slightly movable), like cartilaginous joints.
3. Diarthrosis (freely movable), like synovial joints.

TMJ: Temporomandibular joint is also known as the Craniomandibular joint bicondylar/mandibular/modified ball and socket/compound joint) or bilateral diarthroidal joint. It is the articulation between the squamous part of the temporal bone and the head of the condyle. It is also considered as a complex joint because it involves two separate synovial joints in which there is a presence of intra-capsular disc or meniscus. So, TMJ is a complex diarthrodial (gliding)-ginglymoid (hing) synovial joint (Fig. 3.3a).

Articular surfaces: The *upper articular surface* is formed by the following parts of the temporal bone (Fig. 3.3b):
a. Articular tubercle.
b. Anterior part of mandibular fossa.

The *inferior articular surface* is formed by the head of mandible.

The articular surfaces are covered with *fibrocartilage*. The joint cavity is divided into upper and lower parts by an intra-articular disc.

Mandibular fossa: Anterior aspect—articular eminence; Posterior non articular fossa is a part of temporal squama and is formed by tympanic plate.

Condyle: Barrel shape; ~20 mm mediolateral and ~10 mm anteroposterior. Perpendicular to ascending ramus of the mandible, oriented 10–30° with frontal plane. Medial pole is more prominent than lateral pole.

Bony surface of condyle and articular part of the temporal bone covered with dense fibrous connective tissues with irregular cartilage like cells. The number of cells increases with age and stress on the joint.

Ligaments: A ligament is the fibrous connective tissue that connects bones to other bones. They do not enter actively into joint function but instead act as passive restraining devices to limit and restrict border movements. Ligaments of TMJ includes (Fig. 3.3c):

1. **Fibrous capsule** is attached above to the articular tubercle, the circumference of the mandibular fossa and the squamotympanic fissure and below to the neck of the mandible. The capsule is loose above the intra-articular disc, and tight below it. The synovial membrane lines the fibrous capsule and the neck of the mandible.

2. **Lateral or temporomandibular ligament** reinforces and strengthens the lateral part of the capsular ligament. Its fibers are directed downwards and backwards. It is attached above to the articular tubercle,

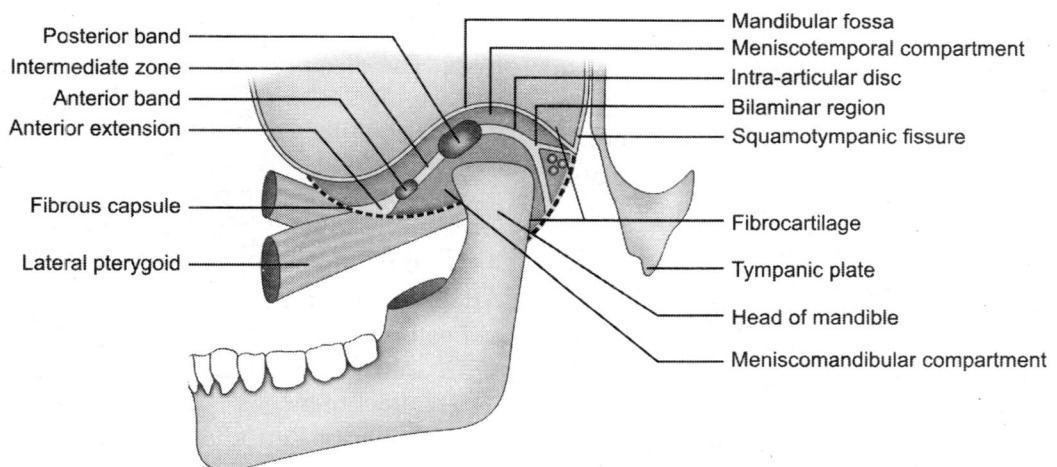

Fig. 3.3a: Temporomandibular joint (TMJ) with all attachments

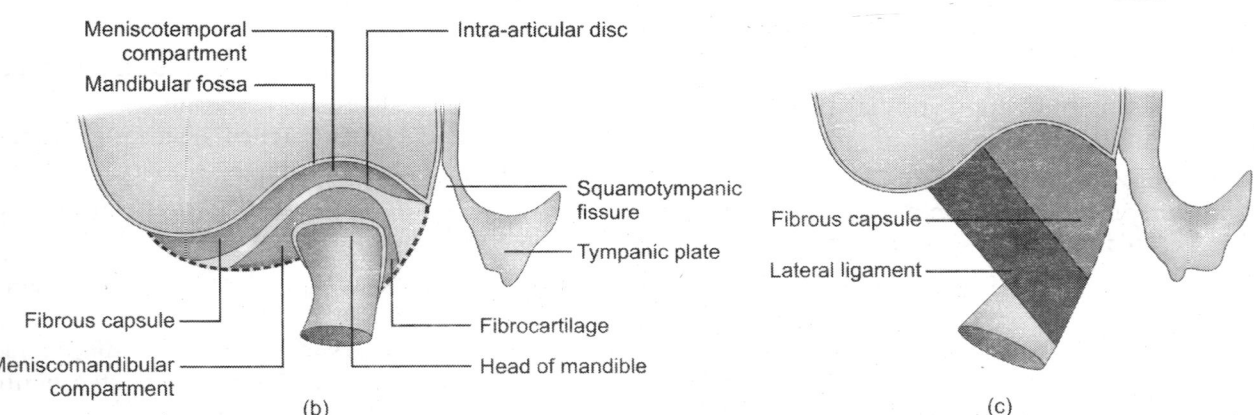

(b)

(c)

Fig. 3.3b and c: Articular disc and its components (L), Lateral ligament of TMJ (R) and below to the posterolateral aspect of the neck of the mandible.

3. **Sphenomandibular ligament (SML)** (*NTR Uni., June 2015*) is an accessory ligament that lies on a deep plane away from the fibrous capsule. It is attached superiorly to the spine of the sphenoid, and inferiorly to the lingula of the mandibular foramen. It is a remnant of the dorsal part of Meckel's cartilage. The ligament is related:
   a. Laterally: To lateral pterygoid muscle; Auriculo-temporal nerve; Maxillary artery.
   b. Medially: To chorda tympani and Wall of pharynx.

4. **Stylomandibular ligament** (*NTR Uni., June 2015*) is another accessory ligament of the joint. It represents a thickened part of the *deep cervical fascia* which separates the parotid and submandibular glands. It is attached above to the lateral surface of the styloid process and below to the angle and adjacent part of the posterior border of the ramus of mandible.

5. **Oto-mandibular ligaments** are:
   a. **Discomalleolar ligament (DML):** Arises from the malleus and runs to the medial retrodiscal tissue of the TMJ.
   b. **Anterior malleolar ligament (AML):** Arises from the malleus and connects with lingula of the mandible via the sphenomandibular ligament.

   These ligaments are implicated in tinnitus associated with TMD.

Synovium/synovial membrane: Synovial tissue is a vascular connective tissue lining the fibrous joint capsule and extending to the boundaries of the articulating surfaces. This lining, along with a specialized synovial fringe located at the anterior border of the retrodiscal tissues, produces synovial fluid, which fills both joint cavities. Synovial fluid is a filtrate of plasma with added mucins and proteins.

Contents of synovial fluid

Cells: Monocytes, lymphocytes, free synovial cells and occasionally PMNs.

Chemical, hyaluronate is a glucosaminoglycans (GAG), gives viscosity to the synovial fluid, draws water and salts to the cavity.

Function of synovial fluid
i. Medium for providing metabolic requirements to the non vascular articular surface of the joint.
ii. Lubricant between articular surfaces during function.

Mechanisms by which synovial fluid lubricates are:
a. Boundary lubrication: Occurs when joint is moved and synovial fluid is forced from one area of cavity into another.
b. Weeping lubrication: Ability of articular surfaces to absorb a small amount of synovial fluid. This is the mechanism by which metabolic exchange occurs.

Articular disc (Fig. 3.3c): The articular disc is a biconcave oval fibrous plate interposed between the condyle and the temporal bone that divides the joint into upper and lower compartments. *Superior cavity* contains mandibular fossa and superior surface of disc; *Inferior cavity* contains mandibular condyle and inferior surface of disc. The upper compartment permits gliding movements and the lower, rotator as well as gliding movements. The disc has a concavo-convex superior surface, and a concave inferior surface. The periphery of the disc is attached to fibrous capsule. It consists of dense collagenous tissue that is avascular, hyaline and devoid of nerve tissues in the central area but has vessels and nerves in the peripheral area. The disc is composed of an anterior extension, anterior thick band, intermediate zone (articular surface), posterior thick zone and bilaminar region. The disc represents the degenerated primitive insertion of lateral pterygoid. It is thicker medially than laterally and shape of disc is determined by morphology of condyle and mandibular fossa. The disc prevents friction between the articular surfaces. It acts as a cushion and helps in shock absorption. It stabilizes the cartilage by filling up the space between articulating surfaces. The proprioceptive fibers present in the disc help to regulates movements of the joint. The disc helps in the distribution of weight across the TMJ by increasing area of contact.

Attachments of disc

a. Posteriorly:
   i. Retrodiscal tissue: highly vascularized posterior attachment.
   ii. Superior Retrodiscal lamina: elastic fibres.
   iii. Inferior Retrodiscal lamina: collagenous fibres.
   iv. Remaining: large venous plexus which fills with blood as condyle moves forward.
b. Anteriorly:
   i. Superior attachment: Articular surface of temporal bone.
   ii. Inferior attachment; Articular surface of condyle. Both composed of collagen fibres
   iii. Between the capsular ligament attachment: Superior lateral pterygoid muscles.

Histology: The articular surfaces are composed of 4 zones: (**Fig. P-1; Color Plate 1**)

1. *Articular zone:* Most superficial layer, adjacent to the joint cavity and forms the outermost functional surface. It is made up of dense fibrous connective tissue and the collagen fibres bundles are oriented

nearly parallel to the articular surface to withstand the forces of movement. It is less susceptible to the effects of aging and has much better ability to repair than hyaline cartilage.

2. *Proliferative zone:* This is composed of undifferentiated mesenchymal tissue. This is responsible for the proliferation of articular cartilage in response to the functional demands.

3. *Fibrocartilagenous zone:* Collagen fibrils are arranged in bundles in a crossing pattern. The fibrocartilage appears in a random orientation providing three dimensional networks that offers resistance against compressive and lateral forces.

4. *Calcified zone:* It is made up of chondrocytes and chondroblasts distributed throughout the articular cartilage. The chondrocytes produce collagen, proteoglycans, glycoproteins, and enzymes that form the matrix.

Relations of Temporomandibular Joint

A. **Lateral**
   a. Skin and fasciae.
   b. Parotid gland.
   c. Temporal branches of the facial nerve.
B. **Medial**
   a. Tympanic plate.
   b. Spine of the sphenoid.
   c. Auriculotemporal and chorda tympani nerves.
   d. Middle meningeal artery (MMA).
C. **Anterior**
   a. Lateral pterygoid.
   b. Masseteric nerve and artery.

D. **Posterior**
   a. Parotid gland.
   b. Superficial temporal vessels.
   c. Auriculotemporal nerve.
E. **Superior**
   a. Middle cranial fossa.
   b. Middle meningeal vessels.
F. **Inferior:** Maxillary artery and vein.

Blood supply: Superficial temporal (posterior, Main supply); Middle meningeal artery (anterior); Internal maxillary artery (inferior); Deep auricular; Anterior tympanic and ascending pharyngeal arteries. The condyle is vascularized through marrow spaces by the inferior alveolar artery. Veins follow the arteries.

Nerve supply: Auriculotemporal nerve, deep temporal and masseteric nerve.

Movements of TMJ (Fig. 3.3d): Movements of TMJ can be palpated by intra-auricular or extra-auricular palpation. These movements can be divided into those occurring between upper articular surface and articular disc, i.e. meniscotemporal (upper) compartment and those between disc and head of mandible, i.e. meniscomandibular (lower) compartment. The various TMJ movements are:

1. **Forward movement** or **protraction** of the mandible: The articular disc glides forwards over the upper articular surface, the head of the mandible moving with it. This movement occurs in meniscotemporal compartment.

2. **Retraction:** The articular disc glides backwards over the upper articular surface taking the head of

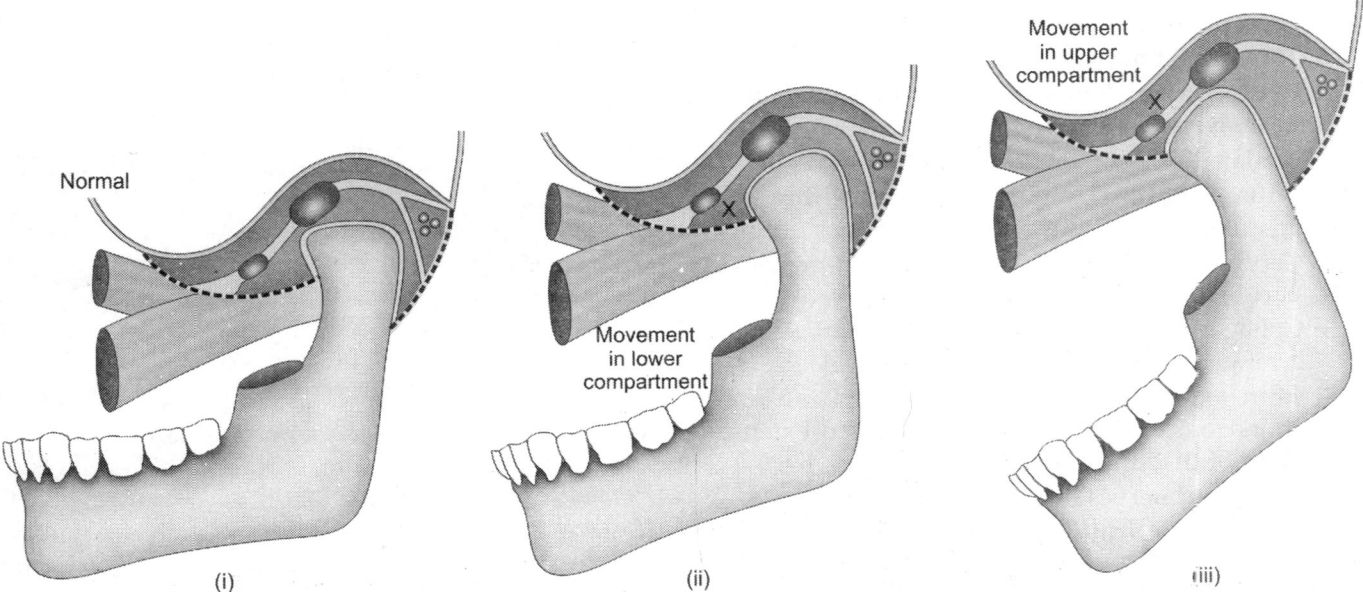

Fig. 3.3d: Movement of TMJ

mandible with it. Mandible rotates around a horizontal axis extending from left to right condyle.

3. **Slight opening of the mouth or depression of the mandible:** The head of the mandible moves on the undersurface of the disc like a hinge in lower compartment. The movement occurs around a vertical axis passing through the condyle and posterior border of ramus of mandible.

4. **Wide opening of the mouth:** Hinge-like movement is followed by gliding of the disc and the head of the mandible, as in protraction. At the end of this movement, the head comes to lie under the articular tubercle.

5. **Closing the mouth** or **elevation of the mandible:** Reverse of that in opening.

6. **Chewing movements:** Involve side to side movements of the mandible. In these movements, the head of right side glides forwards along with the disc as in protraction, but the head of the left side merely rotates on a vertical axis. As a result of this, the chin moves forward and to left side. Alternate movements of this kind on the two sides result in side to side movements of the jaw.

Age changes

A. **Condyle**
1. Stop growing at 20 years of age with continuous adaptation response.
2. Condylar head decreases in convexity and in condylar height.
3. Resorption is more on lateral aspect than medial.
4. Condyle becomes flattened.
5. Fibrous capsule becomes thicker with chondroid changes.
6. Osteoporosis of underlying bone.
7. Thinning or absence of cartilaginous zone.

B. **Articular layer:** Vascular at birth and becomes progressively fibrous.

C. **Articular disc**
1. Initially flat and highly vascular, with aging vascularity decreases and disc becomes fibrous.
2. Central part thins with anterior and posterior part becoming thicker.
3. Collagen fibres become coarse and dense and get arranged in three dimensional networks.
4. Thin articular disc with hyalinization and chondroid changes leads to decreased extensibility of disc and capsule.
5. Decreased nerves in disc and capsule.

D. **Synovial membrane:** Synovial folds and villi increases and becomes fibrotic with thick basement membrane. Also decrease in synovial fluid formation leading to loss of lubrication.

E. **Blood vessels and nerves:** Thickened walls of blood vessels and decrease in number of nerves.

Applied Clinical Anatomy

1. During the surgical exposure through a preauricular approach, surgeon should protect the temporal branch of facial nerve.

2. Incising and reflecting the capsule usually lead to the cutting of nerve fibres, which may result in postoperative analgesia and relief from pain.

3. **TMJ disorders** (*Gujarat Uni., June 2018*): Table 3.3 shows classification of TM disorders (TMDs).

4. **Dislocation of mandible** occurs during excessive mouth opening as the head of condyle slips into the infratemporal fossa, leading to inability to close

Table 3.3: Classification of TMDs

Articular disorders (intra-articular)
Congenital or developmental disorders
Condylar hyperplasia
First and second branchial arch disorders
Idiopathic condylar resorption
Degenerative joint disorders
Inflammatory capsulitis, synovitis, polyarthritides (rheumatoid arthirits, psoriatic arthriris, ankylosing spondylitis, reiter syndrome, gout)
Non-inflammatory: Osteoarthritis
Disk derangement disorders
Displacement with reduction
Displacement without reduction (closed lock)
Perforation
Infection
Neoplasia
Temporomandibular hypermobility
Dislocation
Joint laxity
Subluxation
Temporomandibular hypomobility
Ankylosis: True ankylosis (bony or fibrous) or pseudo-ankylosis
Postradiation fibrosis
Trismus
Trauma
Contusion
Fracture
Intracapsular hemorrhage
Masticatory muscle disorders (extra-articular)
Local myalgia
Myofascial pain disorder
Myofibrotic contracture
Myositis
Myospasm
Neoplasia

the mouth. Reduction can be done by depressing the jaw with the thumbs placed on the last molar teeth, with downward, backward and upward pressure.

5. **Derangement of articular disc** may result from any injury, like over closure or malocclusion leading to clicking/crepitus and pain.

6. **During TMJ surgery,** the 7th nerve and auriculotemporal nerve should be preserved carefully as they have close relation with joint.

Myofascial pain dysfunction syndrome (MPDS): MPDS is a pain disorder in which unilateral pain is referred from the trigger point in myofascial structures, to the muscles of head and neck. *Trigger points* are localized tender areas within taut bands of skeletal muscles when stimulated by macro/micro traumatic injury. Palpation of trigger points gives a positive '*Jump sign*'. It is characterized by masticatory muscle tenderness (lateral pterygoid > temporalis > medial pterygoid > masseter); Limited opening of mandible (<37 mm); Joint sounds; Seen more commonly in females (F: M; 3:1).

Etiology

1. Tooth muscle theory: Occlusal interference causes an altered proprioceptive feedback, leading to incoordination and spasm of muscles of mastication.
2. Prosthetic problems: Faulty prosthesis, over closure, bilateral loss of molar teeth, increased vertical dimensions.
3. Malocclusion: Oral habits (clenching, grinding of teeth), anxiety.
4. Psycho-physiologic theory: Masticatory muscle spasm causes MPDS, degenerative arthritis and contracture arthritis.
5. Steep angulations of articular eminence.

Pathophysiology: Micro/macro trauma to muscles increased tone of musculature → muscle fatigue and accumulation of metabolic byproducts like lactic acid, prostaglandins, bradykinin, histamines, which lowers pH → involves a psychogenic component which modifies pain and complicates the treatment.

Diagnosis is by Laskin's cardinal symptoms of MPDS:

1. Pain or discomfort anywhere about the head or neck.
2. Limitation of motion of the jaw.
3. Joint noises—grating, clicking, snapping.
4. Tenderness on palpation of the muscles of mastication.

Negative characteristics:

1. Absence of clinical, radiographic or biochemical evidence of organic changes in TMJ.
2. Lack of tenderness in TMJ area when palpated via external auditory meatus.

Associated symptoms: Neurologic (tingling, numbness, blurred vision, twitches, lacrimation); Gastrointestinal tract (nausea, vomiting, diarrhea, constipation, indigestion); Musculoskeletal (fatigue, tension, tiredness, and weakness); Otologic (tinnitus, ear pain, dizziness, vertigo, diminished hearing).

Treatment

1. Mild analgesics
2. Splint or mouth guard
3. An anxiolytic at bedtime
4. Physical therapy like transcutaneous electrical nerve stimulation (TENS)

Q. 4. Write a short note on infratemporal fossa.
(HP Uni., May 2018)

Ans. The infratemporal fossa is an inverted square pyramid irregularly shaped cavity in the face.

Boundaries

Anteriorly: Posterolateral surface of maxillary sinus.
Laterally: Ramus of mandible.
Medially: Medial pterygoid and tensor veli palatini muscle.
Inferiorly: Medial pterygoid muscle.
Anteromedially: Lateral pterygoid muscle.
Posteriorly: Styloid process and tympanic part of temporal bone.

Embryology: Mandible and maxillary artery are formed from first pharyngeal arch. Bones forming its boundaries are derived from mesenchyme of neural crest cells and undergo membranous ossification.

Blood supply: Maxillary artery and its branches.

Venous: Pterygoid plexus, retromandibular vein.

Nerves: Mandibular n. and its branches, otic ganglion.

Muscles: Lateral pterygoid muscle, medial pterygoid muscle, tensor veli palatini and levator veli palatini.

Surgical Considerations

1. Accidental incision of ICA can result in profuse hemorrhage and rapid death. One technique employed by surgeons to confirm whether a visible vessel is the internal or external carotid artery involves the temporary blocking of the vessel and checking the pulse of the superficial temporal artery. Pulselessness of this artery confirms that the external carotid is blocked.

2. The classic lateral approach to the infratemporal fossa involves beginning with a posterior auricular incision.
3. The anterior approach involves utilizing the airspace of the maxillary sinus.

Applied Clinical Anatomy

1. Pathology found in this region tends to spread posteriorly due to anterior, medial, and lateral bony barriers present in the infratemporal fossa.
2. Symptoms include trismus, paresis of mastication muscles, numbness or loss of taste sensation from the tongue, anesthesia of the gums, or speech articulation difficulties.
3. Neoplastic tumors rhabdomyosarcoma, liposarcoma, fibrosarcoma, meningioma, hemangioma, and peripheral nerve sheath tumors arising from any of the nerves in this region.
4. Schwannomas and neurofibromas are typically found between the pterygoid muscles due to the location of the lingual and inferior alveolar nerves in this region.
5. Hemangiomas arising from the pterygoid venous plexus can occur between the lateral pterygoid and temporalis muscles.
6. Tumors found in the nasopharynx and sphenoid sinus are known to spread to the infratemporal fossa.
7. Meningiomas can spread to the infratemporal fossa through the foramen ovale and often push the lateral and medial pterygoids apart.
8. Due to the continuity of the infratemporal fossa with the inferior parapharyngeal space, larger neoplasms have the potential to spread to this region.
9. Infections in the infratemporal can spread to the cavernous sinus and cause cavernous sinus thrombosis.

Q. 5. Discuss in detail the muscles of mastication. Add a note on applied aspects.

(KUHS, June 2013; UHSR, April 2015; AHSUC, May 2017; RGUHS; Nov. 2017; NTR Uni., June 2016; TNMGR, June 2016; RGUHS, July 2016; AHSUC, July 2016; RUHS, June 2017; Sumandeep Uni., May 2018; MUHS, June, Dec. 2018)

Q. Write a short note on secondary muscles of mastication.

(HNBG Uni., June 2016; HP Uni., April 2019; (Sumandeep Uni. April 2015)

Ans. The muscles of mastication (MOM) move the mandible during mastication and speech.

Development: The muscular system develops from intra embryonic mesoderm. Muscle tissues develop from embryonic cells called myoblasts. Muscles of mastication are derived from 1st brachial arch (mandibular arch). They are supplied by the mandibular nerve which is the nerve of that arch.

They are:
I. **Main (primary) muscles:** Temporalis, masseter, lateral pterygoid, medial pterygoid.
II. **Accessory (secondary) muscles:** Buccinator, suprahyoid muscles (digastric muscle, mylohyoid muscle, and geniohyoid muscle), and infrahyoid muscles (sternohyoid, sternothyroid, thyrohyoid and omohyoid muscle).

Strap muscles are composed of the suprahyoid and infrahyoid muscles are located on the side of the neck bilaterally, primarily function to raise and depress the hyoid bone and larynx. The strap muscles also assist with depression of the mandible when opening the mouth against an opposing force. *Buccinator* is a facial expression muscle that helps in mastication by keeping food pushed back within the oral cavity.

Primary muscles of mastication:
1. **Masseter:** Quadrilateral in shape covers lateral surface of mandible (Fig. 3.5a).
   Origin
   a. Superficial layer (largest): Anterior two-third of lower border of zygomatic arch and adjoining zygomatic process of maxilla.
   b. Middle layer: Anterior two-third of deep surface and posterior one-third of lower border of zygomatic arch.
   c. Deep layer: Deep surface of zygomatic arch.
   Fibers
   a. Superficial fibers pass downward and backwards at 45°.
   b. Middle and deep fibers pass vertically downwards.
   Insertion
   a. Superficial layer: Lower part of lateral surface of ramus of mandible.

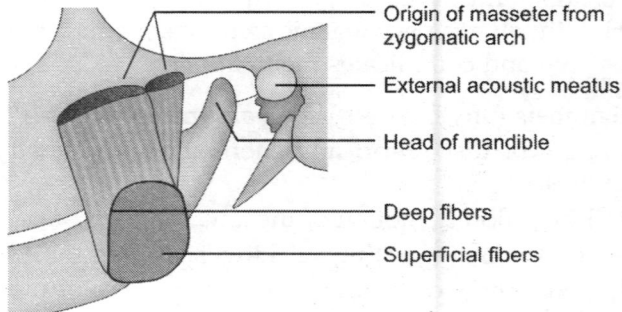

Origin of masseter from zygomatic arch

External acoustic meatus

Head of mandible

Deep fibers

Superficial fibers

Fig. 3.5a: Origin and insertion of masseter muscle

b. Middle layer: Middle part of ramus.

c. Deep layer: Rest of the ramus of mandible.

Nerve supply: Masseteric nerve.

Action: Elevates mandible to close the mouth to bite.

2. **Temporalis:** Fan-shaped. Fills the temporal fossa. (Fig. 3.5b)

Origin: Temporal fossa, (excluding zygomatic bone) and temporal fascia.

Fibers: Anterior fibers run vertically, middle obliquely and posterior horizontally. All converge and pass through gap deep to zygomatic arch.

Insertion: Margins and deep surface of coronoid process and Anterior border of ramus of mandible.

Nerve supply: Deep temporal branches from anterior division of mandibular nerve.

Actions

1. Elevates mandible.

2. Helps in side to side grinding movements.

3. Posterior fibers retract the protruded mandible.

3. **Lateral pterygoid:** Short and conical (Fig. 3.5c).

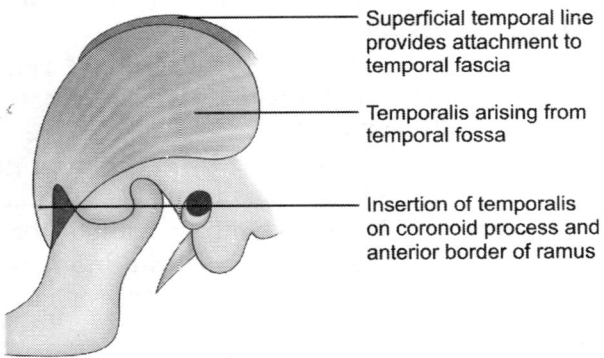

Superficial temporal line provides attachment to temporal fascia

Temporalis arising from temporal fossa

Insertion of temporalis on coronoid process and anterior border of ramus

Fig. 3.5b: Origin and insertion of temporalis muscle

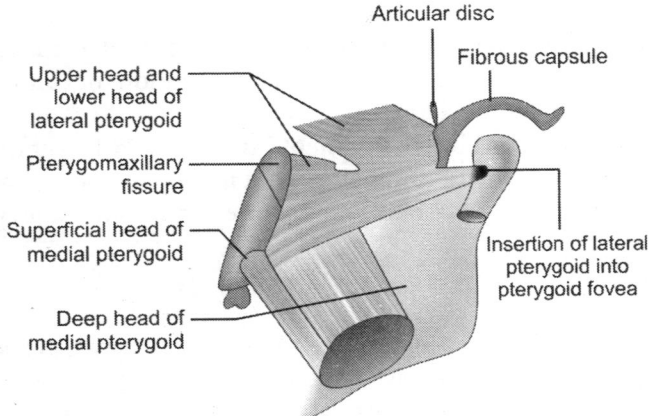

Articular disc

Fibrous capsule

Upper head and lower head of lateral pterygoid

Pterygomaxillary fissure

Superficial head of medial pterygoid

Insertion of lateral pterygoid into pterygoid fovea

Deep head of medial pterygoid

Fig. 3.5c: Origin and insertion of lateral and medial pterygoid muscle

Origin

a. Upper head (small): Infratemporal surface and crest of greater wing of sphenoid bone.

b. Lower head (larger): Lateral surface of lateral pterygoid plate.

Fibers: Run backwards and laterally and converge for insertion.

Insertion

a. Pterygoid fovea on the anterior surface of neck of mandible.

b. Anterior margin of articular disc and capsule of temporomandibular joint.

Nerve supply: A branch from anterior division of mandibular nerve.

Actions

1. Depress mandible to open mouth, with suprahyoid muscle.

2. Lateral and medial pterygoids protrude mandible.

3. Left lateral pterygoid and right medial pterygoid turn the chin to left side as part of grinding movements.

Relations of Lateral Pterygoid

Superficial: Masseter, ramus of mandible, tendon of the temporalis, maxillary artery.

Deep: Mandibular nerve, middle meningeal artery, sphenomandibular ligament, deep head of the medial pterygoid.

Structures emerging at the upper border: Deep temporal nerves, masseteric nerve.

Structures emerging at the lower border: Lingual nerve, inferior alveolar nerve, middle meningeal artery passes upwards deep to it.

Structures passing through the gap between the two heads: Maxillary artery enters the gap. The buccal branch of the mandibular nerve comes out through gap. The pterygoid plexus of vein surrounds the lateral pterygoid.

4. **Medial pterygoid:** Quadrilateral in shape (Fig. 3.5c).

Origin:

a. Superficial head (small slip): Maxillary tuberosity and adjoining bone.

b. Deep head (large): Medial surface of lateral pterygoid plate and adjoining process of palatine bone.

Fibers: It runs downwards, backwards and laterally.

Insertion: Medial surface of angle and adjoining ramus of mandible.

Nerve supply: Nerve to medial pterygoid.

Actions

1. Elevates mandible.
2. Help protrude mandible.
3. Right medial pterygoid with left lateral pterygoid turn the chin to left side.

Relations of Medial Pterygoid

Superficial relations: The upper part of muscle is separated from the lateral pterygoid muscle by lateral pterygoid plate, lingual nerve, and inferior alveolar nerve. Lower down the muscle is separated from the ramus of mandible by the lingual and inferior alveolar nerves, the maxillary artery, and the sphenomandibular ligament.

Deep relations: Tensor veli palatini, superior constrictor of pharynx, styloglossus, and stylopharyngeus attached to the styloid process.

Muscles Producing Movements (Fig. 3.5d)

1. **Depression:** Lateral pterygoid muscle. Digastrics, geniohyoid and mylohyoid muscles help when mouth is opened wide or against resistance. Gravity has passive role.
2. **Elevation:** Masseter, anterior vertical and middle oblique fibres of temporalis and the medial pterygoid muscles of both sides (antigravity muscles).
3. **Protrusion:** Lateral and medial pterygoids, superficial oblique fibers of masseter.
4. **Retraction:** Posterior horizontal fibers of the temporalis and deep vertical fibres of masseter
5. **Lateral or side to side movements:** For example, turning the chin to left side produced by left lateral pterygoid and right medial pterygoid and vice versa.

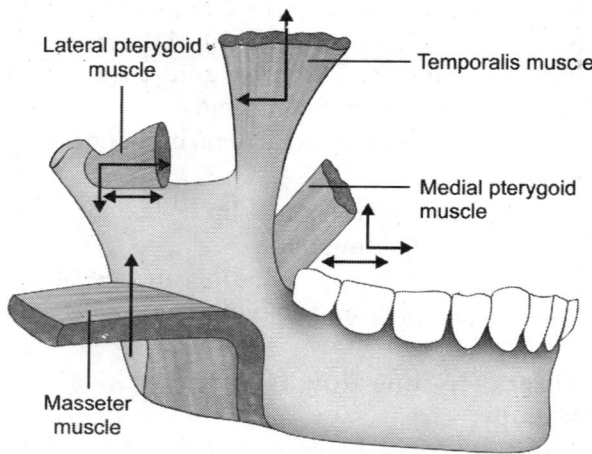

Fig. 3.5d: Masticatory muscle producing movements of mandible

Applied Clinical Anatomy

1. MOM can be tested by asking the patient to clench his teeth repeatedly and then palpating temporalis and masseter.
2. The muscle that commonly undergoes hypertrophy in bruxism is masseter.
3. Trismus following inferior alveolar nerve block is mostly due to involvement of medial pterygoid muscle.
4. Classification of disease of muscle:
   a. Primary myopathies: Dystrophy, myotonias, hypotonia, myasthenia, myositis, metabolic defects, miscellaneous (amylcidosis, contracture, degeneration)
   b. Secondary: Atrophy; Hypertrophy; Endocrine; Infection.
5. Trismus can be a symptom of masseter space tumor or infection.
6. Average jaw opening during chewing is between 16–20 mm.
7. Average lateral displacement on chewing is between 3 mm and 5 mm.
8. Masticatory forces: Average maximum sustainable biting force is 756N (170 pounds).
   Molar region: 400–890N; Premolar region: 222–445N; Cuspid region: 133–334N; Incisor region: 89–111N (20–55 pounds)
9. Tetanus (lock jaw): Caused by exotoxin of gram positive bacillus *Clostridium tetani.*
10. Bruxism: Jaw clenching, with or without forcible excursive movements, where the intensity of the clenching dictates the severity (or lack of) grinding.
11. Clenching: It can occur as brief rhythmic strong contractions of the jaw muscles during eccentric lateral jaw movements, or in maximum intercuspation.
12. Temporal tendonitis: Due to chronic strain from the temporalis muscle pulling on the tendon that attach to the mandible.
13. Stylomandibular ligament strain: sharp to aching pain in the region behind the jaw bone and below the ear, due to bad bite or from a traumatic injury.

4. TONGUE AND PALATE

Q. 1. Describe the tongue. Add notes on its blood supply, nerve supply, lymphatic drainage, microscopic structure and embryonic development.

(TNMGR, Sept. 2009, June 2016; MUHS, May 2011; KUHS, Jan. 2014; MUHS, Dec. 2018)

Q. Write a short note on taste buds.

(TNMGR, May 2019)

Ans. The tongue is a muscular organ situated in the floor of the mouth. It is associated with the functions of taste, speech, mastication, deglutition and cleansing of mouth.

Part: The tongue has:

1. A root.
2. A tip: A body, which has curved upper surface or dorsum; an inferior surface.

The **root** is attached to the styloid process and soft palate above, and to mandible and the hyoid bone below. In between it is related to geniohyoid and mylohyoid muscles.

The **tip** of the tongue forms the anterior free end which, at rest, lies behind the upper incisor teeth.

The **dorsum** is divided into oral and pharyngeal parts by a V-shaped sulcus terminalis. It is divided into (Fig. 4.1a):

a. *Oral part* or anterior two-thirds.
b. *Pharyngeal part* or posterior one-third, by a faint V-shaped groove, the *sulcus terminalis*. The two limbs of the 'V' meet at a median pit, *foramen caecum*. They run laterally and forward up to the palatoglossal arches. *Foramen caecum* represents the site from which the thyroid diverticulum grows down in the embryo.
c. Posterior most part.

Oral or papillary part of the tongue is placed on the floor of the mouth. In front of the palatoglossal arch, each margin shows 4–5 vertical folds called the *foliate papillae*.

The superior surface of the oral part shows a median furrow and is covered with papillae which make it rough.

Inferior (ventral) surface is confined to oral cavity and is covered with a smooth mucous membrane, which shows a median fold called *frenulum linguae* (Fig. 4.1b). *Glands of Blandin-Nuhn* (anterior lingual

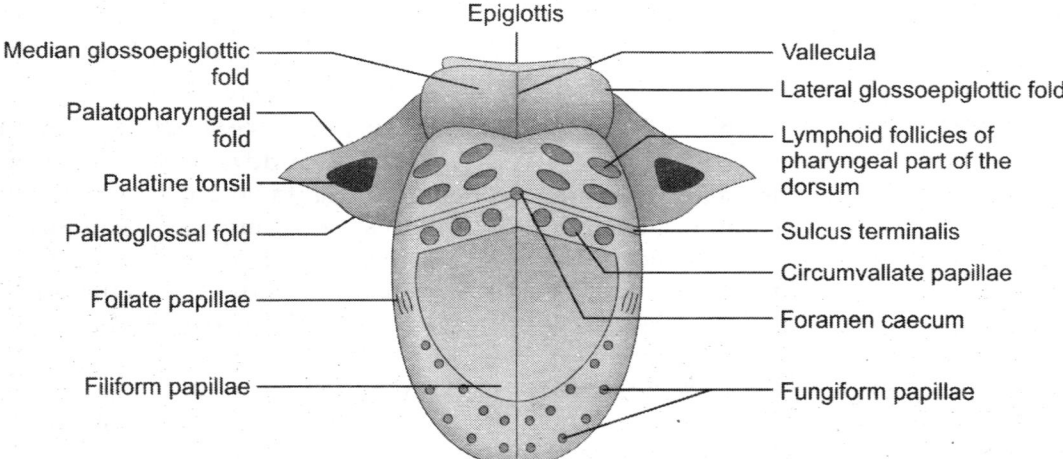

Fig. 4.1a: Dorsum of tongue showing papillae, epiglottis and palatine tonsil

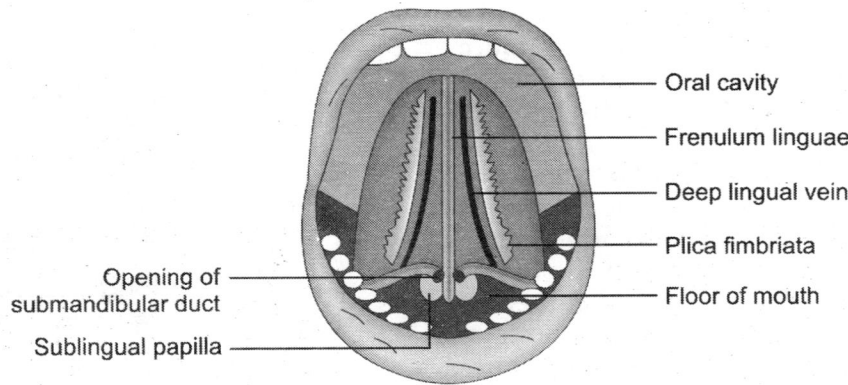

Fig. 4.1b: Ventral surface of tongue

glands/apical glands) are deeply seated seromucous glands located near the tip on each side of frenulum linguae, covered by bundle of muscle fibres derived from styloglossus and longitudinalis inferior. They are between 12–25 mm in length and 8 mm wide and each opens by 34 ducts on the under surface of the tongue's apex. On the either side of the frenulum, there is a prominence produced by the deep lingual veins. More laterally there is a fold called the plica fimbriata that is directed forwards and medially towards the tip of the tongue.

Pharyngeal or **lymphoid** part of the tongue lies behind the palatoglossal arches and the *sulcus terminalis*. Its posterior surface (the base of the tongue), forms the anterior wall of the oropharynx. The mucous membrane has no papillae, but has many *lymphoid follicles* that collectively constitute the **lingual tonsil**. Mucous glands are also present.

Posteriormost part of the tongue is connected to the epiglottis by three folds of mucous membrane. These are *median glossoepiglottic fold* and the right and left lateral *glossoepiglottic folds*. On either side of the median fold, there is a depression called the *vallecula*. The lateral folds separate the vallecula from the piriform fossa.

Functions of tongue: Deglutition, taste sensation, speech, self cleansing, mastication.

Papillae of the tongue (*RGUHS, June 2006*): These are projections of mucous membrane or corium which give the anterior two-thirds of the tongue its characteristic roughness. These are of the following types:

I. **Vallate or circumvallate papillae:** They are large in size, 1–2 mm in diameter and are 8–12 in number. They are situated immediately in front of the *sulcus terminalis*. Each papilla is a cylindrical projection surrounded by a circular sulcus. The walls of the papilla have taste buds (maximum taste buds).

II. **Fungiform papillae:** They are more near the tip and margins of tongue, but some of them are also scattered over the dorsum. These are smaller than the vallate papillae, but larger than the filiform papillae. Each papilla consists of a narrow pedicle and a large rounded head. They are distinguished by their bright red color.

III. **Filiform papillae or conical papillae:** They cover the presulcal area of the dorsum of the tongue, and give it a characteristic velvety appearance. They are the smallest and most prevalent of the lingual papillae. Each is pointed and covered with keratin; the apex is often split into filamentous processes.

IV. **Foliate papillae** are present at the lateral border just infront of circumvallate papillae. They are leaf shaped, short vertical folds.

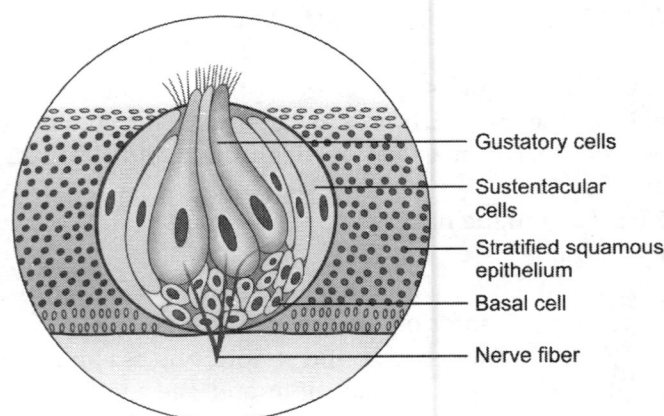

Fig. 4.1c: Structure of taste bud

Taste buds (Fig. 4.1c) are sensory receptors of taste. The sensation of taste is called Gustation. They are located on the surfaces of papillae except filiform papillae. Taste sensations are sour, sweet, salty, bitter and recent one is ***Umami*** (***Umami*** is from Japanese word which means 'pleasant savory taste'. Glutamate receptors in human tongue are source of this taste. This is mostly found in fish, meats, mushrooms, cheese, spinach etc.)

Muscles of the Tongue (*UHSR, April 2014; TNMGR, Oct. 2017*): A middle fibrous septum divides the tongue into right and left halves. Each half contains four intrinsic and four extrinsic muscles (Fig. 4.1d).

A. **Intrinsic muscles:** Occupy the upper part of the tongue and are attached to the submucous fibrous layer and to the median fibrous septum. They alter the shape of the tongue.

1. Superior longitudinal: It lies beneath the mucous membrane. It shortens the tongue and makes its dorsum concave.

2. Inferior longitudinal: A narrow band lying close to the inferior surface of the tongue between the

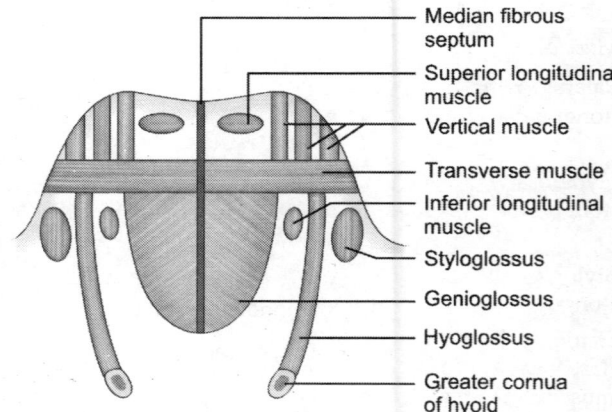

Fig. 4.1d: Tongue muscles and their arrangement

genioglossus and the hyoglossus. It shortens the tongue and makes its dorsum convex.

3. **Transverse:** It extends from the median septum to the margins. It makes the tongue narrow and elongated.
4. **Vertical:** Found at the borders of the anterior part of the tongue. It makes the tongue broad and flattened.

B. **Extrinsic muscles:** Connect tongue to mandible via genioglossus; to the hyoid bone through hyoglossus; to the styloid process via styloglossus, and palate via palatoglossus. These are described as (Table 4.1):

Arterial supply: Lingual artery (dorsal lingual, sublingual, deep lingual arteries), ascending palatine, tonsillar and ascending pharyngeal artery.

Venous drainage: Deep lingual vein (largest and principal vein of the tongue), venae comitantes accompanying the lingual artery and hypoglossal nerve. All the veins unite at posterior border of hyoglossus to form the lingual vein which ends in IJV.

Lymphatic drainage

1. **Tip** of tongue: Bilaterally to submental lymph nodes.
2. **Right and left halves** of anterior two-third: Unilaterally to Submandibular nodes.
3. Posterior most part and posterior one-third: Bilaterally into upper deep cervical lymph nodes.

The whole lymph finally drains to the **jugulo-omohyoid nodes** (*lymph nodes of the tongue*).

Nerve Supply

a. **Motor nerves:** All the intrinsic and extrinsic muscles, except palatoglossus, are supplied by *hypoglossal nerve* (CN XII). Palatoglossus is supplied by cranial root of *accessory nerve* through pharyngeal plexus.

b. **Sensory nerves**
Lingual nerve: General sensation.
Chorda tympani: Taste for anterior two-third of tongue except circumvallate papillae.
Glossopharyngeal nerve: Both general sensation and taste for posterior one-third of tongue including circumvallate papillae.
The posterior most part of the tongue is supplied by *vagus nerve* through internal laryngeal branch.

Microscopic structure of the tongue (Fig. P-2; Color Plate 1):

1. The bulk of tongue is made up of striated muscle.
2. The mucous membrane consists of layer of connective tissue, lined by stratified squamous epithelium. On the oral part, it is thin, forms papillae. On the pharyngeal part, it is rich in lymphoid follicles.

Applied Clinical Anatomy

1. *Glossitis* is usually a part of generalized ulceration of the mouth. In certain anemias, the tongue becomes smooth due to atrophy of the filiform papillae.
2. The presence of a rich network of lymphatics and of loose areolar tissue in the substance of tongue is responsible for enormous swelling of the tongue in *acute glossitis*.
3. The undersurface of the tongue is a good site along with the bulbar conjunctiva for observation of jaundice.
4. Injury to hypoglossal nerve produces paralysis of the muscles of the tongue on the side of lesion.
   a. **Infranuclear lesion:** Gradual atrophy and muscular twitching of the affected half of tongue.
   b. **Supranuclear lesion:** Paralysis without palsy, tongue becomes stiff, small and moves sluggishly.

Table 4.1: Extrinsic muscles of tongue with their origin, insertion and action

Muscles	Origin	Insertion	Action
Palatoglossus (tongue elevator)	Oral surface of palatine aponeurosis	Descends in the palatoglossal arch to side of tongue at the junction oral and pharyngeal parts	Pulls up the root of tongue, approximates palatoglossal arches, closes the oropharangeal isthmus
Hyoglossus (tongue depressor)	Whole length of greater cornua and lateral part of body of hyoid bone	Side of tongue between styloglossus and inferior longitudinal muscle of tongue	Depresses tongue, makes dorsum convex, and retracts the protruded tongue
Styloglossus (tongue retractor)	Tip and part of anterior surface of styloid process	Into the side of tongue	Pulls tongue upwards and backwards
Genioglossus (fan-shaped, bulky muscle) (tongue protruder) 'Life-saving muscle'	Upper genial tubercle of mandible	Upper fibers into the tip of tongue Middle fibers into dorsum Lower fibers into hyoid bone	Retracts the tongue Depresses the tongue Pulls the posterior part of tongue forwards and protrude the tongue forwards

5. In unconscious patients, tongue may fall back and obstruct the air passages. This can be prevented either by lying the patient on one side with head down ('**tonsil position**') or by keeping the tongue out mechanically.

6. **Lingual tonsil** in the posterior one-third of tongue forms part of Waldeyer's ring.

7. Carcinoma of the tongue is quite common. The affected side is removed surgically along with all the deep cervical lymph nodes.

8. Sorbitrate is taken sublingually for immediate relief from angina pectoris.

9. Genioglossus is called '**safety muscle of the tongue**' because if it is paralyzed, the tongue will fall back on the oropharynx and block the air passage.

Q. 2. Describe the development of tongue with a note on its anomalous development.

(CDER-AIIMS, May 1990; TNMGR, March 2008, May, Oct. 2019; KUHS, June 2013; RUHS, May 2018; Gujarat Uni., April 2019; UHSR, April 2019)

Ans. Development of the tongue (Fig. 4.2) starts in 4th month of IUL. Tongue develops in relation to the pharyngeal arches in the floor of the developing mouth. Each pharyngeal arch arises as a mesodermal thickening in the lateral wall of the foregut and then it grows ventrally to become continuous with the corresponding arch of the opposite side. The medialmost parts of the mandibular arches proliferate to form two *lingual swellings*, partially separated from each other by another midline swelling, *tuberculum impar*. Another midline swelling is seen in relation to the medial ends of 2nd, 3rd, and 4th arches, called hypobrachial eminence. The eminence soon shows a subdivision into a cranial part related to 2nd and 3rd arches (called the *copula*) and a caudal part related to 4th arch. The caudal part forms the epiglottis.

Anterior two-thirds of tongue is formed by fusion of *tuberculum impar* and two *lingual swellings* thus derived from the mandibular arch.

Posterior one-third of tongue is formed from the cranial part of the hypobrachial eminence (copula). In this situation, the 2nd arch mesoderm gets buried below the surface and 3rd arch mesoderm grows over it to fuse with mesoderm of 1st arch. Posterior one-third of tongue is thus formed by 3rd arch mesoderm.

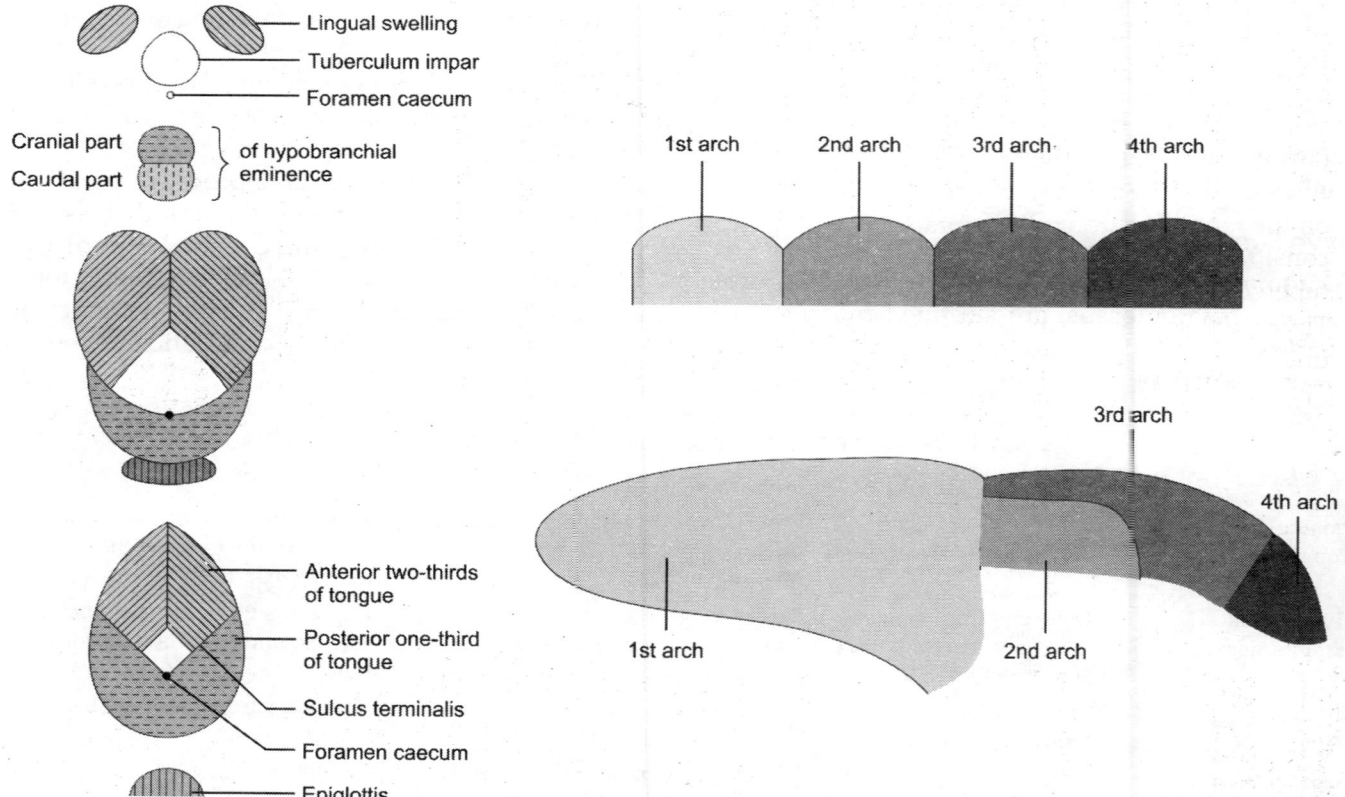

Fig. 4.2: Development of various parts of tongue

Posteriormost part of tongue is derived from 4th arch. In keeping with its embryological origin, anterior two-thirds of tongue is supplied by lingual branch of mandibular nerve, which is post-trematic nerve of 1st arch and by chorda tympani (pretrematic nerve of 1st arch); posterior one-third is supplied by glossopharyngeal nerve; most posterior part of tongue is supplied by superior laryngeal nerve, which is nerve of 4th arch.

Musculature of tongue is derived from occipital myotomes and is supplied by hypoglossal nerve, which is the nerve of these myotomes.

Epithelium of the tongue is at first made up of a single layer of cells. Later it becomes stratified and papillae become evident. Taste buds are formed in relation to the terminal branches of the innervating nerve fibers.

Connective tissue develops from local mesenchyme.

Developmental anomalies of the tongue
1. The tongue may be too large (**macroglossia**) or too small (**microglossia**). Very rarely the tongue may be absent (**aglossia**).
2. The tongue may be bifid because of non-fusion of the two lingual swellings.
3. The apical part of the tongue may be anchored to the floor of the mouth by an overdeveloped frenulum. This condition is called **ankyloglossia** or **tongue-tie**. It interferes with speech. Occasionally, the tongue may be adherent, to the palate (**ankyloglossia superior**).
4. A rhomboid-shaped smooth zone may be present on the tongue in front of the foramen caecum. It is considered to be the result of persistence of the tuberculum impar.
5. Thyroid tissue may be present in the tongue either under the mucosa or within the muscles.
6. The surface of the tongue may show fissures.

7. Remnants of the thyroglossal duct may form cysts at the base of the tongue.

Q. 3. Write a note on hyoglossus muscle and its relations. *(TNMGR, Feb. 2005; KUHS, Dec. 2012, June 2013)*

Ans. Hyoglossus is an extrinsic muscle of tongue. For origin, insertion and action of hyoglossus muscle, refer to Table 4.1.

Relations of hyoglossus muscle (Fig. 4.3): It has a free anterior border; free posterior border; lateral/superficial surface; medial/deep surface.

Along anterior border: a. 3rd part of lingual artery, b. Genioglossus.

In front of hyoglossus: a. Sublingual salivary gland, b. Sublingual branch of lingual artery.

Posterior border
a. Glossopharyngeal nerve.
b. Stylohyoid ligament.
c. 1st part of lingual artery.
d. Middle constrictor of pharynx.

Superficial or lateral surface
a. **Two muscles:** Mylohyoid and styloglossus.
b. **Two nerves:** Lingual nerve and hypoglossal nerve.
c. **Two glands:** Superficial and deep part of the submandibular gland.
d. **Two submandibular structures:** Submandibular ganglion and submandibular duct.

Deep or medial
a. Inferior longitudinal muscle of tongue.
b. Genioglossus.
c. Middle constrictor of the pharynx.
d. Glossopharyngeal nerve.
e. Stylohyoid ligament.
f. Lingual artery.

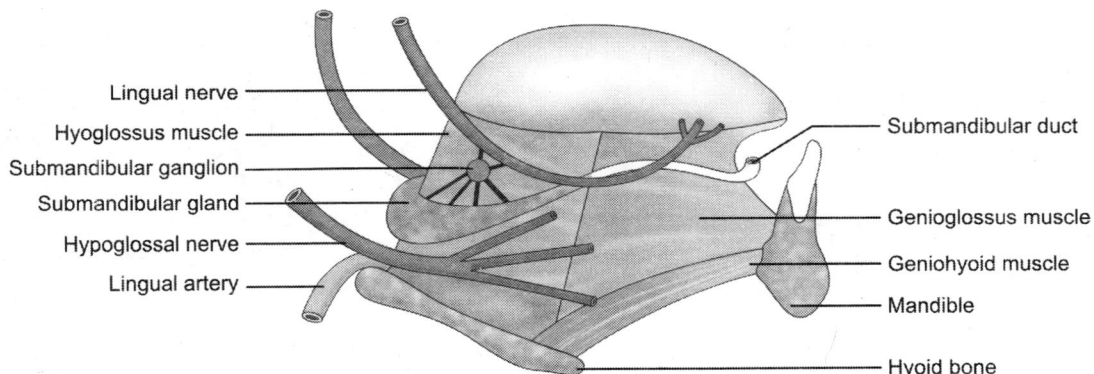

Fig. 4.3: Hyoglossus muscle and its relation

Q. 4. Write a short note on soft palate.

(TNMGR, April 1997)

Ans. It is a movable muscular fold, suspended from the posterior border of hard palate. It separates nasopharynx from oropharynx. Soft palate has **two surfaces**, anterior and posterior; and **two borders**, superior and inferior.

Anterior (oral) surface is concave and is marked by a median raphe.

Posterior surface is convex, and is continuous superiorly with floor of the nasal cavity.

Superior border is attached to posterior border of hard palate, blending on each side with pharynx.

Inferior border is free and bounds pharyngeal isthmus.

From its middle, there hangs a conical projection, called *uvula* (Latin *small grape*). From each side of base of uvula, two curved folds of mucous membrane extend laterally and downwards.

Anterior fold (*palatoglossal arch* or *anterior pillar of fauces*): It contains palatoglossus muscle and reaches side of the tongue forming lateral boundary of oropharyngeal isthmus.

Posterior fold (*palatopharyngeal arch* or *posterior pillar of fauces*): It contains palatopharyngeus muscle and forms posterior boundary of tonsillar fossa, and merges inferiorly with lateral wall of pharynx.

Structure: Soft palate is a fold of mucous membrane containing the following parts (Fig. 4.4):

Palatine aponeurosis: Flattened tendon of tensor veli palatini forms the fibrous basis of the palate. Near the median plane, aponeurosis splits to enclose musculus uvulae.

Levator veli palatini and **palatopharyngeus** lie on the superior surface of palatine aponeurosis.

Palatoglossus lies on the inferior surface of palatine aponeurosis.

Muscles of the soft palate (*CDER-AIIMS, April 2017*): Table 4.4.

Nerve supply

1. **Motor nerves:** All muscles of soft palate **except** tensor veli palatine are supplied by the pharyngeal plexus (the fibres are derived from cranial part of accessory nerve through vagus). The tensor veli palatine is supplied by medial pterygoid nerve (branch of mandibular nerve).
2. **General sensory nerves:** Middle and posterior lesser palatine nerves; Glossopharyngeal nerve.
3. **Special sensory or gustatory nerves:** Lesser palatine nerves.
4. **Secretomotor nerves:** Lesser palatine nerves.

Passavant's ridge: Some of the upper fibers of the palatopharyngeus pass circularly deep to the mucous membrane of the pharynx, and form a sphincter internal to superior constrictor at the level of hard palate. These fibers constitute *Passavant's muscle* which on contraction raises a ridge called the *Passavant's ridge* on the posterior wall of the nasopharynx. When soft palate is elevated it comes in contact with this ridge, the two together closing the pharyngeal isthmus between oropharynx and nasopharynx. *Passavant's muscle* is best developed in case of cleft palate as this compensate for the deficiency in the palate.

Movements and functions of the soft palate

1. It isolates the mouth from the oropharynx during chewing, so that breathing is unaffected.
2. It separates the oropharynx from the nasopharynx by locking into Passavant's ridge during the second stage of swallowing, so that food does not enter the nose.

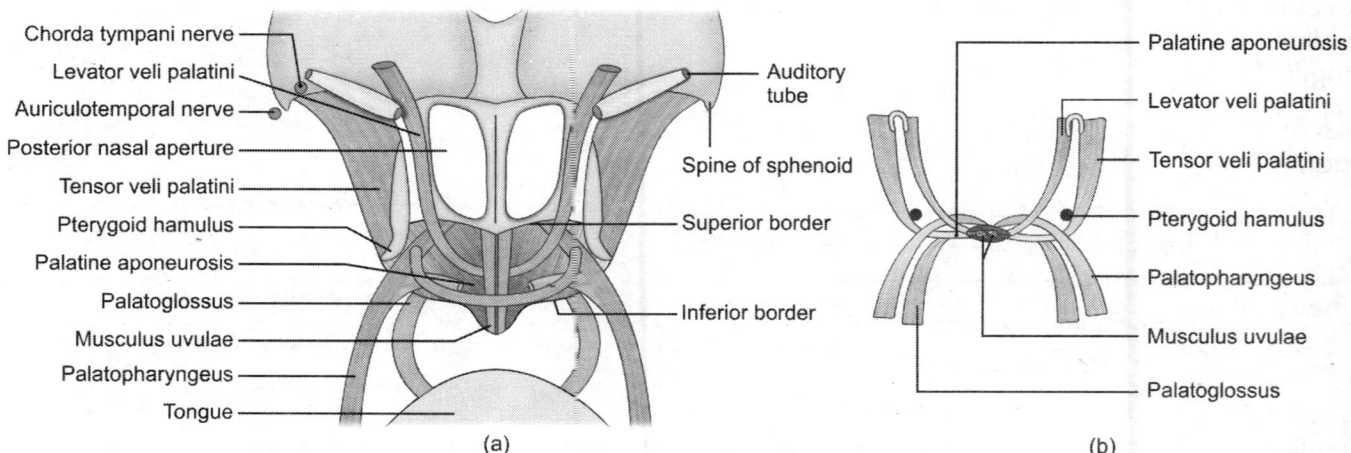

Fig. 4.4: Soft palate and muscle attachments

Table 4.4: Muscles of the soft palate

Muscles	Origin	Insertion	Actions
Tensor veli palatini (tensor palati): Thin, triangular muscle	Lateral side of auditory tube and greater wing and scaphoid fossa auditory tube	Posterior border of hard palate and inferior surface of palate	Tightens the soft palate. Opens auditory tube
Levator veli palatini (levator palati) Cylindrical muscle	Inferior aspect of auditory tube, and inferior surface of petrous temporal bone	Upper surface of the palatine aponeurosis	Elevates soft palate and closes pharyngeal isthmus Opens the auditory tube
Musculus uvulae Longitudinal strip	Posterior nasal spine Palatine aponeurosis	Mucous membrane of uvula	Pulls up the uvula
Palatoglossus	Oral surface of palatine aponeurosis	Side of the tongue, at the junction of oral and pharyngeal part	Pulls up the root of the tongue, closes oropharyngeal isthmus
Palatopharyngeus consist of two fasciculi	Anterior fasciculus: From posterior border of hard palate Posterior fasciculus: From palatine aponeurosis	Posterior border of lamina of thyroid cartilage Wall of the pharynx and its median raphe	Pulls up the wall of the pharynx and shortens it during swallowing

3. By varying the degree of closure of the pharyngeal isthmus, the quality of voice can be modified and various consonants are correctly pronounced.
4. During sneezing, the blast of air is appropriately divided and directed through the nasal and oral cavities without damaging the narrow nose.
5. During coughing, it directs air and sputum into the mouth and not into the nose.

Blood Supply

Arteries: Greater palatine artery; Ascending palatine artery; Palatine artery.

Veins: Pterygoid and tonsillar plexuses of veins.

Lymphatics: Upper deep cervical and retropharyngeal lymph nodes.

Applied clinical anatomy: Paralysis of soft palate in lesions of vagus nerve produces: Nasal regurgitation of fluids, nasal twang in the voice, flattening of the palatal arch and deviation of uvula to normal side (opposite).

Q. 5. Write about development of hard and soft palate and its anomalies. *(TNMGR, March 2007; KUHS, June 2013; RUHS, June 2014; NITTE Uni., April 2016)*

Q. Describe the development of palate and discuss the etiology of cleft lip and palate. *(Sumandeep Uni., April 2015; June 2016; UOK, June 2019)*

Ans. The palate is structure that interposes between oral and nasal cavities. Development of palate starts between 5th and 9th weeks of IUL. It develops from two parts (Fig. 4.5a):

Primary palate or intermaxillary segment (future premaxilla): It is formed by fusion of two medial processes with frontonasal process.

Secondary palate: The formation commences between 7–8th weeks and complete around the 3rd month of gestation.

Three outgrowths appear in the oral cavity. These are:
1. The two palatal processes.
2. The nasal septum.

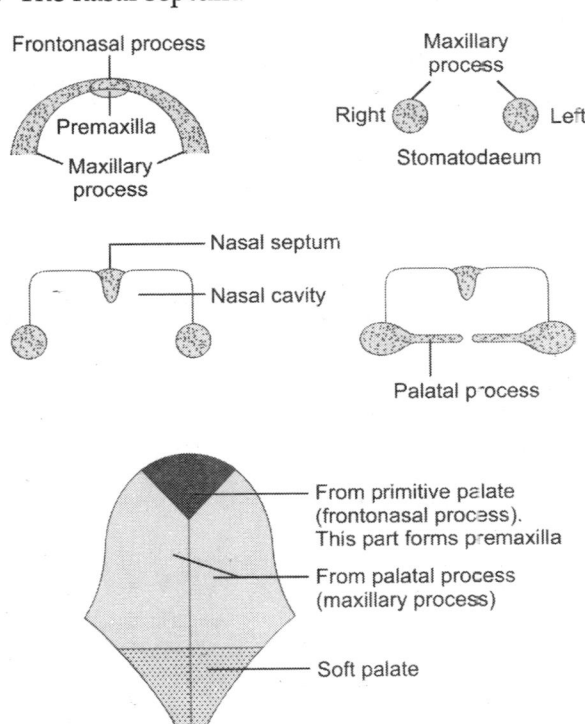

Fig. 4.5a: Development of palate (hard and soft)

Each palatal process fuses with the posterior margin of the primary palate. The two palatal processes fuse with each other in the midline. Their fusion begins anteriorly and proceeds backwards. The medial edges of the palatal processes fuse with the lower edge of the nasal septum, thus separating two nasal cavities from each other and from the mouth.

At a later stage, the mesoderm in the palate undergoes intra-membranous ossification to form the **hard palate**. However, ossification does not extend into the most posterior portion, which remains as the **soft palate**. The part of the palate derived from the fronto-nasal process forms the **premaxilla**, which carries the incisor teeth.

Developmental anomalies *(TNMGR, April 2012)*:

Cleft palate: It is a congenital defect caused by non-fusion of the right and left palatal processes. It may be of different degrees. In the least severe types, the defect is confined to the soft palate. In the most severe cases, the cleft in the palate is continuous with harelip. These may be unilateral or bilateral (Fig. 4.5b).

Uranoschisis: Cleft hard palate.

Staphyloschisis: Cleft soft palate.

Etiology *(CDER-AIIMS, May 2014)*: The etiology is multifactorial in nature.

- Genetic factors: Syndromic, non-syndromic (isolated) forms, chromosomal aberrations and single gene mutations.

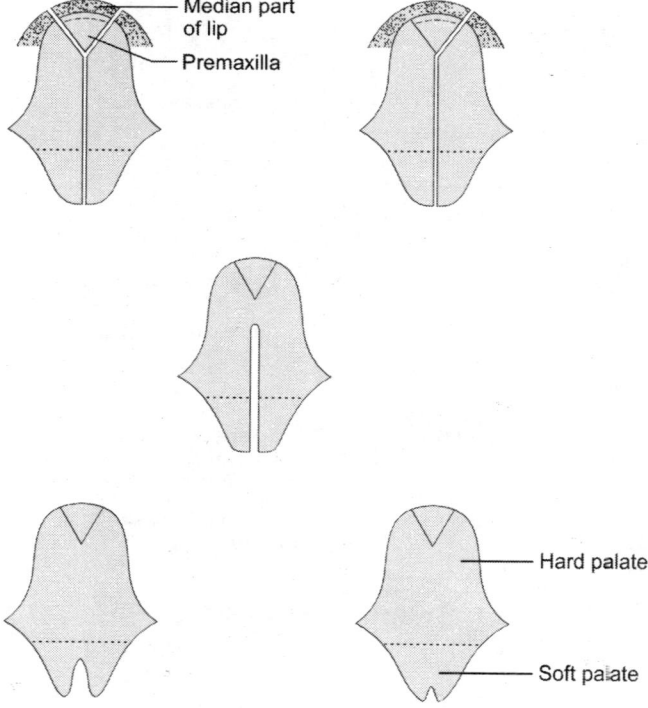

- Environmental factors: Folic acid deficiency in pregnancy, teratogenic drugs, child born to mothers suffering from diabetes mellitus or phenylketonuria, high grade fever during pregnancy, early amniotic rupture.

Primary cleft: This cleft is before the mark of the incisive foramen and therefore in the primary palate. The mesenchyme in the lateral palatine shelves does not merge with the primary palate or intermaxillary segment as it is also known. The most common types of primary cleft include the unilateral cleft lip, the unilateral cleft alveolus, the unilateral cleft lip and primary cleft palate and the bilateral cleft lip and primary palate.

Secondary cleft: The secondary clefts occurs posterior to the incisive foramen in the secondary palate. The lateral palatine shelves don't fuse to one another and there is a gap running down the midline of the roof of the mouth. Secondary clefts include clefts in the soft palate, unilateral clefts in the soft and hard palate and bilateral clefts in the soft and hard palate.

Complete cleft: In a complete cleft, the lip, the primary palate and the secondary palate are all affected and are all part of one big cleft. The nasal septum, the primary palate and the lateral palatine shelves all fail to fuse together in that order. This lack of development results in either a unilateral cleft lip and cleft palate or a bilateral cleft lip and cleft palate.

Q. 6. Write a short note on development of palatine tonsil. *(TNMGR, March 2007)*

Ans. The palatine tonsil development begins in 3rd month of IUL (on each side) in relation to the lateral part of 2nd pharyngeal pouch. The endoderm lining the pouch undergoes considerable proliferation. At 4th month, epithelium proliferate to form solid endodermal buds growing into underlying mesoderm, these buds give rise to tonsillar stroma. Central cells of the buds later die and slough, converting the solid buds into hollow tonsillar crypts. Lymphocytes collect in these crypts. Follicles of lymphoid tissue begin to collect around buds in the 5th month of IUL. The intratonsillar cleft or tonsillar fossa is believed to represent a persisting part of 2nd pharyngeal pouch. Similar epithelial proliferations and aggregations of lymphoid tissue give rise to tubal tonsils, lingual tonsil and pharyngeal tonsils. Origin of lymphoid tissue in tonsils takes place:

1. Old theory: From the blood or surrounding connective tissue, creep in and form follicles round the glandular endodermal buds.

Fig. 4.5b: Types of cleft palate

2. Gulland's theory (most accepted): Epithelial endo-dermal cells which form the glandular buds of the tonsil, give rise to broods of lymphoid cells.

Q. 7. Write a short note on palatine tonsil.

(TNMGR, April 1995; Feb. 2005)

Ans. Palatine tonsil (**the tonsil**) (Latin—*swelling*) occupies tonsillar sinus or fossa between the palato-glossal and palatopharyngeal arches. It has **two surfaces,** medial and lateral; **two borders**, anterior and posterior and **two poles**, upper and lower (Fig. 4.7).

Medial surface: Covered by stratified squamous epi-thelium continuous with that of the mouth, has 12 to 15 crypts. The largest of these is called intratonsillar cleft, which is semilunar in shape and parallel to dorsum of tongue. It represents the internal opening of 2nd pharyngeal arch.

Lateral surface: Covered by a sheet of pharyngobasilar fascia and forms the hemi-capsule of tonsil. It is loosely attached to the muscular wall of the pharynx, formed by the superior constrictor and styloglossus, but anteroinferiorly the capsule is firmly adherent to side of tongue (suspensory ligament of tonsil) just in front of the insertion of the palatoglossus and the palatopharyngeus muscles. This firm attachment keeps the tonsil in place during swallowing. Tonsillar artery enters the tonsil by piercing the superior constrictor.

The palatine vein or external palatine or para-tonsillar vein descends from palate in the loose areolar tissue on the lateral surface of the capsule.

The bed of the tonsil is formed from within out-wards by:
a. Pharyngobasilar fascia (capsule).
b. Superior constrictor and palatopharyngeus muscles.
c. Buccopharyngeal fascia.
d. Styloglossus.
e. Glossopharyngeal nerve.
f. Facial artery with tonsillar and ascending palatine branches.
g. Internal carotid artery.

Anterior border: Related to palatoglossal arch with its muscle.

Posterior border: Related to the palatopharyngeal arch with its muscle.

Upper pole: Related to soft palate and **lower pole**, to tongue.

Plica triangularis is a triangular vestigial fold of mucous membrane covering anteroinferior part of tonsil.

Plica semilunaris is a semilunar vestigial fold of mucous membrane that may cross the upper part of tonsillar sinus.

Microscopic structures (*TNMGR, June 2016*) (**Fig. P-3; Color Plate 1**)

Oral/medial aspect is covered by non-keratinized stratified squamous epithelium, which extends into the substance of tonsil in the form of tonsillar crypts. Crypts greatly increase the contact surface ~295 cm². The lymphocytes lie on the sides of crypts in the form of

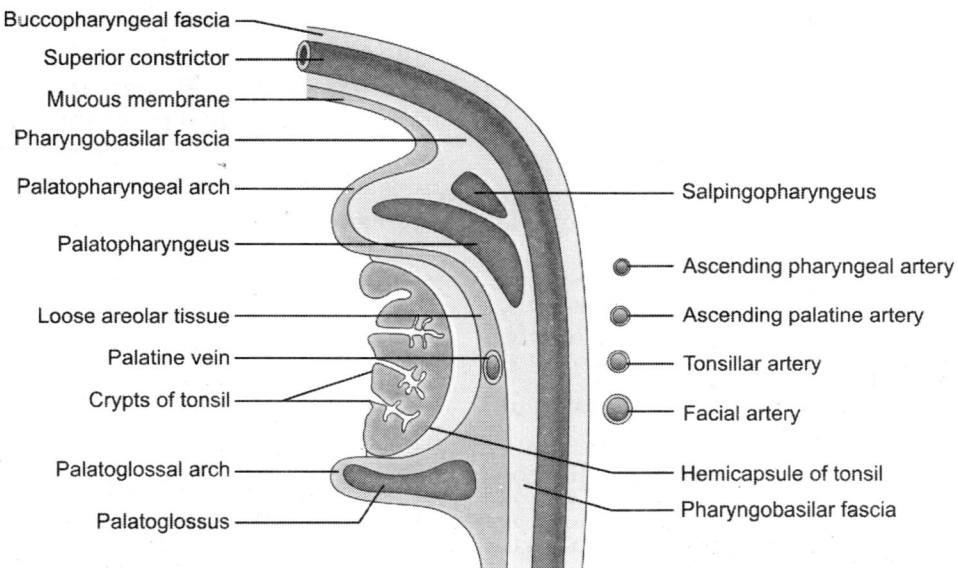

Fig. 4.7: Palatine tonsil and its relations

nodules. The structure is not differentiated into cortex and medulla. There are four lymphoid compartments:
   a. Reticular cell/crypt epithelium; b. Extrafollicular area; c. Mantle zone of lymphoid follicles; d. Germinal centre of lymphoid follicle.

Numerous mucous glands open into the crypts

Arterial supply: Tonsillar branch of facial artery (main), ascending palatine branch of facial artery, dorsal lingual branches, ascending pharyngeal branch of ECA, greater palatine branch of the maxillary artery.

Venous drainage: Peritonsillar plexus → lingual and Pharyngeal veins → IJV.

Lymphatic drainage: Jugulodigastric node.

Nerve supply: Glossopharyngeal and lesser palatine nerves.

Applied Clinical Anatomy

1. Importance of tonsillar bed:
   a. Capsule: Because of the septa, tonsil is not easily separated from its capsule.
   b. Loose areolar tissue: One can easily dissect the tonsil by separating the capsule from muscle through this loose connective tissue.
   c. Glossopharyngeal nerve: This nerve can be injured if the tonsillar bed is violated.
2. *Weber's glands:* Tubular mucous glands located at upper pole of tonsils.
3. Referred Otalgia in tonsillitis is through tympanic branch of glossopharyngeal nerve.
4. Acute infection of tonsil is classified as: a. Acute catarrhal; b. Acute follicular; c. Acute parenchymatous; d. Acute membranous.
5. Chronic tonsillitis is sequelae of recurrent episodes of acute tonsillitis for >12 weeks. Types include: a. follicular; b. parenchymatous; c. fibroid
6. *Irwin-Moore sign:* Pressure on anterior pillar expresses frank pus or cheesy material, seen in chronic tonsillitis.
7. **Peritonsillar abscess** or **Quinsy** is a collection of pus in peritonsillar space due to recurrent tonsillitis. Typical feature is muffled and thick speech *"hot potato voice"*.
8. A rare complication of quinsy is jugular vein thrombosis leading to Lemierr's syndrome.
9. *Tonsillolith* or tonsillar concretions: Formation of calculus/stone in tonsils.
10. Tonsillar cyst: Due to blockage of tonsillar crypts.

5. PARANASAL SINUSES

Q. 1. Describe the paranasal air sinuses.
(TNMGR, April 2012; Sumandeep Uni. April 2013; HNBG Uni., May 2015; KUHS, June 2016; TNMGR, May 2018)

Ans. Paranasal sinuses (PNS) are air filled spaces present within some bones around the nasal cavities. These are:
1. Frontal sinus
2. Maxillary sinus
3. Sphenoidal sinus
4. Ethmoidal sinus

All of them open into the nasal cavity through its lateral wall.

Function
- To make the skull lighter decreasing the relative weight of the skull.
- Increasing the resonance of the voice.
- Providing a buffer against facial trauma.
- Insulating sensitive structures from rapid temperature fluctuations in the nose.
- Humidifying and heating inspired air.
- Immunological defense.

Development of paranasal sinuses: Development of PNS is heralded by appearance of series of ridges or folds on lateral nasal wall at approximately 8th week of IUL, known as *ethmoturbinals*.
- 1st ethmoturbinal: Ascending portion forms agger nasi; descending portion forms uncinate process.
- 2nd ethmoturbinal: Middle turbinate.
- 3rd ethmoturbinal: Superior turbinate.
- 4th and 5th ethmoturbinals: Fuse to form supreme turbinate.
- **Frontal sinus** originates from anterior pneumatization of the frontal recess into the frontal bone. The frontal sinus does not appear until the age of 5 to 6 years old.
- **Sphenoid sinus** develops during 3rd month of IUL; nasal mucosa invaginates into posterior portion of cartilaginous nasal capsule to form a pouch-like cavity. During 2nd and 3rd year of life, cartilage is resorbed and cavity becomes attached to body of sphenoid. By 6th or 7th year of life, pneumatization of sphenoid sinus progresses and by 12th year, pneumatization is complete.
- **Maxillary sinus** is first to develop in utero. Maxillary sinus shows a biphasic growth pattern, with growth at 3rd and 7–18 years of age.

- **Ethmoid sinuses** are comprised of 3–4 air cells at birth; by the time an individual reaches adulthood, they consist of 1–15 aerated cells.

Frontal sinus: Frontal sinus lies in the frontal bone deep to super ciliary arch, superior to orbit. Typical volume at adult stage is 4–7 ml. It extends upward above the medial end of the eyebrow, backward into the medial part of roof of the orbit. It opens into middle meatus of nose at anterior end of hiatus semilunaris either through infundibulum or through fronto nasal duct. The right and left sinuses are usually unequal in size and rarely one or both may be absent. The sinuses are better developed in males than in females; rudimentary or absent at birth and well developed between 7–8 years of age, but reach full size only after puberty.

Arterial supply: Supraorbital and supratrochlear artery.

Venous drainage: Supraorbital and superior ophthalmic vein.

Lymphatic drainage: Submandibular lymph nodes.

Nerve supply: Supraorbital and supratrochlear nerve.

Important anatomical structures are:

- **Frontal recess:** Drainage space between frontal sinus and semilunar hiatus bounded by posterior wall of agger nasi cell, lamina papyracea, and middle turbinate.
- **Frontal sinus infundibulum:** Space that drains into the frontal recess that is located superior to agger nasi cells.
- **Frontal cells:** Anterior ethmoid cells that pneumatize frontal recess. They are four types as classified by Bent and Kuhn:

Type I: Single cell above agger nasi cell but below the floor of frontal sinus.

Type II: Multiple cells above agger nasi, may extend into frontal sinus.

Type III: Single large cell that extends supraorbitally through floor of frontal sinus.

Type IV: Single isolated cell that is contained within frontal sinus.

Sphenoid sinus: The right and left sphenoidal sinuses lie within the body of sphenoid bone. They are separated by a septum and are usually unequal in size. Each sinus opens into the sphenoethmoidal recess located within the superior meatus of corresponding half of the nasal cavity. The typical adult size is 0.5 to 8 ml. Each sinus is related superiorly to optic chiasma and hypophysis cerebri; and laterally to ICA and cavernous sinus.

Arterial supply: Posterior ethmoidal and internal carotid arteries.

Venous drainage: Pterygoid venous plexus and cavernous sinus.

Lymphatic drainage: Retropharyngeal nodes.

Nerve supply: Posterior ethmoidal nerve, orbital branches of pterygopalatine ganglion.

Important anatomical structures: Carotid artery and optic nerve are located adjacent to lateral wall of the sinus.

Q. 2. Write a short note on ethmoid air sinuses.
(TNMGR, Oct. 2000; June 2016)

Ans. Ethmoidal sinuses are numerous (total volume of 2 to 3 ml) small intercommunicating spaces which lie within the labyrinth of the ethmoid bone.

Subgroups

1. **Anterior ethmoidal sinus:** 1–11 air cells. It opens into anterior part of hiatus semilunaris of nose. It is supplied by anterior ethmoidal nerve and vessels and drain into submandibular lymph nodes.
2. **Middle ethmoidal sinus:** 1–7 air cells. It opens into middle meatus of nose. It is supplied by anterior ethmoidal vessels and nerve and orbital branches of pterygopalatine ganglion and drain into submandibular lymph nodes.
3. **Posterior ethmoidal sinus:** 1–7 air cells. It opens into superior meatus of nose. It is supplied by posterior ethmoidal vessels and nerve and orbital branches of pterygopalatine ganglion and drain into the retropharyngeal lymph node.

The complex ethmoidal labyrinth can be reduced into a series of lamellae based on embryologic precursors.

1. 1st lamella is *uncinate process*.
2. 2nd lamella corresponds to *ethmoid bulla*.
3. 3rd lamella is known as ***basal or ground lamella*** of middle turbinate. It serves as division of anterior and posterior ethmoids. Anterior part inserts vertically into *crista ethmoidalis*; middle portion attaches obliquely into *lamina papyracea*; posterior third attaches to lamina papyracea in horizontal fashion.
4. 4th lamella is *superior turbinate*.

Agger nasi cell: the most anterior of anterior ethmoid cells, found anterior and superior to middle turbinate attachment to lateral wall.

Ethmoid bulla: Largest of anterior ethmoid cells that lie above infundibulum.

Haller cells: Ethmoid air cells that extend laterally over medial aspect of roof of maxillary sinus.

Onodi cells: Lateral and posterior extensions of posterior ethmoid cells.

Q. 3. Discuss in detail anatomy and applied importance of maxillary air sinuses.

(BFUHS, Nov. 2002; KLE Uni. Jan.2009; HNBG Uni., May 2015; NTR Uni., May 2019)

Ans. The maxillary sinus is a large cavity in the body of maxilla under the eyes and is largest of all the sinuses. It is pyramidal in shape, with its base directed medially towards lateral wall of nose and apex directed laterally into zygomatic process of maxilla. Typical volume at adult stage is 15 ml (Fig. 5.3).

1. It opens into middle meatus of nose usually by two openings one of which is closed by mucous membrane (into the lower part of *hiatus semilunaris*). The large bony hiatus of the sinus is reduced to 3–4 mm in the articulated skull by following bones.
   a. From above, by uncinate process of ethmoid and descending part of lacrimal bone.
   b. From below, by inferior nasal concha.
   c. From behind, by perpendicular plate of palatine bone.
2. **Size:** Avg. size—height: 3.7 cm; Width: 2.5 cm; Anteroposterior depth: 3.7 cm.
3. Its *roof* is formed by floor of orbit and is traversed by infraorbital nerve.
4. The *floor* is formed by alveolar process of maxilla and lies about 1.2 cm below level of floor of nose. (lower border of ala of nose).

Development: Refer Que. 5.1

Processes of maxilla

1. **Zygomatic process:** A pyramidal lateral projection on which anterior, posterior and superior surfaces of maxilla converge.
2. **Frontal process**
   a. **Frontal process** articulates with nasal margin of frontal bone, nasal bone, and lacrimal bone.
   b. **Lateral surface** is divided by a vertical ridge, anterior lacrimal crest, which gives attachment to lacrimal fascia and medial palpebral ligament.
   c. **Medial surface** forms part of the lateral wall of nose. From above downwards, the surface presents following features:
      i. Uppermost area articulates with ethmoid.
      ii. Ethmoidal crest.
      iii. Atrium of the middle meatus.
      iv. Conchal crest.
      v. The inferior meatus of the nose with nasolacrimal groove.
3. **Alveolar process**
   1. The alveolar process bears sockets for roots of upper teeth.
   2. Buccinator arises from posterior part of its outer surface.
   3. A rough ridge, *maxillary torus*, is sometimes present on inner surface opposite the molar sockets.
4. **Palatine process**
   1. Palatine process is a thick horizontal plate projecting medially from lowest part of nasal surface.
   2. Inferior surface is concave, and two palatine processes form anterior three-fourths of bony palate.

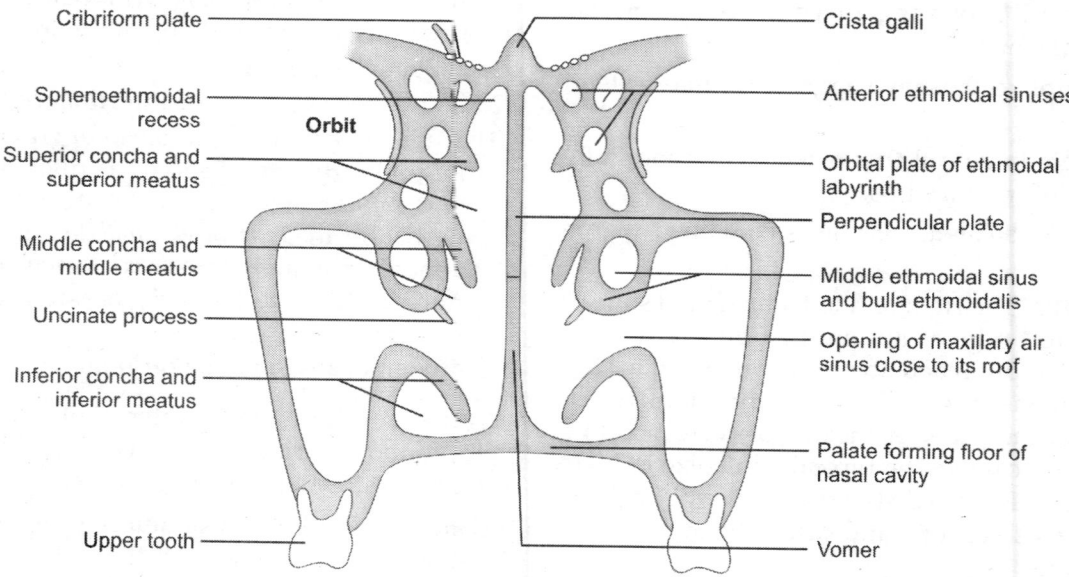

Fig. 5.3: Maxillary sinus and its opening

Cribriform plate — Crista galli

Sphenoethmoidal recess — Orbit — Anterior ethmoidal sinuses

Superior concha and superior meatus — Orbital plate of ethmoidal labyrinth

Middle concha and middle meatus — Perpendicular plate

Uncinate process — Middle ethmoidal sinus and bulla ethmoidalis

Inferior concha and inferior meatus — Opening of maxillary air sinus close to its roof

Upper tooth — Palate forming floor of nasal cavity

Vomer

3. Superior surface is concave from side to side and forms part of floor of nasal cavity.

4. Medial border is raised superiorly into nasal crest. Groove between nasal crests of two maxillae receives lower border of *vomer*.

5. Posterior border articulates with horizontal plate of palatine bone.

6. Lateral border is continuous with the alveolar process.

Arterial supply: Facial, Infraorbital and Greater palatine arteries (FIG).

Venous supply: Facial vein, pterygoid plexus of veins.

Nerve supply: Anterior and middle superior alveolar branches from infraorbital nerve and posterior superior alveolar branches from maxillary nerve.

Lymphatics: Submandibular lymph nodes.

Applied Clinical Anatomy

1. Infection of the sinus is known as *sinusitis*, characterized by headache, persistent thick purulent discharge from the nose.

2. Maxillary sinus is most commonly involved in this. It may be infected from nose or caries tooth. The frontal and maxillary sinuses may be involved in allergies.

3. Drainage of the sinus is difficult because its ostium lies at a higher level than its floor. So the sinus is drained surgically by making opening near to floor by antrum puncture or by *Caldwell-Luc operation*.

4. **Carcinoma of maxillary** sinus arises from the mucosal lining, majority in maxillary sinus, more common in men. Symptoms depend on the direction of growth:
   a. Invasion of the orbit: Propotosis, diplopia, facial pain, and numbness of the skin over maxilla.
   b. Invasion of the floor: Bulging and ulceration of the palate.
   c. Forward growth: Obliterates the canine fossa, swelling of the face.
   d. Backward growth: Severe pain in upper teeth.
   e. Growth in medial direction: nasal obstruction, epistaxis, and epiphora.
   f. Growth in lateral direction: Swelling on face, and palpable mass in labio-gingival groove.

5. Frontal sinusitis and ethmoiditis can cause edema of lid secondary to infection of sinuses.

6. Pain from ethmoid sinus may be referred to forehead as both are supplied by ophthalmic nerve.

7. Pain of maxillary sinusitis may be referred to maxillary teeth and infraorbital skin as all these are supplied by the maxillary nerve.

6. CRANIAL NERVES

Q. 1. Enumerate the cranial nerves. Write a note on trigeminal nerve. *(TNMGR, Oct. 2000, 2012; Pacific Uni., May 2011; NTR Uni., June 2017; TNMGR, May 2019)*

Ans. Cranial nerves: The cranial nerves provide afferent and efferent (sensory, motor, and autonomic) innervations to the structures of head and neck. Cranial nerves are composed of the neural processes associated with distinct brainstem nuclei and cortical structures.

Trigeminal nerve *(UOK, June 2019)*: CN V is the largest cranial nerve, developing from 1st brachial arch. It provides sensory fibers to four parasympathetic ganglia: ciliary, pterygopalatine, otic and submandibular. It has two nuclei:

1. **General somatic afferent column (sensory):** This column has three nuclei. These are (Fig. 6.1):
   - **Spinal nucleus:** It takes pain and temperature sensations from most of the face area which relay here. The crossed fibers are called **trigeminal lemniscus** which goes to ventroposteromedial nucleus of thalamus for another relay, to finally terminate in lower part of postcentral gyrus.
   - **Superior sensory nucleus:** Fibers carrying touch and pressure relay in this nucleus. Remaining path is same as of spinal nucleus.
   - **Mesencephalic nucleus:** This nucleus extends from pons till midbrain. It receives proprioceptive impulses from muscles of mastication, temporomandibular joint and teeth.

2. **Branchial efferent column (motor):** The nucleus of 5th nerve is situated at the level of upper pons. The fibers of motor nucleus supply muscles derived from 1st branchial arch.

Course: It is attached to the ventral surface of pons by a large sensory root and small motor root. The motor root lies ventromedial to sensory root. The two roots pass forward to trigeminal ganglion in middle cranial fossa.

Sensory components of 5th nerve (CN V): Sensation of pain, temperature, touch and pressure from skin of face, mucous membrane of nose, most of tongue, PNS, travel along axons. Their cell bodies lie in trigeminal ganglion or semi-lunar ganglion or gasserian ganglion. It lies at apex of petrous temporal bone in a dural cave, **Meckel's cave.** Peripheral processes of the ganglion cells form three nerves. The central processes of trigeminal ganglion form sensory root. Ascending fibers end in superior sensory nucleus. Descending fibers end in spinal nucleus of 5th nerve.

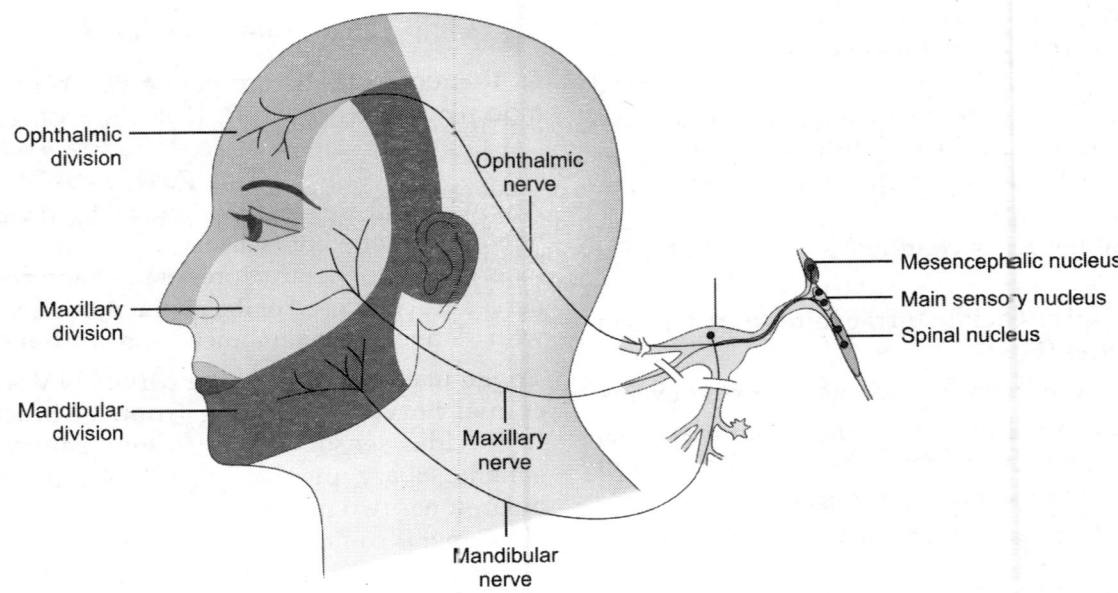

Fig. 6.1: Trigeminal nerve and its branches

Ophthalmic nerve fibers end in inferior part, **maxillary nerve** fibers end in middle part and **mandibular nerve** fibers terminate in upper part of spinal nucleus.

Proprioceptive fibers from muscles of mastication, extraocular muscles and facial muscles bypass 5th ganglion to reach unipolar cells of mesencephalic nucleus.

Motor component: The motor nucleus receives impulses from the right and left cerebral hemispheres, red nucleus and mesencephalic nucleus. Fibres of motor root supply four muscles of mastication and tensor veli palatine, tensor tympani, mylohyoid and anterior belly of digastrics.

Trigeminal nerve/cranial nerve (V) (Gujarat Uni., April 2019) comprises three branches, ophthalmic V1, maxillary V2 and mandibular V3 (Fig. 6.1).

A. **Ophthalmic nerve (V1):** It is sensory. Its branches are:
   1. **Frontal**
      a. Supratrochlear: Upper eyelid, conjunctiva, lower part of forehead.
      b. Supraorbital: Frontal air sinus, upper eyelid, forehead, scalp till vertex.
   2. **Nasociliary**
      a. Posterior ethmoidal: Sphenoidal air sinus, posterior ethmoidal air sinuses.
      b. Long ciliary: Sensory to eyeball.
      c. Nerve to ciliary ganglion.
      d. Infratochlear: Both eyelids, side of nose, lacrimal sac.
   e. Anterior ethmoidal:
      I. Middle and anterior ethmoidal sinuses.
      II. Medial internal nasal.
      III. Lateral internal nasal.
      IV. External nasal: Skin of ala of vestibule and tip of nose.
   3. **Lacrimal:** Lateral part of the upper eyelid; conveys secretomotor fibers from zygomatic nerve to lacrimal gland.
B. **Maxillary nerve (V2):** (UHSR, April 2010; RGUHS, July 2017)
   1. In middle cranial fossa: Meningeal branch.
   2. In pterygopalatine fossa:
      a. Ganglionic branches.
      b. Zygomatic:
         I. Zygomaticotemporal.
         II. Zygomaticofacial.
      c. Posterior superior alveolar.
   3. In infraorbital canal:
      a. Middle superior alveolar.
      b. Anterior superior alveolar.
   4. On face: Infraorbital.
      a. Palpebral
      b. Labial
      c. Nasal.

Mandibular nerve (V3) (UOK, July 2014)

Development: The trigeminal nerve is derived from 1st pharyngeal arch. The development follows in three stages. First, a pioneer neurite emerges and a nerve

Table 6.1a: Cranial nerves and their functions

Number	Name	General function*	Specific function
I	Olfactory	S	Smell
II	Optic	S	Vision
III	Oculomotor	M, P	Motor to four of six extrinsic eye muscles and upper eyelid; parasympathetic: constricts pupil, thickens lens
IV	Trochlear	M	Motor to one extrinsic eye muscle
V	Trigeminal	S, M	Sensory to face and teeth; motor to muscles of mastication (chewing)
VI	Abducens	M	Motor to one extrinsic eye muscle
VII	Facial	S, M, P	Sensory: Taste; motor to muscles of facial expression; parasympathetic to salivary and tear glands
VIII	Vestibulocochlear	S	Hearing and balance
IX	Glossopharyngeal	S, M, P	Sensory: Taste and touch to back of tongue, motor to pharyngeal muscles; parasympathetic to salivary glands
X	Vagus	S, M, P	Sensory to pharynx, larynx, and viscera; motor to palate, pharynx, and larynx; parasympathetic to viscera of thorax and abdomen
XI	Accessory	M	Motor to two neck and upper back muscles
XII	Hypoglossal	M	Motor to tongue muscles

*S, sensory; M, somatic motor, P. parasympathetic

Table 6.1b: Cranial nerves examination (BFUHS, May 2017)

Cranial nerve	Examination
I Olfactory	Sense of smell for common odors
II Optic	Visual acuity (Snellen types ± ophthalmoscopy); nystagmus Visual fields (by confrontation) Pupil responses to light and accommodation
III Oculomotor	Eye movements Pupil responses
IV Trochlear	Eye movements
V Trigeminal	Sensation over face ± corneal reflex ± taste sensation Motor power of masticatory muscles; jaw jerk
VI Abducens	Eye movements
VII Facial	Motor power of facial muscles Corneal reflex ± taste sensation
VIII Vestibulocochlear	Hearning (tuning fork at 256 Hz) Balance
IX Glossopharyngeal	Gag reflex Taste sensation
X Vagus	Gag reflex
XI Accessory	Motor power of trapezius and sternomastoid
XII Hypoglossal	Motor power of tongue

forms, later neurites fasciculate with this. Upon reaching the inside surface of the cement gland, the neuritis separate and penetrate holes in the basal lamina. Finally, the neurites grow between the cells they will innervate and form free nerve endings.

Blood supply: a. Superolateral branch of the basilar artery, b. Peduncular cerebellar branch of the anterior inferior cerebellar artery, c. Trigeminocerebellar artery.

Surgical consideration: Surgical interventions for trigeminal neuralgia are: non-destructive and destructive. The goal of non-destructive surgery is to alleviate nerve compression by removing any structure that may be impinging on the nerve. Destructive procedures aim to disrupt the trigeminal nerve completely so that pain is no longer transmitted by the nerve. The result of a destructive procedure is the irreversible loss of sensation of affected side of the face.

Applied Clinical Anatomy

1. Injury to ophthalmic nerve—loss of corneal blink reflex.
2. Injury to maxillary nerve—loss of sneeze reflex.
3. Injury to mandibular nerve—loss of jaw jerk reflex.
4. Peripheral lesions involving sensory portion of the trigeminal at any point distal to the pontine exit can produce ipsilateral pain and/or varying degrees of anesthesia.
5. Central lesions: Lesions of sensory cortex will produce a raised threshold to pain and temperature on the opposite side of the face.
6. Thalamic lesions: Contralateral hypesthesia and hyperpathia of face.
7. Midpontine lesions: Ipsilateral decrease in tactile sensation of face and ipsilateral paralysis of masticatory muscles.
8. Spinal tract and nucleus lesion: Ipsilateral pain and temperature sensation is lost.

9. Damage to mandibular division: Atrophy and flaccid paralysis of muscles of mastication.
10. Spasm of masticatory muscles is seen with tetanus and strychnine poisoning.
11. **Trigeminal neuralgia/Tic Douloureux/Fothergill disease:** Trigeminal neuralgia is defined as sudden, unilateral, severe, brief, often described as burning or shock-like, recurring pain in the distribution of one or more branches of the CN V. The most commonly it is caused by nerve compression. Diagnosis is typically made based on the clinical presentation alone once other possible causes such as postherpetic neuralgia or dental issues are ruled out. The first-line treatment is carbamazepine, and second-line medications include lamotrigine, oxcarbazepine, phenytoin, gabapentin, pregablin, and baclofen and surgical (peripheral injections, peripheral neurectomy, cryotherapy and thermo-coagulation).

Q. 2. Write a short note on infraorbital nerve.

(TNMGR, April 1998)

Ans. Infraorbital nerve (IAN), continuation of maxillary nerve, enters the orbit through inferior orbital fissure. It then runs forwards on floor of orbit or roof of maxillary sinus, at first in infraorbital groove and then in infraorbital canal remaining outside periosteum of orbit. It emerges on face through infraorbital foramen and terminates by dividing into palpebral, nasal and labial branches. The nerve is accompanied by infra-orbital branch of third part of maxillary artery and accompanying vein.

Branches

1. **Posterior superior and middle superior alveolar nerve** arises in the infraorbital groove, runs in the lateral wall of the maxillary sinus, and supplies the upper premolar teeth.
2. **Anterior superior alveolar nerve** arises in the infraorbital canal, and runs in a sinuous canal having a complicated course in the anterior wall of the maxillary sinus. It supplies upper incisors and canine teeth, maxillary sinus, and antero-inferior part of the nasal cavity.
3. **Terminal branches** (emerges from infra-orbital foramen)—**palpebral, nasal and superior labial** supply skin of medial cheek, lateral nose, mucosa of anteroinferior nasal septum, upper lip and cheek.

Applied Clinical Anatomy

1. The nerve is a risk of injury with orbital blowout fractures.

2. This nerve is also commonly implicated in trigeminal neuralgia.

Q. 3. Describe the nuclei of origin, course, relations, distribution and applied anatomy of mandibular nerve.

(TNMGR, April, Oct. 2013, 2019; KUHS, June 2013; MAHE, April 2014; RGUHS, May 2015; SGT Uni., July 2016; Sumandeep Uni., May 2018)

Q. Write a short note on lingual nerve.

(RGUHS, Nov. 2011)

Q. Write a short note on inferior alveolar nerve.

(TNMGR, Oct. 1996, 1999, Nov. 2001, Oct. 2003, March 2008; Oct., 2018; RGUHS, April 2007; KUHS, Jan. 2014)

Ans. Mandibular division (V3) is the largest of three divisions of the trigeminal nerve. It has both sensory and motor fibers. It is the nerve of the first branchial arch and supplies all structures derived from the mandibular or first branchial arch.

Course and relations: Mandibular nerve begins in the middle cranial fossa through a large sensory root and a small motor root. **Sensory root** arises from the lateral part of the trigeminal ganglion and leaves the cranial cavity through the foramen ovale. **Motor root** lies deep to the trigeminal ganglion and to sensory root. It also passes through the foramen ovale to join the sensory root just below the foramen thus forming the main trunk. The main trunk lies in the infratemporal fossa, on the tensor veli palatini, deep to the lateral pterygoid. After a short-course, the main trunk divides into a small anterior trunk and a large posterior trunk.

Branches (Fig. 6.3)

From main trunk: Meningeal branch/nervous spinosus; Nerve to the medial pterygoid.

From anterior division: Buccal nerve (sensory); Masseteric; deep temporal nerve; Nerve to the lateral pterygoid.

From the posterior division: Auriculotemporal nerve; Lingual nerve; Inferior alveolar nerves.

Meningeal branch or nervus spinosus: Duramater of middle cranial fossa and mastoid cells.

Nerve to medial pterygoid: Medial pterygoid from the deep surface, tensor palatine and tensor tympanic muscles.

Buccal nerve: Skin of cheek and mucous membrane related to the buccinators, labial aspect of gums of molar and premolar teeth.

Masseteric nerve: Deep surface of masseter, TMJ.

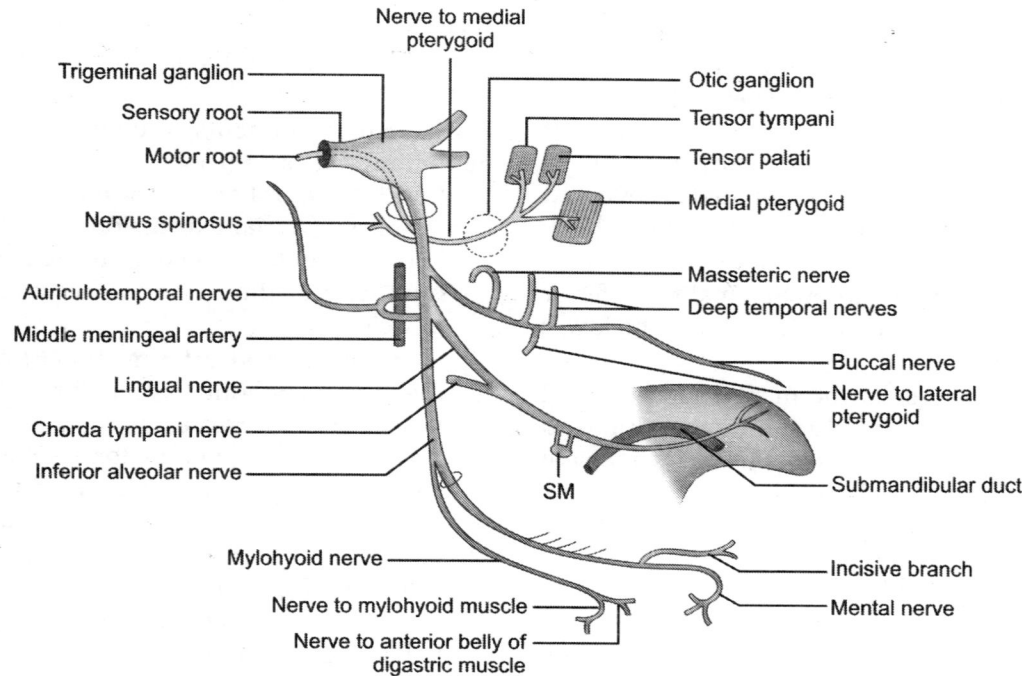

Fig. 6.3: Mandibular nerve and its branches

Deep temporal nerves: These are two nerves, anterior and posterior, supplies the deep surface and anterior of the temporalis.

Nerve to lateral pterygoid: It enters the deep surface of the muscle.

Auriculotemporal nerve: It arises by two roots:

Superior root—comprises sensory fibers.

Inferior root—carries secretory-motor parasympathetic fibers, originating from CN IX, to the parotid gland.

Both the roots runs backwards, encircle the middle meningeal artery and unite to form a single trunk. Auricular part of the nerve supplies skin of the tragus; and upper parts of the pinna, external acoustic meatus and the tympanic membrane. **Temporal part** supplies skin of temple. Auriculotemporal nerve also supplies parotid gland and TMJ.

Lingual nerve (Fig. 6.3): Lingual nerve is one of the two terminal branches of the posterior division of the mandibular nerve. It is sensory to anterior two-thirds of tongue and to floor of mouth.

Course and relations: It begins 1 cm below the skull, runs first between tensor veli palatine and lateral pterygoid and then between lateral and medial pterygoids. About 2 cm below the skull, it is joined by chorda tympani nerve. Emerging at lower border of lateral pterygoid, the nerve runs downwards and forwards between ramus of mandible and medial pterygoid. Next it lies in direct contact within the mandible, medial to the third molar tooth between the origins of the superior constrictor and mylohyoid muscles. It soon leaves the gum and runs over the hyoglossus deep to the mylohyoid. Finally, it lies on the surface of the genioglossus deep to the mylohyoid. Here, it winds around the submandibular duct and divides into its terminal branches.

Applied Clinical Anatomy

1. Entrapment of lingual nerve can cause numbness and loss of taste from anterior two-thirds of tongue, loss of sensation from lingual gingiva, and pain with speech disorders.
2. Smoking can cause loss of non-noxious thermal stimuli, due to degeneration of the thermoreceptors. The sensation of mechanical or painful thermal stimuli remains intact.

Inferior alveolar nerve (KUHS, Jan. 2014): It is the larger terminal branch of the posterior division of the mandibular nerve. It runs vertically downwards lateral to medial pterygoid and to sphenomandibular ligament. It enters mandibular foramen and runs in mandibular canal. It is accompanied by the inferior alveolar artery.

Branches (Fig. 6.3)

a. **Mylohyoid branch** contains all the motor fibers of the posterior division. It arises just before the inferior alveolar nerve enters the mandibular foramen. It pierces the sphenomandibular ligament with the mylohyoid artery, runs in the mylohyoid groove, and supplies the mylohyoid muscle and the anterior belly of the digastrics.

b. While running in the mandibular canal the inferior alveolar nerve gives branches that supply the lower teeth and gums.

c. **Mental nerve** emerges at the mental foramen and supplies the skin of the chin, and the skin and mucous membrane of the lower lip. Its incisive branch supplies the labial aspect of gums of canine and incisor teeth.

Applied Clinical Anatomy

1. Dentists not achieving complete mandibular nerve anesthesia is a common problem due to many anatomical variations.

2. Temporomandibular joint dysfunction (TMD) is caused by a group of conditions that cause pain and joint dysfunction in the jaw, joint and muscles that control jaw movement.

3. The auriculotemporal nerve may be damaged during TMJ surgery, which may cause parasthesia of the auricle and the ear region.

4. Trigeminal neuralgia is commonly seen with damage to the mandibular branch.

5. Classical trigeminal neuralgia is due to vascular compromise of the trigeminal nerve root.

6. Secondary trigeminal neuralgia is due to major neurological diseases such as multiple sclerosis or tumors with possible involvement of the mandibular nerve branches.

7. *Tonic tensor tympani syndrome* results in ear pain, fluttering sensations, or fullness of the ear due to increased activity of the tensor tympani muscle.

Q. 4. Describe the intra-cranial, intra-petrous and extra-cranial course, branches and clinical importance of the facial nerve. (KUHS, Dec. 2012; MUHS, Oct. 2013; MAHE, June 2016; UOK, 2016; MUHS, June 2017; NTR Uni., May 2019; TNMGR, Oct. 2019)

Ans. Facial nerve (CN VII/7th), the nerve of 2nd branchial arch, is the '**Queen of the face.**' It arises from brain stem and extends posteriorly to abducens nerve and anteriorly to the vestibulocochlear nerve. It courses through facial canal in temporal bone and exits through stylomastoid foramen after which it divides into terminal branches at the posterior edge of the parotid gland.

Functional components: The facial nerve carries both motor and sensory fibers.

1. **Special visceral or branchiomotor efferent (SVE):** Muscles of facial expression and elevation of the hyoid bone, the stapedius muscle, the stylohyoid muscle, and the posterior belly of the digastric muscle.

2. **General visceral efferent (GVE)** or parasympathetic preganglionic motor fibres: They leave the facial nerve as greater petrosal nerve and chorda tympani nerve. Secretomotor to submandibular and sublingual salivary glands, lacrimal glands, and glands of nose, palate and pharynx.

3. **General visceral afferent (GVA):** Afferent impulses from submandibular and sublingual salivary glands, lacrimal glands, and glands of nose, palate and pharynx.

4. **Special visceral afferent fibers (SVA):** Taste sensation from anterior two-thirds of tongue except from vallate papillae and from palate. Its fibers travel with lingual nerve and chorda tympani.

5. **General somatic afferent fibers (GSA):** Innervate pinna of the ear and the external acoustic meatus by forming the auricular nerve together with the vagal nerve.

   Nuclei: The fibers of the nerve are connected to four nuclei situated in the lower pons.
   1. Motor nucleus or branchiomotor.
   2. Superior salivatory nucleus or parasympathetic.
   3. Lacrimatory nucleus is also parasympathetic.
   4. Nucleus of the tractus solitarius which is gustatory and also receives afferent fibers from the glands.

Motor nucleus lies deep in reticular formation of lower pons. The part of the nucleus that supplies muscles of upper part of face receives corticonuclear fibers from motor cortex of both right and left sides. In contrast, part of nucleus that supplies muscles of lower part of face receives corticonuclear fibers only from opposite cerebral hemisphere.

Development: The facial nerve is derived from the second branchial arch.

Course and relations (Fig. 6.4a): The facial nerve exits the brain stem from its venterolateral surface at the cerebellopontine angle.

A. **Intracranial course:** The facial nerve is attached to the brainstem by two roots, motor and sensory. The sensory root is also called the **nervus intermedius.**

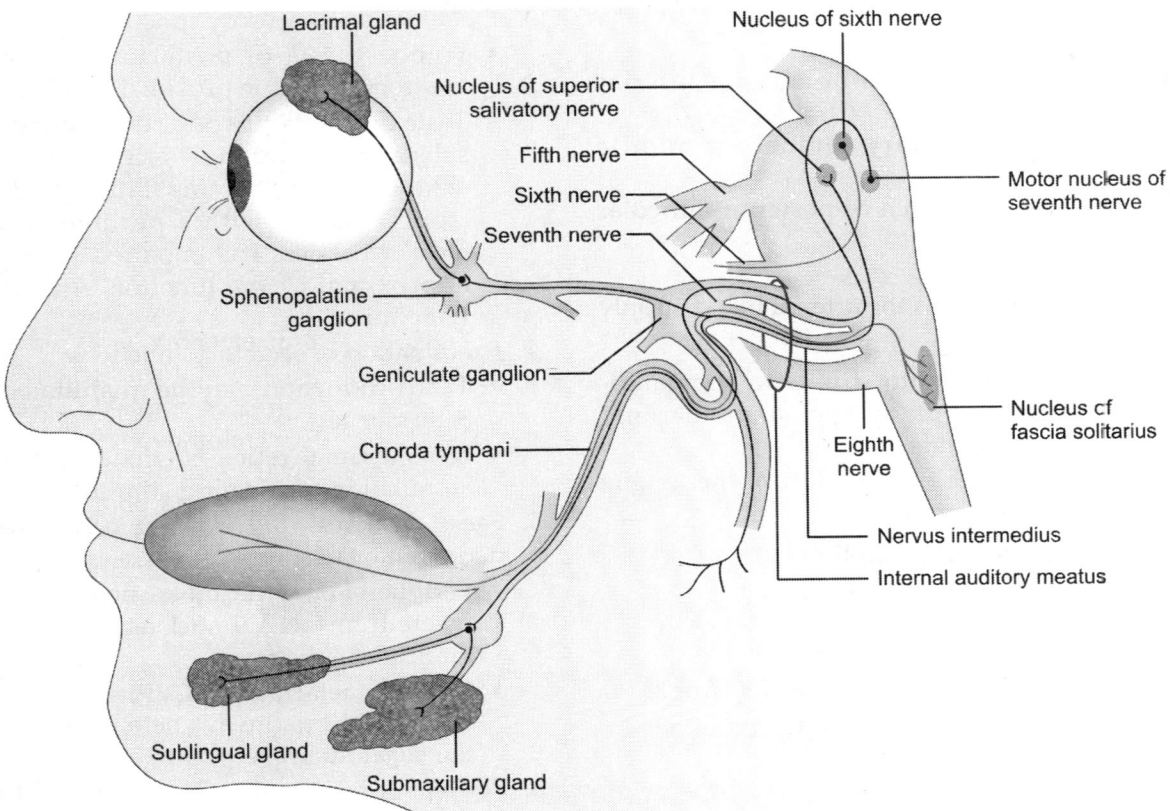

Fig. 6.4a: Facial nerve and its branches

The two roots of the facial nerve are attached to the lateral part of the lower border of the pons. The two roots run laterally and forwards with the eighth nerve to reach the internal acoustic meatus. In the meatus, motor root lies in a groove on eighth nerve, with sensory root intervening. At bottom of meatus, the two roots fuse to form a single trunk, which lies in the petrous temporal bone. Within the canal, course of the nerve can be divided into three parts by two bends:

First part is directed laterally above the vestibule.

Second part runs backwards in relation to the medial wall of the middle ear, above the promontory.

Third part is directed vertically downwards behind the promontory. The facial nerve leaves the skull by passing through the stylomastoid foramen.

B. **Intratemporal part:** The intratemporal part of the facial nerve begins when the facial nerve, together with intermediate nerve, passes through internal auditory meatus of temporal bone to enter the facial canal within petrous part of temporal bone. After synapsing on geniculate ganglion, facial nerve gives

rise to the first branch; the greater petrosal nerve. The greater petrosal nerve joins the deep petrosal nerve to form **nerve of the pterygoid**.

Second branch of facial nerve running in the facial canal is the **nerve to stapedius muscle. Chorda tympani** nerve is last branch of facial nerve within facial canal and at the same time, the terminal extension of the intermediate nerve. It runs through the ossicles in the middle ear and exits the tympanic cavity at the petrotympanic fissure where it joins the lingual nerve, which is itself a branch of the trigeminal nerve.

a. **Extracranial course:** The extratemporal part of the facial nerve begins when the facial nerve leaves the cranium through the stylomastoid foramen. As the facial nerve exits, it gives GSA fibers to the pinna of ear and external auditory meatus and SVE fibers to the posterior belly of digastric, stylohyoid, the superior and inferior auricular, and occipitalis muscles. Thereafter, the facial nerve divides at the end of the posterior edge of the parotid gland into the terminal branches (temporal, zygomatic, buccal, mandibular, cervical)

Blood supply
- Anterior inferior cerebellar artery
- Labyrinthine artery (branch of anterior inferior cerebellar artery)
- Superficial petrosal artery (branch of middle meningeal artery)
- Stylomastoid artery (branch of posterior auricular artery)
- Posterior auricular artery.
- Venous drainage parallels the arterial blood supply

Chorda tympani: It carries:
a. **Preganglionic secretomotor fibers** to submandibular ganglion for supply of submandibular and sublingual salivary glands.
b. **Taste fibers** from anterior two-third of the tongue except circumvallate papillae.

Posterior auricular nerve: It supplies:
a. Auricularis posterior.
b. Occipitalis.
c. Intrinsic muscles on the back of auricle.

Digastric branch: Posterior belly of the digastric.

Stylohyoid branch: It supplies stylohyoid muscle.

Temporal branches:
a. Auricularis anterior.
b. Auricularis superior.
c. Intrinsic muscles on the lateral side of the ear.
d. Frontalis.
e. Orbicularis oculi.
f. Corrugator supercilii.

Zygomatic branches: Orbicularis oculi.

Buccal branches: Buccinators.

Marginal mandibular branch: Muscles of lower lip and chin.

Cervical branch: Platysma.

Applied Clinical Anatomy

1. Testing of facial nerve branches: *(BFUHS, May 2017)*
   - Temporal branches: Patient is asked to frown and wrinkle his or her forehead.
   - Zygomatic branches: Patient is asked to close their eyes tightly.
   - Buccal branches: Puff-up cheeks (buccinator).
2. Examination of reflexes:
   - Corneal reflex: Afferent limb of the reflex is mediated by CN V1.
   - Stapedius reflex: Impedance audiometry can record the presence or absence of stapedius muscle contraction to sound stimuli above hearing threshold.

3. Examination of sensory functions:
   - Hypoesthesia of posterior wall of external auditory meatus in proximal facial nerve lesions.
   - Taste on anterior two-thirds of tongue: Use four substances for testing—sucrose (sweet), sodium chloride (salty), quinine (bitter), and citric acid (sour). Patient with a peripheral pattern of facial weakness has impaired taste; the lesion is proximal to the junction with the chorda tympani.
4. Examination of secretory functions:
   - Tear production may be quantitated with the Schirmer test.
   - Nasolacrimal reflex is elicited by mechanical stimulation or chemical stimulation.
5. Facial weakness (*BFUHS, May 2017*): Two types of neurogenic facial nerve weakness:
   - Peripheral or lower motor neuron—lesion anywhere from CN VII nucleus in pons to terminal branches in the face.
   - Central facial palsy (CFP)—lesion involving upranuclear pathways before they synapse on the facial nucleus.
6. Peripheral facial palsy: There is flaccid weakness of all the muscles of facial expression on the involved side, both upper and lower face, and the paralysis is usually complete.
   - Palpebral fissure is open wider than normal and there may be inability to close eye (lagophthalmos).
   - *Bell's phenomenon:* Attempting to close involved eye causes a reflex upturning of the eyeball.
   - *Levator sign of Dutemps and Céstan:* Patient look down, and then close the eyes slowly the upper lid on the paralyzed side moves upward slightly.
   - *Negro's sign:* Eyeball on the paralyzed side deviates outward and elevates more than the normal one when the patient raises her eyes.
   - *Bergara-Wartenberg sign:* Loss of the fine vibrations palpable with the thumbs or fingertips resting lightly on the lids as the patient tries to close the eyes as tightly as possible.
   - *Platysma sign of Babinski:* Asymmetric contraction of the platysma, less on the involved side, when the mouth is opened.
7. **House-Brackmann grading system of facial nerve palsy:**
   - Grade I: Normal.
   - Grade II: Mild dysfunction, slight weakness on close inspection, normal symmetry at rest.

- Grade III: Moderate dysfunction, obvious but not disfiguring difference between sides, eye can be completely closed with effort.
- Grade IV: Moderately severe, normal tone at rest, obvious weakness or asymmetry with movement, incomplete closure of eye.
- Grade V: Severe dysfunction, only barely perceptible motion, asymmetry at rest.
- Grade VI: No movement.

8. Damage to the facial nerve can have various etiologies including iatrogenic, trauma, stroke, idiopathic Bell's palsy, neoplasm or granulomatous meningitis (Fig. 6.4b).

   a. **Supranuclear lesion:** Occurs as a result of damage to UMN of the facial nerve. the supranuclear innervation is bilateral to the muscles of the upper part of the face and contralateral to the muscles of the middle and lower part of the face.

   b. **Nuclear or infranuclear lesion:** Lesions that involve the facial motor nucleus or the infranuclear portion of the facial nerve result in complete paralysis of all the facial muscles on the ipsilateral side.

   c. **Lesion of ventral pons:** Ipsilateral facial plegia, palsy of lateral rectus muscle (abducens nerve), contra lateral hemiplegia (corticospinal fibers).

   d. **Lesion of pontine tegmentum:** Ipsilateral facial plegia, contra lateral hemiplegia, paralysis of conjugate gaze to the side of the lesion.

   e. **Lesion at cerebello pontine angle:** Ipsilateral facial plegia, decreased secretion of saliva and tears, hyperacusis and loss of taste (ageusia) in anterior two-thirds of ipsilateral part of tongue.

   f. **Facial canal between the internal acoustic meatus and the geniculate ganglion:** Ipsilateral facial plegia, decreased secretion of saliva and tears, hyperacusis and ageusia to anterior two-thirds of ipsilateral part of tongue.

   g. **Facial canal between geniculate ganglion and nerve to the stapedius muscle:** Ipsilateral facial plegia ↓ salivary secretion, ageusia to anterior two-thirds of ipsilateral part of tongue, hyperacusis.

   h. **Facial canal between nerve to stapedius and leaving of chorda tympani:** Ipsilateral facial plegia ↓ salivary secretion, ageusia to anterior two-thirds of ipsilateral part of tongue.

   i. **After giving the branch of chorda tympani:** Ipsilateral facial plegia.

9. '*Crocodile tears syndrome*,' also known as *Bogorad syndrome*, is shedding of tears while eating or drinking in patients recovering from Bell's palsy (*gustatory lacrimation*).

10. *Ramsay Hunt syndrome* is characterized by facial paralysis, herpetiform vesicular eruptions, and vestibulocochlear dysfunction. Vesicular eruptions may occur over the ear, face, and neck down to the shoulder.

11. *Melkersson-Rosenthal syndrome* is characterized by facial paralysis, episodic facial swelling, and a fissured tongue (scrotal tongue or lingua plicata).

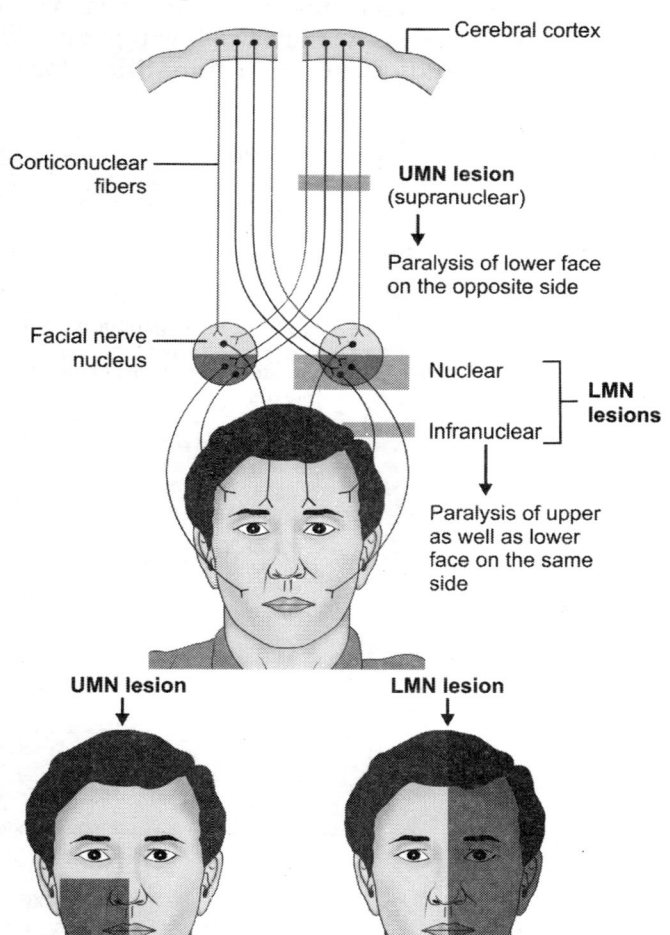

Fig. 6.4b: Damage to facial nerve at various levels

Q. 5. Write a note on glossopharyngeal nerve.
(RGUHS, Nov. 2011; TNMGR, April 2012)

Ans. The glossopharyngeal nerve is the 9th cranial nerve (CN IX). It originates from the medulla oblongata and terminates in the pharynx.

Functional components: The glossopharyngeal nerve carries sensory, efferent motor and parasympathetic fibers.

a. **Special visceral efferent fibers** (branchial motor): Arise in nucleus ambiguous and supply the stylopharyngeus muscle.

b. **General visceral efferent fibers** (preganglionic/visceral motor): Arise in inferior salivary nucleus, then travel with the tympanic nerve through the foramen ovale and travel to otic ganglion, from where postganglionic fibers supply to the parotid.

c. **General visceral afferent fibers** (visceral sensory): They are peripheral processes of cells in the inferior ganglion of the nerve. They carry general sensations from pharynx, carotid body and carotid sinus to the ganglion. The central processes convey these sensations to the nucleus of the solitary tract.

d. **Special visceral afferent fibers** (general sensory): They are peripheral processes of cells in the inferior ganglion of the nerve. They carry sensations of taste from the posterior one-third of the tongue including circumvallate papillae to the ganglion. The central processes convey these sensations to the nucleus of the solitary tract.

e. **General somatic afferent fibers:** They are peripheral processes of cells in the inferior ganglion of the nerve. They carry general sensations (pain, touch, temperature) from the posterior one-third of the tongue, tonsil, and pharynx. The central processes convey these sensations to the nucleus of the spinal tract of trigeminal nerve.

Development: The glossopharyngeal nerve derives from third pharyngeal arch.

Course (Fig. 6.5):

Intracranial: The fiber arises at the level of medulla oblongata. It is attached at the base of brain in posterolateral sulcus, and then exits skull via jugular foramen, where tympanic nerve branches to give parasympathetic innervations to parotid gland.

Extracranial: Superior ganglion (small) is a detached part of inferior ganglion. Inferior ganglion carries cell bodies of all the sensory fibers. It enters the pharynx through the interval between constrictor muscles, splitting into its other branches—lingual, pharyngeal, and tonsillar.

Branches and distributions

1. Tympanic nerve (*nerve of Jacobson*): Middle ear, auditory tube, mastoid antrum and cells.
2. Lesser petrosal nerve: Secretomotor for parotid gland.
3. Carotid branch/*Sinus nerve (Hering's nerve)*: Carotid sinus (baroreceptors) and carotid body (chemoreceptors).
4. Pharyngeal branches: Mucous membrane of pharynx.

5. Stylopharyngeal nerve: Stylopharyngeus.
6. Tonsillar branches: Tonsil, soft palate, palatoglossal arch.
7. Lingual branches: Taste and general sensations from posterior one-third of the tongue.

Clinical Applied Anatomy

1. Paralysis of nerve leads to:
   a. Dysphagia, impaired gustation over the posterior one-third of tongue and palate.
   b. Reduced sensation over the posterior one-third of tongue, palate, and pharynx.
   c. Loss of carotid sinus reflex.
   d. Absent gag reflex.
   e. Parotid gland secretory dysfunction loss of reflex contraction of muscle of pharynx and loss of taste sensation.

2. **Glossopharyngeal neuralgia:** It consists of episodic, unilateral sharp pain in posterior throat, tonsils, base of tongue, and inferior to angle of mandible that can last from seconds to minutes, triggered by mandibular actions, mainly swallowing, chewing, coughing, and yawning. Idiopathic glosso-

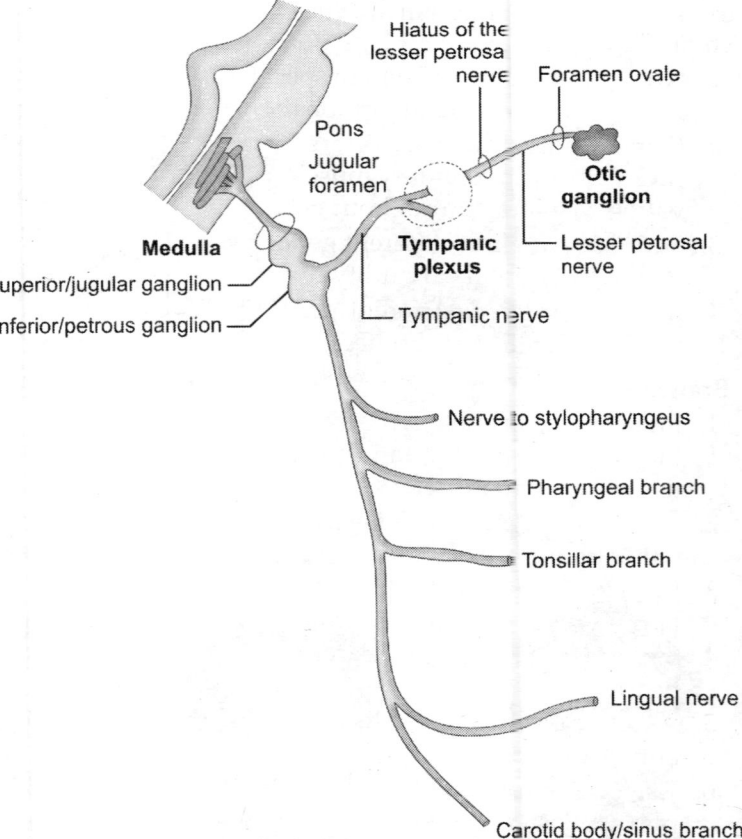

Fig. 6.5: Glossopharyngeal nerve and its branches

pharyngeal neuralgia is caused by compression of cranial nerve IX by a vessel or dysfunction of the central pons, whereas secondary glossopharyngeal neuralgia can result from trauma, neoplasm, infection of the throat, surgery, or malformations. Carbamazepine is most often the first medication used in therapy, and if it achieves partial pain relief, a second medication can be added. Also, low dose selective serotonin reuptake inhibitors (SSRIs) can be useful. If pharmacologic treatments fail, other options include microvascular decompression (MVD), percutaneous radiofrequency neurolysis and gamma knife radiosurgery.

3. **Glossopharyngeal nerve dysfunction following carotid endarterectomy:** Transection of this nerve during surgery causes glossopharyngeal nerve paresis, which can cause symptoms such as dysphagia and dysphonia.

Q. 6. Write a note on vagus nerve.

Ans. The vagus nerve (CN X) is the longest cranial nerve in the body, containing both motor and sensory functions in both the afferent and efferent regards. The vagus nerve has its origin in medulla oblongata and exits skull via jugular foramen. Nucleus associated with vagus nerve:

1. Nucleus ambiguous: Efferent special visceral (ESV); mediate swallowing and phonation.
2. Dorsal motor nucleus: Efferent general visceral (EGV) fibers; involuntary muscle control and innervation to glands throughout gastrointestinal tract.
3. Superior ganglion: Afferent general somatic innervation to external ear and tympanic membrane.
4. Inferior ganglion: Afferent general visceral fibers to carotid and aortic bodies.

Branches

1. Pharyngeal branches: Form pharyngeal plexus; innervate pharyngeal and palate muscles (except tensor palatine muscle).
2. Superior laryngeal nerve: a. Internal: Mucosa superior to glottis; b. External: Cricothyroid muscle.
3. Recurrent laryngeal nerve: All laryngeal musculature except cricothyroid muscle.
4. Superior cardiac nerve: Parasympathetic fibers to heart.
5. Anterior bronchial: Anterior pulmonary plexus; anterior lung.
6. Posterior bronchial nerve: Posterior pulmonary plexus; Posterior lung.
7. Esophageal branches: Esophageal plexus.
8. Gastric branches: Stomach.
9. Celiac branches: Pancreas, spleen, kidneys, adrenals and small intestine.

Embryology: The vagus nerve arises from the fourth branchial arch.

Blood supply: Middle meningeal artery, common carotid artery and branches, a posterior meningeal artery, internal thoracic arteries, bronchial arteries, and esophageal arteries.

Applied Clinical Anatomy

1. The vagus nerve is commonly tested clinically by asking the patient to open their mouth and say 'ah,' this should cause elevation of the uvula.
2. Gag reflex should not be used as a clinical exam as there can be a bilateral loss of gag reflex in a healthy patient.
3. If there is hoarseness with a normal gag reflex and palatal elevation, this indicates a lesion of recurrent laryngeal nerve.
4. Vagus nerve stimulation technique is approved to treat epilepsy and depression; treatment of obesity.
5. Stimulation of larynx provides reflexes including cough, apnea, and effects on the cardiovascular system such as bradycardia and hypotension.
6. Central lesions of the vagus nerve can cause: dysphagia, dysarthria and hoarseness; Uvula deviation (towards the opposite side of the lesion); and transient parasympathetic effects.

Q. 7. Write a note on accessory nerve.

Ans. Accessory nerve (CN XI) nerve supplies the sternocleidomastoid and trapezius muscles. It has two parts.

1. Cranial part (smaller): Arises from cells in the nucleus ambiguous and distributed with vagus nerve. This portion innervates the pharyngeal muscles.
2. Spinal part: Arises from a long column of nuclei situated in the ventral part of the medulla and extending to the fifth cervical segment or lower, then leave through the jugular foramen with the vagus nerve. The nerve descends in the neck near the jugular vein and supplies the sternocleido mastoid and trapezius muscles, joined by motor or sensory contributions from the upper cervical nerves.

Applied Clinical Anatomy

1. Supranuclear lesions cause moderate, often transient, impairment of function of the sternocleido-mastoid and trapezius muscles, due to the bilateral innervation.

2. In the spinal cord the nuclei can be involved in amyotrophic lateral sclerosis, syringomyelia, polio, and intraspinal tumors.

3. **Wallenberg's syndrome:** Due to occlusion of vertebral or posterior inferior cerebellar artery producing infarction of medullary tegmentum, with deficits of V, IX, X, and XI.

4. **Vernet's syndrome:** Due to compression of nerves IX, X, and XI all together in jugular foramen.

5. **Villaret's syndrome:** Due to lesions occurring in the posterior retroparotid space.

Q. 8. Write a short note on hypoglossal nerve.
(TNMGR, April 1997, 2000; RGUHS, Nov. 2011)

Ans. The hypoglossal nerve is the 12th cranial nerve (cranial nerve XII). It is mainly an efferent nerve for the tongue musculature. The nerve originates from the medulla and travels caudally and dorsally to the tongue.

Development: Hypoglossal nerves originate from the somatic efferent column of the brainstem, by fusion of ventral root fibers of 3–4 occipital nerves. These nerve fibers grow from the hypoglossal nucleus and branch into small hypoglossal nerve roots leaving the ventrolateral side of the medulla which converges again to form the CN XII common trunk. They grow rostrally until contact with the tongue muscles.

As the neck develops, hypoglossal nerve gradually extends upward.

Function components/nuclear columns

1. **General somatic efferent column:** The fibers arise from the hypoglossal nucleus which lies in the medulla, in the floor of fourth ventricle deep to the hypoglossal triangle.

2. **General somatic afferent column:** The nucleus is spinal nucleus of V cranial nerve where proprioceptive fibers from tongue end

Nucleus: The hypoglossal nucleus lies in the floor of fourth ventricle beneath the hypoglossal triangle. Connection of the nucleus with opposite pyramidal tract forms supranuclear pathway of the nerve. It is also connected to cerebellum, reticular formation of medulla, sensory nuclei of V nerve and the nucleus of tractus solitarius.

Course and relations (Fig. 6.8)

1. In their **intraneural course**, hypoglossal nerve's course starts from hypoglossal nuclei pair in lower medulla. The two nerves travel laterally and ventrally from the respective nucleus. The nerve splits in two before exiting the medulla and passes through the hypoglossal canal in the occipital bone of the skull.

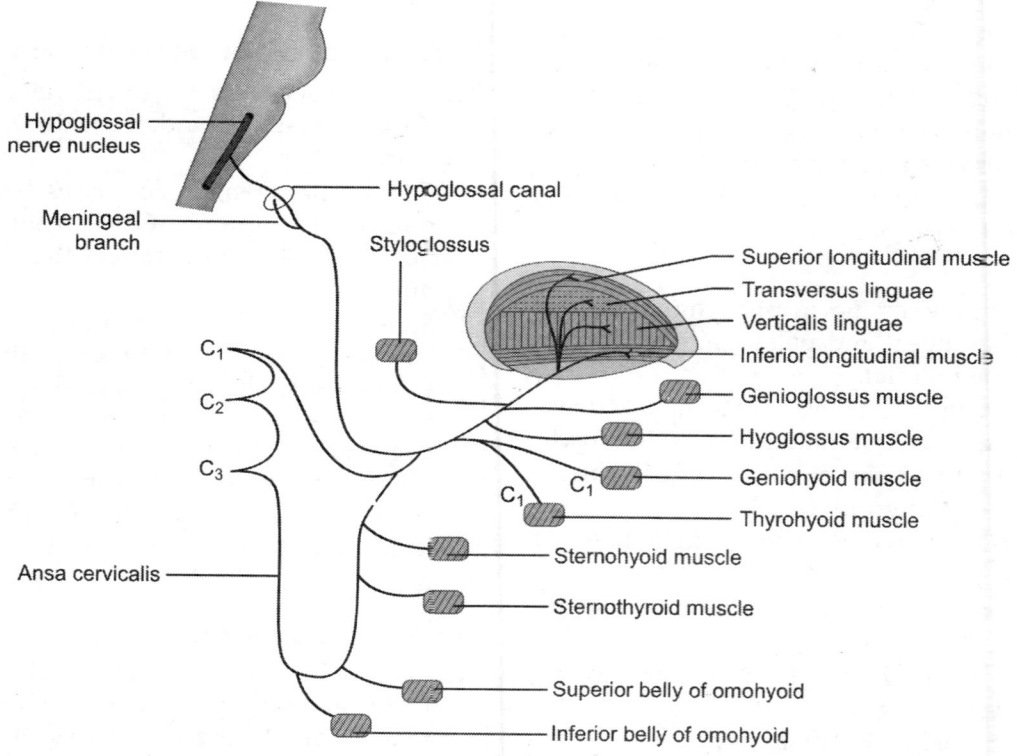

Fig. 6.8: Hypoglossal nerve and its distribution

2. During **extracranial course**, nerve first lies deep to the internal jugular vein, but soon inclines laterally between the internal jugular vein and the internal carotid artery in front of the vagus. Then the nerve travels above the hyoid bone and in between the mylohyoid and hyoglossus muscles before branching to the various parts of the tongue musculature.

Branches and distribution: Branches supply extrinsic and intrinsic muscles of tongue. Only extrinsic muscle, palatoglossus is supplied by fibers of cranial accessory nerve through vagus and pharyngeal plexus.

Branches of the hypoglossal nerve containing fibers of nerve C1: These fibers join the nerve at the base of the skull.

1. Meningeal branch: Bone and meninges in anterior part of posterior cranial fossa.
2. Descending branch: Continues as descends hypoglossi or upper root of ansa cervicalis.
3. Branches are also given to thyrohyoid and geniohyoid muscles.

Applied Clinical Anatomy

1. Clinical examination: Examining hypoglossal nerve involves observation of tongue.
2. Hypoglossal nerve lesions:
   a. Supranuclear lesions: No atrophy, uncoordinated tongue with slow but spastic tongue movements.
   b. Infranuclear and nuclear lesions cause weakness of the tongue but additionally cause ipsilateral atrophy.
   c. Unilateral lesions are not typically a serious problem.
   d. Bilateral lesions can cause profound difficulty with speech and swallowing.
3. Hypoglossal nerve in neurologic disorders:
   a. Progressive bulbar palsy and advanced amyotrophic lateral sclerosis (ALS): Severe tongue atrophy and glossoplegia.
   b. Neck–tongue syndrome: Pain on one side of upper neck or back of the head, usually involved with rapid rotation of neck along with pain in ipsilateral side of tongue. The cause is strain/pressure on the C2 nerve. As the C2 nerve route is involved with hypoglossal nerve route, tongue pain can result.
4. Obstructive sleep apnea: In obstructive sleep apnea (OSA), the decrease in muscle tone of the genioglossus muscle causes the tongue to retract and impede airflow into the trachea.

Q. 9. Write a short note on pterygopalatine ganglion.
(TNMGR, April 1998; KUHS, Jan. 2014)

Ans. Pterygopalatine or sphenopalatine ganglion or **Meckel's ganglion,** or **nasal ganglion** is the largest parasympathetic ganglion, suspended by two roots of maxillary nerve. Functionally, it is related to cranial nerve 7th. It is also called the **ganglion of 'Hay fever'.** The pterygopalatine ganglion is a structure that is morphologically formed during the third trimester of fetal life, with its neurons derived from Schwann cell precursors.

Roots

- **Sensory root** is from maxillary nerve. The ganglion is suspended by two roots of maxillary nerve.
- **Sympathetic root** is from postganglionic plexus around internal carotid artery. The nerve is called deep petrosal. It unites with greater petrosal to form **nerve of pterygoid canal** (*Vidian nerve*). The fibers of deep petrosal do not relay in the ganglion.
- **Secretomotor root** is from greater petrosal nerve arises from geniculate ganglion of cranial nerve 7th. These fibers relay in the ganglion.

Branches (Fig. 6.9):

1. For lacrimal gland: The postganglionic fibers pass through zygomatic branch of maxillary nerve. Theses fibers hitch hike through zygomaticotemporal nerve into the communicating branch between zygomaticotemporal and lacrimal nerve, then to the lacrimal nerve for supplying the lacrimal gland.
2. Nasopalatine nerve: Secretomotor fibers to both nasal and palatal glands.
3. Palatine branches: Sensory and secretomotor fibers to mucous membrane and glands of soft palate and hard palate.
4. Nasal branches: Glands and mucous membrane of nasal septum.
5. Orbital branches: For the orbital periosteum.
6. Pharyngeal branches: For the glands of pharynx.

Rusu et al. (2009) has described four morphological variants

1. Type A (10%): A partitioned structure with superior partition receiving Vidian nerve.
2. Type B (55%): A single structure with superior part (base) of pterygopalatine ganglion receiving Vidian nerve.
3. Type C (15%): A single structure with inferior part (tip) of pterygopalatine ganglion receiving Vidian nerve.
4. Type D (20%): A partitioned structure with inferior partition receiving Vidian nerve.

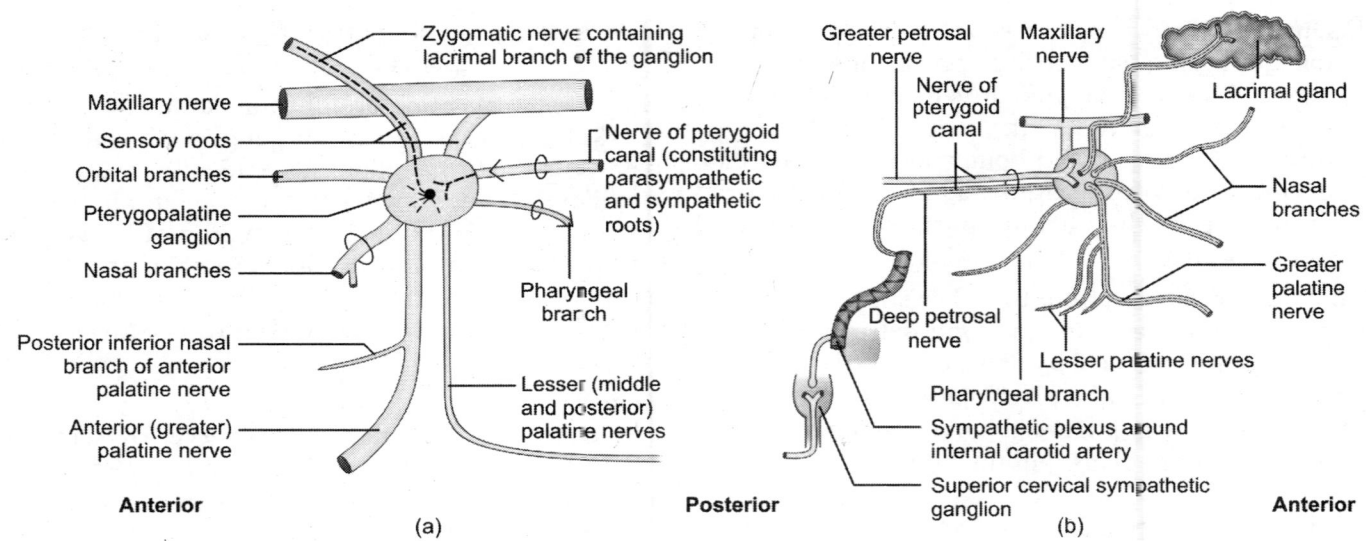

Fig. 6.9: Connections and branches of pterygoid ganglion

Applied Clinical Anatomy

Pterygopalatine ganglion is theorized to be a component for a group of headache disorders classified as trigeminal autonomic cephalalgias (TACs) which present as unilateral headaches with ipsilateral autonomic features (lacrimation, rhinorrhea, nasal congestion, eyelid edema, and ptosis).

Q. 10. Write a short note on otic ganglion.
(RGUHS, Oct. 2010)

Ans. It is parasympathetic ganglion which relays secretomotor fibers to parotid gland. Topographically, it is intimately related to mandibular nerve, but functionally it is a part of glossopharyngeal nerve. It is 2–3 cm in size, and is situated in infratemporal fossa, just below foramen ovale.

Connections and branches

Motor or parasympathetic root is formed by lesser petrosal nerve.

Sympathetic root is derived from plexus on middle meningeal artery. It contains postganglionic fibers arising in superior cervical ganglion. The fibers pass through the otic ganglion without relay and reach parotid gland via auriculotemporal nerve. They are vasomotor in function.

Sensory root comes from auriculotemporal nerve and is sensory to the parotid gland. Other fibers passing through the ganglion are as follows:

1. Nerve to medial pterygoid gives a motor root to ganglion which passes through it without relay and supplies medially placed tensor tympani muscles.

2. Chorda tympani nerve is connected to otic ganglion and also to nerve of pterygoid canal. These connections provide an alternative pathway of taste from anterior two-thirds of tongue.

Q. 11. Write a short note on submandibular ganglion.
(RGUHS, 2007)

Ans. This is a parasympathetic peripheral ganglion. It is a relay station for secretomotor fibers to submandibular and sublingual salivary glands. Topographically, it is related to lingual nerve, but functionally, it is connected to chorda tympani branch of facial nerve.

Connections and branches (Fig. 6.11):

1. **Secretomotor fibers** pass from lingual nerve to ganglion through the posterior root. These are preganglionic fibers that arise in superior salivatory nucleus and pass through nervus intermedius till facial nerve, chorda tympani and lingual nerve to reach ganglion.

   Postganglionic fibers for **submandibular gland** reach the gland through five or six branches from ganglion.

   Postganglionic fibers for **sublingual and anterior** lingual glands re-enters lingual nerve through anterior root and travel to gland through distal part of lingual nerve.

2. **Sympathetic fibers** are derived from plexus around facial artery. It contains postganglionic fibers arising in the superior cervical ganglion. They pass through submandibular ganglion without relay and supply vasomotor fibers to submandibular and sublingual glands.

3. **Sensory fibers** reach the ganglion through lingual nerve.

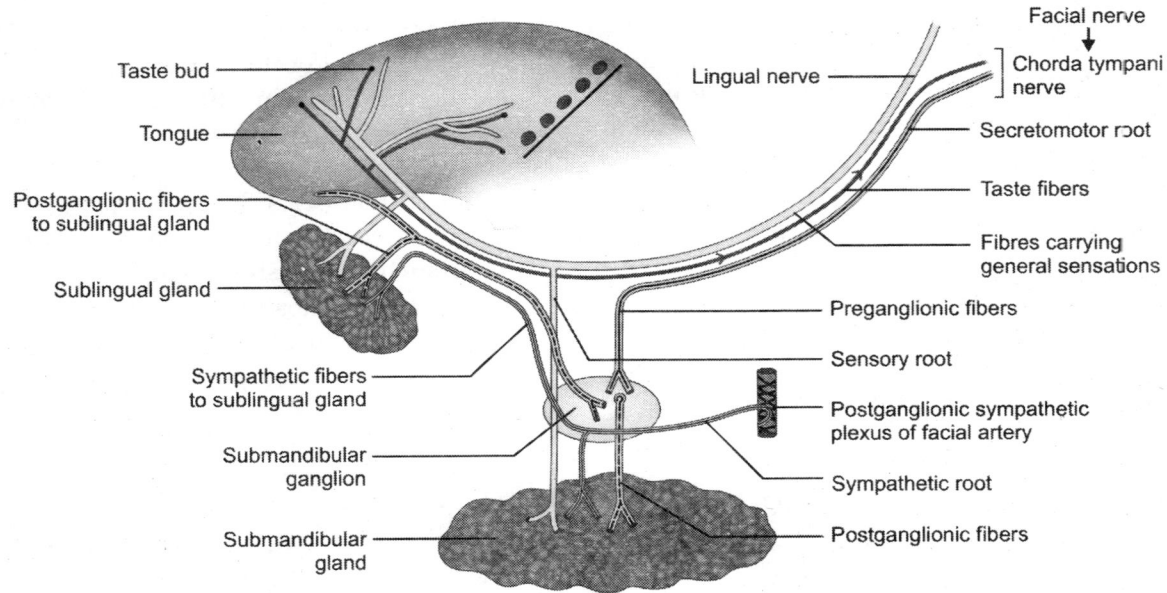

Fig. 6.11: Submandibular ganglion and its connections

Q. 12. Write a short note on trigeminal ganglion.
(TNMGR, March 2008)

Ans. Trigeminal ganglion/Gasserian ganglion is the sensory ganglion of trigeminal nerve. The ganglion is crescentric or semi-lunar in shape. It lies in the trigeminal impression on the anterior surface of petrous temporal bone, in trigeminal or Meckel's cave.

Relations:

Medially: Internal carotid artery, posterior part of cavernous sinus.

Laterally: Middle meningeal artery.

Superiorly: Parahippocampal gyrus.

Inferiorly: Trigeminal nerve (motor root); greater petrosal nerve; petrous temporal bone (apex); foramen lacerum.

The central process of ganglion cells forms large sensory root of trigeminal nerve. The peripheral processes of ganglion cells form three divisions of the trigeminal nerve.

Blood supply: ICA, middle meningeal artery, accessory meningeal artery, and meningeal branch of ascending pharyngeal artery.

Q. 13. Write a short note on brachial plexus.
(TNMGR, April 2012)

Ans. The brachial plexus is a major network of nerves transmitting signals responsible for motor and sensory innervation to upper extremities. The plexus originates as an extension from ventral rami of C5 through T1 spinal nerves. The plexus consists of roots, trunks, divisions, cords and branches.

Development: By the start of 5th week of IUL, human embryo develops forelimbs and hind limbs which are observed as 'paddle-shaped' buds. The buds of forelimbs are located to pericardial swelling posteriorly at the level of fourth cervical somites down to level of first thoracic somites. This is the stage where peripheral nerves are developed from growing brachial plexus into mesenchyme of developing upper limb, while spinal nerves are developed to both dorsal and ventral aspects of limb in the form of segmental bands.

A. **Roots:** These are constituted by anterior primary rami of spinal nerves C5, 6, 7, 8 and T1 with contributions from anterior primary rami of C4 and T2. The roots are located behind scalenus anterior. The origin of plexus may shift by one segment upward or downward, resulting in a prefixed or post-fixed plexus, respectively. In a prefixed plexus, the contribution by C4 is large and that from the T2 is often absent. In a post-fixed plexus, the contribution by T1 is large, T2 is always present, C4 is absent and C5 is reduced in size. The roots join to form trunks as follows.

B. **Trunks:** Roots C5 and C6 join to form **upper trunk**. Root C7 forms **middle trunk**. Roots C8 and T1 join to form **lower trunk**. They are located in lower part of posterior triangle of neck.

C. **Divisions of the trunks:** Each trunk divides into ventral and dorsal divisions (which ultimately supply anterior and posterior aspects of the limb). These divisions join to form cords. They are located behind clavicle.

D. **Cords:**
   i. Lateral cord is formed by union of ventral divisions of upper and middle trunks.
   ii. Medial cord is formed by ventral division of lower trunk.
   iii. Posterior cord is formed by union of dorsal divisions of all three trunks.

E. **Branches:**
   a. **Branches of the roots:**
      i. Nerve to serratus anterior (C5–C7).
      ii. Nerve to rhomboideus (C5).
   b. **Branches of the trunks:**
      i. Suprascapular nerve (C5, 6)
      ii. Nerve to subclavius (C5, 6)
   c. **Branches of the cords:**
   1. **Branches of lateral cord:**
      i. Lateral pectoral (C5–C7).
      ii. Musculocutaneous (C5–C7).
      iii. Lateral root of median (C5–C7).

2. **Branches of medial cord:**
   i. Medial pectoral (C8, T1).
   ii. Medial cutaneous nerve of arm (C8, T1).
   iii. Medial cutaneous nerve of forearm (C8, T1).
   iv. Ulnar (C7, C8, T1).
   v. Medial root of median (C8, T1).
3. **Branches of posterior cord:**
   i. Upper subscapular (C5, C6).
   ii. Nerve to latissimus dorsi (C6–C8).
   iii. Lower subscapular (C5, C6).
   iv. Axillary (C5, C6).
   v. Radial (C5–C8, T1).

Applied Clinical Anatomy

1. **Erb-Duchenne palsy** (*Waiter's tip syndrome*) is due to lesion in upper brachial plexus, C5 and C6 spinal nerves.
2. **Klumpke's paralysis** is result of lesion in lower brachial plexus, C8 and T1 spinal nerves.
3. Axillary nerve lesion can alter sensation of lateral arm.
4. Median nerve lesion alters sensation of lateral 3 and a half digits and lateral palm with motor weakness for wrist.

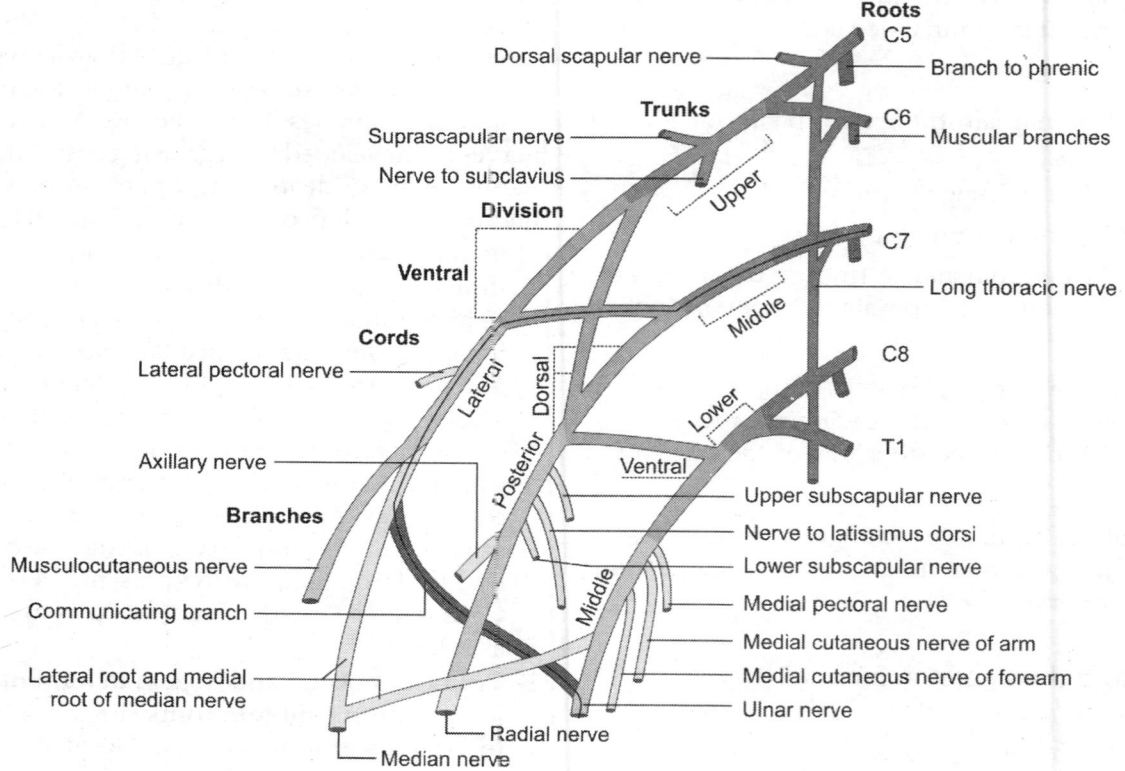

Fig. 6.13: Branchial plexus

5. *Saturday night palsy* is due to injury to radial nerve, characterized by a wristdrop brought about by the weakened supination and loss of sensory function on the posterior arm, forearm, and dorsum of thumb.

6. *Claw hand sign* and radial deviation are seen in ulnar nerve lesion, affecting the medial 1 and a half digit and median palm sensation followed by weakness in wrist flexion.

7. GLANDS–SALIVARY, THYROID AND PARATHYROID GLANDS

Q. 1. Discuss the topographical anatomy of the parotid gland and its development. How is its secretory activity regulated?
(Bangalore Uni., Jan. 1992; Gujarat Uni., Oct. 2004; TNMGR, March 2010; BFUHS, Oct. 2005; KUHS, July 2012; PAHER, May 2015; NTR Uni., June 2017, May 2019)

Ans. The parotid (*Para* = around; *otic* = ear) is the largest of all salivary glands, weighing around 25 g. It is situated below the external acoustic meatus (EAM), between ramus of mandible and sternocleidomastoid (SCM). A part of this forward extension is often detached, and is known as **accessory parotid** and it lies between zygomatic arch and parotid duct.

Capsule of parotid gland (Fig. 7.1a): The investing layer of deep cervical fascia forms a capsule for gland. *Superficial lamina* (parotidomassetric fascia), thick and adherent to the gland, is attached above to the zygomatic arch. *Deep lamina* is thin and is attached to styloid process, mandible and tympanic plate, angle, and posterior border of ramus of mandible. A portion of deep lamina, extending between styloid process and mandible, is thickened to form *stylomandibular ligament*, which separates parotid gland from submandibular salivary gland.

External features: The gland resembles a three-sided pyramid. The apex of the pyramid is directed downwards. The gland has four surfaces (Fig. 7.1b):
1. Superior (base of the pyramid).
2. Superficial.
3. Anteromedial.
4. Posteromedial.
   The surfaces are separated by three borders:
   1. Anterior.
   2. Posterior.
   3. Medial/pharyngeal.

Relations: The *apex* overlaps posterior belly of digastric and adjoining part of carotid triangle. The cervical branch of facial nerve and two divisions of retromandibular vein emerge through it.

Surfaces: The **superior surface** or base forms upper end of gland which is small and concave. It is related to:
a. Cartilaginous part of the external acoustic meatus.
b. Posterior surface of the temporomandibular joint.
c. Superficial temporal vessels.
d. Auriculotemporal nerve.

Superficial surface is the largest of four surfaces. It is covered with:
a. Skin.
b. Superficial fascia with anterior branches of great auricular nerve, preauricular lymph nodes, posterior fibers of platysma and risorius.
c. Parotid fascia.
d. Deep parotid lymph nodes.

Anteromedial surface is grooved by posterior border of the ramus of the mandible. It is related to:
a. Masseter.
b. Lateral surface of TMJ.
c. Posterior border of ramus of the mandible.
d. Medial pterygoid.
e. Emerging branches of facial nerve.

Posteromedial surface is molded to mastoid and styloid processes and structures attached to them. It is related to:
a. Mastoid process, sternocleidomastoid and posterior belly of digastric.
b. Styloid process with structures attached to it.

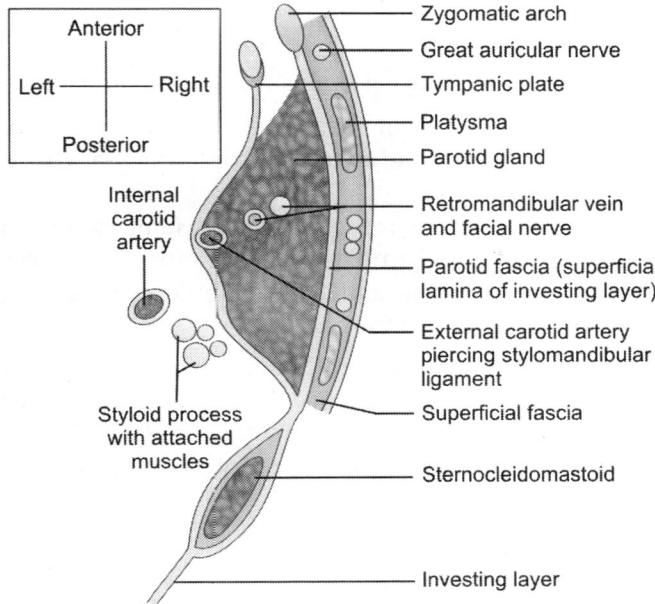

Anterior

Left — Right

Posterior

Internal carotid artery

Styloid process with attached muscles

Zygomatic arch
Great auricular nerve
Tympanic plate
Platysma
Parotid gland
Retromandibular vein and facial nerve
Parotid fascia (superficial lamina of investing layer)
External carotid artery piercing stylomandibular ligament
Superficial fascia
Sternocleidomastoid

Investing layer

Fig. 7.1a: Capsule of parotid gland

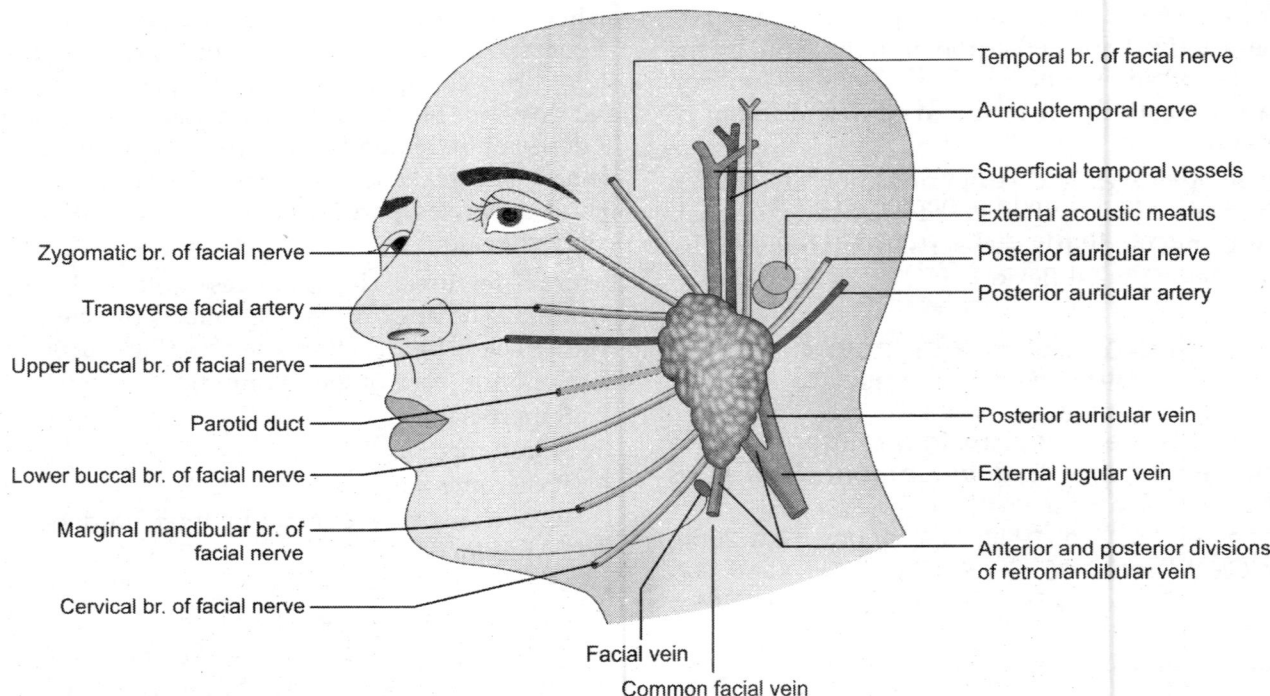

Fig. 7.1b: Parotid gland and various structures emerging from it

c. External carotid artery, facial nerve and internal carotid artery.

Borders (Fig. 7.1b)

Anterior border separates superficial surface from anteromedial surface. The following structures emerge at the border.
a. Parotid duct.
b. Terminal branches of the facial nerve.
c. Transverse facial vessels.
d. Accessory parotid gland.

Posterior border separates superficial surface from posteromedial surface. It overlaps sternocleidomastoid.

Medial edge or pharyngeal border separates anteromedial surface from posteromedial surface. It is related to lateral wall of pharynx.

Structures within the parotid gland: From medial to lateral side, these are as follows: (Fig. 7.1b)
  i. **Arteries:** ECA, maxillary artery, superficial temporal artery, transverse facial artery.
 ii. **Veins:** Retromandibular vein, superficial temporal and maxillary veins.
iii. **Nerves:** Facial nerve and its terminal branches (temporal, zygomatic, buccal, marginal mandibular and cervical) radiating like a goose foot from anterior border of gland, this pattern of branching is called *"Pes anserinus"*.
 iv. **Parotid lymph nodes.**

Parotid duct/Stenson's duct (Dutch anatomist 1638–86): It is thick-walled and is about 5 cm long. It emerges from middle of anterior border of the gland. It runs forwards and slightly downwards on the masseter. Its relations are: (Fig. 7.1b)

Superiorly:
a. Accessory parotid gland.
b. Upper buccal branch of the facial nerve.
c. Transverse facial vessels.

Inferiorly: Lower buccal branch of the facial nerve.

At superior border of the masseter, it turns medially and pierces: Buccal pad of fat, buccopharyngeal fascia, buccinators.

The duct runs forwards for a short distance between buccinator and oral mucosa. Finally, the duct turns medially and opens into buccal vestibule, opposite the maxillary 2nd molar tooth.

Blood supply: External carotid artery and its branches (superficial temporal artery (STA) and maxillary artery). The veins drain via retromandibular vein into the external jugular vein (EJV) and internal jugular vein (IJV).

Nerve supply:
a. **Parasympathetic nerves** are secretomotor. They reach gland through auriculotemporal nerve. **Preganglionic fibers** begin in inferior salivatory

nucleus; pass through glossopharyngeal nerve, its tympanic branch, tympanic plexus and lesser petrosal nerve and relay in *otic ganglion*. **Postganglionic fibers** pass through auriculotemporal nerve and reach the gland.

b. **Sympathetic nerves** are vasomotor and are derived from plexus around middle meningeal artery.

c. **Sensory nerves** to the gland come from auriculotemporal nerve, but parotid fascia is innervated by sensory fibers of great auricular nerve (C2, C3).

d. Facial nerve courses through parotid gland without supplying any structure in it.

Lymphatics: Parotid nodes ⟶ Upper deep cervical nodes.

Parotid lymph nodes: They are present between superficial fascia and deep to deep fascia over the gland. They drain:

   i. Temple.
   ii. Side of the scalp.
  iii. Lateral surface of the auricle.
   iv. External acoustic meatus.
   v. Middle ear.
   vi. Parotid gland.
  vii. Upper part of the cheek.
 viii. Parts of the eyelids and orbit.

Applied Clinical Anatomy *(UOK, July 2017)*

1. Parotid gland variations include accessory parotid gland, ectopic parotid tissue, parotid duct duplication, congenital agenesis.

2. Sialadenitis is due to inflammation of the salivary gland caused by obstruction and infection by bacteria, viruses, or stones.

3. **Parotid swellings** are very painful due to the unyielding nature of the parotid fascia.

4. **Mumps** is an infectious disease of the salivary glands caused by a specific virus.

5. A **parotid abscess** may be caused by spread of infection from the opening of parotid duct in the oral cavity.

6. **Parotid abscess** is best drained by horizontal incision/making multiple small holes below the angle of mandible, known as *Hilton's method*.

7. During **parotidectomy**, the facial nerve is preserved by removing the gland in two parts, superficial and deep separately. The plane of cleavage (*Patey's faciovenous plane*) is defined by tracing the nerve from behind forwards.

8. **Mixed parotid tumor** is a slow growing lobulated painless tumor without any involvement of facial nerve. Malignant change of such a tumor is indicated by pain, rapid growth, fixity with hardness, involvement of facial nerve and enlargement of cervical lymph nodes.

9. **Parotid calculi (sialolithiasis)** may get formed within parotid gland or in its duct.

10. After **parotidectomy**, occasionally, there may be regeneration of secretomotor fibers in auriculotemporal nerve which join great auricular nerve. This causes stimulation of sweat glands and hyperemia in area of its distribution, thus producing redness and sweating in area of skin supplied by nerve. This clinical entity is called *Frey syndrome* (*auriculotemporal syndrome*).

Q. 2. Write about submandibular and sublingual salivary glands.

    (Bangalore Uni., Jan. 1992; TNMGR, Oct. 2000)

Ans. Submandibular salivary gland (*see* Fig. 4.3): This is a large salivary gland, situated in anterior part of digastric triangle. The gland is of the size of walnut, weigh around 15–20 g and roughly J-shaped, being indented by posterior border of mylohyoid which divides it into a larger part superficial to muscle, and a small part lying deep to muscle. The gland is partially enclosed between two layers of deep cervical fascia. The superficial layer of fascia covers inferior surface of the gland and is attached to base of mandible. The deep layer covers medial surface of gland and is attached to mylohyoid line of mandible.

Superficial part: This part fills digastric triangle. Superiorly, it extends deep to mandible up to mylohyoid; inferiorly, it overlaps stylohyoid and posterior belly of digastrics.

Relations:

Inferior surface is covered by:
a. Skin.
b. Platysma.
c. Cervical branch of facial nerve.
d. Deep fascia.
e. Facial vein.
f. Submandibular lymph nodes.

Lateral surface is related to:
a. Submandibular fossa.
b. Medial pterygoid.
c. Facial artery.

Medial surface is related to:
a. Mylohyoid muscle, nerve and vessels.
b. Hyoglossus muscle.
c. Styloglossus muscle.

Deep part: This part is small in size. It lies deep to mylohyoid, and superficial to hyoglossus and styloglossus. Posteriorly, it is continuous with superficial part round the posterior border of mylohyoid. Anteriorly, it extends up to posterior end of sublingual gland.

Relations: Present in between mylohyoid and hyoglossus:

Laterally: Mylohyoid muscle.

Medially: Hyoglossus muscle.

Above: Lingual nerve with submandibular ganglion.

Below: Hypoglossal nerve.

Submandibular duct: (Wharton's Duct, English scientist; 1614–73): It is thin walled, and is about 5 cm long. It emerges at anterior end of deep part of gland and runs forwards on hyoglossus, between lingual and hypoglossal nerves. At the anterior border of hyoglossus, duct is crossed by lingual nerve. It drains into oral cavity at sublingual caruncle. The sublingual caruncle is a papilla located medial to sublingual gland and lateral to each side frenulum linguae.

Blood supply: Submental artery (branch of facial artery) and sublingual artery (branch of lingual artery)

Venous supply: Common facial vein, lingual vein ⟶ IJV.

Lymphatic drainage: Submandibular lymph nodes **(3 to 6).**

Nerve supply: Submandibular ganglion. These branches convey:
a. Secretomotor fibers.
b. Sensory fibers from the lingual nerve.
c. Vasomotor sympathetic fibers from the plexus on the facial artery.

Applied Clinical Anatomy *(Sumandeep Uni. April 2015):*

1. **Neoplasia:** Adenoid cystic and mucoepidermoid carcinomas are most common malignancies.
2. **Sialolithiasis:** Salivary stones may cause swelling of duct or gland, causing a colicky periprandial pain.
3. **Sialadenitis:** Sialadenitis is salivary gland inflammation caused by infection and obstruction or microorganisms (bacteria or mumps virus).
4. **Sialadenosis:** Sialadenosis is a benign, noninflammatory enlargement of submandibular glands. It is a more common presentation in patients with malnutrition, bulimia or diabetes, advanced liver disease.

Sublingual Salivary Glands (Fig. 2.4b)

This is the smallest of the three salivary glands. It is almond-shaped and weighs about 3–4 g. It lies above mylohyoid, below the mucosa of floor of mouth, medial to sublingual fossa of mandible and lateral to genioglossus. About 15 ducts emerge from the gland. Most of them open directly into floor of the mouth on summit of sublingual fold, rest joins submandibular duct. The *ducts of Rivinus,* a group of excretory ducts, drain sublingual gland. These ducts empty along an elevated ridge called *plica fimbriate* formed by sublingual folds, which are oblique to frenulum linguae bilaterally. The largest sublingual excretory duct called sublingual *duct of Bartholin,* joins Wharton's duct near sublingual caruncle on each side of lingual frenulum.

Relations:

Front: Sublingual salivary gland of opposite side.

Behind: Deeper part of submandibular gland.

Above: Mucous membrane of mouth.

Below: Mylohyoid muscle.

Lateral: Sublingual fossa.

Medial: Genioglossus muscles.

Blood supply: Sublingual and submental arteries.

Venous supply: Sublingual vein → Lingual vein → IJV.

Lymphatic drainage: Submandibular lymph nodes **(3 to 6).**

Nerve supply: Similar to that of the submandibular gland.

Applied Clinical Anatomy

1. **Ranula:** It is a mucocele of the sublingual gland caused by local trauma that damages sublingual gland allowing mucous to collect. The ranula presents as a fluctuant, swollen mass at floor of the mouth with a bluish tint.
2. **Neoplasia:** Adenoid cystic carcinoma and mucoepidermoid carcinoma count as the most common sublingual gland malignancies reported.
3. **Sialolithiasis**
4. **Sialadenitis**
5. The use of interferential current stimulation has been investigated for patients who suffer from dry mouth.

Q. 3. Write about development of salivary glands.
(TNMGR, Sept. 2007)

Ans. The salivary glands develop as outgrowths of the buccal epithelium. The outgrowths are at first solid and are later canalized. They branch repeatedly to form the duct system. The terminal parts of duct system develop into secretory acini (Fig. 7.3).

Parotid gland: Salivary glands development begins at around 6–8 weeks when reciprocal interactions between the epithelium and adjacent mesenchyme initiate thickening of oral ectoderm. The glands develop via process of branching morphogenesis of epithelium. The terminal buds at end of branched ductal structures become acini at 14 weeks. The parotid is first to begin its formation. The outgrowth for the parotid gland arises in relation to line along which maxillary and mandibular processes fuse to form the cheek. It is generally considered to be ectodermal. By 13–16 weeks, the basal lamina surrounds the epithelium, and myoepithelial cells are thought to begin to appear at this stage. After 16 weeks, striated and intercalated ducts can be noticed. The glands stop developing at 28 weeks, marking the point at which acini produce secretory products. The glands are fully functional at birth.

Submandibular gland develops after the parotid gland in the 6th week of IUL. The striated and intercalated ducts develop by 16 weeks, and acinar cells predominate by 24 weeks. The outgrowths for the submandibular and sublingual glands arise in relation to linguo-gingival sulcus. They are usually considered to be of endodermal origin

Sublingual gland develops later than other major salivary glands as it first appears in 8th week of IUL. Initially, the sublingual gland develops laterally to submandibular gland before transitioning to a position anterior and superior to submandibular gland when development is complete.

Q. 4. Write a note on histology of salivary glands.

(*KUHS, Jan. 2014; Sumandeep Uni., April 2015*)

Ans. Salivary glands are tubule-alveolar glands (racemose glands) **(Fig. P-4a, b; Color Plate 1 and Fig. P-4c; Color Plate 2)**.

In the **parotid gland**, the cells of secretory element, the alveoli are made up of entirely serous cells (homocrine gland). The serous acini are small and round with basophilic stain. Pyramidal cells line the acini. Nuclei are round and basal.

In the **submandibular gland**, the secretory cells are both serous and mucous (heterocrine gland). Pyramidal cells line the acini. Some mucous acini are covered by serous *demilunes of Gianuzzi*.

In the **sublingual gland**, predominantly mucous secretory cells are present. Mucous acini are larger, light stained and variable in size. Typical *demilunes of Gianuzzi* on one side of mucous acini. Nuclei of acini are flattened and peripheral.

Q. 5. Write a short note on thyroid gland.

(*TNMGR, March, 2002*)

Ans. Thyroid gland (*shield like*) is an endocrine gland with rich blood supply situated in the lower part of the neck. It consists of right and left lobes that are joined to each other by isthmus. A third, *pyramidal lobe*, may project upwards from the isthmus (or from one of the lobes). Occasionally, a fibrous or fibromuscular band (*levator glandulae thyroidea*) descends from body of hyoid bone.

Situation and extent (Fig. 7.5a):

1. The gland lies against vertebrae C5–C7 and T1, embracing the upper part of trachea.
2. Each lobe extends from middle of thyroid cartilage to 4th or 5th tracheal ring.

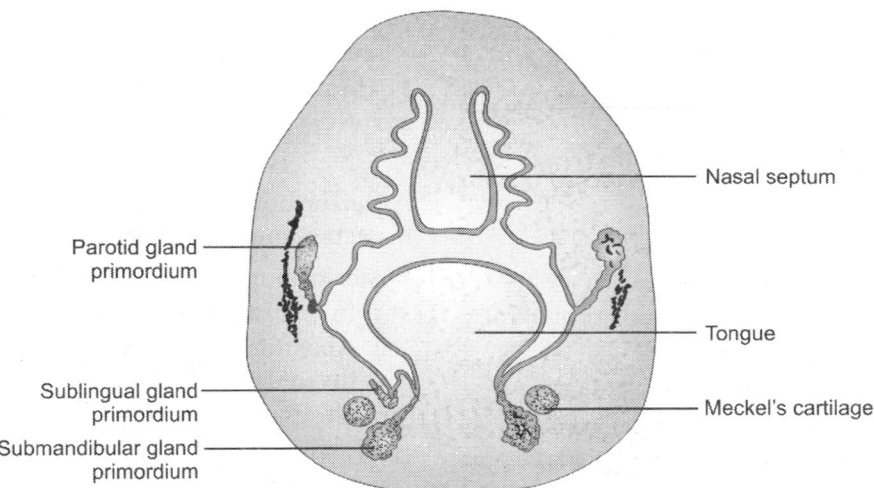

Fig. 7.3: Development of salivary glands from the epithelial lining of the primitive stomodeum (9-week old embryo)

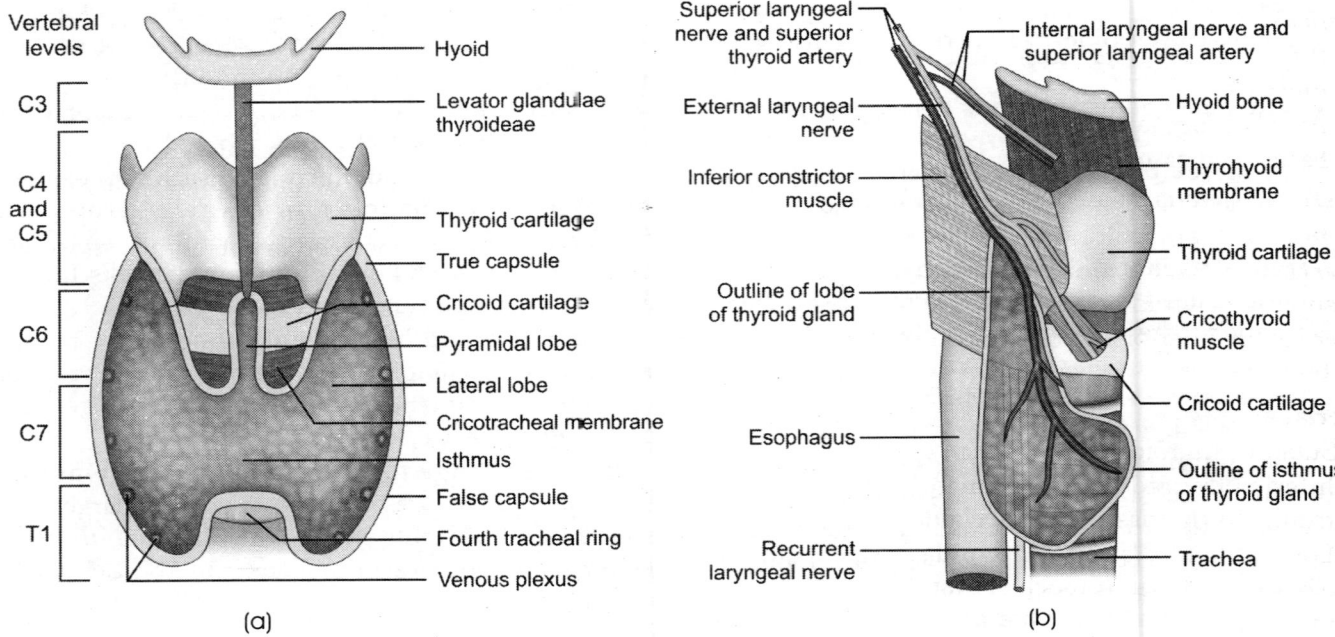

Fig. 7.5: Thyroid gland location, its capsule (a) and its relation (b)

3. The isthmus extends from second to fourth tracheal ring.

Dimensions and weight: Each lobe measures about 5 cm × 2.5 cm × 2.5 cm, and the isthmus 1.2 cm × 1.2 cm. On an average, the gland weighs about 25 g, larger in females, increases in size during pregnancy and menstruation.

Capsules of thyroid (Fig. 7.5a):
1. **True capsule:** It consists of peripheral condensation of connective tissue of the gland. A dense capillary plexus is present deep to capsule.
2. **False capsule:** It is derived from pretracheal layer of deep cervical fascia. It is thin along the posterior border of the lobes, but thick on the inner surface of the gland where it forms a suspensory *ligament of Berry*, which connects the lobe to the cricoid cartilage.

Parts and Relations (Fig. 7.5b): The lobes are conical in shape having:
a. An apex.
b. A base.
c. Three surfaces: Lateral, medial and posterolateral.
d. Two borders: Anterior and posterior.

Apex is directed upwards and slightly laterally. It is limited superiorly by the attachment of sternothyroid muscle to oblique line of thyroid cartilage and is related to superior thyroid artery and external laryngeal nerve.

Base is at level with the 4th or 5th tracheal ring, related to inferior thyroid artery and recurrent laryngeal nerve.

Lateral or **superficial surface** is convex, and is covered by:
  i. Sternohyoid
  ii. Superior belly of the omohyoid
  iii. Sternothyroid
  iv. Anterior border of the sternocleidomastoid.

Medial surface is related to:
  i. **Two tubes:** Trachea and esophagus.
  ii. **Two muscles:** Inferior constrictor and cricothyroid.
  iii. **Two nerves:** External laryngeal and recurrent laryngeal.

Posterolateral or **posterior surface** is related to the carotid sheath and overlaps the common carotid artery.

Anterior border is thin and is related to the anterior branch of superior thyroid artery.

Posterior border is thick and rounded. It is related to:
  i. Inferior thyroid artery.
  ii. Anastomoses between the superior and inferior thyroid arteries.
  iii. Parathyroid glands.
  iv. Thoracic duct (only on the left side).

Isthmus has **two surfaces**, anterior and posterior and **two borders**, superior and inferior.

Anterior surface is covered by:
   i. Right and left sternothyroid and sternohyoid muscles.
   ii. Anterior jugular veins.
   iii. Fascia and skin.

Posterior surface is related to the 2nd to 4th tracheal rings.

Upper border is related to anastomosis between right and left superior thyroid arteries.

Lower border: Inferior thyroid veins leave the gland at this border.

Arterial supply

1. Superior thyroid artery (branch of ECA).
2. Inferior thyroid artery (branch of thyrocervical trunk which arises from subclavian artery).
3. Lowest thyroid artery (**Thyroidea ima artery**): In 3% of individuals (branch of brachiocephalic trunk or directly from arch of aorta).
4. Accessory thyroid arteries (branch of tracheal and esophageal arteries).

Venous drainage: The thyroid is drained by:
- *Superior thyroid vein* → IJV
- *Middle thyroid vein* → IJV
- *Inferior thyroid vein* → Left brachiocephalic vein
- *A 4th thyroid vein of Kocher* may emerge between middle and inferior veins → IJV.

Lymphatic drainage

Upper part: Upper deep cervical lymph nodes, pre-laryngeal nodes.

Lower part: Lower deep cervical nodes, pretracheal and paratracheal nodes.

Nerve Supply: Superior, middle and inferior cervical ganglia (all vasoconstrictor)

Histology: The gland is made up of two types of secretory cells **(Fig. P-5; Color Plate 2):**
a. *Follicular cells:* They are present in the lining of follicle of the gland, secrets tri-iodothyronin and tetra-iodothyronine (thyroxine) which stimulates basal metabolic rate and somatic and psychic growth of the individual. During active phase the lining is columnar, during resting phase it is cuboidal. Follicles contain the colloid (the hormone) in their lumina.
b. *Parafollicular cells (C cells):* They are fewer, light cells and lie in between the follicles. They secrete the thyrocalcitonin and tend to produce hypocalcaemia (opposite to effects of parathormone).

Development: The thyroid develops from a median endodermal thyroid diverticulum, which grows down in front of the neck from floor of primitive pharynx (foramen caecum), just caudal to tuberculum impar. The lower end of diverticulum enlarges to form the gland. The rest of the diverticulum remains narrow and is known as **thyroglossal duct**. The position of upper end is marked by foramen *caecum* of tongue, and lower end often persists as pyramidal lobe. The gland becomes functional during third month of development.

Applied Clinical Anatomy

1. Any swelling of the thyroid gland (goitre) moves with deglutition should be palpated from behind.
2. Removal of thyroid (thyroidectomy) with true capsule may be necessary in hyperthyroidism.
3. In subtotal thyroidectomy, the posterior parts of both lobes are left behind to avoids risk of removal of parathyroid.
4. During thyroidectomy, superior thyroid artery is ligated near the gland to save external laryngeal nerve, and inferior thyroid artery is ligated away from the gland to save recurrent laryngeal nerve.
5. Hypothyroidism causes cretinism in infants and myxoedema in adults.
6. Benign tumors of the gland may displace and even compress the neighboring structures, like the carotid sheath, trachea, etc.
7. Malignant tumors tend to invade and erode the neighboring structures.
8. *Ectopic thyroid tissue* can present with varying symptoms depending on its location.
   a. *Lingual ectopic **thyroid** tissue:* Dysphagia, bleeding, dyspnea.
   b. *Suprahyoid and infrahyoid **thyroid** tissue:* Midline mass in the neck.
   c. *Intratracheal or intralaryngeal **thyroid** tissue:* Respiratory obstruction.
   d. *Intraesophageal **thyroid** tissue:* Dysphagia.
   e. *Pyramidal lobe, aortic, pericardial, and cardiac **thyroid** tissue:* Asymptomatic.

Q. 6. Write a short note on parathyroid glands.

Ans. The **parathyroid glands** are endocrine **glands** located at posterior medial aspect of thyroid gland. There are four individual small and round **glands** that divide into pairs (superior and inferior). The **parathyroid glands** have two distinct types of cells: chief cells and the oxyphil cells.

- *Chief cells:* The chief cells manage secretion of **parathyroid** hormone (PTH).

- *Oxyphil cells:* The purpose of these cells is not entirely understood. They are larger than chief cells and seem to increase in number with age.

Function: When the calcium levels in the blood decrease, **parathyroid** gland releases a hormone called parathormone or **parathyroid** hormone (PTH). When secreted, PTH effects select target organs; which are the kidneys, intestine and the skeletal system.

Embryology: Inferior **parathyroid** originates from 3rd pharyngeal pouch, and superior **parathyroid** arises from 4th pharyngeal pouch.

Blood Supply and Lymphatics

The thyroid gland and the **parathyroid** gland share the same blood supply.

Parathyroid veins → Thyroid vein plexus.

Parathyroid lymphatic: Deep cervical and paratracheal lymph nodes.

Nerves: Cervical ganglia of thyroid gland.

Applied Clinical Anatomy

1. **Hyperparathyroidism:** Due to overactivity of the **parathyroid** gland.
   a. *Primary:* Due to direct gland alterations like benign tumor, hyperplasia, or even **parathyroid** cancer. Excess secretion of the PTH will present with hypoglycemia, osteoporosis, osteitis fibrosa cystica and hypertension.
   b. *Secondary:* Due to reduced calcium levels in the blood like inadequate vitamin D intake or chronic renal failure.
   c. *Tertiary:* This occurs after prolonged secondary hyperparathyroidism.
2. **Hypercalcemia:** Hypercalcemia can be the result of an overactive parathyroid gland. Symptoms can range from being non-existent to severe.

3. **Hypoparathyroidism:** Due to a reduced activity of the gland.
   a. *Primary:* There is a gland failure which results in a decrease in PTH secretion.
   b. *Secondary:* This occurs when there is surgical removal/injury of parathyroids.

---

8. INTRACRANIAL VENOUS SINUSES

Q. 1. Name the venous sinuses of the cranium (dura mater).   (TNMGR, Sept. 2008; BFUHS, May 2011)

Ans. Dural venous sinuses are a group of sinuses or blood channels formed by dura mater, lined by epithelium with no muscle in their walls and valveless. These venous sinuses receive venous blood supply from the brain, meninges and bones of the skull. They communicate with veins outside the skull through *emissary veins.*

A. **Paired venous sinuses** (Fig. 8.1):
   1. Cavernous sinus.
   2. Superior petrosal sinus.
   3. Inferior petrosal sinus.
   4. Transverse sinus.
   5. Sigmoid sinus.
   6. Sphenoparietal sinus.
   7. Petrosquamous sinus.
   8. Middle meningeal sinus/veins.

B. **Unpaired venous sinuses:**
   1. Superior sagittal sinus.
   2. Inferior sagittal sinus.
   3. Straight sinus.
   4. Occipital sinus.
   5. Anterior intercavernous sinus.
   6. Posterior intercavernous sinus.
   7. Basilar plexus of veins.

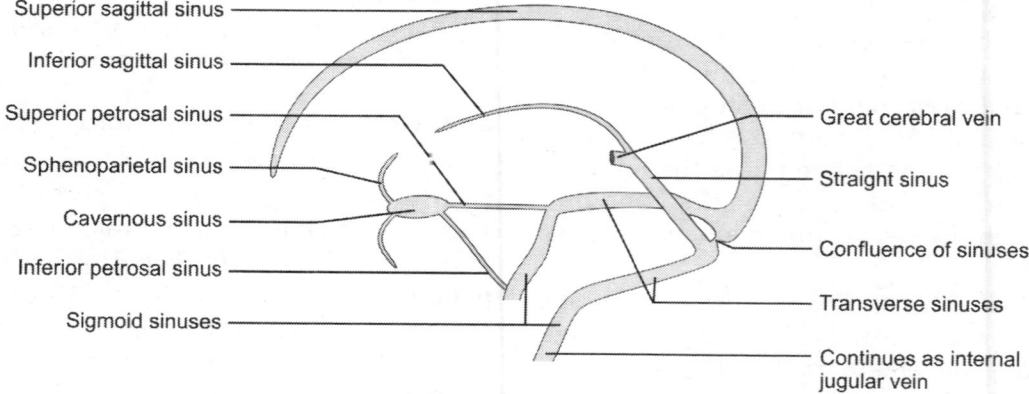

Fig. 8.1: Intracranial venous sinuses

Development: Major dural venous sinuses, such as the superior petrosal sinus was derived from pro-otic veins; while cavernous sinus originated from vena capitis medialis.

Tributaries:

1. **Bridging veins**: Cerebral and cerebellar veins which cross subdural space to drain into superior sagittal vein.
2. Emissary veins that progress through skull allowing communication between intracranial and extracranial contents.
3. Diploic veins which drain blood between inner and outer layers of skull bones (diploe).
4. Meningeal veins collect blood from meninges.
5. Arachnoid granulations for CSF returning to venous circulation.

Applied Clinical Anatomy

1. All dural venous sinuses are valveless, allowing pathogens and neoplastic cells to travel to different parts of brain.
2. **Dangerous triangle** of face is a triangular area bounded by medial angle of eyes, sides of nose and upper lip as its boundaries. It serves as the passage for pathogens from the face into the brain via the cavernous sinuses (cavernous sinus thrombosis).

Q. 2. Write a short note on relations and tributaries of the cavernous sinus. *(TNMGR, April 2000, 2019)*
Ans. A cavernous sinus is a large venous space situated in middle cranial fossa, on either side of body of sphenoid bone. Its interior is divided into a number of spaces by trabeculae. The floor and medial wall is formed by endosteal dura mater and lateral wall is formed by meningeal dura mater. This sinus is about 2 cm long and 1 cm wide; extends anteriorly up to medial end of superior orbital fissure and posteriorly up to apex of petrous temporal bone.

Relations: (Fig. 8.2) *(KUHS, Dec. 2017)*
A. **Structures outside the sinus:**
   a. **Superiorly:** Optic tract, optic chiasma, olfactory tract, ICA, anterior perforated substance.
   b. **Inferiorly:** Foramen lacerum, junction of body and greater wing of sphenoid bone.
   c. **Medially:** Hypophysis cerebri, sphenoidal air sinus.
   d. **Laterally:** Temporal bone with uncus.
   e. **Below laterally:** Mandibular nerve.
   f. **Anteriorly:** Superior orbital fissure, apex of the orbit.
   g. **Posteriorly:** Apex of petrous temporal, crus cerebri of midbrain.
B. **Structures in the lateral wall of the sinus (from above downward):**
   a. Oculomotor nerve.
   b. Trochlear nerve.
   c. Ophthalmic nerve.
   d. Maxillary nerve.
   e. Trigeminal ganglion.
C. **Structures passing through medial aspect of sinus:**
   a. ICA with venous and sympathetic plexus.
   b. Abducent nerve.

Tributaries (incoming channels)

From the orbit:
a. Superior ophthalmic vein.
b. Inferior ophthalmic vein.
c. Central vein of retina.

From the brain:
a. Superficial middle cerebral vein.
b. Inferior cerebral veins (from temporal lobes)

From the meninges:
a. Sphenoparietal sinus.
b. Frontal trunk of middle meningeal vein.

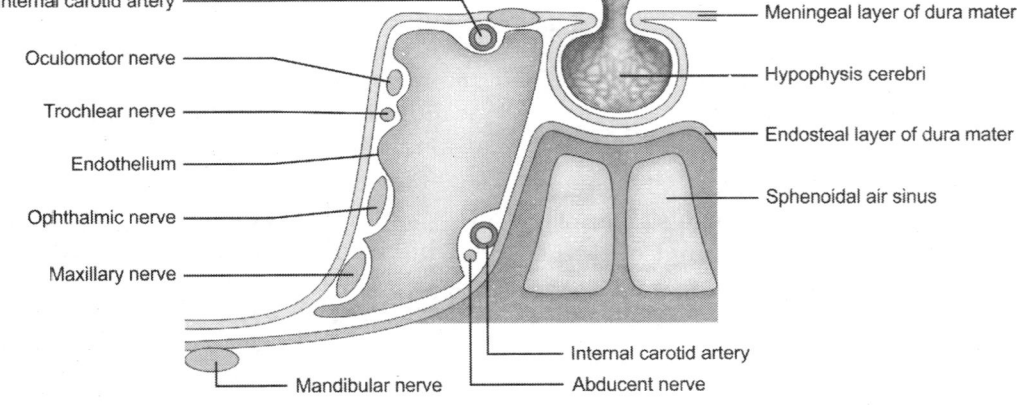

Internal carotid artery — Oculomotor nerve — Trochlear nerve — Endothelium — Ophthalmic nerve — Maxillary nerve — Mandibular nerve — Internal carotid artery — Abducent nerve — Meningeal layer of dura mater — Hypophysis cerebri — Endosteal layer of dura mater — Sphenoidal air sinus

Fig. 8.2: Cavernous sinus and its relations

Distributaries (draining channels)

a. Transverse sinus: Through superior petrosal sinus.

b. Internal jugular vein: Through inferior petrosal sinus and plexus around ICA.

c. Pterygoid plexus of veins: Through emissary veins.

d. Facial vein: Through superior ophthalmic vein.

e. Right and left cavernous sinuses communicate with each other through anterior and posterior inter-cavernous sinuses and basilar plexus of veins.

All these communications are valveless. (i.e. blood can flow in either direction).

Applied Clinical Anatomy

1. **Thrombosis of cavernous sinus** may be caused by infection in dangerous area of face, nasal cavity and paranasal sinuses. Symptoms includes severe pain in the eye and forehead; paralysis of muscle supplied by 3, 4, 6 cranial nerves; marked edema of eyelid, cornea, and root of nose; exophthalmos.

2. **Pulsating exophthalmos:** Due to head injury, a communication may be produced between cavernous sinus and internal carotid artery, leading to protruding eyeball, which is pulsatile with each heart beat.

3. **Cavernous sinus syndrome** is a medical emergency and life-threatening disorder that presents with different symptoms depending on what structure is affected. A severe lesion involving the entire sinus will present with total ophthalmoplegia, due to CN III, IV, and VI injury, accompanied with fixed and dilated pupils due to compression of the superficial parasympathetic fibers of the CN III. **Cavernous sinus syndrome** can lead to Horner's syndrome when the sympathetic plexus around the internal carotid is damaged. When CN V1 and CN V2 are involved, sensory loss in the face, scalp, maxilla, nasal cavity, sinuses, and palate occurs.

Q. 3. Write a short note on sagittal sinus.

(TNMGR, Oct. 2011)

Ans. Sagittal sinus is a midline vein without valves or tunica muscularis that courses along the falx cerebri, draining many of the cerebral structures surrounding it. There are two types of sagital sinus:

A. **Superior sagittal sinus** (Fig. 8.1): It occupies the upper convex attached margin of the falx cerebri. It is triangular in cross section and begins anteriorly at crista galli and ends near internal occipital protuberance, turning to right side to continue with right transverse sinus. This sinus receives tributaries from:

1. Superior cerebral veins.
2. Parietal emissary veins.

3. Venous lacunae.

4. A vein from nose.

B. **Inferior sagital sinus** (Fig. 8.1): It is a small channel lies in posterior two-thirds of lower, concave, free margin of falx cerebri. It ends by joining great cerebral vein to form straight sinus.

Blood supply

Most significant draining vessel is:

a. *Vein of Trolard:* connects superficial middle cerebral vein and superior sagittal sinus.

b. *Rolandic vein:* Drains primary motor and sensory cortices of the brain.

c. *Bridging veins:* Connect superior sagittal sinus between two leaves of dura mater.

d. *Emissary veins*

Applied Clinical Anatomy

1. Thrombosis of superior sagital sinus may be caused by infection from nose, scalp and diploe. This leads to increased intracranial tension, delirium, convulsions, paraplegia.

2. Meningiomas may develop due to its intimate proximity to the falx cerebri.

3. Dural AV fistulas are aberrant, abnormal connections between dural arteries and veins leading to a high-pressure intracranial vascular system prone to hemorrhage.

4. The superior sagittal sinus is a vital structure that is involved in a variety of potentially life-threatening conditions such as papilledema, cryptogenic stroke, seizures, or change in mental status.

Q. 4. Write a note on falx cerebri.

(TNMGR, April 2001)

Ans. The meningeal dura mater invaginates between brain regions to form dural partitions: Falx cerebri, falx cerebelli, tentorium cerebelli, and sellar diaphragm. The falx cerebri is a large sickle-shaped fold of dura mater occupying the median longitudinal fissure between two cerebral hemispheres. The falx cerebri separates cerebral hemispheres and provides channels, known as *dural sinuses*, for blood and cerebral spinal fluid to drain. It has:

A. **Two ends:**
   a. Anterior end: Narrow, attached to crista galli.
   b. Posterior end: Broad, attached along the median plane to upper surface of the tentorium cerebelli.

B. **Two margins** (Fig. 8.4):
   a. Upper margin: Convex and is attached to lips of sagital sulcus.
   b. Lower margin: Concave and free.

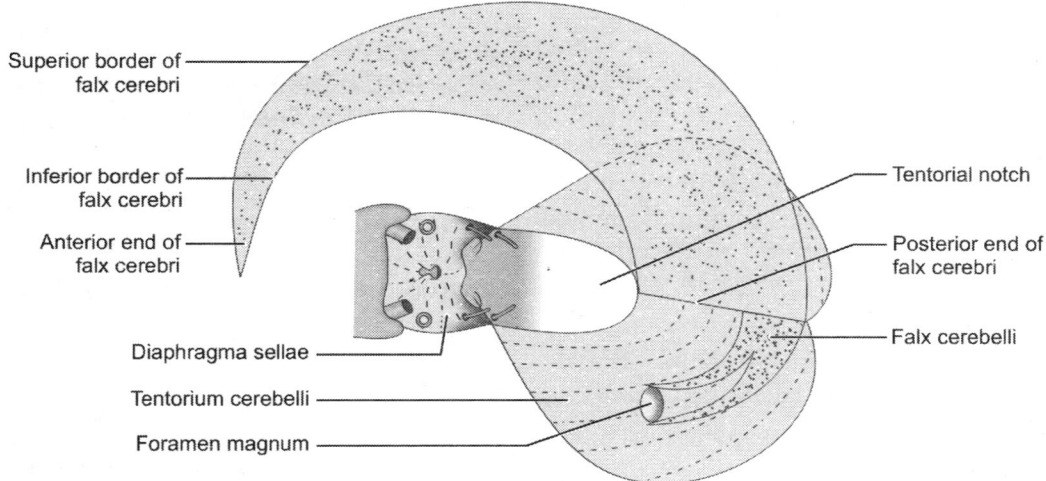

Fig. 8.4: Falx cerebri (superior and inferior)

C. **Two surfaces:** Right and left surfaces; each of which is related to medial surface of corresponding cerebral hemisphere.

Three important venous sinuses are present in relation to this fold. *Superior sagital* sinus lies along the upper margin; *inferior sagital* sinus along the lower margin and *straight sinus* along the line of attachment of falx to tentorium cerebelli.

Development: The three meningeal layers derive from the meninx primitiva, which is meningeal mesenchyme. The arachnoid and pia forms from leptomenix (neural crest cells) and dura mater from pachymeninx (mesoderm). The dura mater forms a single layer of protection around the developing spinal cord but forms a double layer around skull, eventually forming periosteal and meningeal dural membranes. As the brain develops, meningeal dural layer invaginates between brain regions forming dural partitions.

Blood supply

a. Anterior part: Ant. meningeal artery (ant. falx artery/ant. falcine artery) (branch of ant. ethmoidal artery)
b. Posterior part: Post. meningeal artery (branch of ascending pharyngeal artery)

Lymphatics: Meningeal lymphatic vessels → Deep cervical lymph nodes.

Nerve supply: Trigeminal nerve, sup. cervical ganglia (sympathetic), dorsal rami of cervical nerve 1, 2, 3, hypoglossal nerve, vagus nerve.

Applied Clinical Anatomy

1. Falx cerebri is site of falcine meningiomas, causing headaches, nausea, and vomiting due to increased intracranial pressure.

2. Frontal contusions can occur due to traumatic brain injury, causing mass effect forcing ipsilateral cingulate gyrus to herniate under falx cerebri leading to subfalcine herniation.

3. Agenesis or partial agenesis of falx cerebri allows cerebral hemispheres to adhere and prevent midline transcallosal surgical access to ventricles.

9. ORAL CAVITY, PHARYNX AND LARYNX

Q. 1. Write a note on oral cavity and discuss innervation of orodental tissue.
(TNMGR, Oct. 2016; HP Uni., May 2017)

Ans. Oral cavity, or **mouth** or buccal **cavity,** consists of several different anatomically different aspects that work together effectively and efficiently to perform several functions.

Oral cavity is surrounded by the lips and is composed of two separate regions, *vestibule,* the area between the cheeks, teeth, and lips, and the *oral cavity proper.* The oral cavity proper is mostly filled with tongue and bounded anteriorly and on the sides by alveolar processes containing **teeth** and posteriorly by isthmus of fauces. Anteriorly, roof formed by **hard palate** and posteriorly by soft palate. The uvula hangs downwards from **soft palate.** The mylohyoid muscles constitute floor of oral cavity proper. A mucous membrane known as **oral mucosa** is composed of stratified squamous epithelium and forms inner lining of mouth. Salivary glands secrete viscous and Mucoid fluid to lubricate and keep oral cavity moist.

Development: The oral cavity is a unique structure in that it forms from both ectodermal and endodermal structures. The development of tongue, palate upper lip and lower lip is described elsewhere.

Blood supply: ECA and its branches.

Tongue: Lingual artery; **Hard palate:** Greater palatine and superior alveolar arteries; **Gingiva and upper dentition:** Alveolar arteries from terminal branches of maxillary artery; **Lips:** Labial branches of facial artery; **Lower dentition and mandible:** Inferior alveolar artery.

Nerve supply:

Oral mucosa, teeth, and supporting structures: Maxillary and mandibular divisions of trigeminal nerve.

Hard palate: Greater palatine and nasopalatine nerves.

Soft palate: Lesser palatine nerve.

Tongue: Hypoglossal nerve, vagus nerve (motor), chorda tympani nerve, lingual nerve, glossopharyngeal nerve.

Cheek: Buccal nerve.

Muscles:

Floor of oral cavity: Mylohyoid and geniohyoid.

Soft palate: Tensor veli palatini, musculus uvulae, levator veli palatini, palatopharyngeus, palatoglossus.

Muscles of tongue.

Applied Clinical Anatomy

Squamous cell carcinoma of the oral cavity (SCCOC): The anatomy of the oral cavity plays a huge role in the surgical management of oral cancers. For premalignant lesions or small superficial cancers, a transoral approach is an option for removal of tumors of the anterior floor of mouth, alveolus, and tongue. Posteriorly located tumors must be treated invasively due to inadequate surgical field exposure.

Q. 2. Write a short note on pharynx.

Ans. The pharynx is a conductive funnel-shaped structure located in the midline of the neck.

Parts

1. **Nasal pharynx:** Located behind posterior nasal apertures with two openings on lateral surface, called **auditory tubes** (*Eustachian tubes or pharyngotympanic tubes*) surrounded by elevations of mucous membrane called *tubal elevations*.
2. **Oral pharynx:** A continuation of oral cavity and functions to pass bolus toward laryngeal **pharynx** below.
3. **Laryngeal pharynx,** located behind inlet (opening) of larynx, receives bolus from the oral **pharynx** and passes it into the esophagus for digestion.

Embryology: During 4th–5th weeks of IUL, whole **pharynx** develops from pharyngeal (branchial) apparatus. The musculature of **pharynx** develops from three pharyngeal arches, i.e. the third, fourth, and sixth arches.

Blood supply: Ascending pharyngeal, tonsillar, maxillary and lingual arteries.

Venous drainage: Pharyngeal veins → IJV

Lymphatics: Deep cervical lymph nodes, retropharyngeal lymph nodes, paratracheal lymph nodes.

There is a ring of lymphoid tissue that is formed by four lymph groups, referred to as the **Waldeyer's ring** (*RUHS, May 2018*). This ring protects the entrance of the GIT and the respiratory tract. It is formed superiorly by the pharyngeal tonsils, also known as adenoids, in the roof of the nasal **pharynx**. The palatine tonsils and tubal tonsils (around the auditory tubes) form the lateral wall of the ring. Inferiorly, the ring forms by the lingual tonsils on the posterior surface of the tongue (Fig. 9.2).

Nerves

Nasal pharynx: Maxillary nerve.

Oral pharynx: Glossopharyngeal nerve

Laryngeal pharynx: Internal laryngeal nerve.

The muscles of the **pharynx** receive motor (efferent) supply from vagus **except** stylopharyngeus muscle, which is supplied by glossopharyngeal nerve.

Muscles

1. **Constrictor muscles:** Superior, middle, inferior and cricopharyngeus.
2. **Longitudinal group:** Stylopharyngeus, palatopharyngeus, and salpingopharyngeus.

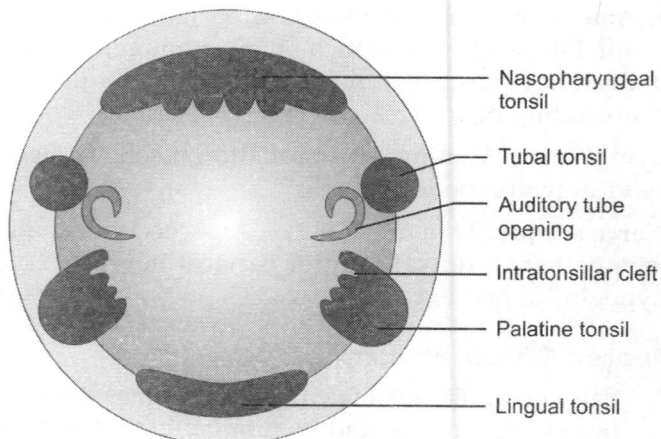

Nasopharyngeal tonsil

Tubal tonsil

Auditory tube opening

Intratonsillar cleft

Palatine tonsil

Lingual tonsil

Fig. 9.2: Waldeyer's lymphatic ring

Applied Clinical Anatomy

1. **Pharyngitis:** The inflammation of the pharynx is also known as 'sore throat.'
2. **Dysphagia:** Inability to swallow properly due to muscle weakness, nerve damage.
3. **Adenoiditis:** Inflammation of adenoid lymph tissues present in upper part of the nasal pharynx.
4. **Sleep apnea:** The muscles of the pharynx can become hypotonic in certain occasions like during sleep. In such a case, they become too weak to prevent the collapse of the airways resulting in difficulty breathing.
5. **Zenker diverticulum:** Its false pouching of weakened pharyngeal mucosa due to its herniation into *Killian dehiscence* (small triangular gap between inferior constrictor and cricopharyngeus) leading to food accumulation.
6. **Cricopharyngeal achalasia:** A rare clinical condition in which the cricopharyngeus muscle does not open appropriately and adequately, can lead to both difficulty swallowing and Zenker diverticulum.

Q. 3. Write about muscles of larynx.

(TNMGR, Oct. 1999)

Ans. The larynx (Latin—*supper windpipe*) is the organ for production of voice or phonation.

In adult male it lies in front of 3rd–6th cervical vertebrae, in children and female, it lies at little higher level. At puberty, male larynx grows rapidly and seen as prominent angle of thyroid cartilage (**Adam's apple**), which makes voice louder and low pitch.

Constituents of larynx

A. **Cartilages:** Larynx contain 9 cartilages; Unpaired (thyroid, cricoid, epiglottis) and paired (arytenoid, corniculate/santorini, cuneiform)
B. Joints: Cricothyroid, cricoarytenoid.
C. **Ligaments and membranes**
   1. Extrinsic: Thyrohyoid membrane, hyoepiglottic ligament, cricotracheal ligament
   2. Intrinsic: Quadrate membrane (vestibular fold and aryepiglotticus fold); conus elasticus or cricovocal membrane (cricothyroid ligament and vocal fold).
D. Cavity of larynx.
E. Mucous membrane of larynx.

Intrinsic muscles of larynx: Table 9.3

Actions

1. Muscles which abduct vocal cords: Posterior cricoarytenoid (**safety muscle of larynx**).
2. Muscles which adduct vocal cords: Lateral cricoarytenoids, transverse arytenoids, cricothyroid, thyroarytenoids.
3. Muscles which tense vocal cords: Cricothyroid.
4. Muscles which relax vocal cords: Thyroarytenoid, vocalis.
5. Muscles which close inlet of the larynx: Aryepiglottic.
6. Muscles which open inlet of larynx: Thyroepiglotticus.

Arterial supply: Superior laryngeal artery, inferior laryngeal artery.

Table 9.3: Intrinsic muscles of larynx with origin and insertion

Muscle	Origin	Fibers	Insertion
Cricothyroid (only muscle outside the larynx) **"Tuning fork of larynx"**	Lower border and lateral surface of cricoid	Backwards and upwards	Inferior cornua and lower border of thyroid cartilage
Posterior cricoarytenoid	Posterior surface of the lamina of cricoid	Upwards and laterally	Posterior aspect of muscular process of arytenoids
Lateral cricoarytenoid	Lateral part of upper border of arch of cricoid	Upwards and backwards	Anterior aspect of muscular process of arytenoid
Transverse arytenoids (unpaired)	Posterior surface of one arytenoid	Transverse	Posterior surface of another arytenoid
Oblique arytenoid and aryepiglotticus	Muscular process of one arytenoid	Oblique	Apex of the other arytenoid
Thyroarytenoid and thyroepiglottic	Thyroid angle and adjacent cricothyroid ligament	Backwards and upwards	Anterolateral surface of arytenoid cartilage
Vocalis	Vocal process of arytenoid cartilage	Forwards	Vocal ligament and thyroid angle

Venous supply: Superior laryngeal vein, inferior laryngeal vein.

Lymphatics: Deep cervical lymph nodes.

Nerve supply

Motor nerves: All intrinsic muscles of larynx are supplied by *recurrent laryngeal nerve* **except** cricothyroid which is supplied by *external laryngeal nerve*.

Sensory nerves

Internal laryngeal nerve → Mucous membrane up to level of vocal folds.

Recurrent laryngeal nerve → Mucous membrane below level of vocal folds.

Lymphatic drainage

Above vocal folds: Anterosuperior group of deep cervical nodes.

Below vocal folds: Posteroinferior group of deep cervical nodes, prelaryngeal nodes.

Development: The developing larynx arises from branchial structures around 4th week of IUL, from 3, 4, and 6 arches.

Applied Clinical Anatomy

1. Vagus nerve damage can lead to a unilateral paresis or paralysis of the vocal fold.
2. Recurrent laryngeal nerve damage can lead to hoarseness or swallowing difficulties.
3. Superior laryngeal nerve damage can lead to an inability to increase pitch.

4. Ischemic damage from the pressure of endotracheal tube can results in apraxia and subsequent scar formation.

10. TRIANGLES OF NECK: FACIAL SPACES, LYMPH NODES

Q. 1. Write a note on digastric triangle.

(TNMGR, April 2001, Sept. 2010)

Ans. The term triangles of the neck describe the divisions created by major muscles in the region. The digastric triangle is also known as submandibular triangle. The area between the body of the mandible and hyoid bone is known as the submandibular region. The superficial structures of this region lie in the submental and digastrics triangles (Fig. 10.1).

Development: 1st , 2nd, and 3rd pharyngeal arches play a role in development.

Boundaries

Anteroinferiorly: Anterior belly of digastric.

Posteroinferiorly: Posterior belly of digastric and stylohyoid.

Superiorly or base: Base of mandible and line joining angle of mandible to mastoid process.

Roof

1. Skin.
2. Superficial fascia, containing:
   a. Platysma.
   b. Cervical branch of facial nerve.

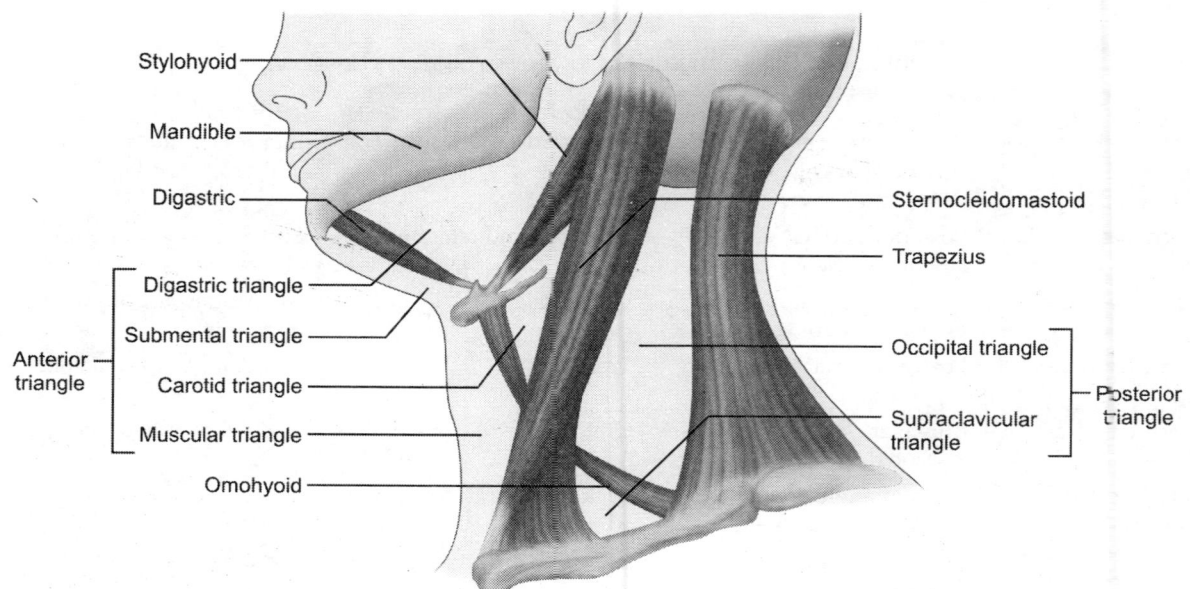

Fig. 10.1: Triangles of neck

c. Ascending branch of transverse or anterior cutaneous nerve of neck.
3. Deep fascia, which splits to enclose submandibular salivary gland.

Floor: Mylohyoid muscle anteriorly and hyoglossus posteriorly.

Contents:

Anterior part of the triangle:
1. Structures superficial to mylohyoid:
   a. Superficial part of submandibular salivary gland.
   b. Facial vein, submandibular lymph nodes and facial artery.
   c. Submental artery.
   d. Mylohyoid nerve and vessels.
   e. Hypoglossal nerve.
2. Structures superficial to hyoglossus:
   a. Submandibular salivary gland.
   b. Intermediate tendon of digastrics and stylo-hyoid.
   c. Hypoglossal nerve.

Posterior part of the triangle:
1. Superficial structures:
   a. Lower part of parotid gland.
   b. External carotid artery.
2. Deep structures:
   a. Styloglossus.
   b. Stylopharyngeus.
   c. Glossopharyngeal nerve.
   d. Pharyngeal branch of vagus nerve.
   e. Styloid process.
   f. Part of the parotid gland.
3. Deepest structures:
   a. Internal carotid artery.
   b. Internal jugular vein.
   c. Vagus nerve.

Applied Clinical Anatomy
1. The most common pathology arising in the submandibular triangle is sialadenitis.
2. Neoplasms of submandibular triangle can be divided into benign and malignant masses.

Q. 2. Describe the carotid triangle of the neck.
(MUHS, April 2014; KUHS, Dec. 2017)

Ans. The carotid triangle is one of the paired triangles in the anterior triangle of the neck.

Boundaries (Fig. 10.1)
Anterosuperiorly: Posterior belly of digastric muscle and stylohyoid.

Anteroinferiorly: Superior belly of the omohyoid.
Posteriorly: Anterior border of sternocleidomastoid muscle.

Roof
1. Skin
2. Superficial fascia containing
   a. Platysma
   b. Cervical branch of the facial nerve
   c. Transverse cutaneous nerve of the neck
3. Investing layer of deep cervical fascia.

Floor: It is formed by parts of:
a. Middle and inferior constrictors of the pharynx.
b. Thyrohyoid membrane.
c. Hyoglossus.

Contents
a. **Arteries:**
   i. Common carotid artery (CCA)
   ii. Internal carotid artery (ICA)
   iii. External carotid artery with branches.
b. **Veins:**
   i. Internal jugular vein
   ii. Common facial vein
   iii. Pharyngeal vein
   iv. Lingual vein
c. **Nerves:**
   i. Vagus nerve
   ii. Superior laryngeal nerve
   iii. Spinal accessory nerve
   iv. Hypoglossal nerve
   v. Sympathetic chain
d. **Carotid sheath with its contents**
e. **Lymph nodes:**
   i. Deep cervical lymph nodes
   ii. Jugulodigastric node
   iii. Jugulo-omohyoid node.

Applied Clinical Anatomy
1. Carotid triangle holds great importance for structures running through the neck; carotid arteries, jugular veins, and vagus and hypoglossal nerves.
2. Carotid triangle houses carotid sinus or bulb containing baroreceptors which are responsible in detecting stretch caused by pressure within a vessel and have a role in maintaining blood pressure (baroreceptor reflex).

Q. 3. Write a note on carotid artery.

Ans. The carotid arteries are the primary vessels supplying blood to brain and face.

Structure: Carotid arteries originate posterior to the sternoclavicular joints. At the level of upper border of thyroid cartilage, common carotid arteries bifurcate into ECA and ICA. This bifurcation point is clinically significant as it serves as a point for location of '**carotid body**' (chemoreceptor) and '**carotid sinus**' (baroreceptor).

Carotid body chemoreceptor is sensitive to decreased PO_2, increased PCO_2, and decreased pH of blood, and is responsible for alerting brain to change respiratory rate.

Carotid sinus baroreceptors respond to changes in the stretch of blood vessel and are responsible for detecting changes and maintaining blood pressure. After its division, the ECA exits sheath to provide oxygenated blood to face and neck, while the ICA continues in carotid sheath to enter carotid canal within temporal bone.

ECA: ECA along with its branches anastomose with branches from contra lateral side, allowing for collateral circulation.

ICAs anastomose with branches of basilar artery to form circle of Willis. At the **circle of Willis**, ICA branches to become middle cerebral artery (MCA) and anterior cerebral artery (ACA). The MCA is responsible for supplying motor and sensory cortices of upper limb and face, as well as Wernicke's area of temporal lobe and Broca's area of frontal lobe. The ACA is responsible for supplying motor and sensory cortices of lower limb. The ophthalmic artery is responsible for blood supply to inner layers of retina, as well as supplying other parts of orbit, meninges, face, and upper nose.

Course of ICA: Four parts: a. cervical, b. petrous, c. cavernous, d. cerebral

The ophthalmic artery branches off cavernous portion of ICA while MCA and ACA are branches of cerebral ICA.

Development: During 4–5th week of IUL, common carotid arteries (CCAs) and proximal ICAs derive from third pharyngeal arch, distal ICA derives from dorsal aorta and ECA derives from CCA via angiogenesis.

Nerves: Glossopharyngeal nerve and vagus nerve.

Applied Clinical Anatomy

1. The common carotid artery can be used to measure the pulse.
2. In the setting of hypovolaemic shock, if only the carotid pulse is palpable, this correlates to a systolic blood pressure of 60–70 mmHg.

Q. 4. Discuss the applied anatomy of various fascial spaces in relations to spread of infection from dental origin. (TNMGR, March 2010; Sumandeep Vidyapeeth, April 2011; UHSR, July 2018; TNMGR, Oct. 2019)

Ans. The fascial spaces in head and neck are the potential spaces between the various layers of fascia normally filled with loose connective tissue and bounded by anatomical barriers, usually of bone, muscle or fascial layers.

Classification

I. Based on mode of involvement: (Fig. 10.4a)
A. **Primary (direct):**
   1. **Maxillary:** a. Canine, b. Buccal, c. Infratemporal
   2. **Mandibular:** a. Submental, b. Submandibular, c. Sublingual, d. Buccal
B. **Secondary (indirect):**
   1. Masseteric; 2. Pterygomandibular; 3. Superior and deep temporal; 4. Lateral pharyngeal; 5. Retropharyngeal; 6. Prevertebral; 7. Parotid.

II. By Grodinsky and Holyoke (1938)
A. Space 1: Space superficial and deep to platysma
B. Space 2: Space behind anterior layer of deep cervical fascia
C. Space 3: 1. Space 3a: Pretracheal space; 2. Space 3b: Viscero-vascular space (*Lincoln's highway*)
D. Space 4: Danger space: Between alar and prevertebral fascia.

III. Based on clinical significance (Scott, 1952):

A. **Suprahyoid spaces:**
   1. Superficial fascial compartment
   2. Floor of the mouth: a. Sublingual space; b. Submandibular space; c. Submental space.
   3. Masticator space: a. Temporal space (superficial/deep); b. Submasseteric space; c. Superficial pterygoid space (Fig. 10.4b)
   4. Parapharyngeal space including deep pterygoid space
   5. Parotid compartment
   6. Paratonsillar space
   7. Space of the body of mandible.

B. **Infrahyoid spaces (Hollinshead, 1958):**
   1. Visceral compartment: a. Pretracheal/previsceral space; b. Retrovisceral space
   2. Visceral space
   3. Other spaces: a. Cavity within carotid sheath; b. Space between two layers of prevertebral fascia.

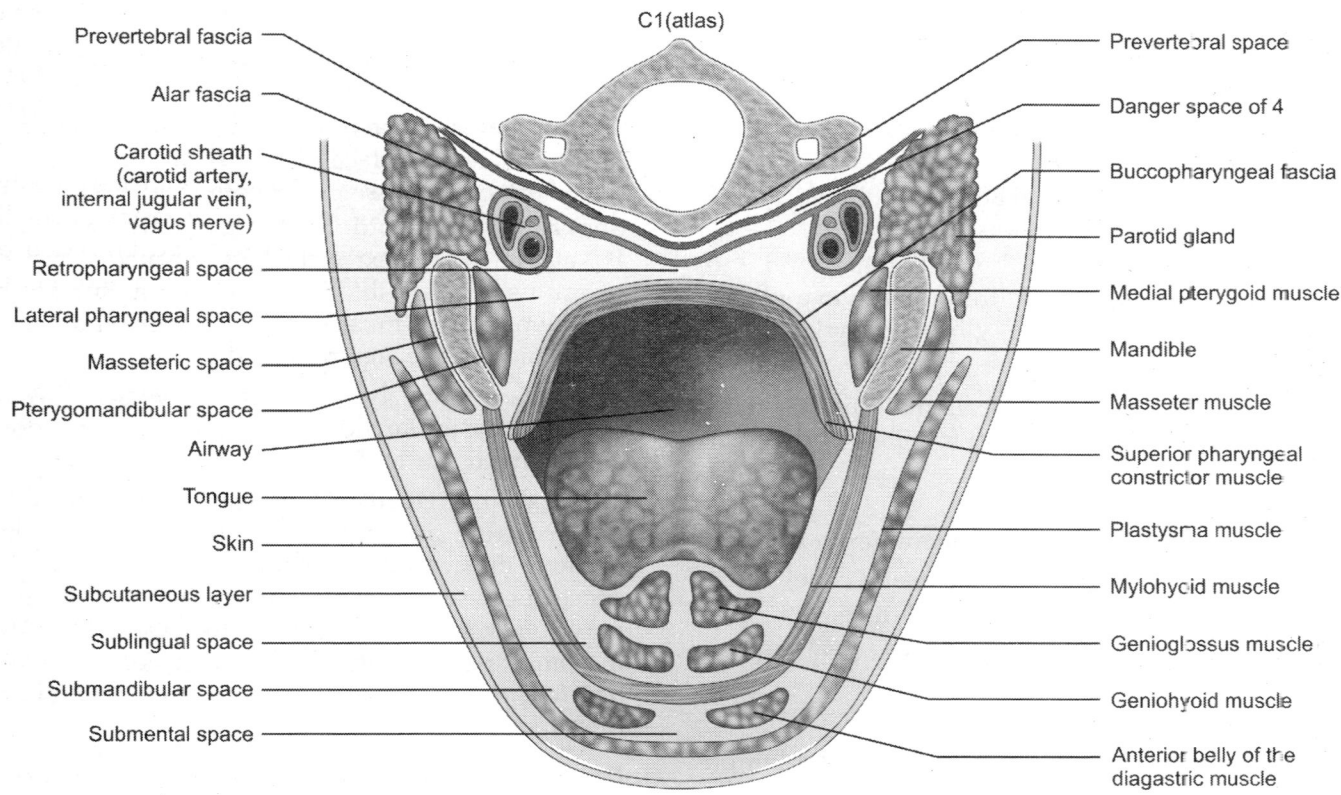

Fig. 10.4a: Fascial spaces seen in oblique transverse section

Labels (left side, top to bottom): Prevertebral fascia, Alar fascia, Carotid sheath (carotid artery, internal jugular vein, vagus nerve), Retropharyngeal space, Lateral pharyngeal space, Masseteric space, Pterygomandibular space, Airway, Tongue, Skin, Subcutaneous layer, Sublingual space, Submandibular space, Submental space

Labels (top center): C1(atlas)

Labels (right side, top to bottom): Prevertebral space, Danger space of 4, Buccopharyngeal fascia, Parotid gland, Medial pterygoid muscle, Mandible, Masseter muscle, Superior pharyngeal constrictor muscle, Plastysma muscle, Mylohyoid muscle, Genioglossus muscle, Geniohyoid muscle, Anterior belly of the diagastric muscle

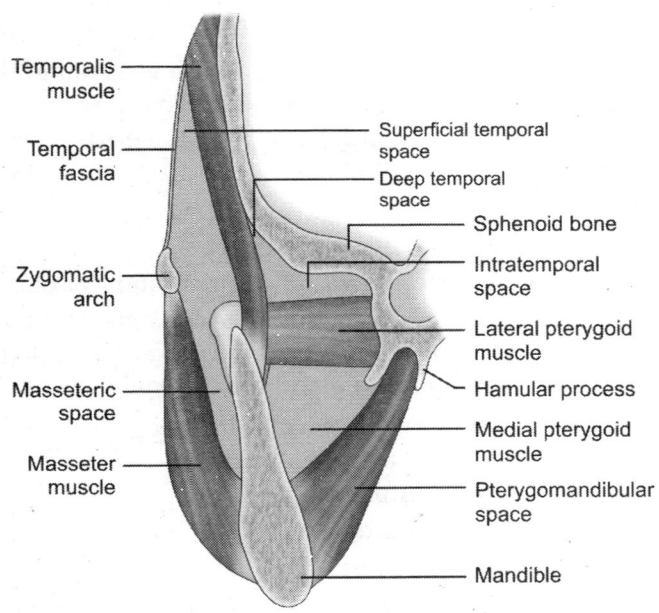

Fig. 10.4b: Fascial spaces associated with mandibular ramus

Labels (left side): Temporalis muscle, Temporal fascia, Zygomatic arch, Masseteric space, Masseter muscle

Labels (right side): Superficial temporal space, Deep temporal space, Sphenoid bone, Intratemporal space, Lateral pterygoid muscle, Hamular process, Medial pterygoid muscle, Pterygomandibular space, Mandible

(A) Suprahyoid spaces
1. Superficial fascial compartment

Subdivisions:

(i) **Canine space:** It overlies the canine fossa of maxilla and underneath levator labii superioris and levator labii superioris alaquae nasi.

(ii) **Buccal space:** It has following boundaries:

Laterally: Skin and subcutaneous tissue.

Medially: Buccinator and buccopharyngeal fascia.

Anteriorly: Labial musculature, posterior border of zygomaticus major, depressor anguli oris.

Posteriorly: Pterygomandibular raphe and anterior edge of masseter muscle.

Superiorly: Zygomatic arch.

Inferiorly: Lower border of mandible.

Contents: Buccal pad of fat, parotid duct, facial artery, buccal branch of facial nerve and mandibular division.

Clinical implications: Canine space may be involved in odontogenic infections and in nasal infections.

2. Floor of the mouth:
(i) **Sublingual spaces:** These are present above the mylohyoid muscle.

Boundaries

Laterally—alveolar process of mandible above mylo-hyoid line.

Medially—genioglossus and geniohyoid.

Roof—mucosa.

Posteriorly—body of hyoid bone, geniohyoid, genio-glossus and styloglossus muscles.

Contents: Deep part of submandibular gland and submandibular duct, sublingual salivary gland, lingual vessels and nerve, glossopharyngeal and hypoglossal nerve.

(ii) Submental space: It is a conical, small anterior, mid-line, single space between anterior bellies of digastric muscles.

Boundaries

Anterosuperiorly—symphysis menti (apex of cone)

Posteroinferiorly—hyoid bone (base of cone)

Superolaterally—anterior bellies of digastrics

Superficially—skin, superficial fascia containing platysma, deep fascia

Deep—mylohyoid muscle

Contents: Anterior jugular vein, submental lymph nodes.

Clinical significance: It may be involved in infections of mandibular incisors causing a swelling at the point of chin.

(iii) Submandibular spaces: These bilateral spaces are located lateral to submental space.

Boundaries

Superiorly—mylohyoid, genioglossus.

Inferiorly—skin, superficial fascia, platysma, deep fascia.

Laterally—mandible.

Anteroinferiorly—anterior belly of digastrics.

Posteroinferiorly—posterior belly of digastric.

Contents: Submandibular salivary gland, submandi-bular lymph nodes, mylohyoid vessels and nerves, facial artery and vein.

Clinical implications: Submandibular space is the most commonly involved space in primary infections of head and neck. Infection may arise from injuries to oral mucosa, submandibular or sublingual gland sialadenitis or infection from roots of mandibular teeth.

3. Masticator space: Space formed by splitting of deep cervical fascia to include ramus of mandible, masseter, medial and lateral pterygoid and that part of temporalis muscle.

Subdivisions

a. **Temporal or zygomaticotemporal space:** It is a superior extension of the masticator space.

b. **Submasseteric space:** It is an inferior extension between lateral surface of ramus of mandible and deep surface of masseteric muscle.

c. **Superficial pterygoid or pterygmandibular space:** It is also an inferior extension between medial surface of ramus of mandible laterally, lateral surface of medial pterygoid muscle inferomedially and lateral pterygoid muscle superomedially.

Contents: Inferior alveolar nerve and vessels, lingual nerve, mandibular nerve, maxillary artery, loose connective tissue and fat.

Clinical significance: Masticator space may be infected from infection of zygoma, temporal bone or lower molar teeth. Infection of pterygmandibular space due to septic needles during the inferior dental nerve block anesthesia. Trauma to mandible involving molar teeth. It has larger area at skull base and has foramen ovale at its roof allowing potential tumor spread.

4. Parapharyngeal space: It is also known as lateral pharyngeal space, peripharyngeal space, pharyngo-masticator space, pharyngomaxillary space, or pterygopharyngeal space. Parapharyngeal space can be divided into:

(i) Lateral pharyngeal space: This space is pyramidal in shape with apex directed inferiorly towards the lesser cornu of hyoid bone and base directed superiorly towards skull base.

Boundaries

Anteriorly—posterior pharyngeal wall.

Posteriorly—vertebrae with ligaments and muscles.

Laterally—deep cervical fascia anteriorly and styloid process with its attached structures posteriorly and deep surface of parotid gland in between.

Medially—midline fibrous septum.

Superiorly—deep pterygoid space, base of skull.

Inferiorly—hyoid bone.

Divisions and contents: This space is subdivided by styloid process into:

a. **Anterior compartment (prestyloid compartment)** contains lymph nodes, ascending pharyngeal and facial arteries, maxillary artery, inferior alveolar nerve, lingual nerve, auriculotemporal nerve and loose areolar tissue.

b. **Posterior compartment (poststyloid compart-ment)** contains carotid sheath with its contents,

9, 11, 12th cranial nerves and cervical sympathetic chain.

Clinical significance: It may receive infection from teeth, submandibular gland, masticator space, parotid space and paratonsillar space. From this space infection can pass to retropharyngeal space and then to superior mediastinum. Medial displacement of the lateral pharyngeal wall and tonsil is a hallmark of parapharyngeal space. Parotid space displaces the parapharyngeal fat anteromedially, masticator space displaces it posteromedially, carotid space → anteriorly, retropharynheal and danger space → anterolaterally.

(ii) **Retropharyngeal space:** This spans from base of skull to mediastinum divided by alas fascia into true retopharyngeal space (anteriorly) and danger space (posteriorly).

Boundaries

Anteriorly—posterior wall of pharynx.

Posteriorly—prevertebral fascia.

Superiorly—base of skull.

Inferiorly—communicates with superior mediastinum.

Clinical significance: It acts as a route through which infection from the mouth and throat can reach the superior mediastinum.

5. Parotid compartment: The parotid gland is completely enclosed in a well defined compartment of deep fascia derived from superficial layer of deep cervical fascia.

Contents: Parotid gland, parotid lymph nodes.

Clinical significance: Infection in this space may be because of infection of gland or lymph nodes and may readily pass deep to parapharyngeal space.

6. Paratonsillar space: This space contains palatine tonsils

Boundaries

Laterally—superior pharyngeal constrictor.

Medially—mucous membrane of anterior and posterior pillar of fauces.

Superiorly—extends into soft palate.

7. Space of the body of the mandible: This space to be formed by attachment of superficial layer of deep cervical fascia to both outer and inner surfaces of the body of mandible.

Boundaries:

Anteriorly—anterior belly of digastric.

Posteriorly—pterygoids.

Inferiorly—fascial layers.

Superiorly—mandible.

Clinical significance: Infection of this space can occur from osteomyelitis secondary to dental infections. Infection may spread by rupture of its wall into the masticator space posteriorly or submandibular space inferiorly.

(B) Infrahyoid fascial spaces

1. Visceral compartment: The area of loose connective tissue surrounding the thyroid gland, trachea and esophagus as a whole was long known as visceral compartment.

(a) Pretracheal space/anterior cervical space
Boundaries

Superiorly—strap muscles and their fascia.

Inferiorly—superior mediastinum.

Laterally—root of the neck.

Clinical importance: This space can get infected from retrovisceral space, around the sides of esophagus and thyroid gland between the levels of upper border of thyroid cartilage and inferior thyroid artery; or directly by anterior perforation of esophagus.

(b) Retrovisceral space
Boundaries

Superiorly—base of skull.

Inferiorly—superior mediastinum.

Clinical importance: This space may be infected by posterior perforation of esophagus or infection of deep cervical lymph nodes.

2. Visceral space: The esophagus is enclosed in a connective tissue sheath continuous above with buccopharyngeal fascia, posterior surface of pharynx and adjacent to surface of thyroid gland and trachea. The visceral space is a potential space which may be imagined to exist between visceral fascia and the organs themselves (may these be trachea or esophagus). Actually, this visceral fascia is firmly united to structures which it covers and the visceral space in the latter sense does not really exist. Also infections lying deep to the fascia on esophagus do not tend to spread within this fascia up and down the esophagus but rather perforate it to reach the visceral compartment.

Q. 5. Describe in detail the structure of lymph node. Add a note on levels of lymph node.

(TNMGR, Sept. 2010; HNBG Uni., May 2017)

Ans. Each cervical lymph node has cortical and medullary regions, and is covered by a fibrous capsule.

Cortex: Consists of lymphocytes which are densely packed together to form spherical lymphoid follicles.

Medulla: Composed of medullary trabeculae, medullary cords and medullary sinuses. Medullary trabeculae composed of dense connective tissue and act as a framework extending from the capsule. The medullary cords and medullary sinuses are composed of reticulum cells. The medullary cords contain mainly plasma cells and small lymphocytes, whilst the medullary sinuses are filled with lymph.

Paracortex: An intermediate area between the cortex and the medulla, where the lymphocytes return to the lymphatic system from the blood circulation.

Blood supply: The main artery enters the lymph node at the hilus, which then branches into arterioles, run along the medullary trabeculae to the cortex where the arterioles further branch into capillaries and supply the lymphoid follicles. The rest of the arterioles run along the trabeculae and reach the capsule where they anastomose with other branches.

Venous supply: Venules converge to form small veins in the cortex which run along the trabeculae of the lymph node and reach the medulla where they further converge to form the main vein. The main vein leaves the lymph node at the hilus (Fig. 10.5).

Classification of lymph nodes
There are about 800 lymph nodes in the body and about 300 lymph nodes are located in the neck. The lymph nodes of the neck are classified by levels: Ia, Ib, II, III, IV, V, VI, VII, VIII, IX, X.

Level I: Mandible superiorly and laterally and hyoid bone inferiorly.

Level Ia: Submental lymph nodes. Drainage: Skin of mental region (chin), middle of lower lip, anterior portion of tongue, floor of mouth.

Level Ib: Submandibular lymph nodes. Drainage: Submental lymph nodes, lower nasal cavity, hard and soft palate, alveolar ridges of maxilla and mandible, skin and mucosa of cheek, upper and lower lips, floor of mouth and anterior tongue.

Level II: Upper jugular lymph nodes: Skull base superiorly and hyoid bone inferiorly (carotid bifurcation), adjacent to the top third of IJV. **Drainage:** Face, parotid gland, level I, retropharyngeal nodes, nasal cavity, entire pharyngeal axis, larynx, external auditory canal, middle ear.

Level III: Middle jugular lymph nodes: Hyoid bone superiorly to cricothyroid membrane inferiorly, adjacent to the middle third of the IJV. **Drainage:** Level II, level V, and partially from retropharyngeal, pretracheal, recurrent laryngeal nodes, base of the tongue, tonsils, larynx, hypopharynx, and thyroid gland.

Level IVa: Lower jugular lymph nodes: Cricothyroid membrane superiorly to clavicle inferiorly, adjacent to the inferior third of the IJV. **Drainage:** Levels III, V, partially from retropharyngeal, pretracheal, recurrent laryngeal nodes, larynx, hypopharynx, and thyroid gland.

Level IVb: Medial Supraclavicular lymph nodes: Continuation of level IVa to the superior edge of the sternal manubrium. **Drainage:** Levels IVa, Vc, pretracheal, recurrent laryngeal nodes, larynx, trachea, hypopharynx, esophagus, and thyroid gland.

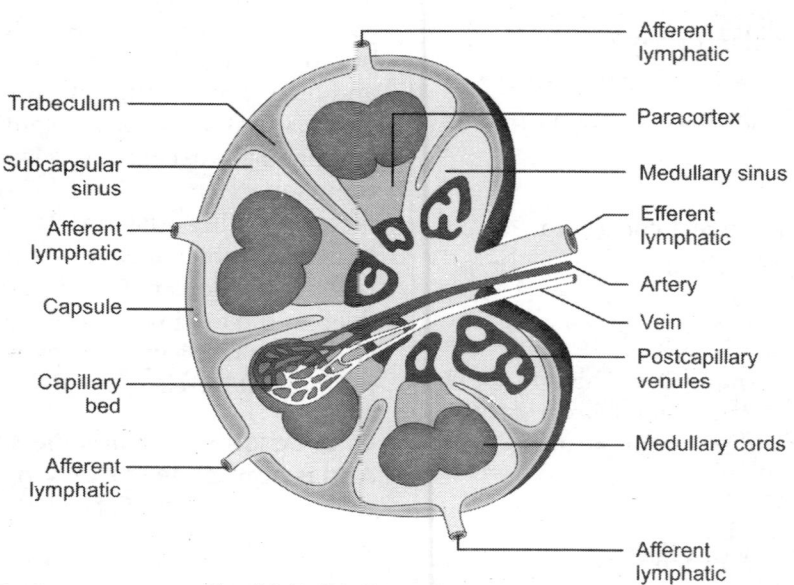

Fig. 10.5: Structure of lymph node

Level Va and Vb: Posterior triangle group: Anterior border of sternocleidomastoid muscle anteriorly and clavicle inferiorly. A virtual plane at the inferior edge of the cricoid cartilage divides this group into upper (Va) and lower (Vb). **Drainage:** Occipital, retro-auricular, parietal scalp nodes, skin of the lateral and posterior neck and shoulder, nasopharynx, oropharynx, and thyroid gland.

Level Vc: Lateral supraclavicular group: Sontinuation of levels Va and Vb; **Drainage:** Levels Va and Vb.

Level VI: Anterior compartment group: Hyoid bone superiorly to suprasternal notch inferiorly.

Level VIa: Superficially-located anterior jugular nodes: Superiorly by inferior edge of level Ib and inferiorly by superior edge of the sternal manubrium. **Drainage:** Integuments of the lower face and anterior neck.

Level VIb: Deeper pre-laryngeal, pre-tracheal, and para-tracheal (recurrent laryngeal) nodes: Superiorly by superior edge of the thyroid cartilage and inferiorly by superior border of sternal manubrium. **Drainage:** Anterior floor of mouth, tip of oral tongue, lower lip, thyroid gland, glottic and supraglottic larynx, hypopharynx, and cervical esophagus.

Level VII: Prevertebral compartment

Level VIIa: Retropharyngeal nodes: Medial and lateral subgroups. **Drainage:** Nasopharynx, eustachian tube, and soft palate.

Level VIIb: Retrostyloid nodes: Level VIIb is bounded superiorly by jugular foramen at base of skull, and inferiorly by inferior edge of lateral process of C1 vertebral body, superior boundary of level II. **Drainage:** nasopharynx.

Level VIII: Parotid group (preauricular, intraparotid, subparotid): Superiorly by zygomatic arch and external auditory canal, and inferiorly by mandibular angle. **Drainage:** Frontal and temporal skin, eyelids, conjunctivae, auricles, external acoustic meatus, tympanum, nasal cavities, root of the nose, nasopharynx, and eustachian tube.

Level IX: Buccofacial group (malar and buccofacial): Superficial nodes on external surface of buccinator muscle. **Drainage:** Nose, eyelids, and cheek.

Level X: Posterior skull group.

Level Xa: Retroauricular and subauricular nodes: Superficial nodes on mastoid process, bounded superiorly by superior edge of external auditory canal, and inferiorly by mastoid tip. **Drainage:** Posterior auricular surface, external auditory canal and adjacent scalp.

Level Xb: Occipital nodes: Superior and superficial continuation of level Va, bounded superiorly by external occipital protuberance, and inferiorly by superior border of level V. **Drainage:** Posterior hairy scalp.

Q. 6. Write a note on cervical chain of lymph nodes.
(RGUHS, 2006; Pacific Uni., May 2015)

Q. Classify lymph nodes and describe the lymphatic drainage of head and neck.
(TNMGR, March 2009, Oct. 2019; KLE Uni., Jan. 2009; MUHS, May 2010; RUHS, June 2017; HP Uni., April 2019; UOK, June 2019)

Ans. Lymph nodes in head and neck are as follows: For detailed drainage, refer to Que. 5.

The entire lymph from the head and neck drains ultimately into the deep cervical nodes.

A. **Deep cervical nodes** form a vertical chain situated along the entire length of the internal jugular vein.
1. **Jugulodigastric node:** It lies below the posterior belly of the digastrics, between the angle of the mandible and anterior border of the sterno-cleidomastoid. It is the main node draining the tonsil.
2. **Jugulo-omohyoid node:** It lies just above the intermediate tendon of the omohyoid, under cover of the posterior border of the sterno-cleidomastoid. It is the main lymph node of the tongue.

Efferents of the deep cervical lymph nodes join together to form the jugular lymph trunks, one on each side. The left jugular trunk opens into the thoracic duct. The right trunk may open either into the right lymphatic duct, or directly into the angle of junction between the internal jugular and subclavian veins.

B. **Peripheral nodes** are arranged in two circles.
   I. **Superficial circle** is made up of the following groups (Fig. 10.5b):
   1. Submental.
   2. Submandibular.
   3. Buccal and mandibular (facial).
   4. Preauricular (Parotid).
   5. Postauricular (mastoid).
   6. Occipital.
   7. Anterior cervical.
   8. Superficial cervical nodes.
   II. **Deep circle (inner)** includes the following: (Fig. 10.6a)
   1. Prelaryngeal.
   2. Pretracheal.
   3. Paratracheal.
   4. Retropharyngeal nodes.
   5. Waldeyer's ring.

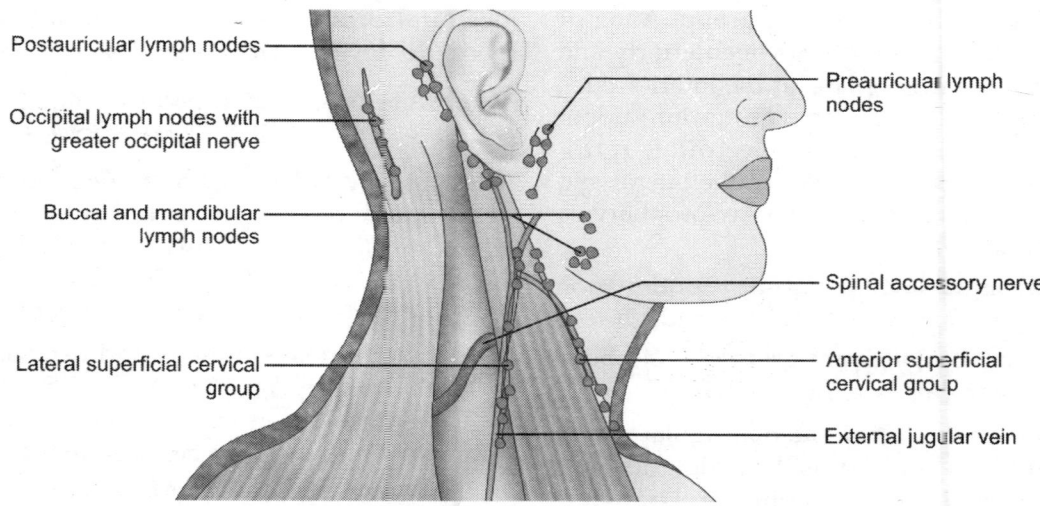

Fig. 10.6a: Superficial group of cervical lymph nodes

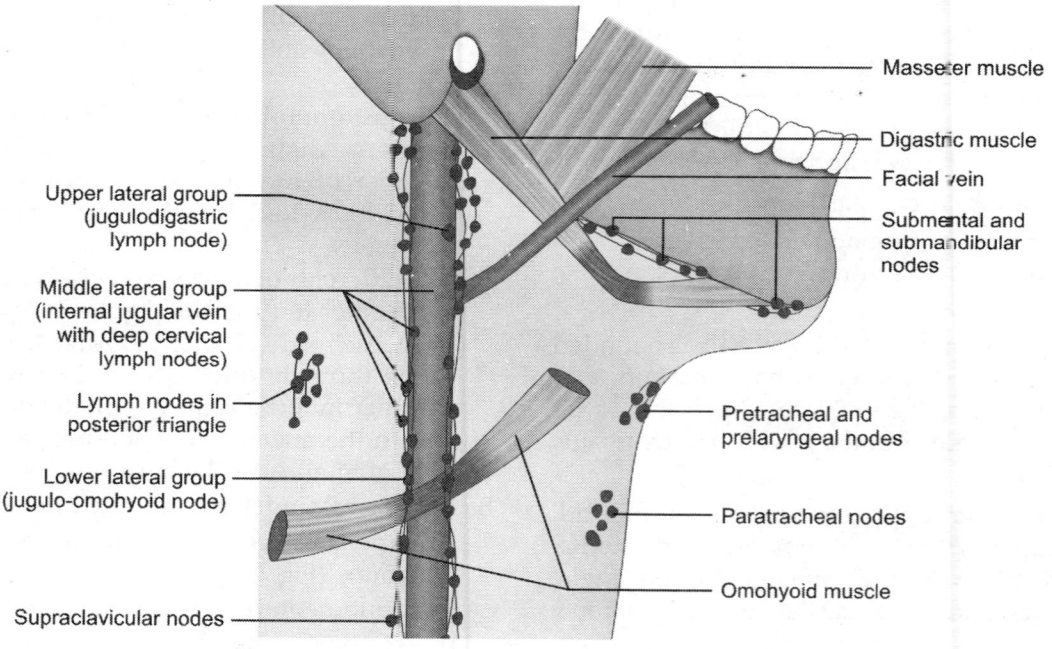

Fig. 10.6b: Deep group of cervical lymph nodes

Q. 7. Write a note on thoracic duct.

(TNMGR, April 2003; KUHS, July 2012)

Ans. The thoracic duct is the largest lymph trunk of the body. It begins in the abdomen from the upper end of the cisterna chyli, traverses the thorax, and ends on the left side of the root of neck by opening into angle of junction between left internal jugular vein and left subclavian vein. Before its termination, it forms an arch at the level of transverse process of vertebra C7 rising 3 to 4 cm above the clavicle. The relations of the arch are (Fig. 10.7):

Anterior: 1. Left common carotid artery, 2. Vagus. 3. Internal jugular vein.

Posterior: 1. Vertebral artery and vein, 2. Sympathetic trunk, 3. Thyrocervical trunk or its branches, 4. Prevertebral fascia, 5. Phrenic nerve, 6. Scalenus anterior.

Apart from its tributaries in the abdomen and thorax, thoracic duct receives: Left jugular trunk, left subclavian trunk, left broncho-mediastinal trunk.

It drains most of the body, **except** for right upper limb, right halves of the head, neck and thorax and superior surface of liver. **Right jugular trunk** drains

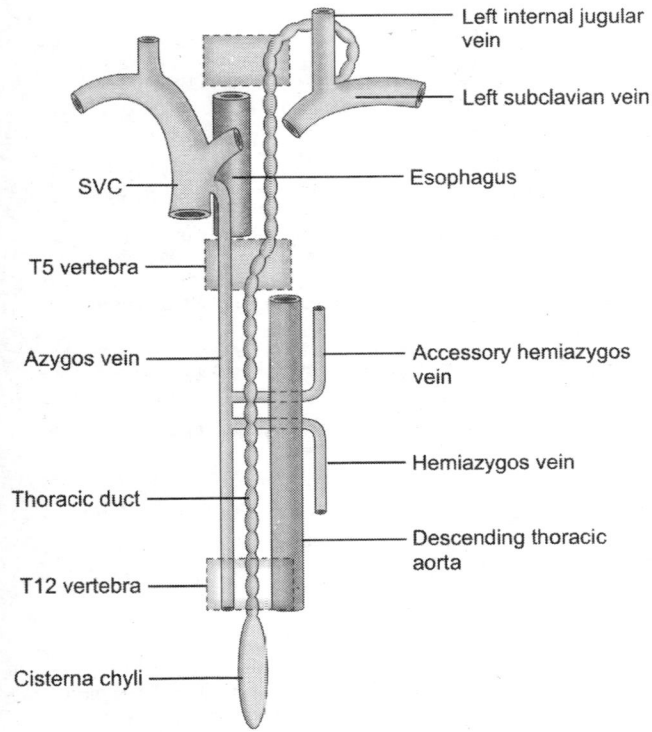

Left internal jugular vein

Left subclavian vein

SVC

Esophagus

T5 vertebra

Azygos vein

Accessory hemiazygos vein

Hemiazygos vein

Thoracic duct

Descending thoracic aorta

T12 vertebra

Cisterna chyli

Fig. 10.7: Thoracic duct and its formation

half of head and neck. **Right subclavian trunk** drains the upper limb, **broncho-mediastinal trunk** drains the lung, half of the mediastinum and parts of anterior walls of thorax and abdomen. On right side, subclavian and jugular trunks may unite to form **right lymph trunk** which ends in a manner similar to the thoracic duct.

Development: During the 6th week of IUL, early lymphatic system is composed of blunt buds near the base of neck. By the end of embryonic period, six lymph sacs form: Cisterna chyli, two jugular lymph sacs, two iliac lymph sacs, and a retroperitoneal lymph sac. The thoracic duct develops from lymphatic trunks on either side of aorta that anastomoses to form a channel from the jugular lymph sacs to the cisterna chyli.

Applied Clinical Anatomy

1. Thoracic duct dysfunction results in chyle accumulation, which may mimic for malignancy.
2. Lymph from organs can drain directly into the thoracic duct without passing a lymph node (skip metastasis).
3. Virchow node (lymph node located at the base of the neck where the duct generally terminates) can be enlarged in cases of malignancy.
4. The long course of the thoracic duct predisposes it to traumatic injury during surgeries.

Q. 8. Describe the deep cervical fascia.

(KUHS, Jan. 2014)

Ans. The deep cervical fascia of the neck was first described in the early 1800s. The deep fascia of the neck is condensed to form the following layers (Fig. 10.8):

1. **Investing layer:** It lies deep to platysma and surrounds the neck like a collar. It forms roof of posterior triangle of neck. It splits to enclose **muscles** (trapezius, sternocleidomastoid), **salivary glands** (parotid and submandibular), and **spaces** (suprasternal, supraclavicular).
2. **Pretracheal fascia:** This fascia encloses and suspends thyroid gland and forms its false capsule. The posterior layer of thyroid capsule forms a thick suspensory ligament for thyroid, known as **ligament of Berry.** The fascia provides a slippery surface for the free movements of trachea during swallowing.
3. **Prevertebral fascia:** It lies in front of prevertebral muscles and forms floor of posterior triangle of neck. Superiorly, it is attached to base of skull. Inferiorly, it extends to mediastinum. The cervical and brachial plexuses lie behind prevertebral fascia. The fascia is pierced by cutaneous branches of cervical plexus. This fascia provides a fixed base for movements of the pharynx, esophagus and carotid sheath during swallowing.
4. **Carotid sheath:** It is the condensation of fibro-areolar tissue around the main vessels of neck. It is formed by pretracheal fascia anteriorly and by prevertebral fascia posteriorly. The contents include common and internal carotid arteries, internal jugular vein and cranial nerve 9th, 11th and 12th. The *ansa cervicalis* is embedded in its anterior wall. The cervical sympathetic chain lies behind.
5. **Buccopharyngeal fascia:** This fascia covers superior constrictor muscle externally and extends on to the superficial aspect of buccinator muscle.
6. **Pharyngobasilar fascia:** This fascia is especially thickened between the upper border of superior constrictor muscle and the base of skull. It lies deep to pharyngeal muscles.

Development: The fasciae are derived from fibromuscular laminae during ontogenesis. The prevertebral lamina develops as an aponeurosis for longus colli muscles. The visceral fascia develops independently of the organs or vessels which they enclose.

Blood supply: By branches of vessels that supply structure which they enclose.

Functions: 1. Serve as guide for muscular movement, 2. As attachment site for some muscles, 3. As supporting structure for viscera.

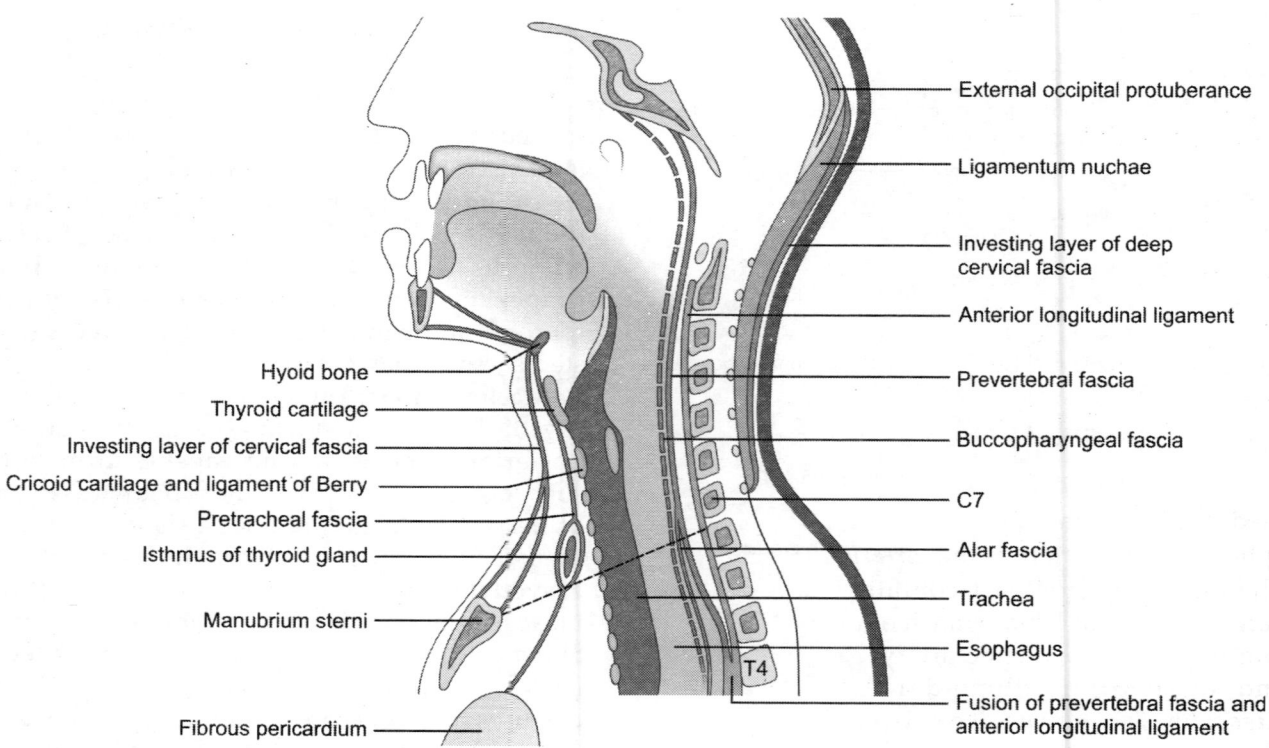

Fig. 10.8: Deep cervical fascia and its layers

Applied Clinical Anatomy

1. The various layers of deep fascia may provide a way for spread of infection.
2. Danger space, lying just posterior to the retropharyngeal, is in free communication with posterior mediastinum and infection can spread inferiorly to the mediastinum.

11. NASAL CAVITY AND ORBITS

Q. 1. Discuss surgical anatomy of nose in detail.
(BFUHS, May 2011; MUHS, April 2011, 2013; HP Uni., June 2016)

Q. Write in detail about the lateral wall of the nasal cavity. (TNMGR, March 2008)

Ans. Nose is a respiratory passage as well as organ of smell (upper one-third).

A. Nasal septum: It is median osseo-cartilaginous partition between two halves of nasal cavity (Fig. 11.1a).

Bony part: Vomer, perpendicular plate of ethmoid, nasal spine of frontal bone, rostrum of sphenoid, and nasal crests of nasal, palatine and maxillary bones.

Cartilaginous part: Septal cartilage, inferior nasal cartilage.

Cuticular part (lower end): Fibro-fatty tissue covered by skin.

The lower margin of septum is called *columella*. The septum has:

a. Four borders—superior, inferior, anterior, posterior.
b. Two surfaces—right and left.

Arterial supply

1. Anterosuperior part: Anterior and posterior ethmoidal arteries.
2. Anteroinferior part **(Little's area)**: Superior labial artery.
3. Posterosuperior part: Sphenopalatine artery.
4. Posteroinferior part: Greater palatine artery.

Venous drainage: Pterygoid venous plexus.

Nerve supply

1. General sensory nerves:
   a. Anterosuperior part: Internal nasal branch.
   b. Anteroinferior part: Anterior superior alveolar nerve.
   c. Posterosuperior part: Medial posterior superior nasal branch.
   d. Posteroinferior part: Nasopalatine branch.
2. Special sensory (olfactory) nerve: Upper part or olfactory area.

Lymphatics: Submandibular (anterior), retropharyngeal and deep cervical lymph nodes (posterior).

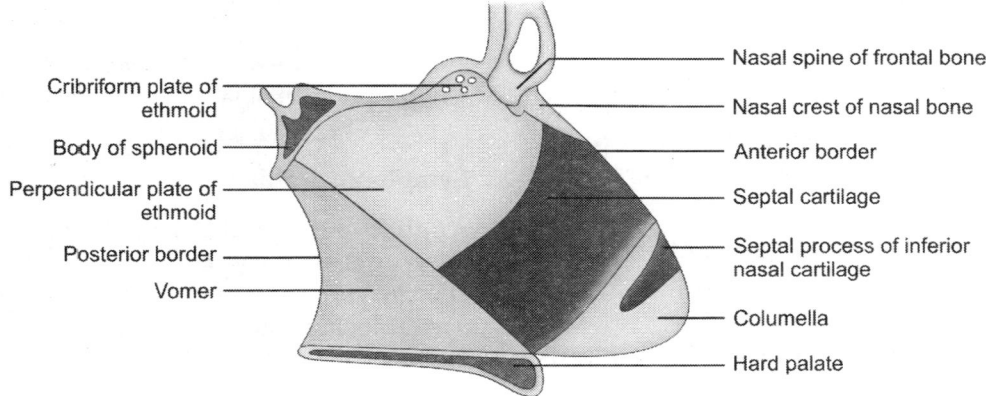

Cribriform plate of ethmoid
Body of sphenoid
Perpendicular plate of ethmoid
Posterior border
Vomer

Nasal spine of frontal bone
Nasal crest of nasal bone
Anterior border
Septal cartilage
Septal process of inferior nasal cartilage
Columella
Hard palate

Fig. 11.1a: Nasal septum and its parts

Applied Clinical Anatomy
1. Sphenopalatine artery is the '*artery of epistaxis*'
2. The anteroinferior part contains anastomoses between superior labial branch of the facial artery, branch of sphenopalatine artery, greater palatine and of anterior ethmoidal artery forming *Kiesselbach's plexus*. This is common site of bleeding from the nose (epistaxis) and is known as *Little's area.*

B. Lateral wall of nose: It is irregular due to the presence of three shelf-like bony projections called *conchae*. The conchae increase surface area of nose for effective air-conditioning of inspired air. The lateral wall separates the nose.
a. From the orbit above, with ethmoidal air sinuses intervening.
b. From the maxillary sinus below.
c. From the lacrimal groove and nasolacrimal canal in front.

Lateral wall can be subdivided into three parts:
a. A small depressed area in anterior part is called the **Vestibule.** It is lined by modified skin containing short, stiff, curved hairs called **vibrissae.**
b. Middle part is known as **atrium** of middle meatus.
c. Posterior part contains the conchae.

Skeleton of the lateral wall is partly bony, partly cartilaginous, and partly made up only of soft tissues as follows:

Bony part is formed from before backwards by following bones (Fig. 11.1b).
1. Nasal
2. Frontal process of maxilla
3. Lacrimal
4. Labyrinth of ethmoid with superior and middle conchae
5. Inferior nasal concha

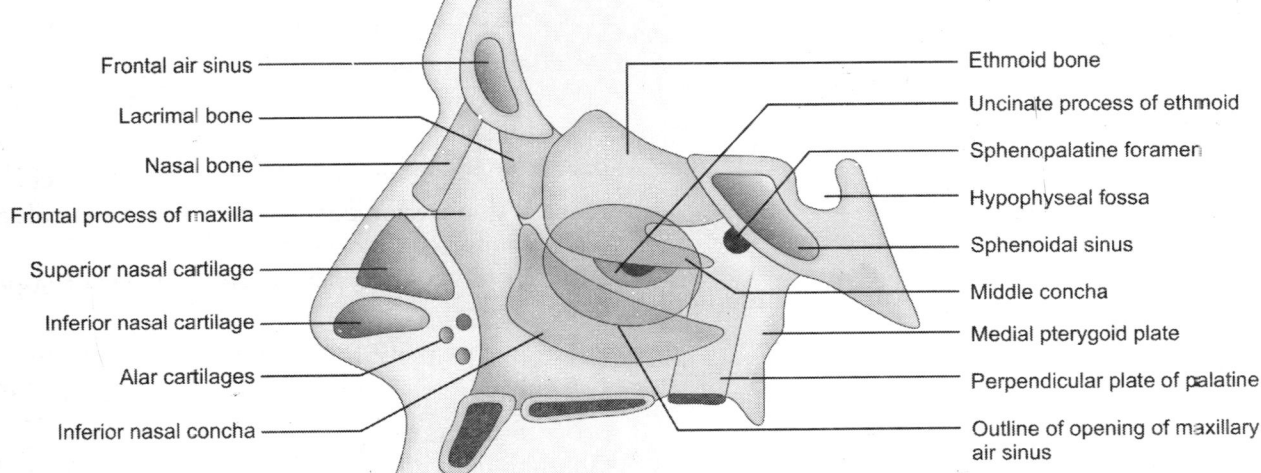

Frontal air sinus
Lacrimal bone
Nasal bone
Frontal process of maxilla
Superior nasal cartilage
Inferior nasal cartilage
Alar cartilages
Inferior nasal concha

Ethmoid bone
Uncinate process of ethmoid
Sphenopalatine foramen
Hypophyseal fossa
Sphenoidal sinus
Middle concha
Medial pterygoid plate
Perpendicular plate of palatine
Outline of opening of maxillary air sinus

Fig. 11.1b: Lateral wall of nose

6. Perpendicular plate of palatine bone together with its orbital and sphenoidal processes.
7. Medial pterygoid plate

Cartilaginous part is formed by superior and inferior nasal cartilage, 3 or 4 small cartilages of ala. *Cuticular lower part* is formed by fibro-fatty tissue covered with skin.

Conchae: The nasal conchae are curved bony projections directed downwards and medially.

a. *Inferior concha* is an independent bone.
b. *Middle concha* is a projection from medial surface of ethmoidal labyrinth.
c. *Superior concha* (smallest) is also projection from medial surface of ethmoidal labyrinth.

Meatuses: Passages beneath the overhanging conchae.

a. *Inferior meatus* lies beneath inferior concha and is the largest. The nasolacrimal duct opens (guarded by lacrimal fold, **Hesner's valve**) into it.
b. *Middle meatus:* Lies beneath the middle concha.
   Ethmoidal bulla is elevation of underlying middle ethmoidal sinuses.
   Hiatus semilunaris is deep semicircular sulcus below the bulla.
   Infundibulum is a short passage at the anterior end of the hiatus.
   The opening of frontal sinus is seen in the anterior part of the hiatus semilunaris. The opening of the anterior ethmoidal sinus is present behind the opening of frontal sinus. Maxillary sinus opening is located in the posterior part of hiatus semilunaris.
c. *Superior meatus:* Lies below the superior concha and shortest and shallowest. Posterior ethmoidal sinus opens here.
d. *Sphenoethmoidal recess* is triangular fossa just above superior concha. Sphenoidal sinus opens here.

Arterial supply: Same as nasal septum

Venous drainage: Facial vein (anteriorly), pterygoid plexus of veins (middle part), pharyngeal plexus of veins (posteriorly).

Nerve supply
1. General sensory nerves
   a. Anterosuperior quadrant: Anterior ethmoidal nerve.
   b. Anteroinferior quadrant: Anterior superior alveolar nerve.
   c. Posterosuperior quadrant: Posterior superior lateral nasal branches.
   d. Posteroinferior quadrant: Anterior palatine branch.
2. *Special sensory nerves* or *olfactory nerves* are distributed to upper part of lateral wall just below the cribriform plate of ethmoid up to superior concha.

Lymphatic drainage: Same as nasal septum.

Applied clinical anatomy: Hypertrophy of mucosa over inferior nasal concha is a common feature of allergic rhinitis which is characterized by sneezing, nasal blockage and excessive watery discharge from the nose.

Q. 2. Write in detail about content of orbit and ocular muscles. *(KUHS, Jan. 2014)*

Q. Describe in detail anatomy of orbit.
(Suamandeep Uni., May 2018)

Ans. The orbits are bony structures of skull that house globe, extraocular muscles, nerves, blood vessels, lacrimal apparatus, and adipose tissue. Each orbit resembles a four-sided pyramid situated one on each side. The long axis of orbit passes backwards and medially. The medial walls of two orbits are parallel (distance between two medial walls ~2.5 cm) and the lateral walls are set at right angles to each other.

Roof: It is concave from side to side and is formed by orbital plate of frontal bone and lesser wing of sphenoid.

Relations:
a. It separates the orbit from anterior cranial fossa.
b. The frontal air sinus may extend into its anteromedial part.

Lateral wall: This is the thickest and strongest of all the walls of the orbit. It is formed by: greater wing of sphenoid bone and frontal process of zygomatic bone.

Relation:
a. Greater wing of sphenoid separates orbit from middle cranial fossa.
b. Zygomatic bone separates it from temporal fossa.

Floor: It slopes upwards and medially to join the medial wall. It is formed by orbital surface of maxilla, orbital surface of zygomatic bone, orbital process of palatine bone.

Relation: It separates orbit from maxillary sinus.

Medial wall: It is very thin. It is formed by frontal process of maxilla, lacrimal bone, orbital plate of ethmoid, body of sphenoid bone.

Relations

a. Lacrimal groove, formed by maxilla and lacrimal bone, separates the orbit from nasal cavity.
b. Orbital plate of ethmoid separates the orbit from ethmoidal air sinuses.
c. Sphenoidal sinuses are separated from the orbit only by a thin layer of bone.

Foramina in relation to the orbit

i. Inferior orbital fissure transmits zygomatic nerve, orbital branches of pterygopalatine ganglion, infraorbital nerve and vessels, and communication between inferior ophthalmic vein and pterygoid plexus of veins.
ii. Infraorbital groove and canal transmit the corresponding nerve and vessels.
iii. Zygomatic foramen transmits zygomatic nerve.
iv. Anterior ethmoidal foramina transmit the corresponding nerves and vessels. Posterior ethmoidal foramina only transmit vessels.

A. Content of orbit

1. Eyeball: Occupies anterior one-third of orbit.
2. Fascia: Orbital (periorbita) and bulbar (fascial sheath of eyeball).
3. Muscles: Extraocular and intraocular.
4. Vessels: Ophthalmic artery, superior and inferior ophthalmic veins and lymphatics.
5. Nerves: Optic, oculomotor, trochlear, abducent, branches of ophthalmic and maxillary nerves and sympathetic nerves.
6. Lacrimal gland.
7. Orbital fat.

Orbital (periorbita): It forms the periosteum of the bony orbit. Due to loose connection to bone, it can be stripped easily. The extensions of this fascia into lower and upper margins of orbit form the *orbital septum*. The extension which bridges the lacrimal groove forms the *lacrimal fascia*.

Bulbar fascia: *Tenon's capsule* forms a thin, loose membranous sheath around eyeball, extending from optic nerve to sclerocorneal junction. Its lower part is thickened and is known as *suspensory ligament of eye or suspensory ligament of Lockwood*.

The sheath is pierced by tendons of extraocular muscles. Its expansions are:

a. *Tubular sheath* covers each orbital muscle.
b. *Medial check ligament* from sheath of medial rectus muscle is attached to lacrimal bone.
c. *Lateral check ligament* from sheath of lateral rectus muscle is attached to zygomatic bone.

Applied Clinical Anatomy

1. The bones of the orbit protect globe of eye as well as other periocular contents.
2. A fracture to orbit can involve contents of orbit and potentially compress nerves or muscles within the orbit.
3. Intracranial lesions can cause damage to optic nerve and associated vessels, central retinal artery, and central retinal vein.
4. Abducent nerve is commonly affected when intracranial pressure increases.

B. Muscles of eye:

I. **Extraocular muscles:** (Fig. 11.2)
  a. Voluntary muscles:
    1. Four recti: Arise from a ***common annular tendon*** or ***tendinous ring of zinn***, attached to

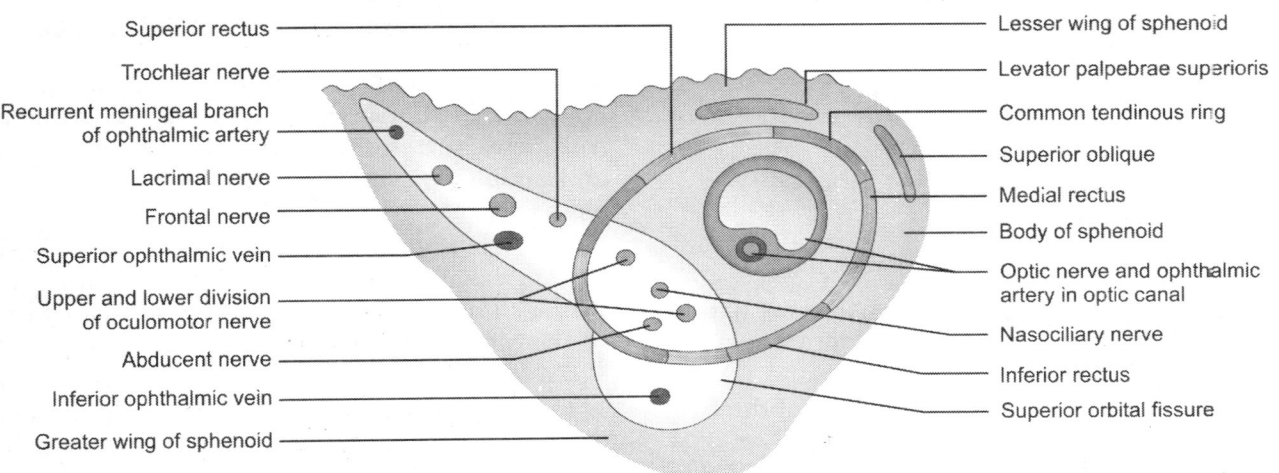

Fig. 11.2: Origin of extraocular muscles

superior orbital fissure and inserted into the sclera: i. Superior rectus; ii. Medial rectus; iii. Inferior rectus; iv. Lateral rectus.

2. Two obliqui:
   i. Superior oblique: Originates from undersurface of lesser wing of sphenoid.
   ii. Inferior oblique: Originates from orbital surface of maxilla.
3. Levator palpebrae superioris elevates the upper eyelid. It originates from orbital surface lesser wing of sphenoid.
b. Involuntary muscles:
   1. Superior tarsal muscle: It elevates the upper eyelid.
   2. Inferior tarsal muscle: It depresses the lower eyelid.
   3. Orbitalis: Its action is uncertain.

Nerve supply:
1. Superior oblique—4th cranial nerve/trochlear nerve (SO_4).
2. Lateral rectus—6th cranial nerve/abducent nerve (LR_6).
3. Remaining extra ocular muscles and part of levator palpebrae superioris—3rd cranial nerve/oculomotor nerve.

Arterial supply: Ophthalmic artery:
a. Central artery of retina: It supplies retina, most of nervous layer.
b. Lacrimal artery: Lacrimal gland, zygomatic bone, muscles of orbit.
c. Anterior ciliary artery: Eyeball
d. Posterior ciliary artery: Coroid and iris.
e. Supraorbital and Supratrochlear: Skin of forehead.
f. Anterior and posterior ethmoidal branches: Ethmoidal air sinuses.
g. Medial and lateral palpebral branches: Eyelids.
h. Dorsal nasal branches: Upper part of nose.

Venous supply: Ophthalmic veins
a. Superior ophthalmic vein.
b. Inferior ophthalmic vein.

Lymphatics: Preauricular lymph nodes.

Actions: Normally, movements of two eyes are harmoniously coordinated. Such coordinated movements are called *conjugate ocular movements*.
1. Medial and lateral recti adduct and abduct the cornea, respectively.
2. Superior and inferior recti cause simple elevation and depression, respectively.
3. Upward rotation or elevation: Superior rectus and the inferior oblique.
4. Downward rotation or depression: Inferior rectus and the superior oblique.
5. Medial rotation or adduction: Medial rectus, the superior rectus and the inferior rectus.
6. Lateral rotation or abduction: Lateral rectus, the superior oblique and the inferior oblique.
7. Intorsion: Superior oblique and the superior rectus.
8. Extorsion: Inferior oblique and the inferior rectus.

Development: Orbital development begins in the 3rd week of IUL. The optic pits appear first as an invagination of diencephalon, eventually forming the orbit after contributions from many different embryonic cell populations. The cranial neural crest cells are generally thought to be the fundamental cells of orbital embryogenesis.

Applied Clinical Anatomy

1. Weakness/paralysis of muscle causes squint/strabismus.
2. In concomitant squint (congenital) there is no diplopia and no limitation of movements.
3. In paralytic type, movements are limited, diplopia and vertigo are present.
4. **Nystagmus:** Involuntary, rhythmical oscillatory movements of eye due to in coordination of ocular muscles.
5. **Phoria:** Turning of an eye in (*esophoria*) or out (*exophoria*) upon occlusion of the opposite eye.
6. Tropias: Sontaneous eye turn in the absence of an ocular occlusion.
7. Amblyopia results when the vision in one of the eyes is reduced because the eye and the brain are not working together properly.

12. STRUCTURE AND FUNCTION OF BRAIN

Q. 1. Write a short note on taste pathways.
(TNMGR, March 2002; RUHS, July 2016)

Ans. Sense of taste (gustation) allows us to separate undesirable or even lethal foods from those that are pleasant to eat.

1. The taste from **anterior two-thirds** of tongue **except** from vallate papillae is carried by chorda tympani branch of facial nerve till the geniculate ganglion. The central processes go to the tractus solitarius in the medulla.
2. Taste from **posterior one-third** of tongue including the vallate papillae is carried by cranial nerve IXth till the inferior ganglion. The central processes also reach the tractus solitarius.

3. Taste from **posterior most** part of tongue and epiglottis travels through vagus nerve till inferior ganglion of vagus. These central processes also reach tractus solitarius.

4. After a relay in tractus solitarius, the solitario-thalamic tract is formed which becomes a part of trigeminal lemniscus and reaches postero-ventro-medial nucleus of thalamus of the opposite side. Another relay here takes them to lowest part of post-central gyrus, which is the area for taste (Fig. 12.1).

Applied Clinical Anatomy

1. Aguesia: Complete loss of taste.
2. Hypoguesia: Partial loss of taste.
3. Dysgeusia: Distortion of taste.
4. Phantom: Aberrant taste.
5. Familial dysautonomia: Taste blindness—genetic.

Q. 2. Write a short note on motor speech area.
(TNMGR, Sept. 2002)

Ans. Primary motor area: It is located in the precentral gyrus, and in anterior part of paracentral lobule on medial surface of cerebral hemispheres. This corresponds to area 4 of Brodmann. Electrical stimulation of primary motor areas elicits contraction of muscles that are mainly on the opposite side of the body. The contra-lateral half of the body is represented as upside down, except the face. The pharyngeal region, tongue is

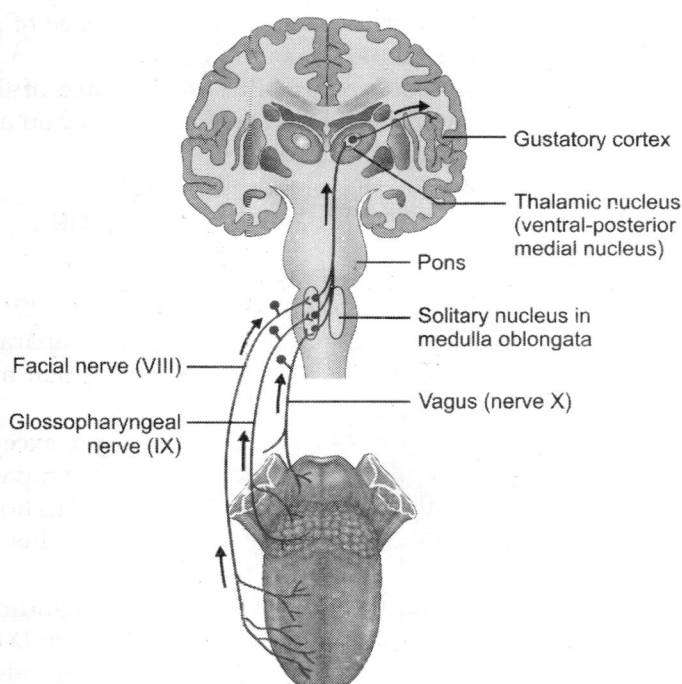

Fig. 12.1: Taste pathways

Gustatory cortex

Thalamic nucleus (ventral-posterior medial nucleus)

Pons

Solitary nucleus in medulla oblongata

Vagus (nerve X)

Facial nerve (VIII)

Glossopharyngeal nerve (IX)

represented in the most ventral and lower part of precentral gyrus, followed by the face, hand, arm, trunk and thigh. The remainder of leg, foot and perineum is on the medial surface of hemisphere in the paracentral lobule.

Premotor area: This area coincides with the Brodmann's area 6 and is situated anterior to motor area in the superolateral and medial surfaces of the hemisphere. The premotor area contributes to motor function by its direct contribution to the pyramidal and other descending motor pathways and by influence on the primary motor cortex.

The premotor and primary motor areas are together referred to as the **primary somato-motor area.**

Supplementary motor area: It is predominantly motor in function. This motor area is in part of area 6 that lies on the medial surface of the hemisphere anterior to paracentral lobule. It differs from main motor area in that its stimulation produces bilateral movements.

Motor speech area (Broca's area): This occupies the opercular and triangular portions of inferior frontal gyrus corresponding to areas 44 and 45 of Brodmann. This is present on left side in 98% of right-handed persons. In 70% of left handers, it is again present in left hemisphere. Only in 30%, it is situated in right hemisphere. It is involved in production and articulation of speech, moves muscles that are required to speak and in analysing grammatical structure of sentences, helps us extract meaning from language.

Frontal eye field: It lies in middle frontal gyrus just anterior to precentral gyrus. It is the lower part of area 8 of Brodmann on the lateral surface of cerebral hemisphere, extending slightly beyond that area. Electrical stimulation of this area causes deviation of both the eyes to the opposite side.

Receptive speech area of Wernicke: This is also known as sensory language area. It consists of auditory association cortex and of adjacent parts of the inferior parietal lobule.

Q. 3. Write a note on circulus arteriosus or circle of Willi's.
(TNMGR, April 2003, 2004)

Ans. Circle of Willi's (circulus arterious) is an arterial polygon (heptagon) formed as the internal carotid and vertebral systems anastomose around optic chiasm and infundibulum of the pituitary stalk in the supra-sellar cistern. It attempts to equalize the flow of blood to different parts of brain and provides a collateral circulation in the event of obstruction to one of its components.

The two anterior cerebral arteries are connected by anterior communicating artery; middle and posterior cerebral arteries of same side are united by the posterior communicating artery.

Branches (Fig. 12.3):

1. **Cortical or external branches** run on the surface of cerebrum, anastomose freely and if these get blocked they give rise to small infarcts.
2. **Central branches** perforate the white matter to supply thalamus, corpus striatum, and internal capsule. These do not anastomose and if these get blocked, they give rise to large infarcts.

The central branches are arranged in six groups:

1. **Anteromedial:** The largest branch is called .the **medial striate** or **recurrent artery of heubner**. It supplies corpus striatum and internal capsule which has motor fibers for face, tongue and shoulder.
2. **Anterolateral:** These are in two groups. The largest branch is called **lenticulostriate** or **Charcot's artery of cerebral hemorrhage**. It supplies internal capsule which has motor fibers for one side of the body.
3. **Posterolateral or thalamogeniculate:** These are also in two groups. They supply thalamus and geniculate bodies.
4. **Posteromedial supply** thalamus and hypothalamus.

Arterial supply of different areas: Cerebral cortex is supplied by branches of all three cerebral arteries.

Middle cerebral is main artery on superolateral surface.

Anterior cerebral artery is chief artery on medial surface.

Posterior cerebral is principal artery on inferior surface.

Applied Clinical Anatomy

1. The circle of Willis perfuses the brain and protects against ischemia.
2. It is one of the most common locations for intracranial aneurysms.
3. **Subclavian steal syndrome/phenomenon:** Vertigo or ataxia precipitated by the exercise of the upper extremity supplied by the stenotic subclavian artery.
4. Moyamoya disease is a chronic vascular disease characterized by bilateral stenosis of the terminal portion of the ICA. This is characterized by *'puff of smoke'* appearance of fine collateral on angiography.

Q. 1. Write a short note on cell cycle. (*TNMGR, 2011*)

Ans. Multiplication of somatic (mitosis) and germ (meiosis) cells is the most complex of all cell functions. Mitosis is controlled by genes which encode for release of specific proteins molecules. Mitosis-promoting protein molecules are cyclins A, B and E. Period between the mitosis is called **interphase**. The cell cycle is the phase between two consecutive divisions. There are four sequential phases in the cell cycle (Fig. 13.1):

1. G_1 **(Premitotic gap) phase** is the stage when messenger RNAs for the proteins and the proteins themselves required for DNA synthesis (e.g. DNA polymerase) are synthesized.
2. **S phase** involves replication of nuclear DNA.

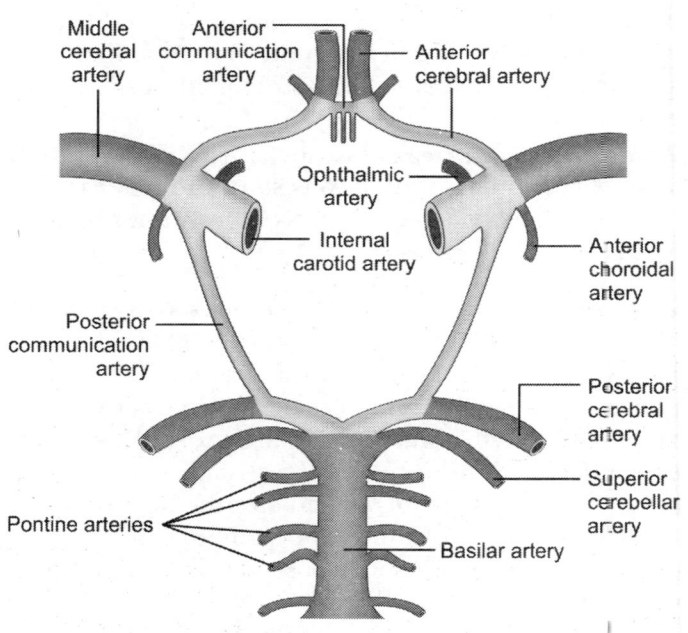

Fig. 12.3: Circle of Willi's and its communications

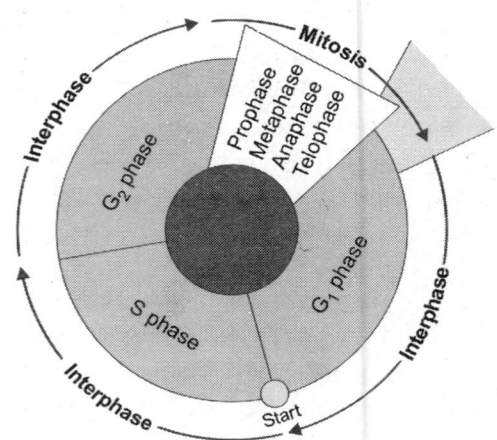

Fig. 13.1: Cell cycle

3. **G$_2$ (Premitotic gap) phase** is the short gap phase in which correctness of DNA synthesized is assessed.
   - **M phase** is the stage in which process of mitosis to form two daughter cells is completed. This occurs in four sequential stages: **Prophase, metaphase, anaphase, and telophase**
4. **G$_0$ phase:** The daughter cells may continue to remain in the cell cycle and divide further, or may go out of the cell cycle into resting phase, called G$_0$ phase.

Q. 2. Write a short note on mitosis.

(*RGUHS, May 2011*)

Ans. The period during which the cell is actively dividing is the phase of mitosis. The period between two successive divisions is called interphase, during which DNA content is duplicated, makes up 90% of a cell's life cycle. In mitosis, the daughter cells have identical number of chromosomes (Fig. 13.1).

1. **Prophase:** The chromatin of the chromosome becomes coiled, rod-like appearance. At the end, two chromatids of a chromosome become distinct which are held together by centromere. The centriole divides and the two daughter centrioles move towards opposite poles of the nucleus and the nuclear membrane disintegrates.
2. **Metaphase:** With the formation of the spindle, chromosomes move to a position midway between the two centrioles, where each chromosome becomes attached to microtubules.
3. **Anaphase:** The centromere of each chromosome splits longitudinally into two so that the chromatids now become independent chromosomes, which moves towards the opposite poles of the spindle.
4. **Telophase:** Two daughter nuclei are formed by appearance of nuclear membranes. Chromosomes gradually elongate and become indistinct. Nucleoli reappear. The centriole is duplicated at this stage or in early interphase.

The division of nucleus is accompanied by division of the cytoplasm.

Clinical Significance of Mitosis

1. Throughout mitosis, certain checkpoints are essential to the continuation of the process. Cancer cells can bypass these checkpoints and divide indefinitely.
2. Individuals can have a somatic or inherited mutation in certain tumor suppressor genes that will increase their risk of developing cancers.

Q. 3. Write in detail about meiosis. (*TNMGR, April 2012*)

Ans. Meiosis consists of two successive divisions called the first and second meiotic divisions. During the interphase preceding the first division, duplication of the DNA content of chromosomes takes place as in mitosis. In meiosis the number of chromosomes is reduced to half the normal number (Fig. 13.3).

First meiotic division

Prophase of the first meiotic division is prolonged and is usually divided into a number of stages as follows:

a. **Leptotene:** The chromosomes become visible (as in mitosis), but the chromatids cannot be distinguished at this stage.
b. **Zygotene:** There are 46 chromosomes in each cell consist of 23 pairs (the X- and Y-chromosomes of a male being taken as a pair). The two chromosomes of each pair come to lie parallel to each other and are closely apposed. This pairing of chromosomes is also referred to as *synapsis* or *conjugation*. The two chromosomes together constitute a bivalent.
c. **Pachytene:** The two chromatids of each chromosome become distinct. The bivalent now has four chromatids in it and is called a **tetrad**. There are two central and two peripheral chromatids—one from each chromosome. The two central chromatids (one belonging to each chromosome of the bivalent) become coiled over each other so that they cross at a number of points (*crossing over*). The site of crossing is called *chiasmata*.
d. **Diplotene:** The two chromosomes of a bivalent now try to move apart. As they do so, the chromatids involved in crossing over 'break' at the points of crossing and the 'loose' pieces become attached to the opposite chromatid. This results in exchange of genetic material between these chromatids.

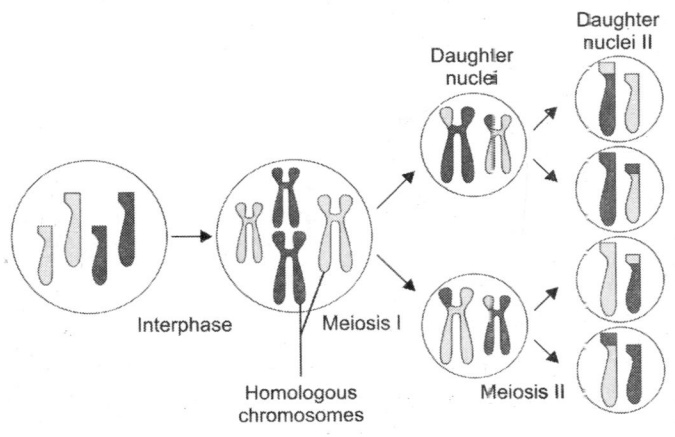

Fig. 13.3: Meiosis and its type

Interphase

Homologous chromosomes

Meiosis I

Meiosis II

Daughter nuclei

Daughter nuclei II

Metaphase: As in mitosis the forty-six chromosomes become attached to the spindle at the equator, the two chromosomes of a pair being close to each other.

Anaphase: There is no splitting of the centromeres; one entire chromosome of each pair moves to each pole of the spindle. The resulting daughter cells, therefore, have twenty-three chromosomes, each made up of two chromatids.

Telophase: Two daughter nuclei are formed. The division of nucleus is followed by division of the cytoplasm.

Second meiotic division

The first meiotic division is followed by a short *interphase*. This differs from the usual interphase in that there is no duplication of DNA. The second meiotic division is similar to mitosis. However, because of the crossing over that has occurred during the first division, the daughter cells are identical in genetic content.

Clinical Significance of Meiosis

1. This provides consistency of chromosome numbers from generation to generation.
2. During the first meiotic division the chromosomes derived from the father and those derived from the mother are distributed between the daughter cells entirely at random.
3. Crossing over, results in cells that have a distinctive genetic content.
4. Clinically, errors in meiosis can create many life-threatening conditions such as Down syndrome, Patau syndrome, Edwards's syndrome, Klinefelter's syndrome, Turner syndrome, Triple X syndrome, and XYY syndrome.

Q. 4. Write a note on germinal layers and their derivatives. *(TNMGR, Oct. 2012)*

Ans. Formation of germ layers: Blastocyst gives rise to the tissue and organs of the embryo, also gives rise to a number of structures that support the embryo and help it to acquire nutrition. At a very early stage in development, the embryo proper acquires the form of a three-layered disc. This is called the **embryonic disc** (also called **embryonic area, embryonic shield or germ disc**). The three germ layers that constitute this embryonic disc are:

1. Endoderm (endo = inside).
2. Ectoderm (ecto = outside).
3. Mesoderm (meso = in the middle).

All tissues of the body are derived from one or more of these layers.

Derivatives of Ectoderm

1. **Lining epithelia:** The epithelium lining of the following is of ectodermal origin:
   a. Skin, including its pigment cells (from neural crest cells).
   b. Mucous membrane of lips, cheeks, gums, part of floor of the mouth, part of palate, nasal cavities and paranasal sinuses.
   c. Lower part of anal canal.
   d. Terminal part of male urethra.
   e. Outer surface of labia minora and whole of labia majora.
   f. Anterior epithelium of cornea, epithelium of conjunctiva, epithelial layers of ciliary body and iris.
   g. Outer layer of tympanic membrane, epithelial lining of membranous labyrinth including the special end organs.

2. **Glands**
   a. **Exocrine:** Sweat glands, sebaceous glands, salivary glands, mammary gland, lacrimal gland.
   b. **Endocrine:** Hypophysis cerebri, adrenal medulla.

3. **Other derivatives**
   a. Hair
   b. Nails
   c. Enamel of teeth
   d. Lens of eye; musculature of iris; ciliary muscles (from neural crest); vitreous
   e. Nervous system (brain and spinal cord) including all neurons, neuroglia (except microglia), and Schwann cells (from neural crest)
   f. Pia-arachnoid (from neural crest)
   g. Branchial cartilage (from neural crest)
   h. Substance of cornea, sclera and choroid (from neural crest).

Derivatives of Endoderm

1. **Lining epithelia:** The following lining epithelia are of endodermal origin.
   i. Epithelium of part of mouth, part of palate, tongue, tonsil, pharynx, esophagus, stomach, small and large intestines and upper part of anal canal.
   ii. Epithelium of pharyngo-tympanic tube, middle ear, inner layer of tympanic membrane, mastoid antrum and air cells.
   iii. Epithelium of respiratory tract.
   iv. Epithelium of gallbladder and extrahepatic duct system; epithelium of pancreatic ducts.
   v. Epithelium of urinary bladder except trigone (mesoderm); female urethra except part of its

posterior wall (mesoderm); male urethra except part of posterior wall of its prostatic part (mesoderm) and except part of the penile urethra lying in glans penis (ectoderm).

vi. Epithelium of greater part of vagina, vestibule and inner surface of labia minora.

2. **Glands**

i. **Endocrine:** Thyroid, parathyroid, thymus, islets of Langerhans.

ii. **Exocrine:** Liver, pancreas, glands in wall of gastrointestinal tract, greater part of prostate (except inner glandular zone) and its female homologues

Derivatives of Mesoderm

1. All connective tissues including loose areolar tissue filling the interstices between other tissues, superficial and deep fascia, ligaments, tendons, aponeurosis, and dermis of skin.
2. Specialized connective tissues like adipose tissue, reticular tissue, cartilage and bone.
3. Dentin of teeth.
4. All muscles (smooth, striated and cardiac) except musculature of the iris (ectoderm) and ciliary muscles (neural crest).
5. Heart, all blood vessels and lymphatics, and blood cells.
6. Kidneys, ureters, trigone of bladder, posterior wall of part of female urethra, posterior wall of upper half of prostatic part of male urethra, and the inner glandular zone of prostate.
7. Ovary, uterus, uterine tubes, upper part of vagina.
8. Testis, epidydimis, ductus deferens, seminal vesicle, ejaculatory duct.
9. Lining mesothelium of pleural, pericardial and peritoneal cavities and of tunica vaginalis.
10. Lining mesothelium of bursae and joints.
11. Substance of cornea, sclera and choroid.
12. Substance of ciliary body and iris.
13. Duramater, pia-arachnoid and microglia.
14. Adrenal cortex.

Q. 5. Write a short note on neural crest cells. Write a short note on the aberrations associated with neural crest cells. *(TNMGR, March 2007, 2016, 2019; RGUHS, Nov. 2011; May 2012; CDER-AIIMS, May 2014; HP Uni., April 2019)*

Ans. The neural crest is a transient embryonic structure in vertebrates that gives rise to most of the peripheral nervous system (PNS) and to several non-neural cell types, including smooth muscle cells of the cardiovascular system, pigment cells in the skin, and craniofacial bones, cartilage, and connective tissue. At the time

when the neural plate is being formed, some cells at the junction between the neural plate and the rest of the ectoderm become specialized (on either side) to form the primordia of the neural crest. With the separation of the neural tube from the surface ectoderm, the cells of the neural crest appear as groups of cells lying along the dorsolateral sides of the neural tube. These neural crest cells soon become free (by losing the property of cell to cell adhesiveness). They migrate to distant places throughout the body (Fig. 13.5).

In subsequent development, several important structures are derived from the neural crest. These are:

1. Neurons of the spinal posterior nerve root ganglia.
2. Neurons of the sensory ganglia of the fifth, seventh, eighth, ninth and tenth cranial nerves.
3. Neurons of the sympathetic ganglia.
4. Schwann cells that form the neurolemmal sheaths of all peripheral nerves.
5. The specific cells of the adrenal medulla.
6. Chromaffin tissue.
7. Pigment cells (melanoblasts) of the skin.
8. Piamater and arachnoidmater.
9. Mesenchyme of the dental papilla and odontoblasts.

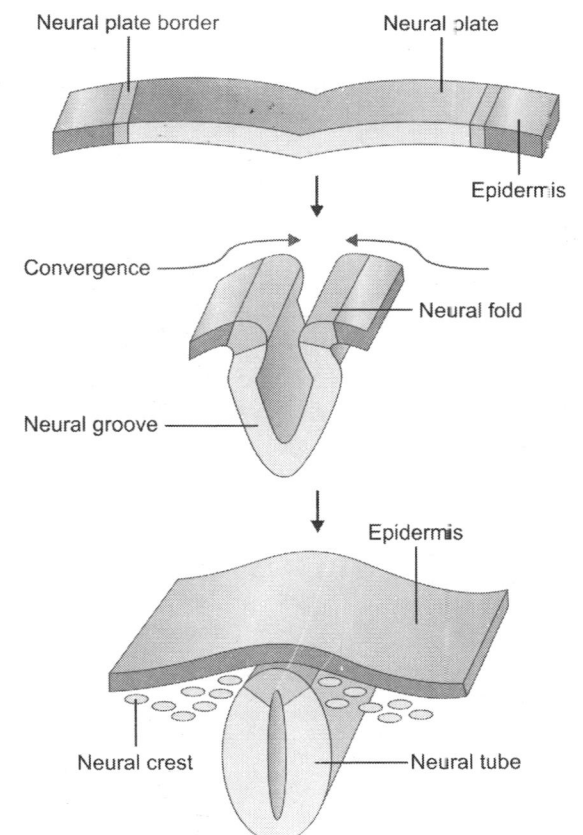

Fig. 13.5: Neural crest cells development and its migration

10. Cells arising from the cranial part of the neural crest migrate into the mesenchyme of the head and neck and influence development of somaitomeres. They play an important role in development of musculature of head and formation of face.

Aberrations: Neurocutaneous syndromes
1. Hirschsprung's disease
2. Riley-Day syndrome
3. Neurofibromatosis I
4. Tuberous sclerosis complex
5. Epidermal nevus syndrome
6. Incontinentia pigmenti (Bloch-Sulzberger syndrome)
7. Incontinentia pigmenti achromians (hypomelanosis of Ito)
8. Neurocutaneous melanosis
9. Sturge-Weber syndrome
10. Klippel-Trénaunay-Weber syndrome
11. Waardenburg syndromes: Types I, II, III, and IV.

Q. 6. Write a short note on Meckel's cartilage.
(CDER-AIIMS, May 1990; TNMGR, March 2007, April 2012)

Ans. It is derived from first branchial arch around 41–45th day of IUL. It extends from the cartilaginous otic capsule to midline or symphysis and provides a template for guiding the growth of the mandible. Major portion of this cartilage disappears and remaining part develops into (*see* Fig. 1.1c):

1. Mental ossicles
2. Incus and malleus
3. Spine of the sphenoid
4. Anterior ligament of malleus
5. Sphenomandibular ligament

The ossifying membrane is located lateral to Meckel's cartilage and its accompanying neurovascular bundle. From this primary centre, the ossification spreads below and around inferior alveolar nerve and its incisive branch and upwards to form a trough for accommodating developing tooth buds. Spread of the intramembranous ossification dorsally and ventrally forms the body and ramus of mandible.

As ossification continues, Meckel's cartilage becomes surrounded and invaded by bone. Ossification stops at the site that will later become the mandibular lingula from where the Meckel's cartilage continues into the middle ear and develops into auditory ossicles. The sphenomandibular ligament which extends from the lingula of mandible to the sphenoid bone also forms a remnant of the Meckel's cartilage.

Q. 7. Write a short note on endochondral and intramembranous ossification. *(TNMGR, April 2012)*

Ans. Bone ossification, or osteogenesis, is the process of bone formation. This process begins between 6–7th weeks of IUL and continues till the age of 25. There are two types of bone ossification (Fig. 13.7).

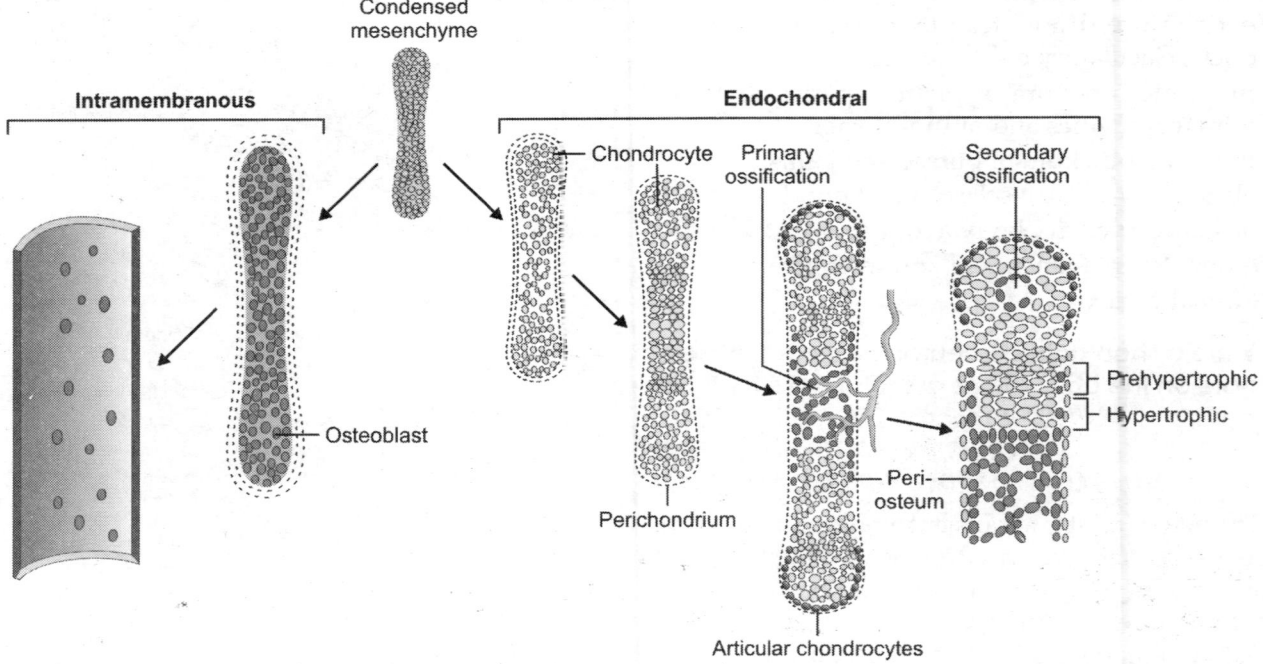

Fig. 13.7: Ossification—(L) intramembranous, (R) endochondral

Intramembranous ossification directly converts mesenchymal tissue to bone and forms flat bones of skull, clavicle, and most of the cranial bones. Mesenchymal cells differentiate into osteoblasts and group into ossification centers. Osteoblasts become entrapped by the osteoid they secrete, transforming them to osteocytes. Trabecular bone and periosteum form cortical bone forms superficially to the trabecular bone. Blood vessels form the red marrow.

Endochondral ossification: It begins with mesenchymal tissue transforming into a cartilage intermediate, which is later replaced by bone and forms remainder of axial skeleton and long bones. Mesenchymal cells differentiate into chondrocytes and form cartilage model for bone. Chondrocytes near center of cartilage model undergo hypertrophy and alter contents of matrix they secrete, enabling mineralization. Chondrocytes undergo apoptosis due to decreased nutrient availability; Blood vessels invade and bring osteogenic cells. **Primary ossification** center forms in diaphyseal region of periosteum called *periosteal collar*. **Secondary ossification** centers develop in epiphyseal region after birth. Development of skeleton can be traced back to three derivatives:

Cranial neural crest cells: These form flat bones of skull, clavicle, and cranial bones (excluding a portion of the temporal and occipital bones).

Somites: These form remainder of axial skeleton.

Lateral plate mesoderm: This forms long bones.

Q. 8. Describe briefly the development of face.
(BFUHS, Nov. 2003; Gujarat Uni., Oct. 2004; TNMGR, Sept. 2009, April 2012; DRMLA Uni., July 2013)

Q. Add a note on the common developmental anomalies.
(Sumandeep Uni., June 2016; CDER-AIIMS, May 2017)

Q. Write a short note on buccopharyngeal membrane.
(RUHS, July 2016)

Ans. After formation of the head fold, the developing brain and the pericardium form two prominent bulging on ventral aspect of the embryo. These bulgings are separated by stomatodaeum. The floor of stomatodaeum is formed by **buccopharyngeal membrane**, which separates it from foregut. Soon mesoderm covering developing forebrain proliferates and forms a downward projection that overlaps upper part of stomatodaeum. This downward projection is called **frontonasal process**.

The pharyngeal arches are laid down in lateral and ventral walls of most cranial part of foregut. The face is derived from following structures that lie around stomatodaeum (Fig. 13.8):

a. Frontonasal process
b. First pharyngeal (or mandibular) arch of each side.

At this stage, each mandibular arch forms lateral wall of stomatodaeum. This arch gives off a bud from its dorsal end. This bud is called **maxillary process**. It grows ventro-medially cranial to the main of the arch which is now called **mandibular process**.

The ectoderm overlying frontonasal process soon shows bilateral localized thickenings, **nasal placodes** induced by underlying forebrain. The placodes soon sink below the surface to form **nasal pits**. The pits are continuous with stomatodaeum below. The edges of each pit are raised above the surface; medial raised edge is called **medial nasal process (MNP)** and lateral edge is called **lateral nasal process (LNP)**.

Lower lip: Mandibular processes of two sides grow towards each other and fuse in midline, forming lower margin of stomatodaeum. The fused mandibular processes give rise to lower lip, and to lower jaw.

Upper lip

1. Each maxillary process now grows medially and fuses, first with lateral nasal process and then with medial nasal process. The medial and lateral nasal processes also fuse with each other. In this way the nasal pits (now called **external nares**) are cut off from stomatodaeum.

2. With considerable growth of maxillary processes, frontonasal process becomes much narrower from side to side, with the result that two external nares come closer together.

3. The stomatodaeum is now bounded above by upper lip which is derived as follows.
   a. The mesodermal basis of lateral part of lip is formed from maxillary process. The overlying skin is derived from ectoderm covering this process.
   b. The mesodermal basis of median part of the lip (called **philtrum**) is formed from frontonasal process. The ectoderm of maxillary process overgrows this mesoderm to meet that of the opposite maxillary process in midline. As a result, skin of entire upper lip is innervated by maxillary nerves.

4. The muscles of face (and lips) are derived from mesoderm of 2nd branchial arch and are therefore supplied by facial nerve.

Nose: The nose receives contributions from frontonasal process, and from medial and lateral nasal processes of right and left sides. External nares are formed when nasal pits are cut off from stomatodaeum by fusion of maxillary process with medial nasal process. The

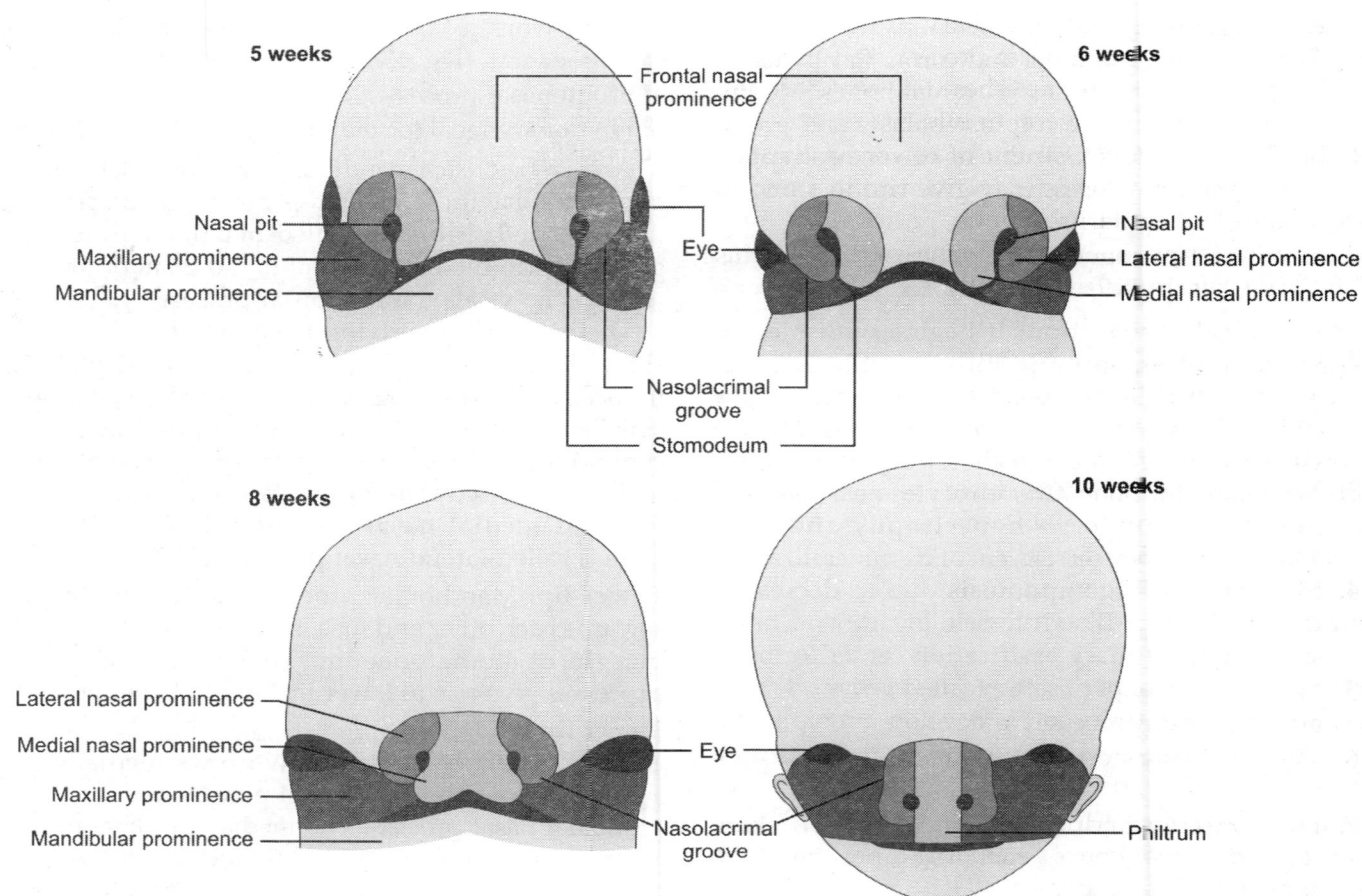

Fig. 13.8: Development of face

external nares gradually approach each other as frontonasal process becomes progressively narrower and its deeper part forms nasal septum. Simultaneously, a groove appears between region of nose and bulging forebrain (which may now be called **forehead**). As nose becomes prominent, external nares come to open downwards instead of forwards.

Cheek

The stomatodaeum bounded above by maxillary process and below by mandibular process. These processes undergo progressive fusion with each other to form cheeks. During formation of upper lip, maxillary process fuses with lateral nasal process. This fusion extends from stomatodaeum to medial angle of developing eye. This line of fusion is marked by a groove called **naso-optic furrow or nasolacrimal sulcus**. A strip of ectoderm becomes buried along this furrow and gives rise to **nasolacrimal duct**.

Eye

The region of eye is first seen as an ectodermal thickening, **lens placodes**, which appear on ventrolateral side of developing forebrain. The lens placode sinks below the surface and is eventually cut off from surface ectoderm. The developing eyeball produces a bulging in this situation. The bulging of eyes is at first directed laterally, and lies in the angles between maxillary processes and lateral nasal processes. The eyelids are derived from folds of ectoderm that are formed above and below eyes, and by mesoderm enclosed within the folds.

External ear

The external ear is formed around dorsal part of first ectodermal cleft. A series of mesodermal thickenings (**tubercles or hillocks**) appear on mandibular and hyoid arches where they adjoin this cleft. The pinna (or auricle) is formed by fusion of these thickenings.

Developmental anomalies of face (*TNMGR, April 2013*)

It has been seen that the formation of various parts of face involves fusion of diverse components. This fusion is occasionally incomplete and gives rise to various anomalies.

1. **Harelip:** The upper lip of the hare normally has a cleft. Hence, the term harelip is used for defects of the lips.

a. When one or both maxillary processes do not fuse with medial nasal process, this gives rise to defects in upper lip. These may vary in degree and may be unilateral or bilateral.

b. Defective development of lowermost part of frontonasal process may give rise to a midline defect of upper lip.

c. When two mandibular processes do not fuse with each other, lower lip shows a defect in midline. The defect usually extends into jaw.

2. **Oblique facial cleft:** Non-fusion of maxillary and lateral nasal process gives rise to a cleft running from medial angle of eye to mouth. The nasolacrimal duct is not formed.

3. **Macrostomia:** Inadequate fusion of mandibular and maxillary processes with each other, leading to an abnormally wide mouth.

4. **Microstomia:** Too much fusion of mandibular and maxillary processes with each other may lead to small mouth.

5. **Lateral facial cleft:** Lack of fusion of mandibular and maxillary processes with each other.

6. The nose may be bifid or one half of it may be absent.

7. **Proboscis:** A cylindrical projection, jutting out form just below the forehead. This anomaly may sometimes affect only one half of the nose.

8. **Cyclops:** Fusion of two eyes leading to single median eye.

9. **Mandibulofacial dysostosis/Treacher Collins syndrome or first arch syndrome:** The entire first arch may remain underdeveloped on one or both sides, affecting lower eyelid (coloboma type defect), maxilla, mandible and external ear. The prominence of cheek is absent and ear may be displaced.

10. **Retrognathia:** Mandible may be small compared to rest of the face resulting in a receding chin.

11. **Agnathia:** Mandible may fail to develop.

12. **Hypertelorism:** The widely separated eyes with broad nasal bridge resulting from presence of excessive tissue in the frontonasal process.

13. The lips may show congenital pits or fistulae. The lip may be double.

Q. 9. Write a note on pharyngeal pouches.

(*TNMGR, April 2001; Oct. 2012; KUHS, June 2013*)

Q. Write a note on pharyngeal arches and their derivatives.   (*MUHS, Dec. 2016; AHSUC, May 2018; TNMGR, Oct. 2019*)

Ans. After the establishment of head fold, foregut is bounded ventrally by pericardium, and dorsally by developing brain. Cranially, it is at first separated from stomatodaeum by buccopharyngeal membrane. When this membrane breaks down, the foregut opens to exterior through the stomatodaeum (future mouth). At this stage, head is represented by the bulging caused by developing brain while pericardium may be considered as occupying the region of future thorax. The neck is formed by elongation of region between stomatodaeum and pericardium, mainly due to appearance of a series of mesodermal thickenings in the wall of cranial—most part of foregut, called **pharyngeal or branchial arches** (Fig. 13.9). In the interval between any two adjoining arches, the endoderm extends outwards in the form of a pouch (**endodermal or pharyngeal pouch**) to meet the ectoderm which dips into this interval as an *ectodermal cleft*.

First arch is called **mandibular arch**; and second is **hyoid arch**. Third, fourth and sixth arches do not have special names. Fifth arch disappears soon after its formation; so that only five arches remain. The following structures are formed in the mesoderm of each arch.

1. **A skeletal element:** This is cartilaginous to begin with. It may remain cartilaginous, may develop into bone, or may disappear.

2. **Striated muscle:** This is supplied by the nerve of the arch.

3. **An arterial arch:** Ventral to the foregut, an artery called *ventral aorta develops*. Dorsal to foregut, another artery called *dorsal aorta*, is formed. A series of arterial arches (**aortic arches**) connect the ventral and dorsal aortae. One such arterial arch lies in each pharyngeal arch.

Each pharyngeal arch is supplied by a nerve. In addition to supplying skeletal muscle of arch, it supplies sensory branches to overlying ectoderm and endoderm.

Derivatives of the skeletal element (Table 13.9)

The cartilage of first arch is called **Meckel's cartilage.** The incus and malleus (of the middle ear) is derived from its dorsal end. The ventral part of cartilage is surrounded by developing mandible, and is absorbed. The part of the cartilage extending from the region of middle ear to mandible disappears but its sheath (perichondrium) forms anterior ligament of malleus and sphenomandibular ligament. Mesenchyme of first arch is also responsible for formation of bones such as maxilla, mandible, zygomatic, palatine and part of temporal bone.

Nerves and muscles of the arches

All the muscles derived from a pharyngeal arch are supplied by nerve of arch. These nerves also innervate

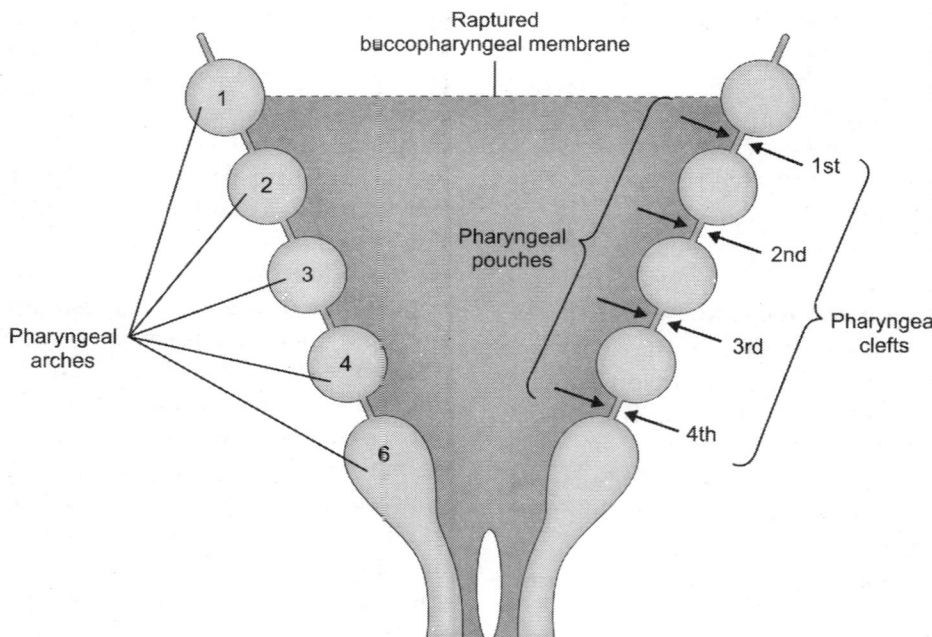

Fig. 13.9: Pharyngeal arches with pouches and cleft

Table 13.9: Derivatives of the skeletal element

Arch	Skeleton	Muscle	Nerve
First (mandibular)	Maxillary process: 1. Upper jaw 2. Palate 3. Dentine Mandibular process give rise to Meckel's cartilage: 1. Malleus 2. Incus 3. Anterior ligament of malleus 4. Sphenomandibular ligament 5. Body of mandible between mental and mandibular foramen 6. Symphysis menti.	1. Medial and lateral pterygoids 2. Masseter 3. Temporalis 4. Mylohyoid 5. Anterior belly of digastric 6. Tensor tympani 7. Tensor palati	1. Mandibular nerve (post-trematic) 2. Chorda tympani (pre-trematic)
Second (hyoid)	It gives rise to Reichert's cartilage: (**five "S"**) 1. Stapes 2. Styloid process 3. Stylohyoid 4. Smaller cornu of hyoid bone 5. Superior part of body of hyoid bone	1. Muscles of face 2. Occipitofrontalis 3. Platysma 4. Stylohyoid 5. Posterior belly of digastric 6. Stapedius 7. Auricular muscles	Facial nerve
Third	Its dorsal part disappears and ventral part forms: 1. Greater cornu of hyoid bone 2. Cuneiform cartilage	1. Stylopharyngeus 2. Superior constrictor of pharynx	Glossopharyngeal nerve
Fourth	1. Thyroid cartilage 2. Cuneiform cartilage	1. Cricothyroid muscle 2. Middle and inferior constrictor of pharynx	Superior laryngeal nerve Muscles of larynx and pharynx
Fifth	Not known (thyroid cartilage may develop)	None	Not known
Sixth	1. Cricoid cartilage 2. Corniculate cartilage 3. Arytenoid cartilage	Intrinsic muscles of larynx except cricothyroid	Recurrent laryngeal nerve

parts of skin and mucous membrane derived from arches. Some of the nerves (e.g. glossopharyngeal) have only a small motor component and are predominantly sensory. The first arch has a double nerve supply. Mandibular nerve is **post-trematic nerve** (nerve of arch itself, which runs along cranial border of arch) of first arch, while chorda tympani (branch of facial nerve) is **pretrematic nerve** (nerve of succeeding arch, which runs along caudal border of arch). These double innervations are reflected in nerve supply of anterior two-thirds of tongue which are derived from ventral part of first arch.

Fate of ectodermal clefts

After the formation of pharyngeal arches, the region of the neck is marked on the outside by a series of grooves, **ectodermal clefts**. Dorsal part of first cleft (between the first and second arches) develops into epithelial lining of *external acoustic meatus*. The **pinna** (or auricle) is formed from a series of swellings or hillocks that arise on the first and second arches, where they adjoin the first cleft. The ventral part of this cleft is obliterated.

Second arch grows much faster than the succeeding arches and comes to overhang them. The space between the overhanging second arch and third, fourth and sixth arches is called **cervical sinus**. The lower overhanging border of second arch fuses with tissues caudal to the arches. The cavity of cervical sinus is normally obliterated. Part of it may persist and give rise to swellings that lie in the neck, along the anterior border of sternocleidomastoid. These are called **branchial cysts**, and are most commonly located just below the angle of the mandible. If such a cyst opens onto the surface, it becomes a *branchial sinus*.

Fate of endodermal pouches

First pouch

a. Its ventral part is obliterated by formation of **tongue**.
b. Its dorsal part receives contribution from dorsal part of second pouch, and together forms a diverticulum known as **tubo-tympanic recess** that grows towards the region of developing ear. The proximal part of this recess gives rise to the **auditory (pharyngo-tympanic) tube**, and the distal part to *middle ear cavity*, including tympanic antrum.

Second pouch

a. The epithelium of ventral part contributes to the formation of the **tonsil**.
b. The dorsal part takes part in the formation of **tubo-tympanic recess**.

Third pouch: Inferior parathyroid glands, and thymus.

Fourth pouch: Superior parathyroid glands, and may contribute to **thyroid gland**.

Fifth or ultimobranchial pouch: A fifth pouch is seen for a brief period during development. It is generally believed to be incorporated into the fourth pouch. The two together forming the **caudal pharyngeal complex**. The superior parathyroid glands arise from this complex. The complex probably also gives origin to the parafollicular cells of the thyroid gland.

Q. 10. Write a short note on primary and secondary cartilages. *(TNMGR, March 2008)*

Q. Write a note on development and role of primary and secondary cartilages in craniofacial development. *(TNMGR, June 2017)*

Ans.

1. **Primary cartilage:** Cartilage of the pharyngeal arches is known as primary cartilage. In this the chondroblasts are surrounded by a cartilaginous matrix, e.g. Meckel's cartilage, cartilages of cranial base.

2. **Secondary cartilage:** It does not develop from the established primary cartilage of the skull. In this, the chondroblasts are not surrounded by a cartilaginous matrix. It is formed after and separate from the primary cartilaginous skeleton, e.g. condylar cartilage, symphysis, ends of clavicle.

14. HUMAN HISTOLOGY

Q. 1. Write a short note on microscopic structure of spleen. *(TNMGR, March 2009)*

Ans. It is the largest lymphoid organ of the body **(Fig. P-6; Color Plate 2)**.

1. It consists of an outermost serous coat derived from peritoneum.
2. Trabeculae arising from the capsule extend into the substance of the spleen.
3. The capsule and trabeculae are made up of fibrous tissue.
4. Trabeculae divide the substance of spleen into lobules.
5. Each lobule contains red and white pulp.
6. The spaces between the trabeculae are composed of reticular network, consisting of reticular cells and macrophages.
7. The interstices of reticulum contain lymphocytes, blood vessels and blood cells.
8. *White pulp* is made up of collection of lymphocytes and plasma cells which are distributed as small ovoid and opaque white areas in the red pulp. The margins of white pulp present dendritic antigen processing cells.

9. *Red pulp* is like a sponge, and is arranged in the form of irregular cords of cells known as **Bilroth's cords**, filled by B- and T-lymphocytes, macrophages, and blood cells and lined by reticular cells.

Q. 2. Write a short note on histology of cartilage.
(TNMGR, Sept. 2008)

Ans. Cartilage is avascular, receives nutrition through diffusion from the nearest capillaries. It is also insensitive to pain and pressure as it has no nerves. Cartilage is surrounded by perichondrium and grows by appositional as well as interstitial growth. It is considered as modified connective tissue, with cells distributed in homogeneous ground substance within which fibers are embedded.

Cartilage cells: Chondrocytes lying in lacunae.

Ground substance: Complex molecules containing proteins and carbohydrates.

Fibres: Type II collagen fibers.

Types of cartilage:

1. **Hyaline cartilage:** It consists of bluish, opalescent tissue which is widely distributed in the body. It is surrounded by perichondrium, which is made of outer fibrous and inner cellular layer. Matrix is homogeneous and cells are arranged in groups surrounded by lacunae **(Fig. P-7a; Color Plate 3)**, e.g. articular cartilage, thyroid cartilage, cricoid cartilage, lower part of arytenoid cartilage, tracheal rings, costal cartilage, bronchial cartilage, and nasal cartilage.

2. **Elastic cartilage:** Perichondrium is absent. The matrix is traversed by thin yellow elastic fibres which anastomose and branch in all directions. Extracellular matrix is metachromatic due to high concentration of glycosaminoglycans. Chondrocytes are present as single cells or in small groups **(Fig. P-7b; Color Plate 3)**, e.g. pinna of external ear, epiglottis, corniculate cartilage, cuneiform cartilage, apex of arytenoid cartilage, auditory tube, and external auditory meatus.

3. **White fibro-cartilage:** Perichondrium is absent. It consists of many regularly arranged collagen fibres like a tendon. It is less cellular than hyaline cartilage and chondrocytes are scattered sparsely all over **(Fig. P-7c; Color Plate 3)**, e.g. intervertebral disc, interpubic disc, menisci of knee joint, articular disc of TMJ, sternoclavicular and inferior radioulnar joints.

Q. 3. Write a short note on histology/microanatomy of bone.
(TNMGR, Sept. 2007, April 2013; HNBG Uni., Dec. 2018)

Ans. Bone is considered as specialized, highly vascular, mineralized connective tissue, with cells distributed in homogeneous ground substance within which collagen fibers and mineral salts are embedded. Bone has:

a. **Cellular component:**
   1. Osteogenic cells: Stem/precursors cells present in inner layer of periosteum.
   2. Osteoblasts: Large basophilic cells with round and eccentrically place nucleus. They secrete collagen fibres and matrix.
   3. Osteocytes: Mature cells present in the matrix. The cytoplasm is less basophilic and the processes radiates in all the directions
   4. Osteoclasts: Large multinucleated cells with eosinophilic cytoplasm. They help in resorption and remodeling of bone.

b. **Matrix:** 40% organic substance (mostly collagen fibres embedded in ground substance), and 60% inorganic substance (mostly inorganic salts of calcium and phosphates).

Histologically: Bones are of two types:

a. **Compact bone:** It is covered by periosteum, consists of outer fibrous and inner cellular layer (osteogenic cell). **Haversian system** is present which has **(Fig. P-8a; Color Plate 3)**:
   1. A centrally placed Haversian canal surrounded by 6–12 concentric lamellae.
   2. Each lamella is formed by collagen fibres and deposited calcium salts.
   3. Lamellae present next to endosteum are called *inner circumferential lamellae.*
   4. Lamellae present adjacent to periosteum are called *outer circumferential lamellae.*
   5. Lamellae present between two Haversian systems are called *interstitial lamellae.*
   6. In between the lamellae, there are lacunar spaces containing osteocytes, with processes into canaliculi, which provide nourishment to osteocytes.
   7. *Volkmann's canal* connects Haversian canal to other Haversian canals as well as with marrow cavity.

b. **Cancellous bone/spongy bone/trabecular bone (Fig. P-8b; Color Plate 4)**
   1. Periosteum is present.
   2. Thin plates of bone tissue known as trabeculae are also present.

3. In between the adjoining trabeculae, there are irregular spaces containing red bone marrow.
4. Osteocytes are present in the lacunae of trabeculae. Osteoblasts and osteoclasts are present at the margins of trabeculae.

Q. 4. Write about histologic picture of lymph node.
(RGUHS, July 2016)

Ans. Each lymph node consists of connective tissue framework and numerous cells **(Fig. P-9; Color Plate 4)**.

Connective Tissue Framework

1. The lymph node is covered by a capsule consisting of mainly of collagen fibers, and some elastic and smooth muscle fibers.
2. Multiple connective tissue septa extend into node from the capsule and divide into lobules.
3. Hilum is occupied by dense fibrous tissue.
4. Fibroblasts are associated with connective tissue framework.

Cells of Lymph Node

1. Rest of the node is occupied by network of reticular fibers filled with lymphocytes, which aggregated to form lymphatic nodules (composed of B-lymphocytes).
2. Lymphatic nodules are present in the outer zone of lymph node, known as cortex.
3. The diffuse lymphoid tissue intervening between nodules is made up of T-lymphocytes.
4. The space between capsule and cortex is known as *subcapsular sinus*.
5. *Medulla* is area around the hilum, inner to cortex, mainly composed of blood vessels and a few lymphocytes.
6. Reticular cells associated with connective tissue framework.
7. Macrophages are present in the lymph sinuses.
8. Endothelial cells lining the blood vessels of lymph nodes.
9. Pericytes and smooth muscle cells present around the blood vessels.

Dental Anatomy and Dental Histology

1. TEETH DEVELOPMENT AND ABNORMALITIES

Q. 1. Discuss in detail the development of tooth.
(TNMGR, March 2010; Guwahati Uni., May 2011; RGUHS, May 2014; Sumandeep Uni., April 2015; MUHS, Dec. 2017)

Q. Add a note on various theories of tooth development. *(NTR, Uni., May 2019)*

Q. Write a short note on enamel organ and its function. *(TNMGR, March 2007)*

Q. Add a note on development disturbances of the enamel. *(Gujarat, Uni., July 2017)*

Ans. Development of tooth is a complex process. Tooth formation starts in 6th week of IUL with formation of primary epithelial band. At about 7th week primary epithelial band divides into a lingual process called **dental lamina** and a buccal process called **vestibular lamina**. All deciduous teeth arises from dental lamina, later permanent successors arise from its lingual extension and permanent molars (accessors) from its distal extension. Tooth germ includes all the formative tissues for tooth and its supporting structures and has three main components:

- Enamel organ: Ectodermal component that gives rise to enamel.
- Dental papilla: Ectomesenchymal component that gives rise to dentin and pulp.
- Dental follicle or dental sac: Ectomesenchymal component giving rise to cementum, periodontal ligament (PDL) and part of alveolar socket.

Stages of Tooth Development (Fig. 1.1)

1. Bud stage
2. Cap stage
3. Bell stage

- Early bell stage.
- Late or advanced bell stage

Bud Stage: Enamel organ is bud shaped with peripheral cuboidal cells and central polyhedral cells. Peripheral cells of enamel organ are separated from ectomesenchymal components by a basement membrane. All the cells are attached to each other by desmosomal junctions. Ectomesenchymal condensation adjacent to enamel organ forms **dental papilla**. Marginal condensation of ectomesenchymal cells enclosing dental papilla and enamel organ is called **dental follicle or dental sac**.

Cap Stage: Enamel organ increases in size and attain shape of a cap by invagination of deep portion of bud. Cells lining the convexity or periphery of the cap are cuboidal in shape and are called **outer enamel epithelium (OEE)**. The cells lining the concave or invaginated portion change to columnar cells, **inner enamel epithelium (IEE)**. Central polyhedral cells transform into network of star-shaped cells called **stellate reticulum**. Dental papilla gets partially enclosed by invaginated portion of enamel organ. Cells of dental papilla undergo proliferation and condensation of ectomesenchymal cells and become more fibrous and denser.

Early Bell Stage: Enamel organ enlarges further and invagination deepens changing shape to that of a bell and four different layers of cells are seen in enamel organ. Cells lining IEE is composed of single layer of tall columnar cells that differentiate to *ameloblasts* (enamel forming cells). **Stratum intermedium (new)** is located between IEE and stellate reticulum and is composed of 2–3 layers of squamous cells. Cells of OEE lining periphery of enamel organ flattens to low cuboidal cells. At cervical region of enamel organ OEE loops inward to join with IEE called **cervical loop**. During early bell stage enamel organ loses its connection to oral ectoderm due to degeneration of dental

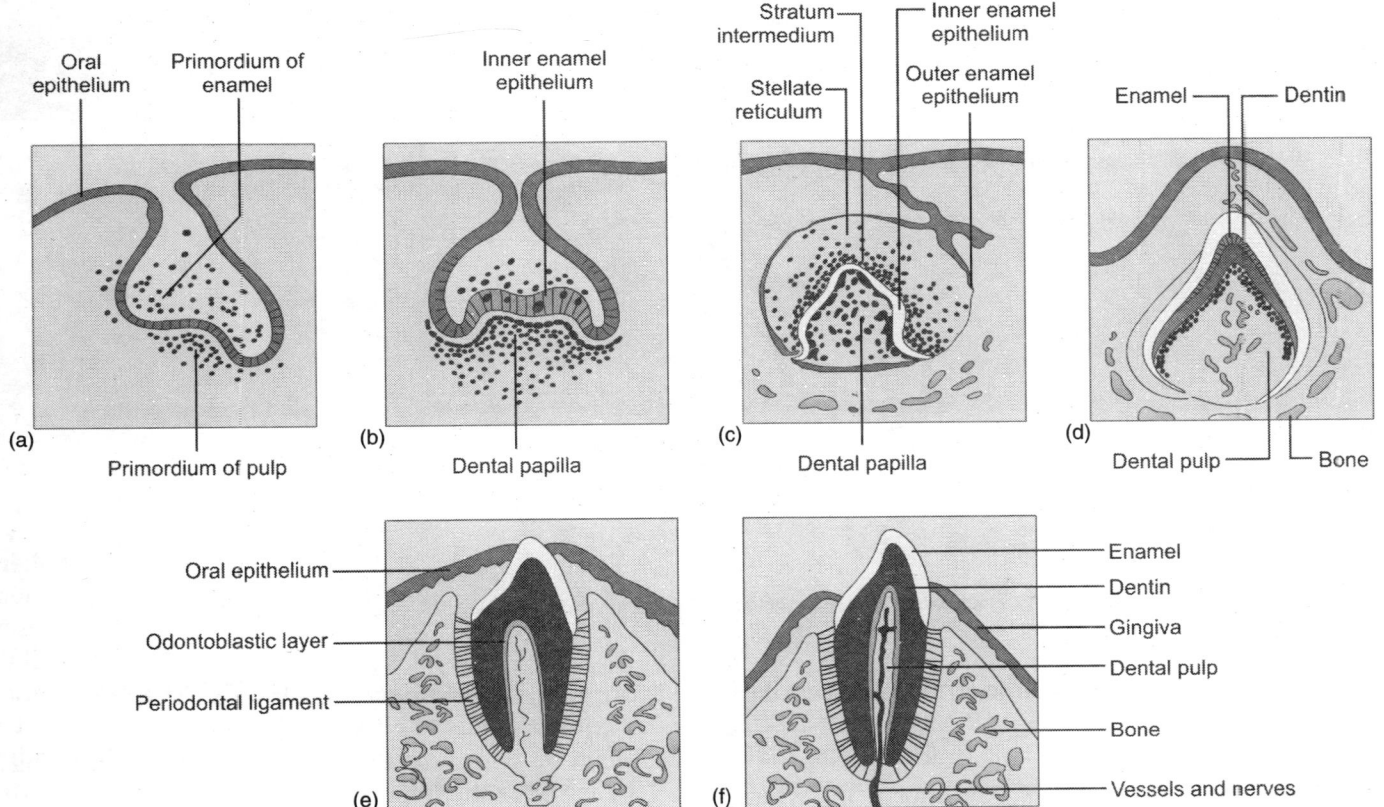

Fig. 1.1: Stages of tooth development: a. Bud stage; b. Cap stage; c. Early bell stage; d. Advanced bell stage; e. Eruption stage; f. Fully formed stage

lamina. Remnants of dental lamina are called **cell rests of serres**. Successional lamina develops at this stage which is the primordium for the permanent successor. Peripheral cells of dental papilla differentiate into *odontoblasts* (dentin forming cells) under the organizing influence of IEE cells. Dental follicle becomes more fibrous with 3 layers, i.e. inner cellular, outer fibrous layer and middle loose connective tissue.

Advanced Bell Stage: Differentiating feature between early and advanced bell stage is formation of hard tissues. Enamel organ shows four different layers, IEE, stratum intermedium, stellate reticulum and OEE. Histological difference from early bell stage are: Hard tissue formation, collapsed stellate reticulum and folding of OEE bringing capillaries of dental follicle nearer to ameloblasts. Dental papilla shows differentiated odontoblast at the periphery.

Q. 2. Write a short note on stellate reticulum.
(RGUHS, April 2006)

Ans. Stellate reticulum/enamel pulp: Polygonal cells located in the center of epithelial organ, between outer and inner enamel epithelium; begin to separate due to water being drawn into enamel organ from surrounding dental papilla as a result of osmotic force exerted by glycosaminoglycans (GAG) contained in ground substance. As a result, the polygonal cells become star shaped but maintains contact with each other by their cytoplasmic process. The spaces in between are filled with mucoid fluid, rich in albumin, giving a cushion-like consistency, protecting the delicate enamel forming cells. The cells in the centre of enamel organ are densely packed and form enamel knot and vertical extension of **enamel knot** is known as enamel cord. Both are temporary structure; act as a reservoir of dividing cells for growing enamel organ (Fig. 1.2).

Functions:
1. It provides elasticity and resistance.
2. Acts as buffer against forces that might distort developing dentinoenamel junction (DEJ).
3. It permits only limited flow of nutritional elements from overlying blood vessels to formative cells.
4. Acts as a shock absorber that may support and protect delicate enamel forming cells.

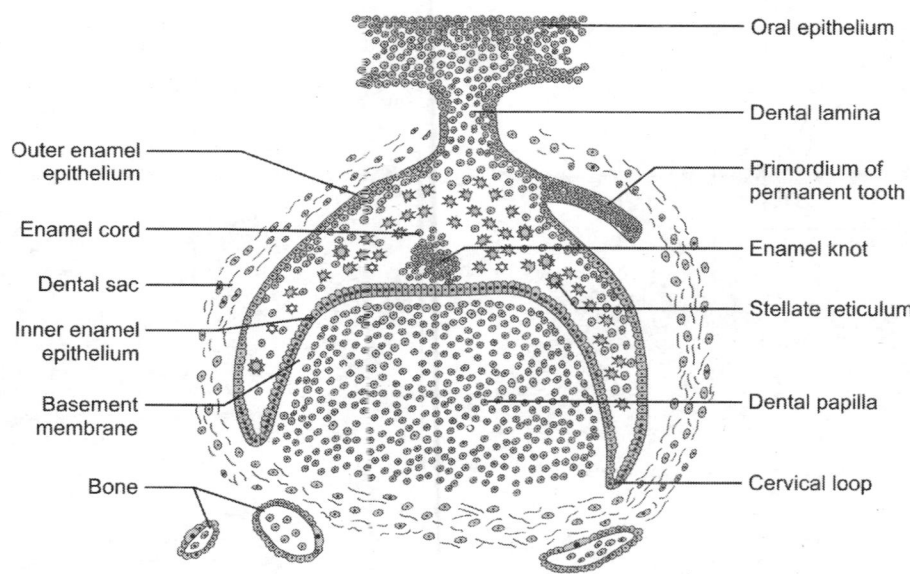

Fig. 1.2: Tooth bud showing star-shaped stellate reticulum, enamel knot and enamel cord

Q. 3. Write a short note on developmental anomalies in tooth morphology.
(TNMGR, Sept. 2007; AHSUC, May 2018)

Ans. Developmental anomalies: An abnormality where pathology starts in embryonic stage of human life before formation of dentition. These include:

1. One or more teeth may be absent. Complete absence is called **Anodontia**.
2. Supernumerary teeth may be present.
3. Individual teeth may be abnormal. They may be too large (**Macrodont**) or too small (**Microdont**).
4. Two (or more) teeth may be fused to each other (**Gemination/Fusion**).
5. **Concrescence:** Union of teeth by cementum only.
6. Dilacerations: Sharp bend in root or crown of tooth.
7. Talon cusp: Accessory cusp projecting from cingulum of incisors.
8. Dense in dente: Invagination in surface of tooth crown before calcification.
9. Dense evaginatus: Proliferation and evagination of an area of IEE during tooth development.
10. Taurodontism: Body of tooth is enlarged at expense of roots.
11. The alignment of the upper and lower teeth may be incorrect (**Malocclusion**). This may be caused by one or more of the above anomalies or by defects of the jaws.
12. Eruption of teeth may be precocious (i.e. too early). Lower incisors may be present at birth (natal/neonatal teeth).
13. Eruption of teeth may be delayed. The third molar frequently fails to erupt.
14. Teeth may form in abnormal situations, e.g. in the ovary or in the hypophysis cerebri.
15. There may be improper formation of the enamel (**Amelogenesis imperfecta**) or dentin (**Dentinogenesis imperfecta**) of the tooth.

Q. 4. Write a short note on theories of tooth eruption.
(TNMGR, Oct. 2012; KUHS, June 2013; RUHS, May 2015; Sumandeep Uni., June 2017; AHSUC, May 2018; DYP Uni., May 2019)

Q. Write a short note on gubernacular cord.
(NTR Uni., May 2018)

Ans. Tooth eruption is defined as the movement of a tooth from its site of development within the alveolar process to its functional position in the oral cavity.

Phases of tooth eruption:

1. **Pre-eruptive phase:** This phase begins in early bell stage and ends at beginning of root formation. Made by deciduous and permanent tooth germs within tissues of jaw before they begin to erupt.
2. **Eruptive phase** (Fig.1.4): It starts with initiation of root formation and made by teeth to move from its position within bone of jaw to its functional position in occlusion. This has intraosseous and extra-osseous compartments.
   a. **Active eruption:** It is gradual appearance of tooth in oral cavity due to axial occlusal movement of tooth.

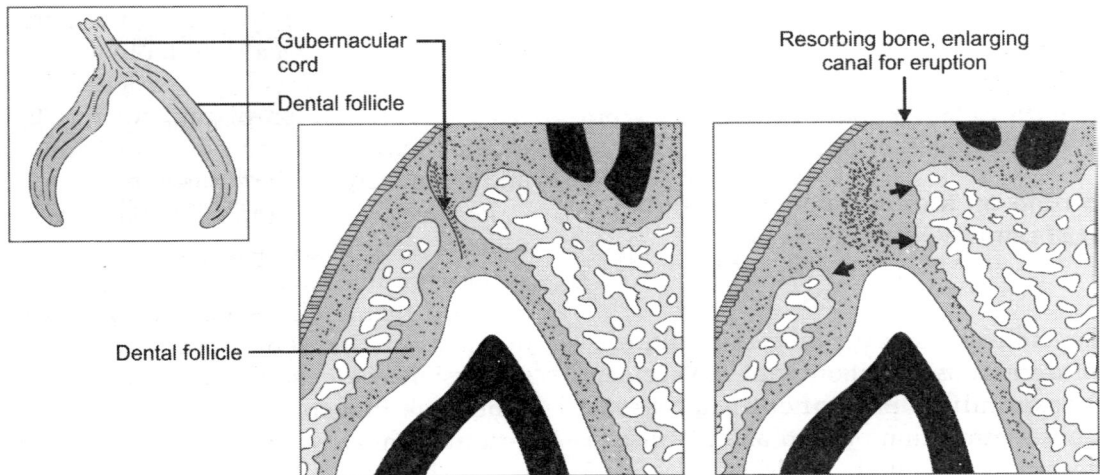

Fig. 1.4: Eruption of tooth through gubernacular cord

b. **Passive eruption:** It happens due to gradual retraction of attachment epithelium from tooth surface.

c. **Gubernacular cord:** As deciduous tooth erupts, permanent tooth germ become situated apically and is entirely enclosed by the bone except for a small canal that is filled with connective tissue and often contains epithelial remnants of the dental lamina known as "**gubernacular cord**".

d. **Gubernacular canal:** Holes noted in a dry skull lingual to primary teeth in jaws that represent openings of gubernacular cord. After removal of any overlying bone there is loss of intervening soft tissue between reduced enamel epithelium covering crown of tooth and overlying oral epithelium.

3. **Posteruptive phase:** Takes place after the teeth are functioning to maintain the position of erupted tooth in occlusion while jaws are continuing to grow and compensate for occlusal and proximal tooth wear.

Mechanism of tooth movements/theories of tooth eruption

1. **Bone remodeling theory (Brash, 1928):** Simultaneous bone deposition and bone resorption in area around tooth causes its axial movement.

2. **Root elongation theory:** The apical growth of roots results in axial directed force that leads to tooth eruption.

3. **Vascular pressure theory (V. Korff, 1935):** Alteration in local vascular supply and increase in local tissue pressure in PDL leads to tooth eruption.

4. **Periodontal ligament traction theory (Thomas, 1967):** The contractility of fibroblasts present in the PDL provides force for tooth eruption.

5. **Pulp constriction theory:** The growth of root dentin and constriction of pulp causes sufficient pressure to move tooth occlusally.

6. **Dental follicle theory (Marks and Cahill, 1984):** Specific cellular changes occurring in and around the follicle leads to tooth eruption.

Factors affecting tooth eruption:

1. **Genetic:** Genetic factors definitely controls tooth emergence, as most of them delay permanent teeth eruption; others are associated with complete failure teeth to erupt.

2. **Gender:** In girls permanent teeth erupt earlier, average 4–6 months than in boys.

3. **Nutrition:** Chronic malnutrition is correlated with delayed teeth eruption.

4. **Preterm birth:** Preterm children have delayed primary and permanent teeth eruption.

5. **Socioeconomic factors:** Children from higher socioeconomic backgrounds show earlier tooth emergence than children from lower socioeconomic classes.

6. **Body height and weight:** The taller and heavier children show early eruption of teeth as compared to children with normal body mass index.

7. **Craniofacial morphology:** Formation and eruption of maxillary teeth, especially molars, are delayed in skeletal Class III patients.

8. **Hormonal factors:** Hypothyroidism, hypopituitarism, hypoparathyroidism, and pseudohypoparathyroidism are associated with delayed permanent teeth eruption. Accelerated dental development

has been noted in association with increased adrenal androgen secretion.

9. **Systemic disease:** Most of the systemic diseases are associated with delayed tooth eruption, except diabetes accelerates tooth eruption.

Q. 5. Write a note on factors influencing shedding and eruption of primary teeth.

(TNMGR, Nov. 1995; March 2009; BBD Uni., April 2014)

Ans. Shedding is the physiologic process resulting in elimination of deciduous dentition with replacement by their corresponding permanent successors. Shedding involves resorption of hard and soft tissue. In soft tissue resorption, apoptotic cell death is involved.

Pressure generated by erupting permanent tooth guides pattern of deciduous tooth resorption. Initially, pressure is against root surface of deciduous tooth and resorption occurs on lingual surface. In mandibular incisors apical positioning of tooth germs does not occur and permanent tooth erupts lingually.

Resorption of deciduous molars Resorption of the roots of deciduous molars first begins on their inner surfaces because early developing bicuspids are found between them. With continued growth of jaws and occlusal movement of deciduous molars, the successional tooth germs lie apical to deciduous molars. When the bicuspids begin to erupt, resorption of deciduous molars is again initiated and continues until roots are completely lost and tooth is shed.

Table 1.5a: Sequence and chronology of deciduous teeth

Jaw	Tooth	Calcification begins (months *in utero*)	Crown completed post-natally (months)	Time of emergence (months)	Root completed (years)	Emergence sequence
Max. (upper)	i^1	3–4 months	2	7–10	2.5	2
	i^2	4 months	2–3	8–11	2.5	3
	c^1	4–5 months	9	16–19	3.5	7
	m^1	4 months	6	12–15	3	5
	m^2	5 months	11	25–28	4	10
Mand. (lower)	i_1	3–4 months	2–3	6–8	2.5	1
	i_2	4 months	3	9–13	2.5	4
	c_1	4–5 months	9	17–20	3.5	8
	m_1	4 months	6	12–16	3	6
	m_2	5 months	10	20–26	3.5	9

Table 1.5b: Sequence and chronology of permanent teeth

Jaw	Tooth	Calcification begins	Crown completed (years)	Time of emergence (years)	Root completed (years)	Emergence sequence
Max. (upper)	I1	3–4 months	4–5	7–8	10	4
	I2	10–12 months	4–5	8–10	10–11	6
	C	4–5 months	6–7	11–13	11–14	12
	P3	1–2 years	6–7	10–12	12–14	8
	P4	2–3 years	7–8	10–12	13–14	10
	M1	At birth	4–5	6–7	9–10	2
	M2	2–3 years	7–8	11–13	15–16	14
	M3	7–9 years	12–16	17–20	18–25	16
Mand. (lower)	I1	3–4 months	3–4	6–7	9	3
	I2	3–4 months	4–5	7–8	9–10	5
	C	4–5 months	5–6	8–10	12–13	7
	P3	1–2 years	6–7	10–12	12–14	9
	P4	2–3 years	7	11–13	14–15	11
	M1	At birth	3–4	6–7	9–10	1
	M2	2–3 years	7–8	11–13	14–15	13
	M3	8–10 years	12–16	17–20	18–25	15

Resorption of cementum and dentine: Resorption involves a loss of organic as well as mineral constituent of matrix and is characterized by presence of osteoclasts.

Resorption of root: Root resorption seems to be initiated and regulated by stellate reticulum and dental follicle of underlying permanent tooth via secretion of stimulatory molecules, i.e. cytokines and transcription factors. The primary root resorption process is regulated in a manner similar to the bone remodeling, involving the same receptor ligand system known as RANK/RANKL (receptor activator of nuclear factor—kappa B/RANK ligand).

Mechanism of resorption and shedding: Pressure from erupting successional tooth and appearance of odontoclasts at site of pressure. Membrane of ruffled borders acts as proton pump → adding hydrogen ions to extracellular region → acidification → mineral dissolution. Increased forces of mastication with increase in jaw size leading to trauma to PDL → degeneration of PDL.

Q. 6. Write a short note on development of root.
(TNMGR, Sept. 2010; KUHS, June 2013)

Q. Write a short note on Hertwig's epithelial root sheath.
(NTR Uni., Aug. 2008)

Ans. The development of the roots begins after enamel and dentin formation has reached the future cemento-enamel junction (CEJ). The enamel organ forms Hertwig's epithelial root sheath (HERS), which molds the shape of roots and initiates radicular dentin formation. HERS consists of outer and inner enamel epithelia only. The cells of inner layer remain short and initiate differentiation of odontoblasts, which forms radicular dentin. Just after this, HERS loses its structural continuity and its remnants persist as epithelial network of strands called **rests of Malassez** (Fig. 1.6).

The root sheath prior to elongation in apical direction forms an epithelial diaphragm, which is a horizontal extension at the future CEJ. Subsequently, epithelial cells disintegrate and move away from surface of dentin so that connective tissue cells come into contact with

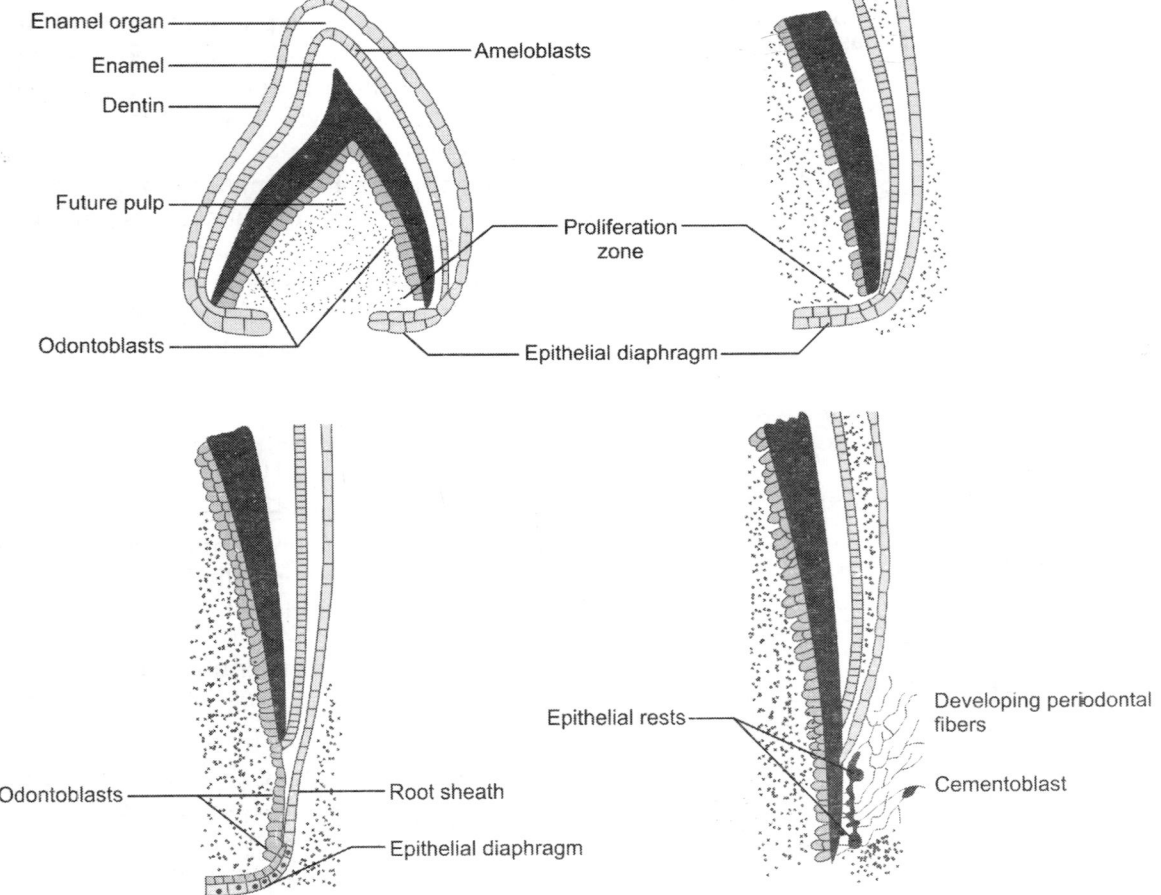

Fig. 1.6: Root formation

outer surface of dentin and differentiate into cementoblasts, that deposit a layer of cementum.

Q. 7. Write a note on anatomy of root apex and its significance. (Sumandeep, Uni., April 2014, 2015)

Ans. The terminal part of a tooth root exhibits four distinct landmarks:

Apical constriction (AC): Apical part of root canal with narrowest diameter. The distance between AC and apical foramen (AF) ranged between 0.4 and 1.2 mm, while its reported location in relation to root apex ranged between 0.5 and 1.01 mm. AC is mostly located either in dentin or at CDJ level and less frequently in cementum. The shape of AC in longitudinal sections has four possible configurations: Single, tapered, multi-constricted and parallel.

Apical foramen (AF): Main apical opening of root canal. Deviation of AF from root apex is common. Average distance between AF and root apex was found to be less than 1 mm.

Roots apex (anatomic and radiographic): Anatomic apex differs from radiographic apex in that former is root end as identified morphologically and latter is identified radiographically. It has been suggested to extend root canal instrumentation to 1 mm short of the radiographic apex, which would ensure closer proximity to position of the AF. However, continuous cementum deposition alters the position of the radiographic apex to the AF (Fig. 1.7).

Cementodentinal junction (CDJ): CDJ is the line of union between dentin and cementum at which pulpal

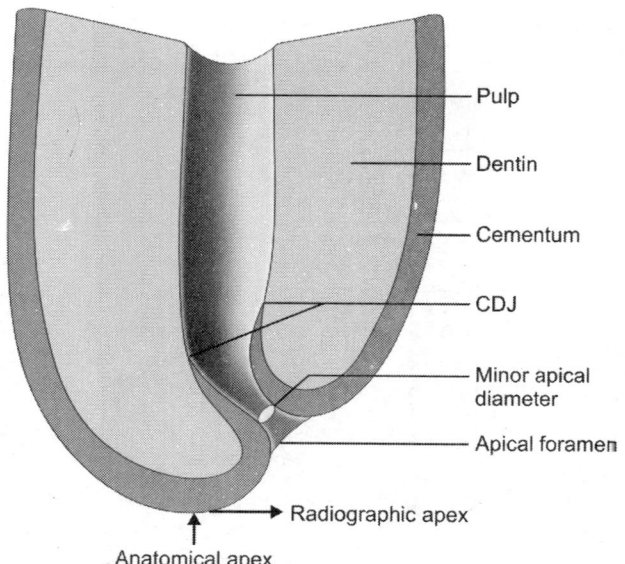

— Pulp

— Dentin

— Cementum

— CDJ

— Minor apical diameter

— Apical foramen

→ Radiographic apex

Anatomical apex

Fig. 1.7: Root apex and its parts

tissue ends and periodontal tissue starts. During tooth development, cementum deposition follows that of dentin, resulting in a line of delineation separating the two tissue types. The CDJ is the ideal termination point for RCT.

Q. 8. Write about theories of mineralization.
(BBD Uni., May 2011;UOK, June 2019)

Ans. Mineralization is deposition of mineral salts in and around organic matrix to make it a calcified structure. The various proposed theories of mineralization are:

1. **Robinson's alkaline phosphatase theory:** The enzyme is responsible for mineralization.
2. **Cartier's theory:** According to Cartier alkaline phosphatase has very little role in mineralization and that ATPase is extremely powerful in inducing mineralization.
3. **White and Hers theory:** White and Hers made surprising discovery that bone and especially dentin still possessed possibility of splitting phosphate easters even ion removing and destroying all the enzymes.
4. **pH of cartilage explaining mineralization:** One of the oldest suggestions for mechanism of mineralization is that pH of cartilage is higher than that of other tissues which would favor precipitation of calcium phosphate.
5. **Seeding mechanism:** According to this mechanism, there are certain substances called seeding or nucleating having resemblance to apatite. These substances act as mould or template upon which crystals are laid down, after which crystallization proceeds automatically. This process is known as **epitaxy.** The following substances have been considered as possible seeding substances: collagen, chondroitin sulphate, lipid substances, phosphoproteins.
6. **Matrix vesicle concept:** Matrix vesicles are organelles of cellular origin that can be observed electron microscopically in the matrix of cartilage, bone, and other hard tissue.

Q. 9. Discuss ectomesenchymal interactions.
(Sharda Uni., July 2016, 2017)

Ans. Epithelial mesenchymal interactions (EMIs) are described as a series of programmed, sequential and reciprocal (complex and multiphase) communications between the epithelium and mesenchyme with its heterotypic cell population, that result in differentiation of one or both cell populations. EMI plays a major role in the following conditions.

1. **In odontogenesis:** Odontogenesis can be described as a complex physiological process of tooth development from ectodermal and mesodermal appendages. Enamel organ derives from ectoderm, whereas dental papillae and dental sac are of mesodermal origin. For the development of teeth, interaction between these ectodermal and mesodermal tissues is essential. Odontoblasts differentiate only in the presence of the enamel epithelium. For EMIs to occur, messenger system is required between epithelium and mesenchyme, which may be: Direct cell–cell communication (cytoplasmic process and gap junctions), matrix vesicles, ions (K^+, Ca^{+2}), extracellular matrix molecules (collagen IV, I, III, fibronectin, tenascin, epithelial cadherin, laminin), hormones and growth factors (bone morphogenetic factor, fibroblast growth factor, epidermal growth factor, TGF), autocrine and paracrine regulators, mRNA, genes (pitx2, p21, Msx2, Lef1, Edar, Lhx6, Lhx7, Dix1, Dix2, Paz9, Gli1, Gli2, Gli3, Barx1 and Runx2)

2. **In dentinoenamel junction:** Enamel originates from epithelial tissue by ameloblast; dentine derives from mesenchymal tissue by odontoblast. The inter-digitation of ameloblasts and odontoblasts is essential for union of dentino-enamel junction (DEJ).

3. **In salivary gland development:** Salivary gland is an epithelial modification and is made up of epithelial components, such as acinar and ductal cells, mesenchymal structures, such as fibrous stroma, vascular elements and a fibrous capsule. Hence, EMIs are required for development of the salivary gland tissue.

4. **In palatogenesis:** During 6th week of palatogenesis, palatal shelves grow rapidly along the vertical plane by proliferating mesenchymal cells, which undergo a sudden elevation to bring them into a horizontal apposition above the flattening tongue followed by fusion of opposing palatal shelves along midline through a series of interactions in cell adhesion molecules. This is considered to be the EMIs in palatogenesis.

5. **In oral cancer:** The new mass of tissue requires angiogenesis for their sustained proliferation and growth. As a consequence of these requirements, epithelial and mesenchymal cells need to have an interactionary signaling mechanism for their growth and proliferation. Basement membrane can be said to maintain the normal histogenesis and morphogenesis of epithelium. In the case of malignant tissue, where there is loss of basement membrane contiguity, normal histogenesis is lost; and the involved epithelial tissue adversely proliferates.

Q. 10. Discuss tooth numbering system.

(UHSR, June 2019)

Ans. There are several **tooth numbering** systems:

1. **Universal Notation System**

   a. *For primary teeth:* Universal system of notation for primary dentition uses 'upper case letters' for each of the primary teeth. The ADA in 1968 officially recommended the "universal" numbering system.

   Right | A B C D E | F G H I J | Left
   Right | T S R Q P | O N M L K | Left

   b. For permanent teeth: Universal system of notation for permanent dentition uses 'numbers' for each of the permanent teeth.

   Right | 1 2 3 4 5 6 7 8 | 9 10 11 12 13 14 15 16 | Left
   Right | 32 31 30 29 28 27 26 25 | 24 23 22 21 20 19 18 17 | Left

2. **Zsigmondy/Palmer Notation System:** In this system, arches are divided into quadrants: ⌐upper right; ⌐upper left; ¬lower right; ⌐lower left.

   a. For deciduous dentition:

   E D C B A | A B C D E
   E D C B A | A B C D E

   b. For permanent dentition:

   8 7 6 5 4 3 2 1 | 1 2 3 4 5 6 7 8
   8 7 6 5 4 3 2 1 | 1 2 3 4 5 6 7 8

3. **Federation Dentaire Internationale (FDI):** Two-digit system, proposed by FDI and is adopted by WHO.

   a. For primary dentition: First digit indicates quadrant: 5 to 8. Second digit indicates tooth within a quadrant, 1 to 5 for primary teeth.

   55 54 53 52 51 | 61 62 63 64 65
   85 84 83 82 81 | 71 72 73 74 75

   b. For permanent teeth: First digit indicates the quadrant: 1 to 4 for permanent dentition. Second digit indicates the tooth within a quadrant: 1 to 8 for permanent teeth.

Upper Right	Upper Left
18 17 16 15 14 13 12 11	21 22 23 24 25 26 27 28
48 47 46 45 44 43 42 41	31 32 33 34 35 36 37 38
Lower Right	Lower Left

2. OCCLUSION AND SKULL BONE DEVELOPMENT

Q. 1. Write about development of occlusion from birth to adolescence. *(BFUHS, May 2010; KUHS, Nov. 2015; HP Uni., May, 2017; April 2019)*

Q. Discuss role of tongue in development and maintenance of normal occlusion. *(DRMLA Uni., July 2008; Gujarat Uni., April 2019)*

Q. Define occlusion. Discuss development of occlusion and malocclusion and factors affecting development of occlusion. *(CDER-AIIMS, Dec. 2016; BVP, June 2018)*

Ans. Occlusion is defined as the contact relationship of the teeth in function or parafunction.

Malocclusion: A condition in which there is a deflection from normal relation of teeth to other teeth in the same arch and/or to teeth in the opposing arch.

Periods of occlusal development:

1. **Pre-dental period:** During this period, neonates have no teeth. It lasts for 6 months after birth. It has following features:
   a. **Gum pads** (Fig. 2.1): The alveolar process at the time of birth is known as **gum pads**. They are horse shoe shape, pink and firm, and develop in two parts: i. Labio-buccal portion; ii. Lingual portion, separated from each other by **dental groove**. Each gum pad is divided into ten segments, each containing deciduous tooth sac, by **transverse grooves**. **Gingival groove** separates gum pad from palate and floor of mouth. **Transverse groove** between canine and first deciduous molar segment is called **lateral sulcus**. Upper gum pad is both wider and longer than lower gum pad. On closing, contact occurs in first molar region, and space exists anteriorly (infantile open bit), which helps in suckling.

   b. **Status of dentition:** Neonates are without teeth for about 6 months. Initially there is crowding of developing teeth, but during first year of life, they grow rapidly, allowing the proper alignment of teeth.

2. **Deciduous dentition period:** From 6 months to 2–3 years.
   The sequence of eruption is: A-B-D-C-E.
   Between 3 and 6 years of age, the dental arch is relatively stable. Other normal features during this period are:
   a. Physiological or developmental spacing in anterior region: **Primate or Simian space** (wider spaces between mesial to maxillary canine and distal to mandibular canine).
   b. Flush terminal plane: Distal surface of maxillary and mandibular deciduous second molars are in same vertical plane.
   c. Deep bite.

3. **Mixed dentition period (6–12 years):** It starts with eruption of first permanent molar (6 years). It has been classified into 3 phases:
   i. **First transitional period (6–8 years):** Emergence of first permanent molar and exchange of deciduous incisors with permanent incisors. The permanent incisors are larger than deciduous, the excess space needed than present is called **incisal liability** (for maxillary 7 mm and for mandibular arch 5 mm). This is compensated by:
      a. Utilization of interdental spaces seen in primary dentition.
      b. Increase in inter-canine width.
      c. Change in incisor inclination.
   ii. **Inter-transitional period:** Both upper and lower arches consist of sets of deciduous and permanent teeth, this phase is relatively stable.
   iii. **Second transitional period (10–12 years):** In this phase, there is replacement of deciduous molars

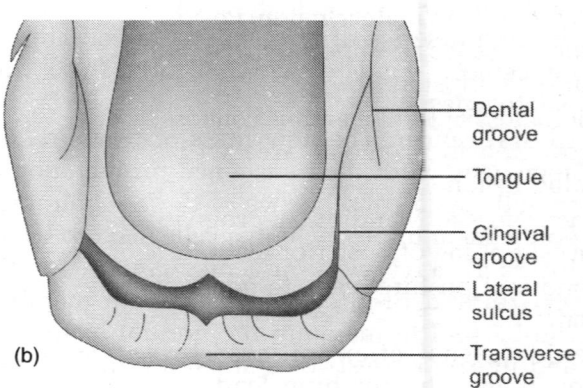

(a) ── Transverse groove
── Lateral sulcus
── Dental groove
── Gingival groove

(b) ── Dental groove
── Tongue
── Gingival groove
── Lateral sulcus
── Transverse groove

Fig. 2.1: (a) Maxillary gum pad; (b) Mandibular gum pad

and canines by premolars and permanent cuspids respectively. The space difference between combined width of deciduous canine and molars and mesiodistal width of permanent canine and premolars (**Leeway space of Nance**) is greater in mandibular arch, which is utilized for mesial drift of mandibular molars.

Ugly duckling stage (Broadbent's phenomenon, 1937): It is transient or self-correcting malocclusion seen in maxillary incisor region between 8 and 9 years of age, seen during the eruption of permanent canines. There is flaring of lateral incisors, maxillary midline diastema.

4. **The permanent dentition period:** The eruption sequence of permanent dentition in maxillary arch:

6-1-2-4-3-5-7 or 6-1-2-3-4-5-7

The eruption sequence of permanent dentition in mandibular arch:

6-1-2-3-4-5-7 or 6-1-2-4-3-5-7

Factors affecting development of occlusion:

A. General factors:
1. Skeletal factors: Conditions that affect jaw growth; pathological, inherited or acquired, trauma or infection
2. Muscle factors: Lip form and activity, tongue size, position and function, adaptive swallowing, thumb sucking, neutral zone.
3. Dental factors: Size of teeth; early loss of teeth leads to over eruption of opposing teeth.

B. Local factors:
1. Aberrant developmental position of individual teeth: Trauma, malposed crown, dilacerated roots.
2. Presence of supernumerary teeth: Supplemental, conical, tuberculated
3. Developmental: Hypodontia affects form and position of teeth and growth of jaw.
4. Upper labial frenum: Median diastema

Role of tongue in malocclusion: Position of tongue and its function plays an important role in development of dental malocclusion.

1. Microglossia: Dental arch is collapsed and reduced. Crowding in premolar area with severe class II malocclusion.
2. Macroglossia: Mandibular prognathism/Class III, buccal tipping of posterior teeth.
3. Abnormal posture leads to generalized spacing of teeth.
4. Genioglossus reflex initiated by large tongue, tonsils, mouth breathing leads to sustained jaw opening → sustained tongue posture → malocclusion

(proclination, open bite, prevention of tooth eruption, posterior open bite, deep overbite).

5. Tongue thrust habit: Proclination of anterior teeth, anterior open bite, bimax dental protrusion, posterior cross bite.

Q. 2. Enumerate various theories of growth.

(UOK, July 2017)

Q. Write a short note on neurotropism.

(UOK, July 2017)

Ans. Growth refers to an increase in size/number (Profitt). **Development** is progress towards maturity (Todd).

Theories of growth:
1. Remodeling theory (Brash): Craniofacial skeletal growth occurs exclusively by bone remodeling.
2. Genetic theory (Brodie, 1941): Growth process is under influence of genetic control and is pre-programmed.
3. Sutural theory (Weinmann and Sicher, 1952): Craniofacial growth occurs at the sutures.
4. Cartilaginous theory (James Scott): Cartilage play primary role in craniofacial growth.
5. Functional matrix theory (Melvin Moss, 1962): Bone growth is influenced by function, as soft tissue grows; both bone and cartilage react and grow in response to soft tissue.
6. Multifactorial theory (Van Limborgh, 1970): Six factors control growth: Genetics, intrinsic growth factors, cartilage, suture, adjacent structures, and muscle function.
7. Enlow's principle of growth: Most of the bones have V-shaped, bone deposition on inner side and resorption in outer surface.
8. Enlow's counterpart principle: Growth in one region of skull influence the growth in others.
9. Neurotrophism (Behrents, 1970): It states that the nerve impulse involving the axoplasmic transport has direct growth potential and has an indirect effect on osteogenic growth by influencing soft tissue growth.

Neurotrophic mechanism:
a. Neuroepithelial tropism: Epithelial growth is normally controlled by release of certain neurotrophic substances by nerve synapses. Lack of this neurotrophic process causes abnormal epithelial growth, orofacial hypoplasia and malformation, etc.
b. Neurovisceral tropism: At the myoblast stage of differentiation, the embryonic myoblasts establish a neural innervation without which further myogenesis usually cannot continue.

c. Neuromuscular tropism: The periosteal matrices generally determine the apparent localized neuro-trophically controlled genomes. The attributing factors that form basis of neurovisceral tropism, e.g. the salivary glands, fat tissue and other organ, regulate the embedded passive position of the skeletal units.

Q. 3. Discuss role of hormone and vitamins in growth and development. *(UOK, July 2017; HP Uni., April 2019)*

Q. Discuss factors affecting growth and development. *(RUHS, May 2018)*

Ans. Factors affecting growth and development

I. Heredity and genetics: Phenotype, characteristics of parents, race, sex, biorhythm and maturation, genetic disorders.

II. Environmental factors: Physical surroundings, social factors.

III. Prenatal environment (maternal nutritional deficiency, endocrine disorders, etc.), postnatal (nutrition, infections, trauma, emotion, etc.)

Hormone:

1. Group 1: Those influencing the skeletal bone growth: Growth hormone, insulin, thyrotrophic hormone.
2. Group 2: Responsible for ossification of long bones: Parathormone.
3. Group 3: Responsible for pubertal growth spurts: Androgens, progesterone and estrogen.
4. Group 4: Prolactin.

Q. 4. Write about prenatal and postnatal growth of cranial base. *(TNMGR, Sept. 2009)*

Ans. Cranial base (also known as base of skull, skull base; Latin: *basis cranii*) is the most inferior part of skull forming the floor of cranial cavity. The cranial base is formed by five bones: Ethmoid, sphenoid, occipital, both frontal and both temporal bones.

A. **Prenatal growth:** The earliest evidence of formation of cranial base is seen in post or late somitic period (4th–8th week of IUL). During this late somitic period mesenchymal tissue derived from primitive streak, neural crest and occipital sclerotomes condense around developing brain. Thus a capsule is formed around the brain called **ectomenix** or ectomeningeal capsule. From around 40th day onwards, this **ectomeningeal capsule** is slowly converted into cartilage which heralds onset of cranial base formation. This occurs in 4 regions.

1. **Parachordal:** Chondrification centers forming around cranial end of notochord.
2. **Hypophyseal:** Cranial to termination of notochord, hypophyseal pouch develops which gives rise to anterior lobe of pituitary gland. On either side of hypophyseal stem, two hypophyseal (post-sphenoid) cartilages develop, which fuse together to form posterior part of body of sphenoid.

   Cranial to the pituitary gland, two presphenoid or trabecular cartilages develop with fuse together and form anterior part of body of sphenoid. Anteriorly, pre-sphenoid cartilage forms mesethmoid cartilage which gives rise to perpendicular plate of ethmoid and crista galli. Lateral to pituitary gland, chondrification centers are seen which form lesser wing (orbito-sphenoid) and greater wing (ali-sphenoid) of sphenoid.
3. **Nasal:** Initially during development, a capsule is seen around nasal sense organ which chondrifies to form cartilages of nostrils.
4. **Otic:** A capsule seen around vestibulo-cochlear sense organs chondrifies and later ossifies to give rise to mastoid and petrous portions of temporal bone.

   The initially separate centers of cartilage formation in cranial base fuse together into a single irregular and greatly perforated cranial base. The early establishment of the various nervous, blood vessels, etc. from and to brain results in numerous perforations or foramina in the developing cranial base. The ossifying chondrocranium meets ossifying desmocranium (cranial vault) to form neurocranium.

   Chondrocranial ossification: The cranial base, which is now in a cartilaginous form, undergoes ossification.

   Occipital bone: Both endochondral and intra-membranous ossification from 7 centers.

   Temporal bone: Both endochondral and intra-membranous ossification from 11 centers.

   Ethmoid bone: This bone shows only endo-chondral ossification from three centers.

   Sphenoid bone: Endochondral and intra-membranous ossification from 15 ossification centers.

   Cranial base or chondrocranium is important as a junction between cranial vault and facial skeleton and is relatively stable during growth compared to cranial vault and face.

B. **Post-natal growth of the cranial base:** The cranial base grows post-natally by complex interaction between the following three growth processes.

1. **Cortical drift and remodeling:** The cranium is divided into a number of compartments by bony elevation and ridges present in cranial base. These elevated ridges and bony partitions show bone deposition, while predominant part of floor shows bone resorption to accommodate growing brain. The foramina that allow passage of nerves and blood vessels undergo drifting by bone deposition and resorption so as to constantly maintain their proper relationship with growing brain.

2. **Elongation at synchondroses:** Most of the bones of cranial base are formed by a cartilaginous process, later replaced by bone. However, certain bands of cartilage remain at junction of various bones, known as synchondroses. The important synchondroses found in cranial base are:

   a. **Sphenooccipital synchondrosis:** It is the cartilaginous junction between sphenoid and occipital bones and considered to be the most important growth site of cranial base. It is believed to be active up to age of 12–15 years. Sphenoid and occipital segments then become fused in midline area by 20 years of age. As endochondral bone growth occurs at spheno-occipital synchondrosis, sphenoid and occipital bones increase in length and width.

   b. **Sphenoethmoid synchondrosis:** This is a cartilaginous band between sphenoid and ethmoid bones. It is believed to ossify by 5–25 years of age.

   c. **Intersphenoidal synchondrosis:** It is a cartilaginous band between 2 parts of sphenoid bone. It is believed to ossify at birth.

   d. **Intraoccipital synchondrosis:** This ossifies by 3–5 years of age.

3. **Sutural growth:** Cranial base has a number of bones that are joined to one another by means of sutures. Some of them include:
   a. Sphenofrontal, b. Frontotemporal, c. Sphenoethmoid, d. Frontoethmoid, e. Frontozygomatic.
   As the brain enlarges during growth, bone formation occurs at the ends of bone.
   Timing of cranial base growth: By birth, 55–60% of adult size is attained; By 4–7 years, 94% of adult size is attained; By 8–13 years, 98% of adult size is attained.

Q. 5. Discuss the prenatal and postnatal growth of maxilla and mandible. *(TNMGR, March 2007; Sept. 2008; UHSR, May 2016; June 2018; BVP, June 2018; NTR Uni., May 2019)*

Q. Write a note on role of condyle in mandibular growth. *(HP Uni., May 2018)*

Q. Write a short note on nasomaxillary complex.
(RHUS, May 2018)

Ans. Around 4th week of IUL, a prominent bulge appears on ventral aspect of embryo corresponding to developing brain. Below the bulge, a shallow depression corresponding to the primitive mouth appears, called **stomodeum**. The floor of stomodeum is formed by the **buccopharyngeal membrane** that separates stomodeum from foregut. Mesoderm covering developing forebrain proliferates and forms a downward projection that overlaps the upper part of stomodeum known as **frontonasal process**. Mandibular arches of both sides form lateral walls of stomodeum, gives off a bud from its dorsal end called **maxillary process**. The ectoderm overlying frontonasal process shows bilateral localized thickenings above stomodeum, **nasal placodes**. These placodes soon sink and form nasal pits. The formation of these **nasal pits** divides the frontonasal process into two parts: a. Medial nasal process, b. Lateral nasal process.

The two mandibular processes grow medially and fuse to form lower lip and lower jaw. As maxillary process undergoes growth, frontonasal process becomes narrow so that the two nasal pits come closer. The line of fusion of the maxillary process and medial nasal process corresponds to nasolacrimal duct.

Development of palate *(MUHS, Dec 2016)*: The palate is formed by contributions of the:
a. Maxillary process.
b. Palatal shelves given off by maxillary process.
c. Frontonasal process.

Ossification of palate: Ossification of palate occurs from 8th week of IUL. This is an intramembranous type of ossification. Palate ossifies from a single centre derived from maxilla. The most posterior part of palate does not ossify, forming **soft palate**. The mid-palatal suture ossifies by 12–14 years.

Development of Maxillary Sinus *(RGUHS, Oct. 2010)*

Prenatal embryology of mandible *(CDER-AIIMS, May 2015)*: About 4th week of IUL, pharyngeal arches are laid down on the lateral and ventral aspects of cranial most part of foregut that lies in close approximation with stomodeum. Initially there are six pharyngeal arches, but fifth one usually disappears. Each of these five arches contains:
1. A central cartilage rod that forms skeleton of arch.
2. A muscular component termed branchiomere.
3. A vascular component.
4. A neural element.

Mandibular process of both sides grows towards each other and fuses in midline forming lower border of stomodeum, i.e. lower lip and lower jaw.

Meckel's cartilage (*UHSR, April 2015*): Meckel's cartilage is derived from 1st branchial arch around 41st and 45th day of IUL. It extends from cartilaginous otic capsule to midline or symphysis and provides template for guiding growth of mandible. A major portion of Meckel's cartilage disappears during growth and remaining part develops into following structures:

1. Mental ossicles, 2. Incus and malleus, 3. Spine of sphenoid bone, 4. Anterior ligament of malleus, 5. Sphenomandibular ligament.

Endochondral bone formation: Endochondral bone formation is seen in 3 areas of mandible:

- **Condylar process** (*CDER-AIIMS, Dec. 2016*): At 5th week of IUL, area of mesenchymal condensation can be seen above ventral part of developing mandible. This develops into a cone-shaped cartilage by 10th week and starts ossification by 14th week and then migrates inferiorly and fuses with mandibular ramus by about 4 months.
- **Coronoid process:** Secondary/accessory cartilages appear in region of coronoid process by 10–14 weeks of IUL. It grows in response to developing temporalis muscle and gets incorporated into intramembranous bone of ramus and disappears before birth.
- **Mental region:** In the mental region, on either side of symphysis, one or two small cartilages appear and ossify in 7th month of IUL to form numbers of mental ossicles in fibrous tissues of symphysis. These ossicles become incorporated into intra-membranous bone when symphysis ossifies completely during the first year of post-natal life.

Postnatal growth of maxilla: Growth of **naso-maxillary complex (NMC)** is produced by:

1. **Displacement:** Growth of cranial base has a direct bearing on NMC as maxilla is attached to cranial base by number of sutures. Primary displacement is seen in forward direction by growth of maxillary tuberosity in posterior direction. Passive/secondary displacement of NMC occurs in downward and forward direction as cranial base grows. This results in whole maxilla being carried anteriorly.
2. **Growth at sutures:** Maxilla is attached to cranium and cranial base by number of sutures. These sutures include:
   a. Frontonasal suture, b. Frontomaxillary suture, c. Zygomaticotemporal suture, d. Zygomatico-maxillary suture, e. Pterygopalatine suture.

These sutures are all oblique and more or less parallel to each other. This allows downward and forward repositioning of maxilla as growth occurs at these sutures. As growth of surrounding soft tissue occurs, maxilla is carried downwards and forward. This leads to opening up of space at sutural attachments, leading to new bone formation on either side of suture and hence overall size of bones increases.

3. **Surface remodeling:** The following are bone remodeling changes that are seen in NMC.
   - Resorption occurs on lateral surface of orbital rim leading to lateral movement of eyeball. To compensate, there is bone deposition on medial rim of orbit and on external surface of lateral rim.
   - Bone deposition occurs along posterior margin of maxillary tuberosity, causing lengthening of dental arch and enlargement of anteroposterior dimension of entire maxillary body. This helps to accommodate erupting molars.
   - Bone resorption occurs on lateral wall of nose leading to an increase in size of nasal cavity. Bone resorption is seen on floor of nasal cavity. To compensate there is bone deposition on palatal side. Thus a net downward shift occur leading to increase in maxillary height.
   - Zygomatic bone moves in posterior direction, achieved by resorption on anterior surface and deposition on posterior surface.
   - Face enlarges in width by bone formation on lateral surface of zygomatic arch and resorption on its medial surface.
   - Anterior nasal spine prominence increases due to bone deposition and resorption from periosteal surface of labial cortex. As a compensatory mechanism, bone deposition occurs on endosteal surface of labial cortex and periosteal surface of lingual cortex.
   - As teeth start erupting, bone deposition occurs at alveolar margins. This increases maxillary height and depth of palate.
   - The entire wall of sinus except mesial wall undergoes resorption. This results in increase in size of the maxillary antrum.

Postnatal growth of mandible (*KUHS, Jan. 2014; CDER-AIIMS, May 2015*)

Basal bone or body of mandible forms one unit, to which is attached alveolar process, coronoid process, condylar process, angular process, ramus, lingual tuberosity and chin.

- **Ramus:** It moves progressively posterior by combination of deposition on the posterior region and resorption on anterior part of ramus.

- **Corpus or body of the mandible:** Displacement of ramus results in conversion of former ramal bone into posterior part of body of mandible.
- **Angle of mandible:** On lingual side of angle of mandible, resorption takes place on postero-inferior aspect and deposition occurs on antero-superior aspect. On buccal side, resorption occurs on anterio-superior part and deposition takes place on postero-superior part. This results in flaring of angle of mandible as age advances.
- **Lingual tuberosity:** It is a direct equivalent of maxillary tuberosity. The combination of resorption in lingual fossa and deposition on medial surface of tuberosity accentuates prominence of lingual tuberosity.
- **Alveolar process:** As teeth erupt, alveolar processes develop and increase in height by bone deposition at margins.
- **Chin:** In infancy, chin is usually underdeveloped. Mental protuberance forms by bone deposition during childhood. Its prominence is accentuated by bone resorption that occurs in alveolar region above it, creating a concavity.
- **Condyle** (*CDER-AIIMS, Dec. 2016, 2018*): Mandibular condyle has been recognized as an important growth site.
  a. It was earlier believed that growth occurs at surface of condylar cartilage by means of bone deposition and hence condyle grows towards cranial base. As condyle pushes against cranial base, entire mandible gets displaced forwards and downwards.
  b. It is now believed that growth of soft tissues including muscles and connective tissue carries mandible forwards away from cranial base. Bone growth follows secondarily at condyle to maintain constant contact with cranial base.
  Condylar growth rate increases at puberty reaching a peak between 12 and 14 years. The growth ceases around 20 years of age.
- **Coronoid process:** Growth of coronoid process follows the 'V' principle. Viewing longitudinal section of coronoid process from posterior aspect, it can be seen that deposition occurs on lingual surface of left and right coronoid process. Although additions take place on lingual side, vertical dimension of coronoid process also increases.

Q. 6. Write a note on growth spurts.

Ans. There are accelerated periods of growth known as growth spurts that occur at specific times during which period of growth shows a definite increase. The physiological alteration in hormone is believed to be the cause for such accentuated growth. The timings of growth spurts differ in boys and girls. The timings of growth spurts are as follows: 1. Just before birth, 2. One year after birth, 3. Mixed dentition growth spurt: Boys: 8–11 years; Girls: 7–9 years, 4. Pre-pubertal growth spurt: Boys: 14–16 years; Girls: 11–13 years.

Importance: Pubertal increments offer best time for orthodontic and orthopaedic treatment.

Q. 7. Write a note on methods of studying growth.
(RGUHS, May 2006; UHSR, May 2007; CDER-AIIMS, May 2015; NITTE Uni., April 2017; HP Uni., May 2017)

Q. Write a short note on growth assessment.
(UHSR, April 2013; AHSUC, May 2018)

Ans. Growth is defined as increase in size or number. According to Profitt:

A. **Measurement approaches:**
  1. Craniometry: It is based on measurements of skull of human skeletal remains. Precise measurements can be made on dry skulls, only for cross sectional studies.
  2. Anthropology: Various landmarks established in studies of dry skull are measured in living individuals by using soft tissue points overlying bony landmarks. Measurements obtained would be of different results. Growth of an individual can be followed over a period of time with repeated measurements.
  3. Cephalometric radiography: It is a standardized radiographic technique in craniofacial region, introduced by Broadbent in 1931. This is based on precise orientation of head before a cephalostat. It allows direct measurement of skeletal dimensions. Disadvantages include two-dimensional representations of structures, technique sensitive and not all measurements are possible.
  4. Comparative anatomy: It is carried out through comparisons with other species.
  5. 3-D Imaging: Computed tomography, CBCT

B. **Experimental approaches:**
  1. Vital staining: It involves administration of dyes to experimental animals. Dyes used are alizarin red 5, tetracycline, trypon blue, and lead acetate.
  2. Autoradiography: It is a technique in which a film emulsion is placed over a thin section of tissue containing radioactive isotope, and then is exposed in dark by radiation. The location of radiation in film indicates site of growth. Commonly used autoradiographic labels are: 3H Thymidine, 3H Proline, Bromodeoxyuridine.
  3. Radioisotopes: Radioisotopes of certain elements are often used *in vivo* markers. When injected into tissue, get incorporated into the developing bone

and can be detected by means of Geiger counter, e.g. Technetium-33, Calcium-45, Potassium-32.

4. Metallic implants: Inert metal pins generally made of titanium are placed in growing bones of skeleton, including face and jaws. These metal pins are well tolerated by skeleton and become permanently incorporated into bone. These serve as reference points to study amount, direction and manner of growth.

5. Natural markers: Certain histological features present in normal bone such as nutrient canals, lines of arrested growth.

Methods of collecting growth data

1. **Longitudinal studies:** These are measurements made of same person or group at regular intervals through time. **Advantages:** Temporary problems are smoothed with time, variability in development within a group is put in proper perspective, and serial comparison makes study of specific developmental pattern of individual possible. **Disadvantages:** Time consuming, expensive, sample loss.

2. **Cross sectional studies:** These are measurements made of different samples or different individuals and studied at different periods. **Advantages:** Quicker, less expensive, statistical treatment of data is easier, studies can be readily repeated, Method can be used in archeological data. **Disadvantages:** Variation in development among individuals within the sample cannot be studied.

3. **Semi-longitudinal studies:** Longitudinal and cross sectional studies can be combined to seek advantages of both. In this way one might compress 15 years of study into 3 years of gathering growth data.

Q. 8. Write about different ways of age estimation.
(UHSR, May 2007)

Q. Write a short note on skeletal maturity indicators.
(DRMLA Uni., July 2013;
BBD, April 2014; Gujarat Uni, June 2018)

Ans. Age estimation is an important factor in biological identification in many forensic fields, such as forensic odontology, forensic medicine, forensic anthropology, and forensic osteology.

Types of age

I. **Chronological age or real age:** It is measured by the calendar.

II. **Height and weight:** Age of a person can be roughly determined from standard charts of height and weight, but is least accurate and reliable.

III. **Skeletal age:** Determined by degree of ossification/development of various bones known to occur at particular time in average individual.

Skeletal maturity indicators

a. **Hand and wrist radiograph:** The hand wrist region is made of numerous small bones. The appearance, ossification and union of these bones from birth to maturity show an orderly sequence of events in predictable schedule pattern. It is indicated when there is marked discrepancy between chronologic and dental age. Methods used are: Atlas method by Greulich and Pyle (1959); Bjork, Grave and Brown method (1976); Julian Singer's Method (1980); Fishman's skeletal maturity indicators (1982); Hagg and Taranger method (1982).

b. **Cervical vertebrae:** Shape of cervical vertebrae changes according to each level of skeletal development. Methods used are: Lamparki's method; Hassel and Farman method.

c. **Tooth mineralization:** Stage of root formation and mineralization has close relation with skeletal maturation of an individual. Methods used are: Nolla's stage of calcification, Goldstein and Tanner method.

d. **Mid-palatal suture ossification.**

IV. **Dental age:** Determined by studying development of various teeth from the time of crypt is visible till the time of root completion.

Dental Age Estimation Methods:

a. **Morphologic/Visual Examination:** Morphological methods are based on assessment of teeth (*ex vivo*). Hence, these methods require extracted teeth for microscopic preparation. Gustafson (1950), Dalitz (1962), Bang and Ramm (1970), Johanson (1971), Maples (1978), Solheim (1993) are a few morphological methods.

b. **Radiographic Examination:** Radiographic assessment of age is a simple, non-invasive and reproducible method that can be employed both on living and unknown dead. Various radiographic images that can be used in age identification are intraoral periapical radiographs, lateral oblique radiographs, cephalometric radiographs, panoramic radiographs, digital imaging and advanced imaging technologies. The radiological age determination is based on assessment of various features as follows:

- Jaw bones prenatally.
- Appearance of tooth germs.
- Earliest detectable trace of mineralization or beginning of mineralization.
- Early mineralization in various deciduous teeth during intrauterine life.
- Degree of crown completion.
- Eruption of crown into oral cavity.

- Degree of root completion of erupted or unerupted teeth.
- Degree of resorption of deciduous teeth.
- Measurement of open apices in teeth.
- Volume of pulp chamber and root canals/ formation of physiological secondary dentine.
- Tooth-to-pulp ratio.
- Third molar development and topography

c. **Histological examination:** Dentin translucency method, incremental lines of cementum.

d. **Biochemical examination:** The biochemical methods are based on the racemization of amino acids. L-aspartic acids are converted to D-aspartic acids and thus levels of D-aspartic acid in human enamel, dentine, and cementum increase with age. Some of the methods are: 1. Helfman and Bada method (1975, 1976), 2. Ritz et al. method (1995).

3. DEVELOPMENT OF DENTAL TISSUES

Q. 1. Explain the formation, structure, chemical composition and physical properties of enamel. Describe the hydroxyapatite crystal.

(UHSR; Sumandeep Uni., April 2014)

Ans. Enamel is a highly mineralized structure covering the anatomic crown of tooth.

A. **Physical properties:**
1. It appears bluish-white or grayish at thick opaque areas and yellow-white at thin areas reflecting underlying dentin.
2. Enamel forms a protective covering of 2–2.5 mm thickness over crown and knife edge thickness at cervical region.
3. It is the hardest calcified tissue in human body, 5–8 KHN.
4. It is selectively permeable.
5. The specific gravity is 2.8.
6. Density decreases from surface of enamel to DEJ

B. **Chemical properties:** Inorganic material: 96%; Organic substance and water: 4%.
   i. **Inorganic contents:** Hydroxyapatite (calcium phosphate), ions (Sr, Mg, Pb, Fl)
   ii. **Protein content:** a. Amelogenin (90%, rich in prolin, histidine, glutamin, leucine); b. Non-amelogenin (10%, protein: Ameloblastin, tuftelin, enamelin)

   Hydroxyapatite crystals: $Ca_{10}(PO_4)_6(OH)_2$; Crystals unite to form enamel rod or prism. Closely packed, long, ribbon-like carbonate crystals, arranged approximately parallel to long axis of rods. It comprises 88–90% of tissue by volume and 95% by weight. Present in form of crystallites; Length: 0.05–1µm; width: 90 µm. Shape is hexagonal in maturing enamel and irregular in matured enamel. It has central core or C-axis of hydroxyl ion around which calcium and phosphorous ions are arranged in form of triangle. During formation, Mg can replace Ca and carbonate can replace hydroxyl ion. Concentration of ions increases from surface of enamel towards dentin, that of fluoride decreases from surface of enamel towards dentin.

C. **Structure:** *(HP Uni., April 2019)*
1. **Enamel rod:** Enamel is composed of enamel rods or prisms (5–12 million). In cross section rods are hexagonal in shape (key hole/paddle shaped). Each enamel rod is built up of segments separated by dark lines. Generally rods are directed at right angles to dentin surface. In deciduous teeth, direction of rods is horizontal in cervical and central parts of crown. Near incisal edge or tip of cusp they gradually increase in oblique direction and almost vertical in cusp tip region. In permanent teeth, in occlusal 2/3rd of crown, direction of rods is oblique. In cervical region rods deviate from horizontal in apical direction.
2. **Rod sheath:** Thin peripheral layer, darker and less calcified than rod.
3. **Gnarled enamel:** This optical appearance of enamel is observed in oblique cut section as bundles of rods seem to interwine more irregular near dentin in region of cusps or incisal edge.
4. **Hunter-Schreger bands:** The regular change in direction of rods produces alternating dark and light strips.
5. **Incremental lines of Retzius:** Successive apposition of enamel during formation produces brownish bands.
6. External manifestations of Retzius striae is known as **Perikymata (imbrication lines)**
7. **Neonatal line:** Accentuated incremental line of Retzius marking the boundary between two portions of enamel of deciduous teeth formed partly before and partly after birth.
8. **Enamel cuticle/Nasmyth's membrane:** Delicate membrane covering the crown of newly erupted tooth.
9. **Enamel lamellae:** Thin leaf-like structures that extend from enamel surface toward DEJ.
10. **Enamel tufts:** Thin ribbon-like structures arising at DEJ and reaching into enamel.
11. **Enamel spindle:** Odontoblast process crossing DEJ into enamel.

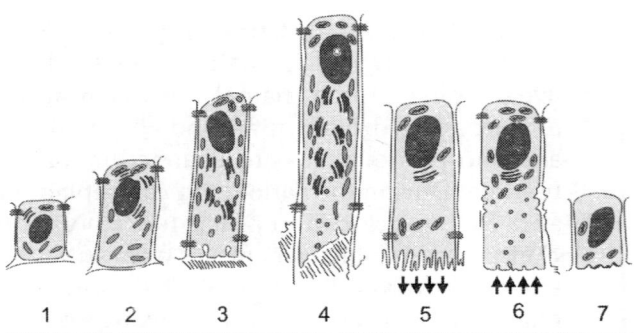

1. Morphogenetic, 2. Inductive, 3. Early secretory, 4. Secretory,
5. Maturation—ruffle-ended, 6. Maturation—smooth-ended, 7. Protective

Fig. 3.1: Life cycle of ameloblasts

D. **Life cycle of ameloblasts** (Fig. 3.1): According to their function, ameloblasts can be divided into following stages:
1. Morphogenic: Short columnar cell with large oval nucleus.
2. Organizing: Cell become longer with reversal of polarity and nutritional stream.
3. Formative: This starts after first layer of dentin is formed, development of Tome's process, key hole pattern of enamel rods.
4. Maturative: Absorption of protein and deposition of minerals, Tome's process disappears.
5. Protective: Radicular dentin formation. HERS breaks mineralized enamel in contact with dental follicle.
6. Desmolytic: IEE stimulates dental follicle to form osteoclast activating factors, epithelia degenerates with tooth eruption.

Q. 2. Write a short note on amelogenins.

(RUHS, June 2017)

Ans. Enamel matrix proteins are generally classified into:
1. Amelogenin group: A 20-kDa hydrophobic protein
2. Enamelin group: A 65-kDa acidic protein and tuftelin.
3. Non-amelogenin, non-enamelin group: Ameloblastin (amelin or sheathlin).

Amelogenins constitute about 90% of total enamel matrix proteins and play a major role in mineralization and morphological changes in enamel. Human amelogenin gene has been located on X-chromosome at Xp22.1–p22.3 and on Y chromosome at Yp11.2.

Basic structure: Amino-terminal domain-A (hydrophobic) and carboxy-terminal domain-B (hydrophilic)
• **Role of amelogenin in enamel formation:** During enamel development and mineralization, secreted amelogenin are lost from tissue by specific proteases

and replaced by mineral ions, calcium and phosphorus, which eventually results in fully mineralized hard and mature enamel.
• **Forensic dentistry:** Females have two identical amelogenin genes present on X-chromosome, whereas males have two different genes, present on both the sex chromosomes.
• **Regeneration of tissues:** Distinct isoforms of amelogenin have also been discovered in places other than enamel-like dentin matrix, odontoblasts, in remnants of Hertwig's root sheath and in periodontal ligament (PDL) cells, long bone cells such as osteocytes, osteoblasts, osteoclasts, some bone marrow cells, and articular cartilage, chondrocytes of articular cartilage and in cell layers of epiphyseal growth plate.
• **Future perspective as tumor markers:** Study of amelogenin gene and protein expression in odontogenesis and odontogenic neoplasms can be used as potentially useful polypeptide for identification of odontogenic epithelial components.

Q. 3. Write a short note on amelogenesis.

(TNMGR, March 2009; BBD Uni., April 2015)

Ans. Amelogenesis or development of enamel consists of two phases:
a. **Formation of enamel matrix:** The ameloblasts begin their secretory activity when a small amount of dentin has been laid down. The projection of ameloblasts into enamel matrix is called ***Tomes process***, gives junction between enamel and ameloblast a **picket fence** or **saw tooth appearance**. Two ameloblasts are involved in the synthesis of each enamel rod. The newly formed enamel matrix has two proteins: Amelogenin and enamelin.
b. **Mineralization and maturation:** Two stages
1. First/primary mineralization stage: Immediate partial mineralization occurs in matrix segment and in interprismatic substance (25–30%).
2. Second maturation stage: Gradual completion of mineralization. It starts from height of crown and progresses cervically. Each rod matures from depth to surface, and sequence of maturing rods is from cusps or incisal edge toward cervical line.

Applied Dental Anatomy

1. Defects in amelogenesis: Amelogenesis imperfecta.
2. Grooves and fissures on the occlusal surfaces are more prone to caries.
3. Lamellae, tufts and spindles may facilitate caries progression.
4. Enamel hypoplasia.

5. Enamel hypocalcification.
6. Fluorosis.

Q. 4. Write a short note on age changes in enamel.
(UOK, 2016; HP Uni., April 2019)

Ans. Age changes in enamel:

1. Attrition or wear of occlusal surfaces and proximal contact points as a result of mastication.
2. Generalized loss of enamel rod ends.
3. Flattening of perikymata.
4. Finally complete disappearance of perikymata.
5. Localized increase of nitrogen and fluorine.
6. Teeth become darker due to increase in organic content and deepening of dentin colour.
7. Increase in resistance to decay.
8. Reduced permeability.
9. Enamel may become harder with age.

Q. 5. Write a short note on events in dentinogenesis with its anomalies.
(RGUHS, Oct. 2010)

Ans. Dentinogenesis is formation of dentin by odontoblasts of mesenchymal origin located at periphery of dental pulp. Dentinogenesis begins when tooth germ reaches bell stage. Dental papilla is the formative organ, separated from IEE by cell free zone. Odontoblasts, dentin forming cells differentiate from ectomesenchymal cells of dental papilla following induction from IEE. Dentinogenesis consists of:

a. **Formation of collagen matrix (predentin):** Dentinogenesis begins at cusp tips after odontoblasts have differentiated and begin collagen production. Odontoblasts change their shape and size and give rise to several processes, which join together and become enclosed in a tubule. Collagen matrix formation continues, till the formation of crown and root formation. Initial dentin deposition along the cusp tips is known as **Korff's fibers**. Odontoblasts secrete both the collagen and other components of extracellular matrix.

b. **Mineralization:** Earliest crystal deposition is in the form of very fine plates of hydroxyapatite on surface of collagen fibrils and in the ground substance, subsequently within fibrils.

Anomalies of dentin formation

1. Dentinogenesis imperfect: Type I (Along with osteogenesis imperfect), II, III (Brandywine type)
2. Dentin dysplasia (rootless teeth): Type I—radicular; Type II—coronal.
3. Regional odontodysplasia (ghost teeth on radiograph).
4. Dens in dente (tooth within tooth).
5. Tetracycline pigmentation.

Q. 6. Write a short note on life cycle of odontoblasts.
(BBD, April 2013)

Ans. Odontoblast is cell of neural crest origin that is a part of outer surface of pulp and its biological function is dentinogenesis. It is the 2nd most prominent cell in pulp. Odontoblast is a large columnar cells arranged in palisading pattern at periphery of pulp rich in rough endoplasmic reticulum (RER), Golgi complex with unidirectional secretory pattern and interconnected by macula adherens and gap junctions. No. of odontoblast = no. of dentinal tubules ($59,000–76,000/mm^2$). Odontoblast deposits 4 μm of dentin/day.

Life cycle: Fig. 3.6

1. **Odontoblast differentiation/preodontoblast stage:** In late bell stage, under the inductive influence of

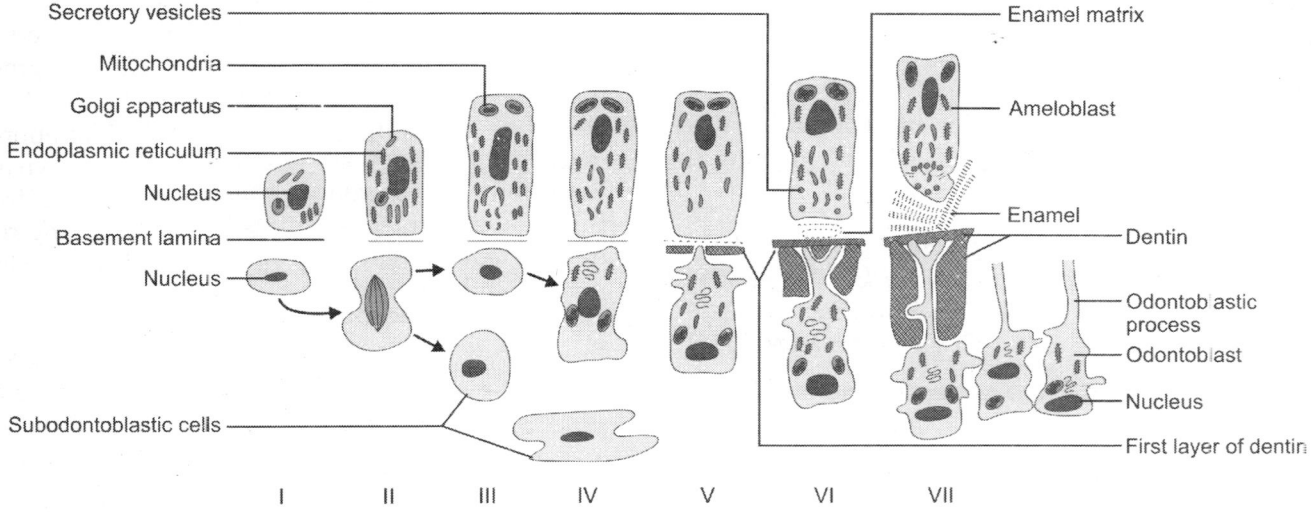

Fig. 3.6: Life cycle of odontoblasts: I–IV: Differentiation stage; V–VII: Formative stage

IEE, peripheral ectomesenchymal cells differentiate into preodontoblasts. They assume columnar shape, aligned as single row along the basement membrane with several projections.

2. **Formative/synthetic/active/secretory stage:** Secretory odontoblasts are aligned along the periphery of pulp. Functionally, it has cell body in which synthesis of proteins occurs and cell process whereby secretion occurs. The first sign of dentin formation is the appearance of distinct, large-diameter collagen fibrils called *von Kroff's fibers* (collagen type III). They originate deep among the odontoblasts; extend toward IEE, and immediately below epithelium.

3. **Quiescent/resting/aged odontoblast stage:** Stubby cells, scanty cytoplasm, dark closed faced nucleus, with absent secretory granules. This stage occurs after completion of circumpulpal dentin. The odontoblast loses most of their protein forming organelles to accommodate the decrease in their function. The fully differentiated and actively secreting odontoblasts decrease slightly in size and the cell process stop to elongate as dentin formation is reduced.

Fate of Odontoblasts: Life span of odontoblasts is equal to that of a viable tooth because once differentiated they cannot undergo further cell division. Resting odontoblasts involved in secondary dentinogenesis is renamed "**odontocytes**" because their function and properties are similar to osteocytes. These odontocytes may participate during reactionary dentinogenesis. Gene DMP1 is involved in differentiation of secretory odontoblasts into odontocytes.

Clinical Significance

1. Pathological differences in functional life of odontoblasts lead to dentinogenesis imperfecta.
2. Shell/thistle-tube teeth: Pre-odontoblasts do not differentiate into odontoblasts.
3. Pulpal obliteration: Odontoblasts do not differentiate into osteocytes.
4. Pink tooth: Outward resorption of dentinal tubules by odontoclasts results in pulpal tissue appearing pink through thin enamel.

Q. 7. Write a short note on age changes in dentin.
(TNMGR, March 2009; Oct. 2012;UHSR, May 2009; HP Uni., May 2015,April 2019; UOK, 2016; Sumandeep Uni., June 2016, 2017; CDER-AIIMS, May 2019)

Q. Write a note on structure of dentin and its clinical significance. *(RGUHS, July 2017)*

Ans. Dentin is the mineralized hard tissue forming main bulk of tooth, covered by enamel in crown and cementum in root.

A. **Physical properties:**
1. Dentin is pale yellow to white in colour.
2. Thickness ranges from 3 to 10 mm.
3. Modulus of elasticity ranges from 15 to 20 GPA.
4. Hardness is 68 KHN.
5. Dentin is less radiopaque than enamel.

B. **Chemical properties:**
Inorganic: 70%; Organic: 20%; Water: 10%

Inorganic: Calcium hydroxyapatite crystals (mainly); Salt: Calcium carbonate, sulphate, phosphate, etc.; trace elements: Cu, Fe, F, Zn.

Organic: Collagen (90%) Type I > III, V; non-collagen matrix proteins (phosphoproteins—phosphoryn; glycoproteins—sialoprotein, osteonectin, osteocalcin; Proteoglycans—chondroitin sulphate enzymes: Acid phosphatase, alkaline phosphatase; Lipids: Phospholipids, glycolipids).

Types of Dentin: (Fig. 3.7a and b)

1. **Primary dentin:** Dentin formed before complete root formation, forms most of the tooth portion. Primary dentin lining pulp chamber is referred as **circumferential dentin**. The outer layer is more mineralized is known as **mantle dentin**.

2. **Secondary dentin:** This is dentin formed after root completion. It is formed at slow rate and contains less number of tubules than primary dentin. It protects pulp from exposure in older teeth.

3. **Tertiary dentin/reparative/reactive/irritation/replacement/adventitious dentin:** This is formed when odontoblasts die during any operative procedure, erosion, dental caries, from newly formed odontoblasts, from underlying undifferentiated perivascular cells in deeper pulpal tissue. It has fewer tubules and more twisted.

Structure of Dentin *(RGUHS, July 2017)*

- Dentinal tubules: It is the unit structure of dentin, forms shallow 'S' shape at middle part of crown, straight at cusp and root portion of tooth. Their density increases towards pulp.
- Periodontoblastic space: Potential space between tubule wall and odontoblastic process contains nerves, collagen fibrils, plasma proteins, glycoprotein and mitochondria.
- Lamina limitans: Organic sheath lining the dentinal tubules.
- Dentinal fluid/dentin lymph: It is ultra-filtrate from pulp capillaries present between dentinal tubules and odontoblastic process.
- Predentin: First formed dentin consists of non-mineralized matrix.

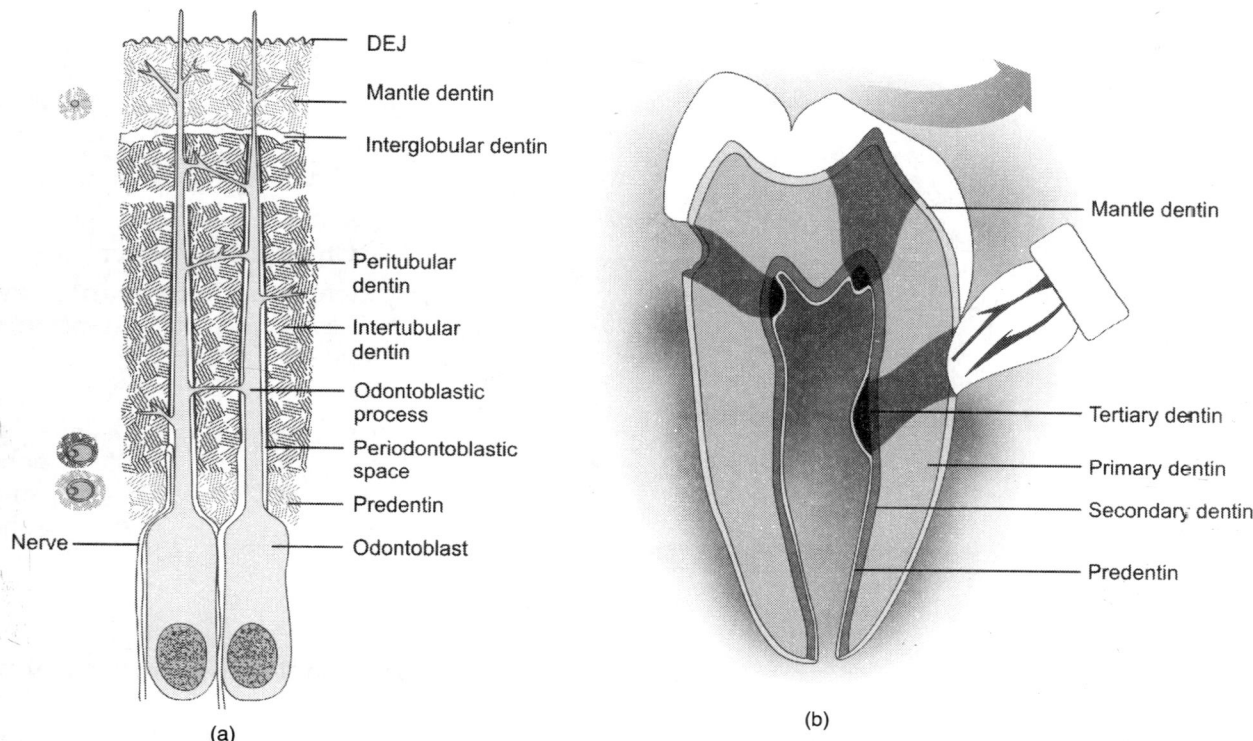

Fig. 3.7: (a) Structure of odontoblasts; (b) Dentin and its types

- **Peritubular dentin:** The wall of dentinal tubules surrounding the odontoblastic process.
- **Intertubular dentin:** The dentin in between dentinal tubules.
- **Interglobular dentin:** Areas of hypomineralization due to failure of fusion of mineral globules.
- **Incremental lines of von Ebner/imbrication lines:** These are fine striations perpendicular to dentinal tubules, due to daily rhythmic deposition of dentin.
- **Lines of Schreger:** Congruence of primary curvatures of dentinal tubules.
- **Granular layer of Tomes':** Smaller areas of interglobular dentin due to interference in mineralization of firstly formed layer of dentin, leading to looping of terminal ends of tubules.
- **Contour lines of Owen:** Accentuated incremental lines due to disturbance in matrix formation.
- **Neonatal lines:** Accentuated incremental lines due to disturbance in calcification, reflects abrupt changes in environment at birth.
- **Dentinoenamel junction (DEJ):** Scalloped interface between dentin and enamel, with convexity towards dentin.

Age Changes:
1. Physiologic secondary dentin formation.
2. Reparative dentin formation.

3. **Dead tracts:** Due to any mechanical injury, odontoblastic process may be lost, which appears black in transmitted light and white in reflected light.
4. **Sclerotic or transparent dentin:** Any external stimulus sometimes leads to increase deposition of collagen fibers and apatite crystals in the tubules, leading to complete obliteration.
5. **Eburnated dentin:** Exposed portion of reactive sclerotic dentine due to slow caries. It is hard, darkened, cleanable and resistant to further caries.

Innervation of dentin:
1. Numerous nerve endings in predentin and inner dentin.
2. Myelinated nerve fibres of pulp (Aδ) reach brain via trigeminal nerve.

Q. 8. Write a short note on dentin hypersensitivity.
(RGUHS, Oct. 2008; TNMGR, March 2011; Oct. 2013; Oct. 2016)

Q. Describe the various theories and management of dentinal hypersensitivity. *(RGUHS May 2015; MUHS, June 2017)*

Ans. The only type of sensation obtained on dentine pulp complex is pain. Theories of dentinal hypersensitivity (Fig. 3.8).

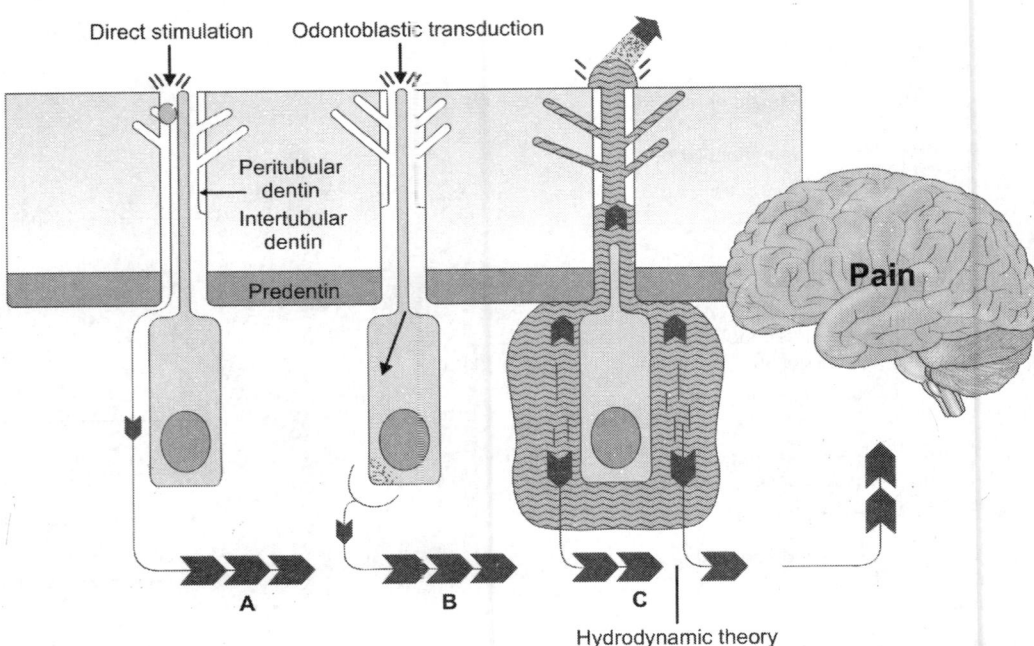

Fig. 3.8: Theories of pain transmission through dentin. A. Direct neural stimulation, B. Transduction theory, C. Hydrodynamic theory

1. **Direct neural stimulation (Scott Stella, 1963):** A stimulus reaches the nerve endings in the inner dentin. This theory assumes that nerve fibers extend to DEJ.

2. **Transduction theory:** This theory presumes that the odontoblasts process is the primary structure excited by the stimulus and impulse is transmitted to the nerve endings in the inner dentin. This is supported by fact that odontoblasts have neural crest in origin.

3. **Fluid or hydrodynamic theory (Gysi 1900, Brannstorm, 1967):** Any stimuli can affect the fluid movements in the dentinal tubules, this fluid movements further stimulates the pain mechanism in the tubules by mechanical disturbances of nerves closely associated with odontoblasts and its process. (most popular).

Management of hypersensitivity: Block the dentinal tubules. Topical fluoride application, fluoride iontophoresis, night guards, restorations, soft tissue grafting, lasers.

Q. 9. Write a short note on pain receptors in dental pulp.   *(TNMGR, April 2012)*

Ans. Sensory nerve fibers of dental pulp are afferent endings of trigeminal cranial nerve. These fibers reach the root canal through apical foramen, going to root pulp in lumps. These lumps are often associated with blood vessels in a collagen sheath, forming neuro-vascular bundle. On approaching subodontoblastic region, fibers form an intricate network known as the *plexus of Raschkow*. After this, myelinated fibers lose their myelin sheath and emerge as free nerve endings. These sensitive fibers act as nociceptors and belong to:

1. **C fibers:** Unmyelinated, sympathetic, found in close association with blood vessels, vasoconstriction and have a low conduction velocity, a smaller diameter, and a higher excitation threshold. They are located deeper than myelinated fibers and are principally activated by heat, causing slow, diffuse, and durable pain. If the pain stimulus intensity increases, the sensory C fibers are recruited and the pain becomes a burning sensation. The C fiber reaction shows that pulp damage is irreversible.

2. **Aδ fibers:** Small myelinated, fast conduction, low stimulation threshold, are superficial (located in pulp and dentin junction), transmit pain directly to thalamus, and generate a sharp and stabbing pain that is easily localized. These characteristics make them the first nerve fibers to react and transmit pain impulse even when there is no irreversible tissue damage.

3. **Aβ fibers:** Large myelinated functionally similar to Aδ fibers but are stimulated at lower electrical threshold. These fibres are located at pulp-dentin border or in close proximity to odontoblast cell body.

4. **Parietal layer of nerves or plexus of Raschkow:** Formed of myelinated and non-myelinated fibers.

Q. 10. Discuss functions of pulp and its response to various stimuli.
(*TNMGR, April 2013; MUHS, June 2017*)

Ans. Pulp is a mass of connective tissue that resides within the center of tooth, directly beneath the layer of dentin. It is a part of "dentin-pulp" complex, and also known as **endodontium.**

Functions of Pulp:

1. **Inductive:** Induces oral epithelium to differentiate into dental lamina and enamel organ.
2. **Formative:** It produces dentin through odontoblasts.
3. **Nutritive:** It nourishes dentin, by means of its rich vascular supply.
4. **Protective:** It responds to various types of stimuli, by forming secondary and tertiary dentin, which increases coverage of pulp.
5. **Defensive or reparative:** It responds to any irritation by forming reparative dentin.
6. **Sensory:** Changes in temperature, vibration and chemical that affect the dentin and pulp.

Response of pulp to stimuli: The pulp is highly responsive to any stimuli. Even a slight stimulus will cause inflammatory cell infiltration, hyperemia or localized abscess. Hemorrhage may be present. The odontoblast layer is either destroyed or greatly disrupted. Compound containing calcium hydroxide induces reparative dentin formation. Closer the restoration to pulp, greater will be the pulp response.

Q. 11. Write a short note on age changes in pulp.
(*TNMGR, March 2009; KUHS, Jan. 2014; Sumandeep Uni., June 2016, 2017; UHSR, May 2017; HP Uni., April 2019*)

Ans. The physiology of pulp has been known to change over time due to the aging process, resulting in distinct phenotypic differences. Compromised circulation and innervation occurs due to increased deposition of secondary dentin at apical root, constricting apical foramen.

1. Decrease in number as well as size of pulp cells with aging.
2. Increase fibrosis and collagen fibers in pulpal tissue.
3. Appearance of atherosclerotic plaques and calcification in pulpal vessels.
4. Progressive mineralization of nerve sheath.
5. Formation of pulp stones or denticles.
6. Formation of diffuse calcifications in pulp chamber.
7. The number of cells in pulp decreases as cell death occurs with age.
8. The volume of pulp chamber decreases with continued deposition of dentin.
9. In some cases, pulp chamber can be obliterated with aging.

Q. 12. Write a short note on calcifications of pulp.
(*TNMGR, Oct. 2012*)

Q. Write a short note on pulp stones.
(*BFUHS, Nov. 2007*)

Ans. Calcification is hardening of tissue by deposition of or conversion into insoluble calcium salts or compounds.

Diffuse calcifications: They appear as irregular calcific deposits in pulp tissue, usually following collagenous fiber bundles or blood vessels. The pulp chamber may appear normal, with these calcifications in roots. These calcifications may be classified as **dystrophic calcifications.**

Pulp stones (Denticles): Nodular, calcified masses appearing in both coronal and root portions of pulp organ. They are usually asymptomatic. **True denticles** are similar in structure to dentin, as they have dentinal tubules. They are rare and usually located close to apical foramen. **False denticles** do not exhibit dentinal tubules. They appear as concentric layers of calcified tissue. Pulp stones may be classified as **free, attached** or **embedded.** Pulp stones may appear close to blood vessels and nerve trunks. Their incidence as well as size increases with age. They are found more commonly in coronal pulp (Fig. 3.12).

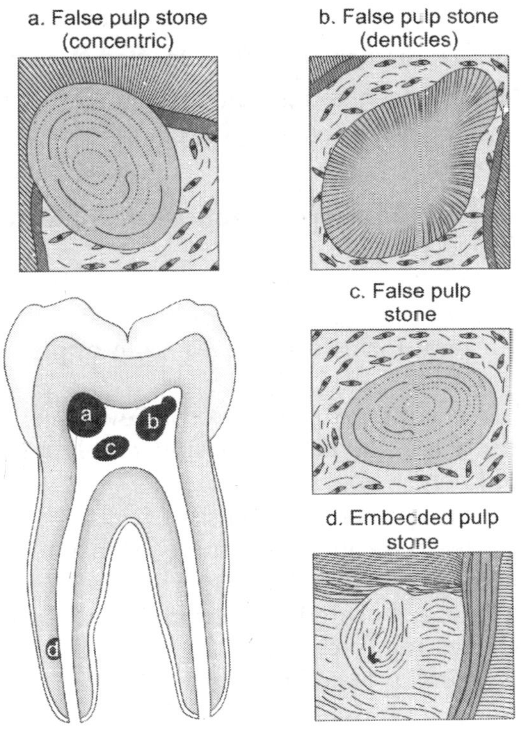

a. False pulp stone (concentric)

b. False pulp stone (denticles)

c. False pulp stone

d. Embedded pulp stone

Fig. 3.12: Pulp stone types and its location

Clinical Significance

1. Presence of pulp stones may alter the internal anatomy of pulp cavity, making access opening of tooth difficult.
2. Pulp stone in large number may indicate chronic irritation of pulp.

Q. 13. Discuss pulpo-dentinal complex as "marriages are made in heaven." *(BBD Uni., April 2014; RGUHS, May 2014)*

Q. Discuss histopathology of dental pulp. *(Sumandeep Uni., April 2015)*

Ans. Dentin and pulp are embryologically, histologically, and functionally the same tissue and therefore are considered as a complex. Both pulp and dentin have a common origin from dental papilla. Structure and response of dentin to injury are largely functions of odontoblasts and other cells in pulp, but these cells are dependent on dentin for their protection and state of differentiation. The embryonic dental papillae are responsible for formation of this coupled tissue. The response of pulp to any restorative material will be influenced by its surrounding dentin also. Dentinal fluid in the tubules, which is continuous with extracellular fluid of pulp, serves as a medium for relaying injurious agents to pulp to induce an inflammatory response.

Pulp: Parts of pulp:

Pulp chamber/coronal pulp: Located in crown of tooth.

Root canal/radicular pulp: Pulp located in root area.

Apical foramen: Opening from pulp at apex of tooth.

Accessory/lateral canal: Extra canal located on lateral portions of root.

Microscopic Zones in pulp (zones from outer to inner zone) (Fig. 3.13):

1. Odontoblastic layer: Lines outer pulpal wall and consists of cell bodies of odontoblast. Secondary dentin may form in this area from apposition of odontoblast.
2. Cell-free zone (zone of Weil): Fewer cells than odontoblastic layer. Nerve and capillary plexus located here.
3. Cell-rich zone: Increased density of cells as compared to cell-free zone and also a more extensive vascular system.
4. Pulpal-core: Located in center of pulp chamber, which has many cells and an extensive vascular supply, similar to cell-rich zone.

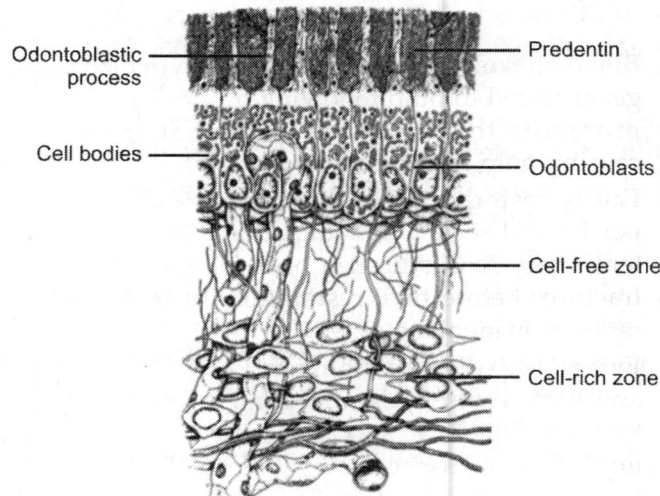

Fig. 3.13: Pulp dentin complex

(labels: Odontoblastic process, Cell bodies, Predentin, Odontoblasts, Cell-free zone, Cell-rich zone)

Contents of the Pulp

1. Cells: Odontoblast, fibroblast, white-blood cells, undifferentiated mesenchymal cells, macrophages and lymphocytes. No fat cell.
2. Fibrous matrix: Mostly reticular fibres and collagen fibres (type I and type III).
3. Ground substance: Act as medium to transport nutrients to cells and metabolites of cell to blood vessels.

Vascularity and nerves of pulp: Pulp organ is extensively vascular with vessels arising from external carotids to superior or inferior alveolar arteries. It drains by same vein.

Nerves: Several large nerves enter apical canal of teeth. This trunks transverse radicular pulp, proceed to coronal area and branch peripherally.

Q. 14. Write about portal of infections in dental pulp. *(Sumandeep Uni., April 2014)*

Ans. The various routes by which the microorganisms reach the pulp are as follows.

1. **Dentinal tubules:** After a carious lesion or during dental procedures, microorganisms may use the pathway in a centripetal direction to reach pulp.
2. **Open cavity:** Direct pulp exposure due to operative procedures, breaks physical barrier imposed by dental structures and leaves pulp in contact with septic oral environment.
3. **Periodontal membrane:** Microorganisms from gingival sulcus may reach pulp chamber through PDL, using lateral channel or apical foramen as pathway.

4. **Blood stream:** A transient bacteremia in blood may get attracted to pulp following trauma or operative procedure that produced inflammation without causing pulp exposure (*anachoresis*).

5. **Faulty restoration:** In obturated tooth with gutta percha and sealer, contamination may occur if the temporary seal is broken or if the tooth structure fractures before final restoration, or if final restoration is inadequate.

6. **Extent:** Microorganisms might reach the principal and/or lateral canals migrating from an infected tooth to a healthy pulp as a consequence of contiguousness of tissues.

Q. 15. Write a short note on cementum.
(TNMGR, Oct. 2013)

Q. Write a short note on histology/ultrastructure of cementum.
(UHSR, 2013; TNMGR, Oct. 2018)

Ans. Cementum is the mineralized dental tissue covering the anatomic roots of human teeth. It is formed by connective tissue cells (cementoblasts) of dental follicles, which comes in the contact of newly formed radicular dentin. It is light yellow in colour and softer than dentin.

Physical Characteristics:
1. Calcified structure whose calcification and hardness is less than dentin.
2. More permeable than dentin.
3. Light yellow in color.
4. Lacks luster and is dark than enamel.
5. Less readily resorbed than bone.
6. Begins at cervical portion of tooth at CEJ and continues to apex.
7. Thickest at apical region and thinnest at CEJ.

Chemical Composition:
1. Organic content and water: 50–55%.
   a. Collagen (type I, III, V, IX), GAGs (chondroitin 4-sulphate, dermatan sulphate).
   b. Non-collagenous proteins: Alkaline phosphatase, bone sialoprotein, fibronectin, osteocalcin, osteonectin, osteopontin, vitronectin, cementum derived attachment protein, insulin like growth factor-I
2. Inorganic content: 45–50%.
   a. Calcium and phosphate as hydroxyapatite.
   b. Trace elements like Cu, F, Fe, Pb, K, Si, Na, Zn. *Cementum has the highest fluoride content.*

Classification
A. **Location:**
   1. Coronal: Formed over enamel covering the crown.
   2. Radicular: On root surface.
B. **Presence/absence of cells:**
   1. Cellular cementum: Secondary cementum formed after tooth reaches occlusal plane, less calcified, contains cementocytes; more frequent on apical half.
   2. Acellular cementum: First formed before tooth reaches occlusal plane, more calcified, devoid of cementocyte; more frequent on coronal half of root.

Histology:
A. **Cells, fibres, ground substance:** Cementoblast (synthesis collagen and organic matrix), cementocytes (present in cellular cementum), cementoclasts (cementum resorption and repair)
B. **Incremental lines of Salter:** Accentuated lines of highly mineralized areas with less collagen due to rhythmic periodic deposition of cementum.
C. **Cementoenamel junction (CEJ):**
   1. Cementum overlaps enamel: 60–65% of the teeth.
   2. Cementum meets enamel in a sharp line: 30% of the teeth.
   3. Cementum and enamel does not meet at all: 5–10% of the teeth.
D. **Cementodentinal junction (CDJ):** Terminal apical area of cementum where it joins internal root dentin.

Functions:
1. It furnishes a medium for attachment of collagen fibers, bind tooth to alveolar bone.
2. It serves as major reparative tissue for root surfaces.
3. It helps in functional adaptation of teeth.

Q. 16. Write a short note on cementogenesis.
(RGUHS, Nov. 2011)

Ans. Cementum formation (cementogenesis) is preceded by deposition of dentin along the inner aspect of HERS. The newly formed dentin comes in contact of connective tissue of dentin follicle, forming cementoblast. Cementoblasts synthesize collagen and protein polysaccharides, which make up cementum matrix. After this, mineralization of matrix starts, by deposition of calcium and phosphate ions present in tissue fluids.

Stages of cementogenesis (Fig. 3.16):

Phase I: Laying down of cementoid tissue (matrix formation)

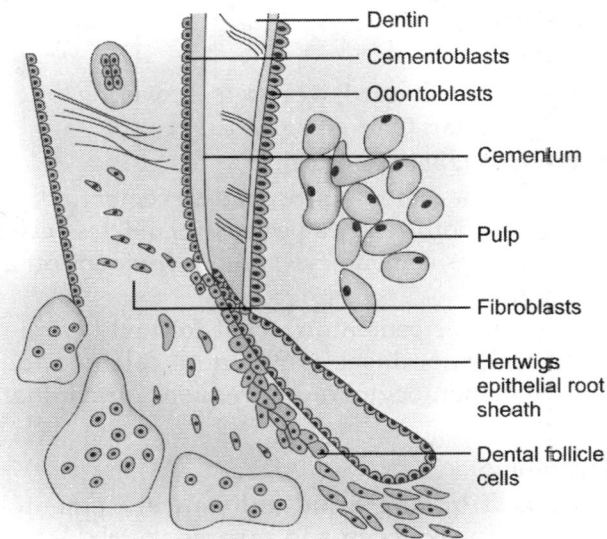

Dentin
Cementoblasts
Odontoblasts
Cementum
Pulp
Fibroblasts
Hertwigs epithelial root sheath
Dental follicle cells

Fig. 3.16: Cementogenesis

Phase II: Mineralization: Apatite crystals are deposited along fibrils.

Cementum formation takes place rhythmically. A thin layer of cementoid is seen on surface of cementum lined by cementoblasts. These fibers are embedded in cementum and attaches tooth to surrounding bone. (*Sharpey's Fibers*)

Cementum is laid down much slowly while the tooth is erupting. This cementum is **acellular or primary**. When tooth comes in occlusion, more cementum forms around the apical 2/3rd of root, which has greater proportion of collagen. The cementoblasts become trapped in lacunae within this matrix. This cementum is called **cellular (secondary)** cementum. The rate of formation of cellular cementum is much more rapid than that of acellular cementum.

Q. 17. Write about role of cementum in health and diseases. (*Suman Vidyapeeth, April 2010*)

Ans. Cementum in health:
1. Cementum is more resistant to resorption than bone.
2. Cementum resorption can occur after trauma or excessive occlusal forces.
3. After resorption the damage is repaired by formation of new cementum.
4. Transverse fracture of the root is repaired by formation of new cementum.
5. In cases of gingival recession, cementum may get hypermineralized.

Cementum in disease:
1. **Developmental anomalies:**
   a. Concrescence: Union of roots by cementum.
   b. Ectopic enamel: Presence of enamel on root cementum.

c. Enamel pearl: Hemispheres of enamel with dentin and pulp present in furcation area.
   d. Cervical enamel projections: Dipping of enamel from CEJ towards bifurcations (mandibular molars).
   e. Hypercementosis: Non-neoplastic deposition of excessive cementum, seen in abnormal occlusal trauma, arthritis, Paget's disease.
   f. Ankylosis: Anatomic fusion of tooth cementum or dentin with alveolar bone.

2. **Regressive alterations of teeth:**
   a. Abrasion: Pathologic wearing of tooth substance by abnormal mechanical process, usually on exposed root surfaces.
   b. Cementicles: Dystrophic calcifications which lie free in periodontal ligament.
   c. Root caries: Soft progressive lesion found anywhere on root surface, that is exposed to oral environment.
   d. Calculocementum: Calculus embedded deeply in cementum.

3. **Due to periodontal pathology:**
   a. Subsurface alteration: Due to gingival inflammation, alterations in structure and composition.
   b. Cervical root resorption.
   c. Bacterial contamination due to exposure to oral environment.
   d. Pathologic granules: Areas of collagen degeneration.
   e. Areas of increased mineralization/demineralization.
   f. Cellular resorption of cementum.

4. **Neoplasms of cementum:**
   a. Benign cementoma.
   b. Periapical cemental dysplasia.
   c. Central cementifying fibroma.
   d. Gigantiform cementum.
   e. Focal cemento-osseous dysplasia

5. **Systemic disease**
   a. Cleidocranial dysplasia: Absence of cellular cementum.
   b. Hypophosphatasia: Absence of cementum.
   c. Hyperpituitarism: Hypercementosis.
   d. Hypothyroidism: External resorption of roots.
   e. Hyperparathyroidism: Loss of lamina dura and root resorption
   f. Paget's disease: Hypercementosis, loss of lamina dura and root resorption

6. In forensic odontology: Age estimation from incremental lines of cementum (acellular cementum).

Q.18. Write a short note on development of periodontal ligament.

(MAHE, Dec. 1997; TNMGR, Sept. 2007; BFUHS, Nov. 2007; UHSR, April 2015, May 2017)

Ans. Development (Fig. 3.18): Enamel organ is surrounded by a condensation of ecto mesenchymal cells called **dental sac**. The part of dental sac immediately close to enamel organ is called **dental follicle**. Once HERS disintegrates leaving behind **epithelial rests of Malassez**, cells of dental follicle come close to surface of newly formed dentin. The dental follicle cells then differentiate into cementoblasts and lay down cementum on dentin on the developing root. The other cells of dental follicle differentiate into fibroblast and lay down fibers and ground substance of periodontal ligament. As crown approaches the oral mucosa during tooth eruption, these fibroblasts become active and start producing collagen fibrils. They initially lack orientation, but they soon acquire an orientation oblique to tooth. The first collagen bundles appear in the region immediately apical to CEJ and give rise to gingivodental fiber groups. As tooth eruption progresses, additional oblique fibers appear and become attached to newly formed cementum and bone. The transseptal and alveolar crest fibers develop when tooth merges into oral cavity. Alveolar bone deposition occurs simultaneously with PDL organization. *Sharpey's fibers* are fewer in number and more widely spaced than those emerging from cementum. At later stage, alveolar fibers extend into middle zone to join lengthening cemental fibers, attain their classic orientation, thickness and strength when occlusal function is established.

Q. 19. Write a short note on periodontal ligament (PDL). Write about its age changes.

(RGUHS, April 2006; TNMGR, March 2010; RUHS, June 2017)

Q. Discuss the architecture variability and clinical considerations with respect to periodontal ligament.

(UHRS, 2013; HP Uni., April 2019)

Ans. The periodontal ligament (PDL) is a specialized connective tissue which occupies the space between root and alveolar bone of tooth socket. Width range is 0.15–0.38 mm, thinnest around middle third of root. (*Hourglass shaped*)

Cells of Periodontal Ligament (PDL):

A. Synthetic cells: Osteoblasts, fibroblasts, cementoblasts.

B. Resorptive cells: Osteoclasts, fibroblasts, cementoclasts.

C. Other cells: Epithelial rests of Malassez, defense cells (mast cells, macrophages, eosinophils).

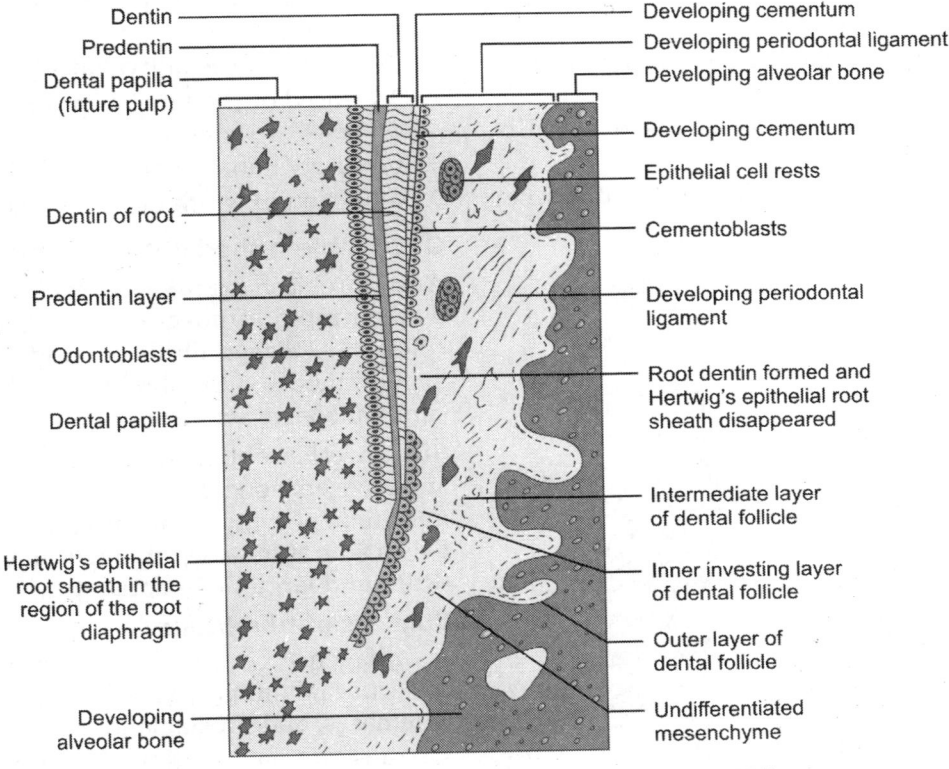

Fig. 3.18: Development of periodontal ligament (PDL)

Extracellular Substances

A. Connective tissue fibers: Collagen fibers (type I, III, XII), oxytalan fibers, reticular fibers, elastic fibers.

B. Ground substance: Proteoglycans (chondroitin sulphate, dermatan sulphate, heparin sulphate, hyaluronic acid), glycoprotein (fibronectin, laminin, tenascin)

Blood supply: Perforating arteries arising from intra-alveolar vessels.

Nerve supply: A and C fibers from trigeminal nerve. These fibers end as:

a. Free nerve ending: Present along the length of root, nociceptors.

b. Ruffini's endings: Appear dendrite and end in terminal expansions among PDL bundle mechanoreceptors.

c. Meissner's corpuscles: Coiled form in mid-region, tactile perception.

d. Encapsulated spindle like endings: Associated with root apex temperature receptor.

Fibers of PDL: Principal fibers consist of individual fibers forming a continuous anastomosing network between tooth (cementum) and bone (Fig. 3.19).

1. **Transseptal group**: Extend interproximally in cementum of adjacent teeth, resist tooth separation, mesial or distal.

2. **Alveolar crest group:** Prevent extrusion of teeth and resist lateral movement.

3. **Horizontal group:** Resist horizontal and tipping forces.

4. **Oblique group:** Largest group, resist apically directed masticatory forces.

5. **Apical group:** Prevent tooth tipping; do not occur on incompletely formed roots.

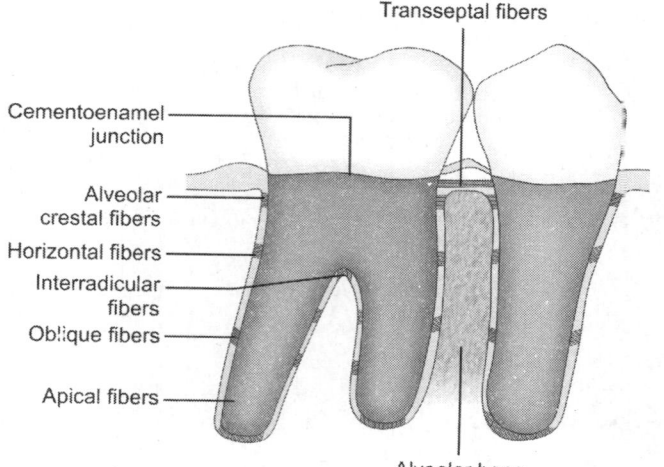

Transseptal fibers
Cementoenamel junction
Alveolar crestal fibers
Horizontal fibers
Interradicular fibers
Oblique fibers
Apical fibers
Alveolar bone

Fig. 3.19: Principal fibers of PDL

6. **Interradicular group:** Resist forces of luxation and rotation, present onto the furcation areas of multirooted teeth.

Functions:

1. Provision of a soft tissue "casing" to protect vessels and nerves from injury by mechanical force.

2. Transmission of occlusal forces to bone.

3. Attachment of the teeth to bone.

4. Maintenance of gingival tissues in their proper relationship to teeth.

5. Resistance to impact of occlusal forces (shock absorption)

6. Formative: Helps in formation of collagen, cementum, and bone.

7. Sensory: PDL transmits sensation of tactile, pressure and pain.

8. Nutritive: Supplies nutrition to cementum, bone and gingiva.

9. Homeostatic.

Age Changes:

1. Reduction in vascularity, elasticity and reparative capacity.

2. Decreased number of fibroblasts with more irregular structure is seen.

3. Decreased collagen synthesis.

4. Decrease in no. of periodontal fibers.

5. The fiber bundles become thicker, broader and more highly organized.

6. Presence of areas of hyalinization.

7. Decreased organic matrix production and epithelial cell rests.

8. Increased amount of elastic fibers.

9. Reduction in width of PDL space.

Q. 20. Write a short note on fibroblasts.

Ans. Fibroblasts are principal cells of PDL characterized by their rapid turnover of extracellular compartment, collagen. Collagen fibrils of bundles are continuously being remodeled by fibroblasts, which are capable of simultaneously synthesizing and degrading collagen.

Structure: Fibroblasts stem from a mesenchymal origin and have an elongated spindle or stellate shape with a multitude of cytoplasmic projections. Within the cytoplasm is an abundance of rough endoplasmic reticulum (RER) and large Golgi apparatus.

Products of fibroblasts

• Collagen type I, III, and IV, proteoglycans, fibronectin, laminins, glycosaminoglycans, metalloproteinases, and prostaglandins.

• Transcription growth factor-alpha and beta (TGF-α and TGF-β), platelet-derived growth factor (PDGF), granulocyte macrophage colony-stimulating factor (GM-CSF), epidermal growth factor (EGF) and tumor necrosis factor (TNF).

- Fibroblasts are known for their plasticity; adipocytes, pericytes, endothelial and epithelial cells, can de-differentiate into fibroblasts.
- They can transform into myofibroblasts, present in both healthy and pathologic tissues and contain features of fibroblasts and smooth muscle cells.

Functions

- Activated fibroblast can be induced by appropriate stimuli from macrophages, lymphocytes, mechanical force, and bacteria.
- In connective tissue remodeling, fibroblasts are capable of synthesis and phagocytosis of collagen and components of extracellular matrix.
- Cytokines produced by fibroblasts have capacity to mediate tissue destruction and stimulate osteoclastic bone resorption.
- Fibroblast-derived proinflammatory mediators and cytokines are implicated in periodontal tissue destruction by promoting fibrosis, granuloma formation or bone resorption.

Q. 21. Write a short note on alveolar bone.
(TNMGR, March 2007; KLE Uni., Dec. 2008; NTR Uni., May 2019)

Q. Write a short note on bone cells.
(TNMGR, Sept. 2010)

Q. Discuss alveolar bone in health and disease.
(UHSR, May 2016; May 2017; HP Uni., May 2017; April 2019)

Ans. Alveolar bone may be defined as that part of maxilla and mandible that forms and supports sockets of teeth. It is also known as **"functional bone"** as it is susceptible to functional changes and is lost after tooth extraction.

Development: Near end of 2nd month of IUL, mandible and maxilla form a groove that opens towards the surface of oral cavity. As tooth germs start to develop, bony septa form gradually and alveolar process starts developing during tooth eruption.

Structure

a. Alveolar bone proper: Thin lamella of bone that surrounds root of tooth and gives attachment to principal fibers of PDL, perforated by multiple openings that carry nerves and blood vessels into PDL, so it is known as **"Cribriform plate."**

b. Supporting alveolar bone: Bone that surrounds alveolar bone proper and gives support to socket.

1. Cortical plates—compact bone, forming inner and outer plates of alveolar processes. Much thicker in mandible than maxilla and thickest in premolar, molar region on buccal side.

2. Spongy bone—fills the area between cortical plates and alveolar bone proper, not found in anterior teeth region.

In health, the distance of 1.5–2 mm is always maintained between alveolar crest and adjacent teeth.

Cells:

1. **Osteoprogenitor cells:** Undifferentiated mesenchymal cells and hematopoietic stem cells divide and transform into osteoblasts and osteoclasts.

2. **Osteoblasts:** Bone forming cells. Formed from multipotent mesenchymal cells. They secrete type I collagen and bone matrix (osteoid). They exhibit a high level of alkaline phosphatase.

3. **Osteoclasts:** Bone resorbing cells. Multinucleated, found in Howship's lacunae, derived from circulating monocytes and local mesenchymal cells.

4. **Osteocytes:** Entrapped osteoblasts in lacunae are called osteocytes. They resorbs surrounding bone to form spaces called *osteocytic lacunae.*

Age changes:

1. More irregular periodontal surface of bone
2. Less regular insertion of collagen fibers.
3. Osteoporosis.
4. Decreased vascularity.

Alveolar bone in disease: Conditions of alveolar bone loss:

1. Extensive gingival inflammation.
2. Trauma from occlusion
3. Systemic conditions: Vitamin D deficiency, diabetes, hyperparathyroidism, etc.
4. Periodontitis/abscess
5. Tooth extraction
6. Overhang restoration
7. Ill fitting prosthesis

Q. 22. Write a short note on bundle bone.
(TNMGR, Sept. 2007)

Ans. The alveolar bone proper consists of lamellated and bundle bone. Bundle bone is that bone in which the principal fibers of the PDL are anchored. The term bundle bone was chosen because the bundles of the principal fibers continue into the bone as Sharpey's fibers. It is characterize by scarcity of fibrils in intercellular substance, which are arranged at right angles to Sharpey's fibers. It contains fewer fibrils than lamellated bone, and therefore, it appears dark in H&E stained sections. The bundle bone contains more calcium salts per unit area than other types of bone tissues, such areas are seen as dense radiopacities (lamina dura), radiographically

Q. 23. Write a short note on lamina dura.
(TNMGR, Oct. 2013)

Ans. Lamina dura (LD) is a radiographic landmark viewed largely on periapical radiographs (PR). The terminology LD (or alveolus) is applied to the thin layer of dense cortical bone, which lines the roots of sound teeth. It appears as a well-defined radiopaque (white) layer in radiograph. The term lamina dura or "hard layer" is derived from the fact that it is more radiopaque than adjacent bone. Presence of LD is an indication of health of teeth. Radiographically it is seen as a thin radiopaque line running around the length of roots. Adjacent to the LD, on tooth side, a thin dark shadow represents the space occupied by periodontal membrane, known as periodontal space. PR has mainly been used to assess both periodontal ligament (PDL) space and LD. The presence or absence of LD and PDL space on radiographs may also be affected by any variations in angulations of X-ray beam. The convexity or concavity of proximal tooth surfaces, the curvature of roots, level of cementoenamel junction and thickness of alveolar bone may also cause variations in thickness and clarity of the LD.

Q. 24. Write a short note on cusp of Carabelli.
(UHSR, June 2017)

Ans. It is accessory lingual cusp located on mesiopalatal cusp of maxillary second deciduous molars and first, second and third permanent molars. It may be unilateral or bilateral, with marked deviation in size. In some cases, accessory cusp is seen occasionally on mandibular permanent or deciduous molar, this is called *protostylid*. Carabelli's trait was found in 1842 by Sir Georg Carabelli. Carabelli's trait is one of the most studied nonmetric traits. The Carabelli's trait has been used as a critical ethnic indicator for several decades, most likely because it can be simply observed in both living individuals and skeletal material, and can, therefore, be used to show major ethnic differences in dentition. Dahlberg's classification is the most commonly applied method for determining degree and expression of Carabelli cusps. (Fig. 3.24). For permanent dentition, Carabelli's trait appears to be generally the most common among the European populations, followed by African populations and American Indians, with lowest prevalence occurring in other Mongoloid races.

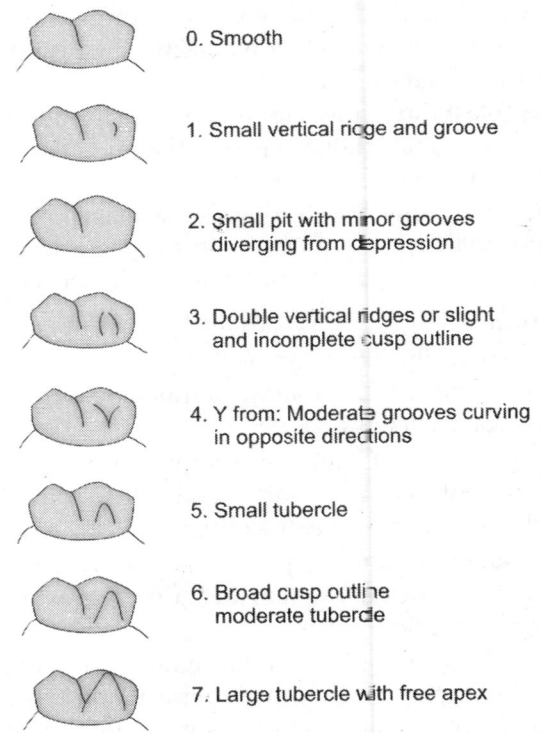

0. Smooth

1. Small vertical ridge and groove

2. Small pit with minor grooves diverging from depression

3. Double vertical ridges or slight and incomplete cusp outline

4. Y from: Moderate grooves curving in opposite directions

5. Small tubercle

6. Broad cusp outline moderate tubercle

7. Large tubercle with free apex

Fig. 3.24: Dahlberg's (1963) scale for the determination of degree and expression of Carabelli cusps

4. ORAL MUCOUS MEMBRANE, GINGIVA AND MISCELLANEOUS

Q. 1. Write a note on oral mucous membrane in health and diseases.   (TNMGR, April 2013)

Q. Write a short note on oral mucosa.
(KLE, June 2007; TNMGR, Oct. 2012)

Q. Describe microanatomy/histology of oral mucosa/ buccal mucosa.   (HNBG Uni., June 2016; MUHS, June 2017)

Ans. It is a protective lining of oral cavity consisting partly of epithelium and partly of connective tissue. Anatomically, it begins at the vermilion border of lip and extends up to a point where the pharynx ends.
Oral mucous membrane in health (Fig. 4.1)
Role of oral mucosa
1. It is protective mechanically against both compressive and shearing forces.
2. It provides barrier to various pathogens.
3. It has a role in immunological defense.
4. Minor salivary glands within the mucosa provide lubrication and buffering as well as secretion of some antibodies.
5. Mucosa is richly innervated, providing inputs for touch, properiception, pain and taste.

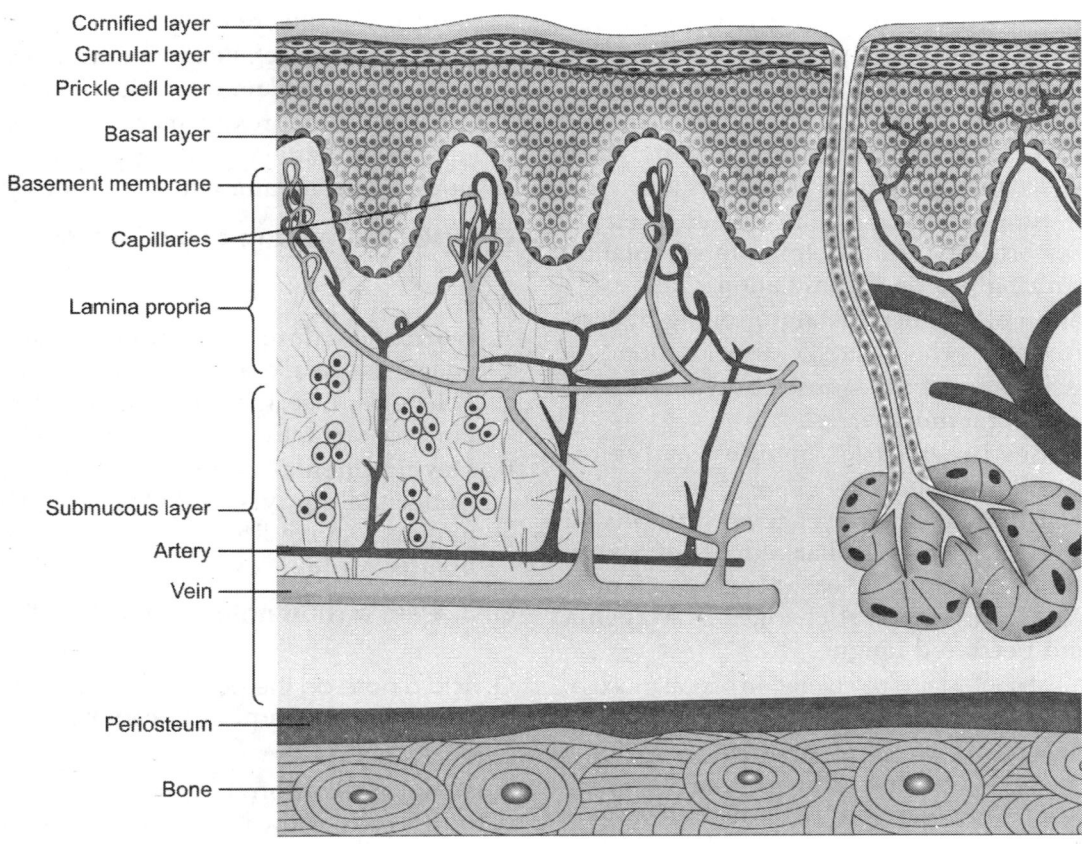

Fig. 4.1: Oral mucous membrane

Labels on figure:
Cornified layer
Granular layer
Prickle cell layer
Basal layer
Basement membrane
Capillaries
Lamina propria
Submucous layer
Artery
Vein
Periosteum
Bone

6. Reflexes such as gagging, salivation are initiated by receptors in the oral mucosa.

Development: Primitive oral cavity develops by fusion of embryonic stomatodaeum with foregut after rupture of buccopharyngeal membrane. Structures from branchial arches like tongue, epiglottis and pharynx covered by epithelium are derived from endoderm. Epithelium covering palate, cheeks and gingiva are of ectodermal in origin.

Oral mucosa can be divided into:

a. **Masticatory mucosa:** Gingiva and hard palate.

b. **Lining or reflecting mucosa:** Lip, cheek, vestibular fornix, alveolar mucosa, floor of mouth, soft palate.

c. **Specialized mucosa:** Dorsum of the tongue, taste buds.

It consists of surface epithelium and underlying connective tissue, lamina propria.

The epithelium: Derived from ectoderm. It can be **keratinized** or **non-keratinized.**

A. Keratinized epithelium consists of four layers:

- Stratum basale: Cells are cuboidal or low columnar, adjacent to basement membrane, most active mitotically.
- Stratum spinosum (prickle cell layer): Spherical or elliptical cells.
- Stratum granulosum: Flat and wide cells, kerato-hyaline granules.
- Stratum corneum (surface layer): Flat cells devoid of nuclei, filled with keratin
  1. Orthokeratinized epithelium: No nuclei in stratum corneum and presents a well-defined stratum granulosum.
  2. Parakeratinized epithelium: Surface cells have pyknotic nuclei; in this stratum corneum and stratum granulosum are absent.

B. Non-keratinized epithelium: In this stratum corneum and stratum granulosum are absent. It includes lips, buccal mucosa, alveolar mucosa, soft palate, ventral surface of tongue, floor of mouth.

The lamina propria: It has
1. Papillar layer: Large finger-like projections.
2. Reticular layer.

Oral mucous membrane in disease: The basic considerations in oral mucosa are variation in tissue colour, dryness, smoothness or firmness and bleeding tendency of gingiva.

1. Periodontal pocket: It is a pathologically deepened gingival sulcus as a response to plaque toxins and subsequent immunologic response.

2. Restorative dentistry: In young patients, when clinical crown is smaller than anatomic crown, it is difficult to prepare a tooth for an abutment or crown.

3. Gingival recession: May result in cemental/root caries and sensitivity of the exposed dentin.

4. Keratinisation of gingiva: Can be achieved by massage or brushing, thus helping in stimulation and minimizing plaque accumulation.

5. Discoloration of gingiva: Metal poisoning by lead or bismuth causes characteristic discoloration.

6. Blood dyscrasias can be diagnosed by characteristic infiltration of oral mucosa.

7. Viral diseases like measles manifest as typical lesions of oral mucosa.

8. Changes of tongue: In scarlet fever, atrophy of lingual mucosa causes peculiar redness of **Strawberry tongue**. Systemic diseases such as vitamin deficiencies lead to typical changes as **Magenta tongue** and **beefy red tongue**.

9. Macule: A flat spot/stain/discoloration of oral mucosa, e.g. amalgam tattoo, nevus, rash of secondary syphilis.

10. Papule: Small rounded pimple-like variably colored, e.g. White variably patterned elevations of lichen planus.

11. Plaque: Slightly raised clearly demarcated area that may be smooth, pebbly cracked or fissured, e.g. leukoplakia, erythroplakia.

12. Vesicle: Small circumscribed elevated blister not more than 5 mm in diameter with covering layer of epithelial cells and containing an accumulation of fluid, e.g. herpes labialis.

13. Pustule: Vesicle predominantly containing pus.

14. Bulla: Large vesicle or blister, e.g. pemphigus and drug reactions. May appear white due to necrosis of epithelium forming pseudomembrane.

15. Ulcer: Sore characterized by loss of epithelium yielding a punched out area, e.g. traumatic ulcers, aphthous stomatitis, cancer and tuberculosis.

16. Fissure: Narrow linear crack of epidermis with an ulcer at its base, e.g. fissured tongue.

17. Erosion: Partial loss of upper layers of epithelium, e.g. toothbrush trauma, erosive lichen planus.

18. Cyst: Cavity lined by epithelium containing fluid or cells, e.g. gingival cyst.

19. Nodule: Localized elevated mass of tissue projecting from surface, e.g. fibroma, mucocele.

20. Tumour: Swelling of part of an organ. Inflammatory, developmental or neoplastic. Carcinoma is a malignant tumour of epithelial cells.

21. Wheal: Pruritic, reddened, edematous papule.

22. Sinus/sinus tract: Leading from underlying cavity cyst or abscess and opening onto surface.

23. Scar: White depressed mark, line or area representing healing after injury, e.g. gingivectomy, apicoectomy, deep inflammation, previous trauma.

Q. 2. Normal variants of oral mucosa.
(NTR Uni., July 2017)

Ans.

A. **Normal anatomic variants:** Linea alba; Leukoedema; Normal oral pigmentation; Lingual tonsils/Foliate papillae; Lymphoid aggregates; Varicosities; Fordyce's granules; Hairy tongue; Fissure tongue

B. **Developmental anomalies:** Fordyce's granules; Congenital lip pits; Ankyloglossia; Cleft lip; Bifid tongue; Double lip; Torus platinus; Torus mandibularis; Multiple exostosis.

Q. 3. Write a short note on keratinization.
(UHSR, May 2016)

Q. Add a note on the consequence of loss of integrity of epithelium-basement complex.
(NTR Uni., May 2018)

Ans. Keratinization/cornification, is a process of cytodifferentiation in which keratinocytes, when proceeding from their postgerminative state (stratum basale) to finally differentiated, become hardened cell filled with protein, constituting a structurally and functionally distinct keratin containing surface layer such as stratum corneum. Keratins that form the intermediate filaments are expressed exclusively in epithelial cells regardless of germ layer origin of these cells and are useful as markers of differentiation. The keratins are broadly divided:

A. **Primary and secondary:**

1. Primary keratins: Synthesized by epithelial cells on a regular basis, e.g. K8/18 in simple epithelia, K5/14 in stratified epithelia.

2. Secondary keratins: Additional keratins produced by epithelial cells, e.g. K7/19 in simple epithelia, K15, and K6/16 in stratified epithelia.

B. **Based on distribution:**

1. Soft keratin: Allows some stretching but returns to normal upon relaxation of tension.

2. Hard keratin: Very little flexibility owing to presence of many cysteine disulfide cross links.

C. **Based on X-ray diffraction pattern:**

1. Alpha
2. Beta
3. Feather keratins
4. Amorphous keratins

D. **Based on amino acid sequence:**
1. Type I family: Keratins numbered from 9–20, acidic.
2. Type II family: Keratins numbered 1–8, basic.

E. **Based on molecular weight:**
1. Low molecular weight keratins: Molecular weight of 40 kDa.
2. Intermediate molecular weight keratins: Molecular weight 40 kDa–57 kDa.
3. High molecular weight keratins: Molecular weight of 57 kDa.

Functions of Keratins

1. Keratins influence architecture and mitotic activity of epithelial cells.
2. Keratins and associated filaments provide a scaffold for epithelial cells and tissues to sustain mechanical stress, maintain their structural integrity, ensure mechanical resilience, to protect against variations in hydrostatic pressure and establish cell polarity.
3. Keratins and its filaments are involved in cell signalling, cell transport, cell compartmentalization and cell differentiation.
4. Keratin filaments influence cell metabolic processes by regulating protein synthesis and cell growth.
5. Keratins are involved in transport of membrane bound vesicles in cytoplasm of epithelial cells.

Keratinization Disorders with Predominant/Associated Oral Lesions

1. **White Sponge Nevus/Cannon's disease/familial white folded dysplasia:** Occurs due to a mutation in gene encoding for K4/13 that is expressed in spinous cell layer of non-keratinized mucosa of oral cavity.
2. **Pachyonychia Congenita (PC) (Greek-thick nails from birth):** Mutation in gene encoding for K6/16 and K17 that typically affects nails and palmo-plantar skin and often oral mucosa, tongue, larynx, teeth and hair.
3. **Dyskeratosis congenita (DC)/Cole-Engmen syndrome/Zinsser-Cole-Engmen syndrome:** Mutation in DKC1 gene, thus disrupting normal maintenance of telomerase.
4. **Hereditary benign intraepithelial dyskeratosis/ Witkop-Von Sallman syndrome**
5. **Darier's disease (keratosis follicularis)**
6. **Pemphigus:** Defects in keratin associated protein, desmosomes.
7. **Keratinizing lesions of oral cavity:** These demonstrate hyperkeratosis on histopathology.
   a. Reactive lesions: Frictional keratosis, smokeless tobacco-induced keratosis, nicotine stomatitis, hairy tongue, hairy leukoplakia

Table 4.3: Distribution of major keratins

Keratin distribution in epithelia	
K5/14	Basal cell layer of both the keratinized and non-keratinized stratified epithelium
K1/10	Keratinized epidermis
K6/16	Spinous cell layer of keratinized mucosa
K4/13	Intermediate layer of non-keratinized epithelium
K19	Basal layer of non-keratinized epithelium
K9	Suprabasal cells of palmar and plantar epidermis
Keratin expression in gingival	
K5/14	Basal cell layer
K19	Basal cell layer of junctional epithelium and gingival margin
K8, 18, 13, 16, 19	Superficial layers of junctional epithelium
K4, 13, 16	Superficial layer of gingival margin
K1/10, K6/16 and K2p	Superficial layers of outer gingival epithelium
Distribution of keratin in the dorsal aspect of the tongue (Dale et al 1990)	
Keratin similar to hair	Posterior portion of filiform papilla
K4/13	Interpapillary region
K4/13 and K1/10	The anterior portion

   b. Immune mediated lesions: Lichen planus, discoid lupus erythematosus, graft versus host disease.
   c. Pre-neoplastic and neoplastic diseases: Actinic cheilosis, leukoplakia, proliferative verrucous leukoplakia, verrucous carcinoma, squamous cell carcinoma.
   d. Infections: Squamous cell papilloma, verruca vulgaris, condyloma accuminatum, molluscum contagiosum and verruciform xanthoma.

Q. 4. Write a short note on biosynthesis of collagen
(Sumandeep Uni., April 2014)

Q. Write a short note on collagen and its degradation. *(TNMGR, March 2009)*

Ans. Collagen (Greek: To produce "Glue") is a major structural protein of extracellular matrix constitutes about 25–30% of protein of mammals. Collagen is fibrous protein that possesses high tensile strength and cannot be stretched. There are at least 12 different types of collagen, each exhibiting certain specific and unique chemical characteristics.

Type I: Skin, bone, scar, tendon, blood vessel, cornea.

Type II: Cartilage, inter-vertebral disc, vitreous body.

Type III: Fetal skin, vessels, granulation tissue.

Type IV: Basement membrane.

Type V: Cell surface, hair, placenta.

Type VII: Beneath stratified squamous epithelia.

Type IX: Cartilage.

Type XII: Tendon, ligaments

Distribution in oral tissues:

1. Alveolar bone: Type I
2. PDL: Type I, III
3. Cementum: Type I
4. Dentin: Type I
5. Pulp: Type I, III
6. Gingiva: Type I, IV
7. TMJ: Type I, II, III

Basic structure: Basic structural unit of collagen is trimer of polypeptides called tropocollagen that forms a triple helix. Tropocollagen is a rod-shaped molecule, 300 nm long and 1.5 nm thick consists of 3 helical polypeptide chains having 1050 amino acids—"α-chains". Peptide bonds are internal-resistant to digestion by proteases. Triple helix is stabilized by hydrogen bonds between the peptide bonds of different chains.

Biosynthesis of collagen: Collagen is one of the proteins that functions outside the cell. Polypeptide precursors of the collagen molecule are formed in fibroblasts, osteoblasts and chondroblasts. These are secreted into extracellular matrix (Fig. 4.4).

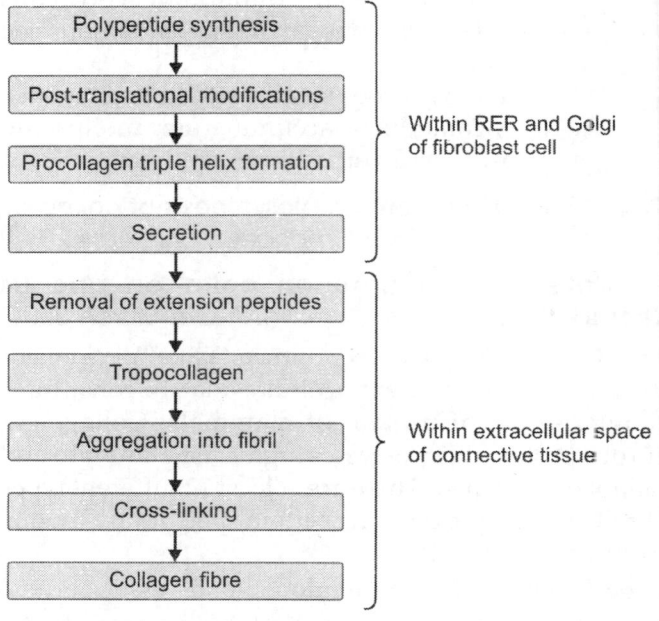

Fig. 4.4: Sequence of collagen synthesis

Degradation: The degradation of collagen is done by enzyme collagenase. Collagenase is secreted as a proenzyme that is activated by specific neutral proteases. Collagenolysis activity takes place outside osteoclast and occurs at a specific site on tropocollagen molecule. The broken fragments of collagen are further decalcified by other proteases.

Conditions associated with defects in collagen synthesis and metabolism:

1. Ehlers-Danlos syndrome
2. Osteogenesis imperfecta
3. Epidermolysis bullosa
4. Dermatosparaxis
5. Alport syndrome
6. Schmid metaphyseal chondrodysplasia
7. Scurvy
8. Menke's disease
9. Lathyrism.

Q. 5. Write a short note on salivary immunoglobulins.
(TNMGR, March 2010)

Ans. The predominant salivary immunoglobulin is secretory IgA or sIgA. It differs from serum IgA in that it exists as an 11S dimer consisting of two IgA molecules joined by a J chain, plus a secretory component, whereas serum IgA exists as a 7S monomer. Secretory IgA is a product of two different cell types where plasma cell synthesize polymeric IgA containing J chain of about 1.5 kD and glandular cell synthesize a glycoprotein secretory component of 7 kD. Secretory component is a receptor for polymeric IgA containing J chain; the IgA binds to secretory component below the tight junction of glandular epithelial cells and is then transported across the luminal surface. The presence of secretory component makes IgA resistant to proteolytic enzymes. Purified salivary IgA and IgG fractions have been found with agglutinating activity against oral isolates of α-hemolytic streptococci.

These immunoglobulins are produced locally by plasma cells in connective tissue stroma of the glands. It is the first line of defense of the host against pathogens which invade mucosal surfaces. Salivary IgA antibodies could help oral immunity by preventing microbial adherence, neutralizing enzymes, toxins and viruses; or by acting in synergy with other factors such as lysozyme and lactoferrin. In addition, low levels of salivary IgA have been presented as a risk factor for upper respiratory infection and have also been associated with an increased risk for periodontal disease and caries.

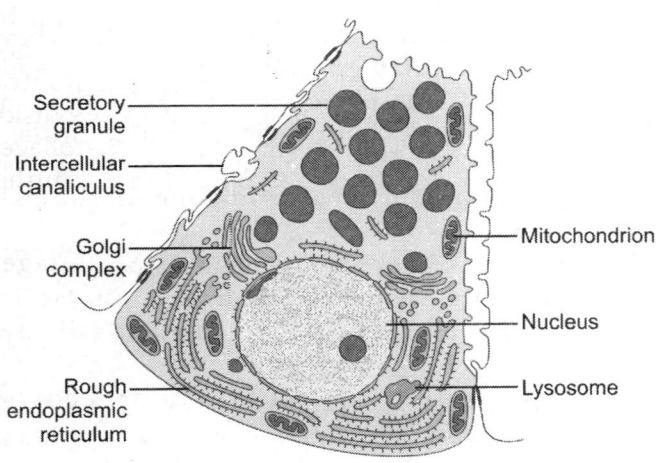

Fig. 4.6: Structure of serous cell

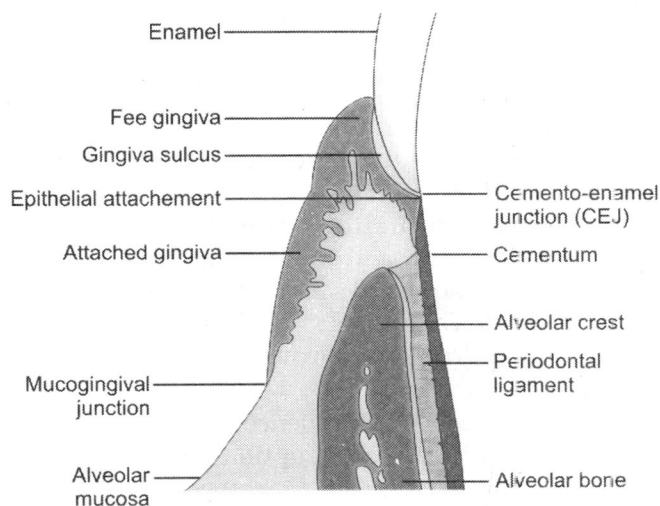

Fig. 4.7: Gingiva and its parts

Q. 6. Write about ultrastructure of serous cell.

(TNMGR, April 2011)

Ans. Serous cells are specialized for the synthesis, storage and secretion of proteins. The typical serous cell is pyramidal in shape, with its broad base resting on thin basal lamina and its narrow apex bordering on the lumen. The spherical nucleus is located in the basal region of the cell; occasionally binucleated cells are observed. There is accumulation of secretory granules in the apical cytoplasm. The basal portion of the cytoplasm is filled with ribosome studded endoplasmic reticulum. Golgi apparatus is located apical or lateral to nucleus. Mitochondria are found throughout the cell. (Fig. 4.6).

Q. 7. Discuss microscopic and macroscopic appearance of gingiva.

(AHSUC, July 2016)

Q. Development of gingival sulcus.

(NTR Uni., May 2019)

Ans. Gingiva is that part of oral mucosa that covers alveolar processes of jaws and surrounds neck of teeth (Carranza).

Functions

A. As part of oral mucosa: It protects supporting tissues from oral environment.

B. As part of peridontium: Its fibres secure against rotational forces; maintain periodontal health by its defense mechanism.

Gingival sulcus: It is shallow crevice around tooth, bounded by surface of tooth on one side and epithelial lining of marginal gingiva on other side. Probing depth is 2–3 mm.

Development of gingival sulcus: After enamel formation completes, the crown is covered with reduced enamel epithelium (REE), which terminates at CEJ. The basal lamina lies in contact with enamel directly. When tooth penetrates oral mucosa, REE fuses with oral epithelium. Shortly the epithelial mass at tip of crown degenerates, resulting exposure of crown in oral cavity. With tooth eruption, this united epithelium condenses along crown and ameloblasts from inner layer of REE become squamous cell with time. The gingival sulcus is formed when tooth erupts into oral cavity. Gradually this united epithelium transforms into junctional epithelium (JE), which occurs in apical direction.

Macroscopic/anatomical structure of gingiva:

1. **Marginal/unattached gingiva:** Terminal edge of gingiva (Fig. 4.7) surrounding the teeth in collar like fashion. *Free gingival groove* is formed by functional folding of free gingival margin during mastication.

2. **Attached gingiva:** It is continuous with marginal gingiva, is firm resilient and tightly bound to underlying periosteum of bone. On facial aspect, it is demarcated from alveolar mucosa by *Mucogingival junction.*

3. **Interdental gingiva:** Pyramidal or "**Col**" shaped, occupies interproximal space below area of tooth contact.

Microscopic structure of gingiva: Stratified squamous epithelium with core of connective tissue made up of collagen fibers and ground substance.

A. **Gingival epithelium:** (UOK, May 2015)

1. **Oral epithelium:** Faces oral cavity; Covers crest and outer surface of marginal gingiva and surface of attached gingiva. On average, oral epithelium is 0.2–0.3 mm in thickness. It is keratinized or parakeratinized or presents various combination.

2. **Sulcular epithelium (SE):** Faces the tooth, lines the gingival sulcus. It is a thin, non-keratinized

stratified squamous epithelium without rete pegs. It extends from coronal limit of JE to crest of gingival margin. It shows many cells with hydropic degeneration. The SE acts as a semi-permeable membrane, not heavily infiltrated by PMNs.

3. **Junctional epithelium (JE):** Provides contact between gingiva and tooth, consists of a collar-like band of stratified squamous non-keratinizing epithelium. The thickness of JE increases with age. JE tapers from its coronal end to its apical termination.

JE is formed by confluence of oral epithelium and REE during tooth eruption. JE is attached to tooth surface (epithelial attachment) by means of an internal basal lamina. It is attached to gingival connective tissue by an external basal lamina.

Attachment of JE to tooth is reinforced by gingival fibers, which brace marginal gingiva against tooth surface. For this reason, JE and gingival fibers are considered functional units referred to as *dentogingival unit*.

Functions: JE firmly attached to tooth surface forming an epithelial barrier against plaque, bacteria; allows access of gingival fluid inflammatory cells, and components of immunologic host defense to gingival margin; JE cells exhibit rapid turnover, contributes to host–parasite equilibrium and rapid repair of damaged tissue.

Cells of gingival epithelium:

1. **Principal cells:** Keratinocytes

2. **Clear cells/non-keratinocytes:** Langerhans cells, Markel's cells, melanocytes, inflammatory cells.

3. **Melanocytes:** These are dendritic cell located in basal and spinous layer of gingival epithelium. They synthesize melanin in organelles: Premelanosomes or melanosomes which contain *tyrosinase* which hydroxylates tyrosine to dihydroxyphenylalanine (DOPA), which in turn is progressively converted to melanin. Melanin granules are phagocytosed and contained within other cells of epithelium and connective tissue called melanophages or melanophores.

4. **Langerhans cells:** These are dendritic cells located among keratinocytes at all supra-basal levels. They belong to mononuclear phagocytes system (reticuloendothelial system) as modified monocytes, derived from bone marrow. They contain elongated granules and are considered macrophages with possible antigenic properties. They have an important role in immune reaction as antigen-presenting cells for lymphocytes. They contain *Birbeck's granules* and have marked adenosine triphosphate activity. They found in oral epithelium of normal gingiva and in smaller amounts in sulcular epithelium; they are probably absent from junctional epithelium of normal gingiva.

5. **Merkel cells:** They are located in deeper layer of epithelium, harbors nerve endings, act as tactile receptors and connected to adjacent cells by desmosomes.

B. **Connective tissue of gingiva** *(UOK, May 2015):* Connective tissue of gingiva is known as **lamina propria**. It has: a. Papillary layer; b. Reticular layer.
Ground substance: Proteoglycans (hyaluronic acid, chondroitin sulfate); glycoproteins (fibronectin, laminin).

Fibres: Collagen type I and IV; reticular; elastic (oxytalan, elaunin and elastin fibers).

Cells: Fibroblast, mast cells, macrophages and eosinophils, plasma cells, lymphocytes and neutrophils.

Blood supply: Supraperiosteal arterioles, vessels of periodontal ligaments, arterioles from crest of interdental septa.

Lymphatics: a. Mandibular incisor gingiva → Submental node; b. Maxillary palatal gingiva → Deep cervical nodes; c. Buccal gingiva of maxilla and buccal and lingual gingiva in mandibular premolar-molar → Submandibular lymph nodes.

Nerve supply: Branches of trigeminal nerve in PDL as: Meshwork of terminal argyrophilic fibers; Meissener tactile corpuscles; Krause end bulbs and encapsulated spidles.

Q. 8. Write a short note on dentogingival unit.
(UHSR, May 2012; HP Uni., April 2019)

Q. Write a short note on gingival fibers.
(MUHS, Dec. 2018; UHSR, May 2019)

Ans. Dentogingival unit comprises junctional epithelium (epithelial attachment), connective tissue and gingival fibres. A term frequently used to describe the dimensions of soft tissues that face the teeth is biologic width of soft tissue attachment. Biologic width of attachment varied between 2.5 mm in normal case and 1.8 mm in advanced disease case. The connective tissue of marginal gingiva is densely collagenous, containing a prominent system of collagen fibres bundle called, gingival fibers, consists of type I collagen (Fig. 4.8).

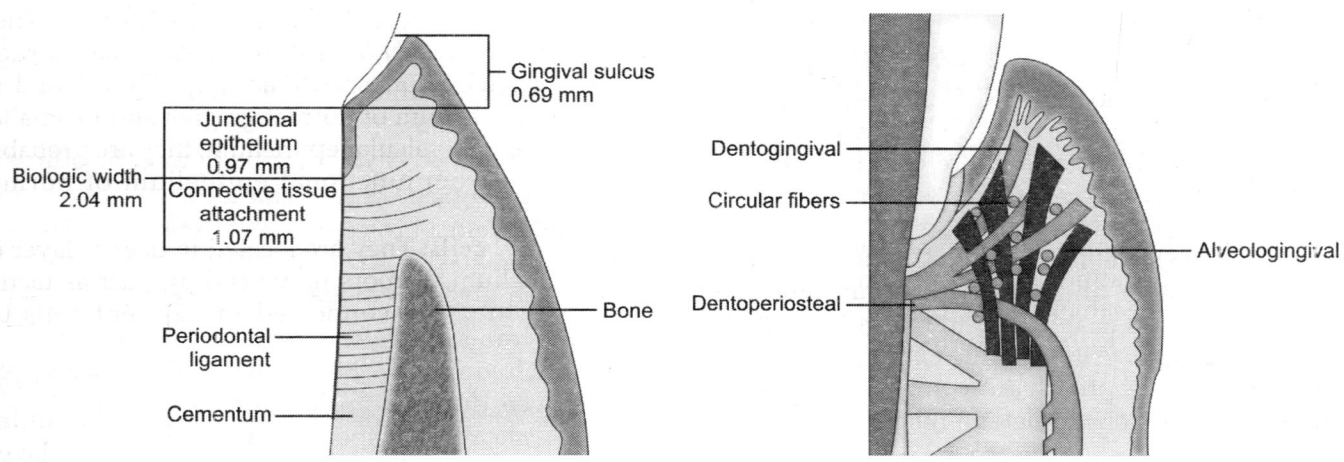

Fig. 4.8: Dentogingival unit

Functions

a. To brace the marginal gingiva firmly against tooth.
b. To provide rigidity.
c. To unite free marginal gingiva with cementum and adjacent gingiva.

Gingival Fibers:

A. Principal:

1. Circular fibers (CF): Run their course in the free gingiva; encircle the tooth in ring-like fashion.
2. Dentogingival fibers (DGF): Embedded in cementum of supra alveolar portion of root, project from cementum in fan-like configuration out into free gingival tissue.
3. Dento-periosteal fibers (DPF): Embedded in cementum of supra alveolar portion of root, but run apically over vestibular and lingual bone crest and terminate in attached gingiva.
4. Transseptal fibers (TF): Extends between supra alveolar cementum of adjacent teeth.

B. Secondary: Periosteogingival, transgingival, intercircular, intergingival, semicircular

Q. 9. Write a short note on gingival crevicular fluid.
(TNMGR, Oct. 2011; UOK, July 2013; RUHS, May 2015; AHSUC, May 2017)

Ans. Gingival crevicular fluid (GCF) is an inflammatory exudate that can be collected at the gingival margin or within the gingival crevice. Gingival crevicular fluid (GCF) can be found in the physiologic space (gingival sulcus), as well as in the pathological space (gingival pocket or periodontal pocket) between the gums and teeth. In the first case it is a transudate, in the second it is an exudate. The constituents of GCF originate from serum, gingival tissues, and from both bacterial and host response cells present in the aforementioned spaces and the surrounding tissues. The collection and analysis of GCF are the noninvasive methods for the evaluation of host response in periodontal disease. These analyses mainly focus on inflammatory markers, such as prostaglandin E2, neutrophil elastase and beta-glucuronidase, and on the marker of cellular necrosis—aspartate aminotransferase. Further, the analysis of inflammatory markers in the GCF may assist in defining how certain systemic diseases (e.g. diabetes mellitus) can modify periodontal disease, and how periodontal disease can influence certain systemic disorders (atherosclerosis, preterm delivery, diabetes mellitus and some chronic respiratory diseases). The gingival fluid is believed to: Cleanse material from the sulcus. Contain plasma proteins that may improve adhesion of the epithelium to the tooth. Possess antimicrobial properties. Exert antibody activity to defend the gingiva.

Clinical Significance

1. Its presence in clinically normal sulcus signifies inflammation.
2. Amount of GCF is proportional to severity of inflammation.
3. GCF follows circadian rhythm more from 6 am to 10 pm.
4. Female sex hormone increases GCF.
5. Drug excreted through GDF like tetracycline, metronidazole may help in local therapy.
6. GCF production is more during healing period after periodontal surgery.
7. Mechanical stimuli increase GCF production.
8. Smoking produces marked but transient increase in GCF.

Q. 10. Write a short note on cell adhesion molecules.
(Sumandeep Uni., April 2015)

Ans. Cell adhesion molecules (CAMs) are glycoproteins located on the cell surface. They are typically transmembrane receptors and are composed of three domains: Intracellular domain with cytoskeleton, transmembrane domain with CAMs, extracellular domain with extracellular matrix. CAMs help cells to stick to each other and to their surroundings. Cell adhesion receptors enable cells to recognize and bind molecules on other cells or in the extracellular matrix. Cell adhesion receptors can form: Homophilic (or homotypic) adhesions or heterophilic (or heterotypic) adhesions.

Types:
1. Cadherins: Calcium-dependent molecules, cell adhesion by forming desmosomes. Subclass: a. Neural, b. Placental, c. Epithelial.
2. Ig super family CAMs: Calcium-independent transmembrane glycoproteins. Subclass: ICAM, VCAM-1 PECAM-1, NCAM.
3. Selectins: Divalent cation dependent glycoproteins. Subclass: a. Endothelial, b. Leukocyte, c. Platelet.
4. Integrins: Large group of heterodimeric glycoproteins, e.g. α and β.
5. Mucins: Group of serine and threonine-rich protein and hydroxyproline enabling post-translational O-glycosylation.

Functions of CAMs:
1. Involvement in inflammation.
2. Tumorigenesis.
3. Establishment of the blood–brain barrier.
4. Involvement in lymphocyte homing.
5. In regulation of apoptosis.

Malfunctioning of CAMs leads to breast cancer, leukocyte adhesion deficiency (LAD) syndrome, and epithelial cell cancer.

Q. 11. Write a note on proteoglycans.
(TNMGR, May 2018)

Ans. "Proteoglycans" (Balaza, 1967): A family of macromolecules composed of one or more Glycosaminoglycans (GAGs) covalently bound to a protein core.

Structure of proteoglycans: GAGs + Core Protein

A. **Glycosaminoglycans:** Principal carbohydrate component of proteoglycans, extend perpendicularly from the core in a brush-like structure. GAGs are composed of repeating disaccharide units of: Uronic acid (D-Glucuronic acid or L-Iduronic acid) and Hexosamine (D-Glucosamine or D-Galactosamine).

GAGs have been classified mainly into:
1. Sulfated glycosaminoglycans: Chondroitin sulfate, dermatan sulfate, heparin and heparin sulfate; keratan Sulfate.
2. Non-Sulfated Glycosoaminoglycans: Hyaluronan

B. **Linkage sugars:** Oligosaccharides.

C. **Core Proteins:** Proteoglycan core proteins range in size from 10–300 KD with one to several hundred attached glycosaminoglycan chains.

Proteoglycan synthesis: Protein core is synthesized in RER with hydrophobic N-terminal leader sequence that is removed during translation of RNA. Addition of GAG occurs after the specific glycopeptide linkage has been formed and later modifications to GAG chains eventually lead to completion of synthetic process. Initiation of GAG chain elongation occurs through sequential addition of sugars that are transported to Golgi and are formed in the cytosol of cell.

Types of Proteoglycans
A. **Based on their GAG composition**
   i. Small dermatan sulfate proteoglycans
   ii. Large aggregating chondroitin sulfate proteoglycans.
B. **Based on location**
   i. Matrix Organizers: 1. Aggrecan, 2. Versican, 3. Perlecan
   ii. Tissue space fillers: Leucine Rice—interstitial proteoglycans (Decorin, Biglycan, Fibromodulin, Lumican)
   iii. Cell surface proteoglycans (or) intracellular proteoglycans of hematopoietic cells: Syndecans, Cd44, Glypicans, Betaglycan, Serglycin

Functions
1. Extracellular matrix proteoglycans and tissue-organizing proteoglycans are principally associated with conferring physicochemical properties to tissues.
2. Large proteoglycans serve to maintain tissue hydration.
3. Smaller extracellular matrix proteoglycans serve important functions in binding to other matrix molecules.
4. Cell surface proteoglycans provide the necessary means for cells to attach to their matrix.
5. Intracellular proteoglycans of hematopoietic cells, important in enzyme packaging in order to prevent non-specific enzymatic activity (or) autolysis of cell.
6. Cell surface proteoglycans and matrix proteoglycan have ability to bind and regulate growth factor activity.

Proteoglycans of Periodontium

1. Gingiva: Chondroitin-4-sulfate + dermatan sulfate (predominant in gingival connective tissue) + hyaluronic acid + heparan sulfate (60% in epithelium)
2. Inflamed gingiva: The gingival proteoglycans in inflammation leading to decrease in dermatan sulfate and increase in chondroitin sulfate, and degradation of their proteoglycan core proteins and hyaluronic acid.
3. Hyperplastic gingiva: There is increased synthesis of proteoglycans.
4. Periodontal ligament: Dermatan sulfate and chondroitin sulfate (mainly). As development progresses, concentration of hyaluronic Acid in PDL decreases and levels of dermatan sulfate and chondroitin sulfate proteoglycans increases.
5. Cementum: Hyaluronan, dermantan sulfate, chondroitin sulfate and keratin sulfate, exclusively in precementum and precementocyte lacunae.
6. Bone: Chondroitin sulfate-4 (major), hyaluronic acid, chondroitin sulfate-6, dermatan sulfate, keratan sulfate, biglycan, decorin (minor)
7. Epithelial attachment: Heparan sulphate (major)
8. Sulcular fluid: Non-inflamed sites: Hyaluronic acid only. Inflammatory sites: Hyaluronic acid, dermatan sulfate, chondroitin sulfate.

Q. 12. Write a short note on osseointegration.
(NTR Uni., May 2018)

Ans. The concept of osseointegration was developed and term was coined by Dr PerIngvar Branemark. It is defined as "Direct structural and functional connection between ordered, living bone and surface of a load carrying implant".

Mechanism: The mechanism involves three phases:
1. Osteoconduction: Migration of osteogenic cell by chemotaxis to surgical sit is known as osteoconduction.
2. New bone formation (osteogenesis):
   a. Stage 1: Osteogenic cells secrets organic matrix.
   b. Stage 2: Organic matrix provides nucleation site for calcium phosphate mineralization.
   c. Stage 3: Growth of calcium phosphate crystal and initiation of collagen fibers assemble.
   d. Stage 4: Calcification of individual collagen fibrils.
3. Bone remodeling: Osteoclastic resorption followed by lamellar bone deposition to maintain health skeletal mass.

Q. 13. Discuss self-protective features of human dentition. *(NTR Uni., May 2018)*

Ans. Protective functional form of teeth includes:

1. **Proximal contact areas:** All teeth contact adjacent teeth at a proximal contact area. Types of proximal contact: Point contact and contact area. Because of contact areas, food will not be packed between teeth causing inflammation to supporting tissues, thereby causing gingivitis and periodontitis. It helps to stabilize dental arches by combined anchorage of all teeth in arch in positive contact with each other.
2. **Interproximal areas (formed by proximal surface in contact):** These triangular shape areas are normally filled with gingival tissues and avoid any food impaction.
3. **Embrasures (spillways):** The curvature formed by two adjacent teeth in an arch from a spillway space.
4. **Height of contours:** Labial and buccal contours at cervical 3rd, and lingual contour at middle 3rd.
5. **Curvature of cementoenamel junction:** Curvature of cervical lines on mesial and distal surfaces.

Q. 14. Write a short note on CPITN. *(UOK, May 2015)*

Ans. Community Periodontal Index of Treatment Needs (CPITN) was developed for joint working family of WHO and FDI by Jukka Ainamo, David Barmes, George Beagrie, Terry Cutress, Jean Martin and Jeniffer Sardo-Infirri in 1982.

Scope and purpose: CPITN procedure is recommended for epidemiological surveys of periodontal health. It provides guidance on planning and monitoring of effectiveness of periodontal care programme and dental personnel required. CPITN records the common treatable conditions, namely periodontal pockets, gingival inflammation, dental calculus and other plaque retentive factors. It does not record irreversible changes such as recession, tooth mobility or loss of periodontal attachment.

Advantages: Simplicity; speed and international uniformity.

Limitations: Partial recording, Exclusion of some important signs of past periodontal breakdown, absence of any marker of disease activity or susceptibility.

Procedure for CPITN
- The dentition is divided into six parts called *sextants*.
- Each sextant is given a score.

- For epidemiological purposes, score is identified by examination of specified index teeth.
- For clinical practice, the highest score in each sextant is identified after examining all teeth.
- Essentially CPITN considers periodontal treatment needs of each sextant with respect to:

  i. No need for care (score 0)
  ii. Bleeding gingivae on gentle probing (score 1)
  iii. Presence of calculus and other plaque retentive factors (score 2)
  iv. Presence of 4–5 mm pockets (score 3)
  v. Presence of 6 mm or deeper pockets (score 4)

Physiology

1. HOMEOSTASIS: FLUID AND ELECTROLYTE BALANCE

Q. 1. Discuss the homeostasis. (*TNMGR, March 2010;*
NTR Uni., June 2015)

Ans. The 'Homeostasis' refers to the maintenance of constant internal environment of the body (homeo = same; stasis = stand or stay).

Role of various systems of the body in homeostasis: Some of the functions in which the homeostatic mechanism is well established are given below:

1. The pH of the extracellular fluid (ECF) has to be maintained at the critical value of 7.4. The tissues cannot survive if it is altered. The respiratory system, blood and kidney help in the regulation of pH.

2. Body temperature must be maintained at 37.5°C. Increase or decrease in temperature alters the metabolic activities of the cells. The skin, respiratory system, digestive system, excretory system, skeletal muscles and nervous system are involved in maintaining the temperature within normal limits.

3. Adequate amount of nutrients must be supplied to the cells. Nutrients are essential for various activities of the cell and growth of the tissues. Digestive system and circulatory system play major roles in the supply of nutrients.

4. Adequate amount of oxygen should be made available to cells for metabolism of nutrients. Simultaneously, CO_2 and other metabolic end products must be removed. Respiratory system is concerned with the supply of oxygen and removal of CO_2. Kidneys and other excretory organs are involved in excretion of waste products.

5. Hormones are essential for metabolism of nutrients and other substances necessary for the cells.

6. Water and electrolyte balance should be maintained optimally; otherwise it leads to dehydration or water toxicity and alteration in osmolality of the body fluids. Kidneys, skin, salivary glands and gastro-intestinal tract (GIT) take care of this.

7. For all these functions, blood must be normal. Only then, it can transport the nutritive substances, respiratory gases, metabolic and other waste products.

8. Skeletal muscles help to protect the organism from adverse surroundings, thus preventing damage or destruction.

9. Central nervous system (CNS) plays an important role in homeostasis. Sensory system detects state of body or surroundings. Brain integrates and interprets pros and cons of these information and commands body to act accordingly through motor system so that body can avoid the damage.

10. Autonomic nervous system (ANS) regulates all vegetative functions of body essential for homeostasis.

Components of homeostatic system: Homeostatic system in body acts through self-regulating devices, which operate in a cyclic manner. This cycle includes four components:

1. Sensors or detectors, which recognize deviation.
2. Transmission of this message to a control center.
3. Transmission of information from control center to effectors for correcting deviation.
4. Effectors, which correct deviation.

Mechanism of action of homeostatic system: The homeostatic system works by feedback system:

1. **Negative feedback**: The system reacts in such a way as to arrest change or reverse direction of change. After receiving a message, effectors send negative feedback signals back to system. Now, system stabilizes its own function and makes an attempt to maintain homeostasis, e.g. secretion of thyroxine.

2. **Positive feedback**: The system reacts in such a way as to increase intensity of change in same direction.

Positive feedback is less common than negative feedback, e.g. during blood clotting, milk ejection reflex, and parturition.

Q. 2. Discuss fluid and electrolyte balance in post-operative polytrauma patient.
(BFUHS, 2006; TNMGR, Sept. 2009, HP Uni., May 2017; NTR Uni., June 2017)

Q. Write a note on postoperative fluid replacement.
(UHSR, June 2017)

Ans. Fluid and electrolyte balance is a term used to describe the balance of input and output of fluids from the body in order to allow metabolic processes to function correctly. Preoperative management of fluids and electrolytes is an essential to provide adequate preoperative stabilization before general anesthesia to prevent hypotension, renal failure, cardiac dysarrythmias and other potential intraoperative complications. Postoperative fluid and electrolyte levels must be closely monitored and managed, if complications develop and alter the expected postoperative course.

Total body water (TBW): Adult male: 60%; Adult female: 55%; Child: 65%; Infant: 75%

TBW decreases with age and obesity. TBW is divided into intracellular and extracellular compartments and is distributed in the body as follows:

Intracellular fluid (ICF) = 40% of body weight (BW); Extracellular fluid (ECF) = 20% of BW; extravascular fluid (EVF)/interstitial fluid = 15% of BW; intravascular fluid (IVF)/plasma = 5% of BW; transcellular fluid (CSF, pleural, synovial, pericardial, urine) = 3.5% of BW.

Sodium and potassium are the principal cations in the body. Sodium is contained primarily in the extracellular fluid and potassium in the intracellular fluid. Chloride is the principle anion in the body and is restricted primarily to the extracellular fluid.

Composition of ECF and ICF

Substance (mEq/L)	ECF	ICF
Na^+	142	10
K^+	5	141
Ca^{2+}	5	<1
Mg^{2+}	3	40
Cl^-	103	4
HCO_3^-	24	6
Phosphate	4	75
Glucose (mg%)	90	0–20

Daily intake of water (70 kg adult): 2000–2500 ml/day
Daily loss of body water: Insensible loss: 700 ml/d (lungs and skin); sensible water loss: 1300–1800 ml (urine, intestinal and sweat)

Fluids: Types—these are categorized by the clinical situation and type of fluid used:

A. **Based on property:**
   1. **Crystalloids:** Molecular weight <8,000 daltons, e.g. Ringer's lactate (Hartmann's solution), normal saline (NS), dextrose-5%, DNS (5% dextrose with 0.9% NaCl), isolytes. Recommended as the initial fluid of choice in resuscitating patients from hemorrhagic shock.
   2. **Colloids:** Molecular weight >8,000 daltons, e.g. albumin (5% and 25%), 10% pentastarch, 10% dextran-40, 6% dextran-70, 10% hexastarch.

B. **Base on use:**
   1. **Maintenance fluids:** Used to meet normal daily requirements in patients unable to consume sufficient water, e.g. dextrose 5% (D5) with 20 mEq/L of KCl.
   2. **Replacement fluids:** Used to acutely replace volume deficits in patients with dehydration, trauma and sepsis, e.g. dextran, Ringer's solution, NS, DNS, isolyte: G, E, M, P.
   3. **Special fluids:** Inj. sodium bicarbonate, mannitol, NS (1.6%, 3%, 5%), Inj. KCl, D25.

Goals of fluid management:
   i. Attain and maintain normal body composition and homeostasis.
   ii. Correct life-threatening imbalances.
   iii. Avoid complications of too rapid correction.
   iv. Integrate fluid and electrolyte therapy with nutritional therapy.

Clinical approach:
1. Identify fluid and electrolyte imbalances and their magnitude.
2. Determine which problems need correction prior to surgery.
3. Determine the daily maintenance of fluids and electrolytes.
4. Anticipate additional losses expected during treatment.
5. Evaluate for renal, cardiac, endocrine and hepatic dysfunction.

Physical evaluation: Clinical signs and symptoms of fluid imbalance:
1. **CNS:** Sleepiness, apathy, slow responses, anorexia, vomiting, decreased tendon reflexes, coma.
2. **GIT:** Progressive decrease in food consumption, nausea, vomiting, refusal to eat, diarrhoea.
3. **CVS:** Orthostatic hypotension, tachycardia, collapsed peripheral and central veins, weak pulse, cold extremities, absent peripheral pulse (deficit).

Increased venous pressure distension of peripheral and central veins, increased cardiac output, loud heart sounds, functional murmurs, high pulse pressure, pulmonary oedema (excess).

4. **Tissues:** Decreased skin elasticity, atonic muscles, sunken eyes, decreased tongue size with longitudinal wrinkles (deficit). Subcutaneous edema, pulmonary crackles (excess).

5. **Metabolic:** Hypothermia.

Body fluid and electrolyte disturbances can be classified as:

I. **Changes in volume:** Hypovolemia; hypervolemia

II. **Changes in concentration:** Hyponatremia; hypernatremia

III. **Changes in composition:** Acid–base imbalance; calcium, magnesium and potassium abnormalities

1. **Hypovolemia:** Decrease in ECF, most common fluid loss, aggravated by general anaesthesia.

Causes: Gastrointestinal loss from vomiting, nasogastric suction, diarrhoea and fistular drainage, soft tissue injury, infections, etc.

Signs and symptoms: Poor skin tugor, dry oral mucosa and axilla, oliguria (<500 ml/d), tachycardia, creatinine >20:1, electrolyte and acid–base imbalance.

Management: Hemorrhage—whole blood transfusion; 6% dextran; 5% albumin; 3.5% Ureabridged gelatin; 1 liter of Ringer's lactate.

2. **Hypervolemia:** Increased in ECF. Iatrogenic or secondary to renal insufficiency, cirrohosis or congestive heart failure (CHF).

Signs and symptoms: Elevated jugulovenous pressure (JVP), shorten breath, pitting edema, electrolyte imbalance.

Management: Diuretics, ↑ oncotic pressure or albumin infusion, dialysis.

Electrolyte abnormalities (*BBD Uni., April 2014; UHSR, May 2016*): Electrolytes are chemical substances that release cations and anions when they are dissolved in water.

1. **Hyponatremia:** Symptomatic when Na^+: <120 mEq/L.

   Causes:

   1. Hyponatremia with normal or elevated osmolarity: Hyperglycemia, hyperlipidemia, hyperprotienemia.

   2. Hyponatremia with increased ECF volume: Glucocorticoid deficiency, vomiting, drugs, hypothyroidism, hypokalemia.

3. Hyponatremia with decreased ECF volume: Gastrointestinal losses, mineralocorticoid deficiency, diuretics, salt losing nephritis.

Clinical signs and symptoms: Lethargy, confusion, seizures, nausea, vomiting, anorexia, muscle cramps, hypothermia.

Treatment: Treat underlying causes.

a. Iso-osmotic: Correct lipids and protein levels.

b. Hyperosmotic: Correct hyperglycemia, discontinue hypertonic fluids.

c. Hypo-osmotic: Na^+ replacements isotonic saline if hypovolemic; Water restriction.

2. **Hypernatremia:** Symptomatic when Na^+ >160 mEq/L

   Causes:

   1. Loss of free water: Inadequate free water intake, loss of water via skin, GIT and renal loss.

   2. Solute loading: Inappropriate, IV replacement, tube feeding, brain stem injuries.

Clinical signs and symptoms: Restlessness, tremors, weakness, delirium, confusion, ataxia, seizures, coma, tachycardia, hypotension, syncope, decreased saliva and tears, dry sticky mucous membrane, red swollen tongue, flushed skin, oliguria and fever.

Treatment: Treating the underlying causes:

a. Hypervolemic: Diuretics

b. Isovolemic: Water replacement

c. Hypovolemic: Isotonic NaCl, then hypotonic saline.

3. **Hypokalemia:** Serum K^+ <3.5. Normal: 3.5–5.5 mEq/L.

   Causes: Decreased dietary intake; increased loss; total parentral excretion; Alkalosis, insulin therapy; dietry loss, medications, hyperaldosteronism.

Clinical signs and symptoms: Dysarrhythmias, T-wave flattening, hypotension, respiratory failure, polyuria, polydypsia, red swollen tongue, decreased saliva and tears, decreased GFR, constipation.

Treatment:

1. Treat underlying causes.

2. K^+ salt orally or IV (oral route is safer). KCl 10–20 mEq/L/hr IV

3. Diet rich in K^+-fruit juices, coffee, milk and animal protein.

4. **Hyperkalemia:** Serum K^+ >5.1 mEq/L

   Causes:

   1. Phlebotomy, hemolysis, thrombocytosis, leucocytosis.

2. Supplements and blood transfusion
3. Decreased renal excretion of K^+.
4. Redistribution to extracellular fluid leading to acidosis, muscle damage and hyperglycemia.

Clinical signs and symptoms: Nausea/vomiting, colic diarrhea, arrhythmia, cardiac arrest, peak T wave, flattened P wave, sine wave formation, weakness, paraesthesia, respiratory failure,

Treatment:

1. Inject 10 ml of 10% calcium gluconate over 1 minute.
2. Inject 50 ml of 50% glucose, monitor plasma glucose.
3. Start infusion of 10–20% dextrose 500 ml, 4–6 h.
4. Calcium resonium 15–30 g orally.
5. If metabolic acidosis is present infuse sodium bicarbonate 1.26%, 500 ml, 6–8 h, until the plasma (HCO_3^-) is in normal range.
6. Correct volume depletion, respiratory acidosis if present.
7. Use haemodialysis/haemofilteration or peritoneal dialysis, if the above fail.

Chloride: Normal intake: 80–140 mEq/24 hr.

5. **Hyperchloremia:** Acidosis, respiratory alkalosis, dehydration, diabetes insipidus, medications like acetazolamides, ammonium chloride, renal tubular acidosis.

6. **Hypochloremia:** Metabolic alkalosis, respiratory acidosis, emphysema, adrenal cortical insufficiency, primary aldosteronism, thiazides, diarrhoea.

Treatment: Treat the underlying cause.

7. **Hypocalcemia:** Serum calcium <8.8 mg/dl (normal = 8.8–10.5 mg/dl)

Causes: Pancreatitis, massive soft tissue infections, renal failure, hypoparathyroidism.

Sign and symptom: Hypotension, anxiety, Psychosis, Paraesthesia, laryngeal spasm, numbness and tingling, tetany, carpopedal spasm, chvostek and trousseau's sign.

Treatment: Acute: IV Calcium: 1 g in D5% or NS; **Chronic:** Oral calcium and Vit. D.

8. **Hypercalcemia:** Serum calcium >10.5 mg/dl

Causes: Hyperparathyroidism, cancer.

Sign and symptom: Hypertension, bradycardia, constipation, anorexia, nephrolithiasis, psychosis, pruritis, weight loss, stupor, coma.

Treatment: Treat the underlying cause.

Postoperative fluid and electrolyte management:

1. Assess losses and gains.
2. Correcting existing deficiencies.
3. For maintenance of water, Na^+ and K^+ are the next necessary to replace in the short-term management of a patient's fluid balance.

Transfusion guidelines:

1. Concomitant disease status may dictate early use of blood products rather than IV fluids replacement in traumatized and surgical patients.
2. The following facts should be considered to take a decision to transfuse a patient: i. Intravascular volume, ii. Duration of anemia and operation, iii. Probability of extended blood loss, iv. Physiologic condition of patient.
3. Healthy patients with hemoglobin >10 g% rarely require preoperative transfusion. Those with <7 g% due to acute anemia will require red blood cell transfusion.
4. With regard to the surgical patients, blood loss during a procedure is based on percent loss of the estimated blood volume (10% in infants and 15–20% in adults).

Q. 3. Write about regulation of acid–base/electrolyte balance. *(TNMGR, Sept. 2008; Oct. 2013)*

Ans. Acid–base balance (body pH) is the proper balance between chemical acids (proton donor) and bases (proton acceptor) in the extracellular fluids.

Regulation of acid-base balance: The body's acid-base balance is normally tightly regulated and kept between 7.35 and 7.45 by:

1. **By acid–base buffer system:** An acid–base buffer system is combination of a weak acid and a base— the salt. Buffer system maintains pH by binding with free H^+.

Types of buffer systems:

I. **Bicarbonate buffer system:** Bicarbonate buffer system is present in ECF (plasma). It consists of carbonic acid (H_2CO_3) which is a weak acid and bicarbonate (HCO_3^-) which is a weak base, in the form of salt, i.e. sodium bicarbonate ($NaHCO_3$).

II. **Phosphate buffer system:** This system consists of a weak acid, dihydrogen phosphate (H_2PO_4) in the form of sodium dihydrogen phosphate (NaH_2PO_4) and base, hydrogen phosphate (HPO_4) in the form of disodium hydrogen phosphate (Na_2HPO_4). Phosphate buffer system is useful in ICF, tubular fluids of kidneys, in red blood cells (RBCs) or other cells. This is more powerful than bicarbonate buffer system.

III. **Protein buffer system:**
   a. Protein buffer systems in plasma: weak acids in the plasma are:
      i. C-terminal carboxyl group, N-terminal amino group and side-chain carboxyl group of glutamic acid.
      ii. Side-chain amino group of lysine.
      iii. Imidazole group of histidine.
   b. Protein buffer system in erythrocytes: Hemoglobin (Hb).

2. **By respiratory mechanism:** Lungs play an important role in maintenance of acid–base balance by removing CO_2 which is produced during various metabolic activities in the body. This CO_2 combines with water to form carbonic acid. Since carbonic acid is unstable, it splits into H^+ and HCO_3^-. Increased H^+ concentration increases pulmonary ventilation (hyperventilation) by acting through chemoreceptor.

3. **By renal mechanism:** Kidney maintains acid–base balance of body by secretion of H^+ and by retention of HCO_3^-.

Disturbances of Acid–Base Status (RUHS, May 2018)

I. **Acidosis:** Reduction in pH ($\uparrow$ in H^+) below normal range. It is produced by either $\uparrow$ in pCO_2 in arterial blood or $\downarrow$ in HCO_3^- concentration.

II. **Alkalosis:** Increase in pH ($\downarrow$ in H^+ concentration) above normal range. It is produced by either $\downarrow$ in pCO_2 in arterial blood or $\uparrow$ in HCO_3^- concentration.

Acid–base disturbances produced by change in arterial pCO_2 are called respiratory disturbances, and those produced by change in HCO_3^- concentration are called metabolic disturbances.

1. **Respiratory acidosis:** During hypoventilation, lungs fail to expel CO_2 (produced in tissues). CO_2 accumulates in blood where it reacts with water to form carbonic acid (**respiratory acid**). Carbonic acid dissociates into H^+ and HCO_3^-. The increased H^+ concentration in blood leads to decrease in pH and acidosis.

   Causes: Hypoventilation: Airways obstruction, lung diseases, respiratory centre depression, neural diseases.

2. **Respiratory alkalosis:** Hyperventilation causes excess loss of CO_2 from the body. Loss of CO_2 leads to decreased formation of carbonic acid and decreased release of H^+.

   Causes: Hyperventilation: Hypoxia, anemia, pulmonary edema, pulmonary embolism, cerebral disturbance, emotional disturbances.

3. **Metabolic acidosis:** Excess accumulation of organic acids in the body, caused by abnormal metabolic processes.

   Causes:
   a. Lactic acidosis: In circulatory shock.
   b. Ketoacidosis: In diabetes mellitus, alcoholic.
   c. Uric acidosis: In renal failure.
   d. Acid poisoning: Ethylene glycol, methanol.

4. **Metabolic alkalosis:** Caused by loss of excess H^+ resulting in increased HCO_3^- concentration.

   Causes:
   a. Vomiting.
   b. Cushing syndrome.
   c. Milk-alkali syndrome.

Clinical evaluation of disturbances in acid–base status anion gap (AG) is an important measure in the clinical evaluation of disturbances in acid–base status. Commonly measured cation is Na^+ and unmeasured cations are K^+, Ca^{2+} and Mg^{2+}. Measured anions are chloride and bicarbonate and unmeasured anions are phosphate, sulfate, proteins (albumin) and other organic anions like lactate. Difference between concentrations of unmeasured anions and unmeasured cations is called **anion gap**. It is calculated as:

Anion gap = $[Na^+] - [HCO_3^-] - [Cl^-]$ = 144 – 24 – 108 mEq/L = 12 mEq/L

Normal value of anion gap is 9–15 mEq/L. It increases when concentration of unmeasured anion increases and decreases when concentration of unmeasured cations decreases.

Arterial Blood Gases (ABG) (HP Uni., Nov. 2018): ABG is a collective term applied to three separate measurements—pH, $paCO_2$, and paO_2 generally made together to evaluate acid–base status, ventilation, and arterial oxygenation. It has following advantages: Aids in establishing diagnosis, guides treatment plan, aids in ventilator management, improvement in acid–base management, allows for optimal function of medications, acid–base status may alter electrolyte levels critical to a patient's status.

Interpretation: By modified Henderson equation: $[H^+] [HCO_3]/paCO_2 = 24$

1. In a normal ABG: pH and $paCO_2$ move in opposite directions; HCO_3^- and $paCO_2$ move in same direction.

2. When the pH and $paCO_2$ change in the same direction, the primary problem is metabolic; when pH and $paCO_2$ move in opposite directions and $paCO_2$ is normal, then the primary problem is respiratory.

3. Mixed disorder—if HCO_3^- and $paCO_2$ change in opposite direction (which they normally should not), then it is a mixed disorder: pH may be normal with abnormal $paCO_2$ or abnormal pH and normal $paCO_2$).

Rules for rapid clinical interpretation of ABG:
1. Look at pH – <7.40 = Acidosis; >7.40 = Alkalosis.
2. If pH indicates acidosis, then look at $paCO_2$ and HCO_3^-
3. If $paCO_2$ is ↑ HCO_3^-, then it is primary respiratory acidosis.
4. If $paCO_2$ ↓ and HCO_3^- is also ↓→ primary metabolic acidosis.
5. If HCO_3^- is ↓, then AG should be examined.
6. If AG is unchanged → Hyperchloremic metabolic acidosis.
7. If AG is ↑→ Wide AG acidosis.
8. If pH indicates alkalosis, then look at HCO_3^- and $paCO_2$
9. If $paCO_2$ is ↓→ primary respiratory alkalosis.
10. If $paCO_2$ ↑ and HCO_3^- also ↑→ Primary metabolic alkalosis.

Q. 4. What are the plasma proteins? What are their functions? *(NTR Uni., May 2005)*

Ans. Plasma proteins help to maintain the colloidal osmotic pressure at about 25 mmHg.

Development:

In embryo: From mesenchymal cells, albumin is synthesized first followed by globulin and other plasma proteins.

In adults: Reticuloendothelial cells of liver (mainly), bone marrow, degenerating blood cells, and spleen. Gamma globulins originate from B lymphocytes, which in turn form immunoglobulins.

Normal Values:
Total proteins: 7.3 g/dl (6.4 to 8.3 g/dl)
Serum albumin: 4.7 g/dl
Serum globulin: 2.3 g/dl (α_1 and α_2, β and γ-globulins)
Fibrinogen: 0.3 g/dl

Albumins/Globulin Ratio: It is an important indicator of some diseases involving liver or kidney. Normal A/G ratio is 1.2:1 to 1.5:1.

Properties of Plasma Proteins
1. **Molecular weight:** Albumin: 69,000; Globulin: 1,56,000; Fibrinogen: 4,00,000
2. **Specific gravity:** 1.026.

3. **Buffer action:** Plasma proteins have 1/6 of total buffering action of the blood.

Functions of Plasma Proteins:
1. **Role in coagulation of blood:** Fibrinogen is essential for the coagulation of blood.
2. **Role in defense mechanism of body:** Gamma globulin acts as antibodies (immunoglobulins).
3. **Role in transport mechanism:** Albumin, α-globulin and β-globulin are responsible for transport of hormones, enzymes, etc.
4. **Role in maintenance of osmotic pressure in blood:** Proteins exerts colloidal osmotic (oncotic) pressure.
5. **Role in regulation of acid–base balance:** Plasma proteins have buffering action.
6. **Role in viscosity of blood:** Plasma proteins provides viscosity to blood, important to maintain blood pressure.
7. **Role in erythrocyte sedimentation rate (ESR):** Fibrinogen increases during acute inflammatory conditions and contributes to increase in ESR.
8. **Role in suspension stability of red blood cells:** During circulation, RBCs remain suspended uniformly in the blood (suspension stability). Globulin and fibrinogen help in the suspension stability of the red blood cells.
9. **Role in production of trephone substances:** Trephone is necessary for nourishment of tissue cells in culture. These substances are produced by leukocytes from plasma proteins.
10. **Role as reserve proteins:** During fasting, inadequate food intake or inadequate protein intake, plasma proteins are utilized by body tissues as the last source of energy.

Q. 5. Discuss regulation of body temperature.
(TNMGR, April 2013; NTR Uni., May 2019)

Ans. The body temperature is regulated by hypothalamus, which sets the normal range of body temperature. The set point under normal physiological conditions is 37°C/98.6°F. Hypothalamus has two centers which regulate the body temperature:

A. **Heat loss center:** Heat loss center is situated in preoptic nucleus of anterior hypothalamus. Stimulation of preoptic nucleus results in cutaneous vasodilatation and sweating. Removal or lesion of this nucleus increases the body temperature.

B. **Heat gain center:** Heat gain is otherwise known as heat production center. It is situated in posterior hypothalamic nucleus. Stimulation of posterior hypothalamic nucleus causes shivering. The removal or lesion of this nucleus leads to fall in body temperature.

Mechanism of temperature regulation:

I. When body temperature increases, the heat loss center brings the temperature back to normal by two mechanisms:

1. Promotion of heat loss: By increasing secretion of sweat and by inhibiting sympathetic centers in posterior hypothalamus. This causes cutaneous vasodilatation.
2. Prevention of heat production: By inhibiting mechanisms involved in heat production, such as shivering and chemical (metabolic) reactions.

II. **When body temperature decreases**: It is brought back to normal by two mechanisms:

1. Prevention of heat loss: Sympathetic centers in posterior hypothalamus cause cutaneous vasoconstriction. This leads to decrease in blood flow to skin so the heat loss is prevented.
2. Promotion of heat production: i. Shivering, ii. Increased metabolic reactions.

Applied Clinical Physiology

1. **Malignant hyperthermia** is rare but is life-threatening event due to certain anesthetic agents.
2. **Serotonin syndrome and neuroleptic malignant syndrome** are due to adverse drug reactions, and present with clinical hyperthermia.
3. **In hyperthyroidism**, core body temperature is raised because basal metabolic rate (BMR) is raised.
4. Hypothermia is seen in diabetes, hypothyroidism, hypoadrenalism, and hypopituitarism.

Q. 6. Write a short note on fever. (TNMGR, Sept. 2007; UHSR, May 2016)

Ans. Fever/pyrexia is defined as a core temperature of 38.3°C or higher, i.e. just above the upper limit of a normal human temperature, irrespective of the cause. (American College of Critical Care Medicine, International Statistical Classification of Diseases, Infectious Diseases Society of America). **Fever** is also defined as a state of elevated core temperature, which is often, but not necessarily, part of the defensive responses of multicellular organisms (host) to the invasion of live (micro-organisms) or inanimate matter recognised as pathogenic or alien by the host. (International Union of Physiological Sciences Commission for Thermal Physiology, 2001)

Classification of fever

Based on the height of body temperature:

1. **Mild/low-grade fever:** Body temperature: 38°C–39°C (100.4°F–102.2°F)
2. **Moderate-grade fever:** Body temperature: 39°C–40°C (102.2°F–104°F)
3. **High-grade fever:** Body temperature: 40°C to 41°C (104°F–105.8°F).
4. **Hyperpyrexia:** Rise in body temperature >41°C (105.8°F).

Based on duration:

1. **Acute fever:** <7 days in duration, e.g. infectious diseases.
2. **Sub-acute fever:** Usually not more than 2 weeks in duration, e.g. typhoid fever, intra-abdominal abscess.
3. **Chronic or persistent fever:** >2 weeks duration, e.g. Chronic bacterial infections, viral.

Causes of fever: Infection (74%), malignancy, tissue ischemia, drug reactions, neurogenic fever, fever associate with endocrinopathies.

Signs and symptoms: Headache, sweating, shivering, muscle pain, dehydration, loss of appetite, general weakness.

Pathophysiology/Mechanism of Fever (Fig. 1.6)

Pyrogens directly or indirectly lead to fever, may be exogenous or endogenous based on their site of production. Exogenous pyrogens are part or whole microorganisms or products of microorganisms such as toxins, e.g. Gram-negative cell wall component lipopolysaccharide (LPS). Endogenous pyrogens are pyrogenic cytokines, e.g. interleukins (IL)-6, IL-1, interferon gamma (INF-γ). Cryogens prevent excessive temperature elevation, include anti-inflammatory cytokines (e.g. IL-10), hormones (e.g. α-melanocyte stimulating hormone, corticotrophin and corticotrophin releasing hormone) and many other neuroendocrine products (e.g. neuropeptide Y, bombesin, and thyroliberin), cytochrome P-450.

Deleterious Effects of Fever

1. Direct cellular damage: Membrane, mitochondrial and DNA damage; Stimulation of excitotoxic mechanisms; Protein denaturation; Cell death.
2. Local effects: Cytokine stimulation; Inflammatory response; Vascular stasis; Extravasation; Edema.
3. Systemic effects: Endotoxaemia; Gut bacterial translocation.

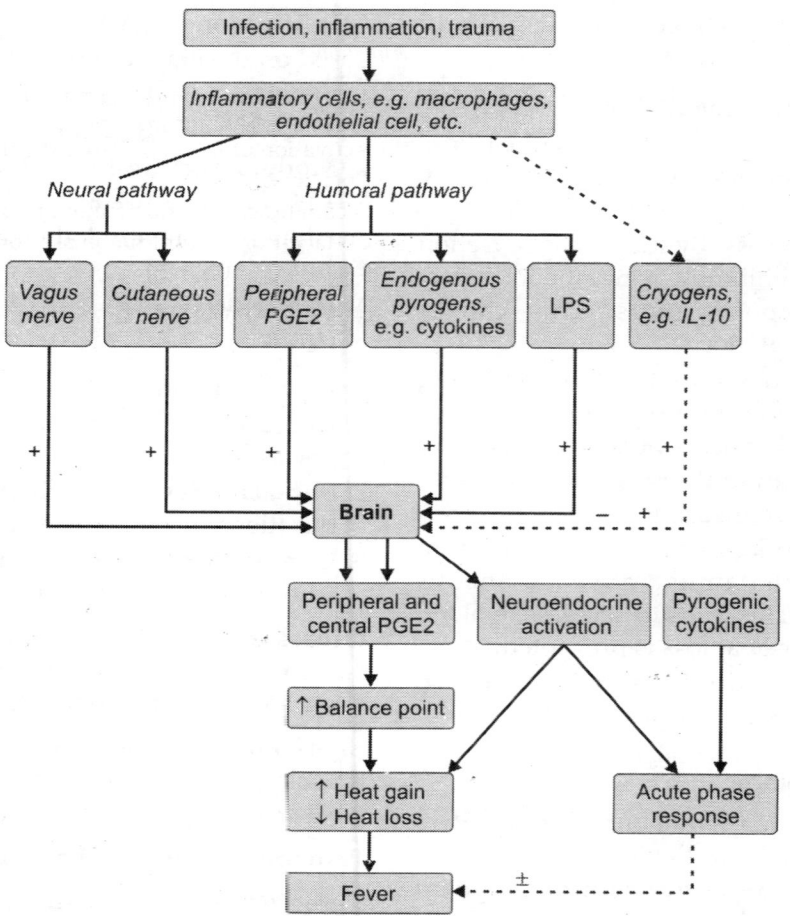

Fig. 1.6: Pathophysiology of fever. LPS=Lipopolysaccharide; +=Activate; ñ=Inhibit

2. BLOOD

Q. 1. What are the factors of coagulation? Describe the coagulation mechanism and the common deficiency factors which commonly occur.

(MAHE, Dec. 1996; PAHER, May 2011; BBD Uni., April 2018;MUHS, July 2018; HP Uni., Nov. 2018; NTR Uni., Oct. 2019)

Q. Describe the hemostatic mechanism of the human body. Add a brief note on hemophilia and von Willebrand's disease.

(TNMGR, March 2010; April 2012, 2013)

Q. Write a note on hemostasis.

(Nagpur Uni., March 1998; BFUHS, May, Nov. 2009; KLE Uni. May 2009; RUHS, June 2017)

Ans. Hemostasis is arrest or stoppage of bleeding. It is defined as the body's physiologic response to vascular endothelial injury, which results in a series of processes that attempt to retain blood within the vascular system through the formation of a clot.

Primary hemostasis: Formation of soft platelet plug, by vasoconstriction, platelet adhesion, platelet activation, and platelet aggregation.

Secondary hemostasis: Formation of fibrinogen into fibrin, by converting soft platelet plug into hard, insoluble fibrin clot.

Clotting Factors: Table 2.1, Clotting factors with functions (International Committee in Nomenclature of Blood Coagulation Factors)

Stages of Hemostasis: It occurs in three stages:

1. **Vasoconstriction:** When blood vessels are cut, endothelium is damaged and the collagen is exposed. The platelets adhere to this collagen, and get activated. The activated platelets secrete serotonin and other vasoconstrictor substances which cause constriction of the blood vessels. The adherence of platelets to the collagen is accelerated by von Willebrand factor.

2. **Formation of Platelet Plug:** The platelets get adhered to the collagen of ruptured blood vessel and secrete

Table 2.1: Clotting factors with functions

Clotting factor		Function
Number	Name	
I	Fibrinogen	Clot formation
II	Prothrombin	Activation of I, V, VII, VIII, XI XIII, protein C, platelets
III	TF	Cofactor of VIIa
IV	Calcium	Facilitates coagulation factor binding to phospholipids
V	Proaccelerin, labile factor	Co-factor of X-prothrombinase complex
VI	Unassigned	—
VII	Stable factor, proconvertin	Activates factors IX, X
VIII	Antihaemophilic factor A	Cofactor of IX-tenase complex
IX	Antihaemophilic factor B or Christmas factor	Activates X: Forms tenase complex with factor VIII
X	Stuart-Prower factor	Prothrombinase complex with factor V: Activates factor II
XI	Plasma thromboplastin antecedent	Activates factor IX
XII	Hageman factor	Activates factors XI, VII and prekallikrein
XIII	Fibrin-stabilising factor	Crosslinks fibrin
XIV	Prekallikrein (F-Fletcher)	Serine protease zymogen
XV	HMWK-(F-Fitzgerald/Flaujac/William factor)	Cofactor
XVI	vWF	Binds to VIII, mediates platelet adhesion
XVII	Antithrombin III	Inhibits IIa, Xa, and other proteases
XVIII	Heparin cofactor II	Inhibits IIa
XIX	Protein C	Inactivates Va and VIIIa
XX	Protein S	Cofactor for activated protein C

HMWK: High molecular weight kininogen; vWF: von Willebrand factor; TF: Tissue factor

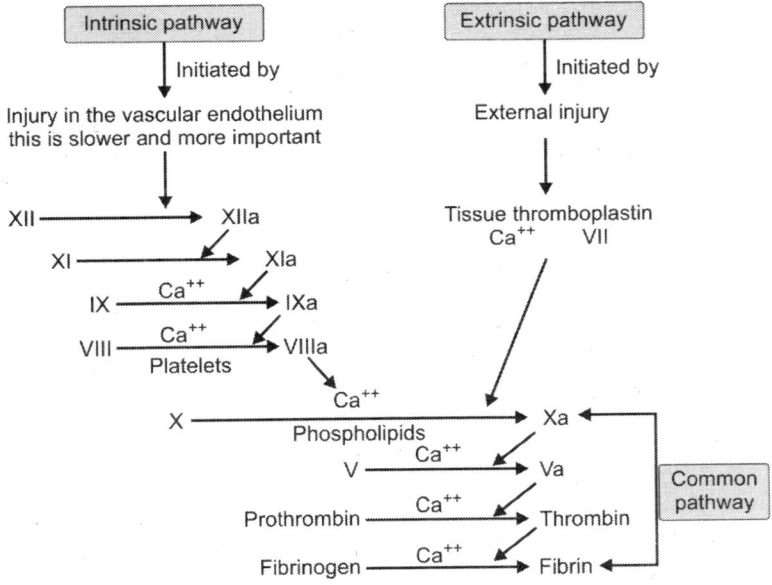

Fig. 2.1: Coagulation pathway

ADP and thromboxane A2. All these platelets aggregate together and form a loose temporary platelet plug which closes the vessel and prevents further blood loss. The platelet aggregation is accelerated by platelet-activating factor (PAF).

3. **Coagulation of Blood:** Coagulation or clotting is defined as the process in which blood loses its fluidity and becomes a jelly-like mass a few minutes after it is shed out or collected in a container.

4. **Clot Retraction**

Stages of blood clotting: In general, blood clotting occurs in three stages:

Stage 1: Formation of prothrombin activator/ prothombinase: Blood clotting commences with the formation of prothrombin activator, which converts prothrombin into thrombin. Prothrombin activator forms by:

i. **Intrinsic pathway/contact activation pathway:** Formation of prothrombin activator is initiated by platelets (Fig. 2.1).

ii. **Extrinsic pathway/tissue factor pathway:** The formation of prothrombin activator is initiated by tissue thromboplastin (Fig. 2.1).

Stage 2: Conversion of prothrombin into thrombin

Stage 3: Conversion of fibrinogen (soluble) into fibrin (insoluble)

Applied Clinical Physiology

1. Deficiencies in protein C and S can lead to hypercoagulable states due to an inability to inhibit factors V and VIII respectively.

2. Prothrombin time (PT) and partial thromboplastin time (PTT) evaluate the time it takes for the extrinsic and intrinsic pathways to take effect, respectively.

3. Vitamin K deficiency can lead to elevated PT and PTT.

4. Heparin is an anticoagulant used in hospital settings for deep venous thrombosis prophylaxis. Heparin binds and activates AT. AT goes on to inactivate thrombin and factor Xa.

5. Warfarin acts by inhibiting epoxide reductase. Epoxide reductase is a critical component in coagulation factor production because it helps recycle vitamin K.

Bleeding disorders: *(UHSR, June 2018)*

1. Hemophilia *(NTR Uni., April 2011)*: Hemophilia is a group of sex-linked inherited blood disorders, characterized by prolonged clotting time. However, the bleeding time is normal. Usually, it affects the males, with the females being the carriers. Because of prolonged clotting time, even a mild trauma causes excess bleeding which can lead to death.

Causes of hemophilia: Hemophilia occur due to lack of formation of prothrombin activator. The formation of prothrombin activator is affected due to the deficiency of factor VIII, IX or XI.

Types of hemophilia:

i. **Hemophilia A or classic hemophilia/bleeder's disease/disease of the Hapsburgs/disease of kings:** Due to deficiency of factor VIII, 85% of people with hemophilia are affected by hemophilia A. X-linked recessive disorder. The gene for factor VIII is located on the long arm of Xq28

Classification: Severe (<1% of Normal); Moderate (1–5% of normal); Mild (>5%–<40% of normal)

ii. **Hemophilia B or Christmas disease:** Due to the deficiency of factor IX, 15% of people with hemophilia are affected by hemophilia B, autosomal recessive disorders. The gene for factor IX is located on Xq27.

iii. **Hemophilia C or factor XI deficiency:** Due to the deficiency of factor XI. It is a very rare bleeding disorder. The gene for factor XI is located on chromosome 4.

Symptoms of hemophilia

i. Spontaneous bleeding.

ii. Prolonged bleeding due to cuts, tooth extraction and surgery, oral hematoma

iii. Hemorrhage in gastrointestinal and urinary tracts.

iv. Bleeding in joints followed by swelling and pain.

v. Appearance of blood in urine (haematuria).

Treatment for hemophilia: Replacement of missing clotting factor, fresh frozen plasma.

2. Purpura: Purpura is a disorder characterized by prolonged bleeding time, with normal clotting time. Characteristic feature is spontaneous bleeding under the skin from ruptured capillaries. It causes small tiny hemorrhagic spots (petechiae/purpuric spots) in many areas of the body. Blood collects in large areas beneath the skin, known as ecchymoses.

3. von Willebrand's disease (vWD) (pseudohemophilia/vascular purpura) *(UOK, July 2017; HP Uni., April 2019)*: vWD is due to deficiency of von Willebrand's factor (vWF), which is a protein secreted by endothelium of damaged blood vessels and platelets. This protein is responsible for adherence of platelets to endothelium of blood vessels during hemostasis after an injury. It is also responsible for the survival and maintenance of factor VIII in plasma. Deficiency of von Willebrand's factor supresses platelet adhesion. It also causes deficiency of factor VIII. This results in excess bleeding, which resembles the bleeding that occurs during platelet dysfunction or hemophilia. The gene for vWF is located on the short arm of 12 chromosomes.

Classification:

a. Type 1: Most common, autosomal dominant, vWF is normal in structure and function with decreased in quantity

b. Type 2: Autosomal dominant, vWF is normal in structure and function.

c. Type 3: Autosomal recessive, vWF is very low or undetectable.

Clinical features: Asymptomatic, epistaxis, mucosal membrane bleeding, menorrhagia, and ecchymoses.

Lab finding: Prolonged bleeding time, reduced vWF concentration, reduced factor VIII activity.

Treatment: Desmopressin, cryoprecipitate, fresh frozen plasma.

4. **Thrombosis or intravascular blood clotting:** Coagulation of blood inside the blood vessels.

Q. 2. Describe RBCs morphology and its variations.
(RGUHS, Nov. 2006; MUHS, June 2011; BFUHS, Nov. 2012; AHSUC, May 2018; Sumandeep Uni., May 2018)

Ans. Normally, the RBCs are disk-shaped and biconcave (dumbbell shaped). The central portion is thinner and periphery is thicker.

Advantages of Biconcave Shape of RBCs

1. It helps in equal and rapid diffusion of O_2 and other substances into the interior of the cell.
2. Large surface area is provided for absorption or removal of different substances.
3. Minimal tension is offered on the membrane when the volume of cell alters.
4. Because of biconcave shape, while passing through minute capillaries, RBCs squeeze through the capillaries very easily without getting damaged.

Normal size

Diameter: 7.2 μ (6.9 to 7.4 μ).
Thickness: At the periphery—2.2 μ and at the center—1 μ.
Surface area: 120 μ².
Volume: 85–90 μ³.

Normal structure: RBCs are non-nucleated; cytoplasm contains heamoglobin, a chromoprotein. Other organelles such as mitochondria and Golgi apparatus are absent in RBC. RBCs do not have insulin receptor. **Cytoskeleton** of RBCs is made up of **actin** and **spectrin**, anchored to transmembrane proteins by means of **ankyrin**. Lifespan is 120 days in peripheral blood.

Variations in size: Anisocytosis

1. Microcytes (smaller cells): Iron deficiency anemia (IDA), thalassaemia.
2. Macrocytes (larger cells): Megaloblastic anemia, liver disease, aplastic anaemia.
3. Anisocytes (cells with different sizes): Pernicious anemia.

Variations in color: Hypochromic: RBCs with an area of pallor that is larger than normal, seen in IDA, anaemia of chronic disease.

Variations in shape: Poikilocytosis: Crenation/echinocytes (shrinkage as in hypertonic conditions); spherocytes (globular form as in haemolytic anaemia); ovalocytes (in IDA); pencil cells (IDA), target cells (hypochromica cells with central spot on Hb, seen in sickle cell disease, thalassemia syndrome); sickle cell (crescentic shape as in sickle cell anemia); acanthocytes (spicules over the surface of cells, in severe liver disease); tear drop/pear shaped (IDA); schistocytes (fragmented RBC, in severe burn).

Variations in structure of red blood cells: Inclusions in RBC: Abnormal structures present in RBCs.

1. **Howell-Jolly bodies**—some nuclear fragments present in cytoplasm of RBCs seen in splenectomy, Sickle cells anaemia.
2. **Cabot rings:** Remnants of nuclear membrane appear as rings or figure of 8 patterns. Seen in dyserthropoiesis.
3. **Heinz bodies:** Denatures Hb near the periphery of cell, seen in G6PD-deficiency.
4. **Siderocytes:** RBC containing non-Hb iron granules. Seen in haemolytic anaemia.
5. **Punctate basophilism:** Striated appearance of RBCs by the presence of dots of basophilic materials (porphyrin). It occurs in lead poisoning.
6. **Goblet ring in red blood cells:** Ring or twisted strands of basophilic material appear in the periphery of RBCs.

RBCs indices:

1. **Mean Corpuscular volume (MCV):** Average volume of single RBC. Normal = 85–90 μ³
2. **Mean Corpuscular Haemoglobin (MCH):** Average weight of hemoglobin in each RBC. normal = 27–33 pg
3. **Mean Corpuscular Haemoglobin Concentration (MCHC):** Amount of Hb expressed as percentage of the volume of RBC. Normal = 30–33%.
4. **Color index:** Ratio of Hb to RBC. Normal = 0.85–1.15.

Q. 3. Classify leukocytes. Give an account of leukopoiesis. Mention normal counts of granulocytes and give their functions.
(TNMGR, Nov. 1995; 2009; PAHER, May 2012)

Q. Discuss role of neutrophils in health and disease.
(UHSR, May 2016; TNMGR, June 2017)

Ans. Leukocytes (White Blood Cells, WBCs) are the mobile units of body's protective system. They are formed partially in bone marrow (granulocytes and monocytes and a few lymphocytes) and partially in lymph tissue (lymphocytes and plasma cells). After formation, they are transported in the blood to different parts of body where they are needed.

Leucopoiesis: The process of development and maturation of WBCs.

Regulation: By feedback mechanism, decresed WBC count releases various growth factors which stimulate bone marrow for more production.

Normal range of WBC: At Birth: 10,000–25000/μl; Infant: 6000–16000/μl; Adults: 4000–11000/μl

Classification of leucocytes:

A. Granulocytes:

  i. **Neutrophils (50–70%, 3000–6000/mm³):** Antimicrobial action, anti-inflammatory action, wound healing, chemotaxis, aggregation of platelets, first line of defense against infection. Life span = >2–5 days.

   Granules of Neutrophils:

   1. Primary (Azurophilic): Myeloperoxidase, acid β-glycerophosphatase, cathepsins, defensins, elastase, proteinase-3 (antimicrobial activity)
   2. Secondary: β$_2$-microglobulin, collagenase, gelatinase, lactoferrin, plasminogen activator (phagocytic and antimicrobial activity).
   3. Tertiary: Gelatinase, collagenase, lysozyme, acetyltransferase, β$_2$-microglobulin.

  ii. **Eosinophils (2–4%, 150–450/mm³):** Destruction of worms, neurotoxic action, prevention of intravascular clotting, acute hypersensitivity reactions. Lifespan= >7–12 days.

  iii. **Basophils (0–1%, 0–100/mm³):** Antimicrobial action, acceleration of inflammatory response. Life span= >12–15 days.

B. Agranulocytes:

  i. **Monocytes (2–6%, 200–600/mm³):** Formation of colony forming blastocytes, aggregation of platelets, chemotaxis, stimulation of phagocytic cells, acceleration of inflammatory response, activation of T-cells. Life span = >2–5 days.

  ii. **Lymphocytes (20–30%, 1500–2700/mm³):** Antimicrobial action, necrosis of tumor, activation of immune system, promotion of inflammation, chemotaxis. Life span = >1/2–1day.

Applied Clinical Physiology

A. **Variations in Leukocyte Count:** Increase in leukocyte count is called **leukocytosis** and decrease in the count is called **leucopenia**.

Physiological variations: Age (more at birth); sex (more in male); diurnal variation (maximum in afternoon); exercise, emotional stress, pregnancy, menstruation, parturition ard after food intake: Increases. Sleep: Decreases slightly.

Pathological Variations

Leukocytosis: Acute bacterial infections, allergy, burns, postoperative period, common cold, tuberculosis, glandular fever.

Leukopenia: Infections by non-pyrogenic organisms, e.g. typhoid fever; viral infections; protozoal infections; starvation and malnutrition, anaphylactic shock, cirrhosis of liver.

Leukemia: The leukemia is characterized by abnormal and uncontrolled increase in leukocyte count more than 10,00,000/mm³.

B. **Neutrophils in disease:** Agranulocytosis, cyclic neutropenia, leukocyte adhesicn deficiency, hypergammaglobulinaemia (Job's syndome), specific granule deficiency, Papillon-Lefèvre syndrome.

Q. 4. Write a short note on blood groups and their significance.   *(TNMGR, March 2008, 2009; March, Sept 2010; RGUHS, Oct. 2010, June 2018)*

Q. Write a note on importance of blood groups in blood transfusion.   *(TNMGR, Sept. 2007; BFUHS, May 2007; HP Uni., May 2018)*

Ans. Blood groups are determined by the presence of antigen in RBC membrane. When blood from two individuals is mixed, sometimes clumping (agglutination) of RBCs occurs due to immunological reactions. Blood groups were discovered by Austrian Scientist Karl Landsteiner in 1901. *Blood transfusion* is a common, safe procedure in which healthy blood is given patient through an intravenous (IV) line inserted in blood vessels.

Landsteiner's Rule: If an antigen/agglutinogen is present on red blood cell membrane of an individual, the corresponding antibody/agglutinin will be absent in the plasma. If an antigen/agglutinogen is absent on the red cell membrane of an individual, the corresponding antibody/agglutinin will be present in the plasma.

ABO system is based on the presence or absence of antigen A and antigen B.

Blood having antigen A belongs to 'A' group. Blood with antigen B and α-antibody belorgs to 'B' group. If both the antigens are present, blood group is called 'AB' group and serum of this group does not contain any antibody. If both antigens are absert, blood group is called 'O' group.

Determination of ABO group: Also called blood grouping, blood typing or blood matching or cross-matching.

Principle of blood typing: Blood typing is done on the basis of agglutination. Agglutination occurs if an antigen is mixed with its corresponding antibody which is called isoagglutinin.

1. **Major crossmatch:** It tests donor cells with recipient's serum to detect antibodies in patient serum.
2. **Minor crossmatch:** It tests donor serum with recipient's cells to detect antibodies in donor serum.

Techniques for crossmarthing: Immediate spin method, saline room temperature technique, anti-globulin compatibility techniques (indirect Coombs' test), albumin addition technique.

Table 2.4: Antigen and antibody present in ABO blood groups

Group	Antigen in RBC	Antibody in serum	% of Indian having the blood group
A	A	Anti-B (β)	23
B	B	Anti-A (α)	33
AB	A and B	No antibody	7
O	No antigen	Anti-A and anti-B	37

Importance of ABO groups in blood transfusion: During blood transfusion, only compatible blood must be used. While transfusing the blood, antigen of the donor and the antibody of the recipient are considered. Thus, RBCs of 'O' group are called '**universal donors**'.

People with AB group are called '**universal recipients**'.

Transfusion reactions due to ABO incompatibility: Transfusion reactions occur due to transfusion error that involves transfusion of incompatible (mismatched) blood. In mismatched transfusion, the transfusion reactions occur between donor's RBC and recipient's plasma. So, if the donor's plasma contains agglutinins against recipient's RBC, agglutination does not occur because these antibodies are diluted in the recipient's blood. But, if recipient's plasma contains agglutinins against donor's RBCs, the immune system launches a response against the new blood cells. Donor RBCs are agglutinated resulting in transfusion reactions.

Rh factor (*NTR Uni., May 2019*): Rh factor is an antigen present in RBC. The persons having D antigen are called 'Rh positive' and those without D antigen are called 'Rh negative'. Among Indian population, 85% of people are Rh positive and 15% are Rh negative. Rh group system is different from ABO group system because antigen D does not have corresponding natural antibody (anti-D). If Rh positive blood is transfused to Rh negative person anti-D is developed in that person. There is no risk of complications if Rh positive person receives Rh negative blood.

Transfusion reactions due to Rh incompatibility: When Rh negative person receives Rh positive blood for the first time, he/she is not affected much, since the reactions do not occur immediately. But Rh antibodies develop within one month and remain in the body forever. So, when same person receives Rh positive blood for the second time, donors RBCs are agglutinated and severe transfusion reactions occur immediately.

Hemolytic disease of fetus and newborn: Erythroblastosis fetalis: It is characterized by abnormal hemolysis of RBCs, due to Rh incompatibility. **Erythroblastosis fetalis** is a disorder in fetus, characterized by the presence of erythroblasts in blood. When a mother is Rh negative and fetus is Rh positive (Rh factor being inherited from father), usually first child escapes complications of Rh incompatibility, as the Rh antigen cannot pass from fetal blood into mother's blood through placental barrier. However, at time of parturition (delivery of child), Rh antigen from fetal blood may leak into mother's blood because of placental detachment. During postpartum period, i.e. within a month after delivery, the mother develops Rh antibody in her blood. When the mother conceives for the second time and if the fetus happens to be Rh positive again, Rh antibody from mother's blood crosses placental barrier and enters fetal blood. Rh antibody which enters the fetus causes agglutination of fetal RBCs resulting in hemolysis with complications like severe anemia, hydrops fetalis, kernicterus.

Prevention or treatment for erythroblastosis fetalis

i. If mother is found to be Rh negative and fetus is Rh positive, anti-D (antibody against D antigen) should be administered to mother at 28th and 34th weeks of gestation, as prophylactic measure. If Rh negative mother delivers Rh positive baby, then anti-D should be administered to mother within 48 hours of delivery.

ii. If the baby is born with erythroblastosis fetalis, treatment is given by means of exchange transfusion.

Other blood groups: Lewis blood group, MNS blood groups, Auberger groups, Diego group, Bombay group, Duffy group, Lutheran group, P group, Kell group, I group, Kidd group.

Blood Transfusion (*NTR Uni., May 2019*): Transfused red blood cells (RBCs) provide three beneficial effects: Circulatory (volume-related), rheological (viscosity-related) and oxygen carriage.

Transfusion triggers: It is defined as that value of haemoglobin (Hb) below which RBC transfusion is indicated. Traditionally, the rule of "10/30" was followed for RBC transfusion, according to which a Hb level of 10 g/dl or a haematocrit of 30% was recommended in surgical patients.

Guidelines for transfusion: Summary of Guidelines by American Society of Anesthesiologists, Society of Critical Care Medicine, American Association of Blood Banks (AABB), American College of Physicians and the British Committee for Standards in Haematology.

1. **Post-operative patients:** In haemodynamically stable post-operative surgical patients, the trigger for transfusion is Hb ≤8 g/dl or presence of symptoms of inadequate oxygen delivery.

2. **Patients in the intensive care unit:**
   - In critically ill normovolaemic patients, transfusion is considered at a Hb level of ≤7 mg/dl with a target of 7–9 g/dl.
   - During early resuscitative phase of severe sepsis if there is evidence of inadequate oxygen delivery to the tissues, blood transfusion is considered to achieve Hb of 9–10 g/dl.
   - In late phases of severe sepsis, guidelines are similar to those for other critically ill patients with target Hb of 7–9 g/dl.
   - Blood transfusion should not be used to assist weaning from mechanical ventilation if Hb is >7 g/dl.

3. **Patients with cardiac disease**
   - In haemodynamically stable patients with cardio-vascular disease transfusion is considered for Hb ≤8 g/dl, or the presence of symptoms of inadequate oxygen delivery.
   - In critically ill patients with stable angina, Hb should be maintained >7 g/dl.
   - In patients suffering from acute coronary syndrome, Hb should be maintained at >8–9 g/dl.
   - Restrictive transfusion strategy (trigger Hb: 7–8 g/dl) is recommended for patients with coronary artery disease.

4. Patients with neurotrauma or neurological diseases
   - In patients with traumatic brain injury, target Hb should be 7–9 g/dl; and in those with additional evidence of cerebral ischaemia, target Hb should be >9 g/dl.

- In patients with subarachnoid haemorrhage, target Hb should be 8–10 g/dl.
- In patients with an acute ischaemic stroke, Hb should be maintained above 9 g/dl.

Blood Product Transfusion

1. **Plasma** is conventionally prescribed to replace coagulation factors in patients receiving massive transfusion (>one blood volume or 70 ml/kg in 24 h or >50% of blood volume in 3 h), for urgent reversal of the effect of warfarin, in known coagulation factor deficiency, and in cases of thrombotic thrombo-cytopaenic purpura. The decision to transfuse is based on both presence of bleeding and abnormal laboratory values of prothrombin time (>1.5), international normalized ratio (>2) and partial thromboplastin time (>2 times). Plasma should not be used to replace intravascular volume.

2. **Platelet** transfusion is usually required in a bleeding patient below a platelet count of 50×10^9/L but rarely above 100×10^9/L. If the values fall between these two, transfusion is considered in case of platelet dysfunction (e.g. clopidogrel therapy), on-going bleeding and surgeries in confined spaces such as eye and brain.

3. **Cryoprecipitate** is used to increase fibrinogen levels in patients with dysfibrinogenaemia and hypo-fibrinogenaemia (fibrinogen <80–100 mg/dl), micro-vascular bleeding in patients receiving massive transfusion when fibrinogen cannot be measured and congenital fibrinogen deficiency.

Techniques of Blood Transfusion: Direct, indirect, whole blood with syringe, whole blood with Kimpton's tube, transfusion with anticoagulants.

Q. 5. Write a note on blood substitutes.
(Sumandeep Uni., April 2015)

Ans. A blood substitute is a substance used to mimic and fulfil some functions of biological blood.

Ideal blood substitutes: It should
1. Oxygen carrying capacity equal or more than that of biological blood.
2. Universal compatibility.
3. Volume expansion.
4. Minimal side effects.
5. Pathogen free.
6. Long shelf life
7. Cost effective.

Types:
A. **Plasma expanders:** They are infusion solutions, expands intracellular volume, e.g. crystalloids (NS, D, RL) and colloids (gelatin, dextran, hydroxyethyl starch, albumin)

B. RBC Substitutes:

1. Modified hemoglobins: Human Hb extracted from outdated blood, e.g. hemoglobin-based oxygen carriers (HBOC).
2. Perflurocarbons (PFC): Synthetic organic compounds, e.g. Oxygent, Oxycyte, PHER-O_2, Perftoran, Fluosol-DA,

Complications: Anaphylaxis, disease transmission, nephrotoxicity, volume overload, electrolyte imbalance.

Q. 6. Write functions and applied aspects of platelets.
(TNMGR, March 2002; April 2012; BFUHS, May 2011; AHSUC, May 2017)

Ans. Platelets are anucleated, discoid in shape with life span of 5–7days.

Noraml range: 150000–400000 µl.

1. **Role in blood coagulation**: By forming intrinsic prothrombin activator.
2. **Role in clot retraction**: By releasing contractile proteins, actin, myosin, thrombosthenin.
3. **Role in prevention of blood loss**: By releasing 5-HT, sealing of damaged blood vessels and formation of temporary plugs.
4. **Role in repair of ruptured blood vessel**: By forming platelet derived growth factors.
5. **Role in defense mechanism**: By agglutination of foreign body.

In addition, the platelet membrane contains large amounts of phospholipids that activate multiple stages in the blood clotting process.

Applied Clinical Physiology: Platelet Disorders

1. **Thrombocytopenia:** Decrease in platelet count. It leads to thrombocytopenic purpura. Thrombocytopenia occurs in: Acute infections, acute leukemia, aplastic and pernicious anemia, chickenpox, smallpox, splenomegaly, scarlet fever, typhoid, tuberculosis.
2. **Thrombocytosis:** Increase in platelet count. It occurs in: Allergic conditions, hemorrhage, bone fractures, surgical operations, splenectomy, rheumatic fever, trauma.
3. **Thrombocythemia:** Persistent and abnormal increase in platelet count. It occurs in: Carcinoma, chronic leukemia, Hodgkin's disease.
4. **Glanzmann's thrombasthenia:** An inherited hemorrhagic disorder caused by structural or functional abnormality of platelets. It leads to thrombasthenic purpura.

Q. 7. Write a short note on composition and functions of blood.
(TNMGR, March 2010; MUHS, June 2011; RGUHS, Nov. 2011; BBD Uni., April 2017; Gujarat Uni., April 2019)

Q. Write a note on blood components.
(BFUHS, May 2011)

Ans. Blood is a vital connective tissue. It is considered as *"Fluid of life"* or *"Fluid of growth"* or *"Fluid of Health"*. Blood contains blood cells which are called formed elements and liquid portion known as **plasma**.

A. Cellular Components (45%):
1. Red blood cells or erythrocytes (RBCs).
2. White blood cells or leukocytes (WBCs).
3. Platelets or thrombocytes.

B. Plasma (55%): Plasma is a straw colored clear liquid part of blood. It contains:
1. Solids (7–8%).
   i. Organic substance: Plasma proteins; amino acids; glucose; fats; hormones; enzymes; non-protein nitrogenous substances.
   ii. Inorganic substances: Sodium; calcium; potassium; magnesium, etc.
2. Water (92–93%).
3. Gases: Oxygen, carbon dioxide, nitrogen.

Serum is the clear straw colored fluid that is left after blood has clotted.

Serum = plasma – fibrinogen.

Functions:

1. **Nutritive function:** Nutritive substances absorbed from gastrointestinal tract (GIT) are carried by blood to different parts of the body for growth and production of energy.
2. **Respiratory function:** It carries oxygen from alveoli of lungs to different tissues and carbon dioxide from tissues to alveoli.
3. **Excretory function:** Waste products formed in tissues are removed by blood and carried to excretory organs like kidney, skin, liver, etc. for excretion.
4. **Transport of hormones and enzymes:** Blood transports hormones and enzymes to their target organs/tissues.
5. **Regulation of water balance:** Water content of blood is freely interchangeable with interstitial fluid. This helps in the regulation of water content of body.
6. **Regulation of acid–base balance:** Plasma proteins and hemoglobin act as buffers and help in regulation of acid–base balance.

7. **Regulation of body temperature:** Because of the high specific heat of blood, it is responsible for maintaining the thermoregulatory mechanism in the body.

8. **Storage function:** Water and some important substances like proteins, glucose, sodium and potassium are constantly required by the tissues. Blood serves as a readymade source for these substances.

9. **Defensive function:** Neutrophils and monocytes engulf bacteria by phagocytosis. Lymphocytes are involved in development of immunity. Eosinophils are responsible for detoxification, disintegration and removal of foreign proteins.

Q. 8. Describe erythropoiesis and factors affecting erythropoiesis.
(TNMGR, March 2008; HNBG Uni., July 2015)

Q. Discuss the development of hematopoietic system from progenitor cells.
(TNMGR, Oct. 2013; UHSR, May 2016)

Ans. Erythropoiesis is the process of the origin, development and maturation of erythrocytes. **Hemopoiesis or hematopoiesis** is the process of origin, development and maturation of all the blood cellular components, occurs during embryonic development and throughout adulthood to produce and replenish the blood system.

The blood cells begin their lives in the bone marrow from a single type of cell called the pluripotential hematopoietic stem cell, from which all the cells of the circulating blood are eventually derived (Fig. 2.8). Then the successive divisions of the pluripotential cells occur to form the different circulating blood cells. As these cells reproduce, a small portion of them remains exactly like the original pluripotential cells and is retained in

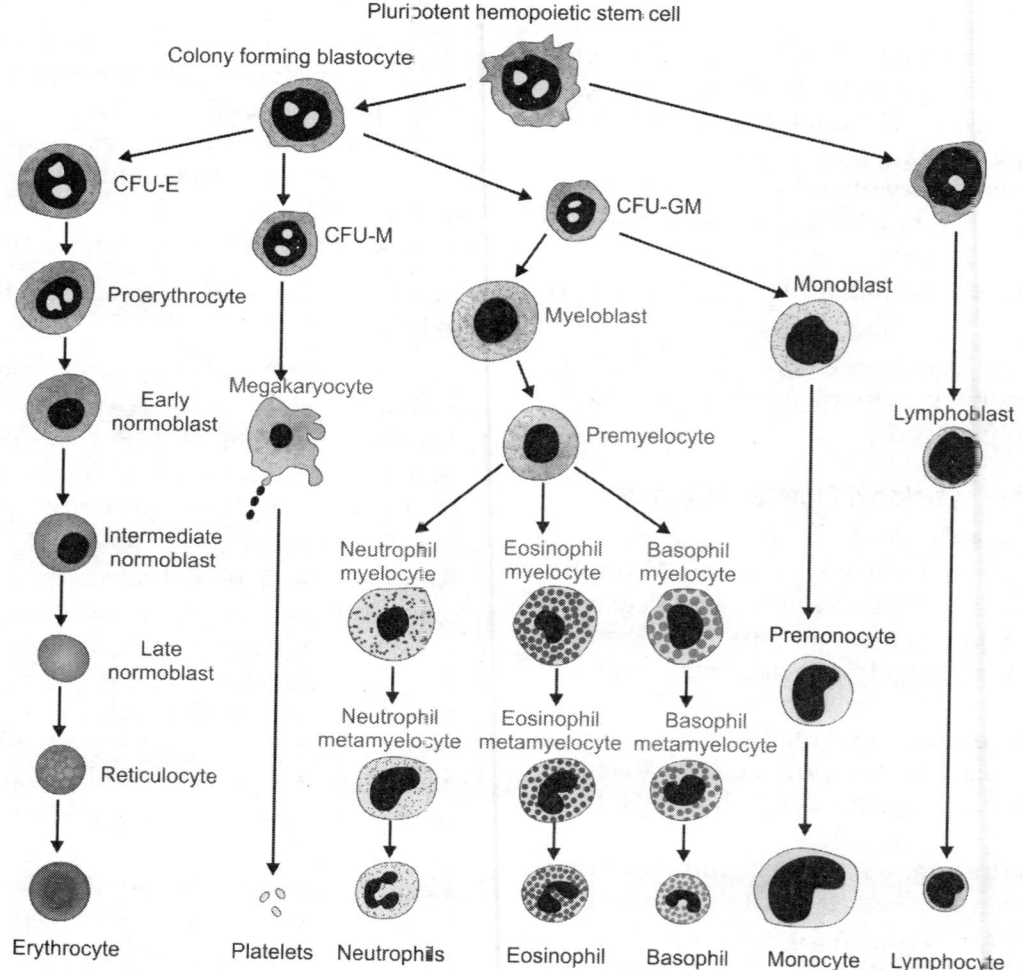

Fig. 2.8: Stages of Hematopoiesis. CFU-E=Colony forming unit-erythrocyte, CFU-M=Colony forming unit-megakaryocyte, CFU-GM=Colony forming unit-granulocyte/monocyte

the bone marrow to maintain a supply of these, although their numbers diminish with age. Most of the reproduced cells, however, differentiate to form the other cell types.

The intermediate stage cells are very much like pluripotential stem cells, even though they have already become committed to a particular line of cells and are called **committed stem cells.**

The different committed stem cells, when grown in culture, will produce colonies of specific types of blood cells. A committed stem cell that produces erythrocytes is called a colony forming unit-erythrocyte (CFU-E).

Factors affecting erythropoiesis

A. **General factors:**
1. **Erythropoietin/hemopoietin/erythrocyte stimulating factors**: Production of proerythroblasts, development and release of matured erythrocytes into blood.
2. **Thyroxine**: It accelerates erythropoiesis.
3. **Growth factors**: Induce proliferation of stem cells. Interleukin-3; interleukin-6; interleukin-11.
4. **Vitamins**: Vitamins B, C, D, E.

B. **Maturation factors:**
1. **Vitamin B12 (cyanocobalamin/Antipernicious factor)**: Essential for synthesis of DNA in RBCs.
2. **Intrinsic factor**: Required for absorption of vitamin B12.
3. **Folic acid**: Essential for synthesis of DNA in RBCs.
4. **Factors necessary for hemoglobin formation**: First class proteins and amino acids, iron, copper, cobalt and nickel, vitamins.

Q. 9. Write about formation of lymph.
(TNMGR, Sept. 2002)

Ans. Lymph is formed from interstitial fluid, due to the permeability of lymph capillaries (Fig. 2.9). When blood passes via blood capillaries in the tissues, 9/10th of fluid passes into venous end of capillaries from the arterial end and remaining 1/10th of the fluid pass into lymph capillaries, which have more permeability than blood capillaries. So, when lymph passes through lymph capillaries, the composition of lymph is more or less similar to that of interstitial fluid including protein content. Proteins present in the interstitial fluid cannot enter the blood capillaries because of their larger size. So, these proteins enter lymph vessels, which are permeable to large particles also.

Composition of lymph: Usually, lymph is a clear and colorless fluid. It is formed by 96% water and 4% solids. Some blood cells are also present in lymph.

Addition of proteins and fats: Tissue fluid in liver and gastrointestinal tract contains more protein and lipid

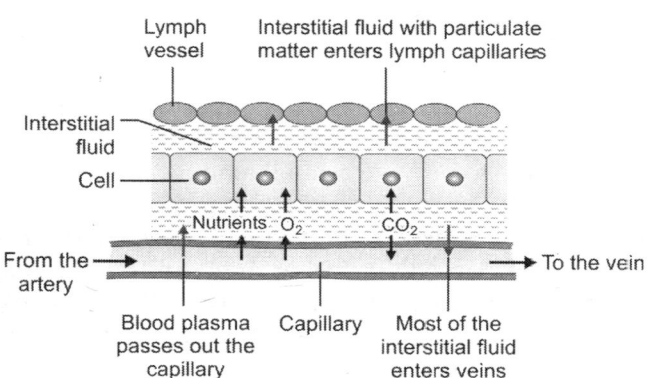
Fig. 2.9: Formation of lymph

substances. So, proteins and lipids enter the lymph vessels of liver and gastrointestinal tract in large quantities.

Concentration of lymph: When the lymph passes through the lymph nodes, it is concentrated because of absorption of water and the electrolytes.

3. CARDIOVASCULAR SYSTEM

Q. 1. Write a note in cardiopulmonary arrest.
(TNMGR, March 2008; BFUHS, May 2008)

Ans. Cardiac arrest is defined as inability of the heart to sustain an effective output. In cardiac arrest circulation ceases or stops and vital organs are deprived of oxygen.

Etiology
1. Cardiac disease
2. Hypoxia
3. Hypotension
4. Hypoglycemia
5. Fainting
6. Drugs: Intravascular injection of adrenalin, sensitivity to local anaesthetics
7. Electrolytic imbalance
8. Vagal reflex mechanism
9. Terminal illness

Diagnosis
1. Absence of pulse in major vessels.
2. Cessation of respiration, absence of breath sounds.
3. Absence of the heart sounds.
4. Pupils may be dilated with sluggish or no reaction to light.
5. Skin may appear pale or cyanosed.
6. In general examination, person is unconscious and not responding to stimuli.

Treatment: Cardiac pulmonary resuscitation (CPR) is most effective, when started immediately.

Q. 2. Write about cardiopulmonary resuscitation.
(TNMGR, March 2009, 2010; HP Uni., July 2011)

Ans. CPR is one of the techniques aimed at maintaining blood flow following cardiac arrest. The goal of CPR is to continue to provide a small amount of blood and oxygen to the tissues to prevent permanent damage till standard care arrives. Outside the hospital, it is the basic life support (BLS). Inside the hospital, it is BSL plus advanced care life support (ACLS) and post-resuscitation life support, called cardiac pulmonary cerebral resuscitation (CPCR).

A. **Basic life support (BLS)** *(BBD Uni., April 2018):* Objective of BLS is to maintain oxygenation in lungs, brain and heart before the ACLS.

1. **Airway:** When victim is unresponsive, the victim must be made to lie supine, on the firm flat surface. The rescuer should be at the victim's side at a distance equal to width of the victim's body and at the level of victim's shoulder.

    Triple maneuver:
    i. Open the mouth—clear the airway.
    ii. Head tilt and chin lift.
    iii. Jaw thrust.

    In case of foreign body airway obstruction, following maneuver can be used:
    i. Back blows should be given on the middle of back of patient. This produces cough reflex.
    ii. Hemlich maneuver consists of manual thrust with the patient breathing, rescuer behind the patient and compressing the patient's chest 6–10 times.
    iii. Finger sweep method.

2. **Breathing:** First determine the presence or absence of breathing by: Placing the ear near the victim's mouth or nose, looking for the chest wall movement, auscultation of the chest for breath sounds.

    Expired air resuscitation:
    i. **Mouth to mouth breathing:** The rescuer uses his expired air oxygen to supply to the victim.
        a. Open the airway with triple maneuver.
        b. Close the victim's nostrils with the thumb and index finger.
        c. Take a deep breath and form a seal with lips around the victim's mouth before exhaling.
        d. Two slow breaths (½ to 2 seconds per puff) are given to provide good chest expansion.
    ii. **Mouth to nose breathing:**
        a. Tilt the victim's head back with one hand over the victim's forehead.
        b. Close the victim's mouth.
        c. Lift the victim's lower jaw with the other hand.
        d. Take a deep breath, form a seal with the lips around victim's nose and blow.
        e. Victim is then allowed to exhale.
    iii. **Mouth to airway breathing:**
        a. Close the victim's nostrils with the thumb and index finger.
        b. Take a deep breath and form a seal with the lips around the victim's mouth before exhaling.
        c. Two slow breaths are given to provide good chest expansion.

3. **Circulation:** If no pulse is palpated one should start external cardiac compression to establish circulation.

    External cardiac compression: These compressions provide circulation as a result of a generalized increased in intrathoracic pressure. When the compressions are accomplished by rescue breathing, the blood supplied to the organ is likely to carry oxygen.
    a. Position the victim, supine on the firm surface.
    b. Locate the lower margin of the victim's rib cage.
    c. Locate the lower part of the sternum, by moving the fingers along the notch, where rib meets the sternum in the centre of the chest wall.
    d. Place the heel of one hand, on the lower half of sternum, with the other hand on the top of first hand.
    e. For adult, sternum should be depressed approximately ½ to 1½ inches.
    f. Duration of the each compression should be 50% of the compression release cycle with a chest compression rate of 80–100 per minute.

    Standard approach to unconscious patient in one rescuer CPR:
    a. Open the airway and deliver slow air breaths.
    b. Perform 18 compressions at the rate of two ventilations.
    c. After 5 cycles of compressions, reevaluate the patient.
    d. Check for return of carotid pulse.
    e. If absent, resume CPR.
    f. With two rescuers CPR, the ratio of compression and ventilation is maintained at 5:1.

B. **Advanced cardiac life support (ACLS):** ACLS helps to evaluate and restore the spontaneous circulatory function.

    First ABCD of ACLS: A—Airway; B—Breathing; C—Circulation; D—Defibrillation

Second ABCD of ACLS: A—Perform endotracheal intubation; B—Assist ventilation; C—Circulatory support, gain IV access, attach monitor, identify rhythm, measure blood pressure, and provide appropriate medication; D—Differential diagnosis, find and treat the cause.

Postcardiac arrest complications:

1. Complications of CPR: Rib fracture, cardiac laceration etc.
2. Ischaemic injury: Renal, cerebral, hepatic, etc.

Outcome of resuscitation: If the arrest time is less than 6 minutes and CPR time is less than 15 minutes, the outcome is satisfactory. If the arrest time exceeds 6 minutes and CPR time exceeds 15 minutes, chances of survival are almost nil.

Q. 3. Write a note on cardiac cycle.

(TNMGR, April 2000, 2001;
HP Uni., July 2011; NTR Uni., June 2017)

Ans. Cardiac cycle is defined as the sequence of **co-ordinated events** taking place in the heart during each beat. Each heart beat consists of two major periods called systole and diastole. During systole, heart contracts and pumps the blood through arteries. During diastole, heart relaxes and blood is filled in the heart.

Events of cardiac cycle:

1. Atrial events
2. Ventricular events

Divisions and duration of cardiac cycle (Fig. 3.3): When the heart beats at a normal rate of 72/minute, duration of each cardiac cycle is about 0.8 second.

Atrial events: Atrial events are divided into two divisions:

1. Atrial systole = 0.11 (0.1) sec.
2. Atrial diastole = 0.69 (0.7) sec.

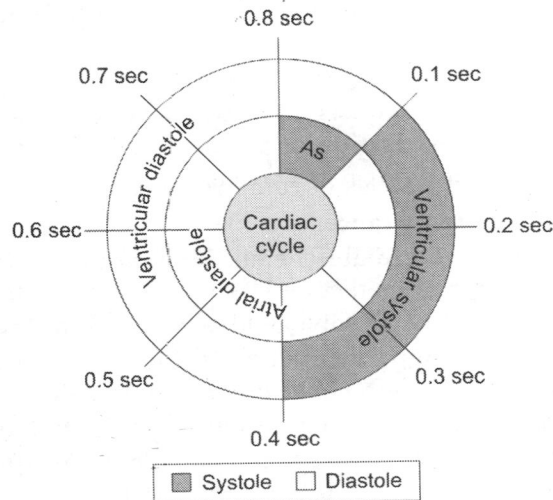

Fig. 3.3: Cardiac cycle

Ventricular events: Ventricular events are divided into two divisions:

1. Ventricular systole = 0.27 (0.3) sec.
2. Ventricular diastole = 0.53 (0.5) sec.

In clinical practice, the term 'systole' refers to ventricular systole and 'diastole' refers to ventricular diastole. Ventricular systole is divided into two subdivisions and ventricular diastole is divided into five subdivisions.

Ventricular systole:

1. Isometric contraction = 0.05 second.
2. Ejection period = 0.22 second.

Ventricular diastole:

1. Protodiastole = 0.04 second.
2. Isometric relaxation = 0.08 second
3. Rapid filling = 0.11 second.
4. Slow filling = 0.19 second.
5. Last rapid filling = 0.11 second.

Atrial systole occurs during the last phase of ventricular diastole. Atrial diastole is not considered as a separate phase, since it coincides with the whole of ventricular systole and earlier part of ventricular diastole.

Q. 4. What is normal cardiac output? Describe the factors regulating cardiac output.

Ans. Cardiac output is the amount of blood pumped from each ventricle. Usually, cardiac output is expressed in three ways:

1. **Stroke volume:** The amount of blood pumped out by each ventricle during each beat. Normal value: 70 ml (60–80 ml).
2. **Minute volume:** The amount of blood pumped out by each ventricle in one minute. Minute volume = Stroke volume × Heart rate. Normal value: 5 L/ventricle/minute.
3. **Cardiac index:** It is defined as the amount of blood pumped out per ventricle/minute/square meter of the body surface area. Normal value: 2.8 ± 0.3 L/m²/min.

Factors maintaining cardiac output:

1. **Venous return:** Venous return is the amount of blood which is returned to heart from different parts of the body. Cardiac output is directly proportional to venous return. Venous return depends upon five factors:
   i. Respiratory pump.
   ii. Muscle pump.
   iii. Gravity.
   iv. Venous pressure.
   v. Sympathetic tone.

2. **Force of contraction:** Cardiac output is **directly proportional** to the force of contraction, provided the other three factors remain constant. According to **Frank-Starling law**, force of contraction of heart is directly proportional to the initial length of muscle fibers, before the onset of contraction. Force of contraction of heart and cardiac output are **directly proportional** to preload. Force of contraction of heart and cardiac output are **inversely proportional** to after load.

3. **Heart rate:** Cardiac output is **directly proportional** to heart rate provided, the other three factors remain constant.

4. **Peripheral resistance:** Peripheral resistance is the resistance or load against which the heart has to pump the blood. So, the cardiac output is **inversely proportional** to peripheral resistance.

Q. 5. Draw and label a normal ECG. Define and describe the different waves of ECG.

(TNMGR, Oct. 2003)

Ans. **Electrocardiography** is the technique by which electrical activities of the heart are studied. **Electrocardiograph** is the instrument (machine) by which electrical activities of the heart are recorded. **Electrocardiogram** (ECG or EKG from electrocardiogram in Dutch) is the record or graphical registration of electrical activities of the heart, which occur prior to the onset of mechanical activities. Normal ECG consists of waves, complexes, intervals and segments.

Waves of Normal ECG: Normal electrocardiogram has the following waves, namely P, Q, R, S and T (Fig. 3.5).

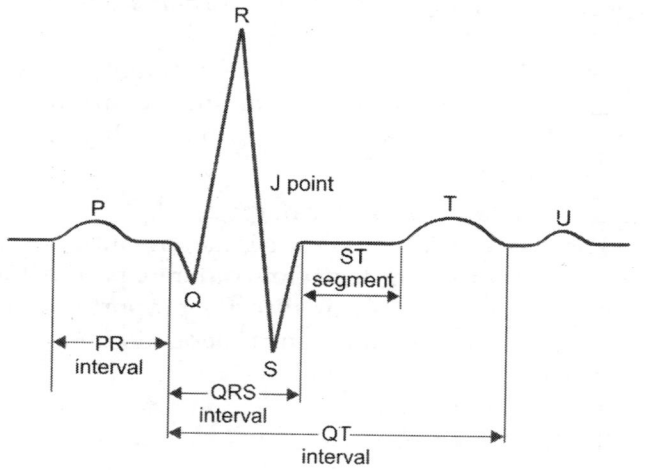

Fig. 3.5: The ECG curve

Major complexes in ECG

1. 'P' wave—atrial complex.
2. 'QRS' complex—initial ventricular complex.
3. 'T' wave—final ventricular complex.
4. 'QRST'—ventricular complex.

1. **'P' wave:** 'P' wave is a positive wave and first wave in ECG. It is produced due to **depolarization** of **atrial musculature**. Normal duration of 'P' wave is 0.1 s. Normal amplitude of 'P' wave is 0.1–0.12 mV.

Clinical significance

1. Right atrial hypertrophy: 'P' wave is tall (>2.5 mm) in lead II. It is usually pointed.
2. Left atrial dilatation or hypertrophy: 'P' wave is tall and broad based or M-shaped.
3. Atrial extrasystole: 'P' wave is small and shapeless.
4. Hyperkalemia: 'P' wave is absent or small.
5. Atrial fibrillation: 'P' wave is absent.
6. Middle AV nodal rhythm: 'P' wave is absent.
7. Sinoatrial block: 'P' wave is inverted or absent.
8. Atrial paroxysmal tachycardia: 'P' wave is inverted.

2. **'QRS' complex:** 'Q' wave is a small negative wave and is continued as tall 'R' wave, which is a positive wave. 'R' wave is followed by a small negative wave, 'S' wave. 'QRS' complex is due to **depolarization** of **ventricular musculature**. 'Q' wave is due to depolarization of basal portion of interventricular septum. 'R' wave is due to depolarization of apical portion of interventricular septum and apical portion of ventricular muscle. 'S' wave is due to depolarization of basal portion of ventricular muscle near atrioventricular ring. Normal duration of 'QRS' complex is 0.08–0.10s.

Clinical Significance

1. Bundle branch block: QRS is prolonged or deformed.
2. Hyperkalemia: QRS is prolonged.

3. **'T' Wave:** 'T' wave is a positive wave. 'T' wave is due to **repolarization** of **ventricular musculature**. Normal duration of 'T' wave is 0.2 s.

Clinical Significance

1. Acute myocardial ischemia: Hyperacute 'T' wave develops. Hyperacute 'T' wave refers to a tall and broad-based 'T' wave, with slight asymmetry.
2. Old age, hyperventilation, anxiety, myocardial infarction, left ventricular hypertrophy and pericarditis: 'T' wave is small, flat or inverted.
3. Hypokalemia: 'T' wave is small, flat or inverted.
4. Hyperkalemia: 'T' wave is tall and tented.

4. **'U' Wave:** 'U' wave is not always seen. It is supposed to be due to **repolarization** of **papillary muscle**.

Clinical Significance

1. Hypercalcemia, thyrotoxicosis and hypokalemia: 'U' wave appears. It is very prominent in hypokalemia.
2. Myocardial ischemia: Inverted 'U' wave appears.

Intervals and segments of ECG

1. **'P-R' Interval:** Interval between onset of 'P' wave and onset of 'Q' wave. It signifies atrial depolarization and conduction of impulses through AV node. Normal duration of 'P-R interval' is 0.18 s and varies between 0.12 and 0.2 s.

Clinical Significance

1. It is prolonged in bradycardia and first degree heart block.
2. It is shortened in tachycardia, Wolff-Parkinson-White syndrome, Lown-Ganong-Levine syndrome, Duchenne muscular dystrophy and type II glycogen storage disease.

2. **'Q-T' interval:** Time interval between onset of 'Q' wave and end of 'T' wave. It indicates ventricular depolarization and ventricular repolarization. Normal duration of Q-T interval is between 0.4 and 0.42 s.

Clinical Significance

1. 'Q-T' interval is prolonged in long 'Q-T' syndrome, myocardial infarction, myocarditis, hypocalcemia and hypothyroidism
2. 'Q-T' interval is shortened in short 'Q-T' syndrome and hypercalcemia.

3. **'S-T' segment:** Time interval between end of 'S' wave and onset of 'T' wave. It is an isoelectric period. The point where 'S-T' segment starts is called *'J' point*. It is junction between QRS complex and 'S-T' segment. Normal duration of 'S-T' segment is 0.08 s.

Clinical Significance

1. Elevation of 'S-T' segment: Anterior or inferior myocardial infarction, left bundle branch block and acute pericarditis. In athletes, 'S-T' segment is usually elevated.
2. Depression of 'S-T' segment: Acute myocardial ischemia, posterior myocardial infarction, ventricular hypertrophy and hypokalaemia.
3. 'S-T' segment is prolonged in hypocalcemia
4. 'S-T' segment is shortened in hypercalcemia.

4. **'R-R' Interval:** Time interval between two consecutive 'R' waves.

   Significance: 'R-R' interval signifies duration of one cardiac cycle. Normal duration of 'R-R' interval is 0.8 s.

Q. 6. Write a short note on heart sounds.

(TNMGR, Oct. 1999)

Ans. Heart sounds are the sounds produced by mechanical activities of heart during each cardiac cycle. Heart sounds are produced by:
1. Flow of blood through cardiac chambers.
2. Contraction of cardiac muscle.
3. Closure of valves of the heart.

Importance of heart sounds: Alteration in heart sounds indicates cardiac diseases involving valves of heart.

I. First heart sound: First heart sound is produced during isometric contraction period and earlier part of ejection period.

Causes:
1. **Valvular factor:** Synchronous closure of atrioventricular valves.
2. **Vascular factor:** Rush of blood from ventricles into aorta and pulmonary artery during ejection period.
3. **Muscular factor:** Myocardial tension and contraction of ventricular muscle.
4. **Atrial factor:** Vibrations produced by atrial systole.

Characteristics: First heart sound is a long, soft and low-pitched sound. It resembles the spoken word '**LUBB**'. The duration of this sound is 0.10–0.17 s.

Applied Physiology

1. **Reduplication of first heart sound:** Splitting of the first heart sound when atrioventricular valves do not close simultaneously (*asynchronous closure*). It occurs in stenosis of atrioventricular valves and atrial septal defect.
2. **Soft first heart sound:** A soft first heart sound is heard in low blood pressure, severe heart failure, myocardial infarction and myxedema.
3. **Loud or accentuated first heart sound:** Mitral stenosis, Wolff-Parkinson-White syndrome and acute rheumatic fever.
4. **Cannon sound:** It is the loud first heart sound that is heard intermittently. It is heard in ventricular tachycardia and complete atrioventricular block.
5. **First heart sound and ECG:** First heart sound coincides with peak of 'R' wave in ECG.

II. Second heart sound: Second heart sound is produced at the end of protodiastolic period due to sudden and synchronous closure of semilunar valves.

Characteristics: Second heart sound is a short, sharp and high-pitched sound. It resembles the spoken word '**DUBB**' (or DUP). Duration of second heart sound is 0.10–0.14 s.

Applied Clinical Physiology

1. **Reduplication of second heart sound:** Due to asynchronous closure of semilunar valves. It occurs during deep inspiration, pulmonary stenosis, right bundle branch block and right ventricular hypertrophy.

2. **Loud or accentuated second heart sound:** During systemic hypertension and coarctation (narrowing) of aorta, pulmonary hypertension.

3. **Soft second heart sound:** In heart failure.

4. **Second heart sound and ECG:** Second heart sound coincides with the 'T' wave in ECG.

III. Third heart sound: Third heart sound is a low-pitched sound that is produced during rapid filling period of cardiac cycle. It is also called **ventricular gallop** or **protodiastolic gallop**, as it is produced during earlier part of diastole. it can be heard only by using microphone.

Causes: Third heart sound is produced by the rushing of blood into ventricles and vibrations set up in the ventricular wall during rapid filling phase.

Characteristics: Third heart sound is a short and low-pitched sound. Duration of this sound is 0.07–0.10 s.

Applied Clinical Physiology

1. **Conditions when third heart sound becomes audible by stethoscope:** In children and athletes, aortic regurgitation, cardiac failure and cardiomyopathy with dilated ventricles. When third heart sound is heard by stethoscope, the condition is called triple heart sound.

2. **Third heart sound and ECG:** Third heart sound appears between 'T' and 'P' waves of ECG.

IV. Fourth heart sound: Normally, the fourth heart sound is an inaudible sound. It becomes audible only in pathological conditions. It is studied only by graphical recording, i.e. by phonocardiography. This sound is produced during atrial systole (late diastole) and it is considered as the physiologic atrial sound. It is also called **atrial gallop** or **presystolic gallop**.

Causes: Fourth heart sound is produced by contraction of atrial musculature and vibrations are set up in atrial musculature, flaps of the atrioventricular valves during systole.

Characteristics: Fourth heart sound is a short and low-pitched sound. Duration of this sound is 0.02–0.04 s.

Applied Clinical Physiology

1. **Conditions when fourth heart sound becomes audible:** Ventricular hypertrophy, long standing hypertension and aortic stenosis. When fourth heart sound is heard by stethoscope, the condition is called triple heart sound.

2. **Fourth heart sound and ECG:** Fourth heart sound coincides with the interval between the end of 'P' wave and the onset of 'Q' wave

V. Cardiac murmur/abnormal heart sound/cardiac bruit: Cardiac murmur is the abnormal heart sound heard by stethoscope along with normal heart sounds, because of the change in the pattern of blood flow.

Q. 7. Write a note on hypertension.
(RGUHS, Nov. 2011; NTR Uni., Oct. 2012)

Ans. Hypertension is defined as persistent high blood pressure. Clinically, when the systolic pressure remains elevated above 150 mm Hg and diastolic pressure remains elevated above 90 mm Hg. it is considered as hypertension. If there is increase only in systolic pressure, it is called **systolic hypertension**.

Pathophysiology: Cardiac output (Heart rate × Stroke volume) × Peripheral resistance = Blood pressure

Types of Hypertension: Hypertension is divided into two types:

1. **Primary or essential hypertension (90%):** Primary hypertension is elevated blood pressure in absence of any underlying disease. It is of two types: i. Benign hypertension, ii. Malignant hypertension.

   Risk factors: Ethnic: Genetic, age, gender, diabetes, overweight, smoking, alcohol, salt intake.

2. **Secondary hypertension (10%):** Secondary hypertension is high blood pressure due to underlying disorders. The different forms of secondary hypertension are:
   i. Cardiovascular hypertension.
   ii. Endocrine hypertension.
   iii. Renal hypertension.
   iv. Neurogenic hypertension.
   v. Hypertension during pregnancy.

Some pregnant women develop hypertension because of **toxemia of pregnancy**. Arterial blood pressure is elevated by the low glomerular filtration rate (GFR) and retention of sodium and water. It may be because of some autoimmune processes during pregnancy or release of some vasoconstrictor agents from placenta or due to the excessive secretion of hormones causing rise in blood pressure. Hypertension is associated with convulsions in eclampsia.

Q. 8. Define the arterial blood pressure and give its normal values. Describe the mechanism which regulates the blood pressure. Add a note on its importance in dentistry.

(TNMGR, April 2000; AHSUC, May 2018)

Q. Write a note on regulation of blood pressure.

(BFUHS, Oct. 2010)

Ans. Arterial blood pressure is defined as the lateral pressure exerted by the column of blood on wall of arteries. Generally, the term 'blood pressure' refers to arterial blood pressure. Arterial blood pressure is expressed in four different terms:

1. **Systolic blood pressure**: Maximum pressure exerted in arteries during systole of heart. Normal systolic pressure: 120 mm Hg (110–140 mm Hg).
2. **Diastolic blood pressure**: Minimum pressure exerted in the arteries during diastole of heart. Normal diastolic pressure: 80 mm Hg (60–80 mm Hg).
3. **Pulse pressure**: Difference between systolic pressure and diastolic pressure. Normal pulse pressure: 40 mm Hg (120 – 80 = 40).
4. **Mean arterial blood pressure**: Average pressure existing in the arteries. It is diastolic pressure plus one-third of pulse pressure.

Determinants of arterial blood pressure:

I. Central factors:

1. **Cardiac output:** Systolic pressure is directly proportional to cardiac output.
2. **Heart rate:** Marked alteration in heart rate affects blood pressure by altering cardiac output.

II. Peripheral factors:

1. **Peripheral resistance:** Diastolic pressure is directly proportional to peripheral resistance.
2. **Blood volume:** Blood pressure is directly proportional to blood volume.
3. **Venous return:** Blood pressure is directly proportional to venous return.
4. **Elasticity of blood vessels:** Blood pressure is inversely proportional to elasticity of blood vessels.
5. **Velocity of blood flow:** Blood pressure is directly proportional to the velocity of blood flow.
6. **Diameter of blood vessels:** Blood pressure is inversely proportional to diameter of blood vessel.
7. **Viscosity of blood:** Blood pressure is directly proportional to viscosity of blood.

Regulation of arterial blood pressure

I. **Nervous mechanism for regulation of blood pressure:** Short-term regulation. Nervous regulation is rapid among all the mechanisms involved in regulation of arterial blood pressure. It operates through **vasomotor system,** by causing vasoconstriction or vasodilatation.

1. **Baroreceptor mechanism:** Baroreceptors (**pressoreceptors**) are situated in the carotid sinus and wall of the aorta and give response to change in blood pressure. *Carotid baroreceptors* are supplied by *Hering n.* (br. of glossopharyngeal n.). *Aortic baroreceptors* are supplied by *aortic n.* (br. of vagus n.). Nerve fibers from baroreceptors reach nucleus of tractus solitarius (NTS), situated adjacent to vasomotor center in medulla oblongata.

   • **When blood pressure increases:** Baroreceptors are activated and send stimulatory impulses to NTS through glossopharyngeal and vagus nerves. It inhibits the vasoconstrictor area and excites vasodilator area. Inhibition of vasoconstrictor area reduces vasomotor tone, causes vasodilatation, resulting in decreased peripheral resistance. Simultaneous excitation of vasodilator center increases vagal tone. This decreases rate and force of contraction of heart, leading to reduction in cardiac output.

   • **When blood pressure decreases:** Fall in blood pressure decreases the pressure in carotid sinus, causing inactivation of baroreceptors. Now, there is no inhibition of vasoconstrictor center or excitation of vasodilator center. Therefore, the blood pressure rises. Since baroreceptor mechanism acts against the rise in arterial blood pressure, it is called **pressure buffer mechanism.**

2. **Chemoreceptor mechanism:** Chemoreceptors are receptors giving response to change in chemical constituents of blood. *Peripheral chemoreceptors* are situated in carotid body and aortic body and influence the vasomotor center. Chemoreceptors in carotid body are supplied by Hering nerve and in aortic body are supplied by aortic nerve.

Function: Whenever blood pressure decreases, blood flow to chemoreceptors decreases, resulting in decreased O_2 and excess of CO_2 and H^+. These factors excite the chemoreceptors, which send impulses to stimulate vasoconstrictor center. Blood pressure rises and blood flow increases.

Sino-aortic mechanism: Mechanism of action of baroreceptors and chemoreceptors in carotid and aortic region constitute sino-aortic mechanism. Nerves supplying the baroreceptors and chemoreceptors are called **buffer nerves** because these nerves regulate heart rate, blood pressure and respiration.

3. **Higher Centers:** Vasomotor center is also controlled by impulses from two higher centers in the brain.

   i. Cerebral cortex: During emotional disturbances, area 13 in cerebral cortex sends impulses to vasomotor center. Vasomotor center is activated, vasomotor tone is increased and the pressure rises.

   ii. Hypothalamus: Stimulation of posterior and lateral nuclei of hypothalamus causes vasoconstriction and increase in blood pressure. Stimulation of preoptic area causes vasodilatation and decrease in blood pressure.

4. **Respiratory Centers:** During the beginning of expiration, arterial blood pressure increases slightly, i.e. by 4–6 mm Hg. It decreases during later part of expiration and during inspiration.

II. **Renal mechanism for regulation of blood pressure—long-term regulation**

Kidneys regulate arterial blood pressure by two ways:

1. **By regulation of extracellular fluid volume:** When blood pressure increases, kidneys excrete large amounts of water and salt, by means of pressure diuresis and pressure natriuresis. This leads to decrease in ECF volume and blood volume.

2. **Through renin-angiotensin mechanism:** When blood pressure and ECF volume decrease, renin secretion from kidneys is increased. It converts angiotensinogen into angiotensin I. This is converted into angiotensin II by ACE (angiotensin converting enzyme). Angiotensin II causes constriction of arterioles in the body, so that the peripheral resistance is increased and blood pressure rises. It causes constriction of afferent arterioles in kidneys, so that glomerular filtration reduces. This results in retention of water and salts, increases ECF volume to normal level. Simultaneously, angiotensin II stimulates adrenal cortex to secrete aldosterone. This hormone increases reabsorption of sodium from renal tubules. Sodium reabsorption is followed by water reabsorption, resulting in increased ECF volume and blood volume.

III. **Hormonal mechanism for regulation of blood pressure:**

Hormones which increase blood pressure:
1. Adrenaline. 2. Noradrenalin. 3. Thyroxine. 4. Aldosterone. 5. Vasopressin. 6. Angiotensin II, III and IV. 7. Serotonin.

Hormones which decrease blood pressure:
1. Vasoactive intestinal polypeptide. 2. Bradykinin. 3. Prostaglandins. 4. Histamine. 5. Acetylcholine. 6. Atrial natriuretic peptide. 7. Brain natriuretic peptide. 8. C-type natriuretic peptide.

IV. **Local mechanism for regulation of blood pressure**

1. **Local vasoconstrictors:** Endothelium-derived constricting factors (EDCF), e.g. endothelins (ET)—ET1, ET2 and ET3.

2. **Local vasodilators:** Local vasodilators are of two types:

   1. Vasodilators of metabolic origin: Carbon dioxide, lactate, hydrogen ions and adenosine.

   2. Vasodilators of endothelial origin: Nitric oxide.

Applied Clinical Physiology

Physiological variation in blood pressure

(NTR Uni., May 2019)

1. **Age:** ↑ with age.
2. **Gender:** In females its low.
3. **Body built:** More in obese.
4. **Diurnal variation:** In early morning, it is low and maximum at noon.
5. **After meals:** It increases.
6. **During sleep:** Generally decreases.
7. **Emotional conditions:** It increases.
8. **After exercise:** Systolic pressure increases, diastolic is not affected.

Pathological increase in: Renal disease, pheochromcytoma, Sympathetic drugs; decrease by relaxants and diuretics.

Q. 9. Write a note on central venous pressure.

(NTR Uni., May 2019)

Ans. Venous pressure is the pressure exerted by the contained blood in the veins. The pressure in vena cava and right atrium is called central venous pressure (CVP). The pressure in peripheral veins is called peripheral venous pressure.

CVP is commonly used as an assessment of hemodynamic status especially in ICU. CVP can be measured using a central venous catheter advanced via IJV and placed in superior vena cava near the right atrium. Normal CVP: 8–12 mm Hg.

Variations of CVP:

Physiological variations: CVP increases in:
1. Changing from standing to supine position.
2. Tilting the body.
3. Forced expiration (Valsalva maneuver).

4. Contraction of abdominal and limb muscles.

5. Effect of gravity during prolonged travelling or standing.

6. Excitement.

Pathological variations: CVP increases in:

1. Low cardiac output.
2. Congestive heart failure.
3. Venous obstruction.
4. Failure of valves in veins.
5. Paralysis of muscles.
6. Immobilization of parts of body.
7. Renal failure.

CVP decreases in: 1. Severe hemorrhage, 2. Surgical shock.

Applied Clinical Physiology

1. Elevated CVP will present clinically as a pulsation of IJV when patient is inclined at 45°.
2. Elevated CVP is indicative of myocardial contractile dysfunction and/or fluid retention.
3. Low CVP is indicative of volume depletion or decreased venous tone.
4. The CVP is consistently used universally to guide fluid resuscitation. The Surviving Sepsis guidelines suggest targeting a CVP between 8 and 12 mmHg during fluid resuscitation.
5. CVP is inversely correlated with tricuspid annular plane systolic excursion (TAPSE) in mechanically ventilated critically ill patients (left ventricular ejection fraction < 55%), thus TAPSE may be used as a surrogate marker of CVP

Q. 10. Write a short note on cyanosis.

(HP Uni., May 2012)

Ans. Cyanosis is defined as the diffused bluish coloration of skin and mucus membrane. It is due to the presence of large amount of reduced hemoglobin in the blood. Quantity of reduced hemoglobin should be at least 5 to 7 g/dL in the blood to cause cyanosis.

Types:

1. **Central cyanosis:** Due to reduced arterial oxygen saturation.

   Features: Generalized cyanosis, extremities are warm to touch, tongue is the best site to check for cyanosis, clubbing

2. **Peripheral cyanosis:** Excessive reduction of oxy-hemoglobin in the capillaries when the flow of blood is slowed.

   Features: Cyanosed extremities are cold to touch, tongue is unaffected.

Etiology: "COLD PALMS"

Peripheral cyanosis: Cold, Obstruction, LVF and Shock, Decreased cardiac output

Central cyanosis: Polycythemia, Altitude, Lung disease, Metsulhemoglobinemia, Shunt.

Management: Cyanosis is a symptom of a disease process. The goal is to treat the underlying condition causing cyanosis.

- Surgical intervention is required for the correction of congenital heart disease causing cyanosis. Oxygen support can be provided to resolve the hypoxia.
- For methemoglobinemia-induced cyanosis, the standard treatment is with methylene blue.
- Exposure to gold or silver salts can also produce cyanosis. The best therapy is to remove the offending agents.

4. RESPIRATORY SYSTEM

Q. 1. Write about mechanism of respiration.

(Sumandeep Uni., June 2017)

Ans. Respiration occurs in two phases, namely inspiration and expiration. During normal quiet breathing, inspiration is active process and expiration is **passive process**.

Muscles of respiration

A. **Inspiratory muscles:** *Primary inspiratory muscles* are diaphragm and external intercostal muscles. *Accessory inspiratory muscles* are sternocleidomastoid, scalene, anterior serrati, elevators of scapulae and pectorals.

B. **Expiratory muscles:** *Primary expiratory muscles* are internal intercostals muscles. *Accessory expiratory muscles* are abdominal muscles.

Inspiration: Diaphragm muscle contracts, increasing thoracic cavity size in the superior-inferior dimension. External intercostal muscles contract, expanding lateral and anterior-posterior dimension. Increased in volume, and decreased in pulmonary pressure, results in air rushing into lungs to fill alveoli. During deep/forced inspirations the accessory muscles are used for more volume expansion of thorax.

Expiration: During quiet expiration (exhalation), the simple elasticity of lungs decreases volume and increases pulmonary pressure, resulting in movement of air out of the lungs. During forced expiration, the contraction of abdominal wall muscles (i.e. obliques and transversus abdominus) further decreases the volume beyond relaxed point and increases pulmonary pressure, so more air moves out.

1. **Movements of thoracic cage:** There is enlargement of thoracic cage by the movements of following structures:
   - **Thoracic lid:** Formed by manubrium sterni and first pair of ribs. It is also called thoracic operculum. Movement of thoracic lid increases the anteroposterior diameter of thoracic cage.
   - **Upper costal series:** Formed by 2nd to 6th pair of ribs. Movement of upper costal series increases anteroposterior and transverse diameter of the thoracic cage. Movement of upper costal series is of two types: i. pump handle movement, ii. bucket handle movement.
   - **Lower costal series:** Formed by 7th to 10th pair of ribs. Movement of lower costal series increases **transverse diameter** of thoracic cage by bucket handle movement.
   - **Diaphragm:** Movement of diaphragm increases vertical diameter of thoracic cage.

2. **Movements of lungs:** Due to the enlargement of thoracic cage, the negative pressure is increased in the thoracic cavity. It causes expansion of lungs. During expiration, thoracic cavity decreases in size and pressure to the preinspiratory position. It compresses the lung tissues so that, the air is expelled out of lungs.

Q. 2. Write a note on respiratory centers.
(TNMGR, Oct. 1999; Feb. 2005)

Q. Write a note on neural control of respiration.
(TNMGR, April 1997; Sumandeep Uni., June 2017)

Ans. Respiratory centers are group of neurons, which control rate, rhythm and force of respiration. These centers are bilaterally situated in reticular formation of the brainstem. The respiratory centers are classified into two groups.

A. **Medullary centers** (Fig. 4.2a)

1. **Dorsal respiratory group of neurons:** They are diffusely situated in **NTS** which is present in upper part of medulla oblongata. All the neurons of this group are **inspiratory neurons** and generate **inspiratory ramp** by virtue of their **autorhythmic property.**
   Function: Dorsal group of neurons are responsible for basic rhythm of respiration.

2. **Ventral respiratory group of neurons:** Ventral respiratory group of neurons are present in **nucleus ambiguous** and **nucleus retroambiguous**, situated anterior and lateral to **NTS**. Ventral respiratory group has both **inspiratory neurons** (centre) and **expiratory neurons** (caudal and rostral area).

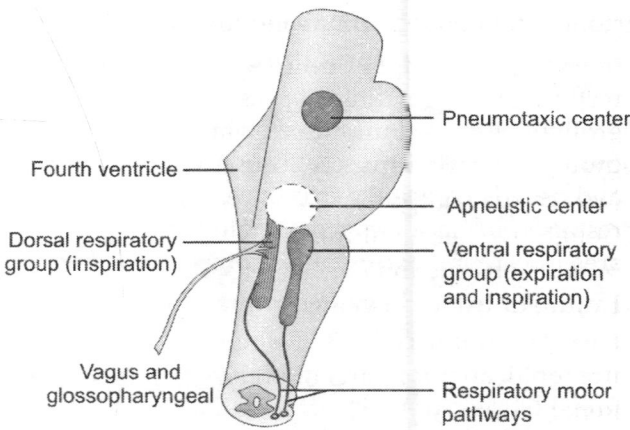

Fig. 4.2a: Location of respiratory centers in brain

Function: Ventral group neurons are inactive during quiet breathing and become active during forced breathing.

B. **Pontine centers**

1. **Apneustic center:** Apneustic center is situated in reticular formation of lower pons.
   Function: Apneustic center increases depth of inspiration by acting directly on dorsal group neurons.
   Apneusis: An abnormal pattern of respiration, characterized by prolonged inspiration followed by short, inefficient expiration.

2. **Pneumotaxic center:** Pneumotaxic center is situated in dorsolateral part of **reticular formation** in **upper pons**. It is formed by neurons of medial **parabrachial** and **subparabrachial nuclei** (**ventral parabrachial** or **Kölliker-Fuse nucleus**).
   Function: To control the medullary respiratory centers, particularly the dorsal group neurons.

Connections of respiratory centers

- **Efferent pathway:** Nerve fibers from respiratory centers leave the brainstem and descend in anterior part of lateral columns of spinal cord. These nerve fibers terminate on motor neurons in the anterior horn cells of cervical and thoracic segments of spinal cord. From motor neurons of spinal cord, two sets of nerve fibers arise:
  1. Phrenic nerve fibers (C3 to C5), which supply the diaphragm.
  2. Intercostal nerve fibers (T1 to T11), which supply the external intercostal muscles.
     Vagus nerve also contains some efferent fibers from the respiratory centers.

- **Afferent pathway:** Respiratory centers receive afferent impulses from:
  1. Peripheral chemoreceptors and baroreceptors via branches of glossopharyngeal and vagus nerve.
  2. Stretch receptors of lungs via vagus nerve.

Factors affecting respiratory centers: (Fig. 4.2b)

1. **Impulses from higher centers:** Higher centers alter respiration by sending impulses directly to dorsal group of neurons. Impulses from anterior cingulate gyrus, genu of corpus callosum, olfactory tubercle and posterior orbital gyrus of cerebral cortex inhibit respiration. Impulses from motor area and sylvian area of cerebral cortex cause **forced breathing**.

2. **Impulses from stretch receptors of lungs:**

   Hering-Breuer reflex: Hering-Breuer reflex is a **protective reflex** that restricts inspiration and prevents overstretching of lung tissues. It is initiated by the stimulation of stretch receptors situated on the wall of the bronchi and bronchioles. Expansion of lungs during inspiration stimulates the stretch receptors and the impulses generated reaches the dorsal group neurons via vagal afferent fibers and inhibits them. Thus, the overstretching of lung tissues is prevented. It operates, only when the tidal volume increases beyond 1,000 ml. This reflex is called **Hering-Breuer inflation reflex**. Reverse of this reflex is called **Hering-Breuer deflation reflex** and it takes place during expiration. During expiration, as the stretching of lungs is absent, deflation occurs.

3. **Impulses from 'J' Receptors of Lungs:** 'J' receptors are **juxtacapillary receptors** which are present on the wall of the alveoli and have close contact with the pulmonary capillaries. These receptors are the sensory nerve endings of vagus and are non-myelinated C type fibers.

   Conditions when 'J' receptors are stimulated i. Pulmonary congestion ii. Pulmonary edema iii. Pneumonia iv. Over inflation of lungs v. Micro-embolism in pulmonary capillaries vi. Stimulation by exogenous and endogenous chemical substances.

   Effect of stimulation of 'J' receptors: Stimulation of 'J' receptors produces a reflex response, which is characterized by **apnea**. Apnea is followed by hyper-ventilation, bradycardia, hypotension and weakness of skeletal muscles.

4. **Impulses from irritant receptors of lungs:** Irritant receptors are stimulated by irritant chemical agents such as ammonia and sulfur dioxide. These receptors send afferent impulses to respiratory centers via vagal nerve fibers. Stimulation of irritant receptors produces **reflex hyperventilation** along with **bronchospasm**.

5. **Impulses from baroreceptors:** Whenever arterial blood pressure increases, baroreceptors are activated and send inhibitory impulses to vasomotor center in medulla oblongata, causing decrease in blood pressure and inhibition of respiration.

6. **Impulses from chemoreceptors:** Chemoreceptors play an important role in the chemical regulation of respiration **(Refer to Q. 3)**.

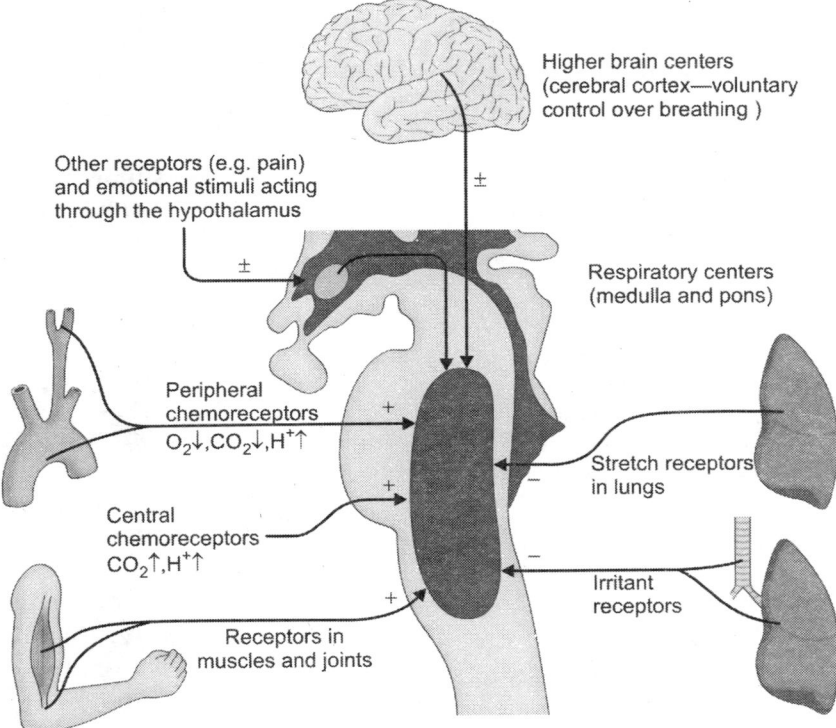

Fig. 4.2b: Factor affecting respiratory centers

7. **Impulses from proprioceptors:** Proprioceptors are stimulated during muscular exercise and send impulses to brain, particularly cerebral cortex, through somatic afferent nerves. Cerebral cortex in turn causes hyperventilation by sending impulses to medullary respiratory centers.

8. **Impulses from thermoreceptors:** Thermoreceptors are of two types, namely receptors for cold and receptors for warmth. When body is exposed to cold or when cold water is applied over the body, cold receptors are stimulated and send impulses to cerebral cortex via somatic afferent nerves. Cerebral cortex in turn, stimulates the respiratory centers and causes hyperventilation.

9. **Impulses from pain receptors:** Whenever pain receptors are stimulated, the impulses are sent to cerebral cortex via somatic afferent nerves. Cerebral cortex in turn, stimulates the respiratory centers and causes hyperventilation.

Applied Clinical Physiology

1. **Ondine's curse:** In conditions like bulbar poliomyelitis, tumors of brain stem, etc. automatic control is lost and voluntary control is present. Death is due to exhaustion.

2. **Sudden infant death syndrome (SIDS):** A type of central sleep apnea due to failure of respiratory centres to produe neural impulses.

3. **Cheyne-Stokes breathing:** Apnea followed by hyperventilation, seen in voluntary hyperventilation, uremia, cardiac failure, brain damage.

4. **Biot's breathing:** Respiration characterized by alternate eupnoea (normal breathing) and apnea, seen in meningitis and diseases affecting medulla.

5. **Kussumaul's breathing:** Rapid and deep breathing without uneasiness, seen in metabolic acidosis.

Q. 3. Write a short note on chemical control of respiration.

(TNMGR, Sept. 2008; Sumandeep Uni., June 2017)

Ans. Chemical mechanism of regulation of respiration is operated through the chemoreceptors. Chemoreceptors are the sensory nerve endings, which give response to changes in chemical constituents of blood. Changes in chemical constituents of blood which stimulate chemoreceptors:

1. Hypoxia (decreased pO_2)
2. Hypercapnea (increased pCO_2)
3. Increased hydrogen ion concentration.

Types of chemoreceptors:

1. **Central/Medullary chemoreceptors:** Central chemoreceptors are situated in deeper part of medulla oblongata. This area is known as **chemosensitive area** and the neurons are called **chemoreceptors**. Central chemoreceptors are connected with respiratory centers, particularly the dorsal respiratory group of neurons through synapses. As pCO_2 increases in blood, it can easily cross the blood–brain barrier and blood cerebrospinal fluid (CSF) barrier and enter the interstitial fluid of brain or CSF. There, the CO_2 combines with water to form carbonic acid. Since carbonic acid is unstable, it immediately dissociates into hydrogen ion and bicarbonate ion. Hydrogen ions stimulate the central chemoreceptors. From chemoreceptors, the excitatory impulses are sent to dorsal respiratory group of neurons, resulting in increased ventilation.

2. **Peripheral chemoreceptors** (Fig. 4.3): Peripheral chemoreceptors are the chemoreceptors present in carotid and aortic region. Hypoxia is the most potent stimulant for peripheral chemoreceptors. Hypoxia

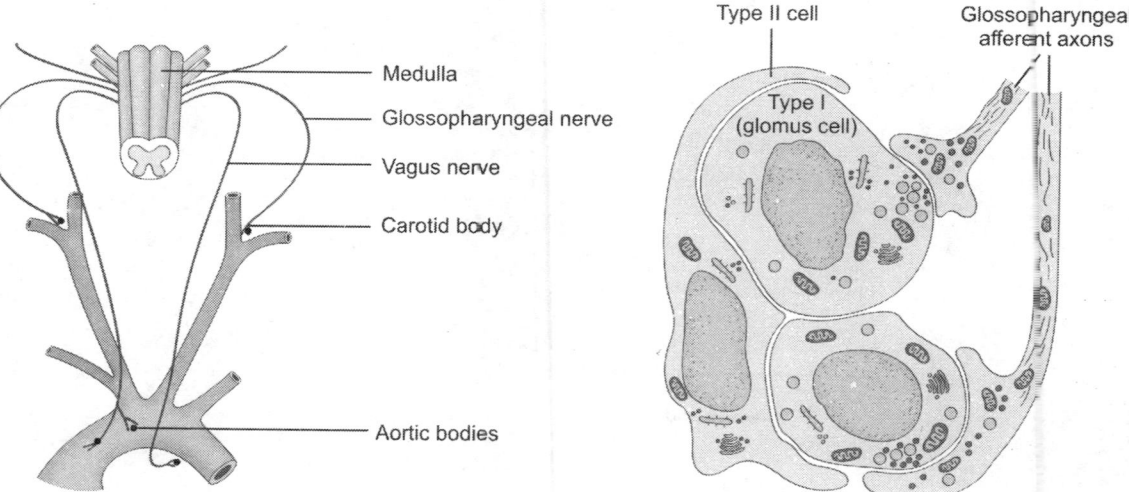

Fig. 4.3: Position of carotid and aortic bodies. (R) Organization of carotid body

causes closure of oxygen sensitive potassium channels and prevents potassium efflux. This leads to depolarization of **glomus cells** (receptor potential) and generation of action potentials in nerve ending. These impulses pass through *aortic* and *Hering nerves* and excite the dorsal group of neurons.

Q. 4. Write a short note on hypoxia.
(Sumandeep Uni., June 2017)

Ans. Hypoxia is defined as reduced availability of oxygen to the tissues.

Classification

1. **Hypoxic hypoxia/arterial hypoxia:** Decreased pO_2 in arterial blood.
   Causes
   i. Low oxygen tension in inspired air-high altitude.
   ii. Respiratory disorders—asthma, emphysema, pneumothorax.
   iii. Cardiac disorders—congestive heart failure.
2. **Anemic hypoxia:** pO_2 in arterial blood is normal but the amount of hemoglobin available to carry O_2 is reduced.
   Causes
   i. Decreased number of RBCs.
   ii. Decreased hemoglobin content in the blood.
   iii. Formation of altered hemoglobin.
   iv. Combination of hemoglobin with gases other than oxygen and carbon dioxide.
3. **Stagnant/ischemic/hypokinetic hypoxia:** Due to low blood flow to tissue; pO_2 and Hb conc. are normal.
   Causes: Congestive cardiac failure, hemorrhage, surgical shock, thrombosis.
4. **Histotoxic hypoxia:** Due to the inability of tissues to utilize oxygen, e.g. cyanide or sulfide poisoning, vitamin B deficiency.

Effects of hypoxia

Immediate effects: Induces secretion of **erythropoietin** from kidney. Initially, increase in rate and force of contraction of heart, cardiac output and blood pressure. Later, there is reduction in the rate and force of contraction of heart. Cardiac output and blood pressure are also decreased. Initially, respiratory rate increases due to chemoreceptor reflex. Later, the respiration tends to be **shallow and periodic**. Finally, the rate and force of breathing are reduced to a great extent due to the failure of respiratory centers. Hypoxia is associated with loss of appetite, nausea and vomiting. Mouth becomes dry and there is a feeling of thirst. **Alkaline urine** is excreted. Individual is depressed, apathetic with general loss of self control. The person becomes talkative, quarrelsome, ill-tempered and rude, loss of consciousness, **coma,** and **leads to death.**

Delayed effects of hypoxia: Person becomes highly irritable and develops the symptoms of mountain sickness, such as nausea, vomiting, depression, weakness and fatigue.

Treatment for hypoxia: Oxygen therapy.

Applied Clinical Physiology

Hyperoxia or oxygen toxicity (*NTR Uni., May 2019*): Extended exposure to above-normal oxygen partial pressures, or shorter exposures to very high partial pressures, can cause oxidative damage to cell membranes leading to the collapse of the alveoli in the lungs. Symptoms include pleuritic chest pain, substernal heaviness, coughing, and dyspnea secondary to tracheobronchitis and absorptive atelectasis which can lead to pulmonary edema. Types:

1. **Acute oxygen toxicity:** CNS toxicity (**Bert effect**): twitching of perioral and small muscles of the hand, facial pallor, 'cogwheel' breathing (due to diaphragmatic twitching), vertigo and nausea, altered behaviour, clumsiness, and finally convulsions result. CNS toxicity is hastened by factors such as raised pCO_2, stress, fatigue and cold.
2. **Chronic oxygen toxicity:** Tracheobronchitis, ARDS and pulmonary interstitial fibrosis.

Prevention and monitoring: The management is purely symptomatic. The abrupt stoppage of oxygen at the onset of toxicity may aggravate the symptoms, the 'oxygen off effect'.

Q. 5. Discuss in detail the causes, prevention and management of acute respiratory distress syndrome.
(TNMGR, April 2012)

Ans. Acute respiratory distress syndrome (ARDS) is clinical syndrome categorized by progressive hypoxemia, dyspnea, and increased work of breathing that is unresponsive to standard respiratory therapy. It is an acute, diffuse pulmonary inflammatory response to either direct or indirect blood borne insults that originate from extrapulmonary pathology.

The **criteria** defining ARDS are:
   i. Hypoxaemia.
   ii. Chest radiograph showing diffuse bilateral infiltrates.
   iii. Absence of a raised left atrial pressure.
   iv. Impaired lung compliance.

Causes:

A. **Inhalational (direct):** Aspiration of gastric contents, toxic gases, pneumonia, blunt chest trauma.
B. **Blood-borne (indirect):** Sepsis, necrotic tissue, multiple trauma, severe burns, major blood

transfusion reaction, anaphylaxis, fat embolism, carcinomatosis.

Pathophysiology: An aggressive inflammatory reaction is triggered by local/systemic events by releasing many mediators into pulmonary and systemic circulations. This results in endothelial damage, causing pulmonary edema and disturbances of the pulmonary and systemic microcirculations. The end result respiratory failure, decreased systemic oxygenation, and ultimately death.

Clinical Features: ARDS developed rapidly, 12–18 hours from insulting injury up to 5 days.

- Restlessness, agitation and hypoxemia.
- Inflammatory pulmonary changes, reduced lung compliance.
- Small tidal volume, increased respiratory rate and increased work of breathing.
- If the patients still able to tolerate → respiratory alkalosis.
- Worsening can occur in a few hours and may need intubation and mechanical ventilation due to respiratory acidosis.

Prevention: It can be accomplished by preventing the infections and injuries that cause it. Even if trauma or infection cannot be prevented, early aggressive treatment may avoid ARDS.

Management
1. **Corticosteroids:** Methylprednisolone (1 mg/kg/day).
2. **Neuromuscular blocking agents:** Cisatracurium (Bolus: 0.1–0.2 mg/kg; continuous: 0.5–10 μg/kg/minute).
3. **Inhaled vasodilators:** Nitric oxide (5–20 ppm).
4. **Exogenous surfactant replacement:** Beractant (100 mg/kg).
5. **β_2-adrenergic agonists:** Salbutamol (15 μg/kg/hour).
6. **Anti-inflammatory agents:** Ketokonazole (200–400 mg).
7. **Antioxidants:** N-acetyl-cysteine (1–10 ml of 20% every 2–6 h).

Q. 6. Write a short note on artificial respiration.
(TNMGR, April 1995; March 2007)

Ans. Artificial respiration is required whenever there is an arrest of breathing, without cardiac failure. Arrest of breathing occurs in the following conditions: Accidents, drowning, gas poisoning, electric shock, anesthesia.

Methods of artificial respiration

A. **Manual methods:** Manual methods are of two types:
1. **Mouth-to-mouth method:** The subject is kept in supine position and the resuscitator (person who give resuscitation) kneels at the side of the subject. By keeping the thumb on subject's mouth, the lower jaw is pulled downwards. Nostrils of the subject are closed with thumb and index finger of the other hand. Resuscitator then takes a deep breath and exhales into the subject's mouth forcefully. Now, a passive expiration occurs in the subject due to elastic recoil of the lungs. This procedure is repeated at a rate of 12–14 times a minute, till normal respiration is restored. Mouth-to-mouth method is the most effective manual method. Only disadvantage is that the close contact between the mouths of resuscitator and subject may not be acceptable for various reasons.

2. **Holger Nielsen method or back pressure arm lift method:** Subject is placed in prone position with head turned to one side. Hands are placed under the cheeks with flexion at elbow joint and abduction of arms at the shoulders. Resuscitator kneels beside the head of the subject. By placing the palm of the hands over the back of the subject, the resuscitator bends forward with straight arms (without flexion at elbow) and applies pressure on the back of the subject. Weight of the resuscitator and pressure on back of the subject compresses his chest and expels air from the lungs. Later, the resuscitator leans back. At the same time, he draws the subject's arm forward by holding it just above elbow. The movements are repeated at the rate of 12 per minute, till the normal respiration is restored.

3. **Schafer's method (prone pressure method):** Resuscitator kneels near patient's waist and put palm on patient's loin (expiration) and bends forward to apply back pressure (inspiration). In this method, inspiration is passive and expiration is active.

4. **Sylvester method (arm lift chest pressure method):** This is performed in supine position. Resuscitator will kneel near patients head, catches patient's wrist and by bending forward will pull patient's arm up, causing inspiration. Then bending forward, resuscitator will put deep pressure on chest with patient's hands, causing expiration.

B. **Mechanical methods:** Mechanical methods of artificial respiration become necessary when the subject needs artificial respiration for long periods. Mechanical methods are of two types:
1. **Drinker method:** The machine used in this method is called iron lung chamber or tank respirator. By using tank respirator, the patient can survive for a longer time, even up to the period

of one year till the natural respiratory functions are restored.

2. **Ventilation method:** Apparatus used for ventilation is called ventilator and it is mostly used to treat acute respiratory failure. Ventilator is of two types:
   a. Volume ventilator.
   b. Pressure ventilator.

Q. 7. Write a short note on cough reflex.
(TNMGR, Nov. 2001)

Ans. Cough is an expulsive reflex that protects lungs and respiratory passages from foreign bodies.

Causes: Irritant: Smokes, fumes, dusts; Diseases: COPD, tumours, etc.; Infections: Influenza.

Mechanism: Cough begins with deep inspiration followed by forced expiration with closed glottis. This increases the intrapleural pressure above 100 mm Hg. Then, glottis opens suddenly with explosive outflow of air at a high velocity. Velocity of the airflow may reach 960 km/hour. It causes expulsion of irritant substances out of the respiratory tract.

Reflex pathway: Cough receptors are situated in pharynx, trachea, bronchi and bronchioles. Afferent fibers pass via vagus, glossopharyngeal and phrenic nerve. The **center for cough** reflex is NTS in medulla oblongata. **Efferent fibers** arising from NTS pass through vagus, phrenic and spinal motor nerves. These nerve fibers activate the primary and accessory respiratory muscles.

5. ENDOCRINE SYSTEM

Q. 1. Describe briefly the importance of endocrine system. *(Bangalore Uni., Jan. 1992)*

Q. Discuss in detail the endocrinal system of human body. Why is pituitary gland called ring master? Add a note on role of parathyroid gland on oral structures and oral health.
(TNMGR, March 2009; PAHER, May 2014; MPMS Uni., July 2017; HP Uni., April 2019)

Ans. Endocrine system functions by secreting some chemical substances called **hormones**. Chemical messengers are the substances involved in cell signaling. Chemical messengers are classified into four types:

1. **Endocrine messengers/(Classical hormones):** A hormone is defined as a chemical messenger, synthesized by endocrine glands and transported by blood to target organs or tissues, e.g. growth hormone and insulin.

2. **Paracrine messengers:** Chemical messengers which diffuse from the control cells to target cells through interstitial fluid, e.g. prostaglandins (PGs) and histamine.

3. **Autocrine messengers:** Chemical messengers that control the source cells which secrete them, e.g. leukotrienes.

4. **Neurocrine or neural messengers:** Neurotransmitters and neurohormones, e.g. acetylcholine (ACh) and dopamine.

Endocrine glands/ductless glands: Glands which synthesize and release the classical hormones into the blood.

Major endocrine glands of the body *(NTR Uni., June 2015)*:

A. **Pituitary gland:**
   1. Anterior pituitary: Growth hormone (GH), thyroid stimulating hormone (TSH), adrenocorticotropic hormone (ACTH), follicle stimulating hormone (FSH), luteinizing hormone (LH), prolactin.
   2. Posterior pituitary: Antidiuretic hormone (ADH) or vasopressin, oxytocin.

B. **Thyroid gland:** Thyroxine (T4), Triiodothyronine (T3), calcitonin.

C. **Parathyroid gland:** Parathormone (PTH).

D. **Pancreas:** Insulin, glucagon, somatostatin, pancreatic polypeptide.

E. **Adrenal gland:**
   1. Adrenal Cortex:
      i. Mineralocorticoids: Aldosterone, 11-deoxy-coticosterone.
      ii. Glucocorticoids: Cortisol, corticosterone.
      iii. Sex hormones: Androgens, estrogen, progesterone.
   2. Adrenal medulla: Catecholamines, adrenaline (epinephrine), noradrenalin (norepinephrine), dopamine.

Pituitary gland or hypophysis (Fig. 5.1) is a small endocrine gland with a diameter of 1 cm and weight of 0.5 to 1 g. It is situated in a depression called 'sella turcica', present in sphenoid bone at the base of skull. It is connected with hypothalamus by pituitary stalk or hypophyseal stalk.

Pituitary gland is divided into two divisions:

1. Anterior pituitary or adenohypophysis: **Ectodermal in origin.**

2. Posterior pituitary or neurohypophysis: **Neuroectodermal in origin.**

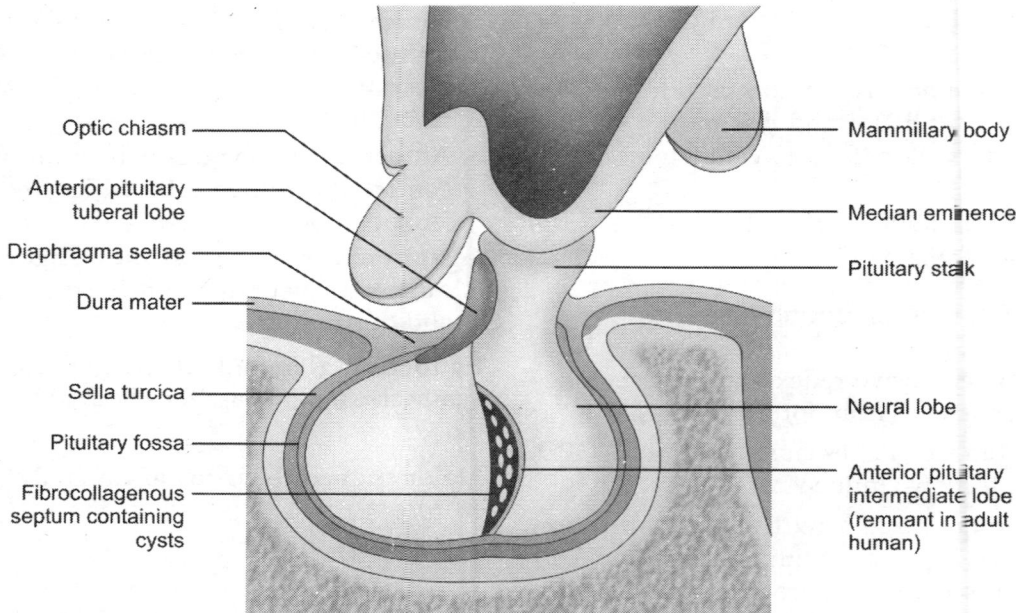

Fig. 5.1: Pituitary gland: Structure and relations

Hormones secreted by anterior pituitary

1. **Growth hormone (GH) or somatotropic hormone (STH):**

   Actions: GH is responsible for the general growth of body. Hypersecretion of GH causes enormous growth of body, leading to **gigantism**. Deficiency of GH in children causes stunted growth, leading to **dwarfism**. It increases size and number of cells by mitotic division. GH causes specific differentiation of certain types of cells like bone cells and muscle cells. GH also acts on metabolism of proteins, lipids and carbohydrates.

2. **Thyroid-stimulating hormone (TSH) or thyro-trophic hormone:** TSH is necessary for growth and secretory activity of thyroid gland.

   I. To increase basal metabolic rate (BMR): Thyroxine increases metabolic activities in most of the body tissues, except brain, retina, spleen, testes and lungs. It increases BMR by increasing oxygen consumption of tissues.

   II. To help in growth of children.

3. **Adrenocorticotropic hormone (ACTH):**

   a. Functions of mineralocorticoids: 90% of mineralocorticoids activity is provided by aldosterone. Aldosterone is very essential for life and it maintains osmolarity and volume of ECF. It is usually called **life-saving hormone** because, its absence causes death within 3 days to 2 weeks. It increases:

   1. Reabsorption of sodium from renal tubules.
   2. Excretion of potassium through renal tubules.
   3. Secretion of hydrogen into renal tubules.

   b. Functions of glucocorticoids: Cortisol or hydrocortisone is more potent and it has 95% of glucocorticoid activity. Cortisol is a **life-protecting hormone** because it helps to withstand stress and trauma in life. Glucocorticoids have metabolic effects on carbohydrates, proteins, fats and water.

4. **Follicle-stimulating hormone (FSH)**

   Actions: In males, FSH acts along with testosterone and accelerates process of spermatogenesis. In females FSH causes secretion of estrogen and promotes conversion of androgens into estrogen.

5. **Luteinizing hormone (LH):**

   Actions: In males, LH stimulates interstitial cells of Leydig in testes. This hormone is essential for the secretion of testosterone from Leydig cells. In females, LH is responsible for ovulation and formation and activation of corpus luteum.

6. **Prolactin:** Prolactin is necessary for the final preparation of mammary glands for production and secretion of milk.

Hormones secreted by posterior pituitary

1. **Antidiuretic hormone (ADH):** Antidiuretic hormone (ADH) is secreted mainly by supraoptic nucleus of hypothalamus and transported to posterior pituitary via nerve fibers of hypothalamo-hypophyseal tract, by means of axonic flow.

   Actions: Retention of water and vasopressor action.

2. **Oxytocin:** Oxytocin causes ejection of milk from the mammary glands. The process by which the milk is ejected from alveoli of mammary glands is called **milk ejection reflex** or **milk letdown reflex**. Oxytocin causes contraction of uterus and helps in the expulsion of fetus.

The action of oxytocin on non-pregnant uterus is to facilitate transport of sperms through female genital tract up to the fallopian tube, by producing the uterine contraction. In males, it facilitates release of sperm into urethra by causing contraction of smooth muscle fibers in reproductive tract.

Applied Clinical Physiology: Disorders of Pituitary Gland

A. **Hyperactivity of anterior pituitary:** i. Gigantism, ii. Acromegaly, iii. Acromegalic gigantism, iv. Cushing's disease

B. **Hypoactivity of anterior pituitary:** i. Dwarfism, ii. Acromicria, iii. Simmond's disease

C. **Hyperactivity of posterior pituitary:** Syndrome of Inappropriate hypersecretion of antidiuretic hormone (SIADH)

D. **Hypoactivity of posterior pituitary:** Diabetes insipidus

E. **Hypoactivity of anterior and posterior pituitary:** Dystrophic adiposogenitalis.

Parathyroid gland: Each parathyroid gland is made up of chief cells and oxyphil cells. Chief cells secrete parathormone (PTH). Oxyphil cells are the degenerated chief cells. Parathormone secreted by parathyroid gland is essential for maintenance of blood calcium level within a very narrow critical level.

Actions:
a. **On blood calcium level:** Primary action of PTH is to maintain blood calcium level within the critical range of 9–11 mg/dl. PTH maintains blood calcium level by acting:
1. **On bone:** Parathormone enhances the resorption of calcium from bones.
2. **On kidney:** PTH increases reabsorption of calcium from renal tubules along with magnesium ions and hydrogen ions. PTH also increases the formation of 1, 25-dihydroxy-cholecalciferol (activated form of vitamin D) from 25-hydroxycholecalciferol in kidneys.
3. **On gastrointestinal tract:** PTH increases absorption of calcium ions from the GIT indirectly, by increasing the formation of 1, 25-dihydroxycholecalciferol in kidneys.

b. **On blood phosphate level:** PTH decreases blood level of phosphate by increasing its urinary excretion. It also acts on bone and GIT.
1. **On bone:** PTH increases phosphate absorption from bones.
2. **On kidney:** Phosphaturic action: PTH increases phosphate excretion through urine.
3. **On GIT:** PTH increases absorption of phosphate from GIT through calcitriol.

Disorders of parathyroid glands
1. **Hypoparathyroidism:** Leads to hypocalcaemia, by decreasing resorption of calcium from bones. Hypocalcaemia causes neuromuscular hyperexcitability, resulting in hypocalcemic tetany. Normally, tetany occurs when plasma calcium level falls below 6 mg/dl.
   a. **Hypocalcemic tetany:** Characterized by violent and painful muscular spasm (spasm = involuntary muscular contraction), particularly in feet and hand. Clinical feature are: Hyper-reflexia, convulsions, carpopedal spasm, laryngeal stridor, cardiovascular changes. Other features: Decreased permeability of cell membrane, dry skin with brittle nails, hair loss, grand mal, petit mal or other seizures, signs of mental retardation in children or dementia in adults.

Latent tetany/subclinical tetany is neuromuscular hyperexcitability due to hypocalcaemia that develops before the onset of tetany. It is characterized by general weakness and cramps in feet and hand. It is associated with: *Trousseau sign* (on inflating the sphygmomanometer cuff above systolic blood pressure for several minutes, there is evidence of muscle spasm, flexion of wrist and metacarpophalangeal joints, hyperextension of fingers, and flexion of thumb on the palm), *Chvostek sign* (mechanical stimulation of the facial nerve leading to twitching of ipsilateral facial muscles), *Erb sign or called Erb-Westphal sign* (increased electrical excitability of the peripheral nerves to the galvanic current).

2. **Hyperparathyroidism (HPT) (TNMGR, March 2007; UHSR, June 2017):** It results in hypercalcemia.

Signs and symptoms of hypercalcemia: Depression of the nervous system, sluggishness of reflex activities, reduced ST segment and QT interval in ECG, lack of appetite, constipation, development of bone diseases such as osteitis fibrosa cystic, development of parathyroid poisoning.

Oral manifestations: Osteoporosis, bone pain and joint stiffness, obliteration of pulp chamber by pulp stone, alterations in dental eruption, loosening and drifting of teeth, malocclusions, spacing of teeth, partial loss of lamina dura, periodontal ligament widening, teeth become sensitive to percussion and mastication, floating teeth delay or cessation of dental development, brown tumor (telltale sign of HPT), generalized bone ratification of jaw, soft tissue calcifications, caries, sialolithiasis, mandibular tori.

Radiographic feature: Osteolytic radiolucent lesion, loss of lamina dura, changes in pattern of trabecular bone of jaws, expansion of cortical bone, root resorption, and displacement of roots.

Q. 2. Write a note on growth hormone.
(*TNMGR, April 2001; April 2013; Oct. 2014*)

Ans. Growth hormone/somatotropin is secreted by somatotropes which are the acidophilic cells of anterior pituitary gland. GH is protein in nature, having a single-chain polypeptide with 191 amino acids. Its molecular weight is 21,500. Basal level of GH concentration in blood of normal adult is up to 300 g/dl and in children, it is up to 500 ng/dl.

Transport: Growth hormone is transported in blood by GH-binding proteins (GHBPs).

Half-life and metabolism: 20 minutes. It is degraded in liver and kidney.

Actions of Growth Hormone

1. **On metabolism:** GH increases synthesis of proteins, mobilization of lipids and conservation of carbohydrates.
   a. On protein metabolism: GH accelerates synthesis of proteins by:
      i. Increasing amino acid transport through cell membrane.
      ii. Increasing ribonucleic acid (RNA) translation.
      iii. Stimulating and increasing transcription of DNA to RNA.
      iv. Decreasing catabolism of protein.
   b. **On fat metabolism:** GH mobilizes fats from adipose tissue. So, the concentration of fatty acids increases in the body fluids.
   c. **On carbohydrate metabolism:** GH helps in conservation of glucose by:
      i. Decrease in **peripheral utilization** of glucose.
      ii. Increase in deposition of glycogen in cells.
      iii. Hypersecretion of GH increases blood glucose level.

2. **On bones:** In embryonic stage, GH is responsible for differentiation and development of bone cells. In later stages, GH increases growth of the skeleton. In bones, GH increases:
   i. Synthesis and deposition of proteins by chondrocytes and osteogenic cells.
   ii. Multiplication of **chondrocytes** and **osteogenic cells** by enhancing intestinal calcium absorption.
   iii. Formation of new bones by converting chondrocytes into osteogenic cells.

Hypersecretion of GH before fusion of epiphysis with shaft of bones causes enormous growth of the skeleton (**gigantism**). Hypersecretion of GH after the fusion of epiphysis with the shaft of the bones leads to **acromegaly**. **Mode of action of GH: Somatomedin:** GH stimulates liver to secrete somatomedin. Somatomedins are of two types:
i. Insulin-like growth factor-I (IGF-I), also called somatomedin C: Role in bones and protein metabolism
ii. Insulin-like growth factor-II: Role in the growth of fetus

Regulation of GH Secretion:

GH secretion is stimulated by: Hypoglycemia, fasting, starvation, exercise, stress, trauma, initial stages of sleep.

GH secretion is inhibited by Hyperglycemia Increased free fatty acids in blood, later stages of sleep.

Hypothalamus regulates GH secretion via three hormones:
1. Growth hormone-releasing hormone (GHRH): It increases the GH secretion by stimulating the somatotropes of anterior pituitary.
2. Growth hormone-releasing polypeptide (GHRP): It increases the release of GHRH from hypothalamus and GH from pituitary.
3. Growth hormone-inhibitory hormone (GHIH) or somatostatin: It decreases GH secretion.

Q. 3. Write a short note on thyroid stimulating hormone.
(*TNMGR, April 2012*)

Ans. Thyroid-stimulating hormone (TSH) is crucial for modulation of thyroid hormone release and growth of thyroid gland. The hypothalamic-pituitary axis regulates TSH release. The hypothalamus releases thyroid-releasing hormone (TRH), which stimulates thyrotrophs of anterior pituitary to secrete TSH. TSH stimulates thyroid follicular cells to release thyroxine, T_4 (80%) and triiodothyronine, or T_3 (20%). T_4 and T_3 can then exert negative feedback on TSH levels with high levels of T_3/T_4 decreasing TSH and low levels of T_3/T_4 increasing TSH levels from anterior pituitary.

Chemistry: TSH is a peptide hormone with one α-chain and one β-chain.

Half-life and plasma level: 60 minutes. Normal plasma level= 2 U/ml.

Actions: TSH increases:

1. Number of follicular cells of thyroid.
2. It causes development of thyroid follicles.
3. Size and secretory activity of follicular cells.
4. Iodide pump and iodide trapping in follicular cells.
5. Thyroglobulin secretion into follicles.
6. Iodination of tyrosine and coupling to form the hormones.
7. Proteolysis of thyroglobulin.

Mode of action: TSH acts through cyclic AMP mechanism.

Q. 4. Write about importance of thyroid hormone in growth.
(BFUHS, May 2011; HP, 2013; RUHS, May 2015; NITTE Uni., April 2017; NTR Uni., June 2017)

Ans. Thyroid hormones are essential for normal growth of tissues, including nervous system.

Actions of Thyroid Hormone

- Required for GH and prolactin production and secretion.
- Required for GH action.
- Increases intestinal glucose reabsorption (glucose transporter); mitochondrial oxidative phosphorylation (ATP production); activity of adrenal medulla (sympathetic; glucose production); induces enzyme synthesis.
- Stimulation of growth of tissues and increased metabolic rate. Increased heat production (calorigenic effect).

Effects on different tissues:

1. **Effects on nutrient sources:**
   - Effects on protein synthesis and degradation: Increased protein synthesis at low thyroid hormone levels; increased protein degradation at high thyroid hormone levels.
   - Effects on carbohydrates: Low doses of thyroid hormone increase glycogen synthesis; high doses increase glycogen breakdown.
2. **Effects on CVS:** Increases heart rate, force of cardiac contractions, stroke volume, cardiac output and up-regulate catecholamine receptors.

3. **Effects on respiratory system:** Increases resting respiratory rate, minute ventilation, ventilatory response to hypercapnia and hypoxia.
4. **Effects on renal system:** Increase blood flow and GFR.
5. **Effects on oxygen carrying capacity:** Increase RBC mass and oxygen dissociation from hemoglobin.
6. **Effects on intermediary metabolism:** Increase glucose absorption from GIT; increase carbohydrate, lipid and protein turnover, downregulate insulin receptors.
7. **Effects in growth and tissue development:** Increases growth and maturation of bone, epidermis, hair follicles and nails, tooth development and eruption, rate and force of skeletal muscle contraction and inhibits synthesis and increases degradation of mucopolysaccharides in subcutaneous tissue.
8. **Effects on nervous system:** Critical for normal CNS neuronal development, enhances wakefulness, and learning capacity, required for normal emotional tone, increase speed and amplitude of peripheral nerve reflexes.
9. **Effects on reproductive system:** Thyroid is required for normal follicular development and ovulation in female, maintenance of pregnancy, normal spermatogenesis in male.

Q. 5. Write a short note on hypothyroidism.
(TNMGR, Oct. 1999; RGUHS, May 2013)

Ans. Decreased secretion of thyroid hormones is called hypothyroidism. Hypothyroidism leads to myxedema in adults and cretinism in children.

1. **Myxedema:** Myxedema is the hypothyroidism in adults, characterized by generalized edematous appearance.

   Causes: Diseases of thyroid gland, genetic disorder or iodine deficiency, deficiency of TSH or TRH. Common cause of myxedema is the autoimmune disease called **Hashimoto's thyroiditis**, which is common in late middle-aged women.

   Signs and symptoms of myxoedema: Swelling of face, bagginess under eyes, non-pitting type of edema, atherosclerosis. Others: Anemia, fatigue, muscular sluggishness, extreme somnolence, menorrhagia and polymenorrhea, decreased cardiovascular functions, increase in body weight, constipation, mental sluggishness, depressed hair growth, scaliness of skin, frog-like husky voice, cold intolerance.

2. **Cretinism:** Cretinism is the hypothyroidism in children, characterized by stunted growth.

   Causes: Congenital absence of thyroid gland, genetic disorder or lack of iodine in the diet.

   Clinical features: Sluggish movements, **croaking sound** while crying, mentally retardation, stunted growth with bloated body, macroglossia, dripping of saliva. Macroglossia produces characteristic **guttural breathing** that may **choke** the baby.

3. **Goiter in hypothyroidism/non-toxic goiter:** Enlargement of thyroid gland without increase in hormone secretion. It can be classifed as:

   i. Endemic colloid goiter.

   ii. Idiopathic non-toxic goiter

Q. 6. Write a short note on sex hormones.

(RGUHS, Nov 2006)

Q. Discuss role of female sex hormone in periodontal disease.

(UHSR, April 2015)

Ans. Adrenal sex hormones are secreted mainly by zona reticularis. Zona fasciculata secretes small quantities of sex hormones. Adrenal cortex secretes mainly the male sex hormones, which are called **androgens**. But small quantity of **estrogen** and **progesterone** is also secreted by adrenal cortex. Androgens secreted by adrenal cortex: Dehydroepiandrosterone, androstenedione, testosterone.

Dehydroepiandrosterone is the most active adrenal androgen. Androgens, in general, are responsible for masculine features of the body. But in normal conditions, the adrenal androgens have insignificant physiological effects, because of the low amount of secretion both in males and females. In **congenital hyperplasia** of adrenal cortex or tumor of zona reticularis, an excess quantity of androgens is secreted. In males, it does not produce any special effect because large quantity of androgens is produced by testes also. But in females, the androgens produce **masculine features**. Some of the androgens are converted into testosterone which is responsible for the androgenic activity in adrenogenital syndrome or congenital adrenal hyperplasia.

Role of female sex hormone in periodontal disease *(BBD Uni., April 2018):* The main sex hormones exerting influence on the periodontium are estrogen and progesterone. Estrogens can influence cytodifferentiation of statified squamous epithelium, and synthesis and maintenance of fibrous collagen. Additionally, estrogen receptors in osteoblast-like cells provide a mechanism for direct action on bone while estrogen receptors in periosteal fibroblasts and periodontal ligament fibroblasts provide a mechanism for direct action on different periodontal tissues. Estrogen, progesterone and chorionic gonadotropin, during pregnancy, affect microcirculatory system by producing following changes: Swelling of endothelial cells and periocytes of the venules, adherence of granulocytes and platelets to vessel walls, formation of microthrombi, disruption of perivascular mast cells, increased vascular permeability and vascular proliferation. Consequently, systemic endocrine imbalances may have an important impact on periodontal pathogenesis, and, vice versa, changes in periodontal conditions might be associated with variations in sex hormone levels. This association is evident in the recent periodontal disease classification which includes the following hormone related disease categories: Puberty-associated gingivitis, menstrual cycle-associated gingivitis and pregnancy-associated gingivitis.

Q. 7. Write a short note on parathormone.

(TNMGR, Sept. 2007; Oct. 2011; RGUHS, Oct. 2010; UHSR, May 2016; RUHS, June 2017)

Ans. PTH secreted by parathyroid gland is essential for the maintenance of blood calcium level within a very narrow critical level. Maintenance of blood calcium level is necessary because calcium is an important inorganic ion for many physiological functions.

Source of secretion: PTH is secreted by the chief cells of the parathyroid glands.

Chemistry: PTH is protein in nature, having 84 amino acids. Its molecular weight is 9,500.

Half-life and plasma level: 10 minutes. Normal plasma level of PTH is about 1.5 to 5.5 ng/dl.

Synthesis: Parathormone is synthesized from the precursor called **prepro-PTH** containing 115 amino acids. First, the prepro-PTH enters the endoplasmic reticulum of chief cells of parathyroid glands. There it is converted into a prohormone called **pro-PTH**, which contains 96 amino acids. Pro-PTH enters the Golgi apparatus, where it is converted into PTH.

Metabolism: Sixty to seventy percent of PTH is degraded by **Kupffer cells** of liver, by means of proteolysis. Degradation of about 20% to 30% PTH occurs in kidneys and to a lesser extent in other organs.

Actions of parathormone: Refer to Q. 1.

PTH and Dental Tissues *(AHSUC, May 2017)*

1. **Effects of PTH on dental bone:** PTH influences bone apposition at the cellular level, increase in the number of osteoblasts, inhibition of osteoblast

apoptosis, and reactivation of the quiescent lining cells to resume the function of matrix formation.

2. **Effects of PTH on the periodontium:** Reduction in periodontitis-associated bone loss and also a reduction in number of inflammatory cells in the marginal gingival area.

3. **Implications in orthodontic treatment:** PTH accelerates tooth movement during orthodontic treatment in the compressed periodontium under mechanical compression.

4. **Effect on implant success:** Increase in formation of cancellous bony trabeculae around the implant and increased the degree of contact between the implants and the bone.

Q. 8. Write a short note on ACTH.

Ans. Anterior pituitary controls the activities of adrenal cortex by secreting adrenocorticotropic hormone (ACTH). ACTH is mainly concerned with the regulation of cortisol secretion and it plays only a minor role in the regulation of mineralocorticoid secretion. ACTH is secreted by the basophilic chromophilic cells of anterior pituitary. ACTH is a single chained polypeptide with 39 amino acids. The daily output of this hormone is 10 ng and the concentration in plasma is 3 ng/dL. Half-life of ACTH is 10 minutes.

Actions:

1. Maintenance of structural integrity and vascularization of zona fasciculata and zona reticularis of adrenal cortex.
2. Conversion of cholesterol into pregnenolone, which is the precursor of glucocorticoids.
3. Release of glucocorticoids.
4. Prolongation of glucocorticoid action on various cells.
5. Mobilization of fats from tissues.
6. Melanocyte-stimulating effect.

Mode of action of ACTH: ACTH acts by the formation of cyclic AMP.

Applied Clinical Physiology

Adrenal Crisis (*BBD Uni., August 2017; DYP Uni., May 2019*): Adrenal crisis, or acute adrenal insufficiency (bronze Addison's disease) is an acute life-threatening condition, considered one of the endocrine emergencies precipitated by an internal or external process in the setting of known or unknown lack of production of the adrenal hormone cortisol.

Etiology: Infections, trauma, pregnancy, surgery, emtional stress, streneous physical activity, thyrotoxicosis, medications.

Primary causes: Etiologies that affect the adrenal gland directly, most notably Addison's disease.

Secondary causes: Due to a disruption of the regulation of cortisol usually from the compromise of the pituitary gland which produces ACTH.

Tertiary causes: Disruption of the hypothalamus which in turn affects ACTH release.

Q. 9. Write a note on Cushing syndrome.

(TNMGR. Oct. 2000)

Ans. Cushing's syndrome is a disorder caused by the body's exposure to an excess of the hormone cortisol.

Causes: Cushing syndrome is due to the hypersecretion of glucocorticoids, particularly cortisol. If it is due to pituitary origin, it is known as **Cushing disease**. If it is due to adrenal origin, it is called **Cushing syndrome**.

Pituitary origin: Increased secretion of ACTH causes hyperplasia of adrenal cortex, leading to hypersecretion of glucocorticoid.

Adrenal origin: Cortisol secretion is increased by:

i. Tumor in zona fasciculata of adrenal cortex.
ii. Carcinoma of adrenal cortex.
iii. Prolonged treatment high dose of exogenous glucocorticoids.

Signs and Symptoms

i. Characteristic feature: Disproportionate distribution of body fat, resulting in:
   a. Moon face.
   b. Torso: Fat accumulation in the chest and abdomen. Arms and legs are very slim in proportion to **torso** (torso means trunk of the body).
   c. Buffalo hump.
   d. Pot belly.
ii. Purple striae: Due to stretching of abdominal wall by excess subcutaneous fat, rupture of subdermal tissues due to stretching, deficiency of collagen fibers due to protein depletion.
iii. Thinning of extremities.
iv. Thinning of skin and subcutaneous tissues.
v. Acanthosis: Darkened skin patches in certain areas such as axilla, neck and groin.
vi. Pigmentation of skin.
vii. Facial plethora: Facial redness.
viii. Hirsutism.
ix. Weakening of muscles because of protein depletion.
x. Bone resorption and osteoporosis.

xi. Hyperglycemia.

xii. Hypertension.

xiii. Immunosuppression resulting in susceptibility for infection.

xiv. Poor wound healing.

Tests for Cushing syndrome

i. Observation of external features.

ii. Determination of blood sugar and cortisol levels.

iii. Analysis of urine for 17-hydroxysteroids.

Treatment for Cushing syndrome: Treatment may include cortisol-inhibiting drugs, surgical removal of pituitary or adrenal tumor, radiation or chemotherapy.

Q. 10. Write about adrenal medulla.

(TNMGR, March 2002)

Ans. Adrenal medulla is the inner part of adrenal gland and made up of interlacing cords of cells known as **chromaffin cells (pheochrome cells or chromophil cells).** Adrenal medulla is formed by two types of chromaffin cells:

1. Adrenaline—secreting cells (90%), 2. Noradrenaline—secreting cells (10%).

Hormones of adrenal medulla: They are amines derived from catechol (**catecholamines**)

1. Adrenaline (Adr) or epinephrine. 2. Noradrenaline or norepinephrine. 3. Dopamine.

Catecholamines are synthesized from amino acid tyrosine in chromaffin cells of adrenal medulla.

Mode of action of adrenaline and noradrenaline-adrenergic receptors: Actions of adrenaline and noradrenaline are executed by binding with receptors called adrenergic receptors, which are present in target organs. Adrenergic receptors are of two types:

1. α-adrenergic receptors (α_1, α_2); 2. β-adrenergic receptors (β_1, β_2)

Actions *(NTR Uni., April 2011):* Circulating adrenaline and noradrenaline have similar effect of sympathetic stimulation.

1. **On metabolism (via α and β receptors):** Adrenaline influences the metabolic functions more than noradrenaline.

   i. General metabolism: Adrenaline increases O_2 consumption and CO_2 removal and BMR (**calorigenic hormone**).

   ii. Carbohydrate metabolism: Adrenaline increases blood glucose level by increasing glycogenolysis in liver and muscle.

   iii. Fat metabolism: Adrenaline causes mobilization of free fatty acids from adipose tissues.

2. **On blood (via β receptors):** Adrenaline decreases blood coagulation time. It increases RBC count in blood.

3. **On heart (via β receptors):** Adrenaline has stronger effects on heart than noradrenaline. It increases overall activity of the heart, i.e.

   i. Heart rate (chronotropic effect).

   ii. Force of contraction (inotropic effect).

   iii. Excitability of heart muscle (bathmotropic effect).

   iv. Conductivity in heart muscle (dromotropic effect).

4. **On blood vessels (via α and β_2 receptors):** Noradrenaline has strong effects on blood vessels. It causes constriction of blood vessels throughout the body via α receptors. So it is called '**general vasoconstrictor**'. Adrenaline also causes constriction of blood vessels. However, it causes dilatation of blood vessels in skeletal muscle, liver and heart through β_2 receptors. So, the total peripheral resistance is decreased by adrenaline.

5. **On blood pressure (via α and β receptors):** Adrenaline increases systolic blood pressure, but it decreases diastolic blood pressure. Noradrenaline increases diastolic pressure.

6. **On respiration (via β_2 receptors):** Adrenaline increases rate and force of respiration.

7. **On skin (via α and β_2 receptors):** Adrenaline causes contraction of arrector pili and increases secretion of sweat.

8. **On skeletal muscle (via α and β_2 receptors):** Adrenaline causes severe contraction and quick fatigue of skeletal muscle. It increases glycogenolysis and release of glucose from muscle into blood. It also causes vasodilatation in skeletal muscles.

9. **On smooth muscle (via α and β receptors):**

   - Catecholamines cause contraction: Splenic capsule, sphincters of GIT, arrector pili of skin, gallbladder, uterus, dilator pupillae of iris.

   - Catecholamines cause relaxation: Non-sphincteric part of GIT (esophagus, stomach and intestine), bronchioles, and urinary bladder.

10. **On CNS (via β receptors):** Adrenaline increases activity of brain. Adrenaline secretion increases during '**fight or flight reactions**' after exposure to stress.

11. Other effects of catecholamines

    i. On salivary glands (via α and β_2 receptors): vasoconstriction $\rightarrow$ increase in salivary secretion.

    ii. On sweat glands (via β_2 receptors): Increase secretion of apocrine sweat glands.

iii. On lacrimal glands (via α receptors): Increase secretion of tears.

iv. On ACTH secretion (via α receptors): Adrenaline increases ACTH secretion.

v. On nerve fibers (via α receptors): Electrical activity is accelerated.

vi. On renin secretion (via β receptors): Increase rennin secretion from juxtaglomerular apparatus (JGA) of kidney.

Regulation of secretion: Adrenaline and noradrenaline are secreted from adrenal medulla in small quantities even during rest. During stress conditions, due to sympathoadrenal discharge, a large quantity of catecholamines is secreted. Catecholamine secretion increases during exposure to cold and hypoglycemia also.

- **Dopamine:** Dopamine is secreted by adrenal medulla. Dopamine is also secreted by dopaminergic neurons in some areas of brain, particularly basal ganglia. In brain, this hormone acts as a neurotransmitter. Injected dopamine produces the following effects:
  1. Vasoconstriction by releasing norepinephrine.
  2. Vasodilatation in mesentery.
  3. Increase in heart rate via β-receptors.
  4. Increase in systolic blood pressure.

Applied Clinical Physiology

1. **Pheochromocytoma:** Hypersecretion of catecholamines caused by tumor of chromophil cells in adrenal medulla. Characteristic feature of pheochromocytoma is hypertension. Other features: Anxiety, chest pain, fever, headache, hyperglycemia, metabolic disorders, nausea, vomiting, palpitation, polyuria, glucosuria, sweating, flushing, tachycardia, weight loss.

2. Deficiency of dopamine in basal ganglia produces nervous disorder called *Parkinsonism*.

Q. 11. Write a short note on neurohormones.
(TNMGR, Sept. 2002; March 2008)

Ans. Neurohormones/neuropeptides/hypothalamic releasing hormone is a chemical substance synthesized and secreted by nerve cell (e.g. hypothalamus) directly into the blood (via hypothalamo-hypophyseal portal system) and transported to target organ (e.g. pituitary) to stimulates or inhibits its secretion, e.g.

1. Thyrotropin-releasing hormone (TRH)/prolactin-releasing hormone
2. Corticotropin-releasing hormone (CRH)
3. Gonadotropin-releasing hormone (GnRH).
4. Growth hormone-releasing hormone (GHRH)/Somatostatin
5. Growth hormone-inhibiting hormone
6. Prolactin-inhibitng hormone/dopamine
7. Oxytocin
8. Vasopressin

Q. 12. Write a note on physiology of regulation of blood glucose level.
(TNMGR, April 1997; Sept. 2007; April 2012; Oct.2019; NTR Uni, May 2019)

Ans. Normal blood glucose level: In early morning, fasting blood glucose (FBS) level is low (70–110 mg/dl). Between 1st and 2nd hour after meals (postprandial), blood glucose level rises to 100–140 mg/dl. Glucose level in blood is brought back to normal at the end of 2nd hour after meals. Among all hormones, insulin reduces blood glucose level and is called **anti-diabetogenic hormone**. Hormones which increase blood glucose level are called **diabetogenic hormones** or **anti-insulin** hormones.

Regulation of blood glucose level:

1. **Role of liver:** When blood glucose level increases after a meal, excess glucose is converted into glycogen and stored in liver. Afterwards, when blood glucose level falls, glycogen in liver is converted into glucose and released into blood.

2. **Role of insulin:** Insulin decreases blood glucose through increased expression of GLUT4 and glycogen synthase, inactivation of phosphorylase kinase (thus decreasing gluconeogenesis), and decreasing expression of rate-limiting enzymes involved in gluconeogenesis.

3. **Role of glucagon:** Glucagon increases blood glucose through increased glycogenolysis and gluconeogenesis.

4. **Somatostatin:** It decreases blood glucose levels through local suppression of glucagon release and suppression of gastrin and pituitary tropic hormones.

5. **Cortisol:** It increases blood glucose by stimulation of gluconeogenesis and by antagonism of insulin.

6. **Epinephrine:** It increases blood glucose levels through glycogenolysis and increased fatty acid release from adipose tissues, which can then be catabolized and enter gluconeogenesis.

7. **Thyroxine:** It increases blood glucose levels through glycogenolysis and increased absorption in intestine.

8. **Growth hormone:** It promotes gluconeogenesis, inhibits liver uptake of glucose, stimulates thyroid hormone, and inhibits insulin.

9. **ACTH:** It stimulates cortisol release from adrenal glands, stimulates release of fatty acids from adipose tissue for gluconeogenesis.

Applied Clinical Physiology

1. **Hyperglycemia:** Diabetes mellitus I and II are characterized by chronically elevated blood glucose levels.
   - Type I: Results from autoimmune destruction of pancreatic β-cells and insulin deficiency and most often in pediatric patients.
   - Type II: Results from peripheral insulin resistance owing to metabolic dysfunction, usually in setting of obesity and is more likely in adulthood

   In both cases, the result is:
   - Osmotic damage: Glucose is osmotically active and can cause damage to peripheral nerves.
   - Oxidative stress: Glucose participates in several reactions that produce oxidative byproducts.
   - Non-enzymatic glycation: Glucose can complex with lysine residues on proteins causing structural and functional disruption.

   Hyperosmolar hyperglycemic state and diabetic ketoacidosis is acute condition due to severely elevated blood glucose level resulting in elevated plasma osmolality which leads to osmotic diuresis (excessive urination) and dehydration.

2. **Hypoglycemia:** Hypoglycemia is most often seen iatrogenically in diabetic patients secondary to glucose-lowering drugs. Symptoms of hypoglycemia:
   - Neuroglycopenic (direct effect on CNS): Fatigue, behavioral changes, seizures, coma, and death.
   - Neurogenic (adrenergic): Anxiety, tremor, and palpitations.
   - Neurogenic (cholinergic): Paresthesias, diaphoresis (excessive sweating), and hunger.

Q. 13. Write about functions of insulin.
(TNMGR, April 1998; April 2012)

Ans. Insulin is the important hormone that is concerned with the regulation of carbohydrate metabolism, blood glucose level, metabolism of proteins and fats.

Glucose Transporters (Glut): Glucose transporters are integral membrane proteins that facilitate transport of glucose across a plasma membrane (Table 5.13).

Insulin is a small protein (5.7 kD) with two polypeptide chains, A and B containing 51 amino acids, joined by two disulfide bonds. It is synthesized in pancreas as inactive single-chain precursor; *preproinsulin* with an amino-terminal "signal sequence." Proteolytic removal of signal sequence and formation of three disulfide bonds produces *proinsulin*, which is later cleaved. After cleavage of the C peptide, mature insulin is formed in the β-granules and is stored in the form of zinc-containing hexamers until secretion.

Functions:
1. **On carbohydrate metabolism:** Insulin is antidiabetic hormone secreted in body. Insulin decreases blood glucose level by:
   i. Facilitating transport and uptake of glucose by cells.
   ii. Increasing peripheral utilization of glucose.
   iii. Increasing storage of glucose by converting it into glycogen (Glycogenesis) in liver and muscle.
   iv. Inhibiting glycogenolysis.
   v. Inhibiting gluconeogenesis.
2. **On protein metabolism:** Insulin facilitates synthesis and storage of proteins and inhibits cellular utilization of proteins.
3. **On fat metabolism:**
   i. Synthesis of fatty acids and triglycerides (Lipogenesis).
   ii. Transport of fatty acids into adipose tissue.
   iii. Insulin promotes storage of fat in adipose tissue by inhibiting enzymes which degrade triglycerides.

Table 5.13: Glucose transporter: Location and functions

	Tissue location	*Function*
Facilitative bidirectional transporters		
GLUT 1	Brain, kidney, colon, placenta, erythrocyte	Uptake of glucose
GLUT 2	Liver, pancreatic B cell, small intestine, kidney	Rapid uptake and release of glucose
GLUT 3	Brain, kidney, placenta	Uptake of glucose
GLUT 4	Heart and skeletal muscle, adipose tissue	Insulin-stimulated uptake of glucose
GLUT 5	Small intestine	Absorption of glucose
Sodium-dependent unidirectional transporter		
SGLT 1	Small intestine and kidney	Active uptake of glucose from lumen of intestine and reabsorption of glucose in proximal tubule of kidney against a concentration gradient

4. **On growth:** Along with growth hormone, insulin promotes growth of body by its anabolic action on proteins. It enhances the transport of amino acids into cell and synthesis of proteins in cells. It also has the protein-sparing effect.

Applied Clinical Physiology:
1. **Hyperinsulinism:** Hypersecretion of insulin due to tumor of β-cells in islets of Langerhans.
2. **Hypoinsulinemia:** Diabetes mellitus.
3. **Insulin resistance** (*Sumandeep Uni., April 2015*): It is defined as reduced sensitivity of peripheral tissues to action of insulin, which is caused by changes in insulin-mediated signaling pathways, and results in systemic hyperglycemia. Causes of insulin resistance include various metabolic aberrations that reduce the capacity of tissues to respond to insulin, e.g. genetic predisposition, hyperinsulinaemia, hyperandrogonism, central obesity, aging, sedentary life, pregnancy, oral contraceptives, glucocorticoid, alcohol and smoking.

6. GASTROINTESTINAL SYSTEM

Q. 1. Write briefly on the composition and functions of saliva and the physiology of its secretion.
(TNMGR, April 1995; PAHER, May 2010; RGUHS, May 2012 UHSR, May 2016; MPMS Uni., July 2017; HP Uni., April 2019)

Q. Write about physiology and mechanism of secretion of saliva. *(TNMGR, March 2009; BFUHS, May 2009, 2010; RUHS, May 2015)*

Q. Discuss the role of saliva in oral health.
(MAHE, Nov. 1999; TNMGR, March 2012)

Ans. Saliva is produced and secreted from salivary glands. The basic secretary units of salivary glands are clusters of cells called acini. Within the ducts, composition of the secretion is altered as sodium is actively reabsorbed; potassium and bicarbonate ion is secreted. Small collecting ducts within salivary glands lead into larger ducts, eventually forming a single large duct that empties into the oral cavity.

Composition of saliva:
A. **Water** 99.5%
B. **Solids** 0.5%
1. **Organic substances:**
   a. **Enzymes:** Amylase, maltase, lingual lipase, lysozyme, phosphatase, carbonic anhydrase, kallikrein.
   b. **Others:** Mucin, albumin, proline rich proteins (PRP), lactoferrin, IgA, IgG, lactate, citrate, uric acid, creatinine, cholesterol, cAMP, blood group antigens, free amino acids, non-protein nitrogenous substance (urea, ammonia).
2. **Inorganic substances:** Na, Ca, K, bicarbonates, Br, Cl, F, PO_4.
3. **Gases:** O_2, CO_2, N.

Properties of saliva
1. Volume: 1000–1500 ml/day and 1 ml/minute. i. Parotid glands: 25%; ii. Submandibular glands: 70%; iii. Sublingual glands: 5%.
2. Reaction: Slightly acidic with pH of 6.35 to 6.85.
3. Specific gravity: 1.002–1.012.
4. Tonicity: Hypotonic to plasma.

Functions of saliva: (CDER-AIIMS, April 2017)
1. **Preparation of food for swallowing:** Mucin of saliva lubricates the bolus and facilitates chewing and swallowing.
2. **Appreciation of taste:** By its solvent action, saliva dissolves solid food substances, which can stimulate the taste buds. Specific zinc-binding salivary protein, gustin mediates taste sensation.
3. **Digestive function:** Saliva has three digestive enzymes.
   • **Salivary amylase:** Salivary amylase acts on cooked or boiled starch and converts it into dextrin and maltose. Salivary amylase cannot act on cellulose.
   • **Maltase:** Maltase converts maltose into glucose.
   • **Lingual lipase:** Lingual lipase hydrolyzes triglycerides into fatty acids and diacylglycerol.
4. **Cleansing and protective functions:** Mucin in saliva helps in phonation as well as food passage and provides for smooth tissue surfaces. Proline-rich glycoprotein with albumin is also an effective lubricant on teeth as part of pellicle, and on mucous membrane.
5. **Maintenance of mucous membrane integrity:** Salivary mucins possess rheological properties which include low solubility, high viscosity, elasticity, and adhesiveness, which enable them to concentrate on oral mucosal surface, where they provide an effective barrier against desiccation and environmental insults and resistant to proteolysis. Second line of defense against protease activity is by cystatins S, an inhibitor of cysteine proteinases, especially cathepsin C. This antiprotease activity is augmented by antileukoprotease, an effective inhibitor of granulocyte elastase and cathepsin G, present in both parotid and submandibular glands.

6. **Soft tissue repair:** The presence of growth factor like epidermal growth factor (EGF), vascular endothelial growth factor (VEGF), transforming growth factor alpha (TFG-α), transforming growth factor beta (TFG-β), nerve growth factor (NGF), fibroblast growth factor (FGF), and insulin-like growth factor (IGF) in saliva may accelerate wound-healing. *Secretory leukocyte protease inhibitor (SLPI)* prevents degradation of proteins involved in connective tissue repair. *Trefoil factor 3 (TFF3)* increases migration of oral epithelial cells, helping in wound healing. *Histatins* also possess wound healing properties by enhancing re-epithelialization process and promoting endothelial cell adhesion. *Opiorphin*, endogenous analgesic, present in saliva; prolongs body's own defenses by preventing breakdown of chemicals that activate opiate receptors that block pain signals from reaching the brain.

7. **Maintenance in ecological balance:** *Human β-defensins* are family of peptides, play key role in maintaining a healthy and dynamic equilibrium across oral mucosal system

8. **Debridement and lavage:** Physical flow of saliva augmented by muscular activity of lips and tongue removes harmful bacteria from teeth and mucosal surfaces.

9. **Aggeregation:** The ability to inhibit bacterial attachment is a major characteristic of secretory IgA system and is the rationale for interest in oral vaccine against caries.

10. **Direct antibacterial property:** Salivary proteins and other components of saliva can interfere with multiplication or killing of bacteria. Due to their positive charge, they bind to negatively charged surface of microbial membranes, forming pores that ultimately result in lethal efflux of vital cell constituents.

- *Lysozyme* can cause lysis of bacterial cells, especially *S. mutans* by interacting with anions of low charge density chaotropic ions (thiocyanate, perchlorate, iodide, bromide, nitrate, chloride, and fluoride), and with bicarbonate.
- *Cathelicidins* are broad-spectrum antimicrobial peptides derived from neutrophils and salivary glands, helps in wound healing, immuno-modulation and angiogenesis.
- *Histatins* have antimicrobial activity against oral microorganisms.
- *Lactoferrin* is bactericidal against bacteria requiring iron for their metabolic processes.
- *Salivary peroxidase* is antimicrobial; effective against *S. mutans* in association with secretory IgA.

- **Mucin** can concentrate all defense force at interface of mucosa and external environment.
- Saliva gets contribution from GCF, which substantiate oral defense system by providing: (a) Serum antibodies against oral bacteria, especially IgG antibodies, (b) phagocytic cells (PMN's) (c) antibacterial products liberated from the phagocytic cells (e.g. lysozyme, lactoferrin, and myeloperoxidase).

11. **Antifungal action:** *Histatin-5* is potent antifungal action primarily against *Candida albicans*. It binds to specific receptors on fungal cell wall and enters into the cell, targets the mitochondria, ultimately disrupting cell homeostasis. Antifungal action of *Statherin* is by inducing *C. albicans* hyphae-to-yeast transition.

12. **Maintenance of oral pH:** In *oral cavity and esophagus*, major regulation of pH is by salivary bicarbonate, level of which varies directly with flow rate. In *bacterial plaque*, bicarbonate, phosphate, and histidine-rich peptides act directly as buffers.

13. **Maintenance of tooth integrity:** The protective function begins immediately after tooth eruption into oral cavity. Interaction with saliva provides a post-eruptive maturation through diffusion of ions such as calcium, phosphorus, magnesium, and fluoride, other trace components into the surface enamel. This maturation increases surface hardness, decreases permeability and increases resistance to caries. Once tooth begins to function in mouth, its *developmental cuticle* or *pellicle* is rapidly worn away and is replaced by a constantly replenished salivary film, *acquired pellicle*. This provides a protective barrier and lubricating film against excessive wear, and diffusion barrier against acid penetration.

14. **Excretory function:** Saliva serves as a route of elimination of many drugs.

15. **Water balance:** Thirst and need for fluid intake sensation results from a diminution in resting secretion and activation of receptors in oral cavity. Thirst satiation and cessation of drinking are initiated by sensory messages passing into brain from taste receptors in mouth.

16. **Hormonal function:** Many hormones like EGF, NGF, and TGF have been found in saliva, which helps in gastric cytoprotection and inhibition of gastric acid secretion.

17. **Saliva and periodontal health:** Saliva plays role in periodontal health by:
   a. **Pellicle and plaque formation:** α-amylase is found in acquired pellicle has role in bacterial adhesion. Saliva helps in supragingival plaque

formation in its *First stage (of deposition of a pellicle or cuticle)* as:

- Bathing of tooth surfaces by salivary fluids which contain abundant proteins.
- Selective adsorption of certain negatively and positively charged glycoproteins which act as an agglutinating base.
- Loss of solubility of adsorbed proteins by surface denaturation and acid precipitation.
- Alteration of glycoproteins by enzymes from bacteria and oral secretions. *Second stage of plaque formation ("bacterial colonization")*:
- Adherence of bacteria to salivary-coated tooth surface.
- Bacteria that adhere to pellicle initially are called "primary" colonizers (*S. sanguis* species followed by *S. mutans*)
- After this "secondary colonizers" adhere to primary bacteria and carve an *"ecological niche"* for themselves.
- In third or maturation stage, saliva continues to provide agglutinating substances and proteins to intercellular matrix and bacterial adhesion continues.
- Salivary proteins and carbohydrates serve as a substrate for metabolic activity of bacteria.

b. **Plaque mineralization and calculus formation:** Salivary proteins such as esterase, pyrophosphates, acid phosphatase and lysozyme play a role plaque mineralization. Salivary calcium, phosphates, magnesium, sodium, and potassium become part of the gel-like consistency of plaque and begin to influence its mineralization and demineralization. Mineral precipitate results from a local rise in degree of saturation of calcium and phosphates in saliva due to (i) increase of pH of saliva (ii) colloidal and particles in saliva which bind to calcium and phosphates making super-saturated solution.

18. **Saliva and dental caries:** Saliva of caries free person has:
    1. Increased rate of flow, increased pH and increased buffering.
    2. Higher calcium, phosphorous, ammonia, ATP and fructose diphosphate.
    3. Increased aldolase, opsonin, and antibacterial activity and O_2 uptake of bacteria.
    4. Higher number of intact leukocytes.
    5. Difference in proportion of epithelial cells to leukocytes.

    The saliva influences caries process by affecting all the three components of *Keye's* *classic Venn diagram* of etiology of caries (tooth, plaque, and substrate). The saliva also affects flow rates and clearance, pH and buffer capacity, calcium phosphate homeostasis and effects on bacterial metabolism. Salivary components which help in this are salivary IgA, lactoferrin, lysozyme and the salivary peroxidase-hypo-thiocyanite system, proline-rich proteins.

19. **Role in speech:** By moistening and lubricating soft parts of mouth and lips, saliva helps in speech.

20. **Regulation of body temperature:** In dogs and cattle, excessive dripping of saliva during panting helps in loss of heat and regulation of body temperature.

Regulation of Salivary Secretion

A. Parasympathetic fibers:

1. **Parasympathetic fibers to submandibular and sublingual glands:** Parasympathetic preganglionic fibers to submandibular and sublingual glands arise from superior salivatory nucleus, situated in pons. Preganglionic fibers run through **nervus intermedius of Wrisberg**, geniculate ganglion, motor fibers of facial nerve, chorda tympani branch of facial nerve and lingual branch of trigeminal nerve and finally reach submandibular ganglion. Postganglionic fibers arising from this ganglion supply submandibular and sublingual glands.

2. **Parasympathetic fibers to Parotid gland:** Parasympathetic preganglionic fibers to parotid gland arise from inferior salivatory nucleus situated in upper part of medulla oblongata. The fibers pass through tympanic branch of glossopharyngeal nerve, tympanic plexus and lesser petrosal nerve and end in otic ganglion. Postganglionic fibers arise from this ganglion and supply parotid gland by passing through auriculotemporal branch in mandibular division of trigeminal nerve.

   Function of parasympathetic fibers: Secretion of saliva with large quantity of water.

B. **Sympathetic fibers:** Sympathetic preganglionic fibers to salivary glands arise from lateral horns of 1st and 2nd thoracic segments of spinal cord. The fibers leave the cord through anterior nerve roots and end in superior cervical ganglion of sympathetic chain. Postganglionic fibers arise from this ganglion and are distributed to salivary glands along the nerve plexus, around arteries supplying the glands.

Function of sympathetic fibers: Secretion of saliva, which is thick and rich in organic constituents such as mucus.

Reflex regulation of salivary secretion:

1. **Unconditioned reflex:** It does not need any previous experience.
2. **Conditioned reflex:** Conditioned reflex is one that is acquired by experience and it needs previous experience. The stimuli for this reflex are sight, smell, hearing or thought of food.

Saliva as diagnostic fluids: Salivary analysis has two main objectives: To identify specific pathologies in patients and monitor change in those patients undergoing treatment. **Biomarker** is defined as any cellular, biochemical, molecular, or genetic alterations which help to recognize and monitor disease susceptibility, progression, resolution, health status and treatment outcome in individuals (Table 6.1).

Advantages:

1. Eliminate potential risk of contracting infectious disease.
2. Non-invasive.
3. Painless and little anxiety in collection process.
4. Simple in collection with a modest trained assistant and applicable in remote areas.
5. Relatively cheap technology.
6. Can be used to study special population where blood sampling is a problem, e.g child, anxious/handicap/elderly patients.
7. In addition, saliva does not clot and can be manipulated more easily than blood.

Limitations:

1. Levels of certain markers in saliva are not always a reliable reflection of levels of these markers in serum.
2. Salivary composition can be influenced by method of collection and degree of stimulation of salivary flow.
3. Variability in salivary flow rate is expected between individuals and in same individual under different conditions.
4. Certain systemic disorders, medications and radiation may affect salivary gland function and consequently quantity and composition of saliva.
5. Proteolytic enzymes of saliva can affect stability of certain diagnostic markers.

Analysis of saliva done for the diagnosis of following:

1. **Hereditary disease:**
   - In cystic fibrosis (CF), there are elevated electrolytes, urea, uric acid, total protein and lipid in submandibular saliva.
   - Early morning salivary levels of 17-hydroxy-progesterone is an excellent screening test for diagnosis of 21-hydroxylase deficiency.
2. **Autoimmune disease:** $\uparrow$concentrations of Na and Cl, IgA, IgG, lactoferrin and albumin, and $\downarrow$ concentration of phosphate are reported in saliva of patients with Sjögren's syndrome.
3. **Renal disease:** Salivary biomarkers associated with end stage renal disease are nitrite, pH, sodium, chloride, uric acid, cortisol, alpha-amylase, and lactoferrin. Salivary phosphate is used as biomarker for hyperphosphatemia.
4. **Cardiovascular diseases:** Salivary biomarkers of cardiovascular diseases include C-reactive protein (CRP), myoglobin, creatinine kinase myocardial band (CK-MB), cardiac troponins (cTn), and myeloperoxidase. Increased levels of salivary lysozyme are associated with hypertension.

3. **Malignancy:**
   - The mRNA levels for specific proteins are elevated in the saliva of head and neck cancer patients.
   - p53 antibodies can be detected in saliva of patients with oral squamous cell carcinoma (OSCC).
   - Elevated levels of salivary defensin-1 are indicative of OSCC.
   - Elevated salivary levels of CA 15-3 detected in patients with untreated and advanced breast.
   - *CA 125* is a tumor associated antigen which is saliva of patients with oral, breast, and ovarian tumors.
   - Fibroblast growth factor 2 (FGF2) and fibroblast growth factor receptor 1 (FGFR1) concentrations in saliva are elevated in patients with salivary gland tumors.
   - Salivary prostate specific antigen is elevated in prostate adenocarcinoma.
   - Salivary cortisol, lactate dehydrogenase, nitrate and nitrite levels are significantly increased in patients of OSCC.
   - Salivary adenosine deaminase (ADA) activity is significantly increased in squamous cell carcinoma of the tongue progressively from stage I to stage III.

4. **Infection:**
   - In children infected with Shigella revealed higher titers of anti-Shiga toxin antibody.
   - PCR-based identification of virus DNA in saliva is a useful method for early detection of HSV-1 reactivation in patients with Bell's palsy.

- Salivary levels of anti-dengue IgM and IgG demonstrated sensitivity of 92% and specificity of 100% in the diagnosis of infection.
- Salivary diagnostic tests have been designed for detection of human papillomavirus by polymerase chain reaction.
- The salivary fungal count analysis provides valuable information in cases of oral candidiasis.

5. **Monitoring of levels of drugs**
   - Saliva may be used for monitoring patient compliance with psychiatric medications.
   - Saliva is useful for monitoring of antiepileptic drugs and anti-cancer drugs.
   - Other drugs that can be identified in saliva are alcohol, amphetamines, barbiturates, benzodiazepines, cocaine, and opioids.
   - Monitoring level of salivary cotinine has proven useful in monitoring compliance with smoking cessation programs.

6. **Monitoring of levels of hormones**
   - Cortisol, steroid hormones can be detected in saliva.
   - Salivary aldosterone was found in patients with primary aldosteronism.
   - Elevated salivary estriol is associated with increased risk of preterm birth.
   - Insulin can be detected in saliva.

7. **In stress:** Chronic stress is associated with increased levels of salivary cortisol and decreased level of salivary IgA and lysozyme. Saliva chromogranin-A and α-amylase are markers of acute stress.

8. **Heavy metal poisoning:** Occupational toxins such as lead and cadmium can also be analyzed from the saliva.

9. **Bone turnover marker in saliva:** Presence of osteocalcin and pyridinoline in saliva can be used to measure bone turnover.

10. **Forensic medicine:** Saliva can potentially be recovered from bite marks, cigarette butts, postage stamps, envelopes and other objects.

11. **Dental caries and periodontal disease:**
    - High numbers of *S. mutans* and Lactobacillus indicate a shift in oral microflora from healthy to more cariogenic.
    - Progress from gingivitis to periodontal disease is determined by genetic susceptibility, and the presence of pathogenic bacteria.
    - People at high risk for periodontal disease can be determined by genetic screening as DNA can easily be isolated from oral epithelial cells.
    - Periodontal diseases have been associated with increased levels of aspartate aminotransferase (AST) and alkaline phosphatase (ALP).
    - Salivary AST can be used as a marker for monitoring periodontal disease.
    - Lower levels of uric acid and albumin in the saliva were associated with periodontitis and diabetes.

12. **Diagnosis of Oral Disease with Relevance for Systemic Diseases:**
    - Quantitative alterations in saliva may be a result of medications. Reduced salivary flows may lead

Table 6.1: *Salivary biomarkers (TNMGR, Oct. 2016; Gujarat Uni., July 2017)*

S. No.	Diseases	Biomarker
1.	Dental caries and periodontal diseases	*Streptococcus mutans* and lactobacilli count. Aspartate aminotransferase, alkaline phosphatase, uric acid, albumin, etc.
2.	Autoimmune diseases (Sjögren's syndrome, multiple sclerosis, sarcoidosis)	Lactoferrin, beta 2 microglobulin, lysozyme C, cystatin C, salivary amylase, carbonic anhydrase, IgA production
3.	Cardiovascular markers	Cardiac troponins, C reactive protein, myoglobin, myeloperoxidase, ICAM-1, CD 40 and salivary lysozyme
4.	Drug level monitoring	Nicotine, cannabinoids, cocaine, phencyclidine, opioids, barbiturates, amphetamines, ethanol, etc.
5.	Forensic evidence	Blood group antigens and DNA testing
6.	Malignancy	Inc. RNA, mi RNA, CCNI, EGFR, FGF19, FRS2, IL 1B, p53, CA15-3, cortisol, lactate dehydrogenase, silver nitrate, etc.
7.	Occupational and environmental medicine	Salivary cortisol, IgA, lysozyme, chromogranin, alpha-amylase, lead and cadmium
8.	Renal diseases	Cortisol, nitrite, uric acid, sodium chloride, pH, alpha-amylase, lactoferrin, salivary phosphate, serum creatinine and glomerular filtration rate.
9.	Psychological research	Salivary amylase, cortisol, substance P, lysozyme, secretory IgG and testosterone.
10.	Bone turnover markers	Interleukin I beta, salivary osteonectin, alkaline phosphatase activity, etc.

to progressive dental caries, fungal infection, oral pain, and dysphagia.

- Increased levels of albumin in whole saliva were detected in patients who received chemotherapy and subsequently developed stomatitis.
- Human salivary proteome can be used in Sjögren syndrome, osteoporosis, rheumatoid arthritis, diabetes, and cancers.

Salivary Proteomics: Proteomics is analysis of the portion of the genome that is expressed by using two-dimensional gel electrophoresis/mass spectrometry and "shotgun" proteomics approaches collectively.

Salivary Transcriptomics: Salivary transcriptome included mRNA molecules that cells use to convey the instructions carried by DNA for subsequent protein production. RNA molecules are elevated in oral cancer tissues are also elevated in saliva, which prompted them to examine the scope and complexity of RNA present in saliva. Other research groups, particularly from forensic sciences, are focusing on multiplex mRNA profiling for the identification of body fluids including saliva.

Artificial Saliva (*NTR Uni., May 2019*):

Composition: Xanthum gum, sodium carboxymethyl-cellulose (CMC), potassium chloride, sodium chloride, magnesium chloride, calcium chloride, di-potassium hydrogen orthophosphate, sodium fluoride, sorbitol, methyl p-hydroxybenzoate, spirit of lemon. CMC is a polymer derived from natural cellulose. It is used in saliva substitute formulation as a thickening agent.

Q. 2. Write a short note on mastication.
(BFUHS, Oct. 2010; AHSUC, May 2018)

Ans. Mastication or **chewing** is the first mechanical process in the **GIT**, by which the food substances are torn or cut into small particles and crushed or ground into a soft **bolus** to increase surface area for the efficient action of digestive enzymes and reduced for swallowing.

Chewing Cycle: A single chewing cycle is usually divided in four phases: *First phase* of chewing cycle is minimum opening. Then jaw moves slowly down-wards followed by *second phase,* i.e. faster opening. Then jaw moves upwards for fast closing, i.e. *third phase.* Closing, i.e. *fourth phase.*

Masticatory Sequence
1. Preparatory period: Food is transported back to the posterior teeth.
2. Reduction period: Food is grounded.
3. Pre-swallowing period: Bolus is formed.

Significance of mastication
1. Breakdown of foodstuffs into smaller particles.
2. Mixing of saliva with food substances thoroughly.
3. Lubrication and moistening of dry food by saliva, so that the bolus can be easily swallowed
4. Appreciation of taste of the food.

Movements of mastication
1. Opening and closure of mouth.
2. Rotational movements of jaw.
3. Protraction and retraction of jaw.

Control of mastication: Action of mastication is mostly a reflex process. It is carried out voluntarily also. The center for mastication is situated in medulla and cerebral cortex. Trigeminal mesencephalic nucleus is sensory nucleus for muscles of mastication. Jaw closing motor neurons are located in the dorsolateral and jaw opening motor neurons are situated in ventromedial divisions of the trigeminal motor nucleus.

Q. 3. Write a note on deglutition. *(BFUHS, Oct. 2010; RGUHS, May 2011; UHSR, April 2013; UOK, July 2017; BBD Uni., April 2018 NTP Uni., May 2018)*

Ans. Deglutition is act of swallowing, through which food or liquid bolus is transported from mouth through pharynx and esophagus into stomach.

Stages of Deglutition:

A. **Oral Stage or First Stage:** Oral stage of deglutition is a voluntary stage. In this stage, the bolus from mouth passes into pharynx by means of series of actions.

1. *Preparatory phase:* In this, food is readied for swallowing by reducing and mixing it with saliva, by the muscles of jaw and oral cavity.
   - Jaw is closed by jaw elevator muscles.
   - Lips maintain a seal under the action of orbicularis oris.
   - Food is returned from the vestibule by contraction of buccinators.
   - Soft palate is lowered and anterior and posterior pillars approximate under the action of palatoglossus and palatopharyngeus muscles.
   - Thus, oral cavity is sealed posteriorly and the airway remains open.
   - Bolus is progressively accumulated on the posterior surface of the tongue, by several cycles of upward and downward movement on the tongue surface.

2. *Oral phase proper:*
   - The first event is mandibular elevation as it is hard to swallow with an open mouth.

- Mandibular elevation assists the suprahyoid muscles in raising the hyoid bone.
- Tip of tongue is elevated towards hard palate by action of genioglossus muscle.
- Blade of the tongue then moves up due to contraction of intrinsic muscles.
- These movements are accompanied by lifting the floor of the mouth under the action of stylohyoid.
- As the bolus reaches back of tongue, soft palate is elevated by tensor and levator veli palatini to protect the nasopharynx.

B. **Pharyngeal Stage or Second Stage:** Pharyngeal stage is an involuntary stage. As the bolus enters the oropharynx, it makes contact with faucial pillars or with the mucosa overlying the posterior pharynx. Pharyngeal phase consists of a sequence of events that ensures that the airway is protected during bolus transport.

- Diaphragmatic contraction is inhibited making simultaneous breathing and swallowing impossible.
- Soft palate is elevated to ensure closure of the nasopharynx.
- Vocal cords start to close to protect the airway, either do the vestibular folds.
- The larynx is closed by the contraction of muscles of laryngeal inlet resembling a draw string purse.
- The larynx is closed under the contraction of suprahyoid muscles, in order to narrow laryngeal inlet and moving it towards the pharyngeal surface of epiglottis.
- As the bolus moves into oropharynx, the epiglottis moves downwards.
- As the food passes over postetrior part of epiglottis, it is diverted into pyriform fossae. Solids tend to go straight over epiglottis, whereas liquids are diverted laterally.

C. **Esophageal Stage or Third Stage:** This phase is involuntary.

- The cricopharyngeus muscle relaxes so the upper oesophageal sphincter opens; bolus is passed on into and through the sphincter and oesophagus by peristalsis.
- Primary peristalsis: Continuation of peristaltic wave initiated in pharynx.
- Secondary peristalsis: Initiated due to distension of esophagus with food and continued till all the food is emptied into stomach.
- Tertiary peristalsis: Irregular, nonpropulsive contractinss involving long segments which occur during emotional stress.

Q. 4. Write a short note on deglutition reflex.
(TNMGR, Sept. 2009; April 2013; NTR Uni., May 2018)

Ans. Though the beginning of swallowing is a voluntary act, later it becomes involuntary and is carried out by a reflex action called **deglutition reflex**. It occurs during pharyngeal and esophageal stages.

Stimulus: When the bolus enters oropharyngeal region, the receptors present in this region are stimulated.

Afferent fibers: Afferent impulses from oropharyngeal receptors pass via glossopharyngeal nerve fibers to deglutition center.

Center: Deglutition center is at the floor of fourth ventricle in medulla oblongata of brain.

Efferent fibers: Impulses from deglutition center travel through glossopharyngeal and vagus nerves (parasympathetic motor fibers) and reach soft palate, pharynx and esophagus. The glossopharyngeal nerve is concerned with pharyngeal stage of swallowing. The vagus nerve is concerned with esophageal stage.

Response: The reflex causes upward movement of soft palate, to close nasopharynx and upward movement of larynx, to close respiratory passage so that bolus enters the esophagus. Now the peristalsis occurs in esophagus, pushing the bolus into stomach.

Applied Clinical Physiology: Disorders of swallowing *(BBD Uni., June 2016)*

1. **Dysphagia:** Difficulty in swallowing affecting any part from mouth to stomach.
2. **Odynophagia:** Painful swallowing.
3. **Globus hystericus:** Sensation of lump lodged in throat.
4. **Phagophagia:** Fear of swallowing as in rabies.
5. **Presbydysphagia:** Swallowing difficulties due to ageing.

Q. 5. Write a short note on gag reflex.
(NTR Uni., June 2017; UHSR, May 2018)

Ans. Gag reflex/pharyngeal reflex is defined as constriction of pharynx but often is associated with more complex behavioral responses, including lowering of the mandible, forward and downward movement of the tongue, and pharyngeal and velar constriction associated with mild coughing. It is induced by touching of base of tongue, soft palate, uvula, or posterior pharyngeal wall with a tongue blade, or finger.

The gag reflex is an innate reflex intended to guard upper respiratory tract and digestive tract from foreign body that might block them.

Etiology:

1. Local factors: Nasal obstruction, deviated septum, postnasal drip, sinusitis.
2. Medical condition: Chronic gastritis, uncontrolled diabetes.
3. Social causes: Heavy smoker and alcoholics, coughing.
4. Psychological factors: Eating disorders, fear, stress, learned response.
5. Iatrogenic factors: Water and suction tubes, local anaesthesia, radiography.
6. Prosthetic factors: Poor retention, surface finish of dentures, overextended/underextended dentures.

Management:

1. **Psychosomatic management:** Relaxation, distraction and desensitization, beavioural modification, sedation and hypnosis, leg lift technique.
2. **Therapeutic management:** Sedative, antihistamine, parasympathetic, analgesics, acupuncture, anticholinergics.
3. **Prosthodontic management:** Finger massage technique, reduction of posterior borders of maxillary dentures, conditioning prosthesis, controlled breathing technique.

Q. 6. Write a short note on digestive enzymes.

(TNMGR, March 2007)

Ans. Digestion is the process of mechanically and enzymatically breaking down food into substances for absorption into the bloodstream. Digestive enzymes belong to hydrolase class and their action is splitting up of large food molecules into their 'building block' components.

A. **Digestive enzymes of saliva:** *(AHSUC, May 2018)*
  1. **Salivary amylase/Ptylin/α-amylase:** Salivary amylase is a carbohydrate-digesting (amylolytic) enzyme. It acts on cooked or boiled starch and converts it into dextrin and maltose.
  2. **Maltase:** Maltase is present in human saliva and converts maltose into glucose.
  3. **Lingual lipase:** It is a lipid-digesting enzyme, secreted from serous glands of posterior aspect of tongue. It hydrolyzes triglycerides into fatty acids and diacylglycerol.

B. **Digestive enzymes of gastric juice:**
  1. **Pepsin:** Pepsin converts proteins into proteoses, peptones and polypeptides.
  2. **Gastric lipase:** Gastric lipase is a tributyrase and it hydrolyzes tributyrin (butter fat) into fatty acids and glycerols.
  3. **Gelatinase:** Degrades type I and type V gelatin and type IV and V collagen into peptides.

4. **Urase:** Acts on urea and produces ammonia.
5. **Gastric amylase:** Degrades starch (but its action is insignificant).
6. **Rennin:** Curdles milk (present in animals only).

C. **Digestive enzymes of pancreatic juice:**
  1. **Trypsin:** It acts on proteins and the end products are proteoses and polypeptides.
  2. **Chymotrypsin:** It acts on proteins and the end products are polypeptides.
  3. **Carboxypeptidases:** It acts on polypeptides and the end products are amino acids.
  4. **Nucleases:** It acts on RNA and DNA and the end products are mononucleotides.
  5. **Elastase:** It acts on elastin and the end products are amino acids.
  6. **Collagenase:** It acts on collagen and the end products are amino acids.
  7. **Pancreatic lipase:** It acts on triglycerides and the end products are monoglycerides and fatty acids.
  8. **Cholesterol ester hydrolase:** It acts on cholesterol ester and the end products are cholesterol and fatty acids.
  9. **Phospholipase A:** It acts on phospholipids and the end products are lysophospholipids.
  10. **Phospholipase B:** It acts on lysophospholipids and the end products are phosphoryl choline and free fatty acids.
  11. **Pancreatic lipase:** It acts on starch and the end products are dextrin and maltose.

D. **Digestive enzymes of intestine/succus entericus:**
  1. **Peptidases:** It acts on peptides and the end products are amino acids.
  2. **Sucrase:** It acts on sucrose and the end products are amino acids.
  3. **Maltase:** It acts on maltose and maltriose and the end products are glucose.
  4. **Lactase:** It acts on lactose and the end products are galactose and glucose.
  5. **Dextrinas:** It acts on dextrin, maltose, maltriose and the end products are glucose.
  6. **Trehalase:** It acts on trehalose and the end products are glucose.
  7. **Intestinal lipase:** It acts on triglycerides and the end products are fatty acids.

Applied Clinical Physiology

1. **Lactose intolerance** results from defective or deficient lactase and can result in bloating, flatulence, diarrhea, and the inability to acquire glucose and galactose from lactose.

2. **Paralytic ileus** is a condition where the normal peristaltic movements of the GIT are inhibited due to abdominal surgery or the use of anticholinergics.

3. **Zollinger-Ellison syndrome** is a condition of excessive gastrin production, which results in excessive hydrochloric acid production, thus leading to ulceration of GIT, discomfort, and hematemesis.

4. **In cystic fibrosis**, pancreatic insufficiency occurs, preventing digestion of proteins, fats, and carbohydrates in the lumen of small intestine.

5. **Cholelithiasis**, results in inability of bile to enter the lumen of duodenum, and, as such, fats are not emulsified.

Q. 7. Write about functions of liver.

(TNMGR, March 2009; RGUHS, May 2011)

Ans. Liver is the largest gland and one of the vital organs of the body.

1. **Metabolic function:** Liver is the organ where metabolism of carbohydrates, proteins, fats, vitamins and many hormones are carried out.

2. **Storage function:** Many substances like glycogen, amino acids, iron, folic acid and vitamins A, B_{12} and D are stored in liver.

3. **Synthetic function:** Liver produces glucose by gluconeogenesis. It synthesizes all plasma proteins and other proteins (except immunoglobulins) such as clotting factors, complement factors and hormone binding proteins. It also synthesizes steroids, somatomedin and heparin.

4. **Secretion of bile:** Liver secretes bile which contains bile salts, bile pigments, cholesterol, fatty acids and lecithin. Bile salts are required for digestion and absorption of fats in the intestine.

5. **Excretory function:** Liver excretes cholesterol, bile pigments, heavy metals, toxins, bacteria and virus through bile.

6. **Heat production:** Liver is the organ where maximum heat is produced.

7. **Hemopoietic function:** In fetus, liver produces blood cells. It produces thrombopoietin that promotes production of thrombocytes.

8. **Hemolytic function:** The senile RBCs are destroyed by Kupffer cells of liver.

9. **Inactivation of hormones and drugs:** Liver catabolizes the hormones, inactivates the drugs.

10. **Defensive and detoxification functions:** Reticuloendothelial cells (Kupffer cells) of liver play an important role in the defense of the body.
    i. Foreign bodies are swallowed and digested by these cells of liver by means of phagocytosis.

ii. Liver produces interleukins and tumor necrosis factors, which activate immune system of body.

iii. Liver cells are involved in removal of toxic property of various harmful substances.

11. **Role in childhood growth:** Liver produces insulin like growth factor-1, which has role on childhood growth.

Q. 8. Write about digestion of proteins.

(TNMGR, Nov. 2001)

Ans. Proteins present in common foodstuffs are:

1. Wheat: Glutenin and gliadin, which constitute gluten.
2. Milk: Casein, lactalbumin, albumin and myosin.
3. Egg: Albumin and vitellin.
4. Meat: Collagen, albumin and myosin.

Digestion of proteins: Enzymes responsible for digestion of proteins are called proteolytic enzymes.

1. **In the mouth:** Saliva does not contain any proteolytic enzymes.
2. **In the stomach:** Pepsin is the only proteolytic enzyme in gastric juice.
3. **In the small intestine:** Most of the proteins are digested in duodenum and jejunum by proteolytic enzymes of pancreatic juice and succus entericus.
   - **Proteolytic enzymes in pancreatic juice:** Pancreatic juice contains **trypsin, chymotrypsin** and **carboxypeptidases**.
4. **Final products of protein digestion:** Amino acids which are absorbed into blood from intestine.

Q. 9. Write about digestion of carbohydrates.

(TNMGR, April 2003)

Ans. Human diet contains three types of carbohydrates:

1. **Polysaccharides:** Large polysaccharides are glycogen, amylose and amylopectin, which are in the form of starch (glucose polymers). Glycogen is available in **non-vegetarian** diet. Amylose and amylopectin are available in **vegetarian diet**.

2. **Disaccharides:**
   i. Sucrose (Glucose + Fructose), is called table sugar or cane sugar.
   ii. Lactose (Glucose + Galactose), is the sugar available in milk.

3. **Monosaccharides:** Mostly glucose and fructose. Others include: Alcohol, lactic acid, pyruvic acid, pectins, dextrins, and carbohydrates in meat.

Digestion of Carbohydrates

1. **In the mouth:** The only amylolytic enzyme presents in saliva is the salivary amylase or ptyalin.

2. **In the stomach:** Gastric juice contains amylase (minor role in digestion).

3. **In the intestine:** Amylolytic enzymes present in small intestine are derived from:
   - **Pancreatic juice:** Pancreatic amylase.
   - **Succus entericus:** Maltase, sucrase, lactase, dextrinase and trehalase.

4. **Final products of carbohydrate digestion:** Mono-saccharides, which are glucose (80%), fructose and galactose (20%).

Q. 10. Write in detail about the calcium and phosphate mechanism. *(BFUHS, Nov. 2011; RGUHS, May 2013; RUHS, May 2015; MUHS, June 2015; HP Uni.,May 2018; April 2019)*

Q. Describe calcium homeostasis and its influence on oral tissues. *(TNMGR, Sept. 2007; March 2008; Oct. 2012; BFUHS, May 2010; HP Uni., May 2013; Gujarat Uni., April 2019)*

Q. Describe the role of hormones in regulations of blood calcium levels. *(Nagpur Uni., 1991; AHSUC, May 2018)*

Ans. Calcium is very essential for many activities in the body such as:

1. Bone and teeth formation.
2. Neuronal activity.
3. Skeletal muscle activity.
4. Cardiac activity.
5. Smooth muscle activity.
6. Secretory activity of the glands.
7. Cell division and growth.
8. Coagulation of blood.

Normal value: In a normal young healthy adult, there is about 1,100 g of calcium in the body. It forms about 1.5% of total body weight. 99% of calcium is present in bones and teeth and rest is present in plasma. Normal blood calcium= 9–11 mg/dl.

Types of calcium:
i. **Diffusible:**
   - Ionized: Found freely in plasma (50%). It is essential for vital functions.
   - Non-ionized: 8–10%
ii. **Non-diffusible** (bound to plasma protein): 40–42% of plasma calcium.

Calcium in bones: Calcium is constantly removed from bone and deposited in bone. Bone calcium is present in two forms:

i. Rapidly exchangeable calcium (exchangeable): Available in small quantity and helps to maintain the plasma calcium level.

ii. Slowly exchangeable calcium (stable): Available in large quantity, and helps in bone remodeling.

Source of calcium

1. **Dietary source:** Whole milk = 10%; Low fat milk = 18%; Cheese = 27%; Other dairy products = 17%; Vegetables = 7%; Others such as meat, egg, grains, sugar, coffee, tea, chocolate, etc. = 21%

2. **From bones:** Besides dietary calcium, blood also gets calcium from bone by resorption.

Daily requirements of calcium: 1–3 years = 500 mg; 4–8 years = 800 mg; 9–18 years = 1,300 mg; 19–50 years = 1,000 mg; >51 years = 1,200 mg; Pregnant ladies and lactating mother = 1,300 mg

Absorption from GIT: Calcium is absorbed from duodenum by carrier mediated active transport and from rest of small intestine, by facilitated diffusion. Vitamin D is essential for its absorption.

Excretion: While passing through the kidney, 98–99% of calcium is reabsorbed from renal tubules (distal convoluted tubules and proximal part of collecting duct) into the blood. Only a small quantity is excreted through urine. In distal convoluted tubule, PTH increases the reabsorption. In collecting duct, vitamin D increases the reabsorption and calcitonin decreases reabsorption.

Regulation of blood calcium level:

1. **Parathormone (PTH):** Increases blood calcium level by mobilizing calcium from bone.

2. **1, 25-dihydroxycholecalciferol (Calcitriol):** It is activated form of vitamin D. Its main action is to increase blood calcium level by increasing calcium absorption from small intestine.

3. **FGF23 (fibroblast growth factor 23):** FGF23 is a 251 amino acid peptide hormone produced by osteoblasts, osteocytes and flattened bone-lining cells. It decreases production of 1, 25-dihydroxycholecalciferol.

4. **Calcitonin:** It reduces blood calcium level mainly by decreasing bone resorption.

5. **Growth hormone:** Increases blood calcium level by increasing intestinal calcium absorption and also increases urinary excretion of calcium.

6. **Glucocorticoids:** Decrease blood calcium by inhibiting intestinal absorption and increasing renal excretion of calcium.

7. **Estrogen:** ↑serum calcium by increasing bone resorption in postmenopausal women.

8. **Insulin:** ↑serum calcium.
9. **Thyroid hormone:** ↑serum calcium.

Factors regulating calcium absorption:

a. Increasing absorption: Acidity, pregnancy, lactation, lactose, arginine, lysine.

b. Decreasing absorption: Oxalates, phytates, high dietary fats and fibers, phosphates, alkalinity, chronic renal failure, alcohol and smoking, lack of exercise.

PHOSPHATE METABOLISM

Phosphorus (P) is an essential mineral that is required by every cell in the body for normal function. Phosphorus is present in many food substances, such as peas, dried beans, nuts, milk, cheese and butter. Inorganic phosphorus (Pi) is in the form of **phosphate** (PO_4).

Importance of phosphate

1. It is an important component of organic substances and intermediates of metabolic pathways.
2. Along with calcium, it forms an important constituent of bone and teeth.
3. It forms a buffer in the maintenance of acid–base balance.

Normal value: Total amount of phosphate in the body is 500–800 g. Though it is present in every cell of the body, 85–90% of body's phosphate is found in the bones and teeth. Normal plasma level of phosphate is 4 mg/dl.

Regulation of phosphate level: Blood phosphate level is regulated mainly by three hormones:

1. **PTH:** Parathormone stimulates resorption of phosphate from bone and increases its urinary excretion. It also increases absorption of phosphate from GIT through calcitriol. The overall action of parathormone decreases plasma level of phosphate.
2. **Calcitonin:** Decreases plasma level of phosphate by inhibiting bone resorption and stimulating urinary excretion.
3. **1, 25-Dihydroxycholecalciferol:** Increases absorption of phosphate from small intestine.
4. **FGF23 (fibroblast growth factor 23):** It increases renal phosphate wasting, decreases production of 1, 25-dihydroxycholecalciferol and lowers serum phosphate.
5. **Growth hormone:** Increases phosphate level by increasing intestinal phosphate absorption.
6. **Glucocorticoids:** Decreases blood phosphate by inhibiting intestinal absorption and increasing renal excretion of phosphate.

Applied Clinical Physiology

1. Deficiency in calcium level during tooth development leads to: Enamel hypoplasia, poorly mineralized dentin, malformed teeth, elongated pulp chambers, anodontia or impacted teeth.
2. Toxic level of calcium leads to milk alkali syndrome.
3. When serum calcium is high, primary hyperparathyroidism and malignancy should be at the top of diagnostic list.
4. When it is low, renal disease, hypoparathyroidism, malabsorption, and vitamin D deficiency should be considered.
5. Chronically abnormal phosphate levels may be caused by renal failure, renal tubular defects, and abnormalities of FGF23 action.
6. Hyperparathyroidism: Painful bones, renal stones, abdominal groans, psychiatric moans.

Q. 11. Write a note on bone remodeling.
(RGUHS, Nov. 2011; TNMGR, Oct. 2016; MUHS, Oct. 2018)

Q. Write a short note on bone metabolism.
(HP Uni., May 2010)

Ans. Bone remodeling is a dynamic lifelong process in which old bone is resorbed and new bone is formed. Usually, it takes place in groups of bone cells called **basic multicellular units** (BMU).

Processes of bone remodeling

Bone resorption-Osteoclastic activity: It involves destruction of bone matrix, followed by removal of calcium by osteoclasts. Osteoclasts attach to the periosteal or endosteal surface of bone resorbing compartment through villi-like membranous extensions by the surface receptors, **integrins**. At the point of attachment, a ruffled border is formed by folding of the cell membrane and resorption occurs by release of substance from membranous extensions of osteoclasts like collagenase, phosphatase, lysosomal enzymes, acids like citric acid and lactic acid.

Bone formation-osteoblastic activity: This is the process which involves the synthesis of collagen and formation of bone matrix that is mineralized. Osteoblasts synthesize and release collagen into the shallow cavity formed after resorption in the bone resorbing compartment. The collagen fibers arrange themselves in regular units and form the organic matrix called osteoid.

Mineralization: Mineralization starts about 10–12 days after the formation of osteoid. First, a large quantity of calcium phosphate is deposited. Afterwards, the hydroxide and bicarbonate ions are gradually added causing the formation of **hydroxyapatite crystals.** The process of mineralization is accelerated by the enzyme alkaline phosphatase, secreted by osteoblast.

The completely mineralized bone surrounds the osteoblast. Now, the synthetic activity of osteoblast is reduced slowly and the cell is converted into osteocytes. Later, the bone is arranged in concentric lamellae on the inner surface of the cavity. At the end of the formation of new bone, the cavity is reduced to form Haversian canal.

Significance of bone remodeling
In children:
1. Thickness of bone increases.
2. Bone obtains strength in proportion to the growth.
3. Shape of the bone is realtered in relation to growth of the body.

In adults:
1. Toughness of bone is maintained.
2. Mechanical integrity of skeleton is ensured throughout life.
3. Blood calcium level is maintained.

Regulation of bone remodeling: Bone remodeling occurs continuously throughout the life. So a balance is maintained always between the bone resorption and bone formation. Apart from the physical stress, a variety of hormonal substances and growth factors are involved in regulation of bone resorption and bone formation.

Applied Clinical Physiology: Diseases of Bone
1. *Osteoporosis:* The loss of bone matrix and minerals leads to loss of bone strength associated with architectural deterioration of bone tissue. Ultimately, the bones become fragile with high-risk of fracture.
2. *Rickets:* Rickets is the bone disease in children characterized by inadequate mineralization of bone matrix. It occurs due to vitamin D deficiency. It causes inadequate mineralization of epiphyseal growth plate in growing bones. This defect produces various manifestations.
   i. Collapse of chest wall: Due to the flattening of sides of thorax with projecting sternum called **pigeon chest, chicken chest or pectus carinatum**.
   ii. Rachitic rosary: A visible swelling where the ribs join their cartilages.
   iii. Kyphosis: Excess curvature of upper back bone with convexity backward.
   iv. Lordosis: Excess forward curvature of back bone in lumbar region.
   v. Scoliosis: Lateral curvature of spine.
   vi. Bowing of hands and legs.
   vii. Enlargement of liver and spleen.
   viii. Tetany in advanced stages.
3. *Osteomalacia:* The rickets in adults is called osteomalacia or adult rickets. It also occurs due to prolonged damage of kidney (renal rickets). The characteristic features of osteomalacia:
   i. Vague pain.
   ii. Tenderness in bones and muscles.
   iii. Myopathy leading to waddling gait (resembles that of duck).
   iv. Occasional hypoglycemic tetany

7. RENAL SYSTEM

Q. 1. Write a note on juxtaglomerular apparatus.
(TNMGR, April 2001; NTR Uni., May 2018)

Ans. Juxtaglomerular apparatus (JGA) is a specialized organ situated near the glomerulus of each nephron (juxta = near). It is formed at the point of contact between nephron's distal tubule and vascular pole of its glomerulus.

Structure of JGA:
1. **Macula densa:** It is the end portion of thick ascending segment before it opens into distal convoluted tubule, situated between afferent and efferent arterioles of nephron. It is formed by tightly packed cuboidal epithelial cells, close to afferent arteriole.
2. **Extraglomerular mesangial cells/agranular cells/ Lacis cells/Goormaghtigh cells:** They are situated in the triangular region bound by afferent arteriole, efferent arteriole and macula densa.
3. **Glomerular mesangial cells/intraglomerular mesangial cells:** Mesangial cells situated in between glomerular capillaries. These cells play an important role in regulating glomerular filtration by their contractile property and are phagocytic in nature. These cells also secrete glomerular interstitial matrix, prostaglandins and cytokines.
4. **Juxtaglomerular cells/Granular cells:** They are specialized smooth muscle cells situated in the wall of afferent arteriole just before it enters the Bowman capsule. These smooth muscle cells are mostly present in tunica media and tunica adventitia of the wall of the afferent arteriole. They form a thick cuff called **polar cushion** or **polkissen** around the afferent arteriole before it enters the Bowman capsule.

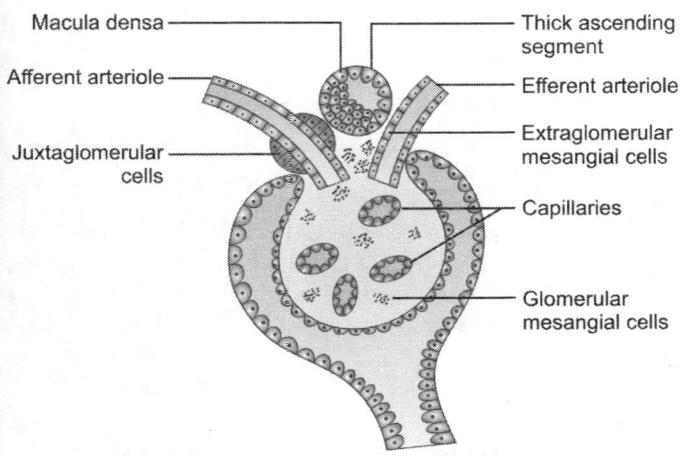

Fig. 7.1: Structure of juxtaglomerular apparatus

Macula densa
Afferent arteriole
Juxtaglomerular cells
Thick ascending segment
Efferent arteriole
Extraglomerular mesangial cells
Capillaries
Glomerular mesangial cells

Functions:

1. **Secretion of hormones:** 1. Renin. 2. Prostaglandin.
2. Secretion of other substances
   - Extraglomerular mesangial cells of JGA secrete cytokines like interleukin-2 and tumor necrosis factor.
   - Macula densa secretes thromboxane A_2.
3. **Regulation of glomerular blood flow and glomerular filtration rate:** Macula densa of juxtaglomerular apparatus plays an important role in the feedback mechanism called **tubuloglomerular feedback** mechanism, which regulates the renal blood flow and glomerular filtration rate.

Q. 2. Write a short note on glomerular filtration.

[TNMGR, April 2003]

Ans. It is the process by which blood is filtered while passing through the glomerular capillaries by filtration membrane. It is the first process of urine formation.

Process of glomerular filtration (ultrafilteration): When blood passes through glomerular capillaries, the plasma is filtered into the Bowman capsule. All the substances of plasma are filtered except plasma proteins. The filtered fluid is called **glomerular filtrate**.

Glomerular filtration rate (GFR): GFR is defined as the total quantity of filtrate formed in all the nephrons of both kidneys in given unit of time. Normal GFR is 125 ml/minute or 180 L/day.

Filtration fraction: It is the fraction of renal plasma, which becomes the filtrate. It is the ratio between renal plasma flow and GFR. Normal filtration fraction varies from 15–20%.

Pressures determining filtration:

1. **Glomerular capillary pressure:** Pressure exerted by blood in glomerular capillaries. It is about 60 mm Hg (45–70 mm Hg). This pressure favors glomerular filtration.
2. **Colloidal osmotic pressure:** Pressure exerted by plasma proteins in the glomeruli (25 mm Hg). It opposes glomerular filtration.
3. **Hydrostatic pressure in Bowman capsule:** Pressure exerted by the filtrate in Bowman capsule (15 mm Hg). It also opposes glomerular filtration.

Net filtration pressure/effective or essential filtration pressure: Balance between pressure favoring filtration and pressures opposing filtration. Net filtration pressure = 60 – (25 + 15) = 20 mm Hg.

Starling hypothesis and Starling forces: It states that the net filtration through capillary membrane is proportional to hydrostatic pressure difference across the membrane minus oncotic pressure difference. All the pressures involved in determination of filtration are called **Starling forces**.

Filtration coefficient: It is the GFR per mm Hg of net filtration pressure.

Factors regulating (affecting) GFR

1. **Renal blood flow:** GFR is directly proportional to renal blood flow.
2. **Tubuloglomerular feedback:** Macula densa is sensitive to this and secretes prostaglandin (PGE_2), bradykinin and renin. PGE_2 and bradykinin cause dilatation of afferent arteriole. Renin induces the formation of angiotensin II, which causes constriction of efferent arteriole. Both lead to ↑ in glomerular blood flow and GFR.
3. **Glomerular capillary pressure:** GFR is directly proportional to this.
4. **Colloidal osmotic pressure:** GFR is inversely proportional to colloidal osmotic pressure.
5. **Hydrostatic pressure in Bowman capsule:** GFR is inversely proportional to this.
6. **Constriction of afferent arteriole:** This reduces blood flow to capillaries, hence ↓ GFR.
7. **Constriction of efferent arteriole:** If efferent arteriole is constricted, ↑ GFR.
8. **Systemic arterial pressure:** Variation in blood pressure >180 mm Hg or <60 mm Hg affects renal blood flow and GFR accordingly.
9. **Sympathetic stimulation:** Initially there is increase in filtration but later it decreases as afferent and efferent arterioles are supplied by sympathetic nerves.
10. **Surface area of capillary membrane:** GFR is directly proportional to this.

11. **Permeability of capillary membrane:** GFR is directly proportional to this.
12. **Contraction of glomerular mesangial cells:** It results in ↓ in GFR.
13. **Hormonal and other factors:**
    - Factors ↑ GFR by vasodilatation: i. Atrial natriuretic peptide, ii. Brain natriuretic peptide, iii. cAMP, iv. Dopamine, v. Endothelial-derived nitric oxide, vi. Prostaglandin (PGE_2).
    - Factors ↓ GFR by vasoconstriction: i. Angiotensin II, ii. Endothelins, iii. Noradrenaline, iv. Platelet-activating factor, v. Platelet-derived growth factor, vi. Prostaglandin (PGF_2).

Applied Clinical Physiology

1. Acute kidney injury is an abrupt increase in serum creatinine.
2. Chronic kidney disease is often irreversible damage and persistent over at least 3 months. Chronic kidney disease is staged on the bases of GFR as follows:

   Stage 1: Normal, >90 ml/min.

   Stage 2: Mild, 60–89 ml/min.

   Stage 3a: Mild to moderate, 45–59 ml/min

   Stage 3b: Moderate to severe, 30–44 ml/min.

   Stage 4: Severe, 15–29 ml/min.

   Stage 5: Failure, <15 ml/min.

Q. 3. Define tubular maximum for glucose (TMG). What is the normal value? Mention the other substances which have tubular maximum.

(TNMGR, Oct. 2003)

Ans. Tubular transport maximum (Tm) is rate at which maximum amount of an actively transported substance is reabsorbed from renal tubule, e.g. **Tm** for glucose is 375 mg/minute.

Threshold level in plasma for substances having Tm value: Renal threshold is the plasma concentration at which a substance appears in urine. Every substance having Tm value has also a threshold level in plasma or blood. Below that threshold level, the substance is completely reabsorbed and does not appear in urine. When the concentration of that substance reaches the threshold, the excess amount is not reabsorbed and, so it appears in urine. This level is called the **renal threshold** of that substance, e.g. renal threshold for glucose is 180 mg/dl. That is, glucose is completely reabsorbed from tubular fluid if its concentration in blood is below 180 mg/dl. So, the glucose does not appear in urine. When the blood level of glucose reaches 180 mg/dl it is not reabsorbed completely; hence it appears in urine.

Table 7.3: Tm for other substances

Substance	Transport maximum
Glucose	375 mg/min
Phosphate	0.10 mM/min
Sulfate	0.06 mM/min
Amino acids	1.5 mM/min
Urate	15 mg/min
Lactate	75 mg/min
Plasma protein	30 mg/min

Q. 4. Write a note on renin-angiotensin system.

(RGUHS, May 2011)

Ans. The renin-angiotensin system (RAS) is composed of three major compounds: Renin, angiotensin II, and aldosterone.

Organs system involved: Kidneys, lungs, systemic vasculature and brain.

Function: RAS functions to elevate blood volume and arterial tone in a prolonged manner. It does this by increasing sodium reabsorption, water reabsorption, and vascular tone.

Mechanism (Fig. 7.4): Within the afferent arterioles of kidney, juxtaglomerular (JG) cells contain prorenin which is secreted constitutively in its inactive form; activation of JG cells (in response to ↓ blood pressure, β-activation, or activation by macula densa cells in response to a decreased sodium load in the distal convoluted tubule) causes cleavage of prorenin to renin,

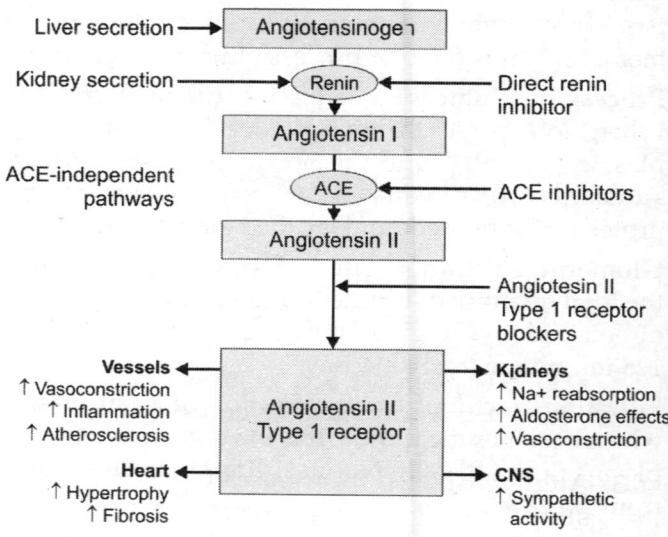

Fig. 7.4: Renin-angiotensin-aldosterone system with mechanism of action of drugs acting on this system

which acts on plasma protein called **angiotensinogen** or **renin substrate** (α_2-globulin), converting it into **angiotensin I**. **Angiotensin I** is converted into **angiotensin II** by angiotensin converting enzyme (ACE) secreted from lungs. **Angiotensin II** is rapidly degraded into **angiotensin III** by **angiotensinases**, which are present in RBCs and vascular beds in many tissues. Angiotensin III is converted into angiotensin IV.

Actions of Angiotensins

1. **Angiotensin I:** Physiologically inactive and serves as precursor of angiotensin II.
2. **Angiotensin II:** Angiotensin II is the most active form. Its actions are:
   - **On blood vessels:** It increases arterial blood pressure directly by vasoconstriction and indirectly by increasing release of noradrenaline from postganglionic sympathetic fibers.
   - **On adrenal cortex:** It stimulates zona glomerulosa of adrenal cortex to secrete aldosterone. Aldosterone acts on renal tubules and increases retention of sodium, which is responsible for elevation of blood pressure.
   - **On kidney:**
     i. Angiotensin II regulates GFR as:
        a. It constricts efferent arteriole, which causes decrease in filtration after an initial increase.
        b. It contracts glomerular mesangial cells leading to decrease in surface area of glomerular capillaries and filtration.
     ii. It increases sodium reabsorption from renal tubules.
   - **On brain:**
     i. It inhibits **baroreceptor reflex** and thereby indirectly increases blood pressure.
     ii. It increases water intake by stimulating thirst center.
     iii. It increases secretion of corticotropin-releasing hormone (CRH) from hypothalamus. CRH in turn increases secretion of ACTH from pituitary.
     iv. It increases secretion of ADH from hypothalamus.
   - **Other actions:** It acts as growth factor in heart and causes muscular hypertrophy and cardiac enlargement.
3. **Angiotensin III:** It increases blood pressure and stimulates aldosterone secretion from adrenal cortex.
4. **Angiotensin IV:** It also has adrenocortical stimulating and vasopressor activities.

Applied Clinical Physiology

1. RAS can be activated inappropriately in many conditions that may lead to development of hypertension, e.g. in renal artery stenosis.
2. Pharmacologically, RAS is frequently manipulated system in management of heart failure, hypertension, diabetes mellitus, and acute myocardial infarction, e.g. ACE inhibitors, angiotensin receptor blockers, and aldosterone antagonists all act to decrease effect of the RAS (Fig. 7.4).

8. CENTRAL NERVOUS SYSTEM

Q. 1. Write a short note on structure of nerve fiber.

Ans. The basic unit of the nervous system is neuron. It consists of 3 main parts (Fig. 8.1):

1. **Nerve cell body/Soma/Perikaryon:** It is constituted by a mass of cytoplasm (neuroplasm), containing a large nucleus, Nissl bodies, neurofibrils, mitochondria and Golgi apparatus. It does not contain centrosome so nerve cell cannot multiply.
2. **Dendrite:** They are short and branched processes of neuron. They are repeatedly branched. They transmit impulses towards nerve cell body.
3. **Axon:** Each neuron has only one axon. It arises from axon hillock of nerve cell body. It transmits impulses away from nerve cell body.

Organization: Many nerve fibers or axons form one bundle or fasciculus. Many fasciculi form a nerve. Two

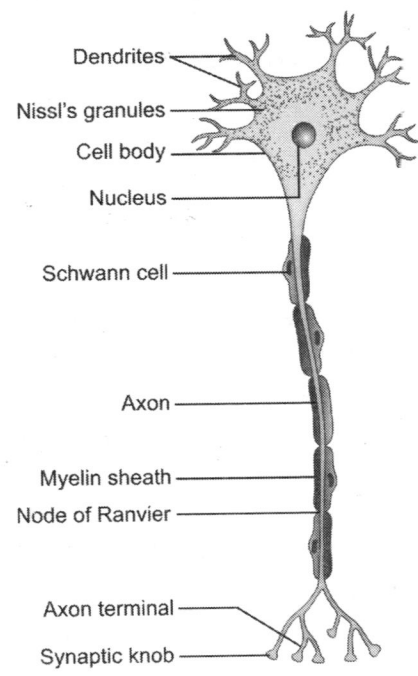

Dendrites
Nissl's granules
Cell body
Nucleus
Schwann cell
Axon
Myelin sheath
Node of Ranvier
Axon terminal
Synaptic knob

Fig. 8.1: Structure of neuron

or more nerves form the nerve trunk. The nerve is covered by epineurium, fasciculus by epineurium, nerve fiber or axon by endoneurium.

Myelin sheath: It is a thick lipoprotein sheath that insulates the myelinated nerve fiber. It is absent at regular intervals known as node of Ranvier. Segment of nerve fiber between 2 nodes is called internode.

Functions:
1. In myelinated nerve fibers, transmission of impulses is called saltatory conduction.
2. Myelin sheath restricts the nerve impulse within single nerve fiber and prevents the stimulation of neighboring nerve fibers.

Neurilemma: It is also called neurilemma sheath or sheath of Schwann. It surrounds the axis cylinder. It contains Schwann cells.

Functions:
i. It serves as covering membrane in non-myelinated nerve fibers.
ii. It helps in formation of myelin sheath in myelinated nerve fibers.

Q. 2. Describe the mechanism of conduction of nerve impulse. *(TNMGR, March 2007; BFUHS, Nov. 2011; HNBG Uni., July 2015)*

Ans. Nerve impulse is an overall physiological change that occurs in a neuron due to mechanical, chemical or electrical disturbance created by a stimulus. Its propagation through axon, synapse and neuromuscular junction is called nerve impulse conduction.

Nerve impulse conduction has three steps:
A. **Polarization/Resting potential** (Fig. 8.2A): A neuron at resting is electrically charged but not conducting. The axoplasm or plasma membrane of a resting neuron is negatively charged as compared to the interstitial fluid. The potential difference measured at this stage is called **resting potential** which is about -70 mV. The interstitial fluid has high concentration of Na^+ (16 times higher outside than inside). Similarly, the axoplasm has high concentration of K^+ (25 times higher inside than outer interstitial fluids).
1. Due to difference in concentration of ions, Na^+ tends to diffuse into the axoplasm and K^+ tends to diffuse outside the axoplasm.

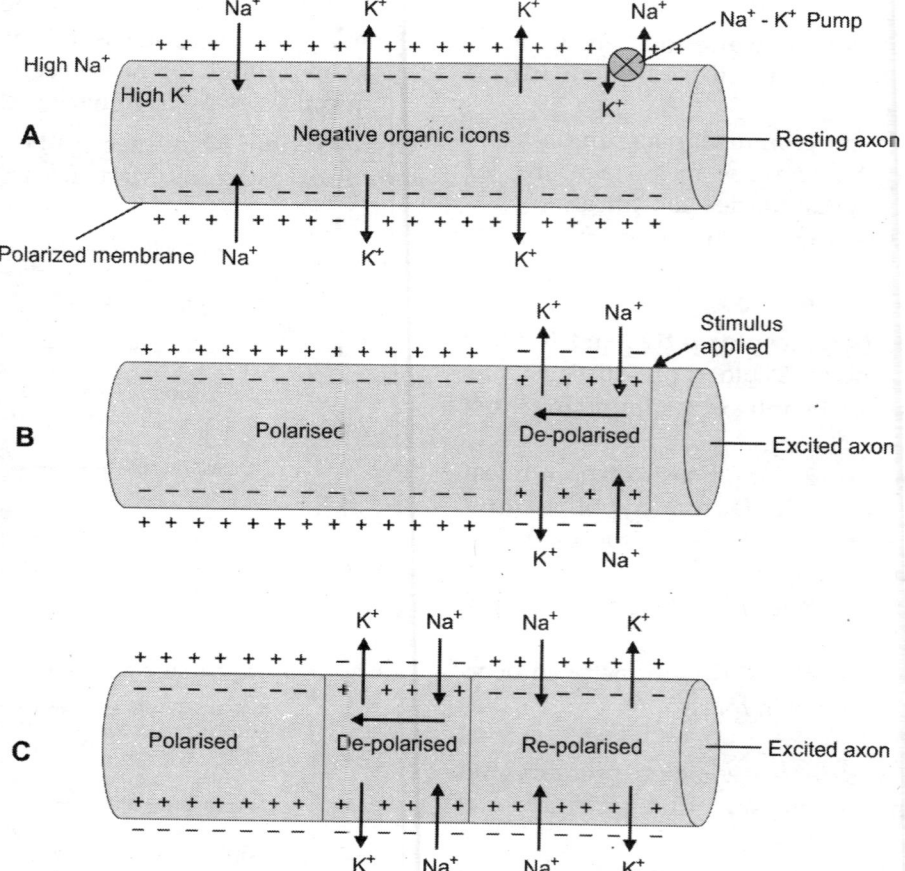

Fig. 8.2: Conduction of nerve impulse. A. Resting potential, B. Action potential, C. Repolarization

2. The membrane of neuron at resting is more permeable to K$^+$ than Na$^+$, So, K$^+$ leaves the neuron faster than Na$^+$ enter the neuron.
3. The difference in permeability results in accumulation of high concentration of cation outside the neuron.
4. This state of resting neuron is called *polarized state* and it is electronegatively charged.

B. **Depolarization/action potential** (Fig. 8.2B): Any stimulus beyond the threshold can initiate an impulse.
  1. When such stimulus is applied in the resting neuron, it opens the sodium channel. Now the permeability of Na$^+$ increases at the point of stimulus causing depolarization.
  2. The diffusion of Na$^+$ increases by 10 times from outside to inside. As a result the axoplasm become positively charges, which is exact opposite to polarized state, so called *depolarized state* or *reverse polarized state*.
  3. The depolarization of membrane stimulates adjacent voltage channel, so the action potential passes as a wave along the length of neuron.

C. **Repolarization** (Fig. 8.2C): When the concentration of Na$^+$ inside axoplasm increases, the permeability to Na$^+$ decreases and the sodium channel starts to close.
  1. The Na-K pump activates, so that Na$^+$ are pumped out and K$^+$ inside until the original resting potential is restored. The process is known as **repolarization** and it starts from the same point from where depolarization starts.

2. The entire process of polarization, depolarization and repolarization occurs within fraction of seconds. Now, again the neuron is read for another impulse.

Saltatory conduction: Saltatory conduction is the form of conduction of nerve impulse in which, impulse jumps from one node to another. Conduction of impulse through a myelinated nerve fiber is about 50 times faster than through a nonmyelinated fiber.

Mechanism of saltatory conduction: Myelin sheath is not permeable to ions. So, the entry of sodium from extracellular fluid into nerve fiber occurs only in the node of Ranvier, where the myelin sheath is absent. It causes depolarization in the node and not in the internode. Thus, depolarization occurs at successive nodes. So, the action potential jumps from one node to another. Hence, it is called saltatory conduction (saltare = jumping).

Q. 3. Write a short note on structure of muscle fibers.

Ans. Human body has more than 600 muscles. Muscles perform many useful functions and help us in doing everything in day-to-day life.
Classification:
a. **Depending upon the presence or absence of striations:** Striated and non-striated
b. **Depending upon the control:** Voluntary and involuntary.
c. **Depending upon the situation:** Skeletal muscle, cardiac muscle and smooth muscle.

Structure of skeletal muscle (Fig. 8.3): Each muscle fiber is cylindrical in shape. Average length of fiber is

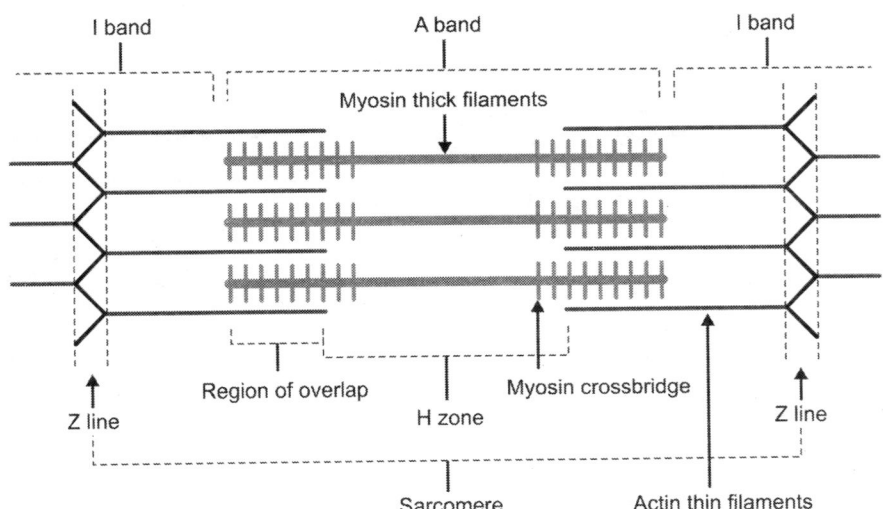

Fig. 8.3: Microscopic structure of muscle

3 cm. Diameter of fiber is 10–100 µ. Muscle is attached to bone through tendon. If tendon is thin, flat and stretched but tough, it is called aponeurosis.

Composition: Skeletal muscle is formed by 75% water and 25% solids. Myoglobin present in sarcoplasm is called myohemoglobin.

Myofibril: They are fine parallel filaments present in sarcoplasm of muscle fibers. They run through entire length of muscle fiber. When myofibrils are arranged in groups, they are called *Cohnhein's areas* or *fields*. Each myofibril consists of two alternating bands: Light band (I band) and dark band (A band). I-band is divided into two portions by means of narrow and dark lines called Z-lines. The portion of myofibril in between two Z-lines is called sarcomere. In the middle of A-band, there is a light area called H-zone. In the middle of H zone lies the middle part of myosin filament. This is called M-line. M-line is formed by myosin binding proteins.

Sarcomere: It is defined as structural and functional unit of a skeletal muscle. It is also called basic contractile unit of the muscle. In relaxed state, average length of each sarcomere is 2–3 µ. It extends between two Z-lines.

Q. 4. Write about molecular mechanism of muscle contraction. *(KUHS, Jan. 2014)*

Q. What is meant by excitation–contraction coupling? Explain the mechanism. *(TNMGR, Oct. 2003)*

Ans. Action potential travels from nerve endings to muscle fibers, causing release of neurotransmitter acetylcholine (ACh). ACh acts on receptor (ACh gated cation channel) and causes large influx of Na^+. Now the action potential travels along muscle fiber similar to nerve and causes release of Ca^{2+} from sarcoplasmic reticulum, which initiates contractile process (actin-myosin slide along each other). Ca^{2+} pumps back into sarcoplasmic reticulum and the contraction ceases.

Mechanism of muscle contraction: It includes:

1. **Excitation–contraction coupling:** When a muscle is excited (stimulated) by the impulses, action potential is generated in the muscle fiber, which spreads over sarcolemma (cell membrane of muscle fibers) and also into the muscle fiber through the 'T' tubules. When the action potential reaches the cisternae of 'L' tubules, these cisternae are excited, releasing calcium ions. The calcium ions move towards the actin filaments to produce the contraction.

2. **Role of troponin and tropomyosin:** Large number of calcium ions, which are released from 'L' tubules during the excitation of the muscle, bind with troponin C. It in turn pulls tropomyosin molecule away from F actin, exposing the active site of F actin. Immediately the head of myosin gets attached to the actin.

3. **Sliding mechanism and formation of actomyosin complex (sliding theory)** (Fig. 8.4) *(NTR Uni., July 2014)*: It is also called **ratchet theory** or **walk along theory**. Sarcomere is the smallest unit of muscle contraction. After binding with active site of F actin, the myosin head is tilted towards the arm so that the actin filament is dragged along with it. The head immediately breaks away from the active site and

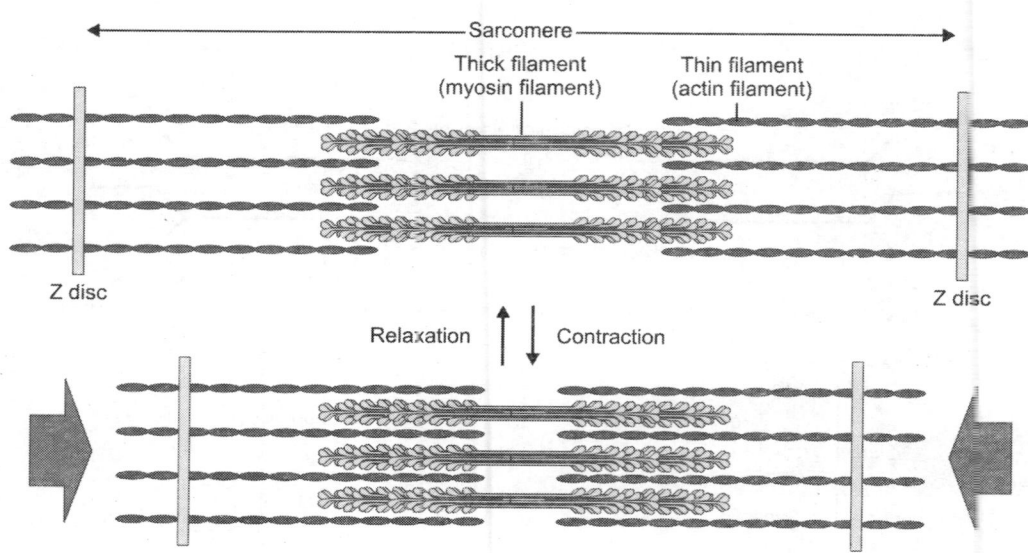

Fig. 8.4: Mechanism of muscle contraction (sliding filament theory)

returns to the original position. Now, it combines with a new active site on the actin molecule, and the tilting movement occurs again. So, the actin filaments of opposite sides overlap and form actomyosin complex. Formation of actomyosin complex results in contraction of the muscle.

Q. 5. Write a short note on neuromuscular transmission.

Ans. It is defined as the transfer of information from motor nerve ending to muscle fiber through neuromuscular junction. This mechanism initiates the muscle contraction by motor nerve impulses.

Events of neuromuscular transmission are (Fig. 8.5):
1. Release of acetylcholine.
2. Action of acetylcholine.
3. Development of endplate potential.
4. Development of miniature endplate potential.
5. Destruction of acetylcholine.
   - **Reuptake process:** It is a process in neuromuscular junction, by which a degraded product of neurotransmitter re-enters the presynaptic axon terminal where it is reused.

Q. 6. Describe the physiology of pain.
(MUHS, June 2010; BFUHS, Oct. 2010; TNMGR, Oct. 2012; Sumandeep Uni., May 2018)

Q. Discuss the types, properties, pathways and mechanism of pain.
(TNMGR, Feb. 2005; March 2010; April 2013; RGUHS, Oct. 2010; June 2018; SGT Uni., May 2019)

Q. Write a short note on orofacial pain.
(MUHS, June 2010; BBD Uni., July 2016)

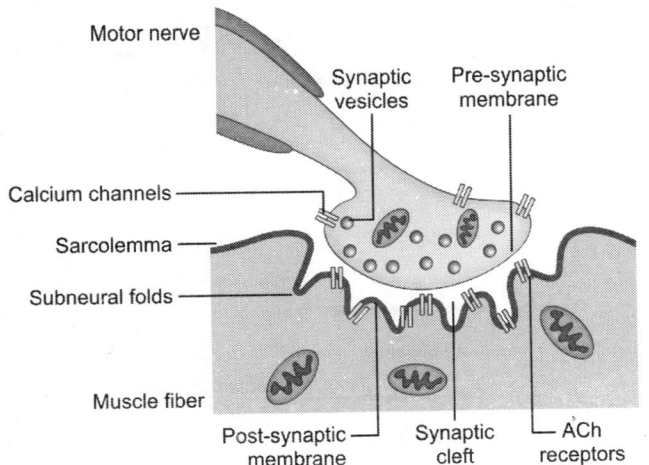

Fig. 8.5: Neuromuscular junction

Q. Write a note on pathway of dental pain.
(TNMGR, April 1995; HP Uni., April 2019)

Ans. Pain is defined as "an unpleasant and emotional experience associated with actual or potential tissue damage, or described in terms of such damage." *(International Association for Study of Pain)*

Benefits of pain sensation:
1. Pain gives warning signal about a problem or threat. It also creates awareness of injury.
2. Pain prevents further damage by causing reflex withdrawal of body from source of injury.
3. Pain forces the person to rest or to minimize activities, enabling rapid healing of injured part.
4. Pain urges the person to take required treatment to prevent major damage.

Classification of Pain

First Classification
A. **Somatic (Somasthetic):**
   1. Superficial: From skin and muocus membrane.
   2. Deep: From muscles/bone/fascia/periosteum.
B. **Visceral:** From viscera/internal organs.

Second Classification
A. Odontogenic: *(NTR Uni., April 2013)*
   1. Pulpal pain: a. Reversible pulpitis, b. Irreversible Pulpitis.
   2. Peripical/periodontal pain: a. Acute apical periodontitis, b. Acute apical abscess
   3. Heterotopic pain (pain felt in an area other than its true site of origin): a. Projected pain (perceived in the anatomic distribution of same nerve that mediates the primary pain), b. Referred pain (perceived in the area innervated by different nerve from one that mediates the primary pain
B. **Non-odontogenic:**
   1. Musculoskeletal: MPDS, TMDs
   2. Neuropathic: Trigeminal neuralgia, glossopharyngeal neuralgia.
   3. Neurovascular: Migraine, cluster headache.
   4. Inflammatory: Allergic sinusitis, bacterial sinusitis.
   5. Systemic disorders: Cardiac pain, herpes zoster
   6. Psychogenic: Munchausen's syndrome.

Pulpal pain/pulpalgia: Increased pulpal pressure due to hyperemia/heat application stimulates the nerve ending, causing pain. $A\delta$ type afferent fibers (myelinated) have low response threshold, transmit sharp, localized pain and respond to cold stimulation. They are extensively distributed in the pulp dentin border, penetrating the inner part of dentin. C fibers (unmyelinated) have higher activation threshold, transmits dull, poorly localized pain and responds to heat stimulation they are located in the pulp proper (Fig. 8.6A).

Process of Pain Physiology

1. Transduction: Pain stimuli are converted to electrical energy. This stimulus sends an inpile across a peripheral nerve fiber.
2. Transmission: Pain stimuli travel via spinothalamic tract through Aδ and C-fibers.
3. Perception: Somatosensory cortex identifies the location and intensity of pain.
4. Modulation: Inhibitory neurotransmitters hinder the pain transmission.

Pathways of pain sensation (TNMGR, Oct. 2012) (Fig. 8.6B)

1. **From skin and deeper structures:** Receptors of pain sensation are the free nerve endings.
   - **First order neurons:** These are the cells in posterior nerve root ganglia, which receive impulses of pain sensation from pain receptors through their dendrites and transmit them to spinal cord.
     a. **Fast pain fibers:** Fast pain sensation is carried by Aδ type afferent fibers which synapse with neurons of *marginal nucleus* in the posterior gray horn.
     b. **Slow pain fibers:** Slow pain sensation is carried by C type afferent fibers, which synapse with neurons of *substantia gelatinosa of Rolando* in the posterior gray horn.
   - **Second order neurons:** These are formed by neurons of *marginal nucleus* and *substantia gelatinosa of Rolando*. Fibers from these neurons ascend in the form of lateral spinothalamic tract.

   a. **Fast pain fibers:** They arise from neurons of *marginal nucleus*, cross midline and ascend to form *neospinothalamic fibers* in lateral spinothalamic tract. These nerve fibers terminate in ventral posterolateral nucleus of thalamus.
   b. **Slow pain fibers:** They arise from neurons of *substantia gelatinosa*, cross midline and run along the fibers of fast pain as *paleospinothalamic fibers* in lateral spinothalamic tract. 1/5th of these fibers terminate in ventral posterolateral nucleus of thalamus and remaining in nuclei of reticular formation in brainstem, tectum of midbrain and gray matter surrounding aqueduct of Sylvius.

   - **Third order neurons:** Third order neurons of pain pathway are the neurons in: Thalamic nucleus, reticular formation, tectum, Gray matter around aqueduct of Sylvius. Axons from these neurons reach sensory area of cerebral cortex (post central gyrus of parietal cortex). Some fibers from reticular formation reach hypothalamus.

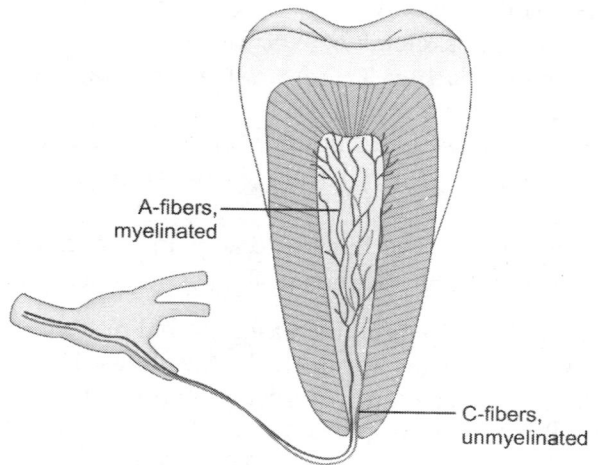

Fig. 8.6A: Distribution of pain receptors in the pulp

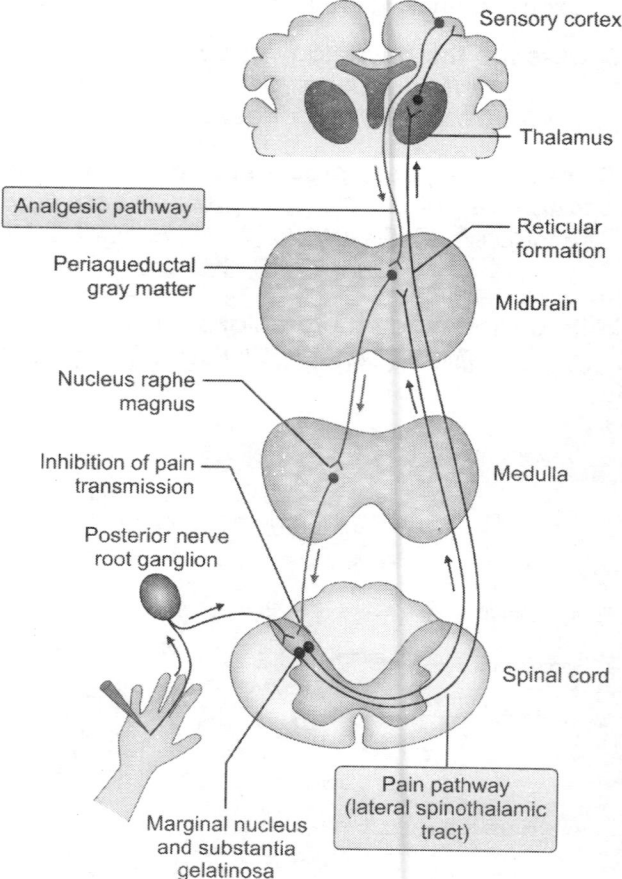

Fig. 8.6B: Pain pathway from skin and other deeper structures

2. **From face:** Pain sensation from face is carried by trigeminal nerve (Fig. 8.6C).

- **Pain perception:** Physioanatomical process by which pain is received and transmitted by neural structures from the end organs or pain receptors, through conductive and perceptive mechanism.
- **Pain reaction:** It represents individual's manifestation of unpleasant reaction and involves complex neuroanatomical and psychological factors.
- *Nociceptors* are receptors sensitive to noxious stimuli. These are the free nerve endings mostly of myelinated fibres. These are found in orofacial skin, oral mucosa, TMJ, peridontium, tooth pulp, periosteum and muscles, etc. These nociceptors are attached to first order neurons of afferents. The two major classes of afferent nerves that provide input to brain are:
  1. **Aδ fibers:** They conduct pain fast or first which is sharp and localized.
  2. **C fibers:** They conduct slow/second pain.

Pain pathways:

1. Ophthalmic division: Skin of parietal, frontal region, eyes, nose, orbit and upper part of nasal cavity.
2. Maxillary divison: Anterior portion of temple, malar, maxillary and nasal cavity, palate, maxillary sinus, maxillary teeth and gums.
3. Mandibular division: posterior temple, tragus, preauricular area, masseter area, mandibular region, anterior two-thirds of tongue, mandibular teeth and gums, masticatory muscles, tensor muscles of soft palate and tympanic membrane.
4. Upper second and third cervical nerves: Superficial structures of head and neck posterior to trigeminal area and below the lower border of mandible, cervical area.
5. Facial nerve: Facial skin in mastoid region, external auditory meatus.
6. Glossopharyngeal nerve: Posterior part of tongue, tonsillar region, tympanic cavity and antrum.

Transmission of impulses in the CNS: Nerves supplying facial and oral tissues carry information of pain through **semilunar or gasserian ganglion,**

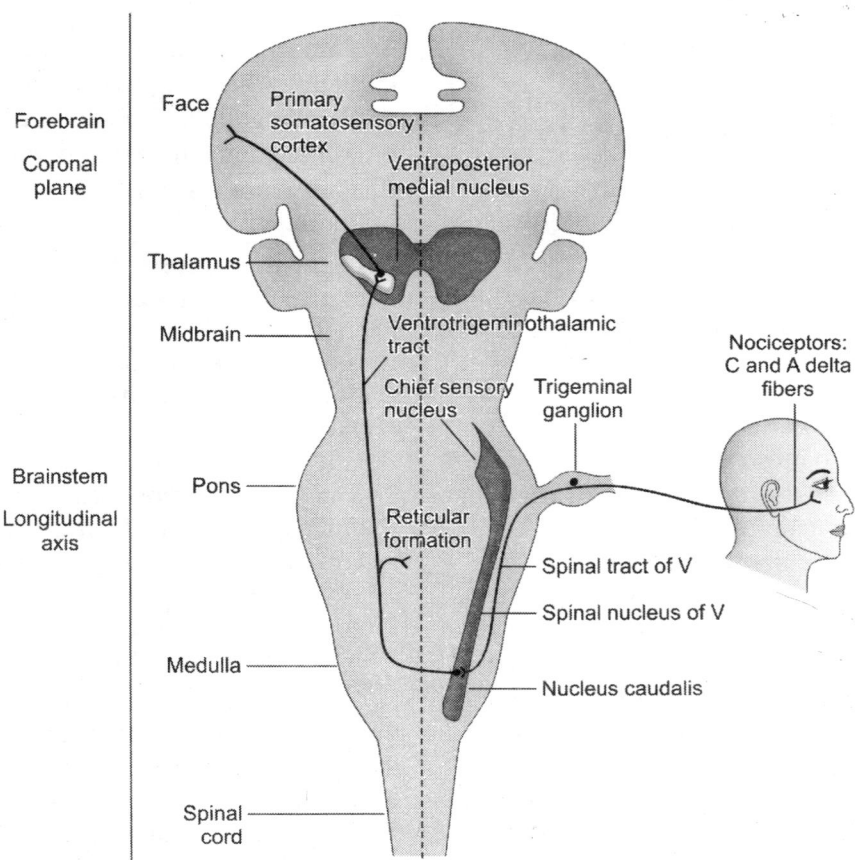

Fig. 8.6C: Pain pathway from oral and maxillofacial region

where primary afferent cell bodies are located. From ganglion, the impulse is mediated by sensory root of the nerve into pons as main sensory nucleus or bifurcates into ascending and descending fibers. The *ascending fibers* convey general tactile sensibility, whereas **descending fibres** convey pain and temperature. Thus pain impulse descends from pons by spinal tract fibres of trigeminal nerve, through medulla, down to the level of second cervical segment, where the tract terminates. Axons of the secondary neurons emerge from spinal nucleus, cross midline and ascend to join with fibres of mesencephalic nucleus to form **trigeminal lemniscus** or **spinothalamic tracts of 5th nerve.** These tracts continue upward and terminate in posteroventral nucleus of thalamus. Here the pain impulse is mediated by secondary connecting neurons that projects from posteroventral thalamus to posterocentral convolutions of the cerebral cortex. Once the impulse reaches thalamus, it is sent to sensory cortex and limbic structure and hypothalamus where it is recognized as pain.

3. **From viscera:** Pain sensation from thoracic and abdominal viscera is transmitted by sympathetic (thoracolumbar) nerves. Pain from esophagus, trachea and pharynx is carried by vagus and glossopharyngeal nerves.

4. **From pelvic region:** Pain sensation from deeper structures of pelvic region is conveyed by sacral parasympathetic nerves.

Visceral pain: Pain from viscera is unpleasant. It is poorly localized.

Causes of visceral pain: Ischemia, chemical stimuli, spasm and over-distention of hollow organs.

Applied Clinical Physiology

1. **Algesia:** Pain sensation.
2. **Analgesia:** Loss of pain sensation.
3. **Hyperpathia:** Threshold for stimulation is increased causing burning pain.
4. **Phantom pain:** Pain in absent limb.
5. **Causalgia:** Spontaneous burning pain long after trivial injuries.
6. **Hyperalgesia:** Hyperalgesia is defined as the increased sensitivity to pain sensation.
7. **Allodynia:** Sensation of pain in response to an innocuous stimulus.
8. **Paralgesia:** Abnormal pain sensation is called paralgesia.
9. **Syringomyelia:** Loss of pain and temperature with sparing of touch and vibration.

10. **WHO analgesic ladder:**
    - **Step 1: Mild to moderate pain.** Non-opioid (paracetamol, aspirin or NSAID) +/– an adjuvant (low dose tricyclic antidepressant/anticonvulsant/muscle relaxant/other NSAIDs)
    - **Step 2: Moderate to severe pain.** Weak opioid (codeine/tramadol) +/– a non-opioid +/– an adjuvant
    - **Step 3: Severe pain.** Strong opioid (morphine/fentanyl/diamorphine) +/– a non-opioid +/– an adjuvant

Q. 7. Define and write about mechanism of referred pain. *(TNMGR, Nov. 1995; Oct. 1996)*

Q. Write about the physiology of referred pain. *(UHSR, May 2016; AHSUC, May 2018)*

Ans. Referred pain is the pain that is perceived at a site adjacent to or away from the site of origin. Deep pain and some visceral pain are referred to other areas. But, superficial pain is not referred.

Examples:

1. Cardiac pain is felt at inner part of left arm and left shoulder.
2. Pain in ovary is referred to umbilicus.
3. Pain from testis is felt in abdomen.
4. Pain in diaphragm is referred to tip of shoulder.
5. Pain in gallbladder is referred to epigastric region.
6. Renal pain is referred to loin.
7. Pain from maxillary sinus is referred to adjacent tooth.

Mechanism of referred pain: When the visceral pain fibers are stimulated, pain from the viscera is conducted through some of neurons that conduct pain signals from the skin and the person has feeling that the sensation originates in the skin itself.

- **Dermatomal rule:** According to *dermatomal rule*, pain is referred to a structure, which is developed from same embryological segment/dermatome from which the pain producing structure is developed. A dermatome includes all the structures or parts of the body, which are innervated by afferent nerve fibers of one dorsal root. For example, heart and inner aspect of left arm originate from same dermatome. So, the pain in heart is referred to left arm.

Neurotransmitters involved in pain sensation and analgesic system:

1. Pain initiators: Glutamate, substance-P, bradykinin, prostaglandin, aspartate.
2. Pain inhibitors: Serotonin, endorphins, enkephalins, dynorphin, glycine, GABA Aδ afferent

fibers, which transmit impulses of fast pain, secrete glutamate. The C type fibers, which transmit impulses of slow pain, secrete substance P.

Analgesia system: Analgesia system means the pain control system. Body has its own analgesia system in brain, which provides a short-term relief from pain. It is also called **endogenous analgesic system**. Analgesic pathway that interferes with pain transmission is often considered as descending pain pathway.

Role of analgesic pathway in inhibiting pain transmission

1. Fibers of analgesic pathway arise from frontal lobe of cerebral cortex and hypothalamus.
2. These fibers terminate in gray matter surrounding third ventricle and aqueduct of Sylvius.
3. Fibers from here descend down to brainstem and terminate on:
   i. Nucleus raphe magnus, situated in reticular formation of lower pons and upper medulla
   ii. Nucleus reticularis, paragigantocellularis situated in medulla
4. Fibers from these reticular nuclei descend through lateral white column of spinal cord and reach the synapses of the neurons in afferent pain pathway situated in anterior gray horn. Synapses of the afferent pain pathway are between:
   i. Aδ type afferent fibers and neurons of marginal nucleus.
   ii. C type afferent fibers and neurons of substantia gelatinosa of Rolando.
5. At synaptic level, analgesic fibers release neurotransmitters and inhibit pain transmission before being relayed to brain.

Q. 8. Elaborate on theories of pain and mode of action of local anaesthetics. *(TNMGR, March 2009; Oct., 2018; RGUHS, Oct. 2010; Sumandeep Uni., June 2017)*

Ans.

1. **Intensity theory:** Stimulation of nerve beyond certain level causes pain, i.e. pain is supposed to be non-specific and depends only on high intensity stimulation.
2. **Specificity theory** (Rene Descartes, 1644): He considered the pain system as a straight through channel from skin to brain. Later Muller postulated the theory of information transmission only by way of the sensory nerves. Von Frey described specific cutaneous receptors, free nerve endings, for mediation of touch, heat, cold and pain. A pain centre was thought to exist within the brain, which was responsible for all overt manifestations of unpleasant experience.
3. **Pattern theory** (Goldscheider, 1894): This theory suggested that particular patterns of nerve impulses that evoke pain are produced by summation of sensory input within the dorsal horn of spinal column. Pain results when the total output of cells exceeds a critical level.
4. **Gate control theory:** Psychologist Ronald Melzack and the anatomist Patrick Wall proposed gate control theory for pain in 1965 to explain the pain suppression. According to them, pain stimuli transmitted by afferent pain fibers are blocked by gate mechanism, i.e. pain pathway and analgesic pathway located at the posterior gray horn of spinal cord. If the gate is opened, pain is felt. If the gate is closed, pain is suppressed.

Mechanism of gate control at spinal level (Fig. 8.8):

1. When pain stimulus is applied on any part of body receptors of pain and other sensations such as touch are also stimulated.
2. When all these impulses reach the spinal cord through posterior nerve root, the fibers of touch sensation (posterior column fibers) send collaterals to neurons of pain pathway, i.e. cells of marginal nucleus and substantia gelatinosa.
3. Impulses of touch sensation passing through these collaterals inhibit release of glutamate and substance P from the pain fibers.
4. This closes the gate and the pain transmission is blocked.

Role of Brain in Gate Control Mechanism

1. If the gates in spinal cord are not closed, pain signals reach thalamus through lateral spinothalamic tract
2. These signals are processed in thalamus and sent to sensory cortex.

Significance of gate control: Gating of pain at spinal level is similar to presynaptic inhibition. It forms the basis for relief of pain through rubbing, massage techniques, application of ice packs, acupuncture and

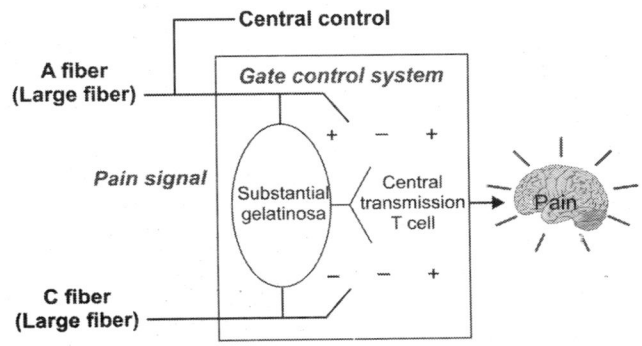

Fig. 8.8: Gate control theory

electrical analgesia. All these techniques relieve pain by stimulating the release of endogenous pain relievers (opioid peptides) which close the gate and block the pain signals.

Q. 9. Write a note on visual pathway.

(TNMGR, April 2001)

Ans. Visual pathway/optic pathway (Fig. 8.9) is the nervous pathway that transmits impulses from retina visual center in cerebral cortex.

Visual receptors: Rods and cones present in retina of eye form the visual photoreceptors. Fibers from here synapse with dendrites of bipolar cells of inner nuclear layer of retina.

First order neurons/primary neurons: Bipolar cells in the retina. Axons from bipolar cells synapse with dendrites of ganglionic cells.

Second order neurons/secondary neurons: Ganglionic cells in ganglionic cell layer of retina. Axons of ganglionic cells form optic nerve. Optic nerve leaves the eye and terminates in lateral geniculate body.

Third order neurons: Third order neurons are in **lateral geniculate body**. Fibers arising from here, reach the visual cortex.

Connections of visual receptors to optic nerve: Two pathways exist between the visual receptors and optic nerve:

1. **Private pathway:** The individual cones in fovea centralis are connected to separate bipolar cells. Each bipolar cell is connected to separate ganglionic cell, namely **midget ganglionic cell**. This pathway

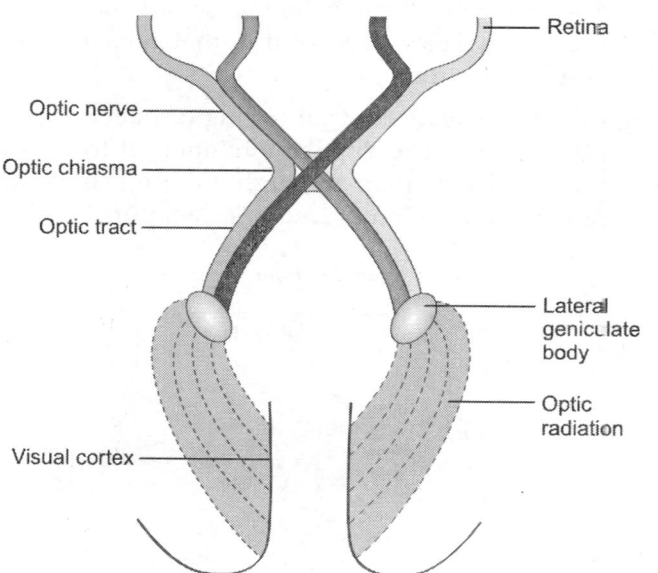

Fig. 8.9: Visual pathway

is responsible for **visual acuity** and **intensity discrimination**.

2. **Diffuse pathway:** A number of cones and rods are connected with a polysynaptic bipolar cell. The bipolar cells are connected to **diffused ganglionic cells**. So, there is great overlapping. This type of pathway is present outside the fovea.

Course of visual pathway: Visual pathway consists of six components:

1. **Optic nerve:** It is formed by axons of ganglionic cells and leaves the eye through optic disk. Fibers from temporal part of retina are in lateral part of nerve and carry impulses from nasal half of visual field of same eye. Fibers from nasal part of retina are in medial part of nerve and carry impulses from temporal half of visual field of same eye.

2. **Optic chiasma:** Medial fibers of each optic nerve cross the midline and join the uncrossed lateral fibers of opposite side, to form optic tract. This area of crossing of optic nerve fibers is called **optic chiasma**.

3. **Optic tract:** This is formed by uncrossed fibers of optic nerve on the same side and crossed fibers of optic nerve from opposite side. All the fibers of optic tract run backward, outward and towards **cerebral peduncle** to reach **lateral geniculate body** in thalamus.

4. **Lateral geniculate body:** Majority of the fibers of optic tract terminate in lateral geniculate body forming **subcortical center** for visual sensation. From here, **geniculocalcarine tract** or **optic radiation** arises. This tract is the last relay of visual pathway.

5. **Optic radiation:** Fibers from lateral geniculate body pass through **internal capsule** and form optic radiation (**geniculocalcarine fibers**) and finally ends in visual cortex.

6. **Visual cortex:** Primary **cortical center** for vision is called visual cortex, which is located on medial surface of occipital lobe. Peripheral retinal representation occupies anterior part and **macular representation** occupies posterior part of visual cortex.

Areas of Visual Cortex and their Function: Three areas are present in visual cortex:

i. Primary visual area (area 17): Concerned with perception of visual impulses.

ii. Secondary visual area (area 18): Concerned with interpretation of visual impulses.

iii. Occipital eye field (area 19): Concerned with movement of eyes.

Applied Physiology

1. Loss of vision in one visual field is known as **anopia**.

2. Loss of vision in one half of visual field is called **hemianopia**.

3. Lesion in one optic nerve will cause **total blindness** or anopia in the corresponding visual field.

4. **Effects of lesion of optic chiasma:** Nature of defect depends upon the fibers involved:
   i. Pressure on uncrossed lateral fibers by aneurysmal dilatation is called **left or right nasal hemianopia**.
   ii. If lateral fibers of both sides are affected, vision is lost in nasal half of both visual fields, causing **binasal hemianopia**.

5. **Effects of lesion of optic tract, lateral geniculate body and optic radiation:** Lesion of optic tract or lateral geniculate body or optic radiation causes **homonymous hemianopia**.

6. **Effects of lesion of visual cortex:** Lesion of upper or lower part of visual cortex leads to inferior or superior homonymous hemianopia.

7. **Oculocardiac reflex (OCR) or Aschner reflex or trigeminovagal reflex (TVR)** *(NTR Uni., Oct. 2011)*: It is defined by a decrease in heart rate (sinus bradycardia) by greater than 20% following globe pressure or traction of the extraocular muscles. This reflex has most notably been depicted during ophthalmologic procedures, facial trauma, regional anesthetic nerve blocks, and during mechanical stimulation.

   Mechanism: Trigeminal nerve serves as sensory afferent limb and vagus nerve comprises efferent limb of OCR.

   Activation of stretch receptors in ocular and periorbital tissues → short and long ciliary nerves conduct impulses → ciliary ganglion → ophthalmic division of trigeminal nerve → Gasserian ganglion → Trigeminal nucleus → internuclear communication between trigeminal sensory nucleus and visceral motor nucleus of vagus nerve → impulses to myocardium at sinoatrial node → activation of vagal motor response.

8. **Oculorespiratory reflex:** Shallow breathing, reduced respiratory rate or respiratory arrest following globe pressure or traction of the extraocular muscles. Its pathways are same as OCR, due to connection between trigeminal nucleus and pneumotactic centre.

Q. 10. Write about division of autonomic nervous system. *(TNMGR, April 2003)*

Ans. Autonomic nervous system (ANS) or **vegetative or involuntary nervous system** is primarily concerned with regulation of visceral or vegetative functions of the body.

Divisions of ANS:

I. **Sympathetic division/thoracolumbar outflow:** Preganglionic fibers from 12 thoracic and first two lumbar segments leave the spinal cord through anterior nerve root and white rami communicantes and terminate in postganglionic neurons situated in **sympathetic ganglia**. Sympathetic division supplies smooth muscle fibers of all visceral organs. **Sympathetic ganglia** are classified into three groups:

A. **Paravertebral/sympathetic chain ganglia:** They are arranged in a segmental fashion along the anterolateral surface of vertebral column forming **sympathetic chains** on either side of spinal cord. They are divided into four groups:

   1. **Cervical ganglia:**
      i. **Superior cervical ganglion:** It is formed by fusion of upper four cervical ganglia. It receives preganglionic fibers from T1. Postganglionic fibers supply blood vessels, glands, etc. It also sends fibers to heart through superior cervical sympathetic nerve and cardiac plexus.
      ii. **Middle cervical ganglion:** It is formed by 5th and 6th cervical ganglia. Preganglionic fibers arise from T1 segment. Postganglionic fibers supply sweat glands, thyroid gland and parathyroid glands. It also sends fibers to heart via middle cervical sympathetic nerve and cardiac plexus.
      iii. **Inferior cervical ganglion:** It is formed by 7th and 8th cervical ganglia. 1st thoracic ganglion fuses with inferior cervical ganglion, forming **stellate ganglion**. It receives preganglionic fibers from T1 segment. It sends postganglionic fibers to heart through inferior cervical sympathetic nerve and cardiac plexus. Postganglionic fibers also form plexus around subclavian artery and its branches.

   2. **Thoracic ganglia:** There are 12 thoracic ganglia on each side. Thoracic ganglia receive preganglionic fibers from thoracic segments of spinal cord. Postganglionic fibers from thoracic ganglia are distributed to **visceral organs** in the **thorax** and **abdomen**.

3. **Lumbar ganglia:** There are 5 lumbar ganglia. Preganglionic fibers for these ganglia arise from L1 and L2. Postganglionic fibers from these ganglia supply abdominal and **pelvic organs**.

4. **Sacral ganglia:** There are 5 sacral ganglia, which receive preganglionic fibers from L1 and L2. Postganglionic fibers from sacral ganglia innervate **blood vessels** and **sweat glands** in lower limb.

   Below sacral level, both sympathetic trunks converge and fuse on the anterior surface of coccyx forming **coccygeal ganglion (ganglion impar)**. It receives preganglionic fibers from L1 and L2. Postganglionic fibers are distributed to abdominal viscera and pelvic region.

B. **Prevertebral or collateral ganglia:** Prevertebral ganglia are situated in thorax, abdomen and pelvis, in relation to aorta and its branches. Prevertebral ganglia are:

   1. Celiac ganglion.
   2. Superior mesenteric ganglion.
   3. Inferior mesenteric ganglion.

   Prevertebral ganglia receive preganglionic fibers from T5 to L2 segments. Postganglionic fibers from these ganglia supply visceral organs of thorax, abdomen and pelvis.

C. **Terminal or peripheral ganglia:** Terminal ganglia are situated within or close to structures innervated by them. Heart, bronchi, pancreas and urinary bladder are innervated by the terminal ganglia.

   Sympathoadrenergic system: Sympathoadrenergic system is a functional and phylogenetic unit that includes sympathetic division and adrenal medulla. Adrenal medulla is a modified sympathetic ganglion. Since adrenal medulla and sympathetic division develop from the same neural crest, their secretions and functions are almost the same.

II. **Parasympathetic division/craniosacral outflow:** Fibers of this division arise from brain and sacral segments of spinal cord.

A. **Cranial outflow:** It arises from brainstem and innervates blood vessels of head and neck and many thoracoabdominal visceral organs. It includes cranial nerves: III, VII, IX, and X.

   Preganglionic fibers arise from neurons situated at two different levels:

   1. Tectal or midbrain outflow (III cranial nerve).
   2. Bulbar level or bulbar outflow (VII, IX and X cranial nerves).

   Preganglionic fibers are longer and reach the postganglionic neurons, which are situated within the organs or close to the organs innervated by these nerves. Preganglionic fibers are myelinated, but postganglionic fibers are non-myelinated.

B. **Sacral outflow:** It arises from the sacral segments of spinal cord and innervates smooth muscles forming walls of viscera and glands such as large intestine, liver, spleen, kidneys, bladder, genitalia, etc. Preganglionic fibers arise from anterior gray horn cells of 2nd, 3rd and 4th sacral segments of spinal cord and form the pelvic nerve (*Nervi erigentes*). Fibers end on postganglionic neurons, which are situated on or near the visceral organs.

   Functions of ANS: ANS plays an important role in maintaining constant internal environment (homeostasis). Almost all visceral organs are supplied by both sympathetic and parasympathetic divisions of ANS and the two divisions produce antagonistic effects on each organ. When the fibers of one division supplying to an organ is sectioned or affected by lesion, the effects of fibers from other division on the organ become more prominent.

Applied Clinical Physiology: Disorders of ANS

1. Inherited: Amyloidosis, porphyrias.
2. Acquired: Diabetes mellitus, uremic neuropathy/chronic liver diseases, vitamin B_{12} deficiency, chemotherapy, HIV, leprosy, Lyme disease, tetanus, rheumatoid arthritis, Sjögren, systemic lupus erythematosus, Parkinson's disease, brain tumors.

Biochemistry

1. CARBOHYDRATES, PROTEINS AND FAT METABOLISM

Q. 1. Write a note on anabolism and catabolism.
(TNMGR, April 2013)

Ans. The entire spectrum of chemical reactions occurring in the living system is collectively referred to as metabolism. Metabolism is divided into two categories:

1. **Catabolism:** The degradative processes concerned with breakdown of complex molecules to simpler ones with a concomitant release of energy. The purpose of catabolism is to trap the energy of biomolecules in the form of ATP (adenosine triphosphate) and to generate substances required for synthesis of complex molecules. Catabolism occurs in three stages:
   a. Conversion of complex molecules into their building blocks: Polysaccharides are broken down to monosaccharides, lipids to free fatty acids and glycerol, proteins to amino acids.
   b. Formation of simple intermediates: The building blocks are degraded to simple intermediates such as pyruvate and acetyl CoA.
   c. Final oxidation of acetyl CoA: Acetyl CoA is completely oxidized to CO_2, liberating NADH and $FADH_2$ that finally get oxidized to release large quantity of energy (as ATP), e.g. β-oxidation, glycolysis, Krebs cycle, oxidative phosporylation.
2. **Anabolism (biosynthesis):** The biosynthetic reactions involving the formation of complex molecules from simple precursors. For synthesis of large variety of complex molecules, the starting materials include pyruvate, acetyl CoA and intermediates of citric acid cycle. Besides the availability of precursors, anabolic reactions are dependent on the supply of energy (as ATP or GTP) and reducing equivalents ($NADPH + H^+$), e.g. acetyl CoA pathway.

Q. 2. Write a short note on homopolysaccharides.
(TNMGR, April 1997)

Ans. Polysaccharides are compound sugars that yield >10 molecules of monosaccharides on hydrolysis. Two types:

a. **Heteropolysaccharides (heteroglycans):** Produce two or more different types of monosaccharide molecules on hydrolysis, e.g. hyaluronic acid.
b. **Homopolysaccharides (homoglycans):** Polysaccharides which are composed of single type of monosaccharides. Various homopolysaccharides are:
   1. **Starch:** Starch is the carbohydrate reserve of plants and is the most important dietary source for higher animals, including man. High content of starch is found in cereals, roots, tubers, vegetables, etc. Starch is a homopolymer composed of D-glucose units held by α-glycosidic bonds. It is known as **glucosin** or **glucan**. Starch consists of two polysaccharide components—water soluble amylose (15–20%) and water insoluble amylopectin (80–85%). Starches are hydrolysed by amylase to liberate dextrins, and finally maltose and glucose units.
   2. **Dextrins:** Dextrins are breakdown products of starch by enzyme amylase. The various intermediates are soluble starch (blue), amylodextrin (violet), erythrodextrin (red) and achrodextrin (no color).
   3. **Dextrans:** Dextrans are polymers of glucose, produced by microorganisms. They are used as plasma volume expanders in transfusion, and chromatography.
   4. **Inulin:** Inulin is a polymer of fructose, i.e. fructosan. It is a low molecular weight polysaccharide easily soluble in water, used for assessing kidney function.
   5. **Agar:** Agar is a polymer of galactose, i.e. galactosans. It is obtained from cell wall of red algae. It becomes gelatinous when dissolved in hot water and cooled.

6. **Glycogen:** It is a carbohydrate reserve in animals (**animal starch**). It is present in high concentration in liver, muscle, brain, etc. Structure of glycogen is similar to that of amylopectin with more number of branches.

7. **Cellulose:** It occurs exclusively in plants. It is a predominant constituent of plant cell wall. Cellulose is composed of $\beta(1 \to 4)$ glycosidic bonds. Cellulose cannot be digested by mammals due to lack of enzyme that cleaves $\beta(1 \to 4)$ glycosidic bonds.

8. **Chitin:** It is a structural polysaccharide found in exoskeleton of some invertebrates. It is composed of N-acetyl-D-glucosamine units held together by $\beta(1 \to 4)$ glycosidic bonds.

Q. 3. Write a short note on mucopolysaccharides.
(TNMGR, Oct. 1996)

Ans. Mucopolysaccharides (MPS)/glycosaminoglycans (GAGs) are heteropolysaccharides made up of repeating units of sugar derivatives, namely amino sugars (N-acetyl glucasamine/N-acetyl galactosamine) and uronic acids (D-glucuronic acid/L-iduronic acid). The presence of sulfate and carboxyl groups contributes to acidity of molecules. Some of the mucopolysaccharides are found in combination with proteins (conjugate proteins) to form mucoproteins (**mucoids or proteoglycans**) when carbohydrate is >protein; and **glycoprotein** when protein is >carbohydrate. The extracellular spaces of tissue consist of collagen and elastin fibers embedded in a matrix or ground substance, predominantly composed of GAGs. GAGs can be classified as:

A. **First classification:**

1. Polycarboxylates: Hyaluronic acid, chondroitin.
2. Polysulfates: Keratan sulfates
3. Polycarboxy-sulfates: Chondroitin 4- and 6-sulfates (previously as chondroitin sulfate A and C, respectively); dermatan sulfates and heparitin sulfates.

B. **Second classification:**

1. Acidic:
   a. Sulfate free:
      i. Hyaluronic acid: Present in synovial fluid, ECM of loose connective tissue. It serve as lubricant and shock absorber. Hyaluronidase depolymerizes it, reducing its viscosity.
      ii. Chondroitin: Present in cornea, cranial cartilages.
   b. Sulfate containing:
      i. Chondroitin sulfate: Principal GAG is ground substance of all tissues and cartilages. Four types—A, B, C, and D.
      ii. Keratan sulfates (1 and 2): Present in costocartilage, cornea, and aorta.
      iii. Heparin: Anticoagulant presents in liver, lungs, thymus, spleen, skin and blood.
      iv. Heparitin sulphate (HS): It is isolated from amyloid liver and spleen of patient with Hurler's syndrome.
2. Neutral: Present in pneumococci capsule, egg protein, acts as blood group substance.

Applied Clinical Aspect

Mucopolysaccharidoses (MPSs) are a group of lysosomal storage diseases, each of which is produced by an inherited deficiency of an enzyme involved in degradation of acid mucopolysaccharides. Over time, these glycosaminoglycans collect in the cells, blood, brain and spinal cord, and connective tissues. These diseases are autosomal recessive, except for mucopolysaccharidosis type II, which is X-linked.

Clinical features: Short stature, hairiness, abnormal development, heavy face with large head, prominent forehead, short nose, and large lips and tongue, intellectual disability, impaired vision/hearing, stiff finger joints and affected arteries or heart valves (Table 1.3).

Treatment: Stem cell transplant (SCT), enzyme replacement therapy (ERT).

Q. 4. Write a short note on glycoproteins.
(TNMGR, March 2007)

Ans. Proteins bound to carbohydrates are called glycoproteins. The carbohydrate content varies from 1–90%. The term glycoprotein is used when the carbohydrates content is less than 4%. The carbohydrate found in glycoproteins include mannose, galactose, N-acetylglucosamine, N-acetylgalactosamine, xylose, L-fucose and N-acetylneuramic acid.

Classification: Three major classes:

1. N-linkage (N-acetylglucosamine to asparagine): Ovalbumin and immunoglobulins.
2. O-linkage (N-acetylgalactosamine to serine): Mucin present in saliva, blood group antigens.
3. Glycosyl-phosphatidyl-inositol (GPI) linkage.

Functions:

1. **As structural molecule:** Collagens.
2. **As lubricant and protective agent:** Mucins
3. **As transport molecules:** Transferrin and ceruloplasmin.
4. **As immunologic molecules:** Immunoglobulins, histocompatibility antigens.
5. **As hormone:** Chronic gonadotropins, TSH.

Table 1.3: Types of mucopolysaccharidoses with subtypes, defective enzymes and oral manifestations

Type	Defective enzyme	Affected GAG	Oral findings
Type IH Hurler syndrome	α-L-iduronidase	Dermatan sulfate, heparin sulfate	Short mandibular rami with abnormal condyle, radiolucent lesions of jaws, macroglossia, peg laterals, spacing of teeth, high-arched palate, hyperplastic gingiva, retarded tooth eruption
Type IS Scheie syndrome	—	—	
Type IHS Hurler-Scheie syndrome	—	—	
Type II Hunter syndrome	Iduronate 2-sulfatase	Dermatan sulfate, heparin sulfate	Short and broad mandible, radiolucent lesions of jaws, flattened TMJ, macroglossia, peg laterals, spacing of teeth, high-arched palate, flattened alveolar ridges, hyperplastic gingiva
Type IIIA Sanfilippo A syndrome	Heparan N-sulfatase	Heparin sulfate	Everted and thick lower lip; upturned upper lip with protruding philtrum
Type IIIB Sanfilippo syndrome	α-N-acetyl-D-glucosaminidase	—	—
Type IIIC Sanfilippo C syndrome	α-glucosaminide-acetyltransferase	—	—
Type IIID Sanfilippo D syndrome	N-acetylglucosamine-6-sulfatase	—	—
Type IVA Morquio A syndrome	N-acetylgalactosamine-6-sulfatase	Keratan sulfate, chondroitan sulfate	Thin, rough and hypoplastic enamel, increased caries incidence
Type IVB Morquio B syndrome	β-galactosidase	Keratan sulfate	
Type VI Maroteaux-Lamy Syndrome	N-acetylgalactosamine-4-sulfatase	Dermatan sulfate	Macroglossia, gingival hypertrophy, delayed tooth eruption
Type VII Sly syndrome	β-glucuronidase	Dermatan sulfate, heparin sulfate, chondroitan sulfate	Macroglossia
Type IX	Hyaluronidase	Hyaluronan	—

6. **As enzyme:** Many, e.g. ALP.
7. **As cell attachment recognition site:** Many, e.g. sperm oocyte, etc.
8. **Antifreeze:** Certain plasma proteins of cold water fish.
9. **Interact with specific carbohydrate:** Lectins, selectins, antibodies.
10. **Receptors:** Proteins involved in hormones and drug action.
11. **Affect folding of certain proteins:** Calnexin, calreticulin.
12. **Regulation of development:** Notch and its analogues.
13. **Hemostasis and thrombosis:** Specific glycoproteins on the surface of platelets.

Q. 5. Write a note on carbohydrate metabolism.
(TNMGR, March 2010; NTR Uni., April 2011)

Ans. Carbohydrates are the first cellular constituents synthesized by green plants during photosynthesis from CO_2 and water on absorption of light. Glucose is the central molecule in carbohydrate metabolism as all major pathways of carbohydrate metabolism are connected with it. Glucose is utilized as a source of energy, it is synthesized from non-carbohydrate precursors and stored as glycogen to release glucose, when the need arises. The other monosaccharides important in carbohydrate metabolism are fructose, galactose and mannose.

Pathways of Glucose Utilization

I. **Major pathways for energy production**
1. **Glycolysis (Embden-Meyerhof pathway):** Oxidation of glucose to pyruvate (aerobic conditions) and to lactate (anaerobic conditions).
2. **Citric acid cycle (Krebs cycle or tricarboxylic acid cycle—TCA):** Oxidation of acetyl CoA to CO_2. Krebs cycle is the final common oxidative pathway for carbohydrates, fats or amino acids, through acetyl CoA.

3. Gluconeogenesis: Synthesis of glucose from non-carbohydrate precursors (e.g. amino acids, glycerol, etc.).
4. Glycogenesis: Formation of glycogen from glucose.
5. Glycogenolysis: Breakdown of glycogen to glucose.

II. **Minor pathways:** For synthesis of other derivatives.
1. **Hexose monophosphate shunt (HMP) (pentose phosphate pathway or direct oxidative pathway):** This pathway is an alternative to glycolysis and TCA cycle for oxidation of glucose (directly to CO_2 and water).
2. **Uronic acid pathway:** Glucose is converted to glucuronic acid, pentoses and, in some animals to ascorbic acid (not in man). This pathway is also an alternative oxidative pathway for glucose.
3. **Galactose metabolism:** The pathways concerned with conversion of galactose to glucose and synthesis of lactose.
4. **Fructose metabolism:** Oxidation of fructose to pyruvate and the relation between fructose and glucose metabolism.
5. **Amino sugar and mucopolysaccharide metabolism:** Synthesis of amino sugars and other sugars for the formation of mucopolysaccharides and glycoproteins.

Q. 6. Discuss glucose metabolism, diabetes mellitus and the clinical implication in the management of a patient with diabetes. *(Pacific Uni., May 2010)*

Q. Write a short note on metabolism of sucrose. *(TNMGR, Sept. 2007)*

Ans. Glycolysis/Embden-Meyerhof pathway (EM pathway) is defined as the sequence of reactions converting glucose (or glycogen) to pyruvate or lactate, with the production of ATP.

Salient features of Glycolysis *(RUHS, May 2018; HP Uni., April 2019)*
1. Glycolysis takes place in all the cells of body.
2. In glycolysis, lactate is the end product under anaerobic condition. In aerobic condition, pyruvate is formed, which is then oxidized to CO_2 and H_2O.
3. Glycolysis is a major pathway for ATP synthesis in tissues lacking mitochondria, e.g. erythrocytes, cornea, lens, etc.
4. Glycolysis is very essential for brain which is dependent on glucose for energy.
5. Glycolysis (anaerobic) may be summarized by the net reaction

$$Glucose + 2ADP + 2Pi \rightarrow 2\ lactate + 2ATP$$

The pathway can be divided into three distinct phases:
A. **Energy investment phase or priming stage:**
1. Glucose is phosphorylated to glucose-6-phosphate by *hexokinase* (extrahepatic) or *glucokinase* (liver and pancreatic β cells).
2. Glucose-6-phosphate undergoes isomerization to fructose-6-phosphate by *phosphohexose isomerase*.
3. Fructose-6-phosphate is phosphorylated to fructose 1,6-bisphosphate by *phosphofructokinase*.
B. **Splitting phase:**
1. Fructose-1,6-bisphosphate is split by *aldolase* into glyceraldehyde 3-phosphate and dihydroxyacetone phosphate.
C. **Energy generation phase:**
1. Glyceraldehydes 3-phosphate is converted into 1,3-bisphosphoglycerate by *glyceraldehyde 3-phosphate dehydrogenase*.
2. 1,3-bisphosphoglycerate is converted to 3-phosphoglycerate by *phosphoglycerate kinase*.
3. 3-phosphoglycerate is converted to 2-phosphoglycerate by *phosphoglycerate mutase*.
4. 2-phosphoglycerate is converted to phosphoenolpyruvate by *enolase*.
5. Phosphoenolpyruvate is converted to pyruvate by *pyruvate kinase*, further lactate dehydrogenase converts pyruvate into lactate.

Production of ATP
1. Under anaerobic condition: 2ATP
2. Under aerobic condition: 6/8 ATP

Regulation of glycolysis: Hexokinase (and glucokinase), phosphofructokinase and pyruvate kinase, catalysing the irreversible reactions regulate glycolysis. These are stimulated by insulin, AMP, fructose-6-phosphate and inhibited by glucagon, ATM, and citrate.

Diabetes mellitus: Diabetes mellitus is a clinical condition characterized by increased blood glucose level due to insufficient or inefficient insulin.

Metabolic changes in diabetes: Diabetes mellitus is associated with several metabolic alterations. Most important among them are:
1. **Hyperglycemia:** Elevation of blood glucose concentration is the hallmark of uncontrolled diabetes. Hyperglycemia is primarily due to reduced glucose uptake by tissues and its increased production via gluconeogenesis and glycogenolysis. When blood glucose level goes beyond renal threshold, glucose is excreted into urine (glycosuria).
2. **Ketoacidosis:** Increased mobilization of fatty acids results in overproduction of ketone bodies which often lead to ketoacidosis.

3. **Hypertriglyceridemia:** Conversion of fatty acids to triacylglycerols and secretion of VLDL and chylomicrons is comparatively higher in diabetics. Further, the activity of enzyme *lipoprotein lipase* is low in diabetic patients. Consequently, the plasma levels of VLDL, chylomicrons and triacylglycerols are increased.

Management of Diabetes

1. **Dietary management:** A diabetic patient is advised to consume low calories, high protein and fiber rich diet. Carbohydrates should be taken in the form of starch and complex sugars. Refined sugars should be avoided. Fat intake should be drastically reduced so as to meet the nutritional requirements of unsaturated fatty acids.

2. **Hypoglycemic drugs:** They promote secretion of endogenous insulin and help in reducing blood glucose level.

3. **Management with insulin:** Short-acting insulins are unmodified and their action lasts for about 6 hours. Long acting insulins are modified ones and act for several hours, which depends on the type of preparation.

Q. 7. Write short note on oxidative phosphorylation.
(TNMGR, Oct. 1999)

Ans. There are two ways of ATP synthesis:

1. **Substarte level phosphorylation:** Direct transfer of phosphate from chemical intermediate to ADP/ GDP forming ATP/GTP, e.g. glcolysis.

2. **Oxidative phosphorylation:** The process of synthesizing ATP from ADP and Pi coupled with electron transport chain (ETC) is known as oxidative phosphorylation. The inner mitochondrial membrane is the site of oxidative phosphorylation.

P:O ratio: P:O ratio refers to the number of inorganic phosphate molecules utilized for ATP generation for every atom of oxygen consumed. P:O ratio represents the number of molecules of ATP synthesized per pair of electrons carried through ETC. The mitochondrial oxidation of NADH has P:O ratio of 3. Oxidation of $FADH_2$ has a P:O ratio of 2.

Sites of oxidative phosphorylation in ETC: There are three reactions in the ETC that are exergonic to result in the synthesis of 3 ATP molecules.

1. Oxidation of $FMNH_2$ by coenzyme Q.
2. Oxidation of cytochrome *b* by cytochrome C_1.
3. Cytochrome oxidase reaction.

Mechanism of oxidative phosphorylation

1. **Chemical coupling hypothesis (Edwards Slater, 1953):** According to this, during course of electron transfer in respiratory chain, a series of phosphorylated high-energy intermediates are first produced which are utilized for synthesis of ATP.

2. **Chemiosmotic hypothesis (Peter Mitchell, 1961):** This mechanism is now widely accepted. The inner mitochondrial membrane is impermeable to protons (H^+) and hydroxyl ions (OH^-). The transport of electrons through ETC is coupled with the translocation of protons (H^+) across the inner mitochondrial membrane (coupling membrane) from the matrix to intermembrane space. The proton gradient developed due to electron flow in respiratory chain is sufficient to result in synthesis of ATP from ADP and Pi. Also the ATP synthase, utilizes proton gradient for synthesis of ATP.

Q. 8. Write a short note on ketone bodies.

Ans. Acetone, acetoacetate and β-hydroxybutyrate are the ketone bodies. Only the first two are true ketones while hydroxybutyrate does not possess a keto group. **Ketone bodies are water-soluble and energy yielding.** Acetone, however, is an exception, since it cannot be metabolized.

Ketogenesis: The synthesis of ketone bodies occurs in liver. The enzymes for ketone body synthesis are located in the mitochondrial matrix. Ketogenesis occurs through following reactions:

1. Two moles of acetyl CoA condense to form acetoacetyl CoA. This reaction is catalysed by *thiolase*, an enzyme involved in final step of β-oxidation.

2. Acetoacetyl CoA combines with another molecule of acetyl CoA to produce β-hydroxy β-methyl glutaryl CoA (HMG-CoA). *HMG-CoA synthase*, catalysing this reaction, regulates the synthesis of ketone bodies.

3. HMG-CoA lyase cleaves HMG-CoA to produce acetoacetate and acetyl CoA.

4. Acetoacetate can undergo spontaneous decarboxylation to form acetone.

5. Acetoacetate can be reduced by a dehydrogenease to β-hydroxybutyrate.

Carbon skeleton of some amino acids (ketogenic) is degraded to acetoacetate or acetyl CoA and, therefore to ketone bodies, e.g. leucine, lysine, phenylalanine, etc.

Utilization: Ketone bodies being water soluble are easily transported from the liver to various tissues. Two ketone bodies—acetoacetate and β-hydroxybutyrate serve as important sources of energy for the peripheral tissues such as skeletal muscle, cardiac muscle/renal cortex, etc. The tissues which lack mitochondria (e.g. erythrocytes) cannot utilize ketone bodies. During prolonged starvation, ketone bodies are the major fuel source for brain and other parts of CNS.

Regulation:

1. Glucagon stimulates ketogenesis.
2. Insulin inhibits ketogenesis.

Ketogenic substance: Fatty acids and amino acids.

Antiketogenic substance: Glucose, glycerol, glucogenic amino acids.

Applied Clinical Aspect

1. **Overproduction of ketone bodies:** When the rate of synthesis of ketone bodies exceeds the rate of utilization, their concentration in blood increases, this is known as **Ketonemia**. Ketonuria is excretion of ketone bodies in urine. The overall picture of ketonemia and ketonuria is commonly referred to as ketosis. Smell of acetone in breath is a common feature in ketosis. Ketosis is most commonly associated with starvation and severe uncontrolled diabetes mellitus.
2. **Ketonuria and weight loss programs:** Appearance of ketone bodies in urine is an indication of active fat metabolism. Some programs designed for body weight loss encourage **reduction in carbohydrate** and total calorie intake until ketone bodies appear in urine.
3. **Ketoacidosis:** Both acetoacetate and β-hydroxybutyrate are strong acids. Increase in their concentration in blood would cause acidosis. Diabetic ketoacidosis is dangerous, may result in coma, and even death, if not treated.

Q. 9. Write a short note on gluconeogenesis.

(TNMGR, March 2009)

Ans. The synthesis of glucose from non-carbohydrate compounds is known as **gluconeogenesis**.

Major substrates for gluconeogenesis are lactate, pyruvate, glucogenic amino acids, propionate and glycerol.

Location of gluconeogenesis: It occurs mainly in the cytosol, in liver and in kidney matrix.

Importance: Glucose supply is absolutely essential for body for a variety of functions:

1. Brain and CNS, erythrocytes, testes and kidney medulla are dependent on glucose for continuous supply of energy.
2. Glucose is the only source that supplies energy to skeletal muscle, under anaerobic conditions.
3. In fasting, gluconeogenesis must occur to meet basal requirements of body and to maintain intermediates of citric acid cycle.
4. Certain metabolites produced in the tissues accumulate in the blood, e.g. lactate, glycerol, pro-

pionate, etc. Gluconeogenesis effectively clears them from the blood.

Gluconeogenesis closely resembles the reversed pathway of glycolysis, although it is not the complete reversal of glycolysis. Essentially 3 (out of 10) reactions of glycolysis are irreversible.

1. Conversion of pyruvate to phosphoenol pyruvate
2. Conversion of fructose-1,6-bisphosphate to fructose-6-phosphate
3. Conversion of glucose-6-phosphate to glucose.

Overall summary of gluconeogenesis or the conversion of pyruvate to glucose is shown below:

$$2\,\text{Pyruvate} + 4\,\text{ATP} + 2\,\text{GTP} + 2\,\text{NADH} + 2\,\text{H}^+ + 6\,\text{H}_2\text{O}$$
$$\rightarrow \text{Glucose} + 2\,\text{NAD}^+ + 4\,\text{ADP} + 2\,\text{GDP} + 6\,\text{Pi} + 6\,\text{H}^+$$

Regulation of gluconeogenesis:

1. Glucagon stimulates gluconeogenesis.
2. Glucogenic amino acids stimulate gluconeogenesis.
3. Acetyl-CoA stimulates gluconeogenesis.

Applied Clinical Aspect

Alcohol inhibits gluconeogenesis due to overconsumption of NAD^+ and excessive production of NADH by alcohol. Alcohol consumption increases the risk of hypoglycemia due to reduced gluconeogenesis.

Q. 10. Write a note on urea cycle.

(TNMGR, Oct. 2003, Aug. 2004)

Ans. Urea is the end product of protein metabolism. The nitrogen of amino acids converted to ammonia, is toxic to body. It is converted to urea and detoxified. Urea is synthesized in liver and transported to kidneys for excretion in urine. Urea cycle is known as **Krebs-Henseleit cycle**.

Urea has two amino ($-NH_2$) groups, one derived from NH_3 and other from aspartate. Carbon atom is supplied by CO_2. Urea synthesis is a five-step cyclic process, with five distinct enzymes. First two enzymes are present in mitochondria while the rest are localized in cytosol. The urea cycle is irreversible and consumes 4 ATP. Two ATPs are utilized for the synthesis of carbamoyl phosphate. One ATP is converted to AMP and PPi to produce arginosuccinate which equals to 2 ATP.

$$NH_4^+ + CO_2 + \text{Aspartate} + 3\,\text{ATP} \rightarrow \text{Urea} +$$
$$\text{Fumarate} + 2\,\text{ADP} + 2\,\text{Pi} + \text{AMP} + \text{PPi}$$

Steps in urea formation:

1. *Carbamoyl phosphate synthase I* catalyses condensation of NH_4^+ with CO_2 to form carbamoyl phosphate.
2. Citrulline is formed from carbamoyl phosphate and ornithine by *ornithine transcarbamoylase*.
3. Arginosuccinate is formed from citrulline with aspartate by *arginosuccinate synthase*.

4. *Arginosuccinase cleaves* arginosuccinate to give arginine and fumarate.

5. *Arginase cleaves* arginine to yield urea and ornithine.

Applied Clinical Aspect

1. **Metabolic disorders of urea cycle:** Metabolic defects associated with urea cycle lead to a build-up in blood ammonia (**hyperammonemia**). Hyperammonemia is toxic to brain and leads to encephalopathy, which can manifest as cerebral edema, vomiting, blurred vision, asterixis, and seizures.

    i. **Ornithine transcarbamylase (OTC) deficiency:** It leads to increased levels of carbamoyl phosphate, which is converted into orotic acid, resulting in increased levels of orotic acid in blood and urine. Orotic aciduria can manifest as orange crystals in diapers.

    ii. **Argininosuccinate synthetase deficiency:** It leads to elevated levels of citrulline.

    iii. **Carbamoyl phosphate synthetase I (CPS I) deficiency:** This disorder is autosomal recessive and is often fatal in infancy.

2. **Blood urea nitrogen (BUN):** In healthy people, normal blood urea concentration is 10–40 mg/dl. Blood urea estimation is widely used as a screening test for evaluation of kidney function.

    i. **Pre-renal:** This is associated with increased protein breakdown, as observed after major surgery, prolonged fever, diabetic coma, thyrotoxicosis, etc.

    ii. **Renal:** In renal disorders like acute glomerulonephritis, chronic nephritis, nephrosclerosis, polycystic kidney, blood urea is increased.

    iii. **Post-renal:** Whenever there is an obstruction in the urinary tract (e.g. tumors, stones, enlargement of prostate gland, etc.), blood urea is elevated. This is due to increased reabsorption of urea from the renal tubules.

    The term 'uremia' is used to indicate increased blood urea levels due to renal failure. Azotemia represents an elevation in blood urea or other nitrogen metabolites which may or may not be associated with renal diseases.

3. **Serum ammonia:** Normal serum ammonia generally ranges from 15–45 m/dl. The serum ammonia level may be elevated in a patient with hepatic dysfunction, urea cycle deficiency, overgrowth of gut flora, protein catabolism, and many other causes.

Q. 11. Write short note on Krebs cycle.
(TNNMGR, March 2009; RUHS, May 2015)

Q. Write a short note on citric acid cycle.
(TNMGR, Nov. 1995)

Ans. The citric acid cycle was proposed by Hans Adolf Krebs in 1937, based on the studies of oxygen consumption in pigeon breast muscle.

TCA cycle—the central metabolic pathway: Krebs cycle is the most important central pathway connecting almost all the individual metabolic pathways (either directly or indirectly).

Location of TCA cycle: Enzymes of TCA cycle are located in mitochondrial matrix, in close proximity to electron transport chain.

Reactions of citric acid cycle:

1. Condensation of acetyl CoA and oxaloacetate by *citrate synthase* forms citryl CoA, which yields citrate.
2. Citrate is isomerized to isocitrate by *aconitase*.
3. Isocitrate is converted to oxalosuccinate then to α-ketoglutarate by *isocitrate dehydrogenase*.
4. α-ketoglutarate is converted to succinyl CoA by *α-ketoglutarate dehydrogenase*.
5. Succinyl CoA is converted to succinate by *succinate thiokinase*.
6. Succinate is converted to fumarate by *succinate dehydrogenase*.
7. Fumarate is converted to malate by *fumarase*.
8. Malate is converted to oxaloacetate by *malate dehydrogenase*.

ATP produced: 12 ATP

Regulation of cycle: Citrate synthase, isocitrate dehydrogenase and α-ketoglutarate dehydrogenase.

Hence, citric acid cycle is the final common oxidative pathway for carbohydrates, fats and amino acids. It utilizes (indirectly) about two-thirds of the total oxygen consumed by the body and generates about two-thirds of the total energy (ATP).

Q. 12. Write a note on essential amino acids.
(TNMGR, Oct. 2012, 2013)

Ans. All proteins are polymers of amino acids (20 in number). Most of the amino acids (except proline) are alpha amino acids, which means that the amino group is attached to the same carbon atom to which the carboxyl group is attached. However, all these 20 amino acids need not be taken in the diet.

Based on the nutritional requirements, amino acids are grouped into:

1. **Essential or indespensable:** They are amino acids which cannot be synthesized by the body and therefore, need to be supplied through diet. They are required for proper growth and maintenance of the individual, e.g. valine, isoleucine, leucine, lysine, methionine, phenylalanine, threonine, tryptophan.

2. **Partially essential or semiessential:** Arginine and histidine can be partly synthesized by adult humans and not by growing children.

3. **Nonessential or dispensable:** Remaining amino acids which can be synthesized by metabolic pathways, e.g. glycine, serine, cysteine, asparagine, glutamine, aspartic acid, glutamic acid, proline and tyrosine.

Q. 13. Write a short note on absorption of fat.
(TNMGR, April 1998)

Q. Write a note on lipid absorption from intestine.
(TNMGR, March 2007)

Ans. Emulsification (dispersion of lipids into smaller droplets due to reduction in the surface tension) is essential for effective digestion of lipids, since enzymes can act only on the surface of lipid droplets. The process of emulsification occurs by three complementary mechanisms:

1. Detergent action of bile salts: Bile salts convert them into smaller particles.
2. Surfactant action of degraded lipids: Surfactants get absorbed to the water–lipid interfaces and increase interfacial area of lipid droplets.
3. Mechanical mixing due to peristalsis: It also helps in emulsification of lipids.

Digestion of lipids by pancreatic enzymes:

1. Degradation of triacylglycerols (fat):
   a. Pancreatic lipase is the major enzyme that digests dietary fats. This enzyme preferentially cleaves fatty acids, forming 2-monoacylglycerol and free fatty acids.
   b. Lipid esterase acts on monoacylglycerols, cholesteryl esters, vitamin esters, etc. to liberate free fatty acids. The presence of bile acids is essential for activity of lipid esterase.
2. Degradation of cholesteryl esters: Pancreatic cholesterol esterase cleaves cholesteryl esters to produce cholesterol and free fatty acids.
3. Degradation of phospholipids: Phospholipases are enzymes responsible for hydrolysis of phospholipids. The products are a free fatty acid and a lysophospholipid.

Lipid/fat Absorption: The major dietary lipids are triacylglycerol, cholesterol and phospholipids. Theories to explain the absorption of lipids are:

1. **Lipolytic theory (Verzar):** Fats are completely hydrolysed to glycerol and free fatty acids. They are absorbed either as soaps or in association with bile salts.
2. **Partition theory (Frazer):** The partially digested triacylglycerols in association with bile salts form emulsions. The lipids are taken up by the intestinal mucosal cells. As per this theory, resynthesis of lipids is not necessary for their entry into circulation.
3. **Bergstrom theory:** This is a more recent and comprehensive theory to explain lipid absorption. According to this, long chain fatty acids are absorbed to the lymph and not to the blood. The primary products obtained from lipid digestion are 2-monoacylglycerol free fatty acids and free cholesterol.

Role of bile salts in lipid absorption: Bile salts form mixed micelles with lipids. The micelles have a disk-like shape with lipids at the interior and bile salts at periphery. The hydrophilic groups of lipids are oriented to outside and hydrophobic groups to inside. In this fashion, bile salt micelles exert a solubilizing effect on the lipids. The mixed micelles serve as the major vehicles for the transport of lipids from the intestinal lumen to membrane of intestinal mucosal cells, the site of lipid absorption. The lipid components are absorbed through the plasma membrane by diffusion. Absorption is almost complete for monoacylglycerols and free fatty acids which are slightly water soluble.

Applied Clinical Aspect

1. **Chyluria:** Due to abnormal connection between urinary tract and lymphatic drainage system of intestine, forming a chylous fistula characterized by passage of **milky urine.**
2. **Chylothorax:** Due to abnormal connection between pleural space and lymphatic drainage of small intestine, resulting in accumulation of lymph in pleural cavity, with milky pleural effusion.
3. **Steatorrhea:** Excretion of fat into faeces due to pancreas disease.

Q. 14. Write a note on β-oxidation of fatty acids.
(TNMGR, Oct. 1996)

Ans. β-Oxidation may be defined as the oxidation of fatty acids on the β-carbon atom. This results in sequential removal of a 2-carbon fragment, acetyl CoA. Fatty acids are oxidized by most of the tissues in the body. However, brain, erythrocytes and adrenal medulla cannot utilize fatty acids for energy requirement. The β-oxidation of fatty acids involves three stages:

I. **Fatty acid activation:** Fatty acids are activated to acyl CoA by thiokinases or acyl CoA synthetases.

The reaction occurs in two steps and requires ATP, coenzyme A and Mg^{2+}.

II. **Transport of acyl CoA into mitochondria:** The inner mitochondrial membrane is impermeable to fatty acids. A specialized carnitine carrier system (**carnitine shuttle**) operates to transport activated fatty acids from cytosol to mitochondria.

III. **β-Oxidation proper:** Each cycle of β-oxidation, liberating a 2-carbon unit, acetyl CoA, occurs in a sequence of four reactions.

1. Acyl CoA undergoes dehydrogenation by an FAD-dependent flavoenzyme, acyl CoA dehydrogenase.
2. Enoyl CoA hydratase brings about hydration of double bond to form β-hydroxyacyl CoA.
3. β-hydroxyacyl CoA dehydrogenase catalyses second oxidation and generates NADH. The product formed is β-ketoacyl CoA.
4. Final reaction in β-oxidation is the liberation of a 2-carbon fragment, acetyl CoA from acyl CoA. This occurs by a thiolytic cleavage catalysed by β-ketoacyl CoA thiolase.

The new acyl CoA, containing two carbons less than the original, re-enter β-oxidation cycle. The process continues till the fatty acid is completely oxidized.

Oxidation of palmitoyl CoA: Palmitoyl CoA undergoes 7 cycles of β-oxidation to yield 8 acetyl CoA. Acetyl CoA can enter citric acid cycle and get completely oxidized to CO_2 and H_2O.

Applied Clinical Aspects

1. **SIDS:** The sudden infant death syndrome (SIDS) is an unexpected death of healthy infants, usually overnight. It is estimated that at least 10% of SIDS is due to deficiency of medium chain acyl CoA dehydrogenase.
2. **Jamaican vomiting sickness:** This disease is characterized by severe hypoglycemia, vomiting, convulsions, coma and death. It is caused by eating unripe ackee fruit which contains an unusual toxic amino acid, hypoglycin A. This inhibits enzyme acyl CoA dehydrogenase and thus β-oxidation of fatty acids is blocked, leading to various complications

Q. 15. Write a short note on lipoproteins.
(TNMGR, April 2012)

Ans. Lipoproteins are molecular complexes of lipids with proteins (conjugated proteins). They are the transport vehicles for lipids in circulation. A lipoprotein is basically consists of neutral lipid core surrounded by a coat shell of phospholipids, apoproteins and cholesterol. The polar portion of phospholipids and cholesterol are exposed on the surface of lipoproteins, which makes it soluble with water (Fig. 1.15). Apolipoproteins/apoprotein are the protein part of lipoprotein, mainly synthesized in liver. Types:

i. **Apo A-I:** It activates lecithin-cholesterol acyl transferase (LCAT). It is the ligand for HDL receptor. It is anti-atherogenic.
ii. **Apo B-100:** It is a component of LDL; it attaches with LDL receptor.
iii. **Apo B-48:** It is the component of chylomicrons.

Classification: Depending on the density (by ultra-centrifugation) or on the electrophoretic mobility, lipoproteins are:

1. **Chylomicrons:** Synthesized in intestine, consist of highest quantity of lipid, least in density and largest in size, transport exogenous triacylglycerol to tissues.
2. **Very low density lipoproteins (VLDL) or pre-beta lipoproteins:** Produced in liver and intestine, responsible for endogenously synthesized triacylglycerols.
3. **Intermediate density lipoproteins (IDL) or broad-beta lipoproteins.**
4. **Low-density lipoproteins (LDL) or beta lipoproteins:** Formed from VLDL in blood circulation, transport cholesterol from liver to other tissues.
5. **High-density lipoproteins (HDL) or alpha lipoproteins:** Mostly synthesized in liver, transport cholesterol from peripheral tissues to liver.
6. **Free fatty acid (FFA) or non-esterified acids-albumin complexes:** Each molecule of albumin can hold about 20–30 molecules of free fatty acids.

Disorders of plasma lipoproteins:

I. **Hyperlipoproteinemias:** Elevation in one or more of lipoprotein fractions.

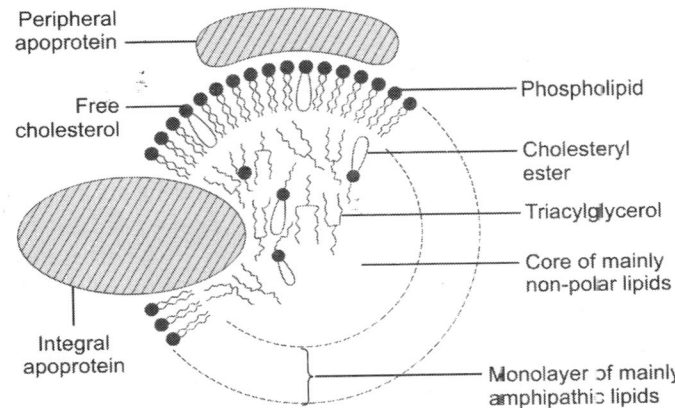

Fig. 1.15: General structure of lipoprotein

1. **Type I:** This is due to familial lipoprotein lipase deficiency, causing increase in plasma chylomicron and triacylglycerol.
2. **Type IIa (hyperbetalipoproteinemia):** This is caused by a defect in LDL receptors. Secondary type IIa hyperlipoproteinemia is observed in association with diabetes mellitus, hypothyroidism, nephrotic syndrome, etc.
3. **Type IIb:** Both LDL and VLDL increase along with elevation in plasma cholesterol and triacylglycerol. This is believed to be due to overproduction of apoprotein B.
4. **Type III (broad-beta disease):** This is characterized by appearance of a broad β-band corresponding to intermediate density lipoprotein (IDL) on electrophoresis.
5. **Type IV:** This is due to overproduction of endogenous triacylglycerols with a concomitant rise in VLDL. It is usually associated with obesity, alcoholism, diabetes mellitus, etc.
6. **Type V:** Both chylomicrons and VLDL are elevated. This is mostly a secondary condition, due to disorders such as obesity, diabetes and excessive alcohol consumption, etc.

II. **Hypolipoproteinemias:** Reduction in one or more of lipoprotein fractions.
1. **Familial hypobetalipoproteinemia:** It is an inherited disorder probably due to impairment in the synthesis of apoprotein B.
2. **Abetalipoproteinemia:** This is a rare disorder due to defect in synthesis of apoprotein B. It is characterized by a total absence of β-lipoprotein (LDL) in plasma.
3. **Familial alpha lipoprotein deficiency (Tangier disease):** The plasma HDL particles are almost absent. Due to this, reverse transport of cholesterol is severely affected leading to accumulation of cholesteryl esters in tissues.

Q. 16. Write a short note on cholesterol, its chemistry and functions.

(TNMGR, April 1997, 2000, March 2007)

Ans. Cholesterol is found exclusively in animals, hence it is called **animal sterol.** The total body content of cholesterol in an adult man weighing 70 kg is about 140 g, i.e. around 2 g/kg body weight. Cholesterol is amphipathic in nature, since it possesses both hydrophilic and hydrophobic regions in the structure.

Structure: Cholesterol has cyclopentano-perhydrophenanthrene ring system. It has A, B, C and D rings. It has 27 carbon atoms; One hydroxyl group on 3rd carbon atom, double bond between 5 and 6 carbon atoms and 8-carbon side chain.

Functions:
1. Cholesterol is a component of membranes and has a modulating effect on the fluid state of the membrane.
2. It is the precursor for the synthesis of all other steroids in body.
3. It is an essential ingredient in the structure of lipoproteins.
4. Fatty acids are transported to liver as cholesteryl esters for oxidation.
5. Cholesterol functions as an insulating cover for transmission of impulses in nerves.
6. Other functions include, its role in membrane structure and function, in synthesis of bile acids, hormones (steroid hormones, glucocorticoids, mineralocorticoids, sex hormones,) and vitamin D.

Sources: Cholesterol is derived from diet, *de novo* synthesis, from hydrolysis of cholesteryl esters.

Cholesterol biosynthesis: All the tissues of the body participate in cholesterol biosynthesis. The largest contribution is made by liver (80%), intestine, skin, adrenal cortex, reproductive tissue, etc. The enzymes involved in cholesterol synthesis are found in the cytosol and microsomal fractions of cell. Acetate of acetyl-CoA provides all the carbon atoms in cholesterol. The reducing equivalents are supplied by NADPH while ATP provides energy. For the production of one mole of cholesterol, 18 moles of acetyl-CoA, 36 moles of ATP and 16 moles of NADPH are required. The synthesis of cholesterol occurs in 5 stages:
1. Synthesis of HMG-CoA
2. Formation of mevalonate (6C)
3. Production of isoprenoid units (5C)
4. Synthesis of squalene (30C)
5. Conversion of squalene to cholesterol (27C)

Regulation of cholesterol synthesis:
1. Feedback control: Increase in the cellular concentration of cholesterol reduces the synthesis of enzyme HMG-CoA reductase.
2. Hormonal regulation: Glucagon and glucocorticoids decrease cholesterol synthesis. Insulin and thyroxine increase cholesterol production.
3. Inhibition by drugs: Compactin and lovastatin reduce cholesterol synthesis.
4. HMG-CoA reductase activity is inhibited by bile acids.
5. Fasting also reduces the activity of this enzyme.

Degradation of cholesterol: Cholesterol is converted to bile acids (excreted in feces), serves as a precursor for synthesis of steroid hormones, vitamin D, coprostanol and cholestanol.

Transport of cholesterol: Cholesterol is present in the plasma lipoproteins in two forms:

1. About 70–75% of it is in an esterified form with long chain fatty acids.
2. About 25–30% as free cholesterol. This form of cholesterol readily exchanges between different lipoproteins and also with the cell membranes.

Clinical importance of serum cholesterol level: In healthy individuals, the total plasma cholesterol is in the range of 150–200 mg/dl. In the new born, it is less than 100 mg/dl and rises to about 150 mg/dl within a year. The women have relatively lower plasma cholesterol which is attributed to hormones-estrogens. Cholesterol level increases with increasing age and in pregnancy.

Applied Clinical Aspects

1. **Hypercholesterolemia:** Increase in plasma cholesterol (>200 mg/dl) concentration. It occurs in: Diabetes mellitus, hypothyroidism (myxoedema), obstructive jaundice, nephrotic syndrome. Hypercholesterolemia is associated with atherosclerosis and CHD.
   - **Bad cholesterol and good cholesterol:** The cholesterol in high concentration, present in LDL, is considered bad due to its involvement in altherosclerosis and related complication. Small dense LDL (sdLDL) is considered to be the most dangerous fraction of LDL associated with CHD. On the other hand, HDL cholesterol is good since its high concentration counteracts atherogenesis.

   Control of hypercholesterolemia:
   i. Consumption of polyunsaturated fatty acids (PUFA).
   ii. Dietary cholesterol: Cholesterol is found only in animal foods and not in plant foods.
   iii. Plant sterols: Certain plant sterols and their esters reduce plasma cholesterol levels.
   iv. Dietary fiber: Fiber present in vegetables decreases cholesterol absorption from intestine.
   v. Avoiding high carbohydrate diet.
   vi. Impact of lifestyles: Elevation in plasma cholesterol is observed in people with smoking, abdominal obesity, lack of exercise, stress, high blood pressure, consumption of soft water etc.
   vii. Moderate alcohol cosumption: The beneficial effects of moderate alcohol intake are masked by the ill effects of chronic alcoholism.
   viii. Use of drugs: Drugs such as lovastatin which inhibit HMG-CoA reductase and decrease

cholesterol synthesis are used. Certain drugs-cholestyramine and colestipol-bind with bile acids and decrease their intestinal reabsorption. Clofibrate increases the activity of lipoprotein lipase and reduces plasma cholesterol and triacylglycerols.

2. **Hypocholesterolemia:** It is seen in hyperthyroidism, pernicious anemia, malabsorption syndrome, hemolytic jaundice, etc.
3. **Type III hyperlipoproteinemia:** This is a genetic disease in which individuals are homozygotic for the apo E-2 ligand resulting in defective clearance of chylomicrons, hypercholesterolemia, and premature atherosclerosis.
4. **Cholelithiasis:** The formation of gallstones occurs if there is either a bile salt deficiency or excess cholesterol secreted into the bile. In hypercholesteremia, gallstones are commonly formed, which can then lead to cholecystitis or ascending cholangitis.

Q. 17. Write a note on glycogen storage diseases.

Ans. The metabolic defects concerned with the glycogen synthesis and degradation are collectively referred to as glycogen storage diseases. The inherited disorders are characterized by deposition of normal or abnormal type of glycogen in one or more tissues (Refer to Table 1.17).

Treatment: Supportive treatment, diet therapy, ERT, genetic counseling and gene therapy

Q. 18. Write a note on lipid storage disease.

Ans. Lipid storage disease is a group of diseases that arise from a deficiency of specific lysosomal hydrolases with a resulting accumulation of the enzyme specific substrate. All are inherited as autosomal recessive except Fabry's disease, which is inherited as X-linked. Glycolipids are derivatives of ceramide (sphingosine bound to fatty acid), hence they are more appropriately known as **glycosphingolipids.** Galactocerebroside and glucocerebroside are the common glycosphingolipids. Galactocerebrosides are major component of membrane lipids in the nervous tissue. Glucocerebroside is an intermediate in the synthesis and degradation of complex glycosphingolipids.

Lipid storage disease (sphingolipidoses):
1. **Gaucher's disease:** This is due to a defect in the enzyme β-glucosidase. As a result, tissue glucocerebrosid levels increase. This disorder is commonly associated with enlargement of liver and spleen, osteoporosis, pigmentation of skin, anemia, mental retardation, etc.
2. **Krabbe's disease:** Defect in enzyme β-galactosidase results in accumulation of galactocerebrosides.

Table 1.17. Glycogen storage diseases

Type	Name	Enzyme defect	Organ involved	Characteristics
0	Lewis disease	Glycogen synthase	Liver	Hypoglycemia, hyperketonemia, early death
I	von Gierke's disease	Glucose-6-phosphatase	Liver, kidney, intestine	Glycogen accumulates in hepatocytes and renal cells, enlarged liver and kidney, hypoglycemia, lactic acidemia, hyperlipidaemia; ketosis, gouty arthritis.
II	Pompe's disease	Lysosomal α-1,4 glucosidase	All organs	Glycogen accumulates in lysosomes in almost all tissues, heart is mostly involved, enlarged liver and heart, nervous system is also affected, early death.
III	Cori's disease (Forbes' disease)	Amylo α-1,6-glucosidase (Debranching enzyme)	Liver, muscle, heart, leucocyte	Branched chain glycogen accumulate, enlarged liver, and kidney, hypoglycemia, lactic acidemia; hyperlipidaemia; ketosis, gouty arthiritis
IV	Anderson's disease (amylopectinosis)	Glucosyl-(4 → 6)-transferase (Branching enzyme)	Most tissues	Glycogen with only a few branches accumulate, cirrhosis of liver, impaired liver function
V	McArdle's disease	Muscle phosphorylase	Skeletal muscle	Muscle glycogen stores very high, but not available during exercise, muscle cramps, blood lactate and pyruvate do not increase after exercise, muscle may get damage due to inadequate energy supply.
VI	Hers' disease	Liver phosphorylase	Liver	Enlarged liver, liver glycogen cannot form glucose, mild hypoglycemia and ketosis.
VII	Tarui's disease	Phosphofructokinase 1	Skeletal muscle, erythrocytes	Muscle cramps due to exercise, blood lactate not elevated, hemolysis occurs.
VIII		Phosphorylase kinase	Liver	Hepatomegaly, glycogen accumulation in liver, hypoglycemia
IX		Phosphorylase kinase	Liver, muscle	Hepatomegaly, glycogen accumulation in liver and muscle, hypoglycemia
XI	Fanconi-Bickel disease	Glucose transporter-2	Liver, kidney	Enlarged liver, and kidney

A total absence of myelin in nervous tissue is a common feature. Severe mental retardation, convulsions, blindness, deafness, etc. are seen. Krabbe's disease is fatal in early life.

3. **Niemann-Pick disease:** It is an inherited disorder due to a defect in enzyme sphingomyelinase. This causes accumulation of sphingomyelins in liver and spleen, resulting in the enlargement of these organs. Victims of Niemann-Pick disease suffer from severe mental retardation, and death may occur in early childhood.

4. **Farber's disease:** A defect in enzyme ceramidase results in Farber's disease. This disorder is characterized by skeletal deformation, subcutaneous nodules, dermatitis and mental retardation. It is fatal in early life.

5. **Tay-Sachs disease:** This is caused by defective enzyme hexosaminidase A, leading to deposition of gangliosides GM2. This is characterized by blindness, mental retardation, death within 2–3 years.

6. **Fabry's disease:** It is caused by defect in enzyme β-galactosidase, leading to deposition of ceramide trihexoside. This causes renal failure, skin rash, pain in lower extremities.

7. **Metachromatic leukodystrophy:** Due to deficiency of enzyme arylsulfatase A, leading to accumulation of sulfogalactosylceramide. This causes mental retardation, psychological disturbances due to demyelination.

Treatment: Supportive treatment, diet therapy, ERT, genetic counseling and gene therapy.

2. ENZYMES, VITAMINS AND MINERALS

Q. 1. Write a short note on competitive inhibition.
(TNMGR, April 1998)

Ans. Enzyme inhibitor (Fig. 2.1): An inhibitor is a chemical agent inhibiting or poisoning enzyme. Enzyme inhibition can be competitive, non-competitive and uncompetitive.

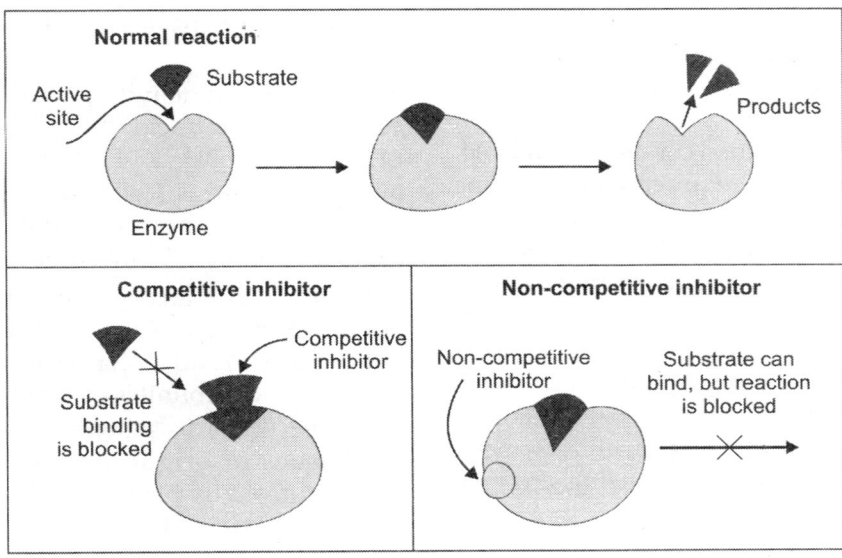

Fig. 2.1: Enzyme inhibition reaction

A. **Competitive inhibition:** In this, the inhibitor (I) closely resembles the real substrate (S) and competes with substrate and binds at active site of enzyme but does not undergo any catalysis. During the reaction, enzyme–substrate (ES) and enzyme–inhibitor (EI) complexes are formed. The relative concentration of the substrate and inhibitor and their respective affinity with the enzyme determine degree of competitive inhibition. The inhibition could be overcome by a high substrate concentration. In competitive inhibition, the K_m is increased but V_{max} is not changed.

Clinical significance:
- Pharmacological action of many drugs may be explained by the principle of competitive inhibition.
- Sulphonamides are commonly employed antibacterial agents. Bacteria synthesise folic acid by combining PABA with pteroyl glutamic acid. Bacterial wall is impermeable to folic acid. Sulpha drugs, being structural analogs of PABA, will inhibit the folic acid synthesis in bacteria, and they die.
- Antimetabolites are usually structural analogues of substrates and thus are competitive inhibitors. They are in use for cancer therapy, gout, etc. The term antivitamins is used for the antimetabolites which block the biochemical actions of vitamins causing deficiencies, e.g. sulphonilamide, dicumarol.

B. **Non-competitive inhibition:** Inhibitor binds at site other than substrate binding site, altering conformation of E. They are mostly used in toxicological applications. In non-competitive inhibition, the K_m is unchanged but V_{max} is reduced.

C. **Uncompetitive inhibition:** Inhibitors bind to ES complex.

Q. 2. Write a note on factors influencing enzymatic reactions. *(TNMGR, April 2007)*

Ans. Activity of enzymes is affected by:
1. **Concentration of enzyme:** As concentration of enzyme is increased, velocity (V_m) of reaction increases.
2. **Concentration of substrate:** Increase in substrate concentration gradually increases enzyme reaction.
3. **Temperature:** V_m of enzyme reaction increases with increase in temperature up to a maximum and then declines (**Bell-shaped curve**).
4. **pH:** Each enzyme has an optimum pH at which the velocity is maximum. Below and above this pH, enzyme activity is much lower and at extreme pH, enzyme becomes totally inactive, e.g. optimum pH for pepsin: 1–2; Alkaline phosphatase: 11
5. **Concentration of products:** Accumulation of reaction products decreases the enzyme velocity (feedback inhibition).
6. **Activators (coenzymes and cofactors):** Some of the enzymes require certain inorganic metal ions. Two categories of enzymes requiring metals for their activity are distinguished.
   a. **Metal-activated enzymes:** Metal is not tightly held by enzyme and can be exchanged easily with other ions, e.g. ATPase (Mg^{2+} and Ca^{2-}).

b. **Metalloenzymes:** These enzymes hold the metals tightly and is not readily exchanged, e.g. alcohol dehydrogenase, carbonic anhydrase contain zinc.

7. **Time:** Under ideal and optimal conditions (like pH, temperature, etc.), the time required for an enzyme reaction is less.

8. **Light and radiation:** Exposure of enzymes to UV, β, γ and X-rays inactivates certain enzymes due to formation of peroxides, e.g. UV rays inhibit salivary amylase activity.

9. **Oxidizing agent:** Oxidizing agents inactivates enzymes.

10. **Antienzyme:** Serum contains certain antienzymes/ antibodies against enzymes decreasing enzyme activity, e.g. antitrypsin, antipepsin.

Q. 3. Write a note on clinical importance of iso-enzymes. *(TNMGR, March 2011)*

Ans. Isoenzymes or **isozymes** are the multiple forms of an enzyme catalyzing the same reaction. They, however, differ in their physical and chemical properties which include structure, electrophoretic and immunological properties, kinetic properties, pH optimum, relative susceptibility to inhibitors and degree of denaturation. Examples:

1. **Isoenzymes of lactic dehydrogenase (LDH):** In health: $LDH_2 > LDH_1$.
   - In myocardial infarction: $LDH_1 > LDH_2$ (12–24 h).
   - In liver diseases: Elevated serum LDH_5.
   - In leukemia and malignancy: Elevated serum LDH_3.
   - In viral meningitis: Elevated serum LDH_1.

2. **Isoenzymes of creatine phophokinase (CPK):** In healthy individuals, isoenzymes CPK_2 (MB) is almost undetectable in serum.
   - Elevated CPK_1: Adenocarcinoma of GIT, carcinoma lung, prostate, testes.
   - Elevated CPK_2 (MB): Myocardial infarction (MI) (6–18 h).
   - Elevated CPK_3: Hypothyroidism, muscular dystrophy.

3. **Isoenzymes of alkaline phosphatase (ALP):** Increase in α_2-heat labile ALP suggests hepatitis, whereas pre β-ALP indicates bone disease.

4. **Acid phosphatase (ACP):** ACP level increases in carcinoma of prostate, tartarate resistant ACP increases in Paget's disases and bone cancer.

5. **Serum amylase:** Increases in disease of salivary gland and pancreas.

Q. 4. Write short note on lactic acid dehydrogenase. *(TNMGR, Oct. 2003)*

Ans. Lactic acid dehydrogenase (LDH) converts lactic acid into pyruvic acid. It has five distinct isoenzymes; LDH_1, LDH_2, LDH_3, LDH_4, LDH_5. They can be separated by electrophoresis (cellulose or starch gel or agarose gel). LDH_1 has more positive charge and fastest in electrophoretic mobility while LDH_5 is the slowest.

Structure: LDH is an oligomeric enzyme made up of four polypeptide subunits. Two types of subunits, namely M (for muscle) and H (for heart) are produced by different genes. M-subunit is basic while H subunit is acidic.

   i. LDH_1 (25%): Its subunit constitution is H_4. Principal tissues of origin are heart and RBC. It is not destroyed by heat.

   ii. LDH_2 (35%): Its subunit constitution is H_3M. Principal tissues of origin are heart and RBC. It is not destroyed by heat.

   iii. LDH_3 (27%): Its subunit constitution is H_2M_2. Principal tissues of origin are brain and kidney. It is partially destroyed by heat.

   iv. LDH_4 (8%): Its subunit constitution is HM_3. Principal tissues of origin are liver and skeletal muscle. It is destroyed by heat.

   v. LDH_5 (5%): Its subunit constitution is M_4. Principal tissues of origin are skeletal muscle and liver. It is destroyed by heat.

Q. 5. Write a short note on chemical messenger. *(TNMGR, March 2007)*

Ans. Chemical messengers are the molecules that are synthesized and secreted by specialized cells.

Classification:

A. **Local chemical messengers:** Chemicals secreted by cells that alter physiological conditions in the vicinity, either acting on same cell (autocrine agents) or adjacent cells (paracrine agents), e.g. histamine.

B. **Neurotransmitters:** Chemicals secreted by neurons, that acts on adjacent target cells, e.g. acetylcholine.

C. **Neuropeptides/neurohormones:** Chemicals secreted by specialized neurosecretory cells and acts on non-adjacent target cells, e.g. neural cells in hypothalamus.

D. **Hormones:** Hormones are conventionally defined as organic substances, produced in small amounts by specific tissues (endocrine glands), secreted into the blood stream to control metabolic and biological activities in the target cells, e.g. insulin.

E. **Pheromones:** Chemical messengers released to the exterior of some animals that affect the behavior of another individual of same species.

Classification of hormone:

A. Based on the chemical structure

1. Protein/peptide hormone: Insulin, glucagon, antidiuretic hormone, oxytocin.
2. Steroid hormone: Glucocorticoids, mineralo-corticoids.
3. Amino acid derivatives: Epinephrine, norepi-nephrine, thyroxine.

B. Based on the mechanism of action

1. Group I hormones: These hormones bind to intracellular receptors to form receptor hormone complexes, which binds to DNA, e.g. estrogen, calcitriol.
2. Group II hormones: These hormones are considered as first messengers, as they bind to cell surface receptors and stimulates release of certain molecules, second messengers, which perform biochemical function, e.g.
   i. Second messenger is cAMP, e.g. ACTH, FSH, glucagon, calcitonin.
   ii. Second messenger is phosphatidyl inositol/calcium, e.g. TRH, gastrin.
   iii. Second messenger is unknown, e.g. growth hormone, oxytocin.

Q. 6. Write a note on vitamins and oral cavity.

(Nagpur Uni., Oct. 2004; TNMGR, March 2008; SGT Uni., May 2019)

Ans. Vitamins may be regarded as organic compounds required in the diet in small amounts to perform specific biological functions for normal maintenance of optimum growth and health of the organism.

Classification:

A. **Water soluble vitamins:**
   1. **B complex:**
      I. **Energy releasing:** Vitamins B_1, B_2, B_3, B_5, B_6, B_7.
      II. **Hematopoietic:** Folic acid (B_9), cyanoco-balamin (B_{12})
   2. **Non-B complex:** Vitamin C.
B. **Fat soluble:** Vitamins A, D, E, K.

A. Vitamin B complex:

1. **Thiamine (vitamin B_1 or anti beri-beri factor or antineuritic vitamin or aneurin):** It has a specific coenzyme, thiamine pyrophosphate (TPP) which is associated with carbohydrate metabolism.
   Biochemical functions:
   i. TPP participate in conversion of pyruvate to acetyl CoA during carbohydrate metabolism.
   ii. TPP also participate in Krebs cycle.
   iii. Transketolase, enzyme required during HMP is dependent on TPP.
   iv. TPP plays an important role in transmission of nerve impulse by acetylcholine synthesis.

Recommended dietary allowance (RDA): 1–1.5 mg/day for adults. 0.7–1.2 mg/day for children. 2 mg/day for pregnant, lactating, old age and alcoholics.

Dietary sources: Cereals, pulses, oil seeds, nuts, yeast, animal foods, etc.

Deficiency symptoms

a. The deficiency of vitamin B_1 results in a condition called **beriberi**. The early symptoms of thiamine deficiency are loss of appetite (anorexia), weakness, constipation, nausea, mental depression, peripheral neuropathy, irritability, etc.
   i. **Wet beriberi:** In this, CVS manifestations are prominent like edema of legs, face, and serous cavities. Death occurs due to heart failure.
   ii. **Dry beriberi:** In this, CNS manifestations are the major features like peripheral neuritis with sensory disturbance leading to complete paralysis.
b. **Wernicke-Korsakoff syndrome (cerebral beri-beri):** Mostly seen in chronic alcoholics, as the body demands of thiamine increase in alcoholism. It is characterized by loss of memory, apathy and rhythmical to-and-fro motion of the eyeballs (**Korsakoff's psychosis**).

Oral manifestations: Hypersensitivity of oral mucosa, pain in tongue, teeth and face, gingiva becomes old rose in color.

2. **Riboflavin (vitamin B_2):** Riboflavin through its coenzymes (flavin mononucleotide, FMN; and flavin adenine dinucleotide-FAD) takes part in variety of cellular oxidation–reduction reactions.
   Biochemical functions:
   i. The flavin coenzymes participate in many redox reactions responsible for energy production.
   ii. The coenzymes are associated with certain enzymes involved in carbohydrate, lipid, protein and purine-metabolisms, besides the electron transport chain.

RDA: For adults—1.2–1.7 mg/day.

Dietary sources: Milk and milk products, meat, eggs, liver, kidney are rich sources.

Deficiency symptoms: Riboflavin deficiency symptoms include cheilosis, glossitis, and dermatitis and anemia. Chronic alcoholics are susceptible to B_2 deficiency.

Oral manifestations: Angular cheilosis, smooth and reddened lips, mushroom shaped fungiform papillae, pebbly or granular tongue, papillary atrophy, patchy and irregular depapillated tongue (**magenta colored tongue**).

3. **Niacin (Vitamin B$_3$):** Niacin or nicotinic acid is also known as *pellagra preventive (PP) factor of Goldberger.* The coenzymes of niacin [nicotinamide adenine dinucleotide (NAD$^+$) and nicotinamide adenine dinucleotide phosphate (NADP$^-$)] can be synthesized by the essential amino acid, tryptophan.

Biochemical functions:
   i. Coenzymes NAD$^+$ and NADP$^+$ are involved in a variety of oxidation–reduction reactions.
   ii. Enzymes belonging to class oxidoreductases are dependent on NAD$^+$ or NADP$^+$.
   iii. NADH is oxidized in electron transport chain to generate ATP.
   iv. NADPH is important for many biosynthetic reactions as it donates reducing equivalents.

RDA: For adults: 15–20 mg, for children: 10–15 mg.

Dietary sources: Liver, yeast, whole grains, cereals, pulses, milk, fish, eggs, vegetables.

Deficiency symptoms: Niacin deficiency results in a condition called pellagra (Italian: Rough skin). This disease involves skin, gastrointestinal tract and central nervous system. The symptoms of pellagra are commonly referred to as '4Ds'.
- **Dermatitis** is usually found in the areas of skin exposed to sunlight. Increased pigmentation around the neck is known as '**Casal's necklace**'.
- **Diarrhea** in the form of loose stools, often with blood and mucus. Prolonged diarrhea leads to weight loss.
- **Dementia** is associated with degeneration of nervous tissue. The symptoms of dementia include anxiety, irritability, poor memory, insomnia.
- **Death**, if not treated.

Oral manifestations: Pellagrous glossitis (painful, scarlet and edematous tongue with loss of filiform and fungiform papillae), oral mucosa becomes fiery red and painful with hypersalivation, fissuring of tongue, inflamed gingiva, corners of lip are pale with fan-like fissuring radiating to perioral region, may leave permanent scars.

Therapeutic uses of niacin (pharmacological doses)
   i. Niacin inhibits lipolysis in adipose tissue and decreases circulatory free fatty acids.
   ii. Triacylglycerol synthesis in liver is decreased.
   iii. Serum levels of LDL, VLDL, triacylglycerol and cholesterol are lowered. Hence niacin is used in the treatment of hyperlipoproteinemia type II b.

4. **Pyridoxine (vitamin B$_6$):** Vitamin B$_6$ is used to collectively represent three compounds, namely pyridoxine, pyridoxal and pyridoxamine (**vitamers of B$_6$**). The active form of vitamin B$_6$ is coenzyme pyridoxal phosphate (PLP).

Biochemical functions:
   i. PLP is closely associated with metabolism of amino acids.
   ii. Synthesis of certain specialized products such as serotonin, histamine, niacin coenzymes from amino acids is dependent on pyridoxine.
   iii. PLP participates in reactions like transamination, decarboxylation, deamination, transsulfuration, condensation, etc.
   iv. PLP is required for the synthesis of δ-amino levulinic acid (precursor for heme synthesis).
   v. PLP is needed for the absorption of amino acids from intestine.
   vi. Adequate intake of B$_6$ is useful to prevent urinary stone formation.

RDA: For adults: 2–2.2 mg/day.

Dietary sources: Animal sources such as egg yolk, fish, milk, meat; vegetable sources include wheat, corn, cabbage.

Deficiency symptoms: Neurological symptoms such as depression, irritability, nervousness, mental confusion, convulsions, peripheral neuropathy, demyelination of neurons, decrease in hemoglobin levels.

Oral manifestations: Glossitis with pain, edema and papillary changes. Initially tongue has scalded sensation followed by reddening and hypertrophy of filiform papillae at tip, margins and dorsum.

5. **Biotin (vitamin B$_7$):** Biotin (**formerly known as anti-egg white injury factor, or vitamin H**) is a sulfur containing B-complex vitamin. It directly participates as a coenzyme in the carboxylation reactions.

Biochemical functions:
   i. Biotin serves as carrier of CO$_2$ in carboxylation reactions.
   ii. As coenzyme, it is involved in gluconeogenesis and fatty acid synthesis.
   iii. Metabolism is dependent on propionyl CoA, leucine.

RDA: For adults: 100–300 μg.

Dietary sources: Liver, kidney, egg yolk, milk, tomatoes, grains, etc.

Deficiency symptoms: Anemia, loss of apetite, nausea, dermatitis, glossitis, depression, hallucinations, muscle pain and dermatitis.

Biotin deficiency is uncommon, since it is well distributed in foods and also supplied by the intestinal bacteria. The deficiency may be associated with: Destruction of intestinal flora due to prolonged use of drugs, or high consumption of raw eggs.

Oral manifestations: Pallor tongue, patch atrophy of lingual papillae.

6. **Pantothenic acid (vitamin B_5):** Pantothenic acid, (formerly known as **chick antidermatitis factor or filtrate factor**) is widely distributed in nature. Its metabolic role as coenzyme A is also widespread.

Biochemical functions:
   i. Coenzyme A is a central molecule involved in metabolism of carbohydrate, lipid and proteins.
   ii. It plays unique role in integrating various metabolic pathways.
   iii. Patothenic acid is involved in formation of fatty acids.

RDA: For adults: 5–10 mg.

Dietary sources: Eggs, liver meat, yeast, milk, etc.

Deficiency symptoms: Burning feet syndrome (pain and numbness in the toes, sleeplessness, fatigue).

7. **Folic acid (vitamin B_9):** Folic acid or folacin (latin word 'folium' means leaf of vegetable) is abundant in vegetables.

Biochemical functions:
   i. Tetrahydrofolate (THF or FH_4), the coenzyme of folic acid is actively involved in one carbon metabolism, amino acid and nucleotide metabolism.
   ii. One carbon metabolism synthesizes purins, pyrimidine, glycine.

RDA: For adults—200 µg/day. During pregnancy—400 µg/day

Dietary sources: Green leafy vegetables, whole grains, cereals, liver, kidneys, yeast, eggs.

Deficiency symptoms: Megaloblastic anemia, neural defects in fetus.

The pregnant women, lactating women, women on oral contraceptives, and alcoholics are also susceptible to folate eficiency. The folic acid deficiency may be due to inadequate dietary intake, defective absorption, use of anticonvulsant drugs and increased demand.

Oral manifestations: Glossitis, fiery red and depapillated tongue, marked chronic periodontitis, loosening of teeth, opportunistic infections.

8. **Cobalamin (Vitamin B_{12}):** Vitamin B_{12} is also known as extrinsic factor (EF) of Castle and antipernicious anemia factor. It is a unique vitamin, synthesized only by microorganisms and not by animals and plants. Vitamin B_{12} is present in diet as bound to proteins and is liberated by enzymes, acid hydrolases, in stomach. The stomach secretes a special protein called intrinsic factor (IF). The cobalamin-IF complex travels through the gut and binds to specific receptors on the surface of mucosal cells of ileum. In mucosal cells, B_{12} is converted to methyl-cobalamin and then transported in circulation as transcobalamins.

Biochemical functions:
   i. It participates in synthesis of methionine from homocysteine.
   ii. It participates in isomerization of methyl-malonyl CoA to succininyl CoA.

RDA: For adults—3 µg/day. For children—0.5–1.5 µg/day. During pregnancy—4 µg/day.

Dietary sources: Foods of animal origin.

Deficiency symptoms: Pernicious anemia (low hemoglobin, reduced RBCs), neuronal degeneration and demyelination of nervous system → symmetrical paresthesia of extremities, alterations of tendon and deep senses and reflexes, unsteadiness in gait, positive **Romberg's sign** (falling when eyes are closed) and positive **Babinski's** sign (extensor plantar reflex).

Oral manifestations: Burning sensations in mouth, tongue, painful swallowing, swollen tongue, pale and fragile buccal mucosa, xerostomia, cheilosis, hemorrhagic gingiva and bone loss.

Q. 7. Write a short note on ascorbic acid.
(TNMGR, April 1995;UHSR, June 2018)

Q. Write a note on vitamin C and oral health.
(RUHS, July 2016)

Ans. Vitamin C or ascorbic acid or antibiotic vitamin is a water soluble vitamin.

Chemistry: Ascorbic acid is a hexose derivative and closely resembles monosaccharides in structure. The acidic property of vitamin C is due to enolic hydroxyl groups. It is a strong reducing agent.

Biosynthesis and metabolism: Many animals can synthesize ascorbic acid from glucose via uronic acid pathway. However, many other primates, guinea pigs and bats cannot synthesize ascorbic acid due to the deficiency of enzyme L-gulonolactone oxidase. Vitamin C is rapidly absorbed from the intestine, it is not stored in the body to a significant extent. Ascorbic acid is excreted in urine as such, or as its metabolites diketogulonic acid and oxalic acid.

Biochemical functions:

1. Collagen formation: Vitamin C acts as a coenzyme in hydroxylation of proline and lysine while proto-collagen is converted to collagen.
2. Bone formation: Bone tissues possess an organic matrix, collagen and inorganic calcium, phosphate, etc.
3. Iron and hemoglobin metabolism: Ascorbic acid enhances iron absorption by keeping it in the ferrous form. Vitamin C is useful in reconversion of methemoglobin to hemoglobin. Degradation of hemoglobin to bile pigments requires ascorbic acid.
4. Tryptophan metabolism: Vitamin C is essential for hydroxylation of tryptophan (enzyme—hydroxylase) to hydroxytryptophan in the synthesis of serotonin.
5. Tyrosine metabolism: Ascorbic acid is required for oxidation of p-hydroxy phenylpyruvate (enzyme—hydroxylase) to homogentisic acid in tyrosine metabolism.
6. Folic acid metabolism: Vitamin C is needed for formation of FH_4 (enzyme—folic acid reductase). Further, in association with FH_4, ascorbic acid is involved in the maturation of erythrocytes.
7. Peptide hormone synthesis: Many peptide hormones contain carboxyl terminal amide which is derived from terminal glycine. Hydroxylation of glycine is carried out by peptidylglycine hydroxy-lase which requires vitamin C.
8. Synthesis of corticosteroid hormones: Adrenal gland possesses high levels of ascorbic acid, particularly in periods of stress.
9. Sparing action of other vitamins: Ascorbic acid is a strong antioxidant. It spares vitamin A, vitamin E, and some B-complex vitamins from oxidation.
10. Immunological function: Vitamin C enhances the synthesis of immunoglobulins (antibodies) and increases phagocytic action of leucocytes.
11. Preventive action on cataract: Vitamin C reduces the risk of cataract formation.
12. Preventive action on chronic diseases: As an anti-oxidant, vitamin C reduces the risk of cancer, cataract, and coronary heart diseases.

Recommended dietary allowance (RDA): Adult—60–70 mg/day. Pregnant and lactation—additional intakes (20–40%).

Dietary sources: Citrus fruits, gooseberry, guava, green vegetables, tomatoes, potatoes (particularly skin).

Deficiency of Vitamin C: Scurvy

Oral manifestations: Scorbutic gingivitis—ulcerative gingivitis, rapid periodontal pocket development, pulp is separated from the dentine and finally teeth are lost. Wound healing may be delayed.

Q. 8. Write a short note on fat soluble vitamins.
(TNMGR, April 2014; BBD Uni., June 2016; HP Uni., July 2018; NTR Uni., May 2019)

Ans. Fat soluble vitamins are A, D, E, K.

1. **Vitamin A** *(BBD Uni., April 2015):* Vitamin A, as provitamin form (retinol) is present in animal. However, its provitamins carotenes are found in plants. The term retinoids is often used to include natural and synthetic forms of vitamin A. Retinol, retinal and retinoic acid are regarded as **vitamers of vitamin A.**

   Dietary retinyl esters are hydrolysed by pancreatic or intestinal brush border hydrolases in the intestine, releasing retinol and free fatty acids. Carotenes are hydrolysed to retinal which is reduced to retinol. In intestinal mucosal cells, retinol is converted to long chain fatty acids, incorporated into chylomicrons and transferred to lymph. The retinol esters of chylomicrons are taken up by liver and stored. Retinol is transported in circulation by plasma retinol binding protein.

   Biochemical functions:
   i. Vitamin A helps in vision.
   ii. Retinol and retinoic acid regulate protein synthesis and involved in cell growth and differentiation.
   iii. Vitamin A is essential to maintain healthy epithelial tissue.
   iv. Retinyl phosphate is required for synthesis of certain glycoproteins required for growth and mucus secretion.
   v. Retinol and retinoic acid are involved in iron transport by synthesizing transferrin.
   vi. Vitamin is needed for proper maintenance of immune system.
   vii. Cholesterol synthesis requires vitamin A.
   viii. Carotenoids function as antioxidants.

   RDA: For adults—600 µg/day

   Dietary sources: Liver, kidney, egg yolk, milk, cheese, fish, yellow and dark green vegetables.

   Deficiency symptoms:
   i. Nightblindness (nyctalopia).
   ii. Xerophthalmia with keratinization of epithelial cells with white triangular plaques on conjunctiva (**Bitot's spots**).

iii. Keratomalacia—destruction of cornea.

iv. Total blindness.

v. Growth retardation.

vi. Sterility in males.

vii. Rough and dry skin.

viii. Increased tendency for stone formation.

Oral manifestations:

i. Defective enamel formation leading to enamel hypoplasia.

ii. Defect in normal tubular structure of dentin.

iii. Increased risk of caries.

iv. Delayed eruption of teeth.

v. Retarded alveolar bone formation.

vi. Hyperplastic and keratinized gingival epithelium.

vii. Increase incidence of periodontal diseases.

viii. Salivary gland undergo typical keratinizing metaplasia.

Hypervitaminosis A: Excessive consumption (>30,000 µg/day). Symptoms include dermatitis, raised intracranial tension, enlargement of liver, skeletal decalcification, tenderness of long bones, loss of weight, irritability, loss of hair, joint pains, etc.

2. **Vitamin D (sunshine vitamin)***(AHSUC, May 2017; NTR Uni., May 2019):* It resembles sterols in structure and functions like a hormone. Ergocalciferol (vitamin D_2) is formed from ergosterol and is present in plants. Cholecalciferol (vitamin D_3) is found in animals. D_2 and D_3 are referred as *vitamers.*

Biochemical functions:

i. Calcitriol increases intestinal absorption of calcium and phosphate.

ii. Calcitriol stimulates calcium uptake for deposition in bone.

iii. Calcitriol decreases excretion and increases reabsorption of calcium and phosphate in kidneys.

RDA: 200 IU.

Dietary sources: Fatty fish, fish liver oils, egg yolk, skin exposure to sunlight.

Deficiency symptoms:

i. Rickets in children—soft and pliable bones, bow-legs, decreased plasma calcitriol, elevated ALP.

ii. Osteomalacia in adults—soft bone, pathological fractures.

iii. Renal rickets—in chronic renal failure, due to decreased synthesis of calcitriol in kidneys.

Oral manifestations:

i. Developmental abnormalities of enamel and dentin.

ii. High risk of caries due to rough surface of enamel.

iii. Mottled, hypoplastic enamel.

iv. High pulp horns, large pulp chamber, delayed closure of root apices.

v. Delayed eruption of teeth.

vi. Altered trabecular pattern of alveolar bone.

vii. Small molars.

viii. Loss of lamina dura.

Hypervitaminosis D: Vitamin D is stored mostly in liver and slowly metabolised. Among all the vitamins, vitamin D is the **most toxic in overdoses** (10–100 times of RDA). Toxic effects of hypervitaminosis D include bone resorption and increased calcium absorption from the intestine, leading to hypercalcemia. Prolonged hypercalcemia is associated with deposition of calcium in many soft tissues such as kidney and arteries, loss of appetite, nausea, increased thirst, loss of weight, etc.

3. **Vitamin E:** Vitamin E (tocopherol) is a naturally occurring antioxidant. It is also known as **antisterility vitamin and vitamin in search of a disease.** Vitamin E is absorbed along with fat in the small intestine. In the liver, it is incorporated into lipoproteins (VLDL and LDL) and transported. Vitamin E is stored in adipose tissue, liver and muscle. The normal plasma level of tocopherol is <1 mg/dl.

Biochemical functions:

i. It is potent antioxidant, prevents non-enzymatic oxidations of various cell components.

ii. It protects polyunsaturated fatty acids from peroxidation reactions.

iii. It is regarded as membrane antioxidant, as it is essential for membrane structure and integrity of cell.

iv. It prevents sterility.

v. It increases synthesis of heme.

vi. It is required for cellular respiration.

vii. It prevents oxidation of vitamin A and carotenes.

viii. It is required for proper storage of creatine in skeletal muscle.

ix. It is required for absorption of amino acids from intestine.

x. It is involved in synthesis of nucleic acids.

xi. It protects liver from damage caused by toxins.

RDA: 10/8 mg/day for male/female, respectively.

Dietary sources: Vegetable oils, meat, milk, butter, eggs.

Deficiency symptoms: Sterility, degenerative changes in muscle, megaloblastic anemia, increased fragility of erythrocytes, neurological symptoms.

Oral manifestation: Loss of pigmentation, atrophic degenerative changes in enamel.

Toxicity of vitamin E: Among all the vitamins, vitamin E is the least toxic.

4. **Vitamin K:** Vitamin K is the only fat soluble vitamin with a specific coenzyme function. It is required for production of blood clotting factors, essential for coagulation. Vitamin K is taken in the diet or synthesized by the intestinal bacteria. Its absorption takes place along with fat (chylomicrons) and is dependent on bile salts. Vitamin K is transported along with LDL and is stored mainly in liver and, to a lesser extent, in other tissues.

Biochemical functions:

i. It brings post-translational modification of blood clotting factors.

ii. Acts as a coenzyme for carboxylation of glutamic acid residues present in proteins.

iii. It is required for carboxylation of glutamic acid residue of osteocalcin.

RDA: 70–140 µg/day

Dietary sources: Cabbage, cauliflower, tomatoes, spinach, egg yolk, meat, liver, cheese.

Deficiency symptoms: Vitamin K deficiency may occur due to its faulty absorption, loss of vitamin into feces and administration of antibiotics. Deficiency of vitamin K leads to lack of active prothrombin in circulation. The result is that blood oozes profusely even for minor injuries. The blood clotting time is increased.

Hypervitaminosis K: Administration of large doses of vitamin K produces hemolytic anemia and jaundice, particularly in infants.

Q. 9. Write about role of trace elements in oral health.
(NTR Uni., Nov. 2007; TNMGR, April 2012; BFUHS, Nov. 2012; PAHER, April 2013)

Ans. Trace elements are chemical micronutrients which are required in minute quantity but play a vital role in maintaining integrity of various physiological and metabolic processes occurring within living tissues.

Classifications:

A. **WHO classification (1973):**

1. Essential elements: Zinc (Zn), copper (Cu), selenium (Se), chromium (Cr), cobalt (Co), iodine (I), manganese (Mn), and molybdenum (Mo).

2. Probably essential elements: Cadmium, nickel, silica, tin, aluminium.

3. Potentially toxic elements: Gold, mercury and lead.

B. **Frieden's categorical classification (1974):**

1. Group I: Basic components of macromolecules (carbohydrates, proteins, and lipids), e.g. C, H, N, O.

2. Group II: Nutritionally important minerals or principal or macroelements. Daily requirement of macroelements is >100 mg/day, e.g. Na, K, Cl, Mg, S, phosphorous.

3. Group III: Essential trace elements or **minor elements** or **microelement** Daily requirement of microelements is <100 mg/day, e.g. Cu, Fe, Zn, Se, Cr, Co, I, Mo.

4. Group IV: Additional trace elements, e.g. cadmium, nickel, silica, tin, vanadium, and aluminium.

5. Group V: These metals are not essential and may produce toxicity in excess amounts, e.g gold, mercury and lead.

1. **Copper:** Copper is the third most abundant trace element with only 75–100 mg of total amount in the human body. It is present as ceruloplasmin (90%), copper–zinc metalloenzyme superoxide dismutase (60%) and loosely bound to proteins and amino acids (40%).

Biological functions:

a. Enzyme cytochrome c oxidase play vital role during aerobic respiration.

b. Superoxide dismutase detoxifies superoxide by converting it into oxygen and hydrogen peroxide.

c. Cu is a component of lysyl oxidase which takes part in synthesis of collagen and elastin. Cu is essential for maintaining strength of skin, hair, blood vessels, epithelial and connective tissue throughout the body.

d. Cu plays role in production of hemoglobin. Ceruloplasmin catalyzes oxidation of iron which is necessary to bind to its transport protein, transferrin.

e. Cu containing enzyme tyrosinase converts tyrosine to melanin.

f. Cu is necessary for synthesis of phospholipids found in myelin sheaths of nerves.

g. Cu is required for production of hormone thyroxine.

h. Cu can act as both an antioxidant and a pro-oxidant.

RDA: For adults—900 mcg/day.

Dietary sources: Oysters, other shell fish, whole grains, beans, nuts, potatoes, organ meats (kidney, liver), dark leafy greens, dried fruits, and yeast.

Role in oral health and diseases:

i. Deficiency of Cu leads to anemia and defective keratinisation in oral cavity.

ii. Deficiency of Cu can lower immunity, resulting infections of the oral cavity.

iii. Bone abnormalities and pain: Loss of trabecular formation with thinning of cortex, osteoporosis due to functional impairment of ascorbate oxidase and lysyl oxidase.

iv. Oral lesions: Serum Cu level is higher in patients with oral potentially malignant disorders and in malignant tumors, due to areca nut chewing.

v. Cu has dental caries-promoting property.

2. **Zinc:** Zn is stored in prostate, parts of eye, brain, muscle, bones, kidney, and liver. It is the second most abundant transition metal in organisms and is only metal which appears in all enzyme classes. In blood plasma, Zn is bound to and transported by albumin (60%) and transferrin (10%).

Biological functions: Zn functions in biology are separated into three main categories: Catalytic, regulatory, and structural roles. It is required for catalytic activity of a large number of enzymes. It plays an important role in immune function, wound healing, protein synthesis, DNA synthesis, and cell division. Zn is required for proper sense of taste and smell. It also supports normal growth and development during pregnancy, childhood, and adolescence. It also possesses antioxidant properties and thus may play a role in speeding up the healing process after an injury. Zn ions are effective antimicrobial agents even at low concentrations.

RDA: For adult—8 mg/day.

Dietary sources: Animal food—meat, milk, and fish.

Role in oral health and diseases (*NTR Uni., April 2007*):

i. In oral cavity, Zn is present naturally in plaque, saliva, and enamel. Low concentrations of Zn can reduce enamel demineralization and modify remineralisation.

ii. Taste disorders: Role of Zn in taste functions is appreciable at taste buds, taste sense nerve transmission, and brain.

iii. Zn deficiency can result in parakeratosis of normally orthokeratinized oral mucosa making it prone for oral and periodontal diseases.

iv. Lower levels of serum zinc is observed in patients with potentially premalignant disorders.

v. As transferrin transports Fe and Zn, level of Zn increases in iron deficiency patients.

vi. Superoxide dismutase has an anticarcinogenic effect in OSMF. Secondly, Zn decreases the activity of Cu containing lysyl oxidase enzyme and thus causes inhibition of cross linkage of collagen peptides. It also plays a significant role in promoting collagen degradation through collagenase and matrix metalloproteinase.

3. **Iron** (*BBD Uni., April 2015*): Iron is the most abundant essential trace element in human body. The total content of iron in the body is about 3–5 g with most of it in blood and the rest in liver, bone marrow, and muscles in the form of heme. Iron is absorbed in the gut from diet. Haemosiderin is a byproduct of metabolism of ferritin and is deposited in cells of reticuloendothelial system.

Factors affecting absorption:

- Iron is absorbed only in its reduced form, i.e. Fe^{2+} (ferrous).
- Ascorbic acid and gastric hydrochloride increase its absorption.
- Iron absorption is decreased by phytic acid, oxalic acid, calcium, Cu, Pb, and phosphorus.

Iron transport: It is transported in the form of transferrin (β-globulin). Transferrin takes up the iron with the help of ceruloplasmin (ferroxidase).

Iron storage: The storage form is ferritin. It is seen in intestinal mucosal cells, liver, spleen and bone marrow. In iron deficiency anemia, ferritin content is reduced.

Excretion: Iron is a one-way element. That is, very little of it is excreted. The regulation of homeostasis is done at the absorption level. Almost no iron is excreted through urine.

i. Feces contains unabsorbed iron as well as iron trapped in the intestinal cells.

ii. Any type of bleeding will cause loss of iron from body.

iii. Upper layers of skin cells are constantly being lost, another route for iron loss from body.

Biological functions:

- Heme is a major iron containing substance in ferrous or ferric state which is present in hemo-globin, myoglobin, and cytochrome.
- Many enzymes are associated with iron, e.g. cytochromes, p450, cytochrome *c* reductase, catalase, peroxidase, xanthine oxidases, tryptophan pyrrolase, succinate dehydrogenase, glucose-6-phosphate dehydrogenase (G-6-PD) and choline dehydrogenase.
- Hemoglobin is major oxygen carrying pigment in RBCs of mammalians.

- It participates in many metabolic cycles such as in energy producing reactions in all cells and activates energy producing oxidizing enzymes.
- It is necessary for synthesis of DNA, RNA, collagen, antibody synthesis.

RDA: For adults—8–18 mg/day.

Dietary sources: Haem iron—liver, meat, poultry, fish; non-haem iron—cereals, green leafy vegetables, legumes, nuts, oilseeds, jaggery, and dried fruits.

Role in oral health and diseases:

i. Oral manifestations of iron deficiency anemia include angular cheilitis, atrophic glossitis, generalized oral mucosal atrophy, candidal infections, pallor, stomatitis and dysphagia.
ii. Significant decrease in serum iron concentrations with elevated total iron-binding capacity has been found in OSMF patients. Also low serum levels of iron have been assessed in oral leukoplakia.
iii. Serum ferritin levels are elevated and serum iron concentrations are decreased with tumor progression in head and neck carcinoma.

4. **Cobalt:** In organic form, it forms an integral part of vitamin B_{12}. Inorganic forms of cobalt are toxic to the human body. Cobalt ions are absorbed within human body through food; respiratory system; skin; and as a component of biomaterials.

Biological functions:

- Vitamin B_{12} contains cobalt in the center of a planar tetrapyrrole corrin ring. Vitamin B_{12} is produced as hydroxocobalamin within bacteria and conversion to methylcobalamin and 5-deoxyadenosylcobalamin (active form) occurs within the body.
- Cyanocobalamin (**fourth vitamer of vitamin B_{12}**) can be metabolized in body to an active coenzyme form and used in food supplements.
- Erythropoietin stimulation is performed by vitamin B_{12} containing cobalt salts.
- Cobalt is necessary for formation of amino acids and various proteins for myelin sheath.
- Cobalt plays a role in generating neurotransmitters.
- Excess of cobalt ions within the body might increase action of thyroid and bone marrow resulting in overproduction of erythrocytes, fibrosis in lungs, and asthma.

RDA: For adults—2.4 mcg/day.

Dietary sources: Fish, nuts, green leafy vegetables, cereals, oats.

Role in oral health:

i. Pernicious anemia due to cobalt deficiency with Hunters' or Moeller's glossitis and shallow ulcers.
ii. Deficiency of cobalt can lead to peripheral neuropathy.
iii. Oral lichen planus and lichenoid reactions have been linked to their exposure to Cr, Co, Ni, and amalgam alloys.

5. **Chromium:** Trivalent Cr is an essential trace element and plays an important role in glucose metabolism. Hexavalent chromium has been classified as carcinogen.

Biological functions: Chromium increases efficacy of insulin and stimulating glucose uptake from muscles and other tissues. Chromium is thought to repress p53, a tumor suppressor protein, whose inactivation through mutations is associated with many types of human cancers.

RDA: For adults—25 mcg/day.

Dietary source: Processed meats, whole grains, and spices.

Role in oral health and diseases: The role of chromium in oral lichenoid reactions has been discussed earlier. Hyperglycemic status of diabetic patients in undiagnosed chromium deficient state may lead to delayed wound healing, suppurative periodontitis, various oral fungal infections, premature periodontal diseases, and hyposalivation.

6. **Selenium:** Selenium is an important component of antioxidant enzymes such as glutathione peroxides and thioredoxin reductase.

Biological functions:

- Selenium has immunomodulating and antiproliferative properties.
- It affects immune response by altering expression of cytokines.
- As glutathione peroxidase, selenium forms part antioxidant defense systems of body.
- Selenoenzyme protein has role in synthesis of triiodothyronine hormone from thyroxine.

RDA: For adults—55 mcg/day.

Dietary source: Liver, kidney, seafood, muscle meat, cereal, cereal products, dairy products, fruits, and vegetables.

Role in oral health and diseases:

i. Decrease in concentrations of selenium results in increased oxidative stress inside body tissues with inadvertent harmful effects like progression of leukoplakia, OSMF, and oral cancer.

ii. Selenium can effectively reduce duration and severity of oral mucositis (Chemotherapy) due to its cytoprotective and antiulcer activity.

7. Molybdenum

Biological functions

- Molybdenum, as a component of molybdoprotein, takes part in formation of active sites for various enzymes (xanthine dehydrogenase/oxidase, aldehyde oxidase, and sulphite oxidase).
- Molybdenum containing enzyme has role in purine catabolism.
- It also influences protein synthesis and growth of the body.
- Molybdenum has an antagonistic effect against copper.

RDA: For adults—45 mcg/day.

Dietary sources: Animal food—liver; vegetables—lentils, dried peas, kidney beans.

Role in oral health and diseases: Boron, vanadium, and molybdenum have a cariostatic effect.

8. **Fluorine:** Fluorine, in the form of fluorapatite crystals, is an important part of organized matrix of hard tissues like bone and teeth. It also stimulates osteoblastic activity.

Biochemical functions

1. Fluoride prevents development of dental caries.
2. Fluoride is necessary for the proper development of bones.
3. It inhibits the activities of certain enzymes. Sodium fluoride inhibits enolase (of glycolysis) while fluoroacetate inhibits aconitase (of citric acid cycle).

RDA: 4 mg/day

Dietary sources: Drinking water, foods (sea fish and cheese), and tea.

Role in oral health and diseases: Low levels of fluoride in drinking water are associated with dental decay. Excessive concentrations of fluoride during calcification stage of the teeth can result in enamel hypoplasia (dental fluorosis).

9. **Iodine:** Iodine is a vital trace element required at all stages of life especially during formative years. Total body contains 25–30 mg of iodine. 80% of the total is stored in the thyroid gland. Iodine level in blood is 5–10 mcg/dl.

Biological functions:

- Iodine is an essential component of thyroid hormones.
- It plays a significant role in functioning of parathyroid glands.

- Iodine plays an important role in general growth and development of body along with maintaining metabolic processes.

RDA: 150 mcg/day.

Dietary sources: Seafoods, cod liver oil, milk, vegetables, cereals.

Role in oral health and diseases:

i. Salivary glands can protect their own cells from peroxidation due to iodine concentrating ability through sodium iodide symporter and peroxidase activity.

ii. Role of iodine in oral immune defense mechanism may be substantiated by high concentration of iodine in thymus.

iii. Hypothyroidism can result in thickening of lips, macroglossia, delayed eruption of teeth.

iv. Hyperthyroidism can result in diffuse brown pigmentation of gingiva, buccal mucosa, palate, and tongue.

Q. 10. Write about deficiency and toxicity symptoms of fluoride. *(TNMGR, April 2015; NTR Uni., Nov. 2017; TNMGR, Oct. 2019)*

Ans. Fluoride is the reduced form (anion) of element fluorine. It is mostly found in bones and teeth due to its affinity to calcium.

Disease states:

A. **Fluoride deficiency:** Dental caries—drinking water containing <0.5 ppm of fluoride is associated with development of dental caries in children.

B. **Fluoride excess:**

I. **Acute fluoride toxicity:** It is due to fluoride intoxication (dose >5 mg/kg) over a short period, causing toxic signs and symptoms, including death. It requires immediate therapeutic intervention and hospitalization. The lethal dose of fluoride 15 mg/kg.

Signs and symptoms: Nausea, vomiting, hypocalcemic tetany, abdominal cramping and pain hyperkalemia, cardiac arrhythmias, convulsions, coma, and death within 4 hours. The toxic effects of fluoride are due to burning the tissues (due to formation of hydrofluoric acid in contact with moisture); impeding nerve function (due to affinity for calcium); cellular poisoning (due to inhibition of enzymes); and impeding cardiac function (due to electrolyte imbalance).

II. **Fluorosis:** It is a crippling disease resulted from deposition of fluorides in the hard and soft tissues of body caused by excess intake of fluoride through drinking water/food products/industrial pollutants over a long period.

1. **Skeletal fluorosis:** An intake of fluoride above 20 ppm is toxic and causes pathological changes in the bones. Hypercalcification increasing the density of bones of limbs, pelvis and spine, is a characteristic feature. The early symptoms include stiffness and pain in the joints. In severe cases, bone structure may change and ligaments may calcify, with resulting impairment of muscles and pain. Constriction of vertebral canal and intervertebral foramen exerts pressure on nerves, blood vessels leading to paralysis and pain. In the advanced stages, individuals are crippled and cannot perform their daily routine work due to stiff joints (genu valgum).

2. **Non-skeletal fluorosis/effects of fluorosis on soft tissues/systems:**
   a. **Gastrointestinal symptoms:** Abdominal pain, excessive saliva, nausea and vomiting.
   b. **Neurological manifestation:** Nervousness and depression, tingling sensation in fingers and toes, excessive thirst and tendency to urinate.
   c. **Muscular manifestations:** Muscle weakness and stiffness, pain in muscle and loss of muscle power.
   d. **Allergic manifestation:** Skin rashes, perivascular inflammation.
   e. **Effects on foetus:** Abortions, stillbirths and children with birth defects.
   f. **Low haemoglobin levels:** Fluoride converts RBCs into echinocytes which undergo phagocytosis and are eliminated from circulation.
   g. **Urinary tract manifestations:** Urine may be much less in volume; yellow-red in color and itching in the region may occur.
   h. **Ligaments and blood vessel calcification:** Soft tissues like ligaments, blood vessels tend to harden and calcify and blood vessels may be blocked.

3. **Dental fluorosis** is a developmental disturbance of dental enamel caused by excessive exposure to high concentrations of fluoride during tooth development. Excessive intake of fluoride is harmful to the body. An intake above 2 ppm (particularly >5 ppm) in children causes mottling of enamel and discoloration of teeth. The teeth are weak and become rough with characteristic brown or yellow patches on their surface.
   - Mild form: Unnoticeable, tiny white streaks or specks in enamel.
   - Severe: Pitted and rough enamel hard to clean.

3. DIET AND NUTRITION

Q. 1. Define diet and nutrition. Discuss the importance of diet in dentistry.
(BFUHS, May 2007; TNMGR, May 2018)

Q. Discuss role of nutrition in prevention of dental diseases. *(UHSR, June 2018)*

Q. Write a note on micro and macronutrients.
(UHSR, April 2019; NTR Uni., May 2019)

Ans. Diet is defined as the types and amounts of food eaten daily by an individual.

Nutrition is defined as the sum of processes by which an individual takes in and utilizes food.

Malnutrition is a pathological state resulting from a relative or absolute deficiency or excess of one or more essential nutrients.

Classification of foods
A. By origin: Animal origin, plant origin.
B. By chemical composition: Proteins, fats, carbohydrates, vitamins, minerals.
C. By predominant function:
   - Body building foods: Protein, milk, meat, poultry.
   - Energy giving foods: Cereals, sugars, roots.
   - Protective foods: Vegetables, fruits, milk.
D. By nutritive value: Cereals and millets, pulses, vegetables, nuts and oilseeds, fruits, animal foods, fats and oils, sugar and jaggery.

Nutrients: Nutrients are organic and inorganic complexes contained in food. Each nutrient has specific functions in the body. They are divided into
a. Macronutrients: Form the main bulk of food.
   - Proteins: 7–15%
   - Fats: 10–30%
   - Carbohydrates: 65–80%
b. Micronutrients: Form the minor portion.
   - Vitamins
   - Minerals

A. Proteins *(BBD Uni., April 2018):* They are complex organic nitrogenous compounds made up of smaller units called amino acids. Their major functions are:

1. Body building.
2. Repair and maintenance of tissues.
3. Synthesis of antibodies, plasma proteins, haemoglobin, enzymes and hormones.
4. The supply energy (4 kcal/g).

RDA: For adults—0.8–1 g/kg.

Dietary sources: Animal sources—milk, meat, egg; vegetable source—pulses, cereals, nuts.

Oral manifestations of protein deficiency: Red, inflamed, depapillated tongue, poor calcification of dentin and matrix, degenerative changes in gingiva and PDL, retarded cementum deposition, increase caries incidence, adverse effects on periodontium cells like fibroblast, osteoblast and cementoblast.

B. Fats/lipids: They are concentrated source of energy. They are classified as:
- Simple lipids—triglycerides (99%).
- Compound lipids—phospholipids.
- Derived lipids—cholesterol.

Functions:
1. They supply energy (9 kcal/g).
2. The carry flavor of food.
3. The add satiety and variety to a meal.
4. They are an integral part of cells and cell membranes.
5. They carry the fat-soluble vitamins.

RDA: 20% of total energy intake.

Dietary sources: Animal sources—ghee, butter, cheese, egg, fat of meat and fish; vegetable sources—groundnut, coconut, mustard; Other sources—rice, wheat, jowar.

Effects on oral health:
- Phospholipids are structural component of cell membrane, enamel and dentin.
- High fat foods reduce dental caries by coating the plaque, thereby preventing fermentable carbohydrates from entering it.

C. Carbohydrates: They are essential in the diet as a source of both glucose and cellulose, the major source of energy. Their major functions are:
1. They supply energy (4 kcal/g).
2. They are essential for the oxidation of fats.
3. They are required for synthesis of non-essential amino acids and ground substance of connective tissues.

4. Glucose is essential for erythrocyte and brain function.

RDA: 130 g/day.

Dietary source: Three main sources of carbohydrates are starches, sugars and cellulose.

Effects on oral health:
- High carbohydrate intake (sucrose) is utilized by bacteria to cause dental caries.

D. Vitamins: They are the substance which must be obtained by dietary means because of lack of capacity to synthesize in the body. They are part of the enzyme system (act either as coenzymes/catalysts for energy-releasing reactions).

E. Minerals: Minerals make up 4% of body weight.

Effects of Nutrition on Oral Tissues

A. **Nutrition and dental caries** *(BBD Uni., April 2017):* The demineralization of enamel and dentin is caused by organic acids that form in dental plaque because of bacterial activity, through anaerobic metabolism of sugars found in the diet. (Based on Vipeholm study which states that time, frequency, consistency and form of food are important factors in causing caries; Turku sugar study concludes that fructose is less cariogenic than sucrose and xyitol is anticariogenic.)

1. Pre-eruptive effects: Malnutrition can cause irreversible changes in teeth that could predispose them to develop caries. Enamel malnutrition, physical and chemical composition, time of eruption, tooth morphology and size are all affected by pre-eruptive nutrient intake. The dental dysplasia is associated with malnutrition. Other effects:
   - An odontoclasia in deciduous dentition.
   - A "yellow teeth" condition seen in permanent teeth.
   - "Infantile melanodontia" in deciduous teeth.
   - A linear hypoplasia of deciduous incisor teeth due to deficiency in Vitamin C or Vitamin A.

2. Post-eruptive effects: The post-eruptive effects of malnutrition (particularly protein deficiency) lead to decreased salivary lysozyme and secretory IgA levels, which leads to increased susceptibility to caries.

B. **Nutrition and periodontal disease** *(UHSR, May 2016):* Periodontal diseases may involve episodic, progressive disruption of several different tissues. The main targets in nutritional deficiency are the epithelial barrier and attachment, PDL, gingival connective tissue, alveolar bone, cellular and humoral immune mechanisms, inflammatory response, composition of gingival fluid. All these are susceptible to nutrient imbalance.

- Vitamin C deficiency can exacerbate existing gingivitis (scorbutic gingivitis).
- Deficiency of vitamins A, C, E and folate has detrimental effects on periodontal health.
- Altered calcium–phosphate in diet causes marked loss of alveolar bone.

C. **Nutrition and oral cancer:** Nutrition plays an important role in etiology of oral and pharyngeal cancers. Malnutrition increases the susceptibility to cancer of head and neck. Foods contain both initiators and modifiers of carcinogenesis.

- Most chemical carcinogens require enzymatic activation, which is significantly influenced by nutritional status and levels of specific nutrients, e.g. by protein or fat intake. Specific nutrient deficiencies may depress these enzymes, thereby reducing body's defence against chemical carcinogens.
- High-protein diets are likely to contain large amounts of animal and other saturated fats and calories. High intakes of saturated animal fats are associated with an increased risk of cancer of mouth and pharynx.
- Malnutrition or anemia reduces the ability of the immune system to counteract neoplastic cells.
- Nutritional factors protect against tumorigenesis by acting as blocking agents, altering metabolism of carcinogen through decreased activation, increasing detoxification, by scavenging the active molecular species of carcinogens to prevent their reacting with target sites in the cell, and by competitive inhibition.
- Vitamin A and retinoid (*BBD Uni., April 2015; HNBG Uni., June 2016*)
  - Inhibits chemically-induced tumors in various tissues.
  - Retinoid are effective in preventing carcinogenesis or in inducing regression of already formed tumors.
  - Have effects on protein kinase C, which influences epidermal growth factor receptors and DNA synthesis inhibition.
  - Retinoid and analogues used topically and systemically in the treatment of oral leukoplakia.
- β-carotene (metabolised to vitamin A)
  - It is an antioxidant and free radical scavenger.
  - Inverse relationship is seen between incidence of oral cancer and dietary availability of β-carotene/retinoid and vitamin C.

- Micronuclei formation in exfoliated buccal cells is reversed by β-carotene supplementation.
- Patients with oral leukoplakia treated with all-trans-retinoic acid, 13-cis-retinoic acid or β-carotene showed reductions in lesion size or stabilization of the leukoplakia.

- Vitamin C
  - Inhibits formation of carcinogenic N-nitroso (nitrosamine) compounds and mutagenecity of certain direct-acting mutagens.
  - Combined vitamins A and C intake is inversely associated with risk for oral cancer.
  - Enhancer of immune responses through effects on phagocytes.
  - Affecter of oxidases involved in detoxification of carcinogens.

- Vitamin E
  - Users have half the risk of developing oral cancer compared to non-users.
  - A free radical scavenger and protects cell membrane from oxidative damage.
  - Blocks nitrosamine formation.
  - Influences humoral and cell-mediated immunity.
  - Increases cell-repair capacity.

- Vitamin B complex: Patients with cancer or precancerous lesions in mouth display signs of vitamin B complex deficiencies.

- Foodstuffs:
  - Risk of cancer of mouth and pharynx is halved in those who eat fruits/vegetables daily.
  - Fish, buttermilk, milk, dairy products and sea food are protective against oral cancer.
  - Frequent consumption of milk, eggs, meat or fish reduces the risk of oral carcinogenesis in smokers and betel-nut chewers.
  - Increased oral cancer risk was observed for vegetable oil and excess animal fat.

Supplementation with iron and vitamins markedly reduced incidence of cancers of mouth, pharynx and oesophagus. Oral mucosal atrophy in iron deficiency states is a predisposing factor in development of oral cancer.

D. **Nutrition and malocclusion** (*BBD Uni., April 2014*): Teeth differentiate early in development and undergo short critical periods of growth. In contrast, jaw bones develop during an extended period of time, undergo a prolonged critical period and achieve their genetic size potential only after the teeth have developed. Because tooth sizes are determined genetically in a much shorter time span, whereas jaw size determination takes longer, a chronic postnatal malnutrition would result in stunted jaw development after the teeth have differentiated. This may result in class I type of malocclusions. Poor tooth alignment and crowding result in increased caries and periodontal disease.

Q. 2. Write a note on diet counseling.

(RGUHS, Nov. 2013; BBD Uni., April 2014)

Ans. Diet counseling is a tailor made individualized nutritional care for encouraging modifications of eating habits to prevent or treat nutrition related illnesses such as dental caries and other dental disorders, cardio-vascular disease, cancer and obesity.

Objectives:

* Conducting an interview, where diet diary forms are introduced with a brief discussion of the purpose of diet counseling.
* Educating patients about the role of sugar in decay process.
* Consumption of acceptable substitutes instead of more cariogenic foods.
* Provision of continuous positive reinforcement.
  A. **Diet and dental caries:** Dental caries is caused by ingestion of fermentable carbohydrates, particularly sucrose. Solid and retentive sucrose containing food are more cariogenic than liquid and non-retentive. The frequency and time of ingestion of foods are also important.

  Diet counseling:
  * Pre-requirements of counseling: Elicit a true response. Phrase the questions correctly. Listen and wait for an answer.
  * Counseling has two types of approaches:
    – Directive: Decisions made by counselor.
    – Non-directive: Patient can make his own decisions (recommended).
  * Guidelines: Gather information. Evaluate and interpret information.
  * Develop and implement a plan of action.
  * Family participation.
  * Follow-up.

  Diet diary: It is a complete record of food items consumed by patient along with its type, quantity, form and frequency in sequential manner. Parents are asked to maintain this record for 6 consecutive days.

  B. **Diet and periodontal disease:** Diets containing sucrose, glucose and other disaccharides can increase plaque mass and facilitate retention and colonization of plaque biofilm which forms a substrate for bacteria to grow leading to perio-dontal diseases.

Diet counseling in periodontal disease:
Step 1: Ascertain dental health diet score and if necessary, demonstrate method for keeping a diet diary.
Step 2: Explain the nutrition-periodontal relation-ship.
Step 3: Assess nutritional status.
Step 4: Prescribe a diet—improve adequacy of diet. Emphasize foods that are particularly beneficial to periodontal tissue—proteins, vitamins C, A, folic acid, calcium, iron and zinc. Encourage elimination of plaque forming sweets and substitution of fibrous foods.

Q. 3. Write a note on balanced diet.

(KLE Uni. Jan. 2009; RGUHS, Oct. 2010; MUHS, June 2010; UHSR, June 2018; HP Uni., April 2019; TNMGR, May 2019)

Ans. Balanced diet or prudent diet is defined as the diet which contains different types of foods, possessing the nutrients—carbohydrates, fats, proteins, vitamins and minerals, in a proportion to meet the requirements of body.

Importance of balanced diet:

* Body organs and tissues need proper nutrition to work effectively.
* Body is more prone to disease, infection, fatigue and poor performance without good nutrition.
* Children with poor diet have the risk of retarded growth and development.

Factors affecting balanced diet: Age, sex, availability of foods, social and cultural habits, economic status, environmental factors like temperature, physical activity, health condition (disease/healthy).

The nutrition expert group, constituted by Indian Council of Medical Research (ICMR) has recommended the composition of balanced diets for Indians. This is done taking into account the commonly available foods in India. Indian balanced diet is composed of cereals (rice, wheat, jowar), pulses, vegetables, roots and tubers, fruits, milk and milk products, fats and oils, sugar and groundnuts. Meat, fish and eggs are present in the non-vegetarian diets. In case of vegetarians, an additional intake of milk and pulses is recommended.

Balanced diet in developed countries: Some people in developed countries consume excessive quantities of certain nutrients. It is recommended that such people have to reduce the intake of total calories, total fat, satu-rated fatty acids, cholesterol, refined sugars and salt. The US Government recommends a daily intake of less than 30% fat against the present 40–50% towards calories.

Recommended dietary allowance (RDA): RDA is the amount of nutrients sufficient for the maintenance of health in nearly all people.

The amounts recommended include:
- A minimal physiological requirement.
- A margin of safety of 30–50% above actual physiologic requirements to allow for individual variation and to provide body stores for times of stress.

The recommendations by the expert committee are:
- Dietary fat should be 20–30% of total daily intake.
- Saturated fats not more than 10% of total energy intake.
- Excessive consumption of refined carbohydrate to be avoided.
- Energy-rich sources such as fats and alcohols consumption to be restricted.
- Salt intake reduced to not more than 5 g/day.
- Protein—15–20% of daily intake.
- Reduced consumption of colas, ketchups, and other foods that supply empty calories.

Food pyramid (*BBD Uni., June 2016; HP Uni., April 2019*): Food guide pyramid is defined as a pyramid-shaped diagram representing the optimal number of servings to be eaten each day from each of the basic food groups which can help to choose a variety of foods to achieve a balanced diet. Food at the base (wide) of the pyramid should be taken in more quantity, as one go higher, the pyramid becomes narrower, hence simultaneously reducing the quantity of food needed (Fig. 3.1).

Basic food group of food guide pyramid:

Group 1: Grain group—bread, cereal, rice and pasta group, e.g. wheat, rolls, tortillas, bagels, pancakes, six servings for children everyday.

Group 2: Vegetable group–vegetable from leaves, stems, roots, flowers, seeds, e.g. tomato, carrot, potato, cabbage, broccoli, peas, greens beans, celery, peppers. Three servings for children everyday.

Group 3: Fruit group—fruit from flowers of different plants, e.g. apple, bananas, citrus (orange, lemon,

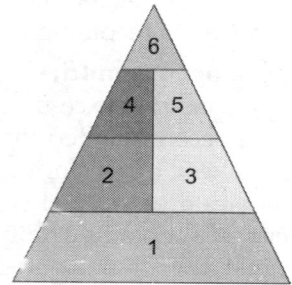

Fig. 3.3: Food guide pyramid with groups

grapefruit), peaches, pears, melons, grapes. Two servings for children everyday.

Group 4: Dairy group—include milk, yogurt and cheeses group. Two servings for children everyday.

Group 5: Protein group—include meat, poultry, fish, eggs, dry beans, nuts, peanut butter group. Two servings for children everyday.

Group 6: Fats, oils, sweet candies, baked goods, sodas, fried foods.

Q. 4. Write about importance of nutrition in an edentulous patient. *(BFUHS, Oct. 2010; AHSUC, May 2017; MUHS, June 2018; HP Uni., April 2019)*

Ans. A major problem of many elderly persons is limited physiological capability to digest and absorb foods, which may be due to:

1. **Physiological factors:** Declines in gastric acidity, nutrient deficiencies, dehydration, reduced kidney function and total body water metabolism, overt deficiency of vitamins, impaired neurological and/or behavioral functions.

2. **Psychosocial factors:** Elders, those living alone, physically handicapped, isolated, with chronic disease and/or restrictive diets, reduced economic status.

3. **Functional factors:** Functional disabilities such as arthritis, stroke, vision, or hearing impairment.

4. **Pharmacological factors:** Prescription drugs, polypharmacy may cause interference with nutrient absorption and utilization.

5. **Xerostomia:** Xerostomia is associated with difficulties in chewing and swallowing.

6. **Sense of taste and smell:** Age-related changes in taste and smell.

7. **Oral conditions:** Periodontal disease and oral infections.

Foods recommended for the elderly: All the nutrients necessary for optimal health can be obtained by eating:

1. Four servings of vegetables and fruits, subdivided into three categories:
   a. Two servings of good sources of vitamin C, such as citrus fruits, salad greens and raw cabbage.
   b. One serving of a good source of pro-vitamin A, such as green and yellow vegetables or fruits.
   c. One serving of vegetables and fruits.

2. Four servings of enriched breads, cereals and flour products.

3. Two servings of milk and milk-based foods, such as cheese.

4. Two servings of meats, fish, poultry, eggs, dried beans, peas, nuts.

5. 2–4 tablespoons of polyunsaturated fats.

Diet recommended for new denture wearer: The use of soft foods is advocated for the next few days and a firm or regular diet can be eaten by the end of the week.

- **First postinsertion day**
  - Vegetable–fruit group—juices.
  - Bread–cereal group—gruels cooked in milk/water.
  - Milk group—fluid milk in any form.
  - Meat group—eggs in eggnogs, pureed meats, meat broths, or soups.
  - The sample menu should contain a glass of milk at least once a day.
- **Second and third postinsertion day**
  - Vegetable–fruit group—juices; tender cooked fruits and vegetables (seedless and skinless)
  - Bread–cereal group—cooked cereals, softened breads boiled, rice, noodles and macaroni.
  - Milk group—fluid milk and cottage cheese.
  - Meat group—ground liver, tender chicken/fish in cream sauce, scrambled eggs, thick soups, etc.
  - Sample menu must include butter/margarine, a glass of milk at least once a day.
- **Fourth day and after:** By fourth day, or as soon as the sore spots have healed, firmer foods can be eaten in addition to soft foods. The sample menu must contain butter or margarine and a glass of milk.

Q. 5. Discuss nutritional assessment of post-surgical patient. *(NTR Uni., May 2008)*

Ans. Surgical procedures and subsequent fasting after admission can cause severe malnutrition quickly in the patients.

Causes of inadequate intake in surgical patient: Weak and anorexic patient, increased metabolic demand, GIT obstruction, cumulative effects of repeated periods of fasting, intestinal failure, low apetite.

Malnutrtion results in delayed wound healing, organ failure, delayed wound healing, and infection. Over-feeding leads to hyperglycemia, increased carbon dioxide, respiratory failure, and hepatic steatosis and hence optimal nutrition is needed.

Nutrtional assessment: Nutritional assessment is based on the findings of a routine history and physical examination.

A. **History:** History of preoperative weight, recent weight loss (or weight gain), loss of appetite, ability to swallow, chronic disease, infection, recent hospitalization, and prior surgery. Unintentional weight loss of >10% body weight within 6 months is to be carefully dealt, and proper nutritional support is indicated in these patients.

Diet history: History of use of dietary supplements, any allergies or food intolerances.

B. **General physical examination:**
- Vital signs and height and weight as BMI.
- General: Loss of subcutaneous fat, any generalized fluid accumulation.
- Head and neck exam: Hair loss, bitemporal wasting, conjunctival pallor, xerosis, glossitis, bleeding or sores on gums and oral mucosa, angular cheilosis or stomatitis.
- CVS: Evidence of heart failure or high-output state
- Neck: Thyromegaly.
- Extremities: Edema, loss of muscle mass.
- Neurologic: Evidence of peripheral neuropathy, reflexes, tetany, mental status.
- Skin: Ecchymoses, petechiae, pallor, pressure ulcers, assessment of surgical wound healing, and signs of surgical site infection.

C. **Investigations:** Anthropometric measurements and laboratory tests.
- **Laboratory tests:** Diagnostic tests including hematological evaluations provide insight into possible causes of oral or other systemic diseases.
  1. Complete blood count should be assessed to aid in determining immune response.
  2. Laboratory data value for electrolytes, serum proteins, trace elements, glucose, lipids, and organ function, blood urea nitrogen/creatinine help to assess overall clinical and fluid volume status.
  3. Iron levels should be measured in the setting of unexplained anemia.
  4. Serum calcium, magnesium, and phosphorous should also be assessed periodically, in the setting of poor oral intake or diarrhea.
  5. Serum albumin and lymphocyte count permit an instant assessment in emergency situations.

Considerations in dental surgery:
- After wisdom tooth removal: After routine 1-day postoperative period patient can go for regular soft, bland diet like any other extractions.
- After dental implants/dentoaleolar surgery/exposure of an impacted tooth, patient should drink plenty of fluids. Avoid hot liquids or food. Return to a normal diet as soon as possible.
- Major jaw surgery:
  - If intermaxillary fixation is done, a liquid diet or blended cooked foods with juice, milk, water, may be advised.
  - After orthognathic surgery, additional calories and nutrients should be added for wound healing.

– Patients with cleft lip and palate require oral liquid nutrition supplements or an enteral tube feeding.

Nutritional Interventions

- **Oral supplementation:** In general, high protein oral supplements, prethickened supplements and puddings.
- **Enteral nutrition:** Enteral nutrition support refers to the provision of calories, protein, electrolytes, vitamins, minerals, trace elements, and fluids through an intestinal route, either orally or via a feeding tube. Tube feeding—enteral nutrition may be delivered in a gastric or postpyloric fashion.
- **Parenteral nutrition:** It is an intravenous solution that contains dextrose, amino acids, electrolytes, vitamins, minerals, and trace elements.
- **Immunonutrition:** Immunonutrition is addition of specific naturally occurring additives to nutritional support, which may modulate inflammation and the associated oxidative stress and lead to an increase, improved immune system function. Immunonutrients include glutamine, arginine, branched-chain amino acids and omega-3 fatty acids, antioxidant, vitamins and minerals.

Q. 6. Write a note on basal metabolic rate.
(TNMGR, Nov. 1995, April 1998; NTR Uni., May 2019)

Ans. Basal metabolism or basal metabolic rate (BMR) or resting metabolic rate (RMR) is defined as the minimum amount of energy required by the body to maintain life at complete physical and mental rest in post-absorptive state (i.e. 12 hours after the last meal).

BMR = Total heat production (kcal per hour)/Body surface area (m²)

Measurement of BMR: Either by apparatus of Benedict and Roth (closed circuit device) or by Douglas bag method (open circuit device).

Normal value of BMR: For an adult man 35–38 cal/m²/hr or 1600 cal/day; For an adult woman 32–35 cal/m²/hr or 1400 cal/day.

A BMR value between –15% and +20% is considered as normal.

Factors affecting BMR

1. **Surface area:** BMR is directly proportional to surface area.
2. **Sex:** Men have higher BMR than women.
3. **Age:** In infants and growing children, BMR is higher. In adults, BMR decreases at the rate of 2% per decade of life.
4. **Physical activity:** BMR increases with regular exercise.

5. **Hormones:** BMR is raised in hyperthyroidism and reduced in hypothyroidism. The other hormones such as epinephrine, cortisol, growth hormone and sex hormones increase BMR.
6. **Environment:** In cold climates, BMR is higher compared to warm climates.
7. **Starvation:** During periods of starvation, BMR decreases up to 50%.
8. **Fever:** Fever causes an increase in BMR (10% increase per 10°C rise in temperature).
9. **Disease states:** BMR is elevated in infections, leukemias, cardiac failure, hypertension, etc. In Addison's disease BMR is marginally lowered.
10. **Racial variations:** The BMR of eskimos is much higher.

Significance of BMR: BMR is important to calculate the calorie requirement of an individual and planning of diets. Determination of BMR is useful for assessment of thyroid function. In hypothyroidism, BMR is lowered (by about 40%) while in hyperthyroidism it is elevated (by about 70%). Starvation and certain disease conditions also influence BMR.

Q. 7. Write a note on caloric values for carbohydrate, fat and proteins.
(TNMGR, March 2007)

Ans. Caloric value/energy density is the amount of heat generated by burning 1 g of foodstuff completely in presence of oxygen. Carbohydrates and fats are completely oxidized in the body; hence their fuel values, measured in bomb calorimeter or in the body, are same. Proteins are not completely burnt in the body as they are converted to products such as urea/creatinine and ammonia, and excreted. Due to this reason, calorific value of protein in the body is less than that obtained in a bomb calorimeter. It must be noted that vitamins and minerals have no calorific value, although they are involved in several important body functions.

Foodstuff	Energy value (cal/g)	
	In bomb calorimeter	In the body
Carbohydrates	4.1	1
Fat	9.4	9
Protein	5.4	4
Alcohol	7.1	7

Specific dynamic action (SDA): It refers to increased heat production following intake of food (thermogenic effect of food) due to expenditure of energy for digestion and absorption of food. SDA can be considered as the activation energy needed for a chemical reaction. This activation energy is to be supplied initially. The values of SDA are—for proteins 30%, for lipids 15%, and for carbohydrates 5%. This means that out of every 100 grams of proteins consumed, the energy available for doing useful work is 30% less than the calculated value. Hence, for a mixed diet, an extra 10% calories should be provided to account for the loss of energy as SDA.

Q. 8. Write a note on protein calorie malnutrition.

(TNMGR, March 2009, Oct. 2013; BBD Uni., April 2014, June 2016; Sumandeep Uni., May 2018)

Ans. Protein calorie/energy malnutrition (PCM/PEM) refers to nutritional disorder where the amount of nutrients taken are less than body requirement characterized by weight loss, edema and retarded growth.

Causes: Worm infestation, infections, failure to increase amount of food intake during growth of child, lack of knowledge on proper preparation of food, early weaning with no proper replacement feeds, diarrhea, poverty.

Types:

1. **Marasmus:** It is severe form of PEM which occurs in children due to inadequate intake of primarily carbohydrates (also proteins and fats) and is characterized by severe weight loss, and stunted growth. Marasmus usually develops between age of 6 months and 1 year in children who have been weaned from breast milk or who suffer from weakening conditions like chronic HIV/AIDS.

   Signs and symptoms:
   - Severe wasting due to decomposition of body fat and tissue.
   - Child looks a little old man or a monkey.
   - Skin is thin flaccid, dry and wrinkled and seems to be too big for the body (baggy pants).
   - Child has good appetite though emaciated.
   - Child looks alert and may cry at the sight of food.
   - Child may have diarrhea due to infection and impaired absorption.
   - Stunted growth due to inadequate intake of carbohydrates.
   - Superficial formy spots on conjunctiva (Bitot's spot), due to vitamin A deficiency.
   - Normal serum proteins and K^+ ion.
   - Increased serum cortisol level.
   - Several vitamin deficiencies occur.

2. **Kwashiorkor:** It is a type of protein energy malnutrition due to inadequate or low proteins in the diet and is characterizes by edema, apathy and moon shaped face. Kwashiorkor is predominantly found in children between 1–5 years of age.

   Signs and symptoms:
   - Pitting edema of feet, ankles and spreading to rest of the body.
   - Child has apathy and is anorexic with moon-shaped face.
   - Dry thin and sparse hair, easily pulled out due to lack of protein.
   - Hyperpigmented skin with epidermis peeling.
   - Temperature may be normal or hypothermic.
   - Distended abdomen and weight loss.
   - Stunted growth due to inadequate intake of food.
   - Delayed puberty due to growth retardation.
   - Impaired immunity.
   - Serum protein is very low, with altered electrolyte balance.
   - Hypokalemia.

3. **Combined marasmus–kwashiorkor:** When the signs and symptoms of both marasmus–kwashiorkor are present.

Management of PEM: WHO management guidelines

1. Intial treatment phase: Treatment of hypoglycemia, hypothermia, dehydration and infections.
2. Rehabilitation phase: It lasts from 2–6 weeks. Mother is trained to continue care at home with dietary supplements.
3. Follow-up phase: Physical, mental and emotional development of the child are monitored after discharge.

Clinical applied aspect: The patients of certain chronic diseases like cancer and AIDS are fequently undernourished, resulting in a codition called cachexia (wasting induced by metabolic stress). This is mainly due to loss of body proteins as a result of hyper-metabolism.

4. BIOCHEMICAL INVESTIGATIONS

Q. 1. Discuss the role of various biochemical investigations in dentistry.

(BFUHS, Nov. 2003; TNMGR, March 2007; Sumandeep Uni., April 2014)

Ans. Laboratory investigations are extension of physical examination in which tissue, blood, urine or other specimens are obtained from patient and subjected to microscopic, biochemical, microbiological or immunologic examination.

Types of laboratory investigations:

A. **Based on location of investigation:** Chair-side or laboratory investigations.

B. **Based on specificity/sensitivity:** Screening tests, diagnostic tests or prognostic tests.

C. **Based on hospital lab services:** Hematology, urine analysis, biochemistry, immunology, cytopathology, histopathology.

1. **Histopathology and cytopathology:** Histopathology is a microscopic examination of tissues, cytopathology is a microscopic study of individual cells or cells types.
   a. **Biopsy:** Biopsy refers to the removal of living tissues for the purpose of microscopic examination.
      Indications:
      1. To establish a diagnosis in case of suspected malignant lesion.
      2. Any chronic non-specific ulcer.
   b. **Exfoliative cytology:** It is a type of screening test with rapid diagnosis.
      Indications: Patient preference, population screening, as an adjunct to biopsy.
   c. **Toluidine blue test:** This test helps in identifying the site for biopsy. The test is performed by painting the suspected area with 2% toluidine blue vital stain, followed by thorough irrigation with water or rinsing with 1% acetic acid to remove the excess dye.
   d. **Chemiluminiscence:** It refers to emission of light from a chemical reaction, e.g. vizilite.
2. **Examination of saliva:** Examination of salivary flow rate, pH, composition.
3. **Caries activity test:** This test mainly provides the information about the individual's susceptibility to caries in future. These include Snyder test, lactobacillus acidophilus count, salivary buffer capacity.
4. **Hematology:** A complete blood count includes:
   a. Total RBCs count (4–5.4 million cells/mm^3)
   b. Hemoglobin concentration (12–16 g/dl)
   c. Packed cell volume (40–50%)
   d. Red cell indices: MCV (82–100 µ^3), MCHC (31–37%) and MCH (26–34 pg).
   e. Total leukocyte count (4000–11000 cells/ mm^3).
   f. Differential leukocyte count: Neutrophil (43–77%), lymphocyte (17–47%), monocyte (0–9%), eosinophil (0–4%), basophil (0–2%).
   g. Peripheral blood smear.

   Other hematological investigations:
   a. Erythrocyte sedimentation rate: 0–10 mm/hour.
   b. Platelet count: 1,50000–450,000/mm^3
5. **Tests for bleeding and coagulation disorders:**
   a. Capillary fragility test/torniquet test/Rumpel-Leede test: This provides information about platelet function.
   b. Bleeding time: Normal—2–6 minutes.
   c. Clotting time: Normal—5–10 minutes.
   d. Platelet count: 1.5–4 lac
   e. Clot retraction time: Normal: 2–24 hours.
   f. Prothrombin time (PT): Normal—11–15 seconds.
   g. Partial thromboplastin time: Normal—35–50 seconds.
   h. International normalized ratio (INR): Normal—0.8–1.2.
   Inference:
   INR <3: Infilteration anesthesia, scaling and root planning.
   INR <2: Block anesthesia, minor surgery, extraction.
   INR <1.5: Major surgery
6. **Serum chemistry:**
   a. Plasma proteins: Normal—6–8 g/dl.
   b. Calcium: 9–11 mg/dl.
   c. Phosphorus: 2–5 mg/dl.
   d. Alkaline phosphatase: 30–110 IU.
   e. Acid phosphatase: Elevated levels in metastatic carcinoma of prostate.
   f. Serum amylase: Increased in mumps, acute pancreatitis.
   g. Blood urea nitrogen: 9–25 mg/dl.
   h. Uric acid: 4–8.5 mg/dl.
   i. Cholesterol: 160–300 mg/dl.
   j. Creatinine: 0.7–1.4 mg/dl.
   k. Serum sodium, potassium, chloride: 135–148 mEq/L; 3.5–5.5 mEq/L; 96–110 mEq/L.
   l. Serum iron, total iron binding capacity: 55–184 µg/mm^3; 250–425 µg/mm^3.
   m. Serum enzymes: SGOT: 8–50 U/L; SGPT: <25 U/L; LDH: 200–400 U/L.
7. **Liver function test:** S. bilirubin (0–1.5 mg/dl), urinary urobilinogen (0.1–1.0 Ehrlich units/2h), bromsulphalein test (normally <6% dye retention), S. cholesterol, ALP, LDH, PT.
8. **Urinalysis:**
   a. Volume.
   b. Color: Light amber.
   c. pH: Slightly acidic.
   d. Specific gravity.
   e. Glucose.
   f. Protein: Normally not present.
   g. Acetone: Its presence indicates ketosis.
   h. Blood: Hematuria.
   i. Sediments: Normally epithelial cells, few leukocytes, erythrocytes (2–3), bacteria, oxalate, phosphate, and urate crystals.
9. Immunology and serology:
   a. Agglutination test.
   b. Latex agglutination test.
   c. Compliment fixation test.
   d. Heterophile agglutination test (Paul-Bunnell test).

e. Monospot test.

f. Immunofluorescence test: Direct, indirect, sandwich technique.

g. Diagnosis of syphilis: Wasserman reaction, Kahn test, reactive plasma reagin test, VDRL test.

10. **Diagnostic skin tests:** Mantoux test → Tuberculosis; Kveim-Siltzbach → Sarcoidosis; Patch tests → Contact dermatitis/stomatitis.

11. **Microbiological examination:** Bacterial smears, cultures and antibiotic sensitivity tests, ELISA.

12. **Examination of the endocrine disorders:**

a. Test for thyroid function: BMR, protein bound iodine (4–8 mg/dl), butanol-extractable iodine (3–7 mg/dl), triiodothyronine uptake test (11.5–19%), S. thyroxin test (4–11 mg/dl), thyroxine binding globulin, pre-albumin, radioactive iodine uptake.

b. Test of pancreatic function:

  • Serum glucose level: Blood glucose levels (random, fasting, post prandial); glucose tolerance test; glycated hemoglobulin (HbA1c) test.

  • Urine glucose examination.

c. Test of parathyroid function.

d. Test of pituitary function.

e. Test of adrenal functions:

  i. Vanillylmandelic acid assay (VMA): 2–10 mg/24 urine sample.

  ii. Urinary 17-hydroxycorticosteroids: Level decreases in Addison's disease.

13. **Nerve and muscle function test:**

a. General sensory perception tests.

b. Reflex testing.

c. Autonomic drug tests.

d. Sweat test of infants nerve conduction test.

e. Electromyography.

f. Muscle biopsy.

g. Blood and urine creatine and creatinine.

h. Serum creatine phophokinase.

i. SGOT.

j. LDH.

Q. 2. Write a short note on liver function test.
(RGUHS, Nov. 2011; TNMGR, June 2017)

Ans. Liver function tests (LFT) are the biochemical investigations to assess the capacity of liver to carry out the functions it performs. The major liver tests can be classified as follows:

1. **Test based on excretory function:** S. bilirubin (0.1–1.2 mg/dl), urine bilirubin, urine and feacal urobilinogen, urine bile salts, dye excretion tests.

2. **Test based on serum enzymes derived from liver:** Determination of transaminases (AST or SGOT, ALT or SGPT), alkaline phosphatase (ALP), 5' nucleotidase (5' NT = 2–15 U/L), γ-glutamyl-transpeptidase (GGT= 9–48 U/L).

3. **Test based on metabolic function:** Galactose tolerance test for carbohydrate metabolism, S. cholesterol for lipid metabolism, S. proteins aminoaciduria for protein metabolism.

4. **Test based on synthetic functions:** Prothrombin time, plasma proteins.

5. **Test based on detoxification:** Hippuric acid synthesis, determination of blood ammonia.

Tests for serum albumin/plasma proteins:

a. Total serum proteins

b. Serum albumin

c. Serum albumin: Globulin ratio

d. Serum protein electrophoresis

e. Prealbumin

f. Procollagen III peptide

g. Ceruloplasmin: 0.2–0.4 g/L

h. α_1-fetoprotein

i. α_1-antitrypsin

Applied clinical aspects: Altered LFTs:

• **Alcohol:** In patients with alcoholism, AST to ALT ratio is generally at least 2:1, showing a high level of AST activity in alcoholic liver disease.

• **Medications:** Acetaminophen causes very high LFTs and liver failure.

• **Viral hepatitis:** Any viral hepatitis in an acute setting can cause increased LFTs.

• **Autoimmune hepatitis:** Patient presents with high LFTs without apparent cause.

• **Hepatic steatosis and non-alcoholic steatohepatitis:** The AST to ALT ratio is generally 1:1. All other labs are usually within normal limits.

• **α1-antitrypsin deficiency:** α1-antitrypsin deficiency predisposes to obstructive pulmonary disease and liver disease (e.g. cirrhosis and hepatocellular carcinoma in children and adults).

Q. 3. Write about the investigatory importance of calcium, phosphate and alkaline phosphatase.
(RGUHS, Nov. 2011)

Ans. Alkaline phosphatase (ALP) is a group of isoenzymes, located on outer layer of cell membrane; they catalyze the hydrolysis of organic phosphate esters present in the extracellular space.

Classification

1. **Tissue specific:** ALP in intestine, placenta, and germinal tissue.

2. **Tissue non-specific types:** ALP circulating in serum (from liver, bone, and kidneys).

Serum ALP levels:
- During childhood and puberty, levels are high.
- Levels decrease in 15–50 year age group, are slightly higher in men than in women, and rise again in old age.
- Positive correlation with body weight and smoking.
- Inverse correlation with height.

Marked elevation of serum ALP: Cholestatic liver disease, biliary obstruction due to cancer, choledocholithiasis, biliary stricture, sclerosing cholangitis, or causes of intrahepatic cholestasis, drug-induced liver injury, chronic rejection of liver allografts, infiltrative liver disease, AIDS.

Moderate elevation (four times higher than normal) **of serum ALP:** Liver cirrhosis, chronic hepatitis, viral hepatitis, CHF, intra-abdominal infections, Hodgkin lymphoma, and osteomyelitis.

Low levels of ALP: Wilson's disease, Zn deficiency, pernicious anemia, hypothyroidism, and congenital hypophosphatasia.

Q. 4. Write about laboratory tests for diabetes mellitus.

(TNMGR, Sept. 2008; NTR Uni., June 2015)

Q. Write a note on glucose tolerance test.

(TNMGR, Oct. 1999; NTR Uni., May 2018)

Ans. Laboratory test for diabetes mellitus includes:
I. **Urine analysis:**
  1. **Detection of urinary glucose (glucosuria):** Normally glucose does not appear in urine until plasma glucose rises above 160–180 mg/dl. This can be detected by Diastix, Benedict's and Fehling's test.
  2. **Ketonuria:** It can be detected by nitroprusside test, Rothera's test.
  3. **Microalbuminuria:** It is the albumin excretion above normality (2.5–25 mg/d) in a 24-hour urine specimen.
II. **Blood biochemistry:**
  1. **Blood glucose estimation:** As per clinical practice recommendations by **American Diabetes Association (2019)**
    a. **Fasting blood glucose (FBG):** Measured after overnight (at least 8 h) fasting.
      Normal: FBG <5.6 mmol/L (100 mg/dl)
      Impaired fasting glucose/prediabetes: FBG— 5.6–6.9 mmol/L (100–125 mg/dl)
      Diabetes: FBG >7.0 mmol/L (126 mg/dl)

  b. **Random (casual) blood glucose:** It is measured without regard to time since the last meal. **Diabetes:** RBG >11.1 mmol/L (>200 mg/dl)
  c. **Glucose tolerance test (GTT):** It measures individual's response to oral glucose load. Procedure of GTT as prescribed by WHO (1999):
    - **Preparation of subject:** The person should have been taking carbohydrate rich diet for at least 3 days prior to test. All drugs known to influence carbohydrate metabolism should be discontinued (for at least 2 days). He/she should be in an overnight (at least 8 h) fasting state.
    - **Procedure:** A fasting blood sample is drawn and urine collected. The subject is given 75 g glucose orally (in 300 ml of water) to be drunk in about 5 minutes. Blood and urine samples are collected at 30 minute intervals for at least 2 hours. All blood samples are subjected to glucose estimation while urine samples are qualitatively tested for glucose.
    - Interpretation of GTT:

	Normal glucose tolerance	Impaired glucose tolerance	Diabetes mellitus
Fasting plasma glucose (mg/dl)	<110	110–125	>126
2 hours after glucose load	<140	140–199	>200

  d. **Glycated hemoglobin (HbA1c) test:** It reflects glycemic control for preceding 8–12 weeks.
    Normal: <5.7%
    Prediabetes: 5.7–6.4%
    Diabetes: >6.5%.
  e. **Serum fructosamine estimation:** It reflects glycemic control for preceding 1–2 weeks. It is indicated when abnormal hemoglobin or hemolytic anemia affects interpretation of HbA1c or in pregnant female.
    Normal = 1.5–2.4 mmol/L.

Q. 5. Write a short note on renal function tests.

(NTR Uni., May 2008; BFUHS, May 2011)

Ans. Renal function tests (RFT) may be divided into four groups.
1. Glomerular function tests: All the clearance tests (inulin, creatinine, urea).
2. Tubular function tests: Urine concentration or dilution test, urine acidification test.

3. Analysis of blood/serum: Estimation of blood urea, serum creatinine, protein and electrolyte.
4. Urine examination: Examination of urine for volume, pH, specific gravity, osmolality and presence of abnormal constituents (proteins, blood, ketone bodies, glucose etc.)

A. **Urine-based test**
1. **Albuminuria:** Urine albumin may be measured in 24-hour urine collections or early morning/random specimens as an albumin/creatinine ratio.
   - Glomerular dysfunction: Presence of albuminuria on two occasions.
   - Chronic kidney disease: Presence of albuminuria for 3 or more months.

   Proteinuria: It is defined as excretion of proteins in urine >300 mg/day.
   - Normal urine protein—up to 150 mg/day
   - In nephrotic syndrome—urine protein >3.5 g/day

2. **Tests of tubular function:**
   - Urine osmolality >750 mOsmol/kg indicates normal concentrating ability of tubules.
   - Water deprivation test: To exclude nephrogenic diabetes insipidus.
   - Ammonium chloride test: To confirm diagnosis of distal renal tubular acidosis.
   - Fanconi's syndrome: Aminoaciduria, glycosuria, phosphaturia and bicarbonate wasting (proximal renal tubular acidosis).

3. **Urine analysis:**
   - **Physical analysis:**
     - Color: Normal urine color → Straw color; Dehydration → Darker color; Red urine → Hematuria or porphyria; Blue urine → Cholera; Orange urine → Fever; Cloudy urine → Pyuria.
     - Specific gravity: Normal—1.003–1.030; ↑ with concentrated urine and ↓ with dilute urine.
     - Odor: Usually light pungent; Aromatic → Volatile fatty acids; Ammonical → Bacterial infection; Fruity → Ketonuria.
     - Volume: Normal—1000–2000 ml/24 h; polyurea due to drugs, diabetes; oligourea (<400 ml/24 h); anurea (<100 ml/24 h) in dehydration, CHF.
     - pH: Normal—6.
   - Biochemical analysis: Dipstick test for presence of protein, glucose, blood, ketones, bilirubin, urobilinogen, nitrite, and leukocyte esterase.
   - Microscopic analysis:
     - Red blood casts: Glomerulonephritis.
     - RBC: Renal injury.
     - White blood cell casts and WBCs: Pyelonephritis.
     - Hyaline casts: Glomerular disease.
     - Crystals: Triple phosphate crystals → Pseudogout; Uric acid crystals → Gout; Oxalate crystals → Ethylene glycol poisoning or 1° and 2° hyperoxaluria; Cystine crystals → Cystinuria.

B. **Serum-based tests**
1. **Glomerular filtration rate:** Normal GFR—90–120 ml/minute.
2. **S. creatinine:** Clearance of creatinine is used to provide an indicator of GFR. Normal—0.6–1.3 mg/dl.
3. **Uric acid:** Normal—3.4–7 mg/dl (M); 2.4–5 mg/dl (F); ↑ in renal failure, nephrolithiasis.
4. **Blood urea nitrogen (BUN):**
   - Increased S. urea (azotemia): Acute and chronic renal failure, upper GI bleeding, dehydration, catabolic states, and high protein diets.
   - Decreased S. urea: Starvation, low-protein diet and severe liver disease.
5. **BUN:** Creatinine ratio: In pre-renal disease: 20:1; In intrinsic renal disease: 10:1.
6. **Cystatin C:** Serum levels of cystatin C are inversely correlated with GFR.

Q. 6. Write a short note on INR. *(BFUHS, Oct. 2011)*
Ans. International normalized ratio (INR) is derived from prothrombin time (PT) which is calculated as a ratio of the patient's PT to control PT standardized for the potency of the thromboplastin reagent developed by the World Health Organization (WHO) using the following formula: INR = Patient PT ÷ Control PT

Normal INR is about 1. In patients taking anticoagulant therapy for atrial fibrillation, INR should be between 2 and 3. For patients with heart valve disorders, INR should be between 3 and 4. But, INR greater than 4 indicates that blood is clotting too slowly and there is a risk of uncontrolled blood clotting.

PT/INR can be prolonged in:
1. Vitamin K antagonist (warfarin) and other anticoagulants like
   - Heparins: Unfractionated or low molecular weight.
   - Direct factor Xa-inhibitor: Rivaroxaban, apixaban, edoxaban
   - Direct thrombin inhibitor: Argatroban, dabigatran.
2. Liver dysfunction.
3. Vitamin K deficiency.
4. DIC.

5. Coagulation factor deficiency in extrinsic pathway.
6. Antiphospholipid antibodies.

Clinical significance: INR level below the target range is associated with increased risk of thrombosis. INR above the therapeutic range is associated with increased risk of bleeding.

Q. 7. Write short note on bilirubinemia.
(TNMGR, Oct. 2000)

Q. Write about classification of jaundice.
(TNMGR, April 2000, Sept. 2002)

Ans. Jaundice (French: *Jaune*—yellow) or icterus is a clinical condition characterized by yellow color of white of the eyes (sclerae), skin and mucous membrane. It is caused by deposition of bilirubin due to its elevated levels in serum (>2 mg/dl).

Hyperbilirubinemia: Increased plasma concentrations of bilirubin (>3 mg/dl) occurs when there is an imbalance between its production and excretion.

Classification of Jaundice

1. **Pre-hepatic/hemolytic jaundice:** This condition is associated with increased hemolysis of erythrocytes, resulting in overproduction of bilirubin beyond the ability of liver to conjugate. It is characterized by:
   i. Elevated serum unconjugated bilirubin.
   ii. Increased excretion of urobilinogen in urine.
   iii. Dark brown color of feces due to high content of stercobilinogen.

2. **Hepatic (hepatocellular) jaundice:** This is caused by dysfunction of liver due to damage to parenchymal cells. This may be attributed to viral infection, poisons and toxins, cirrhosis of liver, cardiac failure, etc. It is characterized by:
   i. Increased levels of conjugated and unconjugated bilirubin in serum.
   ii. Dark colored urine due to excessive excretion of bilirubin and urobilinogen.
   iii. Increased activities of alanine transaminases (ALT/SGPT) and aspartate transaminase (AST/SGOT).
   iv. Patients pass pale, clay colored stools due to absence of stercobilinogen.
   v. Affected individuals experience nausea and anorexia.

3. **Post-hepatic/obstructive (regurgitation) jaundice:** This is due to an obstruction in bile duct that prevents passage of bile into intestine. This is caused by gallstones, tumors (head of pancreas), biliary stricture, etc. It is characterized by:
   i. Increased concentration of conjugated bilirubin in serum.
   ii. S. ALP is elevated as it is released from the cells of damaged bile duct.
   iii. Dark colored urine and clay/gray colored feces.
   iv. Impaired fat digestion with steatorrhea.
   v. Patients experience nausea and gastrointestinal pain.

4. **Jaundice due to genetic defects:**
   i. **Neonatal/physiological jaundice:** Physiological jaundice (transient, resolve in first 10 days) is caused by increased hemolysis coupled with immature hepatic system. The activity of enzyme UDP-glucuronyltransferase is low in newborn. In some infants, serum uncojugated bilirubin is highly elevated, which can cross the blood–brain barrier. This results in **hyperbilirubinemic toxic encephalopathy or Kernicterus** (yellow staining of deep nuclei of basal ganglia) that causes mental retardation. In some neonates, blood transfusion may be necessary to prevent brain damage. Phototherapy (photoisomerization) deals with exposure of jaundiced neonates to UV light, the toxic native unconjugated bilirubin gets converted into a non-toxic isomer namely lumirubin. Lumirubin can be easily excreted by the kidneys in the unconjugated form.
   ii. Crigler-Najjar syndrome type I: This is also known as congenital non-hemolytic jaundice. It is a rare disorder and is due to a defect in the hepatic enzyme UDP-glucuronyltransferase. Generally, the children die within first 2 years of life.
   iii. Other inherited disorder of bilirubin metabolism: Gilbert's syndrome, Crigler-Najjar type-II, Lucey-Driscoll syndrome, Dubin-Johnson syndrome, Rotor's syndrome.

Q. 8. Write a short note on hemoglobin.
(TNMGR, Sept. 2009)

Ans. Hemoglobin (Hb) is the red blood pigment, exclusively found in erythrocytes. The normal concentration of Hb in blood in males is 14–16 g/dl and in females 13–15 g/dl. Hemoglobin performs two important biological functions concerned with respiration:
1. Delivery of O_2 from lungs to tissues.
2. Transport of CO_2 and protons from tissues to lungs for excretion.

Structure of hemoglobin: Hb (Mol. wt. 64,450) is a conjugated protein, containing globin-apoprotein part and heme-non-protein part (prosthetic group). Hemoglobin is a tetrameric allosteric protein.
   i. **Structure of globin:** Globin consists of four polypeptide chains of two different primary structures

(monomeric units). The common form of adult hemoglobin (HbA₁) is made up of two α-chains and two β-chains. Each α-chain contains 141 amino acids while β-chain contains 146 amino acids. The four subunits of hemoglobin are held together by non-covalent interactions primarily hydrophobic, ionic and hydrogen bonds. Each subunit contains a heme group.

ii. **Structure of heme:** Heme contains a porphyrin molecule, namely protoporphyrin IX, with iron at its center. Protoporphyrin IX consists of four pyrrole rings to which four methyl, two propionyl and two vinyl groups are attached.

Other forms of hemoglobin:

   i. $HbA_2 : \alpha_2\delta_2$

   ii. $HbF : \alpha_2\gamma_2$ (fetal Hb)

   iii. $HbAlc : \alpha_2\beta_2$-glucose

Binding of O_2 to hemoglobin: One molecule of hemoglobin (with four hemes) can bind with four molecules of O_2. This is in contrast to myoglobin (with one heme) which can bind with only one molecule of oxygen. In other words, each heme moiety can bind with one O_2.

Applied Clinical Aspect

Hemoglobinopathies: It is a term used to describe the disorders caused by the synthesis of abnormal hemoglobin molecule or the production of insufficient quantities of normal hemoglobin or rarely both.

1. **Thalassemia:** Thalassemias are disorders caused by reductions or absence of globin chain synthesis.

  a. **α-thalassemia** occurs with reduced production of α-globin subunits. Four subtypes:

    i. **α-thalassemia minima/silent carrier:** Due to one gene depletion and has no significant hematologic consequences.

    ii. **α-thalassemia minor:** Due to two gene deletion, causes mild microcytic, hypochromic anemias.

    iii. **Hemoglobin H (HbH) disease:** Due to three gene deletions, causes moderate to severe microcytic, hypochromic anemia, causing accumulation of β-globin subunits that combine to form β-tetramers (HbH).

    iv. **Hemoglobin Bart's disease (Hb Bart's):** Due to four gene deletions, and is incompatible with life. Hb Bart has a high O_2 affinity and does not allow its release to body tissues, leading to severe hypoxia and death of infant (*hydrops fetalis*).

  b. **β-thalassemia** occurs with reduced production of β-globin subunits. Two subtypes:

    i. **β-thalassemia minor:** Due to one gene mutation, no hemolysis.

    ii. **β-thalassemia major:** Due to two gene mutations, ineffective erythropoiesis and extravascular hemolysis causing severe microcytic, hypochromic anemia.

2. **Porphyria:** Porphyrias are a group of hereditary or acquired disorders caused by defective heme synthesis resulting in collection of potentially toxic heme precursors.

   i. **Porphyria cutanea tarda (PCT)** is a chronic hepatic porphyria caused by deficient activity of uroporphyrinogen decarboxylase, resulting in accumulation of porphyrinogens within hepatocytes. Clinically, cutaneous photosensitivity and hyperpigmentation are characteristic.

   ii. **Acute intermittent porphyria (AIP)** is an acute hepatic porphyria causing deficient activity of porphobilinogen deaminase. The result is accumulation of neurotoxic metabolites including ALA and porphobilinogen. Patients can present with abdominal pain, nausea, vomiting, constipation, fever, tachycardia, and hypertension. Neurotoxic effects include autonomic instability, peripheral neuropathy, neuropathic pain, and psychological disturbances.

3. **Sickle cell trait and disease:** The most common abnormal variant of hemoglobin is HbS (sickle cell hemoglobin). HbS results from a substitution of 6th amino acid in the β-globin subunits (replacement of glutamic acid with valine). Heterozygous individuals have a mutation in only one of the two β-chains, resulting in sickle cell trait. Homozygous individuals have mutations in both β-chains, resulting in sickle cell disease. When deoxygenated, HbS causes deformation of erythrocytes from a biconcave disc, to a crescent or "sickle" shape. This change in shape causes damage to erythrocyte membranes, premature destruction of erythrocytes, and chronic hemolytic anemia. Sickled erythrocytes can obstruct blood flow and cause tissue hypoxia, which can cause severe ischemic pain or even stroke.

Q. 9. Write a short note on prostaglandins.

(TNMGR, Oct. 1999)

Ans. Prostaglandins (PGs) are derivatives of a 20-carbon fatty acid, namely prostanoic acid, hence known as prostanoids. This has a cyclopentane ring (formed by carbon atoms 8–12) and two side chains, with carboxyl group on one side. Prostaglandins differ in their structure due to substituent group and double bond on cyclopentane ring.

Synthesis: Arachidonic acid is the precursor for most of prostaglandins in humans. It occurs in endoplasmic reticulum in the following stages.

1. Release of arachidonic acid from membrane bound phospholipids by *phospholipase A$_2$*.
2. Oxidation and cyclization of arachidonic acid to PGG$_2$ which is then converted to PGH$_2$ by a reduced glutathione dependent *peroxidase*.
3. PGH$_2$ serves as immediate precursor for synthesis of a number of PGs, including prostacyclins and thromboxanes.

The above pathway is known as cyclic pathway of arachidonic acid. In linear pathway of arachidonic acid, leukotrienes and lipoxins are synthesized.

Degradation of PGs: Lung and liver are the major sites of PGs degradation.

Biochemical actions: PGs act as local hormones in their function.

1. Regulation of blood pressure: PGs like PGE, PGA and PGI$_2$ are vasodilator in function.
2. Inflammation: PGE$_1$ and PGE$_2$ induce inflammation due to arteriolar vasodilation.
3. Reproduction: PGE$_2$ and PGF$_2$ are used for medical termination of pregnancy and induction of labor.
4. Pain and fever: It is believed that pyrogens promote PGs biosynthesis leading to formation of PGE$_2$ in hypothalamus. PGE$_2$ along with histamine and bradykinin cause pain.
5. Regulation of gastric secretion: In general, PGE inhibit gastric secretion. PGs are used for treatment of gastric ulcers.
6. Influence on immune system: Macrophages secrete PGE which decreases immunological functions of B- and T-lymphocytes.
7. Effects on respiratory function: PGE is a bronchodilator, whereas PGF acts as bronchoconstrictor.
8. Influence on renal functions: PGE increases GFR and promotes urine output. Excretion of Na$^+$ and K$^+$ is also increased by PGE.
9. Effects on metabolism: PGE decreases lipolysis, increases glycogen formation and promotes calcium mobilization from the bone.
10. Platelet aggregation and thrombosis: Prostacyclins (PGI$_2$) inhibit platelet aggregation. Thromboxanes (TXA$_2$) and prostaglandin E$_2$ promote platelet aggregation and blood clotting that might lead to thrombosis.

Q. 10. Write a short note on inborn errors in tyrosine metabolism. *(TNMGR, Oct. 2003)*

Ans. Several enzyme defects in phenylalanine/tyrosine degradation leading to metabolic disorders.

1. Phenylketonuria: Phenylketonuria (PKU) is the most common metabolic disorder in amino acid metabolism. It is due to deficiency of hepatic enzyme, *phenylalanine hydroxylase*, caused by an autosomal recessive gene. This enzyme deficiency impairs synthesis of tetrahydrobiopterin required for action of phenylalanine hydroxylase. The net outcome is that phenylalanine is not converted to tyrosine. Due to disturbances in routine metabolism, phenylalanine is diverted to alternate pathways, resulting in the excessive production of phenylpyruvate, phenylacetate, phenyllactate and phenylglutamine. All these metabolites are excreted in urine in high concentration in PKU. Phenylacetate gives the urine a mousy odour.

Biochemical manifestations
   i. Effects on CNS: Mental retardation, failure to walk or talk, failure of growth, seizures and tremor, low IQ (< 50).
   ii. Effect on pigmentation: Hypopigmentation causing light skin color, fair hair, blue eyes, etc.

Diagnosis:
• **Guthrie Test:** Screening the newborn babies for increased plasma levels of phenylalanine (PKU, 20–65 mg/dl; normal—1–2 mg/dl).
• **Ferric chloride test:** Phenylketones in urine give a green color in this test.
• **DNA probes:** Prenatal diagnosis of PKU.

Treatment: Maintenance of plasma phenylalanine concentration within the normal range by selecting foods with low phenylalanine content. In seriously affected PKU patients, treatment includes administration of 5-hydroxytryptophan and DOPA to restore the synthesis of serotonin and catecholamines.

2. **Tyrosinemia type II (Richner-Hanhart syndrome):** This disorder is due to defect in the enzyme tyrosine transaminase. The result is blockade in the routine degradative pathway of tyrosine. Accumulation and excretion of tyrosine and its metabolites, *p*-hydroxyphenylpyruvate, *p*-hydroxyphenyllactate, *p*-hydroxyphenylacetate, N-acetyltyrosine and tyramine are observed. Tyrosinemia type II is characterized by skin (dermatitis) and eye lesions and, rarely, mental retardation.

3. **Neonatal tyrosinemia:** The absence of the enzyme *p*-hydroxyphenylpyruvate dioxygenase causes neonatal tyrosinemia. This is mostly a temporary condition and usually responds to ascorbic acid.

4. **Alkaptonuria (black urine disease):** Alkaptonuria is a autosomal recessive disorder, defective enzyme is homogentisate oxidase in tyrosine metabolism. Homogentisate accumulates in tissues and blood and is excreted into urine. Homogentisate, on

standing, gets oxidized to give black or brown color (coke in color urine).

Biochemical manifestations: Oxidized product of homogentisate, alkapton, gets deposited in connective tissue, bones and various organs (nose, ear, etc.) resulting in a condition known as ochronosis.

Diagnosis: Change in color of urine on standing to brown or dark has been the simple traditional method to identify alkaptonuria. The urine gives a positive test with ferric chloride and silver nitrate. Benedict's test employed for detection of glucose and other reducing sugars, is also positive with homogentisate.

Treatment: Consumption of protein diet with relatively low phenylalanine content is recommended.

5. **Tyrosinosis or tyrosinemia type I:** This is due to deficiency of enzymes fumarylacetoacetate hydroxylase and/or malylacetoacetate isomerase. It causes liver failure, rickets, renal tubular dysfunction and polyneuropathy. Tyrosine, its metabolites and many other amino acids are excreted in urine. In acute tyrosinosis, infant exhibits diarrhea, vomiting, and 'cabbage-like' odor. Death may occur due to liver failure within one year. For the treatment, diets low in tyrosine, phenylalanine and methionine are recommended.

6. **Albinism:** Albinism is an inborn error, due to lack of synthesis of pigment melanin. It is an autosomal recessive disorder. The most common cause of albinism is defect in tyrosinase, enzyme responsible for synthesis of melanin.

   Clinical manifestations: Sensitive to sunlight, Increased susceptibility to skin cancer, photophobia.

7. **Hypopigmentation:** Oculocutaneous albinism is due to mutations in tyrosinase gene. Vitiligo and leukoderma are important among the localized hypopigmentation disorders.

8. **Hawkinsinuria:** This rare condition, is characterised by failure to thrive and metabolic acidosis in infancy. After the first year of life the condition appears to be asymptomatic. Early weaning from breastfeeding seems to precipitate the disease. Identification of urinary hawkinsin or 4-hydroxy-cyclohexylacetate is diagnostic.

5. DNA, RNA AND MISCELLANEOUS

Q. 1. Write a note on structure of DNA.
(NTR Uni., Nov. 2007)

Ans. DNA (deoxyribonucleic acid)—a polymer of deoxyribos nucleotides is found in chromosomes, mitochondria and chloroplasts and carries the genetic information.

Components of nucleotide: Base [Nitrgenous: Purines—adenine (A) and guanine (G), pyridmidines—thymine (T), cytosine (C)]; Sugar (deoxyribose), phosphate (1-3, hydrolysed to provide energy to form phosphodiester bond).

Structure: A DNA molecule consists of two long polynucleotide chains composed of four types of nucleotide subunits. Each of these chains is known as a DNA chain, or a DNA strand. Hydrogen bonds between the base portions of the nucleotides hold the two chains together. The structure of DNA is right handed double helix (James Watson and Francis Crick, 1953) with 10 nucleotide pairs/helical turn. Each spiral strand, composed of a sugar phosphate backbone and attached bases, is connected to a complementary strand by hydrogen bonds between paired bases, adenine (A) with thymine (T) by two bonds; guanine (G) with cytosine (C) by three bonds (Fig. 5.1).

RNA: Ribonucleic acid (RNA) is polymer of purine and pyrimidine nucleotide linked by phosphodiester bonds. RNA is single stranded, sugar is ribose, purine is adenine and guanine and pyrimidine are cytosine and uracil (U).

Q. 2. Write a note on protein synthesis.
(UHSR, June 2018; HP Uni., April 2019)

Ans. Protein synthesis involves transcription of DNA to mRNA which is translated into protein with the help of ribosomes.

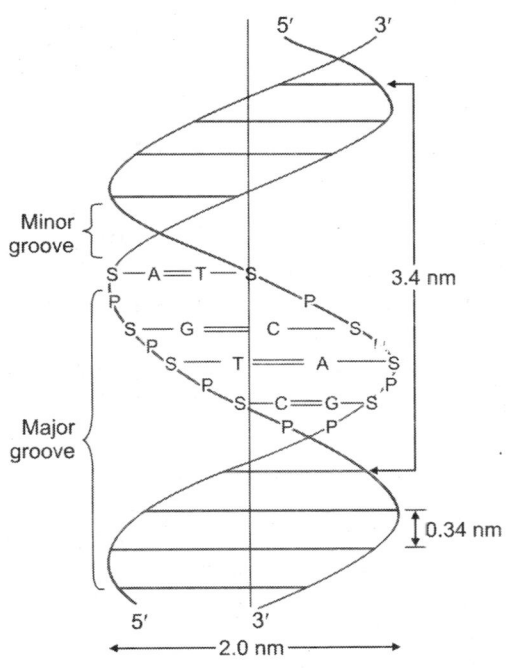

Fig. 5.1: Structure of DNA (Watson and Crick Model of DNA)

A. **Transcription process:** Transcription is achieved by DNA dependent RNA polymerases (RNAP).

1. Initiation of transcription:
   i. DNA helix partially unwinds and RNAP binds with promoter site on DNA and moves forward.
   ii. When it reaches the appropriate site on the gene, first nucleotide of mRNA attaches to the initiation site on RNAP. This becomes 5' end of mRNA.
2. Elongation process:
   i. RNAP moves along DNA template, incorporated new nucleotides in mRNA, one by one, according to the base pairing rule. Thus, A in DNA is transcribed to U in mRNA; T to A; G to C and C to G.
   ii. Synthesis of mRNA is from 5' to 3' end.
3. Termination of transcription: Specific signals are recognized by termination protein, the Rho factor. When it attaches to DNA, RNAP cannot move further.
4. Post-transcriptional processing: mRNA formed and released from DNA template is known as primary transcript or heteronuclear mRNA. It undergoes extensive editing to become the mature mRNA. Modifications are:
   i. Poly-A tailing at 3' end.
   ii. 5' capping by guanosine triphosphate.
   iii. Removal of introns and splicing of exons.
   iv. Primary transcript contains coding regions (exons) interspersed with non-coding regions (introns).
   v. These intron sequences are cleaved and exons are spliced (combined together) to form the mature mRNA molecule.

B. **Translation process:** The translation is a cytoplasmic process. mRNA is translated from 5' to 3' end. The chain growth is from amino terminal to carboxyl terminal. The process of translation has five phases:

1. Activation of amino acids:
   i. Enzyme aminoacyl tRNA synthetases activate the amino acids.
   ii. Amino acid is first activated with the help of ATP. Then carboxyl group of the amino acid is esterified with 3' hydroxyl group of tRNA.
2. Initiation of protein synthesis:
   i. First AUG triplet after the marker sequence is identified by ribosome as start codon. In eukaryotes, the first amino acid incorporated is methionine (AUG codon).
   ii. tRNA carrying methionine and 40S ribosomal subunits are combined; then mRNA binds to form 48S initiation complex.
   iii. 48S initiation complex now binds with 60S ribosomal unit to form the full assembly of 80S ribosome.
   iv. The whole ribosome contains two receptor sites for tRNA molecules. 'P' site or peptidyl site carries the growing peptide chain. 'A' site or aminoacyl site carries the new incoming tRNA with the amino acid to be added next.
3. Elongation process of translation:
   i. A new aminoacyl tRNA comes to 'A' site. The next codon in mRNA determines the incoming amino acid.
   ii. α-amino group of incoming amino acid in 'A' site forms a peptide bond with carboxyl group of peptidyl tRNA occupying 'P' site.
   iii. Translocation process: At this time, tRNA fixed at 'P' site does not carry any amino acid and is therefore released from the ribosome. Then the whole ribosome moves over the mRNA through the distance of one codon (3 bases). The peptidyl tRNA is translocated to the 'P' site.
   iv. Now, 'A' site is ready to receive another aminoacyl tRNA.
4. Termination process of translation
   i. After successive addition of amino acids, ribosome reaches terminator codon sequence (UAA, UAG or UGA) on mRNA. Since there is no tRNA bearing the corresponding anticodon sequence, the 'A' site remains free.
   ii. The releasing factor (RF) hydrolyses peptide chain from tRNA at the P site.
5. Post-translational processing:
   i. Conversion of pro-insulin to insulin by proteolytic cleavage.
   ii. Gamma carboxylation of glutamic acid residues of prothrombin, under the influence of vitamin K.
   iii. Hydroxylation of proline and lysine in collagen with the help of vitamin C.
   iv. Glycosylation: Carbohydrates are attached to serine or threonine residues.

Inhibitors of protein synthesis:
   i. Reversible inhibitors: Tetracyclins, chloramphenicol, erythromycin.
   ii. Irreversible inhibitors: Streptomycin.

Q. 3. Write a short note on osmosis.

(BBD Uni., April 2014)

Ans. Osmosis is the spontaneous net movement of a solvent like water, across a semi-permeable membrane from a less concentrated solution into a more concentrated one, thus equalizing the concentrations on each side of the membrane. Osmosis is passive transport, meaning it does not require energy to be applied.

Diffusion involves solvent and solute particles to move to equalize concentrations from lower to higher concentrations. It mainly occurs in gaseous state or within gas molecules and liquid molecules and usually does not need water for movement.

Hypertonic: Solution with higher concentration or more solute.

Hypotonic: Solution with lower concentration or less solute.

Isotonic: When both solutions have equal concentration.

Osmotic pressure: It is the pressure that would have to be applied to a pure solvent to prevent it from passing into a given solution by osmosis.

Osmotic gradient: Difference in concentration between two solutions on either side of a semi-permeable membrane.

Types

Reverse osmosis: It is a separation process that retains the solute on one side and allows pure solvent to pass to other side, by applying a pressure in excess of the osmotic pressure.

Forward osmosis: Osmosis may be used directly to achieve separation of water from a solution containing unwanted solutes.

Biological importance of osmosis:
1. Fluid balance of different compartments of body is maintained due to osmosis.
2. Osmosis significantly contributes to regulation of blood volume and urine excretion.
3. Isotonic solution of NaCl or glucose is commonly used in IV transfusion in hospitals for treatment of dehydration, burns, etc.
4. Purgatives withdraw water from body, preventing intestinal water absorption.
5. High blood glucose concentration causes osmotic diuresis resulting in loss of water, electrolytes and glucose in urine.
6. Edema due to hypoalbuminemia is caused by reduced osmotic pressure of plasma.
7. Hypertonic solutions of salts ($NaCl$, $MgSO_4$) are used to reduce pressure of CSF.
8. Isotonic solutions are used for washing wounds.

Q. 4. Write a short note on spectrophotometry.

Ans. Spectrophotometry is a method in which absorption or transmission properties of a material is quantitatively measured as a function of wavelength as each compound absorbs or transmits light over a certain range of wavelength.

This method is based on two laws of light absorption by solutions:
- Lambert's law states that "the proportion of light absorbed by a medium is independent of the intensity of incident light".
- Beer's law maintains that "the absorbance of light is directly proportional to concentration of absorbing medium and the thickness or path length of the medium".

Spectrophotometer is an instrument that measures amount of photons absorbed by a sample after it is passed through its solution. Spectrophotometer can be classified:
A. Based on type of beam used:
   1. Single beam spectrometer.
   2. Double beam spectrometer.
B. Based on wavelength used:
   1. Visible spectrophotometer: Uses visible range (400–700 nm).
   2. UV spectrophotometer: Uses UV range (130–400 nm).
   3. IR spectrophotometer: Uses infra red range (700–5000).

Basic components of spectrophotometer: Light source, optical system/wavelength selector, sample container, light detector, output—signal processor and readout.

Applications:
- Concentration measurement.
- Detection of impurities.
- Elucidation of structure of organic compounds.
- Chemical kinetics.
- Detection of functional group.
- Molecular weight determination.
- In dentistry, for measurement of color shade.

Q. 5. Write a short note on centrifugation.
(NTR Uni., April 2012)

Ans. Centrifugation is a technique of separating substances from a solution according to their size, shape, density, viscosity of the medium and rotor speed by the application of centrifugal force.

Principle: Centrifuge works using the sedimentation principle, where the centripetal acceleration causes denser substances and particles to move outward in the radial direction and objects that are less dense are displaced and move to the center.

Types of centrifuge:

Low speed or clinical centrifuge: 4000–5000 rpm, used for sedimentation of RBCs.

High speed: of 15,000–20,000 rpm.

Ultracentrifuges: 65,000 rpm; used for preparative and analytical work.

Applications:

- To separate two miscible substances.
- To analyze the hydrodynamic properties of macro-molecules.
- Purification of mammalian cells.
- Fractionation of subcellular organelles.
- Separation of urine and components in forensic and research laboratories.
- Aids in the separation of proteins using purification techniques.

Q. 6. Write a short note on gel electrophoresis and its applications. *(NTR Uni., May 2019)*

Ans. Electrophoresis is defined as the migration of charged particle through a solution under the influence of an external electrical field.

Factors affecting electrophoresis: Rate of migration of a solute in an electric field depends on the following factors:

- Net charge on the particle.
- Mass and shape of the particles.
- pH of the medium.
- Strength of electric field.
- Properties of supporting medium.
- Temperature

Electrophoresis unit:

1. Media:
   a. Buffers: They carries the applied current, establishes pH, determine the electrical charge on the solute, e.g. barbitone buffer, phosphate buffer, *Tris* borate EDTA.
   b. Support media: It provides the matrix in which separation takes place, e.g. filter paper, cellulose acetate membrane, agar/agarose gel, starch gel and polyacrylamide gel.
2. Electrophoretic chamber:
   Types of electrophoresis:
   a. Zone electrophoresis: Paper electrophoresis, gel electrophoresis, thin layer electrophoresis, cellulose electrophoresis.
   b. Moving boundary electrophoresis: Capillary electrophoresis, isotachophoresis, isoelectric focusing, immune electrophoresis.
   Gel electrophoresis: Types based on media used:
   a. Agarose gel electrophoresis: Agar is used as support media.

b. Starch gel electrophoresis: Potato starch is used as support media.
c. Polyacrylamide gel electrophoresis (PAGE): Polyacrylamide is used as support media. It is the most widely used technique of electrophoresis.

Stains used are: Ethidium bromide, silver or coomassie blue dye.

Types of PAGE:

1. **SDS-PAGE:** In this sodium dodecyl sulphate, an amphoteric surfactant is used. It denatures protein by binding to protein chain, exposing normally buried region and coating the protein chain with surfactant molecules. In this method, separation is based on molecular weight.
2. **Native PAGE:** Original type, the separation is based on charge, size and shape of macromolecules. It is used for separation and purification of mixture of proteins.

Applications:

1. Used for estimation of molecular weight of proteins and nucleic acids.
2. Purification of isolated proteins.
3. Monitoring changes of protein content in body fluids.
4. DNA sequencing.
5. Electrophoresis in combination with autoradiography is used to study the binding of iron to serum proteins.
6. Used for analysis of terpenoids, steroids and antibiotics.
7. For testing purity of thyroid hormones by zone electrophoresis.
8. Paper chromato-electrophoresis is used to separate free insulin from plasma proteins.
9. It is used for diagnosis of various diseases of kidney, liver and CVS.
10. Electrophoresis is also used for separation of carbohydrates and vitamins.
11. Quantitative separation of all fractions of cellular entities, antibiotics, RBC, enzymes, etc. is possible.

Q. 7. Write a note on bone morphogenetic protein. *(NTR Uni., Oct. 2013)*

Ans. Bone morphogenetic proteins (BMPs) are a group of growth factors and cytokines which has ability to induce formation of bone and cartilage and play role in differentiation, proliferation, growth inhibition, and arrest of maturation of a wide variety of cells, depending on the cellular microenvironment and interactions with other regulatory factors.

Mechanism of action: When BMPs bind to cell surface receptors on mesenchymal cell, a BMP signaling cascade is activated and sent to cell nucleus via specific proteins. This results in expression of genes that lead to synthesis of macromolecules involved in cartilage and bone formation, and the mesenchymal cell becomes chondrocyte or osteoblast.

Chemical structure of BMPs: BMPs are members of TGF-β (transforming growth factor-β) super family, a large family of growth factors. At their carboxy-terminal ends, BMPs posses a region containing seven cysteine residues. BMPs are synthesized inside the cell in a precursor form with a hydrophobic stretch of 50–100 amino acids. Prior to secretion, BMPs consists of a signal peptide, pro-domain, and mature peptide. The mature BMP derives from the carboxy terminal region by proteolytical cleavage and are secreted as either heterodimers or homodimers.

Classification of BMPs: The human genome encodes 20 BMPs. Three subclasses:

Subclass A: BMP-2 and BMP-4.

Subclass B: BMP-5, BMP-6, and BMP-7 (osteogenic protein-1), and BMP-8 (OP-2).

Subclass C: BMP-3 (osteogenin)

Factors affecting BMPs activity:

1. **Synergistic factors:** Fibroblast growth factor, TGF, PGE_1, glucocorticoids, vitamin D.

2. **Antagonists factors:** Fibroblast growth factor (high dose)

BMPs in wound healing: BMPs directly affect wound healing process in the following sequential phases:

Injury → Inflammatory response → Complement activation → Extravasation and cell signaling

Proliferation → Granulation tissue → Binding of growth factors to collagens.

Remodeling → Activation of resorption → Formation of osteoclasts resorptive pits.

BMPs in periodontal regeneration:

- BMP-2: Osteogenesis; induces expression of cementum attachment protein in PDL.
- BMP-3: Blocks BMP-2-mediated differentiation of osteoprogenitor cells into osteoblasts.
- BMP-4: Osteoinductive; plays role in bone metabolism, stimulates superoxide production and exert proinflammatory effects on endothelium.
- BMP-6: Stimulates all osteogenic markers in mesenchymal stem cells.
- BMP-7: Role in transformation of mesenchymal cells into bone and cartilage; induces all of genetic markers of osteoblast differentiation in many cell types.
- BMP-9: Potent osteogenic growth factor; possess the capability to promote osteogenesis and chondrogenesis.

Microbiology

CHAPTER 5

1. IMMUNITY AND HYPERSENSITIVITY

Q. 1. Write a note on acquired immunity.
(TNMGR, April 1995; Oct. 2018)

Ans. Immunity is defined as resistance exhibited by the host towards injury caused by microorganisms and their products.

Types:

I. **Innate/natural/native immunity:** It is resistance to infections that an individual possess by virtue of genetic and constitutional make up. It is not affected by prior contact with microorganism. It is classified as species, racial and individual immunity.

Mechanisms: Anatomical barrier, physiochemical barrier, phagocytic barrier and inflammatory barrier.

II. **Acquired/specific immunity** *(UHSR, April 2015)*: It is resistance acquired by an individual during life. Two types:

1. **Active/adaptive immunity** *(UHSR, April 2015)*: Resistance developed by an individual as a result of an antigenic stimulus, by formation of antibodies and immunologically active cells. This develops after a latent period and is long-lasting. Secondary response is quicker, and profound (immunological memory). It is of two types:

   a. **Natural active immunity:** It results from clinical or sub-clinical infection by a microbe and usually long lasting. Immunity following bacterial infection is generally less permanent than following viral infections, e.g. immunity against poliovirus, chickenpox.

   b. **Artificial active immunity:** It is the resistance induced by vaccines, e.g:
   - **Bacterial vaccines:** Live (BCG vaccine for TB); killed (cholera vaccine); subunit (typhoid Vi antigen); bacterial products (tetanus toxoid).
   - **Viral vaccines:** Live (oral polio vaccine—Sabin); killed (injectable polio vaccine—salk); subunit (hepatitis B vaccine).

2. **Passive immunity** *(TNMGR, April 2000; BBD Uni., April 2015)*: Resistance that is transmitted passively to a recipient in a 'readymade' form. The recipient's immune system plays no active role, as preformed antibodies are administered. There is no latent period, and the protection being effective immediately after passive immunization. The immunity is transient, usually lasting for days or weeks. No secondary response occurs and this is less effective in protection.

   a. **Natural passive immunity:** It is resistance passively transferred from mother to baby, predominantly through placenta.

   b. **Artificial passive immunity:** It is resistance passively transferred to a recipient by administration of antibodies. Agents used are hyperimmune sera, convalescent sera and pooled human γ-globulin. Passive immunization is indicated for immediate and temporary protection in a non-immune host faced with the threat of an infection, and for treatment of some infections.

Q. 2. Discuss structure and functions of T-cells in adoptive immune response.
(NTR Uni., April 2013; UOK May 2015).

Ans. Adoptive immunity is of two types:

A. Antibody mediated immunity (AMI) or humoal immunity: Mediated by B-cells.

B. Cell mediated immunity (CMI) or cellular immunity: Medited by T-cells.

T-cells: T-cells are derived from thymus and mediate CMI. They constitute 65–80% of circulating pool of small lymphocytes and found in inner subcortical regions of lymph nodes with longer lifespan than B cells.

Types of T cells:
1. **T helper cells** (T_H cells/CD4$^+$)(65%): They are found in thymic medulla, tonsils and blood. They express CD4 protein on their surface. They become activated when a non-peptide-binding portion of MHC class II molecules are expressed on the surface of APCs. Activated TH cells differentiate into many subtypes (T_H1, T_H2, T_H3, T_H17, or T_{FH}) which secrete cytokines that regulates the active immune system. Main functions are:
   - Help in antigen specific activation of B cells and effector T cells.
   - Th-1 cytokines activate cytotoxic inflammatory and delayed hypersensitivity reactions.
   - Th-2 cells help in production of interleukins which encourage production of antibodies (IgE).
   - Th-2 cytokines are associated with regulation of strong antibody and allergic response.
2. **Cytotoxic T cells** (T_c cells/CD8$^+$): They are found in bone marrow and gut lymphoid tissue. They recognize a nonpeptide-binding portion of MHC class I molecules (present on the surface of nearly all cells of body). They kill virus-infected cells, allograft cells, tumor cells.
3. **Memory T cells:** Memory cells live for many years or have the capacity to reproduce them, so the secondary response is enhanced and is greater than primary response. They are activated by small quantities of antigens and produce greater amounts of interleukins. They have two subtypes: Central memory T cells (T_{CM}-cells) and effector memory T cells (T_{EM}-cells). Memory cells may be either CD4$^+$ or CD8$^+$.
4. **Regulatory T cells (Treg/suppressor):** They are crucial for maintenance of immunological tolerance. Their major role is to shut down T cell-mediated immunity toward the end of an immune reaction and to suppress auto-reactive T cells that escaped the process of negative selection in thymus.

   Two types: Naturally occurring Treg cells (thymus) and adaptive Treg cells.
5. **Natural killer T cells (NKT):** NKT cells bridges the adaptive immune system with innate immune system. NKT cells recognize glycolipid antigen presented by a molecule called CD1d. Once activated, these cells can perform functions of both T_H and T_C cells.
6. **Gamma delta T cells:** They represent small subset of T cells that possess a distinct T cell receptor (TCR) on their surface. (2% of total T cells).

T cell receptor/TCR: Consists of two polypeptides: Alpha and beta, and they are associated with CD3 proteins.

B cells play a major role in AMI, formed in bone marrow. They do not require thymus for maturation. B cells have many molecules on its surface which act as Ag, e.g. IgM, IgD, B220, MHC-II, CR-1, CD40, etc. T cells cause their activation to form Ab.

Q. 3. Write a short note on immunoglobulins.
(Bombay Uni., Oct. 1985; TNMGR, March 2011; HP Uni., May 2017)

Ans. Immunoglobulin (Ig) is a glycoprotein that is made in response to an antigen and can recognize and bind to antigen that caused its production.

Basic structure (RUHS, May 2018) (Fig. 1.3): Immunoglobulin is composed of 4 polypeptide chains (2 heavy-H; 2 light-L: Kappa and lambda), linked by disulphide bonds. Each heavy and light chain is subdivided into constant (amino terminal) and variable region (carboxy terminal). On proteolytic digestion, peptide bonds are broken, producing 2 identical fragments called Fab (antigen binding) and other is called Fc (fraction crystallizable).

Based on physiochemical and antigenic nature of H chain, immunoglobulins are: IgG (gamma), IgA (alpha), IgM (Mu), IgD (delta) and IgE (epsilon).

1. **IgG:** Major serum immunoglobulin (80%). It has molecule weight of 150,000 (7s). It has half-life of 23 day. Sub-classes of IgG: IgG1, IgG2, IgG3, IgG4, each possessing a distinct type of gamma chain.
   Biological functions:
   - IgG1, IgG3, IgG4: Cross placenta and protects fetus.
   - IgG3: Activates complement.
   - IgG1, IgG3: Binds Fc receptor on phagocytic cells and mediate opsonization.
2. **IgA:** IgA (10–15%) is the major immunoglobulin in colostrum, saliva and tears. It has half-life of 6–8 days. It occurs in two forms: **Serum IgA**

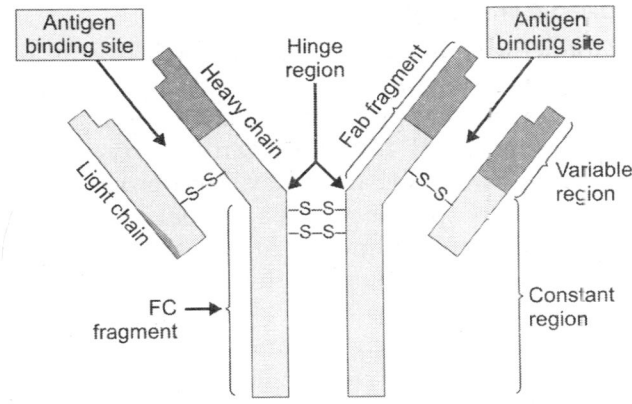

Fig. 1.3: Structure of immunoglobulins

(monomer) and **secretory IgA** (dimer, J-chain and secretory piece).

Biological functions:
- Provide local immunity and immune elimination.
- Provide immunity to newborn through breast milk.
- Activates compliment by alternate pathway.
- Promote phagocytosis and intracellular killing of microorganism.

3. **IgM:** It is (5–10%) polymer of five monomeric units, held together by disulphide bonds and 'J' chain with molecular weight of 900000–1000000 (*millionaire molecule*). It has half life of 5 days. It is mostly present intravascularly and cannot cross placenta. Its presence indicates recent infection. It is the major antibody receptor on the surface of unstimulated B lymphocytes and acts as receptors for antigen.

Biological functions:
- It agglutinates bacteria.
- It activates complement system by classical pathway.
- It causes opsonization and immune hemolysis.
- Earliest immunoglobulin to be synthesized by fetus.

4. **IgD:** It resembles IgG structurally (0.2%). It is mostly intravascular. It has half life of 3 days. It also occurs on the surface of unstimulated B lymphocytes.

5. **IgE (reagin antibody):** Its half-life is 2 days, resembles to IgG, heat labile, mostly extra-vascular and does not cross placenta. It is chiefly produced in the lining of respiratory and intestinal tracts.

Biological functions:
- It mediates immediate hypersensitivity reaction and Prausnitz Kustner reaction.
- It is responsible for symptoms of anaphylactic shock, hay fever and asthma.

Applied Clinical Aspect

- **Monoclonal Ab** (NTR Uni., Nov. 2007): Monoclonal antibodies (mAb) are antibodies that are identical because they are produced by one type of immune cell. Monoclonal antibodies can be very useful in treating cancer because they can be designed to attack a very specific part of a cancer cell, e.g. murin (tositumomab), chimeric (rituximab), humarized (trastuzumab), human (panitumumab). Monoclonal antibodies are also being developed to control infectious diseases. e.g. malaria, influenza and AIDS.
- **Polyclonal Ab:** Polyclonal antibodies are antibodies that are derived from different cell lines.

Q. 4. Define antigen and antibody. What are antigen–antibody reactions? (TNMGR, March 2009)

Ans. Antigen (Ag) or immunogen is a large organic molecule capable of stimulating production of specific antibody(Ab) with which it may reacts specifically and in an observable manner. Immunogenicity is the ability to induce a humoral and/or cell mediated immune response. Antigenicity is the ability to combine specifically with the final products of immune response (i.e. secreted Ab and/or surface receptors on T cells)

- **Antigen determinants (epitopes):** Portion of Ag which can be specifically recognized by Ab or antigenic receptor of lymphocytes. Epitopes can be: Conformational or linear; T cell or B cell type.
- **Paratope:** Combining site on the antibody molecule corresponding to epitope.
- **Adjuvant:** Substances that are non-immunogenic alone but enhance the immunogenicity of any added immunogen.
- **Super-antigen:** These are group of antigens that result in excessive polyclonal activation of T cells resulting in hyperactivation of immune system and subsequent massive release of active cytokines, e.g. staphylococcal enterotoxin, streptococcal pyrogenic exotoxin.

Classification of Antigens

A. **Based on immunogenicity:**
   1. Complete Ag: Contains both immunogenicity and antigenicity.
   2. Incomplete Ag/haptens: Contains only antigenicity, e.g. cardiolipin Ag.
B. **Based on chemical nature:** Proteins, polysaccharides, nucleic acid, lipids.
C. **Based on need of T cells:** Thymus dependent (TD-Ag), thymus independent (TI-Ag)
D. **Based on origin:**
   1. Exogenous Ag, e.g. bacteria, viruses, fungi, etc.
   2. Endogenous Ag, e.g. blood group Ag, HLA.

Antibody (Ab): These are substances which are formed in serum and tissue fluids in response to an Ag and react with that Ag specifically and in observable manner. Chemically they are globulins (immunoglobulins). They constitute 20–25% of total serum proteins and are mainly synthesized by plasma cells (Fig. 1.3).

Antigen–antibody reactions (Ag–Ab reactions) (NTR Uni., May 2019): Ag–Ab reactions are interactions between Ag and specific Ab in an observable manner and form the basis of antibody-mediated immunity (humoral). These reactions can be used for detection and quantification of either Ag or Ab. These reactions occur in three stages:

- **Primary stage:** Initial reaction involves formation of Ag–Ab complex, without any visible effect. The reaction is rapid, reversible, can be detected by use of markers such as radioactive isotopes, fluorescent dyes.
- **Secondary stage:** This is the stage of demonstrable event such as precipitation, agglutination, lysis of cells, killing of live antigens, neutralization of toxins, fixation of complement and enhancement of phagocytosis.
- **Tertiary reactions:** Chain of reactions leading to neutralization or destruction of injurious Ag or to tissue damage, e.g. humoral immunity against infectious diseases, allergy and immunological diseases.

Features of Ag–Ab reactions:

1. Ag–Ab reaction is specific.
2. Entire molecule of Ag and Ab react and not the fragments.
3. There is no denaturation of Ag or Ab.
4. Only surface Ag participates in reactions.
5. The combination is firm but reversible.
6. Both Ag and Ab participate in formation of agglutinates or precipitates.
7. Ag and Ab can combine in varying proportions.

Uses of Ag–Ab reactions:

- *In vivo:* Forms basis of immunity against infectious diseases.
- *In vitro* (serological reactions): For diagnosis of infections; helpful in epidemiological studies; for identification of enzymes; detection and quantification of Ag or Ab.

Types of Ag–Ab reactions:

1. Precipitation or flocculation reaction: Ring test, slide test, tube test, immunodiffusion, electroimmunodiffusion.
2. Agglutination reaction: Slide agglutination, tube agglutination, antiglobulin (Coombs') test, passive agglutination test.
3. Complement fixation test: Indirect complement fixation test, conglutinating complement absorption test, immobilization test.
4. Neutralization test: Virus neutralization test, toxin neutralization test.
5. Immunofluorescence: Direct and indirect immunofluorescence.
6. Radioimmunoassay.
7. ELISA.
8. Chemiluminescence immunoassay.
9. Immunoelectroblot techniques.

Human complement system *(BBD Uni., April 2015)*: Complement refers to a system of factors which occur in normal serum and are activated characteristically by antigen–antibody interaction and subsequently mediate a number of biological consequences.

Properties:

1. Complement is present in sera of all mammals.
2. Complement as a whole is heat labile.
3. Constitutes 5% of normal serum protein.
4. These proteins are not immunoglobulins and their concentrations in serum do not increase after immunization.
5. Binds only with Ag–Ab complex, not to free Ag or Ab.

Components: It is a complex of nine different fractions called C1 to C9.

Synthesis: In liver, blood monocytes, tissue macrophages, fibroblasts and epithelial cells of GIT and genitourinary tract.

Activation:

A. **Stages of Activation:**
1. Formation of C3 convertase.
2. Formation of C5 convertase.
3. Formation of membrane attack complex.

B. **Pathways of activation:**
1. Classical pathway: Ab dependent (C1); Activated by formation of immune complex (Ag–Ab complex).
2. Alternative or properdin pathway: Ab independent (C3); cell surface substances like lipopolysaccharides, fungal cell wall and viral envelop activate the complement.
3. Lectin pathways (mannose binding lectin pathway): Ab-independent (C4) but resembles classical pathways. It is activated when circulating lectin binds to mannose residues on glycoprotein.

Inhibitors: C1 esterase, S protein.

Biological effects:

1. It mediates immunological membrane damage.
2. It amplifies the inflammatory response.
3. Participates in pathogenesis of hypersensitivity reactions.
4. It exhibits antiviral activity.
5. It interacts with coagulation, kinin and fibrinolytic system.

Q. 5. Write a short note on defense mechanism of the body. *(TNMGR, March 2010)*

Q. Write a short note on defense mechanism of the oral cavity. *(RGUHS, April 2007)*

Ans. Types of defense mechanism of the body:

A. **Non-specific (innate) defense mechanism:**
1. First-line defense mechanism: External defense.
2. Second line defense: Internal defense

B. **Specific dense mechanism:** Third line defense mechanism: Humoral and cell-mediated response.

1. **First-line/external defense:**
   a. **Intact skin:** Provides physical barrier to microbes, acidic pH discourage growth, sweat and sebaceous glands secretions kill microbes.
   b. **Eye:** Tears wash away irritating substances, lysozyme kills many bacteria.
   c. **Mucous membr. ne:** Saliva washes microbes from teeth and mucous membrane.
   d. **Respiratory system:** Mucous traps microbes, cilia sweep away trapped microbes.
   e. **Gastrointestinal system:** Stomach acid kills microbes. Normal bacteria in intestine keep check on invading microbes.
   f. **Genitourinary system:** Urine washes microbes from urethra.

2. **Second line/internal defense mechanism:**
   a. **Phagocytic cells:** Main function of phagocytic cells (neutrophils, monocytes, macrophages, natural killer cells) is chemotaxis, ingestion and microbial killing.
   b. **Molecular defense:** Complement proteins causes lysis, opsonization, activation of inflammatory response and clearance of immune complexes. Cytokines are TNF, chemokines, interleukins (IL), interferon (IFN).
   c. **Inflammatory process:** Mediators of inflammation restricts the spread of pathogen until a specific adaptive response is activated.
   d. **Blood clotting:** Blood clotting mechanism helps in formation of clot at site of damaged vessel.
   e. **Fever:** Fever helps body to fight bacterial infections by stimulating body defense.

3. **Third line of defense mechanism:** This is highly specific against particular pathogens. Lymphocyte (B and T cells) plays major role.

   Organs involved—primary/central—bone marrow, thymus; **secondary/peripheral—**spleen, lymph nodes, tonsils, adenoids, and appendix.
   a. Humoral defense *(BBD Uni., April, 2018; NTR Uni., May 2019)*: It is produced when the body synthesizes specific Ig molecules called Ab.

B-lymphocytes give rise to memory cells and plasma cells. Plasma cells are responsible for production of Ab, which interacts with T cells. Humoral defense is made up of:
   1. Immunoglobulins.
   2. Complement system.
   b. **Cell-mediated immune defense** *(HP Uni., May 2017)*: T cells are primarily responsible for cellular immunity.

Stages of Immune Response

1. Primary response: Recognition stage → Proliferation stage → Response stage → Effector stage.
2. Secondary Response (anamnestic): In immunized individual, memory cells elicit rapid response.

Defense mechanism of oral cavity: It can be divided into:

I. **Intact oral mucosa and oral lymphoid tissue:** Intact oral mucosa is barrier against microorganism (keratin barrier). This forms a primary structure barrier between internal and external environment and protects against entry of noxious substance and prevent loss of fluids. In lamina propria, there are lymphoid cells which combat penetrating microorganism. Intra-oral lymphoid aggregation (Waldeyer's ring) functions along with extra-oral lymph node for the protection of oral cavity as whole.

II. **Role of GCF:** GCF contains IgG, IgA, IgM; complement C3, C4, C5 and C3 proactivator which has role in both humoral and cell-mediated immunity. GCF also contains albumin, lysosomal enzymes, lysozyme, collagenase, macrophages, lipoproteins and glycoproteins, hence substantiating the oral immune system.

III. **Role of gingival epithelium:** Prevents bacterial adhesion by constantly shedding keratinocytes into the oral cavity and protecting against invasion by keratin component.

IV. **Role of connective tissue:** Connective tissue of periodontium is highly vascular, facilitating vascular leukocyte emigration in response to infection.

V. **Role of saliva:** Saliva has mechanical cleansing effect in oral cavity. Saliva also has non-specific and specific immune components:
   1. **Non-specific components:** Lysozyme, peroxidase, and lactoferrin.
   2. **Specific components:** Secretory IgA.

VI. **Vascular components:** Platelets are involved in formation of platelet plug, whenever there is injury to oral tissues.

VII. **Inflammation:** Inflammation causes dilation of blood vessels with inflammatory exudates at the site of injury, more the injury more is the inflammation and more likely the infection is localized.

VIII. **Gag reflex:** Gag reflex is normal, health, defense mechanism, prevents entry of foreign body into trachea by altering shape of pharynx.

IX. **Role of tongue:** Tongue acts as a barrier, protecting the deeper tissues from mechanical damage. It also prevents entry of microorganisms. It can reach all parts of oral cavity by virtue of its movement, removing food debris from gums, vestibule, and floor of mouth.

X. **Pain as protective mechanism:** Pain perception is protective as patient experience pain; he/she tries to withdraw the oral tissues from offending stimuli.

XI. **Miscellaneous factors:** Various other factors which play role in oral defense mechanism are:
1. Adaptive capacity of muscles to protect TMJ.
2. TMJ remodeling.
3. Protective functions of TMJ.
4. Dentinal factors like dentinal pain, tubular secretion, reparative dentin.
5. Cough reflex.
6. Mutually protected occlusion.

Applied clinical aspect: Immune disorders

1. **Allergy and asthma:** Immune response to substance which is usually not harmful, due to release of IgE.
2. **Immunodeficiency disorders:** Primary—X-linked agammaglobulinea, severe combined immunodeficiency; secondary—HIV.

Q. 6. Write a note on immunological aspects of dental caries. *(NTR Uni. June 2015)*

Ans. Dental caries is bacterial in origin, infectious in nature and transmissible. Mutans group of microorganisms are the etiological agents. Two prominent species in humans are *Strep. mutans* and *Strep. sorbinus*.

Molecular pathogenesis of dental caries: Formation of mutans streptococcal dental plaques is the primary requisite for the initiation of pathogenic processes. Three phases:

- **Initial attachment:** Acquired pellicle present on tooth surface influence bacterial colonization. Pellicle binding proteins present on mutans streptococci are responsible for initial attachment.
- **Accumulation:** Mutans streptococci accumulate on teeth by synthesis of extracellular glucose polymers from sucrose. Glucosyltransferase (GTF) is extra-cellular enzyme constantly produced by mutans streptococci.
- **Acid formation and cavitation:** Metabolism of various saccharides results in excretion of significant amounts of lactic acid as a metabolic product, which will cause demineralization resulting in carious lesion.

Immonologic control of caries: Major source of salivary Ig is the salivary secretions which produce secretory IgA (1–3%). Saliva also contains humoral immunoglobulins IgG and IgM from GCF. Cellular components of immune system such as lymphocytes, macrophages and neutrophils are present in gingival sulcus. There are two possible ways the antibodies might control bacterial growth:

- Salivary immunoglobulins may act as specific agglutinins interacting with bacterial surface receptors and inhibiting colonization and subsequent caries formation. They might also inactivate surface GTF.
- Antibodies might opsonize bacteria leading to phagocytosis by lymphocytes.

Q. 7. Write a note on caries vaccine and their role in prevention of dental caries. *(NTR Uni., April 2007; TNMGR, May 2019)*

Ans. Vaccines are immunobiological substances designed to produce specific protection against given disease. They may be prepared from live modified organisms, inactivated or killed organisms, cellular fractions, toxoids or combinations of these.

S. mutans possess various cell surface substances including adhesins, glucosyltransferse (GTFs), and glucan binding proteins (GBP).

Mechanism of action:
- Vaccine inactivates surface glucosyltransferases, which reduce synthesis of extracellular glucans resulting in reducing plaque formation.
- Secretory IgA from salivary glands due to direct immunization of gut-associated lymphoid tissue (GALT) may prevent mutans streptococci from adhering to enamel surface. It also prevent formation of dextran by inhibiting activity of glucosyltransferases.

Types of caries vaccine:
1. Sub-unit vaccine: It contains structural elements of either adhesions or glucosyltransferases.
2. Recombinant vaccine (attenuated expression vectors): They target vaccine to lymphoid tissue for mucosal response.
3. Conjugate vaccine: Conjugation of peptide components with bacterial polysaccharides.

Routes of administration: Oral/mucosal (intranasal, tonsillar, minor salivary gland, rectal), systemic (s.c.), active (gingivo-salivary), passive dental immunization.

Passive immunization: Monoclonal antibodies (to *S. mutans* cell surface antigen I/II), bovine milk and whey, (bovine milk and whey-containing polyclonal IgG antibodies), egg-yolk antibodies (formalin killed whole cells and cell-associated GTFs), transgenic plants (genetically-modified tobacco plant).

Adjuvants and delivery systems for caries vaccines: Synthetic peptides, coupling with cholera toxin subunits, fusing with salmonella, microcapsules and microparticles, liposomes.

Advantage: Prevents caries in children, can be incorporated to universal immunization programme, provide lifelong immunity.

Adverse effects: Cross reaction with human heart tissue, hypersensitivity reactions, microbial resistance.

Q. 8. Write a note on immunization for medical professionals. *(NTR Uni., May 2018)*

Ans. Medical professionals/healthcare workers (HCWs) include physicians, nurses, emergency medical personnel, dental professionals, laboratory technicians. They are at risk for exposure to serious, deadly diseases.

Recommended Vaccines for HCWs

1. **Hepatitis B:** If previously unvaccinated, give a two-dose (Heplisav-B) or three-dose (Engerix-B or Recombivax HB) series, IM For HCWs, who perform tasks that may involve exposure to blood or body fluids, obtain anti-HBs serologic testing 1–2 months after second dose (for Heplisav-B) or third dose (for Engerix-B or Recombivax HB).

2. **Influenza:** Give one dose of influenza vaccine annually. Inactivated injectable vaccine is given IM, except when using the intradermal influenza vaccine. Live attenuated influenza vaccine (LAIV) is given intranasally.

3. **MMR (measles, mumps, rubella):** For HCW without serologic evidence of immunity or prior vaccination, give two doses of MMR, 4 weeks apart, subcutaneously.

4. **Varicella (chickenpox):** For HCW, who has no serologic proof of immunity, prior vaccination, or diagnosis, give two doses of varicella vaccine, 4 weeks apart, subcutaneously.

5. **Diphtheria, pertussis, tetanus:** Give one dose of DPT as soon as feasible to all HCWs who have not received DPT previously and to pregnant HCW with each pregnancy. Give DPT boosters every 10 years thereafter, IM.

6. **Menigococcal:** Give both meningococcal conjugate and serogroup B meningococcal vaccine (IM) to microbiologists who are routinely exposed to isolates of *Neisseria meningitidis*, with booster dose at every 5 years.

Q. 9. Write a short note on hypersensitivity reactions. *(TNMGR, Oct. 2012; MUHS, June 2017; BBD Uni., April 2018; HP Uni., April 2019)*

Ans. Hypersensitivity refers to excessive, undesirable (damaging, discomfort-producing and sometimes fatal) reactions produced by the normal immune system.

I. **Type I (immediate, anaphylactic, IgE or regain dependent):** IgE antibodies are fixed on the surface of tissue cells (mast cells and basophils) in sensitized individuals, to which the antigen combines, leading to release of vasoactive amines. These occur in two forms:

1. Anaphylaxis *(UHSR, June 2017; RUHS, May 2018; RGUHS, June 2018):* It is an acute, potentially fatal, systemic form of type I hypersensitivity. The term anaphylaxis (ana—without, phylaxis-protection) was coined by Richet (1902). The clinical effects are due to smooth muscle contraction and increased vascular permeability. Tissues or organs predominantly involved in anaphylactic reaction are known as 'target tissues' or 'shock organs'.

Symptoms and signs: Itching, flushing of skin, difficulty in breathing, nausea, vomiting, abdominal pain, diarrhea, blood in stool, acute hypotension, loss of consciousness and death.

Causes: Injections of antibiotics or other drugs, insect stings.

Treatment: Adrenaline (SC or IM) 0.5 ml (1 in 1000 solution).

Mechanism: Cytotropic IgE antibody, which binds to cells, releasing their granules, which acts as pharmacological mediators:

i. **Primary mediators:** Pre-formed, e.g. histamine, serotonin, chemotactic factors.

ii. **Secondary mediators:** Newly formed, e.g. slow reacting substance of anaphylaxis (SRSA), PGs, platelet activating factor (PAF) and cytokines.

- **Anaphylactoid reaction** *(RGUHS, Nov. 2011):* Intravenous injection of peptone, trypsin and certain other substances provoke a clinical reaction resembling anaphylactic shock known as 'Anaphylactoid reaction.'

2. **Atopy:** Atopy is chronic or recurrent, non-fatal localized form of type I hypersensitivity. The term 'atopy' refers to naturally occurring familial hypersensitivities of human beings, typified by hay fever and asthma. The antigens commonly involved in atopy are characteristically inhalants (pollen, house dust) or ingestants (egg, milk). Predisposition to atopy is genetically determined, probably linked to MHC genotype. Symptoms of atopy are caused by release of pharmacologically active substances following combination of Ag and cell-fixed IgE. Clinical expression of atopic reactions is usually determined by the portal of entry of Ag: Conjunctivitis, rhinitis, gastro-intestinal symptoms and dermatitis.

II. **Type II (cytotoxic or cell stimulating):** It involves activation of complement by IgG or IgM binding to an antigenic cell, the antigenic cell is lysed, e.g. antibody-mediated thrombocyto-penia, agranulocytosis, hemolytic anemia, etc.

Treatment: Anti-inflammatory agents and immunosuppressive agents.

III. **Type III (immune complex or toxic complex disease):** The damage is caused by Ag-Ab complex (immune complex), which may precipitate in and around small blood vessels, causing damage to cells or on membranes, interfering with their function, e.g. incompatible blood transfusion, hemolytic disease of newborn, autoimmune hemolytic anaemia, myasthenia gravis, pemphigus vulgaris. Two types:

1. **Arthus reaction:** It is a local manifestation of generalized hypersensitivity, in which the tissue damage is due to formation of Ag–Ab precipitates causing complement activation and release of inflammatory molecules. This leads to increased vascular permeability and infiltration of the site with neutrophils. Leukocyte–platelet thrombi are formed that reduce the blood supply and lead to tissue necrosi, e.g. farmer's lung.

2. **Serum sickness:** This is a systemic form of type III hypersensitivity. The clinical syndrome consists of fever, lymphadenopathy, splenomegaly, arthritis, glomerulonephritis, endocarditis, vasculitis, urticarial rashes, abdominal pain, nausea and vomiting, appearing 7–12 days following injection. The pathogenesis involves formation of immune complexes which get deposited on endothelial lining of blood vessels in various parts of body, causing inflammatory infiltration. Plasma concentration of complement falls due to massive complement activation and fixation by Ag–Ab complexes. Serum sickness differs from other types of hypersensitivity reaction in that a single injection can serve both as sensitizing dose and shocking dose.

Treatment: Antiinflammatory agents.

IV. **Type IV (delayed type or cell mediated)** (RUHS, May 2018; UHSR, June 2019): Ag activates specifically sensitized CD4, CD8 T cells, leading to secretion of lymphokines, with fluid and phagocyte accumulation. Type IV hypersensitivity is involved in pathogenesis of many autoimmune and infectious diseases and granulomas due to infections and foreign antigens. Mechanisms of damage in delayed hypersensitivity include T lymphocytes and monocytes and/or macrophages. Cytotoxic T cells (Tc) cause direct damage, whereas helper T (T_H1) cells secrete cytokines which activate cytotoxic T cells and recruit and activate monocytes and macrophages, which cause the bulk of the damage. Major lymphokines involved in delayed hypersensitivity reaction include monocyte chemotactic factor, interleukin-2, interferon-gamma, TNF alpha/beta, etc. Two types:

1. **Tuberculin (Mantoux) type:** When a small dose of tuberculin (Ag) is injected intra-dermally in a sensitized individual, an indurated inflammatory reaction develops at the site within 48–72 hours. It provides useful indication of cell-mediated immunity to bacilli.

2. **Contact dermatitis type:** This type of reaction develops (48–72 hours) when allergen comes in contact of skin of sensitized individual. The lesions vary from macules and papules to vesicles. Hypersensitivity is determined by "Patch test".

3. **Granulomatous type:** Granuloma develops due to persistent Ag or foreign body response, leading to hardening at site within 21–28 days, e.g. leprosy.

Treatment of delayed hypersensitivity: Corticosteroids and other immunosuppressive agents.

Q. 10. Discuss the importance of immune complexes in dental diseases. *(TNMGR, Oct. 1999; April 2012)*

Ans. Deposition of immune complexes is a major feature of a wide range of human disease.

- **Composition of immune complex:** The complexes which result in disease usually have a molecular weight >500,000 and comprise both immuno-globulins and antigens.
- **Complex deposition:** In immune complex disease (ICD), complexes become deposited in synovial membrane of joints, walls of blood vessels (kidney and skin mostly).
- **Events following deposition of immune complex** (Flowchart 1.9): When antibodies become fixed to antigens, the Fc portions of their heavy chains become 'activated' and may then either attract non-immune (uncommitted) circulating lymphocytes ('B' cell) or activate the complement cascade. Both can lead to tissue damage when the complex has been deposited.

Clinical features of ICD: Generalized lymphadeno-pathy, glomerulonephritis (hypertension, albuminuria, oliguria, haematuria, edema), cutaneous vasculitis (maculopapular rash, leg ulcers, purpura), Raynaud's phenomenon, arthritis, hepatitis, myositis and myocarditis, generalized urticaria.

Diseases associated with deposition of immune complexes:

1. **Generalized:** Rheumatoid arthritis, systemic lupus erythematosus (SLE), poststreptococcal nephritis, malarial nephritis, hypersensitivities to drugs such as penicillin, virus infections.
2. **Localized:** Farmer's lung, pigeon fancier's lung, Erythema nodosum, insect bites, postmeasles encephalitis, rubella arthritis, and gonococcal arthritis.

Diagnosis of immune complex disease:
1. Serum: Hypo-complementaemia and presence of complement conversion products.
2. Tissue biopsy by immunofluorescent staining techniques.

Treatment of ICD:
1. Steroids (prevents release of proteolytic enzymes, affect platelet and complement).
2. Antihistamines (block actions of some of vasoactive amines).
3. Heparin should be used early in disease process, prevents fibrin deposition.
4. Other drugs: Immunosuppressive drugs, by infusing antibody, or by giving further antigen with adjuvant.

2. MICROFLORA OF ORAL CAVITY

Q. 1. Write a short note on oral microbial flora.
(Bangalore Uni., Jan. 1992; Sumandeep Uni., June 2016; TNMGR, AHSUC, May 2018; HP Uni., April 2019)

Ans. The mixture of organism regularly found at any anatomical site is referred to as normal flora (indigenous microbiota). The presence of nutrients, epithelial debris and secretions makes the oral cavity a favorable habitat for plethora of organism.

- **At birth:** The oral cavity is sterile, but rapidly becomes colonized from environment. *Strep. salivarious* make up 98% of total oral flora until the appearance of teeth (6–9 months). Anaerobic

Flowchart 1.9: Sequence of events following immune complex deposition

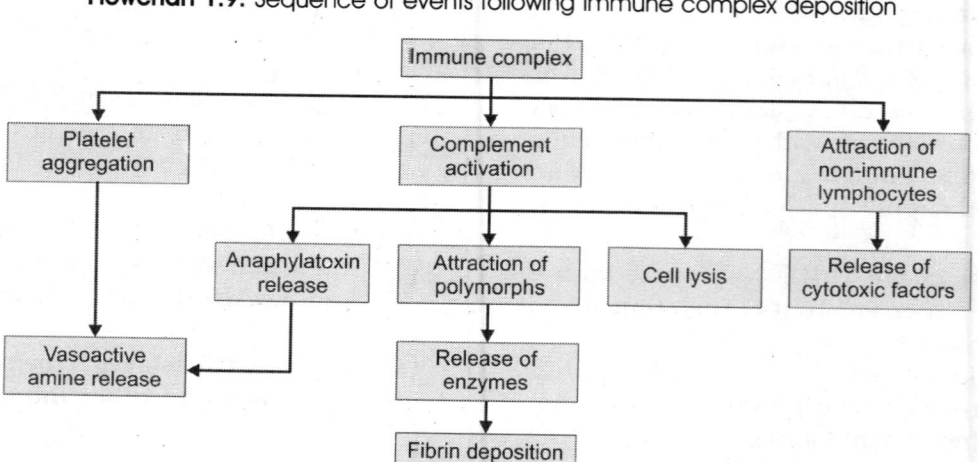

fusiform bacilli found in infants mouths younger than 2 months. Fusiform bacilli increase in number during 4–8 months. *Peptostreptococcus* appears in 5 months old infants.

- **Mouth of 1-year-old child:** Eruption of teeth leads to colonization by *Strep. mutans* and *S. sanguinis* and persist as long as teeth remains. Other strains of streptococci adhere to gums and cheeks. Less commonly are lactobacilli, Actinomyces, Prevotella, fusobacteria, *Nocardia, Candida, Bacteroids, Corynebacterium, Leptotrichia* and coli forms.
  - Crypts of tonsils have anaerobic micrococci, microaerophilic and anaerobic streptococci, vibrios, fusiform bacilli, *Corynebacterium species, Actinomyces, Leptothrix, Mycoplasma, Neisseria* and *Bacteriophage.*
- **In adolescence:** With eruption of permanent teeth, there is increase in anaerobic forms like *Bacteroids, Leptotrichia, Fusobacteria,* and *Spirochetes* and *Vibrio.*

Benefits of Normal Flora

1. Normal flora gets nutrients and habitat from host, this make difficult for non-indigenous microorganisms to get established.
2. Normal flora synthesises some vitamins which are absorbed by host.
3. Normal flora contributes to immunity of host by inducing secretory IgA.
4. Oral bacteria produce inhibitory substances against non-indigenous microorganisms.

Q. 2. Write a note on microbiology of dental caries.
(TNMGR, April 1998, Oct. 2019 MUHS, May 2012)

Q. Why dental caries is infectious and transmissible disease? *(TNMGR, April 2012)*

Ans. Dental caries (disease of civilization) is a chronic endogenous infection caused by normal oral commensal flora. Vertical transmission from mother to child has been suggested as the main pathway for mutans streptococci acquisition. The microflora of dental caries is Gram-positive bacteria, facultative aerobic bacteria and later on, when the lesion depth increases anaerobic and proteolytic bacteria appear. In the process of dental caries initiation, *S. mutans* have been implicated, whereas lactobacillus is implicated in caries progression.

Types of caries	Microorganisms
Pit and fissure	Mutans streptococci, *S. sanguinis*, *Lactobacilli* spp., *Actinomyces* spp.
Smooth surface	Mutans streptococci, *S. salivarius*
Root surface	*A. israelii, Actinomyces naeslundii,* mutans streptococci
Deep dentinal caries	*Lactobacilli* spp., *A. naesulundii,* other filamentous rods.

Q. 3. Write a short note on Gram-positive cocci.
(TNMGR, April 2013)

Ans. Gram-positive cocci include *Staphylococcus* (catalase-positive), which grows clusters and *Streptococcus* (catalase-negative), which grows in chains (Table 2.2). Staphylococci are further subdivided into coagulasepositive (*S. aureus*) and coagulase-negative (*S. epidermidis* and *S. saprophyticus*) species. *Streptococcus* bacteria are divided into *Strep. pyogenes* (group A), *Strep. agalactiae* (group B), Enterococci (group D), *Strep. viridans,* and *Strep. pneumonia.*

Table 2.2: Gram-positive cocci with their predominant site

Gram-positive cocci	Location/infection
Staph. aureus, epidermidis, sapropyticus	Buccal mucosa/angular cheilitis
Strep. mitis, oralis, parasanguinis, sanguinis	Dental plaque, tongue, cheek/dental caries
Strep. pneumonia	Upper respiratory tract
Strep. salivarius	Saliva and tongue dorsum
Strep. vestibularis	Vestibular mucosa
Strep. constellatus, intermedius, anginosus	Gingival crevice/dentoalveolar infections
Strep. mutans	Dental plaque, carious tooth
Gemella morbillorum	In peridontium
Strep. pyogenes	Oropharynx of neonates
Enterococcus spp.	Oral cavity and intestine
Stomatococcus (facutative anerobes)	Tongue, gingival crevice/opportunistic
Micromonas micros, Finegoldia magnus (anaerobs)	Teeth (carious dentin)/periodontal and dentoalveolar abscess

Q. 4. Write a short note on *Streptococcus viridans*.
(TNMGR, March 2008; HP Uni., April 2019)

Ans. Streptococci are Gram-positive, non-motile, non-spore forming, catalase-negative cocci that occur in pairs or chains. Most streptococci are facultative anaerobes, and some are obligate anaerobes. Streptococcus can be classified as:

1. **α-hemolytic:** Partial hemolysis, green color, e.g. pneumonia and viridans.
2. **β-hemolytic:** Complete hemolysis, clear, e.g. pyogenes (group A), agalactiae (group B).
3. **γ-hemolytic:** No hemolysis, e.g. enterococcus (*E. faecalis* and *E. faecium*) (group D).
   - *Streptococcus viridans* are optochin resistant and bile resistant and has no capsule. It includes *Strep. mutans, Strep. sanguinis,* and *Strep. anginosus. Streptococcus viridans* (oral streptococci), is normal commensal in the mouth, upper respiratory tract, skin and genital tract. They are ordinarily non-pathogenic but can cause disease occasionally. In persons with pre-existing cardiac lesions, they may cause bacterial endocarditis, *S. sanguinis* being most often responsible. Following tooth extraction or other dental procedures, they cause transient bacteremia and get implanted on damaged or prosthetic valves or in a congenitally diseased heart, and grow to form vegetations. Prophylactic antibiotic cover is advisable in such persons before tooth extraction or similar procedures.
   - *Sterp. mutans* (*TNMGR, April 2011*) is important in causation of dental caries. It breaks down dietary sucrose, producing acid and a tough adhesive dextran (insoluble polysaccharides). The acid damages dentine and the dextran bind together food debris, epithelial cells, mucus and bacteria to form dental plaques, which lead to caries. It is homofermentive and more aciduric than other streptococci. *S. mutans* does not colonize the mouth of infants prior to eruption of teeth. It disappears from the mouth after complete extraction of teeth. Infants get infected from their parents. Based on nucleic acid base content, it has been divided into five genotypes: *S. mutans, S. rattus, S. sobrinus, S. cricetus, S. ferus. S. mutans* has been divided into eight serotypes 'a' to 'h'. The specific antigen for each serotype represents cell wall constituents, which are chemically characterized as polysaccharides. It utilizes sucrose for its energy requirements and results in formation of lactic acid. The primary habitats for *S. mutans* are mouth, pharynx, and intestine.
   - **Dental caries and *Strep. mutans*** (*Sharda Uni., May 2016*): *Strep. mutans* causes—adherence to enamel surfaces; produces acidic metabolites; build up glycogen reserves and has ability to synthesize extracellular polysaccharides (EPS) in the presence of sucrose, fructose and glucose. The production of large quantities of EPSs from sucrose is an important factor of *S. mutans* cariogenicity. *S. mutans* and *Strep. sobrinus* have a central role in the etiology of dental caries, because these can adhere to enamel salivary pellicle and to other plaque bacteria. Mutans streptococci and lactobacilli are strong acid producers and hence cause an acidic environment creating the risk for cavities. Usually, the appearance of *S. mutans* in the tooth cavities is followed by caries after 6–24 months.

Q. 5. Discuss morphology, culture characteristics and pathogen potential of *Porphyromonas gingivalis*.
(NTR Uni., April 2012; Oct. 2013)

Ans. *Porphyromonas gingivalis* appears to be one of the prime etiological agents in the pathogenesis and progression of the inflammatory events of periodontal disease. *P. gingivalis* is non-motile, asaccharolytic, Gram-negative rod like, obligate anaerobe and it forms black-pigmented colonies on blood agar plates. It has an absolute requirement of iron for its growth.

Major habitat of *P. gingivalis* is subgingival sulcus of oral cavity. It relies on fermentation of amino acids for energy production (a property required for its survival in deep periodontal pocket). *P. gingivalis* serves as the secondary colonizer of dental plaque, adhering to primary colonizers.

Virulence factors: Factors which enable pathogen to adhere, colonize, invades host tissue, evade host defenses and induce tissue destruction. *P. gingivalis* has:

1. Enzymes (hyaluronidase, chondroitin sulphatase) and capsule: Decrease phagocytosis for invasion, chemotaxis inhibitors.
2. Lipopolysaccharides: Bone resorption, immunoglobulin proteases.
3. Fimbriae, exopolysaccharide, outer membrane proteins: Adhesion or attachment to host outer membrane.
4. Collagenase, trypsin-like protease, gelatinase: Degradation of plasma protease inhibitors, destruction of periodontal tissue.
5. Aminopeptidase: Degradation of iron transport protein.

Plaque microflora: Once the bacteria are adhered to follicle, subsequent growth leads to bacterial accumulation and increased plaque mass. Dental plaque growth depends on growth via adhesion of new bacteria and multiplication of attached bacteria. Initial bacteria that colonize the pellicle surface are mostly gram positive facultative microorganisms such as *Actinomyces viscosus* and *Strep. sanguinis*, as the plaque matures, secondary colonization of *Prevotella intermedia*, *Capnocytophaga*, *P. gingivalis* takes place.

Q. 6. Write a note on microflora in infected root canal. *(RGUHS, Nov. 2017; Gujarat Uni., June 2018)*

Ans. Endodontic infections have a polymicrobial nature, with obligate anaerobic bacteria conspicuously dominating the microbiota in primary infections.

A. **Intraradicular infections:**
1. Black pigmented Gram-negative anaerobic rods *(Bacteroides melaninogenicus)*: *Prevotella* (*P. intermedia, P. nigrescens, P. tannerae, P. denticola*), *Porphyromonas* (*P. endodontalis* and *P. gingivalis*).
2. *Fusobacterium*: *F. nucleatum, F. periodonticum*.
3. Spirochetes *(Treponema)*: *T. denticola, T. parvum, T. maltophilum*.
4. Gram-positive anaerobic rods: Pseudoramibacter alactolyticus, *Actinomyces* spp., *Propionibacterium propionicum*, *Olsenella* spp., and *Eubacterium* spp.
5. Gram-positive cocci: *Parvimonas micra* (*Peptostreptococcus micros*), *Strep.* spp. (*Strep. anginosus, Strep. mitisi, Strep. sanguinis, E. faecalis*).
6. Other bacterial spp.: *Campylobacter* spp., *Veillonella parvula, Eikenella corrodens, Neisseria mucosa, Centipeda periodontii, Capnocytophaga gingivalis, Bifidobacterium dentium*, anaerobic lactobacilli.
7. Fungi: *Candida* spp.
8. Viruses: Viruses cannot survive in a necrotic root canal.

B. **Extraradicular infections:** Mostly anaerobic bacteria like *Actinomyces* spp., *P. propionicum*, *Treponema* spp., *P. endodontalis, P. gingivalis, Treponema forsythia, Prevotella* spp., *F. nucleatum*.

C. **Bacteria persisting intracanal disinfection procedures and after root canal treatment (failed treatment)** *(UHSR, June 2018)*: Gram-negative anaerobic rods (*F. nucleatum, Prevotella* spp. and *Campylobacter rectus*). Gram-positive bacteria (Streptococci: *Strep. mitis, Strep. gordonii, Strep. anginosus, oralis*; Lactobacilli—*L. paracasei, L. acidophilus*; Staphylococci; *E. faecalis*; *Parvimonas*

micra; P. alactolyticus; Propionibacterium spp.; *Actinomyces* spp. *Bifidobacterium* spp. and *Eubacterium* spp.), yeasts (*C. albicans*).

- **Faecalis** *(Gujarat Uni., April 2019; TNMGR, Oct., 2019)* is identified as the species most commonly recovered from root canals undergoing retreatment, in cases of failed endodontic therapy and canals with persistent infections. *E. faecalis* are Gram-positive cocci and facultative anaerobes. They are normal intestinal organisms and may inhabit oral cavity and gingival sulcus. *E. faecalis* has many distinct features which make it an exceptional survivor in the root canal:
  - Survive in presence of several medications and irrigants.
  - Form biofilms in medicated canals.
  - Invade and metabolize fluids within dentinal tubules and adhere to collagen.
  - Convert into a viable but non-cultivable state.
  - Acquire antibiotic resistance.
  - Survive in extreme environments with low pH, high salinity and high temperatures.
  - Endure prolonged periods of starvation.
- **Biofilm** *(TNMGR, May 2018; SGT Uni., May 2019)*: Biofilm is defined as a community of micro colonies of microorganisms in an aqueous solution that is surrounded by a matrix made of glycocalyx.

Development of biofilm: Bacteria can form biofilms on any surface that is bathed in a nutrient-containing fluid. The three major components involved in biofilm formation are bacterial cells, a solid surface and a fluid medium. Biofilm formation occurs in three stages as given below.

Stage 1: Adsorption of inorganic and organic molecules to solid surface occurs, leading to the formation of conditioning layer.

Stage 2: Adhesion of microbial cells to conditioned layer. The bacteria substrate interaction occurs in three phases:
- Phase 1: Transport of microbe to substrate surface which is mediated by fimbriae, pili, flagella and glycocalyx.
- Phase 2: Initial non-specific microbial-substrate adherence.
- Phase 3: Specific microbial substrate adherence phase.

Stage 3: Development of biofilm and biofilm expansion occur. In this stage, monolayer of microbes attracts secondary colonizers forming microcolony, and this collection leads to final structure of biofilm.

- **Endodontic biofilms** *(TNMGR, June 2017):* Root canal environment favors the biofilm formation. Endodontic bacterial biofilms can be categorized as:
  1. Intracanal biofilms: Microbial biofilms formed on root canal dentin of infected tooth.
  2. Extraradicular biofilms: Root surface biofilms formed on root (cementum) surface adjacent to root apex of infected teeth, e.g. in asymptomatic periapical periodontitis, chronic apical abscesses with sinus tracts.
  3. Periapical biofilms: They are isolated biofilms found in periapical region of endodontically infected teeth.
  4. Biomaterial-centered infections: It occurs when bacteria adhere to an artificial biomaterial (gutta percha) surface and form biofilm structures. These biofilms can be intraradicular or extraradicular.

Q. 7. Write about role of anaerobic microorganism in maxillofacial infection. *(TNMGR, Sept. 2008; RGUHS, Oct. 2010)*

Ans. Depending on oxygen requirement, microorganism can be classified as:

- **Obligate aerobes** require O_2 for growth.
- **Obligate anaerobes (aerophobes)** do not need or use O_2 as a nutrient. Obligate anaerobes live by fermentation, anaerobic respiration, bacterial photosynthesis, or methanogenesis.
- **Facultative anaerobes** (or **facultative aerobes**) *(NTR Uni., June 2015)*: These organisms can switch between aerobic and anaerobic types of metabolism. Under anaerobic conditions, they grow by fermentation or anaerobic respiration, but in presence of O_2 they switch to aerobic respiration.

- **Aerotolerant anaerobes** are bacteria with an exclusively anaerobic type of metabolism but they are insensitive to presence of O_2. They live by fermentation alone whether or not O_2 is present in their environment.

Microorganism associated with various maxillofacial infections are (Table 2.7):

1. **Chronic periodontitis:** *P. gingivalis, aggregatibacter actinomycetemcomitans, P. intermedia, Tannerella forsythia, Campylobacter rectus,* and fusobacteria.

   In aggressive periodontitis: *A. actinomycetemcomitans, P. gingivalis, Parvimonas micra, C. rectus, Treponema lecithinolyticum,* and *Selenomonas.*

2. **Periapical and endodontic infections:**
   - Primary endodontic infection: Gram-negative anaerobes and Gram-positive anaerobes. Presence of Gram-negative anaerobic bacilli and anaerobic Gram-positive cocci is associated with acute signs and symptoms.
   - Secondary endodontic infections and refractory periapical lesions: *Prevotella, Peptostreptococcus, Eubacterium, Propionibacterium,* and *Enterococcus.*

3. **Periimplantitis:** Strict anaerobes, such as *Porphyromonas, Prevotella, Tannerella, Parvimonas, Fusobacterium,* staphylococci, enteric Gram-negative bacteria, enterococci, yeasts, *Pseudomonas* and *Enterobacteriaceae.*

4. **Chronic osteomyelitis:** In hematogenous origin, enteric rods and staphylococci; In chronic osteomyelitis, mixed infections with *Fusobacterium, Porphyromonas, Prevotella, Parvimonas, Eikenella, Actinomycetes* and staphylococci.

Table 2.7: List of anaerobic microorganisms associated with oral cavity

Microorganisms	Infected areas
Gram-negative rods	
Bacteroides spp. *Fusobacterium* spp., *Centipeda periodonti, Selenomonas* spp.	Peridontium
Porphyromonas spp.	Peridontium, oral cavity
Prevotella spp.	Peridontium, periodontal and endodontic lesions
Leptotrichia buccalis	Oral mucosa
Gram-negative cocci	
Veillonella spp.	Tongue and saliva
Gram-positive rods	
Actinomyces spp.	Dental plaque, calculus
Bifidobacterium dentium	Dental plaque
Eubacterium spp.	Gingival tissues
Gram-positive cocci	
P. niger, Peptostreptococcus spp.	Subgingival areas

Table 2.8: ASEPSIS wound scoring system

ASEPSIS criteria	Points
Additional treatment	
Antibiotics	10
Drainage of pus (local anesthesia)	5
Debridement of wound (general anesthesia)	10
Serous discharge*	Daily 0–5
Erythema*	Daily 0–5
Purulent exudate*	Daily 0–10
Separation of deep tissues*	Daily 0–10
Isolation of bacteria	10
Stay as in patient >14 days	5

*Given score only on 5 of 7 days. Highest weekly score used.

Category of infection: Total score 0–10 = Satisfactory healing; 11–20 = Disturbance of healing; 20–30 = Minor wound infection; 31–40 = Moderate wound infection; > 40 = Severe wound infection.

5. **Facial cellulitis of dental origin:** Gram-positive aerobic-facultative aerobic cocci, Gram-negative anaerobic bacilli, *Prevotella, Porphyromonas* spp., *Bacteroides* spp., *Fusobacterium* spp., *Eubacterium* spp., *Veillonella* spp., oral streptococci, and staphylococci.

6. **Lemierre's syndrome:** *F. necrophorum, F. nucleatum, F. gonidia forum,* and *F. varium, Prevotella, Bacteroides, Peptostreptococcus* and methicillin resistant *S. aureus.*

7. **Deep head and neck infections:** Mixed aerobic-anaerobic infections; *Porphyromonas, Fusobacterium, Prevotella, Peptostreptococcus,* oral streptococci. In case of fistulization of neck infection: Coagulase-negative staphylococci > methicillin-resistant.

Q. 8. Write a note on microbiology of wound infection.

(TNMGR, March, 2002; BBD Uni., Aug. 2014; NTR, Nov. 2017)

Ans. Wound infection (surgical site infections) is defined as an infection caused by physical injury of skin/mucous membrane as a result of penetrating trauma, breaking its continuity and allowing organisms to gain access to tissues. Wound infections are caused by:

- Direct contact: Transfer from surgical equipment/hands of surgeons or nurses.
- Airborne dispersal: Surrounding air contaminated with microorganisms.
- Self-contamination: Physical migration of patient's own endogenous flora to surgical site.

Most wound infections manifest within a week of surgery. *Strep. pyogens* and clostridial infections appear within 1–2 days. Staphylococcal infections typically take 4–5 days. Gram-negative bacillary take 6–7 days.

Non-surgical sites of wound infections include infection cut down, umbilical stumps, ulcers and burns. *Pseudomonas aeruginosa* is the most important cause of infection in burns (Table 2.8).

3. BACTERIOLOGY

Q. 1. Add a note on different culture media and methods. *(TNMGR, March 2008)*

Ans. Culture media *(UHSR, May 2016)*: It is a special medium containing nutrients and physical growth parameters, used to grow different kind of microorganism for the purpose of identifying and studying them.

Basic composition: Energy source; source of Carbon, nitrogen, sulfur, phosphorus; mineral salts; pH (7.2–7.4); accessory growth factors; water.

Classification of culture media:

A. Based on consistency: Solid (blood agar), liquid (nutrient broth), semisolid (sulfide indole motility medium).

B. Based on oxygen requirement: Aerobic and anaerobic.

C. Based on ingredients: Simple (nutrient broth, nutrient agar), complex (blood agar), synthetic/defined media (peptone water), semi-defined media (simple peptone water medium), special media (enriched-blood agar; enrichment—tetrathione broth; selective Lowenstein Jenson medium; differential MacConkey's medium; transport media—Stuart's medium).

- **Culture methods:** Culture methods employed depend on the purpose for which they are intended. Purpose of culture methods include: To isolate bacteria in pure culture, to demonstrate their properties, to obtain sufficient growth for Ag preparation, for bacteriophage and bacteriocins susceptibility, to determine antibiotic sensitivity, to estimate viable counts and maintain stock cultures. Various culture methods are:

1. Streak culture/surface plating method.
2. Lawn or carpet method.
3. Stroke culture method.
4. Stab culture method.
5. Pour plate method.
6. Liquid culture method.
7. Anaerobic culture methods.

- **Anaerobic culture methods** (*TNMGR, April 2013*): Used to isolate anaerobic bacteria, which grow in absence of O_2 but grow in presence of CO_2 (20%). Process of creating anaerobic condition is called anaerobiosis.

Methods of achieving anaerobiosis:

1. Production of vacuum: Incubate the culture in vacuum desiccators.
2. By using anaerobic chambers: McIntosh and Fildes jar, GasPak jar.
3. Displacement of oxygen with other gases such as hydrogen, nitrogen, helium, or carbon dioxide by use of candle jar.
4. Chemical method: By using alkaline pyrogallol which adsorbs oxygen, by using mixture of chromium and sulphuric acid (Rosenthal method).
5. Biological methods: By incubating with aerobic bacteria, germinating seeds or chopped vegetables.
6. By using reducing agents: 1% glucose, 0.1% thioglycolate, 0.1% ascorbic acid and 0.05% cysteine, e.g. Robertson's cooked meat medium (cooked meat particles are used as reducing agents); thioglycolate broth medium.
7. Others: By using semisolid agar (0.05–0.2%), which prevents convention of air.

Q. 2. Write a short note on Gram's stain.
(TNMGR, Oct. 2011, 2013)

Ans. It was developed by Danish bacteriologist, Hans Christian Gram in 1884.

Solution Used: Primary stain (crystal violet); mordant (Gram's iodine); decolorizer (acetone/alcohol); counter stain (neutral red/safranine).

Principle: It is based on the principle that some bacteria are capable of retaining crystal violet stain within them in spite the action of decolorizing agent (Gram-positive bacteria), whereas some fail to do so (Gram-negative bacteria).

Procedure:

1. The fixed smear is covered with crystal violet solution and kept as such for 30–60s.
2. By holding the slide at downward angle, the stain is poured off. Iodine solution is poured over the smear to get rid of remaining stain and smear is covered with fresh iodine solution for 60s.
3. Iodine is washed with 70% acetone/alcohol by simultaneous tilting the slide from side to side till color ceases to come out of preparation (10–20s).
4. Smear is washed with water and stained with counter stain for 20–30s. The slide is dried for examination.

Control: On the same slide, smears should be prepared from *Staph. aureus* (Gram-positive), *Escherichia coli* (Gram-negative) to act as control.

Inference: Gram-positive bacteria, yeast cells—dark purple; Gram-negative bacteria, epithelial cells—pale to dark red.

Characteristics seen in Gram stained smear: Shape, arrangement, stain reaction, quantity, special character, additional structures.

Structures not seen on the Gram stained smear: Flagella, fimbria, nuclei, capsules.

Applications of Gram stains

- Used to guide initial therapy until definitive identification of microorganism is obtained.
- Morphology of stained bacteria can sometimes be diagnostic.
- Sometimes the Gram stain is the only clue to the nature, variety and relative proportion of infecting organism.
- Aids in interpretation of culture reports

Q. 3. Write a note on Gram-negative bacterial cell wall.
(TNMGR, Oct. 2003)

Ans. The bacterial cell wall is a complex, mesh-like structure, essential for maintenance of cell shape and structural integrity. When placed in a hypertonic solution, cytoplasm loses water by osmosis and shrinks while the cell wall retains its original shape and size (**bacterial ghost**). Bacterial cell wall is 10–25 nm thick and account for about 20–30% of the dry weight of cell. Chemically, it is composed of mucopeptide (**peptidoglycan or murein**) scaffolding formed by N-acetyl glucosamine and N-acetyl muramic acid molecules alternating in chains, cross-linked by peptide chains. The cell wall carries bacterial antigens that are important in virulence and immunity.

- **Gram-positive bacterial cell wall** (Fig. 3.3a): Cell wall has simpler chemical nature, mainly composed of peptidoglycan (50–90%) and large amount of teichoic acids.
- **Gram-negative bacterial cell wall** (Fig. 3.3b): It is multilayered and complex in nature. The Gram-negative cell wall is composed of a thin, inner layer of peptidoglycan and an outer membrane consisting of molecules of phospholipids, lipopolysaccharides (LPS), lipoproteins and surface proteins. Outer membrane contains LPS in its outer leaflet and phospholipids in inner leaflet. LPS consists of three regions.
  - **Region I:** Polysaccharide portion determining O antigen specificity (Boivin antigen).
  - **Region II:** Core polysaccharide.
  - **Region III:** Glycolipid portion (lipid A), responsible for endotoxic activities-pyrogenicity, lethal effect, tissue necrosis, anti-complementary activity, B cell mitogenicity, immunoadjuvant property and antitumour activity.

Porins exist in outer membrane, which act like pores for particular molecules. There is a space between peptidoglycan layer and secondary cell membrane called the **periplasmic space**. S-layer is directly attached to outer membrane.

Q. 4. Write a short note on bacterial toxins.

(UOK, June 2019)

Ans. Bacterial toxins are soluble antigens, secreted by pathogenic bacteria, which can modulate cellular functions by selectively targeting number of signaling pathways within host cell in order to tilt the balance in bacteria favor. There are two types of bacterial toxins.

- **Endotoxins** *(RGUHS, Nov. 2012)*: Endotoxins are the integral part of the cell walls of Gram-negative bacteria, and are liberated when bacteria are disintegrated (lysed). Cell wall of Gram-negative bacteria contains lipopolysaccharides (LPS). All endotoxins can produce same signs and symptoms like chills, fever, weakness, general aches, blood clotting and tissue death, shock, and even death. Toxicity is associated with lipid component (lipid A) and immunogenicity is associated with poly-saccharide components. Endotoxins are heat stable, but some powerful oxidizing agents such as super oxides, peroxide and hypochlorite can neutralize them. Organisms that produce endotoxins include *Salmonella typhi, Proteus* spp., *Pseudomonas* spp., etc.
- **Exotoxins** *(RGUHS, Nov. 2012)*: These are proteins released into extracellular environment by Gram-positive and some Gram-negative bacteria. They are denatured by heat; acid, proteolytic enzymes and have a high biological activity. They have entero-toxic, cytotoxic, hemolytic and neurotoxic effect. They are highly toxic and fatal to animals in very small doses. They are highly antigenic, stimulate formation of antitoxin. Antitoxin neutralizes the toxin and converted to toxoid by formalin. Toxoid is nontoxic but antigenic, e.g. tetanus toxoid.

Q. 5. Write a short note on microbial resistance and its clinical relevance.

[TNMGR, April, 2013; NTR Uni., May 2019]

Ans. Drug resistance or antimicrobial resistance is the reduction in effectiveness of a drug in curing a disease, i.e. the bacteria is not killed or their growth is not stopped. The bacteria acquire drug resistance by:

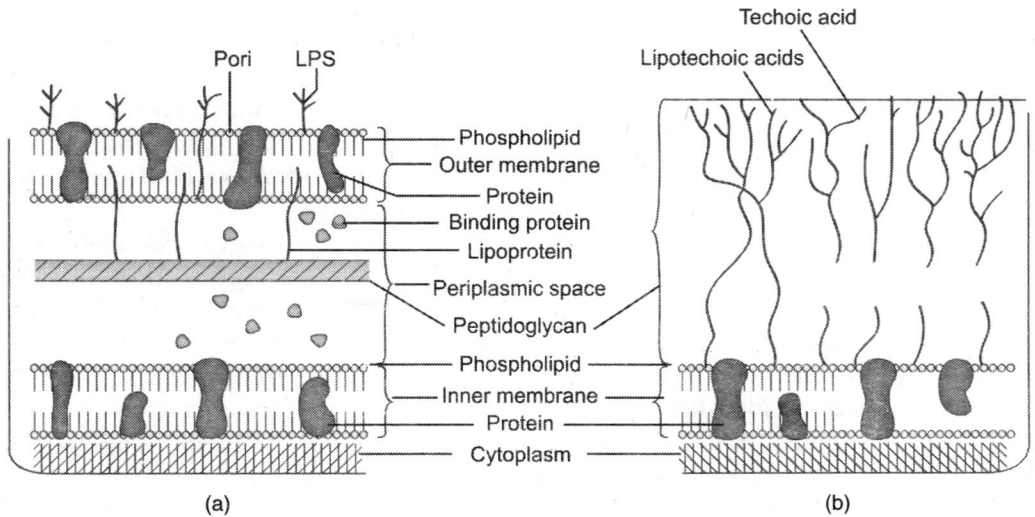

Fig. 3.3: Bacterial cell wall. (a) Gram-positive; (b) Gram-negative

A. **Intrinsic (natural):** Lack of target, drug blocked from entering into cell.

B. **Acquired:** Genetic methods:

1. **Chromosomal methods/mutational resistance:**
   a. Stepwise mutation: Resistance is achieved by series of stepwise mutation, as seen with penicillin.
   b. One step mutation: Mutants differ widely in resistance as seen with streptomycin.

2. **Extrachromosomal methods/genetic transfer resistance:**
   a. Transfer of r-genes from one bacterium to another by conjugation, transformation and transduction (by a bacteriophage).
   b. Transfer of r-genes between plasmids within bacterium: Resistance transfer factor (RTF)—resistance is plasmid mediated and the whole plasmid [RTF + resistance determinant (r)] is known as R factor. This transfer is by transposons and integrons.

Q. 6. Write a note on toxins produced by staphylococci.
(HP Uni., April 2019)

Ans. Staphylococci (Greek: Bunch of grapes) are Gram-positive, non-motile, facultative anaerobic, catalase positive and cluster forming microorganism.

Virulence factors

A. **Cell wall structures:** Peptidoglycan, capsule, protein A, clumping factor.

B. **Coagulase:** Staphylokinase, DNAase, phosphatase, lipase, phospholipase, hyaluronidase, serokinase, protease.

C. **Extracellular/Cytolytic toxins:**
1. Hemolysins:
   a. **α-hemolysin:** It is protein inactivated at 70°C, but reactivated paradoxically at 100°C. α-toxin is less active against human RBCs. It is also leucocidal, cytotoxic, dermonecrotic, neurotoxic and lethal.
   b. **β-hemolysin:** It is a sphingomyelinase, hemolytic for sheep cells. It exhibits a "**hot-cold phenomenon**".
   c. **γ-hemolysin:** It is composed of two separate proteins, necessary for hemolytic activity.
   d. **δ-hemolysin:** It has a detergent like effect on cell membranes of erythrocytes, leucocytes, macrophages and platelets.

2. **Leucocidin (Panton-Valentine toxin):** Kills WBCs by producing holes in cell membranes.

3. **Enterotoxin:** Responsible for staphylococcal food poisoning by acting directly on autonomic nervous system.

4. **Toxic shock syndrome toxin (TSST)** is a potentially fatal multisystem disease presenting with fever, hypotension, myalgia, vomiting, diarrhea, mucosal hyperemia and erythematous rash.

5. **Exfoliative (epidermolytic) toxin:** This is responsible for staphylococcal scalded skin syndrome (exfoliative skin diseases—outer layer of epidermis gets separated from underlying tissues). The severe form of this disease is known as **Ritter's disease** in newborn and **toxic epidermal necrolysis (TEN)** in older patients. Milder forms are **pemphigus neonatorum** and **bullous impetigo.**

Q. 7. Write a short note on toxins of Streptococci.
(TNMGR, April 2003; HP Uni., April 2019)

Ans. Streptococci are Gram-positive, catalase negative, aerobic cocci forming pairs or chains.

Virulence factors

A. **Capsule:** Non-immunogenic.

B. **Surface Ag:** M-protein, fimbriae, C-carbohydrates, hyaluronic acid, C5a protease.

C. **Cytolytic toxins:**
1. **Hemolysin:** Streptococci produce two hemolysin:
   a. **Streptolysin 'O':** Antigenic, oxygen labile, cardiotoxic and leucotoxic. Antistreptolysin 'O' (ASO) appears in sera following streptococcal infection.
   b. **Streptolysin 'S':** Non-antigenic, oxygen stable, and is responsible for hemolysis seen around streptococcal colonies on the surface of blood agar plates.

2. **Pyrogenic exotoxin (erythrogenic/dick/scarlatinal toxin):** This produces scarlet fever (**streptococcal pyrogenic exotoxin**). Three types: A, B and C.

3. **Exoenzymes:**
   a. **Streptokinase (Fibrinolysin):** Digestion of fibrin clots.
   b. **Streptodornase (DNAase):** Depolymerisation of DNA.
   c. **Nicotinamide Adenine Dinucleotidase (NADase/diphosphopyridine nucleotidase):** Releases nicotinamide from NAD and is leucotoxic.
   d. **Hyaluronidase:** Breaks down hyaluronic acid of connective tissues.

4. **Serum opacity factor:** A lipoproteinase produced by M types of *Strep. pyogenes*, which produces opacity when applied to agar gel containing horse or swine serum.

Q. 8. Write a short note on Vincent's organism.

(TNMGR, April 1995)

Ans. *Borellia* (*Treponema*) *vincentii* is called **Vincent's organism.** It forms symbiotic combination with fusiform bacillus. It is motile spirochete, which is longer and coarser than the treponemes. It is 5–20 μm long and 0.2–0.6 μm wide with 3–8 coils of variable size. It is easily stained with dilute carbol fuchsin and is Gram negative. It is a normal mouth commensal, but under predisposing conditions, gives rise to ulcerative gingivostomatitis or oropharyngitis (**Vincent's angina/ Plaut-Vincent/ANUG/trench mouth**).

Laboratory diagnosis: Smears are made directly from the lesions and stained with dilute carbol-fuchsin, which shows both spirochetes and fusiform bacilli along with pus cells.

Q. 9. Write a short note on C. diphtheriae.

(TNMGR, April 1998)

Ans. *Corynebacterium diphtheriae* (**Klebs-Loeffler bacillus**) is non-motile, non-capsulated club-shaped Gram-positive bacillus. When it is stained with **Loeffler's methylene blue**; the granules take up a bluish purple color and hence called **metachromatic granules** (**volutin** or **Babes Ernst granules/polar bodies**). The bacilli are arranged in a characteristic fashion in smears (**Chinese letter or cuneiform arrangement**).

Cultural characteristics: The usual media for cultivation are Loeffler's serum slope, tellurite blood agar, McLeod's media and Hoyle's media at 37°C and pH 7.2. It is an aerobe and a facultative anaerobe. Colonies are at first small, circular white opaque discs but enlarge on continued incubation and may acquire a distinct yellow tint. Based on morphology on tellurite agar, bacilli are:

i. Gravis: Daisy head colony.
ii. Intermedius: Frog's egg colony.
iii. Mitis: Poached egg colony.

Toxin: Diphtheria toxin is a protein and is extremely potent. Toxigenicity of diphtheria bacillus depends on the presence of corynephages (tox+). Non-toxigenic strains may be rendered toxigenic by infecting them with β-phage (**Lysogenic or phage conversion**).

Resistance: Cultures may remain viable for one or more weeks at 25–30°C. It is readily destroyed by heat in 10 min. at 58°C and in one min. at 100°C. It is more resistant to the action of light, desiccation and freezing. It is susceptible to penicillin, erythromycin and broad spectrum antibiotics.

Antigenic structure: Diphtheria bacilli are antigenically heterogeneous. By agglutination, gravis strains have been classified into 13 types, intermedius into 4 types and mitis into 40 types.

Q. 10. Write a short note on diphtheria.

(TNMGR, April 2000)

Ans. Diphtheria is most commonly an infection of upper respiratory tract and causes fever, sore throat, and malaise. A thick, gray–green fibrin membrane (**pseudomembrane**) often forms over the site of infection as a result of bacterial growth, toxin production, necrosis of underlying tissue, and host immune response. Incubation period in diphtheria is commonly 3–4 days. The site of infection may be faucial, laryngeal, nasal, otitic, conjunctival, genital-vulval, vaginal or prepucial and cutaneous. According to clinical severity, diphtheria may be classified as:

1. **Malignant or hypertoxic:** Severe toxemia with marked adenitis (**bull neck**) and death due to circulatory failure.
2. **Septic:** Leads to ulceration, cellulitis and gangrene around the pseudomembrane.
3. **Hemorrhagic:** Characterized by bleeding from the edge of membrane, epistaxis, conjunctival hemorrhage, purpura and bleeding tendency.

Complication: Asphyxia, Acute circulatory failure, Postdiphtheritic paralysis, sepsis.

Mechanical complications of diphtheria are due to pseudomembrane, while the systemic effects are due to toxin.

Laboratory diagnosis:

1. Smear examination of swab.
2. Culture of swab.
   - *In vivo tests:* Subcutaneous test and intracutaneous test.
   - *In vitro test:* Elek's gel precipitation test and tissue culture test.

Prophylaxis: Immunization:

- **Active immunization:** Diphtheria toxoid + Tetanus toxoid + Pertussis vaccine as DTP/DPT/triple vaccine.
- **Passive immunization:** 500–1000 U of antidiphtheritic serum (ADS), SC
- **Combined immunization:** First dose of adsorbed toxoid on one arm, while ADS is given on the other arm.

Treatment: ADS (20,000–100000 U) stat, when a case is suspected as diphtheria. Penicillin is drug of choice. Erythromycin is more active than penicillin in carriers.

Q. 11. Write a note on tetanus and its prophylaxis.

(TNMGR, Oct. 2000)

Ans. Tetanus is an acute bacterial disease caused by neurotoxin tetanospasmin elaborated by *Clostridium tetani* and characterized by prolonged contraction of skeletal muscles. *C. tetani* is a Gram-positive, obligate anaerobes, and flagellate organism, whose spores survive in soil and cause infection by contaminating wounds.

Causes: Injury, especially puncture wound; surgical operations; local suppuration; septic abortion; unsterile injection.

Pathophysiology *(TNMGR, April 2003):* Tetanus toxin is taken up into terminals of lower motor neurons and transported axonally to the spinal cord and/or brainstem. Here the toxin moves trans-synaptically into inhibitory nerve terminals, where vesicular release of inhibitory neurotransmitters becomes blocked, leading to disinhibition of lower motor neurons and muscle rigidity and spasms ensue.

Symptoms: Hyperactivity of voluntary muscles in the form of rigidity (tonic, involuntary contraction of muscles) and spasms (shorter lasting muscle contractions that can be elicited by stretching of the muscles or by sensory stimulation → **Reflex spasms**). Typical features of tetanus are trismus/lockjaw, risus sardonicus, dysphagia, neck stiffness, abdominal rigidity, and opistotonus. In addition, general muscle ache, focal flaccid paralysis, diplopia, nystagmus, vertigo, pain and allodynia may occur.

Tetanus is categorized as:

- **Generalized:** Affects muscles of whole body and lead to opistotonus (backward arching of columna due to rigidity of extensor muscles of neck and back), respiratory failure and death.
- **Neonatal:** Generalized form in children <1 month.
- **Local:** Cephalic—tetanus is localized to head region.

Incubation period is variable from 2 days to several weeks (commonly 3–21 days). Fatality rate varies from 15–50%.

Laboratory diagnosis: The diagnosis is clinical. Demonstration of *C. tetani* by microscopy, culture or by animal inoculation.

Treatment and Prophylaxis

1. **Wound cleaning:** Removal of foreign bodies, necrotic tissue and blood clots, to prevent an anaerobic environment favorable for *C. tetani*.
2. **Antibiotics:** Metronidazole (500 mg) TDS, or penicillin (100,000–200,000 IU/kg/day) IV for 7–10 days.
3. **Immunization:**
   - **Passive immunization:** Antitetanus serum (1500 IU, SC/IM) soon after receiving any tetanus prone injury.
   - **Active immunization:** Tetanus toxoid is given either alone or along with diphtheria toxoid and pertussis vaccine as triple vaccine.
   - **Combined immunization:** Tetanus immune globulin (TIG) injection at one site, along with first dose of toxoid at contra lateral site, followed by second and third doses of toxoid at monthly intervals.

Q. 12. Write a short note on *Mycobacterium tuberculosis*.

Ans. *M. tuberculosis* is a straight, Gram-positive, acid fast bacillus. It is an obligate aerobe. The most widely used media is Lowenstein-Jensen medium without starch. Other media include Dorsat, Tarshis, Loeffler and Pawlowsky. On solid media it forms dry, rough, raised irregular colonies with a wrinkled surface. They are creamy white, becoming yellowish or buff colored on further incubation. They are not heat resistant, being killed at 60°C in 15–20 min. They are relatively resistant to chemical disinfectant. Test used to identify *M. tuberculosis* are niacin test, aryl sulphatase test, neutral red test, catalase-peroxidase test, amidase test, nitrate reduction test. The mode of infection is by direct inhalation of aerosolized bacilli contained in droplet nuclei of expectorated sputum.

Q. 13. Write a short note on nosocomial infections.

(TNMGR, Oct. 2011)

Ans. Nosocomial infection or hospital acquired infection (HAI) is defined as "An infection occurring in a patient in hospital or other health care facility in whom the infection was not present or incubating at the time of admission".

Factors influencing HAI: Long hospital stay, use of indwelling catheters, failure to wash hands, over use of antibiotics, mechanical ventilation, intravenous catheter.

Microorganism involved: 60% cases are caused by aerobic Gram-negative rods, 30% by Gram-positive cocci, remaining 10% by viruses, fungi and parasites. Most common are *Staph. aureus*, *E. coli*, coagulase negative *Staph.*, *Enterococcus* spp., *P. aeruginosa*, *Enterobacter* spp., *Candida*, *Proteus mirabilis*.

Most common HAI: Surgical wounds, urinary tract infection, respiratory infection, wound and skin infection, gastrointestinal infections, eye infections, Miscellaneous: Hepatitis B virus, HIV.

Routes of transmission: Contact spread (direct or indirect), airborne spread, oral route, parenteral route, self infection.

Prevention

1. Provisions of sterile instruments, dressings, surgical gloves, face masks, theatre clothing and fluids.
2. Thorough handwashing and use of gloves by medical staff.
3. Preoperative disinfection of patient's skin.
4. Use of antiseptics for irrigation of wound site.
5. Rational antibiotic prophylaxis.
6. Proper investigation of nosocomial infection and treatment of patients and carriers.

Q. 14. Write a short note on common anaerobic infections. *(TNMGR, March 2007)*

Ans. Anaerobic infections are usually endogenous and are caused by tissue invasion by bacteria normally present on respective body surfaces. These are typically polymicrobial.

Precipitating factors are trauma, tissue necrosis, impaired circulation, hematoma formation or presence of foreign body.

Anaerobic infections as per site:

1. CNS: Brain abscess.
2. Ear, nose, throat: Chronic sinusitis, otitis media, orbital cellulitis.
3. Mouth and jaw: ANUG, dental abscess, cellulitis, abscess and sinus of jaw.
4. Respiratory: Aspiration pneumonia, lung abscess, empyma.
5. Abdominal: Hepatic abscess, appendicitis, peritonitis, wound infection after colorectal surgery.
6. Female genitalia: Wound infection following genital surgery, tubovarian abscess, and septic abortion.
7. Skin and soft tissue: Infected sebaceous cyst, axillary abscess, cellulitis, diabetic ulcer, gangrene.

Clinical features: Production of foul or putrid odor, pronounced cellulitis, toxemia, fever.

Laboratory diagnosis:

1. Specimen collection and transport: By using tissue biopsy or aspiration. Swabs are transferred in Stuart's transport medium.
2. Direct microscopy.
3. Culture: Colony morphology, pigmentation and fluorescence helps in identification of anaerobes.
4. Antibiotic sensitivity tests.

Treatment: Surgical drainage along with antimicrobial therapy (clindamycin and metronidazole, penicillin G).

4. VIROLOGY

Q. 1. Write a short note on viral inclusion bodies. *(TNMGR, Nov. 2001)*

Ans. Inclusion bodies are structures with distinct size, shape, location and staining properties that can be demonstrated in virus infected cells under light microscope. They represent degenerative changes produced by viral infections and hence their presence helps in diagnosis. They are generally acidophilic and can be seen as pink structures when stained with Giemsa or eosin methylene blue stains. Some viruses (e.g. adenovirus) form basophilic inclusions.

Classification:

A. **Cytoplasm (intracytoplasmic):**
  1. **Negri bodies:** Eosinophilic inclusions in brain cells seen in rabies.
  2. **Guarnieri bodies:** Smaller multiple inclusions seen in vaccinia (smallpox) virus.
  3. **Bollinger bodies:** Large inclusions seen in fowl pox virus.
  4. **Molluscum bodies:** Very large inclusions (20–30 µ) seen in molluscum contagiosum.

B. **Nucleus (intranuclear):**
  1. **Cowdry type A:** Variable size and granular appearance, seen in herpes virus, yellow fever virus.
  2. **Cowdry type B:** More circumscribed and multiple, seen in adenovirus, poliovirus.

C. **Both types:** Measles virus.

Q. 2. Write about viral infections of the oral cavity. *(MAHE, Dec. 1996; TNMGR, Oct. 1999; NTR Uni., Oct. 2011; Sumandeep Uni., April 2015)*

Ans. Viral infections typically present with abrupt onset and association of solitary or multiple blister or ulcerations. Concomitant general symptoms such as fever, malaise, and lymphadenopathy are observed in a few viral conditions. Common viral infection of oral cavity are:

1. **Herpes simplex infections:** Herpes gingivostomatitis, herpes labialis.
2. **Herpes-Zoster infection:** Chickenpox, herpes zoster.
3. **Coxsackie virus infection:** Herpangina, hand, foot and mouth disease, acute lymphonodular pharyngitis.
4. *Cytomegalovirus* **infection:** Foot and mouth disease.
5. **Human papillomavirus infection:** Squamous papilloma, verruca vulgaris, condyloma acuminatum, molluscum contagiosum.

6. **Epstein-Barr virus infection:** Infectious mononucleosis, hairy leukoplakia.

7. **Human immunodeficiency virus:** AIDS.

Q. 3. Write a short note on herpes simplex virus.
(TNMGR, April 1995, 2013)

Ans. Herpes simplex virus (HSV) is a kind of enveloped virus with icosahedral core surrounded by a lipoprotein envelope with linear double-stranded DNA. HSV is large in size (120–200 nm), second in size only to poxviruses. Capsid surrounds DNA core and over the capsid is tegument (a protein-filled region). Nuclear membrane derived lipid bilayer containing viral glycoproteins.

Classification:

1. **α-herpesvirinae:** HSV-1, HSV-2, varicella-zoster virus (VZV).

2. **β-herpesvirinae:** *Cytomegalovirus* (CMV), *human herpesvirus* type 6 (HHV-6), *human herpesvirus* type 7 (HHV-7).

3. **γ-herpesvirinae:** Epstein-Barr virus (EBV), *human herpesvirus* type 8 (HHV-8).

There are two types of HSV:

1. **HSV-1:** Usually isolated from lesions in and around the mouth and is transmitted by direct contact or droplet spread (above waist), e.g. acute gingivostomatitis, recurrent herpes labialis (cold sores), keratoconjuctivitis (keratitis), encephalitis. Recurrent HSV-1 of lips is known as **herpes labialis. Herpetic whitlow/herpetic paronychia:** Herpes infection of fingers.

   Herpes gladiaotorum/scrumpox: Vesicular lesion on head, neck and trunk. **Eczema herpeticum Kaposi's varicelliform eruption:** Widespread herpes of skin.

   Keratoconjuctivitis: Infection of eyes.

2. **HSV-2:** Responsible for majority of genital herpes infections, transmitted venerally (below waist), e.g. herpes genitalis, neonatal herpes, aseptic meningitis.

Pathogenesis: Humans are the only natural hosts and sources of infection are saliva, skin lesions or respiratory secretions. The virus enters through defects in skin or mucous membranes and multiplies locally with cell-to cell spread. Virus enters cutaneous nerve fibers and is transported intra-axonally to the ganglia where it replicates. The virus remains latent in the ganglia, to be reactivated, to cause recurrent oral and genital ulcers.

Reactivation: By triggering factors—fever, UV exposure, common cold, fatigue, stress, trauma, cancer therapy, immunosuppression, HIV, GI upset, pregnancy, menstruation.

Laboratory diagnosis:

- Cell culture is the gold standard test.
- Cytology: Scrapings from base of lesion smeared and stained with Wright, Giemsa (Tzanck smear) stain shows multinucleated giant cells and intranuclear inclusion body.
- Direct fluorescent Ag detection test: Specimen incubated with fluorescein labeled HSV type specific monoclonal Ab-positive cells appears green.
- PCR-based DNA detection is the most sensitive method.
- Serological methods: Primary HSV-IgM titers followed by IgG titers (seroconversion). In recurrent HSV-IgG titers only.
- Biopsy.

Treatment:

1. Pain control and supportive care.
2. Definitive therapy: Acyclovir, famciclovir, valacyclovir. Idoxyuridine used topically in eye and skin infection.

Q. 4. Write a short note on varicella-zoster virus.
(NTR Uni., Nov. 2017)

Ans. Varicella-zoster virus (VZV) is an exclusively human virus that belongs to the α-herpesvirus family.

Primary infection leads to acute varicella or 'chickenpox', usually from exposure either through direct contact with a skin lesion or through airborne spread from respiratory droplets.

Primary varicella presents as a disseminated pruritic rash that often starts on the face and spreads down the trunk, with relative sparing of the hands and soles of the feet; mucosal involvement can occur. The symptoms usually resolve within 7–10 days. Complications such as hepatitis, pancreatitis, pneumonitis, and encephalitis are infrequent but can be life-threatening.

After initial infection, VZV establishes lifelong latency in cranial nerve and dorsal root ganglia, and can reactivate years to decades later as **herpes zoster** or 'shingles'. It most often presents as a painful vesicular rash that involves ≤2 adjacent unilateral dermatomes. Presentations may vary as patients may present with pain as a prodrome to the development of lesions. It can present as **herpes zoster ophthalmicus** (trigeminal ganglion) or **Ramsay-Hunt syndrome** (**herpes zoster oticus**—geniculate ganglion)

Risk factors: Patients with previous VZV disease, older transplant recipients, patient on immunosuppressive drugs.

Diagnosis: PCR, direct fluorescent assays (DFA)—methods of choice, viral culture and serologic test.

Treatment: Acyclovir (800 mg) 5 ×/day; valacyclovir 1 g, 3 ×/day; Famciclovir (500 mg) 3 ×/day.

Q. 5. Write about prophylaxis for the control of hepatitis B virus infection.

(TNMGR, Aug. 2004; RUHS, May 2018)

Ans. General prophylaxis for the control of hepatitis B virus infection consists of avoiding risky practices like promiscuous sex, injectable drug abuse and direct or indirect contact with blood, semen or other body fluids of patients and carriers (Table 4.5).

I. **Pre-exposure prophylaxis:** Three dose schedule of hepatitis B vaccine: 0 → 1 month → 6 months.

For adolescent (11–15 years): 2 dose schedule: 0 → 4/6 months.

- **Precautions for HBV positive patient:** Follow universal precautions. Patients should be scheduled at the end of the list. Operators and assistants should wear two pair of gloves, plastic gown, cap mask, protective eyewear. High volume suction should be used; rubber dam should be applied to minimize formation of aerosols. All used instruments should be packed in a labeled plastic wrap. After procedure, all pieces of equipment and surfaces should be cleaned and decontaminated with disinfectant (0.5% Na hypochlorite).

II. **Post-exposure prophylaxis:** It refers to preventive medical treatment started immediately after exposure to diseases causing viruses, to prevent infection and development of diseases.

- Immediate care to exposure site: Wash wounds and skin with soap and water. Flush mucous membranes with water.

- Determine the risk of exposure: Type of fluid (body fluids, saliva, potentially infectious fluids or tissue); type of exposure (percutaneous injury, mucous membrane or non-intact skin exposure).

- Initiation of hepatitis B vaccine within 12–24 h of an exposure. The vaccine should not be given later than 14 days post-exposure. The three doses of hepatitis B vaccine are given at 0, 1–2 months, and 6 months.

- Hepatitis B antibodies should be obtained 1–2 months after completion of third dose of vaccine.

Two types of products are used.

1. Hepatitis B vaccine: It provides long-term protection against HBV infection, and is recommended for pre-exposure and post-exposure prophylaxis.

2. HBIG: Provides temporary protection (i.e. 3–6 months) and is only indicated in some post-exposure settings.

Q. 6. Write about modes of transmission of hepatitis B infection.

(TNMGR, March 2007)

Ans. Blood of the carriers and patients is the most important source of hepatitis B infection. The virus may also be present in other body fluids such as saliva, breast milk, semen, vaginal secretions, urine, bile and feces.

1. **Transfusion of carrier blood (horizontal transmission):** Most widely known mode of infection. Other includes shared syringes, needles, razors, acupuncture, tattooing.

2. **Congenital (vertical transmission):** Quite common for carrier mothers; risk is high if mother is HBeAg positive.

3. **Sexual transmission:** More important particularly in promiscuous homosexual.

Table 4.5: Post-exposure prophylaxis schedule

Vaccination/Ag response status of exposed patient	Status of source patient		
	HBsAg positive	HBsAg negative	HBsAg status unknown
Unvaccinated/non-immune	HBIGX1; initiate HB vaccine schedule	Initiate HB vaccine schedule	Initiate HB vaccine schedule
Previously vaccinated, known responder	No treatment	No treatment	No treatment
Previously vaccinated, known non-responder	HBIGX1 and initiate revaccination or HBIGX2	No treatment	No treatment; if high-risk source—treat as if source were positive HBsAg positive
Previously vaccinated, response unknown	Single vaccine booster dose	No treatment	— Do —
Still undergoing vaccinated	HBIGX1; complete schedule	Complete schedule	Complete schedule

Q. 7. Write a short note on human immunodeficiency virus (HIV). *(TNMGR, Sept. 2009; NTR Uni., May 2018)*

Ans. HIV virus belongs to lentivirus subgroup of family Retroviridae.

Structure (Fig. 4.7): HIV is a spherical enveloped virus, 90–120 nm in size. The nucleocapsid has an outer icosahedral shell and an inner cone-shaped core, enclosing the ribonucleoproteins. The genome is composed of two identical single stranded, positive sense RNA copies along with reverse transcriptase enzyme.

Viral genes and antigens: Genome of HIV contains three structural genes—gag, pol, env. The products of these genes act as antigens.

A. **Genes coding for structural proteins:**
1. gag gene: Determines the core and shell of virus. It is expressed as precursor protein-p55 which further cleaves into p15, p18, p24.
2. pol gene: Codes for polymerase reverse transcriptase and other enzymes. It further cleaves into p31, p51, p66.
3. env gene: Determine the synthesis of envelope glycoprotein gp160, which further cleves into gp120—forms surface spikes, gp41-transmembrane anchoring protein.

B. **Non-structural and regulatory genes:** tat; nef; rev; vif; vpu; vpx; vpr; LTR.

HIV is highly mutable virus with frequent antigenic variations. It is thermo labile, being inactivated in 10 min. at 60°C and in sec. at 100°C. It may survive for 7 days at room temperature, in dried blood.

HIV is inactivated in 10 min. by treatment with 50% ethanol, 35% isopropanol, 0.5% lysol, 0.3% hydrogen peroxide, and 10% household bleach. The standard recommendation is hypochlorite solution (0.5%). For contaminated instruments 2% glutaraldehyde is useful.

Q. 8. Write a note on post-exposure prophylaxis for HIV.

Ans. Post-exposure prophylaxis (PEP) for HIV (National AIDS Control Organization—NACO guidelines) consists of following steps.

1. **First aid:** Immediately clean the wound with water and soap.
2. **Counseling:** Exposed persons should receive appropriate information about what PEP is about and the risk and benefits of PEP in order to provide informed consent.
3. **Risk assessment:** Risk of exposure to be assessed at the earliest as mild, moderate or severe exposure. PEP needs to be started as soon as possible after the exposure and within 72 hours.
   a. **Mild exposure:** Exposure of mucous membrane/non-intact skin with small volume.
   b. **Moderate exposure:** Exposure of mucous membrane/non-intact skin with large volume or percutaneous superficial exposure with solid needle.
   c. **Severe exposure:** Percutaneous exposure with large volume.
4. **Relevant laboratory investigations:** A baseline rapid HIV testing should be done before starting PEP.
5. **Provision of short-term drug therapy** (Table 4.8): PEP should be given for at least 4 weeks. There are two types of regimens:
   • Basic regimen: Two-drug combination
   • Expanded regimen: Three-drug combination
6. **Follow-up and support:** Whether or not PEP prophylaxis has been started, follow-up is indicated to monitor for possible infections and provide psychological support.

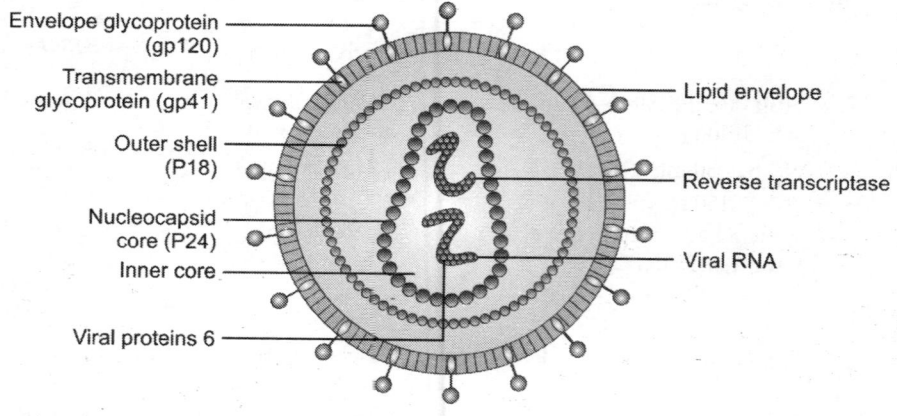

Envelope glycoprotein (gp120)
Transmembrane glycoprotein (gp41)
Outer shell (P18)
Nucleocapsid core (P24)
Inner core
Viral proteins 6
Lipid envelope
Reverse transcriptase
Viral RNA

Fig. 4.7: Structure of HIV

Q. 9. Write a short note on needlestick injuries.

(UHSR, June 2018)

Ans. Needlestick injuries (NSIs) are the most common source of occupational exposures to blood and the primary cause of blood-borne infections of HCWs.

Risk factors for NSIs:
- Overuse of injections and unnecessary sharps.
- Lack of supplies: Disposable syringes, safer needle devices, and sharps-disposal containers.
- Inadequate or short staffing.
- Recapping of needles after use. (Most common cause of NSI).
- Passing instruments from hand to hand in the operating suite.
- Lack of awareness of hazard and lack of training.

Determinants of transmission of infection: The risks of transmission of infection from an infected patient to the HCW following a NSI are: Hepatitis B (3–10%), hepatitis C (3%), HIV (0.3%). Factors that increased risks of transmission of HIV include a deep wound, visible blood on the device, a hollow-bore blood-filled needle, use of device to access an artery or vein, and high-viral-load status of the patient.

PEP for HIV has reduced risk of transmission of HIV following NSI by 80%.

Control measures: Primary prevention of NSIs is achieved through elimination of unnecessary injections and elimination of unnecessary needles.

1. Substitute injections by administering medications through another route, such as tablet, inhaler, or transdermal patches.
2. Jet injectors may substitute for syringes and needles.
3. Engineering controls such as needles that retract, sheathe, or blunt immediately after use.
4. Administrative controls such as policies and training programs aimed to limit exposure to the hazard, e.g. universal precautions, a commitment to HCW safety, a needlestick prevention committee, an exposure control plan, and consistent training.
5. Work practice controls: Include no re-capping, placing sharps containers at eye level and at arm's reach, checking sharps containers on a schedule and emptying them before they're full, and establishing the means for safe handling and disposing of sharps devices before beginning a procedure.
6. Personal protective equipment (PPE): Barriers and filters between the worker and hazard, e.g. eye goggles face shields, gloves, masks, and gowns.
7. Post-exposure measures: Every HCW who sustains a NSI should have access to postexposure prophylaxis (PEP).

5. MYCOLOGY

Q. 1. Write a short note on *Candida albicans*.

(TNMGR, Nov. 1995)

Ans. *C. albicans* is an opportunistic fungal pathogen that is responsible for candidiasis in human hosts.

Table 4.8a: HIV PEP evaluation

Exposure	Status of source		
	HIV+ and asymptomatic	*HIV+ and symptomatic*	*HIV status unknown*
Mild	Consider two-drug PEP	Start two-drug PEP	Usually no PEP or consider two-drug PEP
Moderate	Start two-drug PEP	Start three-drug PEP	— Do —
Severe	Start three-drug PEP	Start three-drug PEP	— Do —

Table 4.8b: Drugs for PEP with dosage

Medication	Two-drug regimen	Three-drug regimen
Zidovudine (AZT)	300 mg BD	300 mg BD
Stavudine (d4T)	30 mg BD	30 mg BD
Lamivudine (3TC)	150 mg BD	150 mg BD
Protease inhibitors	—	**1st choice:** Lopinavir/ritonavir (LPV/r) 400/100 mg BD or 800/200 mg OD with meals.
		2nd choice: Nelfinavir (NLF) 1250 mg BD or 750 mg TDS with empty stomach.
		3rd choice: Indinavir (IND) 800 mg TDS and drink 8–10 glasses of water daily.

Note: If protease inhibitor is not available and third drug is indicated, use efavirenz (EFV 600 mg OD).

C. albicans grow in several different morphological forms, ranging from unicellular budding yeast to true hyphae with parallel side wall. *C. albicans* is a unicellular, oval-shaped diploid fungus (a form of yeast). Typically, *C. albicans* live as harmless commensals in gastrointestinal and genitourinary tract, but overgrowth will lead to Candidiasis, that can affect areas such as skin, genitals, throat, mouth, and blood.

Transmission: *C. albicans* is usually transmitted from mother to infant through childbirth, and remains as part of a normal human's microflora.

Virulence factors: Cell adhesions, degradative enzymes (proteinases, aspartyl proteases, and phospholipases).

Symptoms: *Candida* infection of skin appears as a clearly defined patch of red, itchy skin, often leaking fluid. Scabs and pustules may be seen around the edge of the rash. Vaginal yeast infection may result in slow leakage of a thick, white, cheese-like substance. The vagina may itch or burn, especially during urination or sex. Pain or discomfort during intercourse is common.

Diagnosis: Diagnosis is most commonly made on the basis of skin's appearance.

- **Microscopy:** A scraping or swab of affected area is placed on a microscope slide. A drop of 10% KOH is added to the specimen, which dissolves skin cells, but leaves *Candida* cells intact, permitting visualization of pseudohyphae and budding yeast cells.
- **Culture:** On culture media, colonies are creamy white, smooth and with a yeast odor. It also forms chlamydospores on corn meal agar cultures at 20°C. A rapid method of identifying *C. albicans* is based on its ability to form germ tubes within 2 hours when incubated in human serum at 37°C (**Reynolds-Braude phenomenon**).

Q. 2. Write a short on media used in mycology.
(TNMGR, March 2007)

Ans. The commonest culture media used in mycology are:

1. **Brain–heart infusion agar:** It is a non-selective fungal culture medium that permits growth of all clinically relevant fungi.
2. **Czapek-Dox agar:** It is used for subculture of *Aspergillus* species for their differential diagnosis.
3. **Inhibitory mold agar:** It is used for dimorphic pathogenic fungi.
4. **Sabouraud's dextrose agar:** It is used for dermatophytes.
5. **Niger seed agar:** It is used for identification of *Cryptococcus neoformans*.

6. **Potato dextrose agar:** It is a relatively rich medium for growing a wide range of fungi.
7. **Corn meal agar:** It is used for growing wide range of fungi, especially members of imperfect fungi, and wood inhibiting fungi.
8. **Water agar:** It is used to grow cellulose destroying fungi and spoilage fungi.
9. **Sabouraud's heart infusion agar:** Primary recovery of saprophytic and dimorphic fungi, particularly fastidious strains.
10. **Potato flake agar:** Primary recovery of saprophytic and dimorphic fungi, particularly fastidious and slow growing strains.

The addition of antibiotics prevents bacterial contamination. Cultures are routinely incubated in parallel at room temperature (22°C) for weeks and at 37°C for days. Identification is based on the morphology of fungus and its colony. Growth characteristics useful for identification are rapidity of growth, color, and morphology of the colony.

6. STERILIZATION AND INFECTION CONTROL

Q. 1. Discuss in detail sterilization and disinfection.
(BFUHS, May 2009; RGUHS, May 2011; MPMS Uni., July 2017; RUHS, AHSUC, HP Uni., May 2018)

Ans. Sterilization is defined as the process by which an article, surface or medium is freed of all living microorganisms either in vegetative or spore state. Sterilization can be achieved by physical, chemical and physiochemical means. Chemicals used as sterilizing agents are called **chemisterilants**. **Disinfection** is the process of elimination of most pathogenic microorganisms (excluding bacterial spores) on inanimate objects. Disinfection can be achieved by physical or chemical methods. Chemicals used in disinfection are called **disinfectants**. **Asepsis** is employment of techniques to achieve microbe-free environment. **Antisepsis** is use of chemicals (antiseptics) to make skin or mucus membranes devoid of pathogenic microorganisms.

A. Physical Agents

1. **Sunlight:** The action is primarily due to UV rays.
2. **Drying:** Drying has deleterious effect on many bacteria.
3. **Dry heat** *(SGT Uni., May 2019):* Dry heat acts by protein denaturation, oxidative damage and toxic effects of elevated levels of electrolytes.
   i. **Flaming:** Inoculating wire, tip of forceps, spatulas in flame, till they become red hot.
   ii. **Incineration:** This is a method of destroying contaminated material by burning them in

incinerator. Articles such as soiled dressings; animal carcasses, pathological material, bedding, etc. should be subjected to incineration. This technique results in the loss of the article, hence is suitable only for those articles that have to be disposed.

iii. **Hot air oven:** Most widely used method of dry heating. Holding period is 1 hour on 160°C in an electrically heated oven. Article sterilized are glassware, forceps, scissors, scalpels, glass syringes, swabs, liquid paraffin, and dusting powder. **Advantages:** It is an effective method of sterilization of heat stable articles; articles remain dry after sterilization; only method of sterilizing oils and powders. **Disadvantages:** Poor penetration; cotton wool and paper may get slightly charred; glasses may become smoky; takes longer time as compared to autoclave.

iv. **COX rapid hear sterilizer:** Used for unwrapped instruments, 190°C for 6 min.

v. **Glass/salt bead sterilizer:** It is a heat transfer device, employed for small instruments such as endodontic files, burs, orthodontic bands for 10–45 s at temperature between 218–246°C.

4. **Moist heat sterilization** (*BBD Uni., April 2014*): Moist heat kills microorganism by coagulation and denaturation of proteins.

A. At temperature <100°C:

• **Pasteurization:** Milk is heated at either 63°C for 30 min. (**holder method**) or 72°C for 15 sec. (**flash process**) followed by cooling quickly to 13°C. Vaccine, serum or body fluids, Lowenstein-Jensen and Loeffler's serum are rendered sterile by this method. Other pasteurization methods include ultra-high temperature (UHT), 140°C for 15 sec. and 149°C for 0.5 sec. This method is suitable to destroy most milk borne pathogens like *Salmonella*, mycobacteria, *streptococci*, *staphylococci* and brucella. Efficacy is tested by phosphatase test and methylene blue test.

B. At temperature 100°C

• **Boiling:** The material should be immersed in water and boiled for 10–30 min., killing most vegetative bacteria and viruses. Some bacterial toxins and spores are resistant to boiling; hence this is not a substitute for sterilization. The killing activity can be enhanced by addition of 2% sodium bicarbonate.

• **Steam under normal pressure:** Koch or Arnold steamer is used. A steamer is a metal cabinet with perforated trays to hold the articles and a conical lid. The bottom of steamer is filled with water and heated. The steam generated sterilizes the articles when exposed for a period of 90 min. Media such as TCBS, DCA and selerite broth are sterilized by steaming. Sugar and gelatin in medium may get decomposed on autoclaving; hence they are exposed to free steaming for 20 min for 3 successive days. This process is known as **tyndallisation** (after John Tyndall) or **fractional sterilization** or **intermittent sterilization**. The vegetative bacteria are killed in the first exposure and spores that germinate by next day are killed in subsequent days.

C. At temperature >100°C

• **Steam under pressure (autoclaving):** The principle of **autoclave** or **steam sterilizer** is that water boils when its vapor pressure equals that of the surrounding atmosphere.

5. **Filtration:** With the help of earthenware, candles, asbestos pads, sintered glass, membrane filters made of cellulose acetate. It is mainly used for heat labile substances, e.g. sera, antibiotics.

6. **Radiation:**

i. **Non-ionizing radiation:** Infrared and UV rays for sterilization of prepacked items (syringes and catheters), entryways, operation theaters, laboratories.

ii. **Ionizing radiation:** Electron beams, gamma rays, cosmic rays (cold sterilization) for plastics, syringes, swabs, catheters, etc.

7. **Ultrasonic and sonic vibrations:** Sound waves of frequency >20,000 cycle/sec. kills bacteria and some viruses on exposing for 1 hour. Killing effect of microwave is largely due to the heat they generate. High frequency sound waves disrupt cells. They are used to clean and disinfect instruments as well as to reduce microbial load.

B. Chemical Agents (*TNMGR, Sept. 2010; BBD Uni., April 2014*): Several chemical agents are used as antiseptics and disinfectants. Chemical agents are useful for heat sensitive materials.

An ideal antiseptic or disinfectant should:

1. Have wide spectrum of activity.
2. Be active in presence of organic matter, acid as well as alkaline media.
3. Have speedy action and high penetrating power.
4. Be stable and compatible with other antiseptics and disinfectants.
5. Not corrode metals, cause local irritation or sensitization.

6. Not interfere with healing and non-toxic.
7. Be cheap and easily available and easy to use.

1. **Alcohols:** Alcohols dehydrate cells, disrupt membranes and cause coagulation of protein. Ethyl alcohol and isopropyl alcohol (60–90%) are most frequently used. They are used mainly as skin antiseptics. Isopropyl alcohol is preferred as it is a better fat solvent, more bactericidal and less volatile. It is used for the disinfection of clinical thermometers. Methyl alcohol is effective against fungal spores and is used for treating cabinets and incubators. **Disadvantages:** Skin irritant, volatile (evaporates rapidly), inflammable.

2. **Aldehyde:** Acts through alkylation of amino-, carboxyl- or hydroxyl group, and probably damages nucleic acids. It kills all microorganisms, including spores.

   • **Formaldehyde:** 40% formaldehyde (formalin) is used for surface disinfection and fumigation of rooms, chambers, operation theatres, biological safety cabinets, wards, sick rooms, etc. **Fumigation** is achieved by boiling formalin, heating para-formaldehyde or treating formalin with potassium permanganate. 10% formalin with 0.5% tetraborate sterilizes clean metal instruments. 2% formaldehyde at 40°C for 20 min. is used to disinfect wool. **Disadvantages:** Vapors are irritating, poor penetration, leaves non-volatile residue, activity is reduced in the presence of protein.

   • **Glutaraldehyde (2%):** This has an action similar to formaldehyde. It is especially effective against tubercle bacilli (20 min. for disinfection; 2-3 hours for sterilization), fungi and viruses. It is less toxic and irritant to eyes and skin than formaldehyde. It can be safely used to treat corrugated rubber anesthetic tubes and face masks, plastic endotracheal tubes, metal instruments and polythene tubing. **Disadvantages:** Glutaraldehyde requires alkaline pH and only those articles that are wettable can be sterilized.

   • **Ortho-phthalaldehyde (OPA):** Glutaraldehyde is made into ring shape by attaching two aldehydes to benzene. It kills non-tuberculous Mycobacteria (NTM, e.g. *M. chelonae*, *M. xenopi*, or *M. massiliense*) more effectively. **Disadvantage:** Gray colorization, if used for a long time and risk of anaphylaxis with cystoscopy.

   • **Peracetic acid (liquid sterilization):** Peracetic acid is formed by treatment of acetic acid with hydrogen peroxide. It destroys bacteria by oxidation. Peracetic acid is also effective in removing organic substances by breaking down the proteins. **Disadvantage:** It can corrode metals.

3. **Dyes:** Dyes are used as skin and wound antiseptic, having bacteriostatic activity with low bactericidal activity.

   1. **Aniline dyes:** More active against Gram-positive organisms, used in microbiology laboratory as selective agents in culture media. They react with acid groups in the cell, e.g. brilliant green, malachite green, crystal violet.

   2. **Acridine dyes:** Most active against Gram-positive organisms than Gram-negative. They impair DNA complexes of organisms and thus destroy reproductive capacity of cell, e.g. proflavine, acriflavine, and euflavine.

4. **Halogens:** They are oxidizing agents and cause damage by oxidation of essential sulphydryl groups of enzymes.

   • Chlorine gas is used to bleach water.
   • Tincture of iodine (2% iodine in 70% alcohol) is an antiseptic.
   • Iodine can be combined with neutral carrier polymers (polyvinylpyrrolidone) to prepare **iodophores** such as povidone-iodine. Iodophores permit slow release and reduce the irritation of antiseptic. For handwashing, iodophores are diluted in 50% alcohol. 10% povidone-iodine is used undiluted in pre- and post-operative skin disinfection.
   • Household bleach can be used to disinfect floors (1:10). In higher concentrations chlorine is used to disinfect swimming pools.
   • Sodium hypochlorite is an oxidant, mainly used as bleach. 0.5% sodium hypochlorite is used in serology and virology, in decontamination of spillage of infectious material (1:10). Sodium hypochlorite is sporicidal when used as 5%.
   • Mercuric chloride is used as a disinfectant.
   • Organic chloramines are used as antiseptics for dressing wounds.
   • Hypochlorous acid is formed by reverse reaction of sodium hypochlorite and H_2O_2. It is bactericidal and active against biofilm.

   Disadvantages: They are rapidly inactivated in the presence of organic matter. Iodine is corrosive and staining. Bleach solution is corrosive and will corrode stainless steel surfaces.

5. **Phenols:** The lethal effect of phenols is by disruption of membranes, precipitation of proteins and inactivation of enzymes.

   • Phenols (carbolic acid) are coal-tar derivatives. They act as disinfectants at high concentration and as antiseptics at low concentrations. They are bactericidal, fungicidal, mycobactericidal (5%) but are inactive against spores and most viruses and are used for disinfection of ward floors, in discarding jars in laboratories and disinfection of bedpans.

- o-phenolphenyl (Lysol 5%) and cresol (1–5%) are active against a wide range of organisms.
- Hexachlorophene is chlorinated diphenyl and is much less irritant.
- Chlorhexidine gluconate solution (20%) is used for preoperative hand and skin preparation and for general skin disinfection. It is also mixed with quaternary ammonium compounds such as cetrimide to get stronger and broader anti-microbial effects (Savlon).
- Chloroxylenol are less irritant and can be used for topical purposes and are more effective against Gram-positive bacteria.
- Triclosan is organic phenyl ether with good activity against Gram-positive bacteria and some gram negative bacteria including *Pseudomonas* and fairly active against fungi and viruses.

Disadvantages: It is toxic, corrosive and skin irritant. Chlorhexidine is inactivated by anionic soaps. Chloroxylenol is inactivated by hard water.

6. **Gases: Chemical vapor (Chemiclav)** *(TNMGR, April 2003)*
   i. **Ethylene oxide (EO):** At normal temperature and pressure, it is a highly penetrating gas with a sweet ethereal smell. Its action is due to alkylating of amino, carboxyl, hydroxyl and sulphydryl group in protein molecules. It is effective against all types of microorganisms including viruses and spores. It is used at relative humidity of 50–60%, at temperature of 55–60°C for 4–6 hours. Since it is highly flammable, it is usually combined with CO_2 (10% CO_2+ 90% EO) or dichlorodifluoro-methane. It is specially used for sterilizing heart--lung machines respirators, sutures, dental equipment, glass, metal and paper surfaces, clothing, plastics, soil, some foods and tobacco. **Disadvantages:** It is highly toxic, irritating to eyes, skin, highly flammable, mutagenic and carcinogenic.
   ii. **Formaldehyde gas:** This is widely employed for fumigation of operation theatres and other rooms.
   iii. **Beta-propiolactone (BPL):** This is a conden-sation product of ketone and formaldehyde with a boiling point of 163°C. It is an effective sporicidal agent, and has broad-spectrum activity. 0.2% is used to sterilize biological products. It is more efficient in fumigation than formaldehyde. It is used to sterilize vaccines, tissue grafts, surgical instruments and enzymes. **Disadvantage:** Poor penetrating power and carcinogenic.
   iv. **Hydrogen peroxide:** It is used at 6% concen-tration to decontaminate instruments, equipments such as ventilators. 3% hydrogen peroxide solution is used for skin disinfection and deodorizing wounds and ulcers. Strong solutions are sporicidal. It acts on the micro-organisms through its release of nascent oxygen. **Disadvantages:** Decomposes in light, broken down by catalase, proteinaceous organic matter drastically reduces its activity.

7. **Surface active agents** *(TNMGR, Oct. 2003):* Sub-stances which alter energy relationship at interfaces, producing a reduction of surface tension. They are classified as:
   1. **Cationic compounds:** They act on phosphate groups of cell membrane and enter the cell. The membrane loses its semi-permeability and the cell proteins are denatured. These com-pounds in the form of quaternary ammonium compounds (QUAT) are markedly bactericidal (more active against Gram-positive organisms); but they have no action on spores, tubercle bacilli and most viruses. The common compounds are: Acetyl trimethyl ammonium bromide (cetavlon or cetrimide) and benzalkonium chloride. These are most active at alkaline pH. Organic matter reduces their action and anionic compounds render them inactive.
   2. **Anionic compounds:** Soaps prepared from saturated fatty acids (such as coconut oil) are more effective against Gram-negative bacilli while those prepared from unsaturated fatty acids (oleic acid) have greater action against Gram-positive and *Neisseria* group of organisms.
   3. **Non-ionic:** Polyoxyethylene, e.g. tween, triton.
   4. **Amphoteric or ampholytic compounds:** Also known as Tego compounds, are active against a wide range of Gram-positive and Gram-negative organisms and some viruses.

8. **Metallic salts:** Salts of silver, copper and mercury are used as disinfectant. They act by precipitation of proteins and oxidation of sulphydryl groups. They are bacteriostatic.
   - 1% Silver nitrate solution is used to prevent ophthalmia neonatorum.

- Silver-sulfadiazine cream is used for wound dressings.
- Zinc chloride is used in mouthwash.
- Copper salts are used as fungicide.

C. Physiochemical Method

- **Mode of action:** Use of steam and formaldehyde is a physiochemical method of sterilization. Saturated steam is used at a pressure of 263 mm (5 lb) at a temperature of 70°C for 1 hour. The air is removed from the autoclave chamber and saturated steam at sub-atmospheric pressure is flushed in. Formaldehyde is then injected with steam in a series of pulses, each of 5–10 minutes.

  Disadvantages: Loss of latent heat due to condensation of formaldehyde.

- **Cold sterilization:** It is sterilization by cold chemical solutions, used for heat sensitive instrument. It can be incorporated as method for chair side disinfection of non-critical instruments and chair side accessories.

  Disadvantages: This is not effective against all microorganisms, sterilization time is too long, e.g. formaldehyde (8% aqueous or in 70% alcohol) for 10 h; glutaraldehyde (2% alkaline) for 10 h; chlorine compounds for 30 min. alcohol compounds for 10 min. or more.

Recent advances in sterilization (*NTR Uni., May 2019*):

Classification

A. Chemical methods: Surfacine, superoxidized water, chlorine dioxide, hydroclave, glutaraldehye, orthophthalaldehyde, endoclens.

B. Physical methods: Pulsed-light sterilization, ultra high pressure sterilization.

C. Physicochemical methods: Gas plasma sterilization.

D. Synergistic methods: Psoralen and UVA, ultrasound and bactericide

- **Surfacine:** Surfacine is a surface coating that kills microorganism on contact, by selectively delivering silver. Used to sterilize medical devices, dental care products, food preparation and packaging. **Disadvantage:** Not active against viruses and very less activity against spores.

- **Super oxidized water:** Broad spectrum disinfectant, prepared by electrolyzing saline solution with titanium coated electrodes at 9 amp. It is active against *M. tuberculosis, M. chelonae,* poliovirus, HIV, MRSA, *E. coli, C. albicans, E. faecalis, P. aeruginosa.* **Advantages:** Basic materials, i.e. saline and electricity are cheap and the end product (water) is not damaging.

- **Chlorine dioxide** (ClO_2): Prepared by reacting hypochlorous acid and sodium or potassium chlorate. It is used for drinking water disinfection. **Advantages:** Alternative to chlorine, better disinfectant activity than chlorine. No odor nuisance. **Disadvantages:** Explosive, causes irritation, watery eyes, expensive.

- **Hydroclave:** Hydroclave is a double-walled (jacketed) cylindrical, pressurized vessel, horizontally mounted, with one or more side or top loading doors, and a smaller unloading door at the bottom. **Advantage:** Sterilizes the waste utilizing steam, much faster and much more even heat penetration than autoclave. Hydrolyses the organic components of the waste such as pathological material. Reduces the waste substantially in weight and volume.

- **Endoclens:** Used for sterilization of flexible endoscopes. It consists of a computer-controlled endoscope reprocessing machine that uses performic acid as a sterilant.

- **Pulsed-light sterilization:** It is a non-thermal method for sterilization that involves use of intense, short duration pulses of a broad spectrum (200–1100 nm) light flashes, 25% in UV range to ensure microbial decontamination. **Advantages:** DNA destruction, quick process, no chemicals used, safe and easy to use. **Disadvantages:** Pulsed light is a surface treatment. The decontaminated areas are those which receive the light pulse. **Applications:** Sterilization of caps, cups, lids and other packaging materials, sterilization of food packaging.

- **Plasma sterilization:** Plasma is defined as an ionized gas with an equal no. of positive and negative ions. Plasma is generated in an enclosed chamber under deep vacuum using radiowaves or microwaves to excite gas molecules (hydrogen peroxide) to produce ionized gas particles. This state renders the articles sterile by denaturing all microorganisms. Arthroscopes, urethroscopes, etc. are sterilized by plasma sterilization.

Advantages:

- The process is at room temperature and hence poses no dangers associated with high temperatures.
- Byproducts are generally water and oxygen.
- Time of treatment is fast.

Disadvantages:

- Weak penetrating power of the plasma.
- Complications arise in presence of organic residue.

- High power consumption.
- Can corrode certain materials.

■ **Synergistic sterilization methods: PUVA (psoralen and UVA):** Psoralen intercalates into DNA and on exposure to ultraviolet (UVA) radiation can form mono adducts and covalent interstrand cross-links (ICL) with thymine, resulting in apoptosis. **Uses:** Sterilization of blood plasma and platelets, it is also active against viruses.

■ **Flash sterilization:** Flash sterilization was originally defined by Underwood and Perkins as sterilization of an unwrapped object in a gravity displacement sterilizer. Flash sterilization is considered acceptable for processing cleaned patient-care items that cannot be packaged, sterilized, and stored before use. It also is used when there is insufficient time to sterilize an item by the preferred package method.

■ **Ozone:** Ozone sterilization is the newest low-temperature sterilization method, suitable for many heat sensitive and moisture sensitive or moisture stable medical devices. Ozone sterilization is compatible with stainless steel instruments. The cycle time is 4.5 hours, at a temperature of 455–505°C.

■ **Chemiclav:** Chemiclav or chemical vapor pressure sterilization is an unsaturated chemical vapor system **(Harvey chemiclav),** operates at 131°C, 20 lb pressure with 30 min. cycle. Carbon steel and other corrosion sensitive instruments can be sterilized without rust. **Disadvantage:** Items sensitive to elevated temperature will be damaged; vapor odor is offensive and requires aeration.

Q. 2. Write a short note on autoclave.
(TNMGR, April 1998; BBD Uni., Aug. 2017)

Ans. Autoclaving is standard sterilization method in hospitals. The autoclave is a tough double-walled chamber in which air is replaced by pure saturated steam under pressure.

Principle: Water boils when its vapor pressure equals that of the surrounding atmosphere. Hence, when pressure inside a closed vessel increases, the temperature at which water boils also increases. Saturated steam has penetrative power. When steam comes into contact with a cooler surface, it condenses to water and gives up its latent heat to that surface. The large reduction in volume sucks in more steam to the area and the process continue till the temperature of that surface is raised to that of the steam. The condensed water ensures moist conditions for killing the microbes present.

Sterilization cycle: For wrapped instruments—121°C for 15–20 min. at 15 lb. For unwrapped instruments **(flash sterilization)**—132°C for 3 min at 27–28 lb.

Application: Dressings, instruments, laboratory ware, media and pharmaceutical products, etc.

Construction and working (Fig. 6.2): A simple auto-clave has vertical or horizontal cylindrical body with a heating element, a perforated try to keep the articles, a lid that can be fastened by screw clamps, a pressure gauge, a safety valve and a discharge tap. The screw caps and cotton plugs must be loosely fitted. The lid is closed but the discharge tap is kept open and the water is heated. As the water starts boiling, the steam drives air out of the discharge tap. When all the air is displaced and steam start appearing through the discharge tap, the tap is closed. The pressure inside is allowed to rise up to 15 lb/inch². At this pressure, articles are held for 15 min., after which the heating is stopped and auto-clave is allowed to cool. Once the pressure gauge shows the pressure equal to atmospheric pressure, the discharge tap is opened to let the air in. The lid is then opened and articles removed.

Precautions: Articles should not be tightly packed, the autoclave must not be overloaded, air discharge must be complete and there should not be any residual air trapped inside, caps of bottles and flasks should not be tight, autoclave must not be opened until the pressure has fallen or else the contents will boil over, articles must be wrapped in paper to prevent drenching, bottles must not be overfilled.

Advantage: Temperature is >100°C, therefore, spores are killed; condensation of steam generates extra heat (latent heat of condensation); condensation also allows

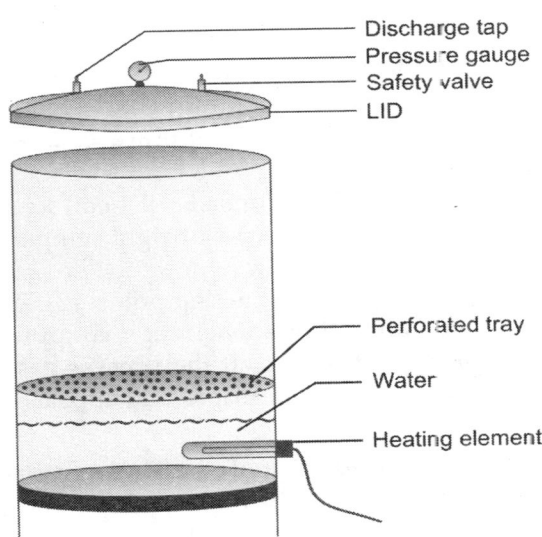

Fig. 6.2: Construction of autoclave

the steam to penetrate rapidly into porous materials; Very effective way of sterilization, quicker than hot air oven; sterilization is verifiable; autoclave is dependable and economical.

Disadvantage: Drenching and wetting of articles may occur, trapped air may reduce the efficacy, takes long time to cool, cannot be used for items that are lacking water.

Types of autoclave

1. **Downward displacement (gravity displacement unit) (N-type):** This is named because of method of air removal in sterilization chamber. It is suitable for solid instruments for immediate use. Two types—vertical type (small) and horizontal type (large).
2. **Positive pressure displacement:** It is an improvement over downward displacement autoclave. Steam is created in a second, separate chamber and held until all the air is displaced in sterilization chamber. The steam is then released into sterilization chamber in a pressurized blast, forcing the air out through the drain hole and starting sterilization process.
3. **Negative pressure displacement (B-type):** In this, once the sterilization chamber door is closed, a vacuum pump removes the air. Steam is created in a second, separate chamber and then released into sterilization chamber in a pressurized blast. It is suitable for wrapped and hollow instrument. (Used in dentistry).
4. **Triple vacuum autoclave:** In this, negative pressure displacement process is repeated three times, hence the name 'triple vacuum' autoclave.

Monitors of sterilization/autoclave

1. **Physical method:** Use of automatic process control, thermocouple and temperature chart recorder to measure accurately the temperature, time and pressure.
2. **Chemical method:** It consists of heat sensitive chemical that changes color at right temperature and exposure time, e.g. Browne's tube no. 1 (black spot) and succinic acid (melting point: 121°C) and Bowie Dick tape. Bowie Dick tape is applied to articles being autoclaved. If the process has been satisfactory, dark brown stripes will appear across the tape.
3. **Biological method:** A spore-bearing organism is added during the sterilization process and then cultured later to ensure that it has been killed, e.g. 10^6 spore of *Geobacillus stearothermophilus*.

Q. 3. Write a note on E-beam sterilization.
[BBD Uni., July 2013]

Ans. Electron-beam (E-beam) sterilization is commonly used for sterilization of medical devices. E-beam sterilization is generally made by use of electron beams that are obtained from accelerator and isotope method. High energy generated is fundamental for an effective sterilization. While 15 min. is sufficient for accelerator method, isotope method (^{60}Co) requires 24 hours.

Mechanism of action: E-beams produce high charge of electrons (continuous or pulsed) generated by e-beam accelerators. These electrons are absorbed by the product to be sterilized, causing changes in chemical and molecular bonds and thus destruction of DNA chain of reproducing cells of bacteria on material.

Advantages:
- It can penetrate variety of products, packaging materials including foils.
- It can cause no damage to sterile seals on packaging.
- It allows control of temperature during irradiation process.
- It has much higher dosing rate than gamma or X-rays.
- It has no residue after sterilization process.
- It has high speed processing.

Disadvantages:
- Less penetration through any material than gamma or X-rays.
- Personnel have to wear protective clothes for the harmful effects of e-beam.

Q. 4. Write a note on methods of sterilization in dentistry.
(TNMGR, Oct. 1999; MUHS, Nov. 2018; NTR Uni., May 2019)

Ans. Accepted methods of sterilization in dentistry:
1. Steam pressure sterilization (autoclave)
2. Chemical vapor pressure (chemiclav): Sterilization by chemical vapor under pressure (131°C, 20 lb, 30 min).
3. Dry heat sterilization (dryclav).
4. Ethylene oxide sterilization (ETC) (Table 6.4).

Disinfection of impression materials *(Sharda Uni., May 2016):* The following four methods of disinfection of impressions:
- **Alginate impression:** 1:10 sod. hypochlorite in a plastic bag for 10 min.
- **Zinc oxide eugenol impression:** 2% glutaraldehyde, iodophores or chlorine compounds.
- **Impression compound:** 1:10 sodium hypochlorite.
- **Elastomeric impression materials:**
  - **Polysulphide and addition silicone:** Glutaraldehyde, iodophore, 0.5% hypochlorite.
  - **Polyether:** Iodophore, 0.5% sod. hypochlorite.

Table 6.4: List of dental equipment along with methods of sterilization

Sr.No.	Equipment	Sterilization method
1.	Dental handpiece	Autoclave (used lubricant spray prior to autoclaving)
2.	Mouth mirrors, probes, tweezers, excavators, chisels, pluggers, carvers, matrix, bands and holders, cartridge syringes.	Autoclave (scrub clean first)
3.	Forceps, elevators, scalpel handles, retractors and other surgical instruments.	Autoclave (scrub clean first)
4.	Sharp instruments	Hot air oven
5.	Syringes	Irradiation
6.	Endodontic files and broaches	Autoclave (may be dipped in alcohol and flamed during treatment)
7.	Glass slab	Swab with tincture of thimerosal, alcohol
8.	Gutta percha cones	Vials containing alcohol, 5.2% sod. Hypochlorite, H_2O_2
9.	Periodontal scalers	Autoclave (scrub clean first)
10.	Air/water spray nozzles	Autoclave; or disinfect with clear phenolic or chlorhexidine in alcohol.
11.	Dental burs (steel)	Disposable, autoclave; ETO for 4–12 h
12.	Tungsten carbide and diamond burs	Treat in ultrasonic bath, then autoclave
13.	Orthodontic bands and wires	Disposable
14.	Orthodontic pliers	Autoclave; or disinfect with clear phenolic or chlorhexidine in alcohol. ETO for 4–12 h; dry heat for 60–120 min at 160°C
15.	Prosthetic trays (metal trays), facebow, bite forks	Autoclave
16.	Plastic trays	Disposable
17.	Tumblers	Disposable. If glass/metal: Washing in hot water with detergent
18.	Gauzes, cotton wool, paper point	Autoclave after wrapping (do not pack tightly)
19.	Linen	Autoclave surgical drapes after wrapping or freshly laundered linen.
20.	Needles for syringe	Disposable
21.	Local anaesthetic cartridges	Sterilized by manufacturer and disposable
22.	Impression compounds, saliva ejectors, sutures and needles	Disposable
23.	Suction tips	Autoclave
24.	Spatula and glass mixing slabs	Wash with hot water and detergent; If contaminated with saliva, then autoclave spatula; disinfect slabs with hypochlorite.
25.	Face masks for general anaesthetic apparatus	Wipe with hypochlorite and wash in clean water before reuse.
26.	Scrubbing brushes	Do not use routinely
27.	Surgery floors	Wash with detergent and dry, daily
28.	General working surfaces	Wash with detergent and dry, daily
29.	Bracket table	Wipe with chlorhexidine in alcohol or in 70% isopropyl alcohol in water, in between patients
30.	Orthodontic bands	Autoclave, dry heat, glass bead
31.	Elastic ligature and chains	2% glutaraldehyde
32.	Arch wires	Autoclave, cold sterilization, dry heat
33.	Lamps	Wipe of dust daily
34.	Cleaning equipment (bucket, mops, clothes, etc.)	Rinse and store dry

- **Wax rim/bites:** Spray wipe of iodophore.
- **Dental casts:** Spraying dental casts with iodophor or chlorine products.

Sterilization in Dental Radiology

1. Routine use of gloves.
2. Contaminated films (exposed) should be kept in separate trays.
3. Film holder should be rinsed in running water to remove saliva.
4. Metallic parts should be autoclaved.
5. Plastic attachments should be kept in chlorhexidine solution.
6. X-ray tube head, exposure selector, timer button and film packets should be wiped with detergents.
7. Tube can be wrapped in disposable plastics.
8. Film packets are discarded in yellow bags.

Implant sterilization: Pre-sterilized with gamma radiation, if need arises for re-sterilization, conventional methods (steam sterilization/dry heat) leaves residue on surface, so preferred method is use of gas plasma.

Q. 5. Write a note on disposal of infectious waste.
(TNMGR, Nov. 2001; NTR Uni., Nov. 2017)

Ans. Infectious waste refers to a waste contaminated with blood and other bodily fluids, cultures and stocks of infectious agents from laboratory work, or waste from patients with infections (by WHO).

1. **Deep burial:** Materials after chemical disinfection are put in deep trenches, covered with lime and filled with soil, safe method for sharps also.
2. **Incineration:** It is safe method for large solid infectious waste like anatomical waste, amputated limbs, and animal carcasses.
3. **Autoclaving (thermal):** Used in laboratories and clinics for disposal of infectious and sharp waste.
4. **Microwave (irradiative):** Useful method of sterilization of small volume infectious waste at the point of generation.
5. **Liquid waste:** Pathological, chemical and toxic liquid waste should be treated with disinfectants and neutralized before flushing into the sewer.

Q. 6. Write a short note on disposal of wastes in dental office.
(UHSR, April 2013; TNMGR, April, 2015)

Ans. Dental practices produce large amounts of waste such as plastic, latex, cotton, glass and other materials, most of them can be contaminated with infected body fluids.

Types of waste generated in dentistry:
- Biomedical waste: Non-anatomic waste and anatomic waste, sharps.
- Silver containing waste: Used fixer solution and unused X-ray films.
- Lead containing wastes: Lead aprons and lead foils inside the X-ray films.
- Mercury containing wastes: Element mercury, scrap amalgam.
- Chemicals, disinfectants and sterilizing agents.

Waste disposal:
1. **Biomedical waste:**
   - **Non-anatomical wastes (blood soaked materials):** Use a yellow biomedical waste bag to collect non-anatomical wastes and then double bag the waste, label the bag with a biohazard symbol. Never throw blood soaked materials into regular garbage or into compost waste and never place them in sharps container.
   - **Anatomical wastes:** Excised tissues, organs, tumors, extracted teeth. Separate the material from other wastes and use a yellow biomedical waste bag to collect the anatomic waste. Double bag the waste and labeled with a bio-hazard symbol and fill the bag till 3/4 levels and tie it tightly and contact a certified biomedical waste carrier (CWC) for disposal.
2. **Silver containing waste:** Spent X-ray fixer used in dental clinics is a hazardous material that should not be easily rinsed in the drain. The fixer with a recovery unit can be mixed with water and developer and disposed down the septic system or sewer after desilvering. The silver should be handed over to the CWC.
3. **Lead containing waste:** Lead foil and lead aprons contain toxin that can result into defilement of soil and groundwater in landfill areas after disposal. They should only be handed over to CWC.
4. **Mercury containing waste:** Dental amalgam particles are a source of mercury that can get into the environment through wastewater, scrap amalgam or vapors. **Vaporous mercury** waste management includes:
   - Store unused elemental mercury in sealed containers.
   - Contact to a CWC for disposal and recycling.
   - Use a 'mercury spill kit' in case of spill of mercury.
   - Unused elemental mercury reacts with silver alloy to form scrap amalgam.
   - Not placing elemental mercury in the garbage.
   - Don't wash elemental mercury in the drain.

For the management of scrap amalgam:
- Mercontainer™ (sponge type) is appropriate to store scrap amalgam.
- Empty amalgam capsules can be disposed in garbage.
- Using certified amalgam separator on the suction lines for removing 95% of contact amalgam before diffusing in sewer system.
- Disposable suction traps should be changed weekly.
- Always use gloves, mask, and glasses while cleaning the suction traps.
- Disposable trap should be placed into a properly labeled container of Merconvap™ solution for proper disposal. After filling it, a CWC should be contacted for recycling or disposal of it. The container must be labeled 'Hazardous Waste: Scrap Amalgam'.

- Premeasured capsules mix only as much amalgam as is required.
- Large pieces of amalgam should be removed manually which are produced and store them in contact amalgam container.
- Appropriate use of amalgam substitutes can be considered.

5. **Sharps:** The sharp wastes should be handled with care. Needles should be mutilated by needle destroyer/cutter, before disposing off syringes. Mutilated needles and other sharp wastes may be kept in puncture proof containers with 1% sod. hypochlorite solution for primary disinfection and after every 2 days, the solution should be changed.

6. **Chemicals, disinfectants, and sterilizing agents:** Staff should be trained in workplace hazardous materials information system (WHMIS) for handling of materials.
   - Steam or dry heat can be use to sterilize dental instruments, whenever it is possible.
   - Non-chlorinated plastic containers should be preferred to decrease environmental impact. Halogenated sterilants have a detrimental effect on environment.
   - Ignitable sterilants should not be poured down the drain as they have potency to explode. Formaldehyde sterilants should also not be disposed down a drain.
   - Directly pouring of sterilants into a septic system may significantly disrupt the bacteria which normally breakdown wastes.

7. **General office waste:** Purchase of products with minimal packaging and use of reusable plastic containers can reduce general waste production. Products made from recycled or partly recycled materials can also be used. Energy-efficient lighting and temperature regulation can limit office energy use. Single-spaced printing and use of both sides of pages can decrease the amount of paper used in dental office.

Q. 7. Write in detail about infection control in dental clinics. *(BFUHS, Nov. 2002; TNMGR, March 2008; UHSR, April 2013; MUHS, Nov. 2017; NTR Uni., May 2019)*

Q. Write a short note on cross infection. *(TNMGR, Sept. 2007; UHSR, May 2012)*

Ans. Infection control refers to all procedures adopted to eliminate factor or factors identified to be responsible for causing infection/cross infection. Cross infection is spread of infection from one source to another, either directly from person to person or indirectly. CDC have given guidelines for infection control in dental practice under universal or standard precautions, which is based on the concept that all blood and body fluids might be contaminated and should be treated as infectious because patients with blood borne infections can be asymptomatic or unaware that they are infected.

Sources of infection in dental office:
- Direct contact with blood, oral fluids, or other infected materials.
- Indirect contact with contaminated objects, environmental surfaces, or equipment.
- Contact of conjunctival, nasal, or oral mucosa with droplets from an infected person and propelled by coughing, sneezing, or talking.
- Inhalation of airborne microorganisms that can remain suspended in air for long periods.

Categories of task in relation to risk
- Category I: Tasks that involved exposure to blood, body fluid or tissues.
- Category II: Tasks that do not involve routine exposure to blood, body fluids or tissues.
- Category III: Tasks that involve no exposure to blood, body fluids or tissues. American Dental Association (ADA) and Occupational Safety and Health Act (OSHA) guidelines advise that all dental office staff in category I and II and dentists be trained in infection control to protect themselves and their patient.

Infection control procedures to be adopted by dental health care personnel (DHCP):

A. **Environmental infection control:** In dental practice a variety of environmental surfaces could become contaminated with patient material during treatment procedure, e.g. light handles, switches, drawer knobs, etc. This can be cleaned by thorough cleaning and by using barrier protection. Floor, walls and sinks should be kept clean by simple cleaning with use of water and detergent.

B. **Personal protection measures.**
   1. **Immunization:** All the DHCPs should be vaccinated against HBV.
   2. **Protective clothing:** Full sleeve lab coat should be worn while treating patients.
   3. **Hand hygiene (washing):** Handwashing should be done before and after treating patient. Types of handwashing agents:
      i. Routine handwash: Water and plain soap.
      ii. Antiseptic handwash: Water and antimicrobial soap.

iii. Antiseptic hand rub: Alcohol-based hand rub.

iv. Surgical antisepsis: Water and plain soap followed by alcohol-based hand rub.

4. **Hand gloves and their correct use:**

i. Before and after use of gloves, hands should be thoroughly washed and dried.

ii. Gloves for medical purpose are intended for single use.

iii. Correct size gloves should be worn.

5. **Mask, protective eyewear and face shield:**

i. Masks are important to prevent droplet infection.

ii. Surgical masks protect the wearer from microorganism generated by water.

iii. Masks should be changed frequently, as they become wet easily.

iv. Majority of surgical masks do not offer adequate protection against tuberculosis.

v. Eyewear/face shields provide protection against splashes of sprays of blood, body fluids.

6. **Avoidance of occupational injuries:** By following safe practices injuries and exposure to patients body fluids should be avoided.

7. **Health status of DHCP:** DHCP monitor their own status, work related illness.

C. **Patient screening:**

1. A thorough and updated medical history, identifying any infective diseases should be recorded.

2. Patient should be encouraged to maintain proper oral hygiene.

3. Protective clothing should be used for the patient.

4. Rubber dam and suction should be used appropriately.

5. Use of preprocedural antimicrobial mouth rinses should be encouraged.

D. **Role of sterilization:** Sterilization and disinfection of patient care items—based on risk of transmission and need of sterilization (Earle H. Spaulding's Classification of instruments):

a. **Critical items:** Penetrates soft tissues/mucous membrane, contact bone, and enters into blood, e.g. surgical instrument, periodontal scalers, scalpel blades, surgical dental burs. They have greatest risk of transmitting infection; therefore they should be sterilized by heat or use sterile single use, disposable devices.

b. **Semicritical items:** Contacts mucous membrane but do not penetrate soft tissue, e.g. mouth mirrors, amalgam condenser, reusable impression trays, dental hand pieces. They should be sterilized by heat or high level disinfectant.

c. **Non-critical items:** Contact intact skin, e.g. radiograph cone, B.P. cuff, facebow, pulse oximeter. They should be cleaned and disinfect using low to intermediate level disinfectant.

- **Sterilization** (Refer to previous Question.)
- **Chemical methods of disinfection:** It is a two step procedure—initial step involves vigorous scrubbing of surfaces and wiping them clean followed by wetting the surface with disinfectant for prescribed time.

Classification of disinfectants:

A. **Based on consistency:** a. Liquid, b. Gaseous.

B. **Based on spectrum of activity:** a. High level, b. Intermediate level, c. Low level

C. **Based on mechanism of action:**

a. Action on membrane (e.g. alcohol, detergent)

b. Denaturation of cellular proteins (e.g. alcohol, phenol)

c. Oxidation of essential sulphydryl groups of enzymes (e.g. H_2O_2, halogens)

d. Alkylation of amino-, carboxyl- and hydroxyl group (e.g. ethylene oxide, formaldehyde)

e. Damage to nucleic acids (ethylene oxide, formaldehyde)

Spectrum of activity of disinfectants

1. **High level disinfection:** Disinfection process that inactivates vegetative bacteria, mycobacteria, fungi, viruses but not bacterial spores, e.g. ETO, glutaraldehyde.

2. **Intermediate level disinfection:** Disinfection process that inactivates vegetative bacteria, most of fungi, mycobacteria and most of viruses but not bacterial spores, e.g. phenolics, halogens.

3. **Low level disinfectant:** Can kill most bacteria, some viruses, and some fungi only, e.g. alcohols, quaternary ammonium compounds.

E. **Other aspects of infection control:**

1. **Dental unit water lines:** Several microorganisms can colonize these water lines, majority of which are common heterotrophic water bacteria.

2. **Dental unit water quality:** Flushing waterline for 2–3 minutes first thing on the Monday is recommended.

3. **Special considerations:** Semicritical equipment attached to waterline should be run to discharge

air or water for a minimum of 20–30 sec. after each patient.

4. **Handling of biopsy specimen:** Each specimen must be placed in a sturdy, leak-proof container with a secure lid.
5. **Dental radiology:** Refer to previous Question.
6. **Dental laboratory material:** Refer to previous Question.
7. **Disposal of clinical waste material and sharps:** Refer to previous Question.
8. **Management of blood spills:** Blood spills should be removed with wearing gloves and other protective wear. Visible organic material should be cleaned with absorbent material. Non-porous surfaces should be cleaned and decontaminated with disinfectant effective against HBV and HIV.

Q. 8. Write a note on hospital waste management.
(RGUHS, May 2011; TNMGR, Oct. 2011; MUHS, Sumandeep Uni., May 2018)

Ans. Hospital waste refers to all waste from hospitals, biological or non-biological that is discarded and not intended for further use. Biomedical waste (BMW) is defined as any waste which is generated during the diagnosis, treatment or immunization of human beings or animals or in research activities pertaining thereto or in the production or testing of biologicals, and including categories mentioned in Schedule I.

Classification of BMW by WHO
A. Non-hazardous (75–90%).
B. Hazardous (10–25%).

1. Infectious (15–18%): Non-sharps, sharps, plastic disposables, liquid wastes.
2. Others (5–7%): Radioactive waste, discarded glass, pressurized containers, chemical waste, cytotoxic waste, incinerator ash.

Sources of BMW: Hospitals, nursing homes, clinics, medical laboratories, blood banks, mortuaries, medical research and training centers, biotechnology units, animal houses.

7. MICROBIOLOGICAL INVESTIGATIONS

Q. 1. Write a short note on immunofluorescence tests.
(RGUHS, May 2011)

Ans. Immunofluorescence is a technique allowing the visualization of a specific protein or antigen in tissue sections by binding a specific antibody, chemically conjugated with a fluorescent dye (fluorescein isothiocyanate (FITC) or Lissamine™ rhodamine). The specific antibodies labeled with FITC makes them glow in apple-green color when observed microscopically under UV light. Immunofluorescence tests are of two types.

1. **Direct immunofluorescence test (DIF)** (Fig. 7.1a): *Principle:* The specific antibodies tagged with fluorescent dye are used for detection of unknown antigen in a specimen. If antigen is present, it reacts with labeled antibodies and fluorescence can be observed under UV light of fluorescent microscope.

Categories of biomedical waste (Schedule I):

Category	Waste category	Treatment and disposal
1.	Human anatomical waste	Incineration; deep burial
2.	Animal waste	Incineration; deep burial
3.	Microbiology and biotechnology waste	Autoclaving/microwaving/incineration
4.	Waste sharps	Disinfection (chemical treatment; autoclaving/ microwaving and mutilation/shredding microwaving)
5.	Discarded medicines and cytotoxic drugs	Incineration
6.	Solid waste (blood/body fluid contaminated items: Cotton, dressings, soiled plaster casts, linen, beddings)	Incineration/autoclaving/microwaving
7.	Solid waste (tubings, catheters, IV sets, etc.)	Disinfection by chemical treatment; autoclaving/ microwaving and mutilation/shredding
8.	Liquid waste	Disinfection by chemical treatment and discharge into drain
9.	Incineration ash	Disposal in municipal landfill
10.	Chemical waste	Disinfection by chemical treatment and discharge into drain for liquids and landfill for solids

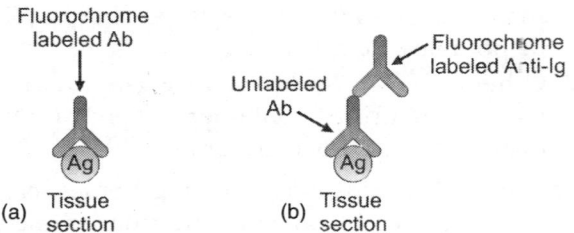

Fig. 7.1: Immunofluorescence tests. a. Direct, b. Indirect

Color coding of bags and categories (Schedule II):

Color coding bags	Waste categories
Yellow	1, 2, 3, 6
Red	3, 6
Blue/white translucent	4, 7
Black	5, 9, 10

Uses:
- It is commonly used for detection of bacteria, viruses or other antigens in blood, CSF, urine, faeces, tissues and other specimens.
- It is a sensitive method to diagnose rabies by detection of rabies virus antigens in brain smears.

Disadvantage: Separate fluorescent conjugate have to be prepared against each antigen.

2. **Indirect immunofluorescence test (IIF)** (Fig. 7.1b): It is used for detection of antibodies in serum or other body fluids.

   Principle: A known antigen is fixed on a slide. The unknown antibody (serum) is applied to the slide. If antibody (globulin) is present in the serum, it attaches to known antigen on the slide. For detection of this Ag–Ab reaction, fluorescin-tagged antibody to human globulin is added. In positive test, fluorescence occurs under UV light.

   Advantages of IIF:
   - It gives an amplification effect—more tag or label ('signal') per molecule of target protein.
   - Requires only one labeled antibody to identify many proteins. Same labeled secondary antibody can be used to bind to ('light up') many different proteins.

   Variants of IIF:
   1. **Salt split technique:** Used to distinguish between sub-epidermal blistering conditions with similar DIF findings. In this, normal skin/mucosa is incubated in 1M NaCl for 48–72 h to split at the level of lamina lucida.
   2. **Antigenic mapping method:** This is used as an adjunct to electron microscopy to differentiate between major forms of epidermolysis bullosa.

3. **Double staining method:**
   Immunofluorescent pattern and their significance:
   - Intercellular deposits between epidermal cells in network pattern: Pemphigus.
   - Intercellular deposits between epidermal cells in network pattern and linear or granular basement membrane zone (BMZ) band: Paraneoplastic pemphigus
   - Linear deposits along BMZ: Pemphigoid, epidermolysis bullosa aquisita
   - Granular deposits along BMZ: SLE
   - IgG, IgM, and C3 deposits in ovoid bodies with ragged fibrin band along BMZ: Lichen planus.

Q. 2. Write a short note on Widal test.

(TNMGR, March 2002)

Ans. Widal agglutination is a serologic technique to aid in diagnosis of typhoid fever. The test is based on demonstrating the presence of agglutinin (Ab) in the serum of an infected patient, against H (flagellar) and O (somatic) antigens of *Salmonella typhi*. Widal test reaction involves use of bacterial suspensions of *S. typhi* and *S. paratyphi* 'A' and 'B', treated to retain only 'O' and 'H' antigens. IgM somatic O antibody appears first and represents the initial serologic response in acute typhoid fever, while IgG flagella H antibody usually develops more slowly but persists for longer.

Procedure of Widal test: Two types:
1. **Slide test:** It is rapid and used as a screening procedure. Using commercially available antigens of *S. typhi*, a drop of suspended antigen is added to an equal amount of previously prepared serum. An initial positive screening test requires the determination of the strength of the antibody. This is done by adding together equal amounts of antigen suspension and serially diluted serum from suspected patient. Agglutinations are visualized as clumps. The result of tests are scored from 0 to 4+, i.e. 0 (no agglutination), 1+ (25% agglutination), 2+ (50% agglutination), 3+ (75% agglutination) or 4+ (100% agglutination).
2. **Tube test:** Equal volumes (0.4 ml) of serial dilutions of serum (from 1/10 to 1/640) and the H and O antigens are mixed in Dreyer's and Felix agglutination tubes, respectively, and incubated in a water bath at 37°C overnight. Control tubes containing Ag and normal saline are set to check for auto-agglutination. The agglutination titers of serum are read. H agglutination leads to formation of **loose, cotton woolly clumps**, while O agglutination is seen

as a disc-like pattern at the bottom of tube. Ag used in test are H and O Ag of *S. typhi* and H antigens of *S. paratyphi* A and B. Results are scored from 0 to 4+ positive agglutination as described above for the slide test. The tube test is useful to clarify erratic or equivocal agglutination reactions obtained by more rapid slide test.

Q. 3. Write about laboratory diagnosis of pulmonary tuberculosis. *(Bombay Uni., Oct. 1985; TNMGR, April 2001)*

Ans. Laboratory diagnosis of tuberculosis is established by testing sputum for demonstrating the bacillus. Sputum is best collected in the morning before any meal for consecutive 3 days. Where sputum is not available laryngeal swabs or bronchial washings may be collected. Currently available diagnostics can be classified as those that:

A. **Direct methods:** Detect actively growing bacilli. These includes:

1. **AFB sputum smear microscopy:** Sputum microscopy is the most reliable method in diagnosis. Smears are dried, heat fixed and stained by Ziehl-Neelsen technique. Under the oil immersion objective, acid fast bacilli are seen as bright red rods while the background is blue, yellow or green depending on the counter stain used. A negative report should not be given till at least 300 fields have been examined taking about 10 minutes. A positive report can be given only if two or more typical bacilli have been seen.

2. **AFB sputum smear with fluorescence microscopy:** When several smears are to be examined daily, it fluorescent microscopy should be used. In this, smears are stained with dyes (auramine phenol or rhodamine), examined under UV illumination, bacilli appear as bright rods against dark background.

3. **Sodium hypochlorite (bleach) microscopy:** Digestion of sputum with household bleach is done before sputum smear preparation and microscopy, to improve the yield of smear microscopy.

4. **Cultures:** Culture is a very sensitive diagnostic technique (gold standard) for tubercle bacilli. The concentrated material is inoculated onto at least two bottles of IUAT-LJ medium. Cultures are examined for growth after incubation at 37°C for 4 days and at least twice weekly thereafter. A negative report is given if no growth occurs after 8–12 weeks. Any growth seen is smeared and stained by ZN staining.

5. **Sensitivity tests:**
   i. Absolute concentration method.
   ii. Resistance ratio method.
   iii. Proportion method.

6. **Animal inoculation:** The concentrated material is inoculated intra muscularly into the thigh of two healthy guinea pigs of 12 weeks old. The animals are weighed before inoculation and at intervals thereafter. Progressive loss of weight is an indication of infection. Infected animals show a positive tuberculin skin reaction.

7. **Nucleic acid technology:** Polymerase chain reaction (PCR) and line probe assay are used as diagnostic techniques.

8. **Immunodiagnosis:** Serological tests are not useful in diagnosis.

B. **Indirect methods:** Detect the immune response against the bacilli indirectly.

1. **Tuberculin skin testing (TST)/Mantoux test:** It involves injecting purified protein derivative (PPD) of *M. tuberculosis* bacillus (MTB) intradermally in the forearm and the resulting reaction is read after 48–72 h. A positive test is considered when 10 mm or more induration is present at the point of injection. Tuberculin test detects only presence or absence of infection, i.e. exposure to MTB or latent TB. The optimal strength of PPD is 2 TU.

2. **Interferon gamma release assay (IGRAs):** This is an *in vitro* assay wherein T cells sensitized with MTB on encountering mycobacterial antigen and culture filtrate protein 10, release interferon-gamma. It has a very high specificity and results can be available within 24 h. **Disadvantages:** Sample drawn should be incubated within 16 h of collection.

C. **Newer methods (indirect):** Volatile organic compounds (VOCs) detection and detection of β-lactamase.

Q. 4. Write a short note on serologic markers for HBV infection. *(TNMGR, Sept 2002)*

Ans. Specific diagnosis of hepatitis B rests on serological demonstration of viral markers.

1. **HBsAg** *(NTR Uni., Oct 2012)*: The first marker to appear in blood after infection (8–12 weeks), being detectable 2–6 weeks before elevation of transaminases and onset of clinical illness. It remains in circulation throughout the symptomatic course of disease. It disappears within 2 months of the start of disease, rarely persists beyond 6 months. When it is no longer detectable, its antibody, anti-HBs appears and remains for very long periods.

2. **HBcAg:** It is not demonstrable in circulation because it is enclosed within HBsAg coat but its antibody; anti-HBc appears in serum a week or two after the appearance of HBsAg. It is the earliest antibody marker to be seen in blood. As anti-HBc remains lifelong, it serves as useful indicator of prior infection with HBV, even after all the other viral markers become undetectable.

3. **HBeAg:** It appears in blood concurrently with HBsAg, or soon afterwards. Circulating HBeAg is an indicator of active intrahepatic viral replication and the presence in blood of DNA polymerase, HBV DNA and virions, reflecting replication and high infectivity. Disappearance of HBeAg is followed by appearance of anti-HBe. (Resolution of infection).

For diagnosis of HBV infection, detection of HBsAg in blood is necessary. The simultaneous presence of IgM anti-HBc indicates recent infection and presence of IgG indicates remote infection. HBeAg provides information about relative infectivity. The presence of anti-HBs without any other serological virus marker indicates immunity following vaccination. Like HBeAg, HBV DNA is also an indicator of viral replication and infectivity. Molecular methods such as DNA hybridization and PCR, used for HBV DNA testing, are highly sensitive and quantitative.

Q. 5. Write a short note on coagulase test.

(TNMGR, April 2003)

Ans. Coagulase is an extracellular enzyme secreted by *Staph. aureus* that converts fibrinogen in plasma into fibrin. Coagulase test is the standard criteria for the identification of *Staph. aureus* isolates from other coagulase negative staphylococci. Coagulase test is done by two methods:

1. **Tube coagulase tests:** This test detects free coagulase. 0.1 ml of a young broth culture or agar culture suspension of isolate is added to 0.5 ml of human or rabbit plasma in a narrow test tube. EDTA, oxalate or heparin may be used as anticoagulant for preparing the plasma. The tubes are incubated in water bath at 37°C for 3–6 hours. If positive, plasma clots and does not flow when tube is tilted.

2. **Slide test:** This detects bound coagulase and is much simpler and usually gives results parallel with the tube test. In this test, isolate is emulsified in a drop of saline on a slide. After checking for absence of auto-agglutination, a drop of human or rabbit plasma is added to emulsion and mixed. Prompt clumping of cocci indicates a positive test.

Q. 6. Classify spirochetes. Describe the clinical features and laboratory diagnosis of syphilis.

(TNMGR, March 2007)

Q. Write a short note on lab diagnosis of syphilis.

(TNMGR, March 2009)

Ans. Spirochetes are elongated motile bacteria twisted spirally along the long axis.

Classification: Human pathogens belong to following three genera:

A. *Treponema:* T. pallidum (syphilis), *T. pertenue* (yaws), *T. carateum* (pinta disease).

B. *Leptospira:* L. interrogans (Weil's disease/*leptospirosis*).

C. *Borrelia:* B. recurrentis (relapsing fever), *B. vincenti* (Vincent's angina), *B. burgdorferi* (Lyme disease).

Clinical features of syphilis:

1. **Primary syphilis:** Hard chancre at the site of entry (painless, avascular, circumscribed, indurated and ulcerated lesion; covered with thick exudate rich in spirochetes), heals spontaneously in days.

2. **Secondary syphilis (most infectious):** Roseolar or papular skin rashes, mucous patches in oropharynx, condylomata at mucocutaneous junctions.

3. **Latent syphilis:** Quiescent stage follows secondary stage.

4. **Tertiary syphilis:** Develop after years, characterized by development of granulomatous lesions (gumma) in skin, bones.

5. **Late tertiary or quaternary syphilis:** Cardiovascular lesions like aneurysm, aortitis; neurosyphilis: Tabes dorsalis or general paralysis of insane.

6. **Congenital syphilis:** Hutchison's triad (keratitis, Hutchinson's teeth, 8th nerve deafness), saddle-shaped nose.

Laboratory diagnosis:

A. **Microscopy:** Tissue fluid from lesions.

1. **Dark ground microscopy:** Exudate is examined under oil immersion with dark-field illumination for typical motile spirochetes.

2. **Direct fluorescent antibody test:** Tissue fluid or exudate is fixed, stained with a fluorescein-labeled anti-treponeme serum, and examined by immunofluorescence microscopy.

B. **Serological tests:**

I. **Reagin antibody tests:** Non-treponemal tests—test for reagin Ab using cardiolipin Ag, used as screening tests for syphilis, e.g. Kahn test, VDRL test, rapid plasma reagin test.

II. **Group specific treponemal tests:** Reiter protein complement fixation test.

III. **Specific *Treponema pallidum* tests:** Measure Ab against *T. pallidum* antigens. The tests are confirmatory for positive result from a non-treponemal test, e.g. *T. pallidum* immobilization (TPI) test, *T. pallidum* hemagglutination Assay (TPHA), fluorescent treponemal antibody absorbed (FTA-ABS) test.

Q. 7. Write a short note on VDRL test.

(TNMGR, Aug. 2004)

Ans. VDRL (veneral disease research laboratory) test is a slide flocculation test used for diagnosis of syphilis.

Principle: Patients suffering from syphilis produce antibodies that react with cardiolipin antigen in a slide flocculation test, which are read using a microscope.

Procedure: In this test, the inactivated serum (serum heated at 56°C for 30 min.) is mixed with cardiolipin antigen on a special slide and rotated for four minutes. Cardiolipin remains as uniform crystals in normal serum but forms visible clumps on combining with reagin antibody. The reaction is read under a low power microscope. By testing serial dilutions, antibody titer can be determined.

Results: Results are reported qualitatively as 'reactive', 'weak reactive' or 'not reactive.' For quantitative reporting, the reciprocal of the end point is given as the titer, for example 'reactive 4 dilution' or 'titer 4.'

VDRL rest can be used for testing CSF also, but not plasma.

Modifications of VDRL test:

1. Rapid plasma reagin (RPR) test: This test is the most popular. It uses VDRL antigen containing fine carbon particles.
2. Automated RPR test: For large scale tests.
3. Automated VDRL–ELISA test: Measure IgG and IgM antibodies separately and is suitable for large scale testing of sera.
4. Unheated serum reagin test.

Q. 8. Write a short note on antibiotic sensitivity test.

(TNMGR, Sept. 1997; April 2015; June 2016; HP Uni., April 2019)

Ans. Antibiotic sensitivity tests refer to vitro testing of bacterial cultures with antibiotics to determine susceptibility of bacteria to antibiotic therapy.

- **Sensitive:** When the infection caused by organism is likely to respond to treatment with that particular antimicrobial agent at recommended dose.
- **Intermediate:** Strains those are moderately susceptible to an antimicrobial agent.

- **Resistant:** An organism is not to respond to a given antimicrobial agent irrespective of dose and location of infection.
- **Minimum inhibition concentration (MIC):** The lowest concentration of antimicrobial agent that inhibits bacterial growth/multiplication.
- **Minimum bactericidal concentration (MBC)/ Minimum lethal concentration (MLC):** The lowest concentration of antimicrobial agent that allows <0.1% of original inoculum to survive.

Uses:
- As a guide for treatment.
- It helps physician in selecting the best antimicrobial agent for patients.
- As an epidemiological tool.
- The emergence of resistant strains of major pathogens (e.g. *Shigella*)
- Continued surveillance of susceptibility pattern of prevalent strains (e.g. staphylococci)

Types:
A. **Diffusion tests:** The drug is allowed to diffuse through a solid medium so that a gradient is established, the concentration being highest near the site of application of drug and decreasing with distance. The test bacterium is seeded on the medium and its sensitivity to drug is determined from inhibition of its growth.

   Methods used for application of the drug:
   i. Ditches or holes cut in the medium.
   ii. By adding to hollow cylinders (heatly cups).
   iii. Filter paper discs, impregnated with antibiotics. (most commonly used.)

1. **Disc diffusion method (Kirby-Bauer test)** uses filter paper discs, 6.0 mm in diameter charged with appropriate concentrations of drugs. A suitable dilution of broth culture or suspension of test bacterium is flooded on the surface of a solid medium (Mueller-Hinton agar or nutrient agar). After drying the plate (37°C for 30 mins), antibiotic discs are applied with sterile forceps. After overnight incubation, the degree of sensitivity is determined by measuring the zones of inhibition of growth around the discs.
2. **Primary disc diffusion method** gives results fast as the swab is directly inoculated uniformly on the surface of a plate and discs applied.
3. **Epsilometer or E-test** uses an absorbent strip with a known gradient of drug concentrations along its length. When the strip is placed on the agar plate seeded with test bacterium, antibiotic diffuse into the medium.

B. **Dilution test:** In this, serial dilutions of drug are prepared and inoculated with test bacterium. Dilution tests are generally employed when the therapeutic dose is to be regulated accurately, for tests on slow growing bacteria, and when small degrees of resistance are to be demonstrated.

1. **Tube dilution method:** Serial dilutions of drug in broth are taken in tubes and a standardized suspension of test bacterium inoculated. After overnight incubation, MIC is read by noting the lowest concentration of drug that inhibits growth.

2. **Agar dilution method:** It is more convenient when several strains are to be tested at the same time. In this, serial dilutions of the drug are prepared in agar and poured into plates.

Q. 9. Write a short note on ELISA.

(TNMGR, March 2002; Sumandeep Uni., June 2016)

Ans. Enzyme-linked Immunosorbent assay (ELISA) is an immunological assay commonly used to measure antibodies, antigens, proteins and glycoproteins in biological samples. In ELISA, an enzyme conjugated with antibody reacts with a colorless substrate to generate a colored reaction product (chromogenic substrate).

Principle of ELISA: ELISA is based on the immuno-chemical principle of Ag–Ab reactions. It is based on the specificity of antigen–antibody complex formation and its detection by a second antibody conjugated with suitable enzyme such as peroxidase.

Enzymes of ELISA: ALP (calf intestine), β-galactosidase (*E. coli*), glucose oxidase (*Aspergillus niger*), G-6-PD (*Leuconostoc mesenteroides*), peroxidase (horseradish).

Technique of ELISA:

- The antibody against the antigen to be determined is fixed on an inert solid such as polystyrene (multi-well titer plates).
- The biological sample containing the protein/antigen is applied on antibody coated surface.
- The antibody binds only to antigen from serum. Other proteins get washed off.
- The second protein specific antibody conjugated with enzyme is added. This binds to antigen forming a complex sticking to plastic surface.
- Enzyme is covalently linked to second protein specific antibody. The enzyme must be assayable and products must be preferably colored product.
- Excess antibody (peroxidase) is washed off. The amount of antibody (peroxidase) conjugate sticking to antibody coated surface is proportional to the amount of antigen and is then determined/assayed by adding substrate.
- Peroxidase converts substrate to color product.
- The color intensity is measured by spectropho-tometer.

In ELISA, the enzyme act on the substrate to produce color in a positive test. It can be used for detection of antigen or antibody. The test can be done in polystyrene tubes (macro ELISA) or polyvinyl microtitre plates (micro ELISA).

Types of ELISA:

1. Sandwich ELISA: It is most frequently used for detecting microbial antigen. It is of two types:

   a. **Single antibody or direct sandwich ELISA:** In this technique, the antibody is immobilized on a microtitre well. The test sample is then exposed to the solid phase antibody to which the antigen (if present) will bind. After the well is washed, a second enzyme linked antibody specific for test antigen is added. The conjugated antibody will react with the antigen held to the solid phase by the first antibody, forming an antibody–antigen–antibody sandwich on the solid phase. After any free second antibody is removed by washing, substrate is added and the colored reaction product is measured.

   b. **Double antibody or indirect sandwich ELISA:** It is used for the detection of antigens. In this, specific antibody is placed in wells of microtitre plate. The antibody is absorbed onto the walls, coating and sensitizing the plate. A test antigen is then added to each well. If antigen reacts with the antibody, the antigen is retained when the well is washed to remove unbound antigen. An antibody enzyme conjugate specific for antigen is then added to each well. The final complex is formed of an outer antibody enzyme, middle antigen, and inner antibody.

2. **Indirect ELISA:** It detects antibodies. For antibody detection, the wells of microtitre plate are coated with antigen. Sera to be tested are added in these coated wells. If antibody (1°) is present in specimen, it binds to coated antigen. To detect this Ag–Ab reaction, a goat antihuman immunoglobulin antibody (2°) conjugated with an enzyme is added. Enzyme conjugated antihuman immunoglobulin binds to antibody. To detect this binding, a substrate is added and enzyme acts on substrate to produce color in a positive reaction. Reading of the test is done by ELISA reader. Substrates are specific for each enzyme. The enzyme (horseradish peroxidase, alkaline phosphatase) gives rise to a color change by adding specific substrate

(o-phenyldiamine dihydrochloride for peroxidase, p-nitrophenyl phosphate for alkaline phosphatase). ALP with this substrate produces a yellow color.

3. **Competitive/inhibition/blocking ELISA:** It measures Ag. In this, positive result shows no color, whereas appearance of color indicates a negative test. There are two specific antibodies, one conjugated with enzyme and other present in serum. Competition occurs between two antibodies for same antigen. A microtitre plate wells are coated with antigen to be measured. Sera to be tested are added to these wells. If antibodies are present, antigen–antibody reaction occurs. To detect this reaction, enzyme labeled specific antibodies are added. These antibodies remain free and washed off during washing. Substrate is added but there is no enzyme to act on it. If serum to be tested is negative for the antibodies, antigen is there to combine with enzyme conjugated antibodies and enzyme acts on substrates to produce color.

Advantages of ELISA

1. Specific and sensitive assay method.
2. Small amount of specimen and single dilution is required to perform the test.
3. Reagents are stable and have longer half-life.
4. The results can be read visually.
5. Large number of specimens can be tested at a time.
6. ELISA can be automated.

Uses of ELISA

1. Screening of donated blood for viral contamination (HIV, HBV, HCV).
2. Estimation of hormone levels (e.g. TSH, T3, T4).
3. Estimation of tumor marker (e.g. HCG, CEA).
4. Detection of infections like HIV antibodies in serum, mycobacterial antibodies in tuberculosis, hepatitis B markers in serum, etc.
5. Detecting allergens in food and house dust.
6. Measuring auto-antibodies in autoimmune disease, e.g. RA factor.
7. Measuring toxins in contaminated food, e.g. enterotoxin of *E. coli* in faeces.
8. Detecting illicit drugs, e.g. cocaine, opiates.

Variations of ELISA: Capture ELISA, Immunometric tests, card method, dipstick method, cylinder or cassette ELISA.

Q. 10. Write a short note on laboratory diagnosis of streptococcal infection. *(TNMGR, Sept. 2002; Sumandeep Uni., June 2016)*

Ans. In acute infections, diagnosis is established by culture while in non-suppurative complications,

diagnosis is mainly based on demonstration of antibodies.

Laboratory diagnosis: Specimen—throat swab, pus swab or exudates are collected.

1. **Microscopy:** Gram-staining of pus/CSF—presence of Gram-positive cocci in chains is indicative of streptococcal infection.
2. **Throat swab culture:** Swab from affected area is collected and are either plated immediately or sent to laboratory in Pike's medium. The specimen should be plated on blood agar and incubated at 37°C anaerobically or under 5–10% CO_2, as hemolysis develops better. Hemolytic streptococci are grouped by Lancefield technique.
3. **Identification:** Rapid diagnostic test kits are available for detection of streptococcal group A antigen from throat swab.
4. **Serology:**
   a. Antistreptolysin O titration:
      - ASO titres >200: Prior streptococcal infection.
      - High levels: Acute rheumatic fever, glomerulonephritis
   b. Antideoxyribonuclease B (anti-DNAase B): Titres >300 are taken as positive.
   c. Streptozyme test: A passive slide hemagglutination test by using erythrocytes sensitized with a crude preparation of streptococci. It is a convenient, sensitive and specific screening test.

Q. 11. Write a short note on Koch's postulates. *(TNMGR, March 2010)*

Ans. Heinrich Hermann Robert Koch (1843–1910) provided remarkable contributions to the field of microbiology. He was a German general practitioner and a famous microbiologist. He identified specific causative agents of tuberculosis, cholera, and anthrax and gave experimental support for the concept of infectious disease.

Koch's postulates are the four steps necessary to confirm if a suspected pathogen is indeed the cause of a disease. Koch's postulates consist of the following four rules:

1. The microorganism must be identified in all individuals affected by the disease, but not in healthy individuals.
2. The microorganism can be isolated from the diseased individual and grown in culture.
3. When introduced into a healthy individual, the cultured microorganism should cause disease.
4. The microorganism must then be re-isolated from the experimental host, and found to be identical to the original microorganism.

Exceptions:
1. Microorganisms those are unable to be cultured on artificial media.
2. Two or more organism work in synergy to cause a disease.
3. Symptoms and disease can be caused by any one of several microbes.

Q. 12. Write a short note on caries activity test.
(NTR Uni., April 2014)

Ans. Caries activity refers to the increment of active lesions over a period of time. Caries susceptibility refers to inherent tendency of the host and target tissue, to be afflicted by caries process. Caries activity test is defined as the test used to predict the probability of developing new or increased carious lesions.

Ideal requirement of caries activity test (Snyder, 1951):
1. Should have sound theoretical basis.
2. Should be simple, easy to perform, inexpensive and adaptable to chair side.
3. Should have maximum correlation with clinical status.
4. Be accurate with respect to duplication of results.

Uses:
1. To determine the need for caries control measures.
2. To act as indicator of patients cooperation.
3. To act as an aid in timing of recall appointments.
4. To aid in the determination of prognosis.

Classification:
A. Tests for evaluating microbiological activity
   1. *Lactobacillus* colony count test.
   2. Dip slide method.
   3. Mutans streptococci colony counts.
   4. Snyder's test.
   5. Alben's test.
   6. Swab test.
B. Tests for evaluating saliva defense
   1. Saliva flow rate.
   2. Viscosity of saliva.
   3. Buffering capacity of saliva.

Q.13. Discuss microbiological tests for diagnosis of fungal infections.
(NTR Uni., May 2019)

Ans. Diagnosis of fungal infections is dependent entirely on the selection and collection of an appropriate clinical specimen for culture. Specimens include skin scrapings, hair, nails, respiratory tract secretions, cerebrospinal fluid (CSF), blood, oral and vaginal specimen, urine, pus, ocular specimen, and tissue bone marrow.

A. **Direct microscopic examination:** These include:
   1. **Unstained preparations with KOH:** Patches from infected sites are examined in a KOH wet mount or gram stain, showing yeast cells of 4–8 µm with budding mixed pseudohyphae.
   2. **Stained preparation with KOH:** To highlight the fungal cell walls, Parker super chrome blue-black ink can be incorporated into the KOH preparation.
   3. **Preparations with calcofluor white and KOH:** Calcofluor White is useful for showing presence of fungal cells in clinical specimens because it binds to polysaccharides. Yeast cells, pseudohyphae, and hyphae display a chalk-white or brilliant apple-green fluorescence.
   4. **Preparation with India ink:** India ink is useful for indicating presence or absence of extracellular polysaccharide capsules of fungal cells. It serves as a negative stain.
   5. **Preparations with PAS stain:** The PAS stain certain polysaccharides found in the fungal cell wall.
   6. **Acid-fast stain procedure for *Nocardia* (modified Kinyoun method):** Acid-fast staining is useful for detecting *Nocardia* species. Some of the filaments stain red with carbol-fuchsin staining, whereas others may appear blue.
   7. **Gram's stain:** Gram's stain is more suited to sections than that to smears.
   8. **Gomori's methenamine silver stain (Grocott's modification):** It is used for demonstration of polysaccharide content on fungus in tissue sections. The aldehydes reduce methenamine silver nitrate complex, resulting in brown-black staining of fungal cell wall.
B. **Culture media:** All fungi require several specific elements for growth and reproduction.
C. **Biochemical tests:** The different biochemical tests are as follows:
   1. **Carbohydrate fermentation:** Yeast is capable of using some but not all sugars as a food source.
   2. **Carbohydrate assimilation:** This test is used for definite speciation of *Candida* and few other fungal microorganisms. In the carbohydrate assimilation test (modified Wickerham method), the carbohydrates used are glucose, maltose, lactose, sucrose, galactose, xylose, trehalose, and cellobiose.
   3. **Rapid urease test:** This test is used to detect the presence of urease enzyme produced by different *Candida* species. Christensen's urea agar slants are used.

D. **Immunological tests:**
  1. **Test for detection of antibodies:** Agglutination of latex-coated particle, immunodiffusion, immune electrophoretic test, radioimmunoassay, and enzyme immunoassay.
  2. **Tests for detection of antigen to *Candida* species:** By enzyme immunoassays, latex agglutination test, ELISA.
  3. **Detection of cell-mediated immunity:** These include *in vivo* tests (skin test), and *in vitro* tests (lymphocyte transformation test).
E. **Other tests:** Detection of fungal metabolites by gas liquid chromatography and enzymatic fluorometric method; molecular biology techniques (DNA probes, RNA profiling, PCR); histopathology.

Q. 14. Write a short note on DNA probes.

(TNMGR, Oct. 2013)

Ans. These are rapid, sensitive and specific diagnostic tools which could be designed because of the following characteristics of DNA:
  i. Double stranded structure.
  ii. Specific base pairing.

The diagnostic reagents comprise of single strand of DNA either from a known organism or synthesized in the laboratory which is conjugated with an easily detectable marker like radioactive isotope or an enzyme. This can be used to identify similar DNA in the test sample since it can combine with single strand of only complementary DNA (hybridization). If the test DNA is present in the sample, it will hybridize with the DNA probe and will become detectable because of the attached marker. Hybridization reaction can be carried out either in the solution or fixed to a solid support such as nitrocellulose or nylon fibers. The latter technique is often called **dot blot, spot blot** or **slot blot**.

Advantages:
- DNA probes are very specific and are used to determine phenotypic markers.
- It has great specificity and sensitivity.
- They are not affected by transport conditions.
- They do not require anaerobic conditions to be maintained.
- They can be done in dead bacteria and they do not depend on bacterial viability.

Disadvantages:
- They are very expensive.
- The minimal detection limits are 10^3–10^5 cells of particular species.
- The chair side diagnosis is not possible.
- The cross reactivity by oligonucleotide probes can occur.
- Antibiotic sensitivity is not possible.

Applications: In detection of those organisms which are difficult to culture in the laboratory. Detection of organism for which diagnostic antigens are not available. These probes provide reliable result in a short time on a large number of specimens.

Microbiological investigations used in diagnosis of periodontal disease *(BBD Uni., July C13)*: Culture methods, direct microscopy, immunofluorescence method, ELISA test, polymerase chain reaction, DNA probe, restriction endonuclease analysis and microbiological kits, etc.

Pathology

1. INFLAMMATION

Q. 1. Define inflammation: List the types, stages and mediators. *(BFUHS, MUHS, May 2009; AHSUC, May 2017; TNMGR, June 2017; HP Uni., May 2017; BBD Uni., April 2018; NTR Uni., May 2019)*

Ans. Inflammation is defined as the local response of living mammalian tissues to injury due to any agent (infectious, immunological, physical, chemical or inert). It is a body defense reaction in order to eliminate or limit the spread of injurious agent, followed by removal of necrosed cells and tissues.

Signs of inflammation: Cardinal signs of inflammation (by Celsus): Rubor (redness); Tumor (swelling); Calor (heat); and Dolor (pain). Fifth sign-functio laesa (loss of function) (by Rudolf Virchow).

Types of inflammation

A. Acute inflammation: It is rapid in onset and is of short duration (<2 weeks). Characteristic features are: Accumulation of fluid and plasma at affected site; intravascular activation of platelets; and polymorphonuclear neutrophils (PMNs) as inflammatory cells. It can be divided into following two events: I. Vascular events. II. Cellular events.

I. **Vascular events** *(UHSR, June 2018)*: Alteration in microvasculature is the earliest response to tissue injury.

a. **Hemodynamic changes**

1. Immediate vascular response is of **transient vasoconstriction** of arterioles. (Initial 3–5 min.)
2. Next is persistent **progressive vasodilatation**, which results in increased blood volume in microvascular bed of the area, responsible for redness and warmth at the site (within 30 min. of injury).
3. Progressive vasodilatation elevates local hydrostatic pressure resulting in transudation of fluid into extracellular space, causing swelling at the local site.

4. **Slowing or stasis** of microcirculation follows which causes increased concentration of RBCs.
5. It is followed by **leucocytic margination** or **peripheral orientation of leucocytes** (mainly neutrophils), along vascular endothelium. These leukocytes then move and migrate through gaps between the endothelial cells into extravascular space (**emigration**).

b. **Altered vascular permeability:** Initially, there is escape of fluid in spaces due to vasodilatation and consequent elevation in hydrostatic pressure (transudate). In inflamed tissues, endothelial lining of microvasculature becomes leakier, resulting in excessive outward flow of fluid into interstitial compartment which is exudative inflammatory edema.

Mechanisms of increased vascular permeability

i. Contraction and retraction of endothelial cells.
ii. Direct injury to endothelial cells.
iii. Endothelial injury mediated by leucocytes.
iv. Leakiness in neovascularisation.

II. **Cellular events:** Cellular phase of inflammation consists of 2 processes:

1. **Exudation of leucocytes:** The changes leading to migration of leucocytes are as follows:
   a. **Changes in formed elements of blood:** Initial increase in blood flow is followed by stasis of blood stream, which leads to changes in normal axial flow of blood. The central stream of cells widens and peripheral plasma zone becomes narrower because of loss of plasma by exudation (**margination**). As a result, neutrophils of central column come close to vessel wall (**pavementing**).
   b. **Rolling and adhesion:** Peripherally marginated and pavemented neutrophils slowly roll over the endothelial cells lining the vessel wall

(**rolling phase**). This is followed by transient bond between leucocytes and endothelial cells becoming firmer (**adhesion phase**).

c. **Emigration:** After sticking of neutrophils to endothelium, the neutrophils get lodged between endothelial cells and basement membrane, cross the basement membrane; escape out into extravascular space (**emigration**). Along with emigration, RBCs also escape through gaps between endothelial cells (**diapedesis**).

d. **Chemotaxis** (*AHSUC, June 2016*): It is chemotactic factor/chemokines mediated transmigration of leucocytes after crossing several barriers to reach interstitial tissues. Examples of chemokines for neutrophils are: Leukotrienes B4 (LT-B4), complement system (C5a and C3a), cytokines (interleukins; IL-8), soluble bacterial products.

2. **Phagocytosis** (*TNMGR, May 2019*): It is defined as the process of engulfment of solid particulate material by cells (cell-eating). There are 2 main types of phagocytic cells: i. Polymorphonuclear neutrophils (PMNs) (**microphage**), ii. Circulating monocytes and fixed tissue mononuclear phagocytes (**macrophages**). Phagocytosis involves 3 steps:

a. **Recognition and attachment:** Phagocytosis is initiated by expression of surface receptors on macrophages which recognize microorganisms. It is further enhanced when the microorganisms are coated with specific proteins (**opsonins**) which establish a bond between bacteria and cell membrane of phagocytic cell, e.g. IgG opsonin, C3b opsonin, lectins.

b. **Engulfment:** This is accomplished by formation of cytoplasmic pseudopods around the particle, enveloping it in a phagocytic vacuole (**phagosome**), which fuses with one or more lysosomes of the cell and form bigger vacuole called **phagolysosome**.

c. **Killing and degradation:** The microorganisms after being killed by antibacterial substances are degraded by hydrolytic enzymes. Disposal of microorganisms can proceed by following mechanisms:

i. **Intracellular mechanisms:** Oxidative bactericidal mechanism by oxygen-free radicals (MPO-dependent and MPO-independent); By lysosomal granules; Non-oxidative bactericidal mechanism.

ii. **Extracellular mechanisms:** Degranulation of macrophages and neutrophils leads to proteolysis outside the cells; Immune-mediated lysis of microbes by cytolysis, antibody-mediated lysis and by cell-mediated cytotoxicity.

Chemical mediators of inflammation (permeability factors/endogenous mediators of increased vascular permeability) (*RUHS, June 2019*): Two types:

I. **Cell-derived mediators**

1. **Vasoactive amines: Histamine and 5-hydroxytryptamine (serotonin):** Vasodilatation, increased vascular permeability, itching and pain; **Neuropeptides** (substance-P, neurokinin A, vasoactive intestinal polypeptide (VIP) and somatostatin): Increased vascular permeability, transmission of pain stimuli.

2. **Arachidonic acid metabolites (eicosanoids)**

    i. **Cyclooxygenase pathway (prostaglandins:** Increased venular permeability, vasodilatation, bronchodilatation, inhibit inflammatory cell function; **Thromboxane** A_2—platelet aggregation; **Prostacyclin**—vasodilatation, inhibits platelet aggregation, resolvins).

    ii. **Lipo-oxygenase pathway** (5-HETE—chemotactic; Leukotrienes—smooth muscle contraction; Lipoxins—counter action of leukotrienes).

    • **Leukotrienes (LT)** are a family of lipid mediators derived from arachidonic acid via the 5-lipoxygenase pathway by the action of lipo-oxygenase. Cysteinyl leukotrienes (cysLTs), LTC4, LTD4, and LTE4, account for the bioactivity originally termed slow-reacting substance of anaphylaxis (SRS-A), whereas LTB4 was identified by its potent chemotactic activity for neutrophils. LTs are a family of biologically active molecules, formed by leukocytes, mastocytoma cells, macrophages, and other tissues and cells in response to immunological and non-immunological stimuli. They exhibit a number of biological effects such as contraction of bronchial smooth muscles, stimulation of vascular permeability, and attraction and activation of leukocytes.

3. **Lysosomal components:** PMNs have 3 types of granules: Primary/Azurophil, Secondary/Specific; and Tertiary; Macrophages: Granules release acid proteases, collagenase, elastase and plasminogen activator.

4. **Platelet activating factor (PAF):** Platelet aggregation, chemotaxis.

5. **Cytokines** (*UHSR, June 2018*): Cytokines are polypeptide substances produced by activated lymphocytes (**lymphokines**) and activated monocytes

(**monokines**). Major cytokines are: Interleukin-1 (IL-1), tumor necrosis factor (TNF)-α and β, interferon (IFN)-γ, and chemokines (IL-8, PF-4). IL-1 and TNF-α are formed by activated macrophages while TNF-β and IFN-γ are produced by activated T cells. Chemokines include IL-8 (released from activated macrophages) and platelet factor-4 from activated platelets, both of which are potent chemo-attractant for inflammatory cells.

   i. **IL-1, TNF-α, TNF-β:** Increased leukocyte adherence, thrombogenicity, elaboration of other cytokines, fibroblastic proliferation and acute phase reactions.

   ii. **IFN-γ:** Activation of macrophages and neutrophils; synthesis of nitric acid synthase.

   iii. **Chemokines** (*HP Uni., April 2019*): IL-8: Chemotactic for neutrophils; Platelet factor-4: Chemotactic for neutrophils, monocytes and eosinophils; MCP-1: Chemotactic for monocytes; and Eotaxin chemotactic for eosinophils.

6. **Free radicals** (oxygen metabolites: Superoxide oxygen, H_2O_2, OH^-): Endothelial cell damage, protease activation; Nitric oxide: Vasodilatation, antiplatelet.

II. Plasma-derived mediators (plasma proteases):
Products of:

1. Kinin system: Bradykinin—smooth muscle contraction, vasodilatation, increased vascular permeability, pain.

2. Clotting system: Fibrinopeptides—increased vascular permeability, chemotaxis for leukocyte, anticoagulant activity.

3. Fibrinolytic system: Plasmin—activation of factor XII—stimulates kinin system to generate bradykinin, splits off complement C3 to form C3a, degrades fibrin to form fibrin split products (FSPs) which increase vascular permeability and are chemotactic to leucocytes.

4. Complement system: Actions of activated complement system in inflammation are:

   i. C3a, C5a, C4a (anaphylatoxins) activate mast cells and basophils to release of histamine.

   ii. C3b is an opsonin.

   iii. C5a is chemotactic for leucocytes.

   iv. Membrane attack complex (MAC) (C5b–C9) is a lipid dissolving agent and causes holes in phospholipid membrane of the cell.

Morphology of Acute Inflammation

1. **Pseudomembranous inflammation:** It is a false membrane formed as part of inflammatory response of mucous surface by combination of denuded epithelium; coagulation of plasma exudes with necrosed epithelium on the surface.

2. **Ulcer:** Ulcers are local defects on the surface of an organ produced by inflammation. In acute stage, there is infiltration by polymorphs with vasodilatation.

3. **Suppuration (abscess formation):** When acute bacterial infection is accompanied by intense neutrophilic infiltrate in the inflamed tissue, it results in tissue necrosis. A cavity is formed containing purulent exudate/pus (**abscess**) and process of abscess formation is known as **suppuration**, e.g.

   i. **Boil or Furuncle:** Acute inflammation via hair follicles in dermal tissues.

   ii. **Carbuncle:** Seen in untreated diabetics and occurs as abscess in dermis and soft tissues of neck.

4. **Cellulitis:** It is diffuse inflammation of soft tissues resulting from spreading effects of substances released by some bacteria.

5. **Bacterial infection of blood**

   i. **Bacteraemia:** Presence of small number of bacteria in blood which do not multiply significantly.

   ii. **Septicemia:** Presence of rapidly multiplying, highly pathogenic bacteria in blood, accompanied by systemic effects.

   iii. **Pyaemia:** Dissemination of small septic thrombi in blood.

Systemic effects of acute inflammation: Fever, leucocytosis, lymphadenitis, shock, DIC, bleeding and death.

Fate of acute inflammation

1. **Resolution:** It means complete return to normal tissue following acute inflammation. This occurs when tissue changes are slight and the cellular changes are reversible.

2. **Healing:** Healing by fibrosis takes place when the tissue destruction in acute inflammation is extensive. But when tissue loss is superficial, it is restored by regeneration.

3. **Suppuration.**

4. **Chronic inflammation:** Persisting or recurrent acute inflammation may progress to chronic inflammation.

B. Chronic inflammation: Chronic inflammation is defined as prolonged process in which tissue destruction and inflammation occur at the same time. It is of longer duration (>2 weeks) and occurs either *de novo* or the causative agent of acute inflammation persists longer. Characteristic feature of chronic inflammation is presence of chronic inflammatory cells, granulation tissue formation, and as granulomatous inflammation.

General features

1. **Mononuclear cell infiltration:** Chronic inflammatory lesions are infiltrated by mononuclear inflammatory cells like phagocytes (circulating monocytes, tissue macrophages, epithelioid cells, multinucleated giant cells) and lymphoid cells. Other chronic inflammatory cells include lymphocytes, plasma cells, eosinophils and mast cells.

2. **Tissue destruction or necrosis:** This is done by activated macrophages which release variety of biologically active substances, e.g. protease, elastase, collagenase, lipase, etc.

3. **Proliferative changes:** Formation of inflammatory granulation tissue followed by healing by fibrosis.

Systemic effects of chronic inflammation: Fever (mild) with loss of weight and weakness, anemia, leucocytosis, elevated ESR, amyloidosis.

Types of chronic inflammation: Histologically, chronic inflammation can be:

1. **Chronic non-specific inflammation:** It is characterized by non-specific inflammatory cell infiltration. Chronic suppurative inflammation is special form, in which infiltration by polymorphs and abscess formation is additional features, e.g. actinomycosis.

2. **Chronic granulomatous inflammation (specific):** It is characterized by formation of granulomas, e.g. tuberculosis, leprosy, etc.

Q. 2. Write a short note on giant cells.
(TNMGR, Sept. 2007)

Ans. Giant cells are multinucleated inflammatory large sized cells formed by fusion of multiple cells such as macrophages, epithelioid cells, monocytes, etc. Various types are:

A. Giant cells in inflammation (Fig. 1.2):

i. **Foreign body giant cells:** These contain numerous nuclei (up to 100) which are uniform in size and shape and resemble the nuclei of macrophages, e.g. chronic infective granulomas, leprosy, tuberculosis.

ii. **Langhan's giant cells:** The nuclei are arranged either around the periphery in the form of horse-shoe/ring, or clustered at the two poles of giant cell, e.g. tuberculosis, sarcoidosis.

iii. **Touton giant cells:** These multinucleated cells have vacuolated cytoplasm due to lipid content, e.g. in xanthoma.

iv. **Aschoff giant cells:** These multinucleate giant cells are derived from cardiac histiocytes and are seen in rheumatic nodule.

B. Giant cells in tumors (Fig. 1.2):

i. **Anaplastic cancer giant cells:** These are larger, have numerous nuclei which are hyperchromatic and vary in size and shape, e.g. soft tissue sarcomas, etc.

ii. **Reed-Sternberg cells:** These are malignant tumor giant cells, generally binucleate, seen in Hodgkin's lymphoma.

iii. **Giant cell tumor of bone:** This tumor of bones has uniform distribution of osteoclastic giant cells spread in stroma.

- **Basophils (mast cells)** *(NTR Uni., Nov. 2007; UOK, July 2012; TNMGR, June 2016):* The basophils comprise about 1% of circulating leucocytes and are morphologically and pharmacologically similar to mast cells of tissue. These cells contain coarse basophilic granules in the cytoplasm and a polymorphonuclear nucleus. These granules are laden with heparin and histamine. Basophils and mast cells

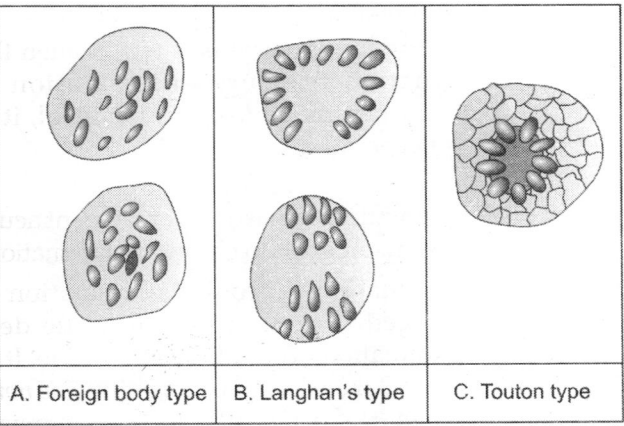

| A. Foreign body type | B. Langhan's type | C. Touton type |

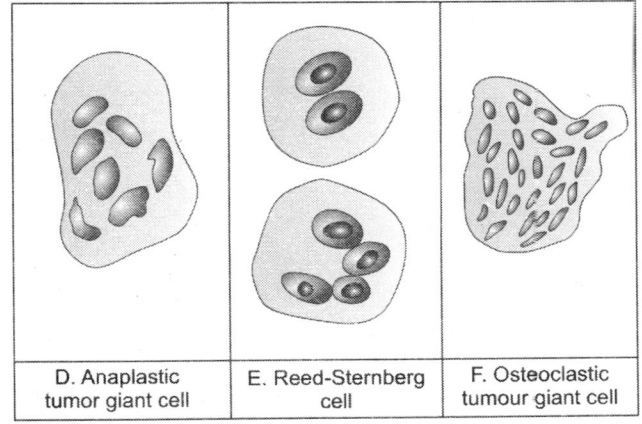

| D. Anaplastic tumor giant cell | E. Reed-Sternberg cell | F. Osteoclastic tumour giant cell |

Fig. 1.2: Various types of giant cells

have receptors for IgE and degranulate when cross-linked with antigen The role of these cells in inflammation are in immediate and delayed type of hypersensitivity reactions; and release of histamine by IgE-sensitized basophils.

- **Plasma cxells** *(NTR Uni., Nov. 2006):* These cells are larger than lymphocytes with more abundant cytoplasm and an eccentric nucleus which has cart-wheel pattern of chromatin. Plasma cells are normally not seen in peripheral blood. They develop from B lymphocytes and are rich in RNA and γ-globulin in their cytoplasm. These cells are most active in antibody synthesis. Their number is increased in following conditions: Prolonged infection with immunological responses (e.g. syphilis, rheumatoid arthritis); Hypersensitivity states; Multiple myeloma.

Q. 3. Write a short note on granulomatous inflammation. *(TNMGR, Nov. 2001)*

Ans. Granulomatous inflammation is characterized by formation of granulomas. **Granuloma** is defined as a circumscribed, tiny lesion (1 mm in diameter), composed predominantly of collection of modified macrophages (**epithelioid cells**), and rimmed at periphery by lymphoid cells. Granuloma formation is a type IV hypersensitivity reaction. It is a protective defense reaction by host but eventually causes tissue destruction because of persistence of poorly digestible antigen.

Pathogenesis of granuloma: Steps in formation of granuloma are:

1. **Engulfment by macrophages:** Macrophages and monocytes engulf the antigen but fail to digest and degrade it, and instead undergo morphologic changes to epithelioid cells.
2. **CD4+ T cells:** Macrophages (APC) present the antigen to CD4+ T lymphocytes. These lymphocytes get activated and elaborate lymphokines (IL-1, IL-2, IFN-γ, TNF-α).
3. **Cytokines:** Activated CD4+ T cells and macrophages form cytokines, e.g.
   i. IL-1, IL-2: Stimulate proliferation of more T cells.
   ii. IFN-γ: Activates macrophages.
   iii. TNF-α: Promotes fibroblast proliferation and activates endothelium to secrete PGs.
   iv. Growth factors (TGF-β, platelet derived growth factor): Stimulate fibroblast growth.

Composition of granuloma *(TNMGR, Sept. 2010)* (Fig. 1.3)

1. **Epithelioid cells:** They are modified macrophages/ histiocytes (epithelial cell-like), with slipper-shaped nucleus, pale staining cytoplasm, hazy outlines and are weakly phagocytic.
2. **Multinucleate giant cells:** Multinucleate giant cells are formed by fusion of adjacent epithelioid cells and may have 20 or more nuclei. These are weakly phagocytic but produce secretory products which help in removing the invading agents.

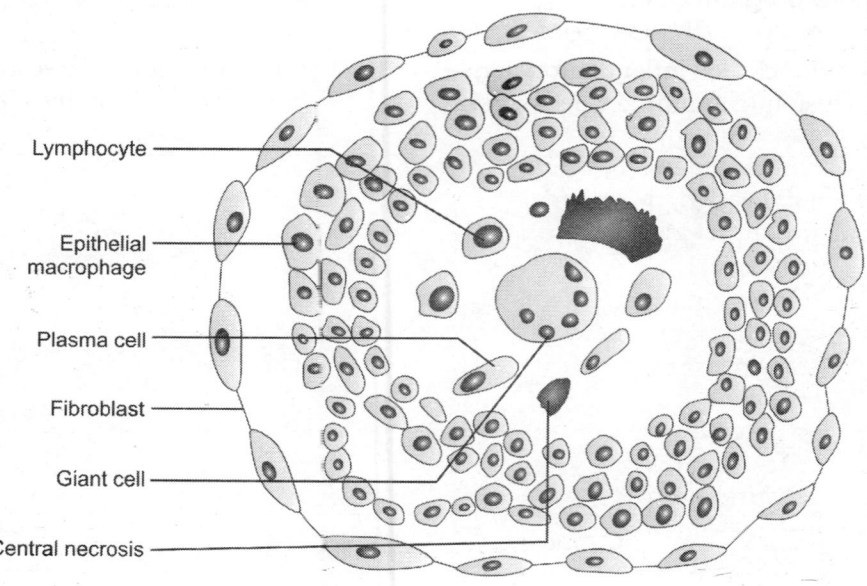

Lymphocyte
Epithelial macrophage
Plasma cell
Fibroblast
Giant cell
Central necrosis

Fig. 1.3: Structure of a typical granuloma

3. **Lymphoid cells:** Lymphocytes are integral to its composition.

4. **Necrosis:** It may be present in some granulomatous conditions, e.g. tuberculosis.

5. **Fibrosis:** It is a feature of healing by proliferating fibroblasts at the periphery of granuloma.

Classical example of granulomatous inflammation is tissue response to tubercle bacilli which is called **tubercle** seen in tuberculosis.

Examples of Granulomatous Conditions

A. **Bacterial:** Tuberculosis, leprosy, syphilis, granuloma inguinale, brucellosis, cat scratch diseases, tularemia, glanders.

B. **Fungal:** Actinomycosis, blastomycosis, cryptomycosis, and coccidiodomycosis.

C. **Parasitic:** Schistosomiasis.

D. **Miscellaneous:** Sarcoidosis, Crohn's disease, silicosis, berylliosis, foreign body granulomas.

Q. 4. Write a short note on primary complex.
(TNMGR, April 2000; BFUHS, May 2011; RUHS, June 2017)

Ans. A. Primary complex/Ghon's complex is the lesion produced in tissue of portal of entry with foci in the draining lymphatic vessels and lymph nodes. Commonly involved tissues for primary complex are lungs, hilar lymph nodes, tonsils, cervical lymph nodes, small intestine and mesenteric lymph nodes. Primary complex consists of 3 components:

1. **Pulmonary component:** Lesion in the lung is **primary focus or Ghon's focus**. It is 1–2 cm solitary area of tuberculous pneumonia located peripherally under a patch of pleurisy, in any part of the lung. *Microscopically*, it consists of tuberculous granulomas with caseation necrosis.

2. **Lymphatic vessel component:** Lymphatics draining the lung lesion contain phagocytes containing bacilli and may develop beaded, miliary tubercles along the path of hilar lymph nodes.

3. **Lymph node component:** Hilar and tracheobronchial lymph nodes are enlarged, matted and show caseation necrosis. *Microscopically*, lesions are characterized by extensive caseation, tuberculous granulomas and fibrosis. Nodal lesions are potential source of re-infection later. In case of primary tuberculosis of alimentary tract due to ingestion of tubercle bacilli, a small primary focus is seen in intestine with enlarged mesenteric lymph nodes producing "**Tabes mesenterica**". Enlarged and caseous mesenteric lymph nodes may rupture into peritoneal cavity and cause "**Tuberculous peritonitis**".

Sequelae of primary complex: Healing by fibrosis and calcification; Progressive spread to other parts; Miliary spread to lungs, liver, spleen, kidneys and brain; Secondary lesions due to reactivation of dormant primary complex.

B. Secondary tuberculosis: The infection of an individual who has been previously infected or sensitized is called **Secondary/Post-primary/Reinfection/Chronic tuberculosis.** The infection may be acquired from: *Endogenous source* such as reactivation of dormant primary complex; or *exogenous source* such as fresh dose of reinfection by the tubercle bacilli.

- **Secondary pulmonary tuberculosis:** The lesions in secondary pulmonary tuberculosis usually begin as 1–2 cm apical area of consolidation of lung, which may develop a small area of central caseation necrosis and peripheral fibrosis. It occurs by haematogenous spread of infection from primary complex to the apex of affected lung. Microscopically, the appearance is typical of tuberculous granulomas with caseation necrosis.

- **Fate of secondary pulmonary tuberculosis**
  1. Lesions may heal with fibrous scarring and calcification.
  2. Lesions may coalesce together to form larger area of tuberculous pneumonia with following pulmonary and extrapulmonary involvements: Fibrocaseous tuberculosis; Tuberculous caseous pneumonia; Miliary tuberculosis.

Q. 5. Write a short note on interleukins.
(NTR Uni., Oct. 2013; TNMGR, Oct. 2016)

Ans. Interleukins (ILs) are a type of cytokine expressed by leukocytes, and many other body cells. Primary function of interleukins is to modulate growth, differentiation, and activation during inflammatory and immune responses. Interleukins consist of a large group of proteins that can elicit many reactions in cells and tissues by binding to high-affinity receptors in cell surfaces. They have both paracrine and autocrine functions.

Clinical Significance

- IL-1 acts on hypothalamus to induce fever; operates on hepatocytes to increase synthesis of specific serum proteins; causes fall in blood pressure or shock in large amounts.
- IL-2 causes suppression of T responses.
- IL-12 overproduction causes allergic disorders.

- IL-19 may be used to induce angiogenesis in ischemic tissue.
- IL-21 may be used in treatment of Th2-mediated allergic diseases.
- IL-26 shows high expression in psoriatic skin lesions, inflammatory bowel disease and in rheumatoid arthritis.
- IL-28 may be sufficient treatment of HCV patients.
- Elevated IL-37 levels are found in SLE.
- IL-38 is correlated with autoimmune diseases and in carcinogenesis.
- IL-39 secreted by activated B cells may be a critical pro-inflammatory cytokine and a potential therapeutic target for the treatment of autoimmune diseases.
- IL-40 expression in several human B cell lymphomas suggests that it may play a role in the pathogenesis of these diseases.
- **Therapy of human diseases with interleukins:** In the immunotherapy of melanoma and renal carcinoma have successfully been used interleukin-2 and interferon-gamma.

Q. 6. Write a short note on hemochromatosis.
(TNMGR, April 2001, March 2010)

Ans. Hemochromatosis is an iron-storage disorder in which there is excessive accumulation of iron in parenchymal cells with eventual tissue damage and functional insufficiency of organs such as liver, pancreas, heart and pituitary gland. It is characterized by triad: Micronodular pigment cirrhosis, diabetes mellitus and skin pigmentation. The term "**Bronze diabetes**" is used on the basis of last two features. Males predominate and manifest earlier than females. Exists in 2 main forms:

1. **Idiopathic (primary/genetic):** An autosomal recessive disorder, associated with overexpression of HFE gene (normally regulates iron absorption) located on chromosome 6 close to HLA gene locus. Here, defect lie at intestinal mucosal level causing excessive iron absorption, or at post-absorption excretion level leading to excessive accumulation of iron.
2. **Secondary (acquired):** This arises secondary to other diseases. Here, the excessive accumulation of iron is due to acquired causes like ineffective erythropoiesis, defective hemoglobin synthesis, multiple blood transfusions and enhanced absorption of iron due to alcohol consumption (**Bantu siderosis**).

Clinical features: Bronze pigmentation of skin, diabetes mellitus, hepatic cirrhosis and carcinoma, cardiac dysfunction, arthropathy, hypogonadism.

Diagnosis: Serum iron, transferrin, ferritin concentration, estimation of chelatable iron stores and liver biopsy.

Q. 7. Write a short note on free radicals.
(TNMGR, April 2012, Oct. 2017)

Ans. Free radical (reactive oxygen radicals/reactive oxygen species) is a type of unstable molecule that is made during normal cell metabolism and can build up in cells, causing damage to other molecules, such as DNA, lipids, and proteins.

Mechanism of oxygen free radical generation: Normally, metabolism of cell involves generation of ATP by oxidative process in which biradical oxygen (O_2) combines with hydrogen atom (H) and forms water (H_2O), by 'four-electron donation' in four steps. These are generated within mitochondrial inner membrane where cytochrome oxidase catalyses O_2 to H_2O reaction.

Oxygen free radicals are the intermediate chemical species having unpaired oxygen in their outer orbit, e.g.

1. Superoxide oxygen (O_2): One electron
2. Hydrogen peroxide (H_2O_2): Two electrons
3. Hydroxyl radical (OH^-): Three electrons
4. Release of superoxide free radical.
5. Nitric oxide (NO).
6. Hypochlorous acid (HOCl).
7. Exogenous sources—tobacco and industrial pollutants.

Cytotoxicity of free radicals: Free radicals are highly destructive to cell since they have electron-free residue and thus bind to all molecules of cell (**oxidative stress**). Free radicals produce membrane damage by: Lipid peroxidation, oxidation of proteins, DNA damage, and cytoskeletal damage.

Conditions with free radical injury: Ischemic reperfusion injury; Ionizing radiation by causing radiolysis of water; Chemical toxicity; Chemical carcinogenesis; Hyperoxia; Cellular aging; Killing of microbial agent; Destruction of tumor cells; Atherosclerosis.

Q. 8. Discuss the nature and pathogenesis of various types of amyloidosis.
(TNMGR, March 2010; RUHS, May 2018)

Ans. Amyloidosis is the term used for a group of diseases characterized by extracellular deposition of fibrillar proteinaceous substance (amyloid), having common morphological appearance, staining properties and physical structure but with variable protein (or biochemical) composition.

Physical and chemical nature of amyloid: Amyloid is composed of 2 types of proteins:

I. **Fibril proteins (95%):** Fibrils have cross-β-pleated sheet configuration which gives characteristic staining properties of amyloid with Congo red and birefringence under polarizing microscopy (β-fibrillosis). These proteins can be categorized as: AL (amyloid light chain); AA (amyloid associated) protein; Other proteins: Transthyretin (TTR), $A\beta_2$-microglobulin ($A\beta_2 M$), β-amyloid protein (Aβ). Immunoglobulin heavy chain amyloid (AH), amyloid from hormone precursor proteins. Amyloid of prion protein (APrP).

II. **Non-fibrillar components (5%):** Amyloid P (AP) component; Apolipoprotein-E (apoE); Sulfated GAGs; α_1-antichymotrypsin; Protein X; Other components—components of complement, proteases, and membrane constituents.

Pathogenesis

1. Pool of amyloidogenic precursor protein is present in circulation in different clinical settings and in response to stimuli.
2. A nidus for fibrillogenesis, to stimulate deposition of amyloid protein is formed. This alteration involves changes and interaction between basement membrane proteins and amyloidogenic protein.
3. Partial degradation or proteolysis occurs prior to deposition of fibrillar protein which may occur in macrophages or reticuloendothelial cells.
4. The non-fibrillar components facilitate in aggregation of proteins and protein folding leading to fibril formation, substrate adhesion and protection from degradation.

Classification

I. Based on cause: Primary and secondary.
II. Based on extent of amyloid deposition: Systemic (generalized) and localized.
III. Based on Histology: Pericollagenous and peri-reticulin.
IV. Based on clinical location: Pattern I, pattern II and mixed.
V. Based on tissue of deposition: Mesenchymal and parenchymal.

A. Systemic (generalized) amyloidosis

1. Primary (AL): Plasma cell dyscrasias.
2. Secondary/reactive/inflammatory (AA): Chronic infections, autoimmune disorders, tumors.
3. Haemodialysis-associated ($A\beta_2M$): Chronic renal failure.
4. Heredofamilial (ATTR, AA, others): Hereditary polyneuropathic, Mediterranean fever.

B. Localized amyloidosis:

1. Senile cardiac (ATTR): Senility.
2. Senile cerebral (Aβ, APrP): Alzheimer's transmissible encephalopathy.
3. Endocrine (hormone precursors): Medullary carcinoma, diabetes mellitus (type 2).
4. Tumour-forming (AL): Lungs, tongue, larynx, skin, and eye.

Staining characteristics

1. **Stain on gross:** Lugol's iodine imparts Mahogany brown colour to amyloid containing area which on addition of dilute sulfuric acid turns blue.
2. **H&E:** Extracellular, homogeneous, structureless and eosinophilic hyaline material.
3. **Metachromatic stains (Rosaniline dyes):** Methyl violet/crystal violet imparts rose-pink coloration.
4. **Congo red and polarized light:** Congo red imparts pink or red color under normal light and characteristic apple-green birefringence by polarizing microscopy.
5. **Fluorescent stains:** Thioflavin-T binds to amyloid and fluoresce yellow under ultraviolet light.
6. **Immunohistochemistry:** Amyloid can be classified by immunohistochemical stains. Most useful in confirmation for presence of amyloid of any type is anti-AP stain.

Diagnosis: Biopsy, *in vivo* Congo red test, other tests: Protein electrophoresis, immunoelectrophoresis of urine and serum, and bone marrow aspiration.

Morphologic features of amyloidosis of organs: *Grossly*, affected organ is usually enlarged, pale and rubbery. Cut surface shows firm, waxy and translucent parenchyma which takes positive staining with iodine test. *Microscopically*, deposits of amyloid are found in extracellular locations, in the walls of small blood vessels producing microscopic changes and effects. Amyloidosis of kidneys is most common and most serious. Amyloidosis of spleen shows two patterns: 1. Sago spleen; 2. Lardaceous spleen. Tongue is the most commonly affected organ of oral cavity with amyloidosis, resulting in macroglossia, followed by gingiva.

Q. 9. What do you understand by the term fibromatosis? Give a brief account of the entities you would include under these headings.

(TNMGR, March 2010)

Ans. Fibromatosis is fibrous overgrowth of dermal and subcutaneous connective tissue, causing tumor-like lesions of fibrous tissue (fibromas) which continue to proliferate actively and may be difficult to differentiate from sarcomas. Generally, they are benign tumors and do not metastasize.

Classification

A. Based on age

1. **Infantile or juvenile fibromatoses:** Fibrous hamartoma of infancy, fibromatosis colli, diffuse infantile fibromatosis, juvenile aponeurotic fibroma, juvenile nasopharyngeal angiofibroma and congenital fibromatosis.

2. **Adult type of fibromatoses:** Palmar and plantar fibromatosis, nodular fasciitis (pseudosarcomatous fibromatosis), cicatricial fibromatosis, keloid, irradiation fibromatosis, penile fibromatosis (Peyronie's disease), abdominal and extra-abdominal desmoids fibromatosis.

B. Based on location

1. **Superficial fibromatosis:** They are usually slow growing, small in size, arising from fascia or aponeurosis, e.g. palmar (Dupuytren's contracture) and plantar (Ledderhose disease) fibromatosis, penile fibromatosis (Peyronie's disease), nodular fasciitis, knuckle pads, fibrous papule of face.

2. **Deep (musculo aponeurotic) fibromatosis:** They are rapidly growing, larger in size, arising from deeper structures, e.g. desmoid tumors, abdominal fibromatosis.

Causes: Trauma, hormonal factors (estrogens), genetic association (trisomy 8, deletion of 5q), secondary to diseases (diabetes, liver disease).

Treatment: Surgery, radiation therapy, drugs (anti-estrogen), chemotherapeutic agents.

2. REPAIR AND DEGENERATION

Q. 1. Write a short note on healing by primary and secondary intention. *(Nagpur Uni., Oct. 2001; TNMGR, March 2008; BBD Uni., Aug. 2017; UHSR, June 2018)*

Q. Define repair and regeneration. Describe the process of healing of a surgical wound.

(TNMGR, Sept. 2010; UHSR, May 2016; RUHS, June 2017; Sumandeep Uni., May 2018; NTR Uni., May 2019)

Ans. Healing is body response to injury in an attempt to restore normal structure and function. Healing involves 2 distinct processes:

A. **Regeneration:** Healing takes place by proliferation of parenchymal cells and usually results in complete restoration of the original tissues.

B. **Repair:** Healing takes place by proliferation of connective tissue elements resulting in fibrosis and scarring.

A. Healing by first intention (primary union) (Fig. 2.1a): Healing of a wound which has following characteristics: i. Clean and uninfected; ii. Surgically incised; iii. Without much loss of cells and tissue; iv. Edges of wound

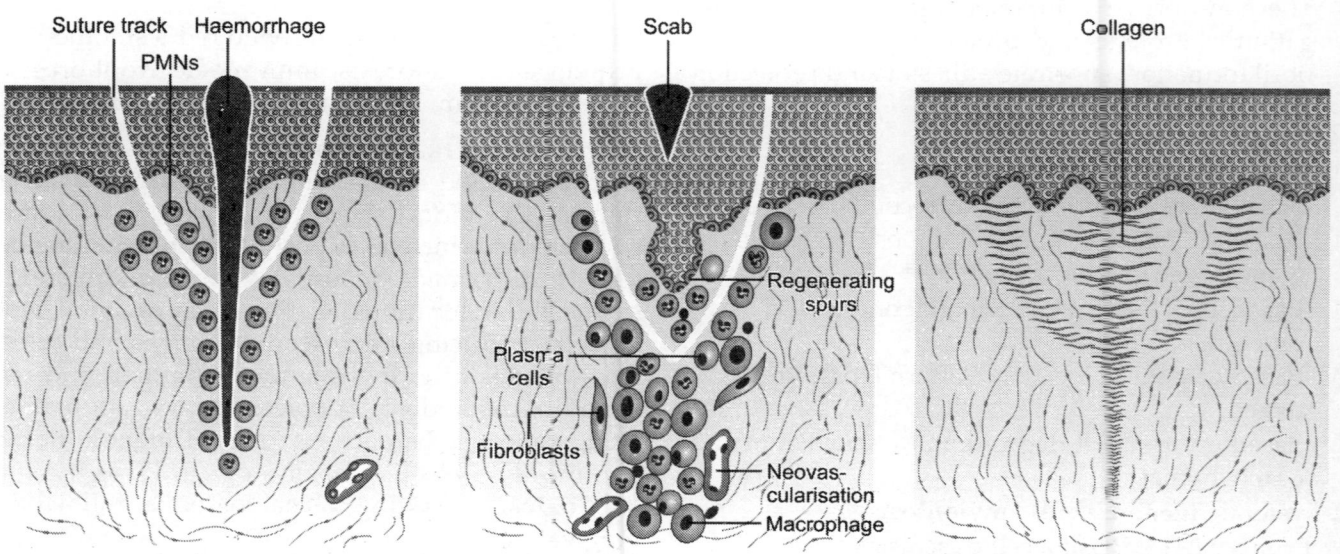

Suture track   Haemorrhage
PMNs
Scab
Collagen
Regenerating spurs
Plasma cells
Fibroblasts
Neovascularisation
Macrophage

Fig. 2.1a: Different stages of healing by primary intention

are approximated by surgical sutures. The sequence of events is as follows:

1. **Initial hemorrhage:** Immediately after injury, the space between the approximated surfaces of incised wound is filled with blood which then clots and seals the wound against dehydration and infection.

2. **Acute inflammatory response:** This occurs within 24 hours with appearance of polymorphs from the margins of incision. By 3rd day, polymorphs are replaced by macrophages.

3. **Epithelial changes:** The basal cells of epidermis from both the cut margins start proliferating and migrating towards incisional space in the form of epithelial spurs. A well approximated wound is covered by a layer of epithelium in 48 hours. The migrated epidermal cells separate the underlying viable dermis from overlying necrotic material and clot, forming scab which is cast off. By 5th day, a multilayered new epidermis is formed which is differentiated into superficial and deeper layers.

4. **Organization:** By 3rd day, fibroblasts also invade the wound area. By 5th day, new collagen fibrils start forming which dominate till healing is completed. In 4 weeks, the scar tissue with scanty cellular and vascular elements, a few inflammatory cells and epithelialised surface is formed.

5. **Suture tracks:** Each suture track is a separate wound and incites the same phenomena as in healing of primary wound. When sutures are removed (7th day), much of epithelialised suture track is avulsed and remaining epithelial tissue in the track is absorbed. However, sometimes suture track gets infected (**stitch abscess**), or epithelial cells may persist in the track (**implantation or**

epidermal cysts). Thus, scar formed in a sutured wound is neat due to close apposition of margins of wound.

B. Healing by second intention (secondary union) (Fig. 2.1b): This is defined as healing of a wound with following characteristics: i. Open with large tissue defect; ii. Extensive loss of cells and tissues; iii. Wound is not approximated by surgical sutures but is left open.

The basic events in secondary union are similar to primary union but differ in having a larger tissue defect which has to be bridged. Hence, healing takes place from the base upwards as well as from the margins inwards. The healing by second intention is slow and results in a large, at times ugly scar. The sequence of events is as follows:

1. **Initial hemorrhage:** As a result of injury, wound space is filled with blood and fibrin clot which dries.

2. **Inflammatory phase:** There is an initial acute inflammatory response followed by appearance of macrophages which clear off debris as in primary union.

3. **Epithelial changes:** The proliferating epithelial cells from both the margins of wound proliferate and migrate into wound in the form of epithelial spurs along with granulation tissue from base, which fills the wound space. Pre-existing viable connective tissue is separated from necrotic material and **clot** on the surface, forming **scab** which is cast off. In time, regenerated epidermis becomes stratified and keratinized.

4. **Granulation tissue** (main bulk): Granulation tissue is formed by proliferation of fibroblasts and neovascularisation from adjoining viable elements. The newly-formed granulation tissue is deep red,

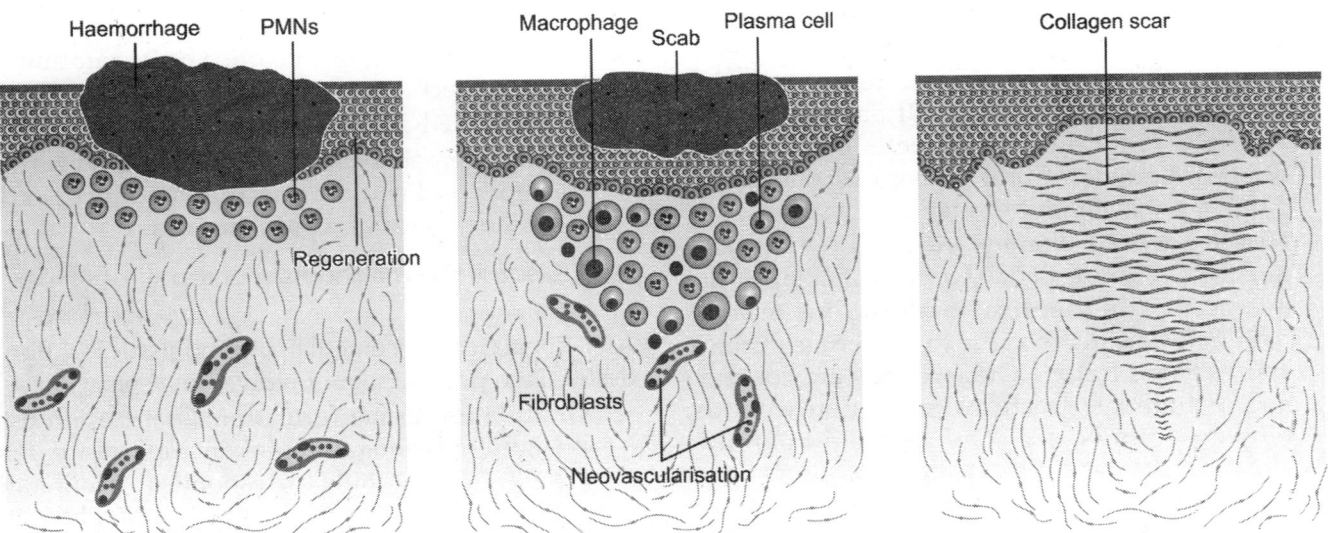

Fig. 2.1b: Different stages of healing by secondary intention

granular and very fragile. With time, the scar on maturation becomes pale and white due to increase in collagen and decrease in vascularity.

5. **Wound contraction:** Contraction of wound is an important feature of secondary healing. Due to action of myofibroblasts present in granulation tissue, the wound contracts to 1/3rd to 1/4th of its original size.

6. **Presence of infection:** Bacterial contamination of an open wound delays the process of healing due to release of bacterial toxins that provoke necrosis, suppuration and thrombosis. Surgical removal of dead and necrosed tissue, debridement, helps in preventing the bacterial infection of open wounds.

Complications of wound healing: 1. Infection of wound. 2. Implantation (epidermal) cyst formation. 3. Pigmentation. 4. Deficient scar formation. 5. Incisional hernia or wound dehiscence. 6. Hypertrophied scars and keloid formation. 7. Excessive contraction. 8. Neoplasia.

- **Repair and Regeneration of Oral Tissues** (HP Uni., April 2019):
  - Regeneration takes place by growth from the same type of tissue that has been destroyed or from its precursors.
  - Repair is to restore the function and tissue continuity but with distortion of normal architecture.
  - Cells responsible for repair and regeneration are: Mesenchymal cells, endothelial cells, macrophages, platelets, and parenchymal cells of injured organs.
  - Growth factors responsible for repair and regeneration are: TGF-β, KGF, EGF, FGF, PDGF, VEGF.
  - Oral tissues use a basic mechanism for repair. Repair of periodontium depends on the degree of damage. If damage is minimal, repair involving scar tissue formation occurs. If damage is more extensive, repopulation of cells in the defect occurs. Wounds of oral mucosa especially the gingiva heals without formation of scar tissue.
  - **Healing of Oral Wounds** (AHSUC, UHSR, NTR, June 2017): Healing of oral wounds after injury has an essentially identical pattern, but may be modified considerably due to numerous intrinsic and extrinsic factors. Oral wounds are common and include jaw fractures, extraction wounds, biopsy wounds, etc. The unusual anatomic situation of oral cavity, teeth protruding from bone, constant inflammation present in gingival tissues, presence of countless microorganisms in a warm, moist medium of saliva all contribute to modify the healing reaction of various oral wounds.
    - **Primary healing** occurs after the excision of a lesion in oral cavity where the pliability of tissues is such that the wound may be drawn together and sutured.
    - **Secondary healing** of an open wound occurs when there is loss of tissue and the edges of wound cannot be approximated. This type of wound is a result of biopsy of a lesion in an area of oral cavity in which the tissues are not pliable and in which the edges cannot be approximated.

Q. 2. Discuss the factors affecting wound healing.
(TNMGR, Sept. 2009; Oct. 2016; AHSUC, May 2018)

Ans. Factors affecting wound healing are:

A. Local factors
1. Infection delays process of healing (most important).
2. Poor blood supply to wound slows healing.
3. Foreign bodies including sutures interfere with healing and cause intense inflammatory reaction and infection.
4. Movement delays wound healing.
5. Exposure to ionizing radiation delays granulation tissue formation.
6. Exposure to ultraviolet light facilitates healing.
7. Type, size and location of injury determines whether healing takes place by resolution or organization.

B. Systemic factors
1. Age: Wound healing is rapid in young.
2. Nutrition: Deficiency of constituents like protein, vitamin C and zinc delays wound healing.
3. Systemic infection delays wound healing.
4. Administration of glucocorticoids has anti-inflammatory effect.
5. Uncontrolled diabetics delay in healing.
6. Hematologic abnormalities like defect of neutrophil functions and neutropenia and bleeding disorders slow the process of wound healing.

Q. 3. Discuss the mechanism of repair of tissues.
(TNMGR, April 1998)

Ans. Repair is replacement of injured tissues by fibrous tissue. Two processes are involved in repair:

1. **Granulation tissue formation:** Granulation tissue is slightly granular and pink in appearance. *Histologically*, each granule corresponds to proliferation of new small blood vessels which are slightly lifted on the surface by covering of fibroblasts and young collagen.

a. **Phase of inflammation:** Following trauma, blood clots at the site of injury. There is acute inflammatory response with exudation of plasma, neutrophils and some monocytes within 24 hours.

b. **Phase of clearance:** Combination of proteolytic enzymes liberated from neutrophils, autolytic enzymes from dead tissues cells, and phagocytic activity of macrophages clear off the necrotic tissue, debris and RBCs.

c. **Phase of ingrowth:** This phase consists of:
   - **Angiogenesis (neovascularisation):** Formation of new blood vessels at the site of injury takes place by proliferation of endothelial cells from the margins of severed blood vessels.
   - **Fibrogenesis:** New fibroblasts originate from fibrocytes as well as by mitotic division of fibroblasts. As maturation proceeds, more and more of collagen is formed while the number of active fibroblasts and new blood vessels decreases. This results in formation of inactive looking scar, called *cicatrisation*.

2. **Contraction of wounds:** The wound starts contracting after 2–3 days and process is completed by 14th day. During this period, wound is reduced by approximately 80% of its original size. Contracted wound results in rapid healing. This occurs because of dehydration, contraction of collagen, and presence of myofibroblasts.

Q. 4. Write a short note on fracture healing.
(TNMGR, March 2008; BFUHS, May 2009; BBD Uni., Aug. 2017; UHSR, June 2018)

Q. Write a note on healing of jaw fracture.
(NTR Uni., May 2019)

Ans. Basic events in healing of any type of fracture are:

A. **Primary union of fractures:** It occurs when the ends of fracture are approximated by application of compression clamps. In these cases, bony union takes place with formation of medullary callus without periosteal callus formation. Patient can be made ambulatory early but there is more extensive bone necrosis and slow healing.

B. **Secondary union:** It is more common process of fracture healing. Secondary bone union is described under the following 3 headings:

I. **Procallus formation** (Fig. 2.4):

1. **Hematoma formation:** Bleeding from torn blood vessels fills the area surrounding the fracture and forms a loose meshwork and fibrin clot which acts as framework for subsequent granulation tissue formation.

2. **Local inflammatory response:** It occurs at the site of injury with exudation of fibrin, polymorphs and macrophages. The macrophages clear away the fibrin, RBCs, inflammatory exudate and debris. Fragments of necrosed bone are scavenged by macrophages and osteoclasts.

3. **Ingrowth of granulation tissue:** It begins with neo-vascularisation and proliferation of mesenchymal cells from periosteum and endosteum. A soft tissue callus is thus formed which joins the ends of fractured bone without much strength.

4. **Callus composed of woven bone and cartilage:** It starts within first few days. The cells of inner layer of periosteum have osteogenic potential and lay down collagen as well as osteoid matrix in the granulation tissue. The osteoid undergoes calcification and is called **woven bone callus**. At times, callus is composed of woven bone as well as cartilage, temporarily immobilizing the bone ends. This

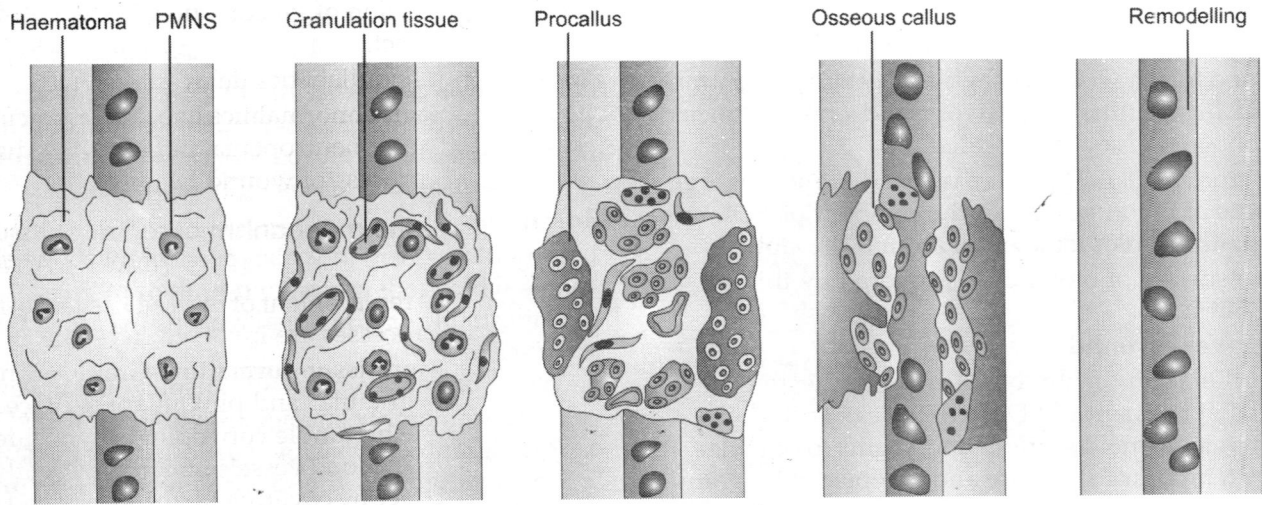

Fig. 2.4: Different stages of fracture healing

Haematoma   PMNS   Granulation tissue   Procallus   Osseous callus   Remodelling

stage is called **provisional callus** or **procallus** formation and is divided into external, intermediate and internal procallus.

II. Osseous callus formation: Woven bone is cleared away by incoming osteoclasts and the calcified cartilage disintegrates. In their place, newly-formed blood vessels and osteoblasts invade; laying down osteoid which is calcified and lamellar bone is formed by developing haversian system concentrically around the blood vessels.

III. Remodeling: During the formation of lamellar bone, osteoblastic laying and osteoclastic removal are taking place, remodeling the united bone ends. The external callus is cleared away, compact bone (cortex) is formed in place of intermediate callus and bone marrow cavity develops in internal callus.

Complications of fracture healing

- **Delayed union:** These result when the calluses of osteogenic tissue of the two fragments fail to meet and fuse or when endosteal formation of bone is inadequate. Local infection and presence of foreign bodies may also result in delayed healing.
- **Non-union** is relatively common in elderly persons, due to lack of osteogenic potential of cells, and in patients with systemic debility, diabetes mellitus, and systemic infection.
- **Fibrous union/pseudoarthrosis arises** as a result of lack of immobilization of damaged bone.
- **Lack of calcification** of newly formed bone in the callus may occur.

Q. 5. Write about healing of tooth socket following dental extraction. *(KLE Uni. Jan. 2009; RGUHS, May 2011; TNMGR, Oct. 2012; BBD Uni., June 2016; HP Uni., May 2017; RUHS, June 2019)*

Ans.

A. Immediate reaction following tooth extraction

1. Blood fills the socket, coagulates, RBCs gets entrapped in the fibrin meshwork and ends of torned blood vessels become sealed off.
2. Within 24–48 hours, there is vasodilation, engorgement of blood vessels in the remnant of PDL and mobilization of leukocytes around the clot.
3. The surface of blood clot is covered by thick layer of fibrin.

B. First week wound

1. Proliferation of fibroblasts from connective tissue cells in remnant of PDL into the clot.
2. This clot forms a scaffold and begins to organize. It is a temporary structure and is replaced by granulation tissue.

3. Peripheral epithelium shows proliferation and crest of alveolar bone shows beginning of osteoclastic activity.
4. Endothelial cell proliferation in PDL signals the beginning of capillary in growth.

C. Second week wound

1. Blood clot becomes organized by growth of fibroblasts growing into fibrin meshwork.
2. New delicate capillaries penetrate to centre of clot.
3. Remnants of PDL undergo degeneration.
4. Extensive epithelial proliferation takes place. In smaller sockets, epithelization may be complete.
5. Margins of alveolar socket exhibit prominent osteoclastic resorption.
6. Fragments of necrotic bone get resorbed.

D. Third week wound

1. Clot becomes completely organized by maturing granulation tissue.
2. Trabeculae of uncalcified bone are formed around the periphery of socket wall.
3. Crest of alveolar bone is rounded off by osteoclastic resorption.
4. Surface of the wound becomes completely epithelized.
5. Early bone is formed by osteoblast derived from pluripotential cells of original PDL.
6. By this time, surface of wound has completely epithelialised.

E. Fourth week wound

1. Continuing bone deposition and remodeling resorption occurs, filling the alveolar socket.
2. The newly formed bone is poorly calcified.
3. Maturative remodeling continues for weeks.

Complication: Alveolar osteitis (dry socket), acutely infected and inflamed alveolus, fibrous healing.

Q. 6. Write a note on biopsy. *(TNMGR, Sept. 2007, April 2012;NTR Uni., May 2019)*

Ans. Biopsy is defined as removal of tissue from living organism for the purposes of microscopic examination and diagnosis. Biopsy also serves as a treatment option for smaller lesions by excising *in toto*.

Indications

1. Any ulcer/growth which persists for >2 weeks or one which fails to respond to therapy.
2. For esthetic or functional reasons in case of benign or reactive lesions.
3. White or red lesions with suspicious appearance and/or in highly suspicious sites in oral cavity.
4. Radiographically suspicious lesions of the jaws.
5. Lesion that has the clinical features of malignancy such as an enlarging mass, tissue friability,

induration on palpation or persistence of mucosal changes, despite removal of local irritants.

6. New or enlarging pigmented lesions with irregular border and non-homogenous coloration.

Biopsy procedure

1. Selection of area to biopsy.
2. Preparation of surgical field.
3. Local anesthesia.
4. The incision.
5. Tissue handling (10% neutral buffered formalin)
6. Suturing.

Methods of obtaining material for microscopic study

1. Surgical excision by scalpel.
2. Surgical removal by cautery or a high-frequency cutting knife.
3. Laser.
4. Removal by biopsy forceps or biopsy punch.
5. Aspiration through a large bore needle.

Types of biopsy (UHSR, May 2016):

1. **Exfoliative cytology** (UOK, July 2013): Exfoliative oral cytology can be defined as the obtention and characterization of cells from the surface of oral mucosa. The cells may be detached naturally or artificially (cytobrush sampling). Characterization is traditionally based on microscopic examination of fixed and stained cell smears. Unfortunately, such methods show low sensitivity in diagnosis of oral cancers, due to inadequate sampling, high risk of procedural errors, and the need for subjective interpretation of findings. Exfoliative cytology is becoming increasingly important in the early diagnosis of oral cancers, as a procedure for obtaining cell samples that can then be analyzed by cytomorphometry, DNA cytometry, and molecular analyses. Exfoliative cytology is a simple and rapid, non-aggressive and relatively painless: it is thus well accepted by patients and suitable for routine application in population screening programmes, for early analysis of suspect lesions, and for pre- and post-treatment monitoring of confirmed malignant lesions.

2. **Oral brush biopsy:** The oral brush biopsy, using a specially devised circular bristled brush, has been designed to access and sample all epithelial layers, in conjunction with basal cell layer and the most superficial portion of lamina propria.

3. **Fine needle aspiration biopsy:** Aspiration or FNA biopsy is performed with a fine needle attached to a syringe. FNA biopsy is a percutaneous (through skin) biopsy. FNA biopsy is typically accomplished with a fine gauge needle (22 gauge or 25 gauge).

FNA is the fastest and easiest method of biopsy, and the results are rapidly available. One disadvantage of FNA is that the procedure only removes very small samples of tissue or cells. If the sample is benign fluid (e.g. a cyst), then the procedure is ideal.

4. **Punch biopsy:** Punch biopsy is typically used by dermatologists to sample skin rashes, moles and other small masses, in a similar way this technique is useful in oral mucosal biopsies. Generally, it is used in an incisional fashion for diagnostic purposes; however, larger punches may be used to excise small lesions. After a local anesthetic is injected, a biopsy punch (3 to 4 mm or 0.15 inch in diameter), is used to cut out a cylindrical piece of mucosa. Punch biopsy is not appropriate for vesiculobullous diseases, as the twisting action would detach the epithelium and prevent proper assessment of the interface between epithelium and connective tissue.

5. **Incisional/diagnostic biopsy:** Incisional biopsy can include the part of a lesion, or part of the affected mucosa plus part of normal mucosa (to show the interface between normal and abnormal mucosa) for purposes of diagnosis. Some lesions are too large to excise initially without having established a diagnosis, or are of such a nature that excision would be inadvisable. In such instances, a small piece is removed for examination.

6. **Excisional biopsy:** Total excision of a small lesion for microscopic study is called excisional biopsy. Excisional biopsy is preferred; if the size of lesion is such that it may be removed along with a margin of normal tissue and the wound can be closed primarily.

7. **Bone biopsy:** Biopsy is usually required to attain a provisional diagnosis, which may need to be confirmed by examination of the full lesion if excision follows. Biopsy may be necessary to differentiate between benign bone tumors, metastatic tumors, degenerative or congenital lesions.

   - **Healing of biopsy wound** (UHSR, June 2018): Healing of a biopsy wound of oral cavity depends upon whether the edges of wound can be brought into apposition, often by suturing, or whether the lesion must fill in gradually with granulation tissue.

Q. 7. Write a short note on healing of root fracture.
(UHSR, June 2017)

Ans. Root fractures are classified as horizontal or vertical. Three healing modalities exist for root fractures: Hard tissue fusion, PDL interposition with and without bone, and non-healing with interposition of granulation tissue owing to coronal pulp necrosis.

Healing following fracture is initiated at the pulpal and periodontal ligament side, creating two types of wound healing response, occurring either independently or competitively of each other. Healing of transverse root fractures involves the union of fracture segments by either hard, calcified tissue or interposition of connective tissue or interposition of bone and connective tissue, or interposition of granulation tissue. A vital pulp and positive pulp sensibility at the time of injury are positively related to faster healing and hard tissue repair of the fracture. Middle-third fractures are considered to have the best prognostic value. The chance of healing with calcified tissue and survival is poorest when the fracture line is very close to the gingival crevice.

Q. 8. Discuss phases of wound healing after implant placement. *(HP Uni., April 2019)*

Ans. Oral implants are of three types, namely endodontic, endosseous, and subperiosteal. Phases of wound healing are:

I. Peri-implant soft tissue healing: Immediately following implant placement, a blood coagulum separates the oral mucosa from implant surface and alveolar bone, which is soon infiltrated by inflammatory cells and the initial mucosal seal is established by formation of fibrin layer at day 4. After 1–2 weeks, migration and proliferation of epithelial cells lead to formation of a junctional epithelium, which lengthens contact interface between implant surface and peri-implant mucosa. Maturation of peri-implant mucosa occurs between 6 and 12 weeks following implant placement and is mainly characterized by formation of a mature epithelial barrier and organization and alignment of collagen fibers.

II. Peri-implant hard tissue healing: Immediately after surgical placement of a dental implant, the peripheral part of implant threads are in close contact with recipient bone, providing implant mechanical stability in early phases of healing. After one week of wound healing, osteoclasts migrate to the site and remnant bone fragments get incorporated in newly formed woven bone. Simultaneously, blood coagulum and granulation tissue are replaced with provisional connective tissue matrix containing fibroblast-like mesenchymal cells, which differentiate into osteoblasts that are able to deposit a collagen fiber matrix that mineralizes. Most of the newly formed woven bone extends from the existing old lamellar bone

(**appositional bone formation or distance osteogenesis**). This bone matrix grows, mineralizes and gradually advances towards the implant surface. Some woven bone has also been found in close contact to the implant surface at distance from existing parent bone bed (**contact osteogenesis**). Wound healing progresses with marked woven bone formation and maturation in such a way that after 4 weeks of healing, it is gradually remodeled and replaced over the course of 1–3 months by lamellar bone. Increases in tissue mineralization occurring over the course of healing are accompanied by rises in bone to implant contact, which allows for the functional loading of implants.

Applied aspects: Pathologic changes of tissues around the implant are referred to as peri-implant disease. Inflammatory changes confined to the soft tissues of implant are called peri-implant mucositis. Progressive bone loss around the implant along with inflammation of the soft tissue is known as peri-implantitis.

Q. 9. Write a note on cellular degeneration. *(Nagpur Uni., 1996; RGUHS, Oct. 2010; TNMGR, April, 2012; NTR Uni., June 2015)*

Ans. Degeneration is defined as deterioration of live cells following injury, with a possibility of injured cells to reverse to normal when the injury is removed. It is morphology of reversible cell injury. Types:

1. Hydropic change: Hydropic change means accumulation of water within the cytoplasm of cell. Other synonyms used are **cloudy swelling** (for gross appearance of affected organ) and **vacuolar degeneration** (due to cytoplasmic vacuolation).

Etiology: Acute and sub-acute cell injury from bacterial toxins, chemicals, burns, high fever, intravenous administration of hypertonic saline, etc.

Pathogenesis: It results from impaired regulation of sodium and potassium at the level of cell membrane.

Morphologic features: *Grossly*, affected organ is enlarged due to swelling; *Microscopically*, it is characterized by: Swollen cells, compressed microvasculature, small clear vacuoles in cells, small cytoplasmic blebs, pale nucleus.

2. Fatty change (steatosis/fatty metamorphosis): It is intracellular accumulation of neutral fat within parenchymal cells (cytosol). Liver is the commonest site for accumulation of fat because it plays central role in fat metabolism.

Etiology: Hyperlipidaemia, liver cell damage.

Pathogenesis: It can occur due to defect at any of the steps involved in normal fat metabolism:

1. Increased entry of free fatty acids into liver.
2. Increased synthesis of fatty acids by liver.
3. Decreased conversion of fatty acids into ketone bodies.
4. Increased α-glycerophosphate causing increased esterification of fatty acids to triglycerides.
5. Decreased synthesis of 'lipid acceptor protein' resulting in decreased formation of lipoprotein from triglycerides.
6. Block in excretion of lipoprotein from liver into plasma.

Morphological features: *Grossly*, liver is enlarged with a tense, glistening capsule and rounded margins. *Microscopically*, there is presence of numerous lipid vacuoles in the cytoplasm of hepatocytes.

3. Hyaline change: Hyaline change is associated with heterogeneous pathologic conditions. It may be intra-cellular or extracellular. **Intracellular hyaline** is mainly seen in epithelial cells, e.g. hyaline degeneration of rectus abdominis muscle (**Zenker's degeneration**) in typhoid fever; Mallory's hyaline in alcoholic liver cell injury; Russell's bodies in rough endoplasmic reticulum of plasma cells. **Extracellular hyaline** is seen in connec-tive tissues, e.g. hyaline degeneration in leiomyomas of uterus; Hyalinised old scar of fibrocollagenous tissues.

4. Mucoid change: Mucin is normally produced by epithelial cells of mucous membranes and mucous glands as well as by some connective tissues like in umbilical cord. Examples of functional excess of epi-thelial mucin: Catarrhal inflammation of mucous membrane; Obstruction of duct leading to mucocele in oral cavity; Cystic fibrosis of pancreas; Mucin-secreting tumors. By convention, connective tissue mucin is termed myxoid (mucus-like), e.g. mucoid or myxoid degeneration in some tumors (myxomas, neuro-fibromas, etc.)

Q. 10. Write a short note on melanin pigment.
(TNMGR, March 2009; NTR Uni., May 2005)

Q. Write a short note on endogenous pigments.
(TNMGR, April 2003)

Ans. Pigments are colored substances present in most living beings including humans.

A. Endogenous pigments: Endogenous pigments are either normal constituents of cells or accumulate under special circumstances, e.g.

1. **Melanin:** It is the brown-black, non-hemoglobin derived pigment normally present in hair, skin, choroid of eye, meninges and adrenal medulla. It is synthesized in melanocytes and dendritic cells of basal cells in epidermis and stored in phagocytic cells (melanophores), in underlying dermis. **Melanocytes** (*NTR Uni., June 2015*) are unicellular dendritic cells reside in basal cell layer of the epidermis and oral epithelium. Primitive melanocytes originate from neural crest of ectoderm. Melanocytes have a round nucleus with a double nucleus membrane and clear cytoplasm lacking desmosomes or attachment plates, but possess long dendritic processes. Melanocytes synthesize melanin in organelles called **melano-somes**. There are four stages in melanosome development:

- Stage I (premelanosomes): They are round, small vesicles with an amorphous matrix.
- Stage II (melanosomes): They have an organized, structured fibrillar matrix and tyrosinase is present but pigment synthesis has not been noted.
- Stage III: Beginning of melanin production takes place at this stage.
- Stage IV: At the last, pigment fills the whole melanosome.

Melanoids are granules of melanoid pigment and are scattered in stratum lucidum and stratum corneum of skin. Melanoid imparts a clear yellow shade to the skin.

Disorders of melanin pigmentation
   i. **Generalized hyperpigmentation:** Addison's disease, chloasma (seen in pregnancy), chronic arsenical poisoning (**raindrop pigmentation of skin**).
   ii. **Focal hyperpigmentation:** Neurofibromatosis and Albright's syndrome (**café au lait spots**), Peutz-Jeghers syndrome, melanosis coli, melanotic tumors, lentigo.
   iii. **Generalized hypopigmentation:** Albinism.
   iv. **Localized hypopigmentation:** Leucoderma, vitiligo, acquired focal hypopigmentation (leprosy, healing of wounds, radiation dermatitis, etc.).

2. **Melanin-like pigments containing diseases:** Alkaptonuria, Dubin-Johnson syndrome.
3. **Haemoprotein-derived pigments:** Haemosiderin, haemozoin, bilirubin, and porphyrins.
4. **Lipofuscin:** Wear and tear pigment.

B. Exogenous pigments: Pigments introduced into the body from outside such as by inhalation, ingestion or inoculation.

1. **Inhaled pigments:** Carbon/Coal dust; silica/stone dust, iron/iron oxide, asbestos and various other organic substances.

2. **Ingested pigments**
   i. *Argyria* due to chronic ingestion of silver compounds, results in brownish pigmentation in skin, bowel, and kidney.
   ii. Chronic lead poisoning produces *blue lines* on teeth at gum line.
   iii. *Carotenaemia* is yellowish-red coloration of skin caused by excessive carotene intake.
3. **Injected pigments (tattooing):** India ink, cinnabar and carbon.
   - **Circumoral pigmentation** (*NTR Uni., June 2003*): Peutz-Jeghers syndrome, McCune-Albright syndrome, Mazabraud disease, Cushing's syndrome, Noonan's syndrome, Leopard syndrome, Laugier-Hunziker pigmentation, Cowden syndrome, Bannayan-Riley-Ruvalcaba, Lhermitte-Duclos syndrome, Cronkhite-Canada syndrome, Primary biliary cirrhosis, Addison's disease, vit. B$_{12}$ deficiency.

Q. 11. Write a short note on metaplasia and dysplasia.
(TNMGR, April 2003; UHSR, April 2015; DYP Uni., May 2019)

Ans. Metaplasia is defined as a reversible change of one type of adult cells to another type of adult cells, in response to abnormal stimuli, and reverts back to normal on removal of stimulus. However, if the stimulus persists for long time, epithelial metaplasia may transform into cancer. **Two types:**

A. Epithelial metaplasia
1. **Squamous metaplasia:** This is more common, due to chronic irritation, e.g.
   i. In bronchus (lined by pseudostratified columnar ciliated epithelium) in chronic smokers.
   ii. In vit. A deficiency, there is squamous metaplasia in nose, bronchi, lacrimal and salivary glands.
2. **Columnar metaplasia:** Transformation to columnar epithelium occurs in few condition, e.g.
   i. Intestinal metaplasia in healed chronic gastric ulcer.
   ii. Columnar metaplasia in Barrett's esophagus.
B. **Mesenchymal metaplasia,** e.g.
   1. **Osseous metaplasia:** It is formation of bone in fibrous tissue, cartilage and myxoid tissue, e.g. Mönckeberg's medial calcific sclerosis; in scar of chronic inflammation.
   2. **Cartilaginous metaplasia:** In healing of fractures, cartilaginous metaplasia may occur due to mobility.

Dysplasia (atypical hyperplasia): Dysplasia means 'disordered cellular development', often accompanied with metaplasia and hyperplasia. Dysplasia occurs most often in epithelial cells. Epithelial dysplasia is characterized by:
1. Increased number of layers of epithelial cells.
2. Disorderly arrangement of cells from basal layer to surface layer.
3. Loss of basal polarity.
4. Cellular and nuclear pleomorphism.
5. Increased nucleo-cytoplasmic ratio.
6. Nuclear hyperchromatism.
7. Increased mitotic activity.

Dysplastic changes often occur due to chronic irritation or prolonged inflammation. On removal of the inciting stimulus, the changes may disappear. In some cases, however, dysplasia progresses into carcinoma *in situ* or invasive cancer.

Q. 12. Write a note on hyperplasia and atrophy.
(NTR Uni., Nov. 2006)

Ans. Cellular adaptations are the adjustments for the sake of survival on exposure to stress. Common forms of cellular adaptive responses are:

I. Atrophy: It is reduction of number and size of parenchymal cells of an organ or its parts.

Causes
A. **Physiologic atrophy.** Atrophy is a normal process of aging in some tissues, which could be due to loss of endocrine stimulation or arteriosclerosis, e.g. atrophy of lymphoid tissue in lymph nodes, appendix and thymus; Atrophy of gonads after menopause.

B. **Pathologic atrophy.** The causes are as under:
1. Starvation atrophy: In this, there is first depletion of carbohydrate and fat stores followed by protein catabolism leading to general weakness, emaciation and anaemia (cachexia), seen in cancer and severely ill patients.
2. Ischemic atrophy: Gradual diminution of blood supply due to atherosclerosis may result in shrinkage of affected organ, e.g. small atrophic kidney in atherosclerosis of renal artery.
3. Disuse atrophy: Prolonged diminished functional activity is associated with disuse atrophy of organ, e.g. wasting of muscles of limb immobilized in cast.
4. Neuropathic atrophy: Interruption in nerve supply leads to wasting of muscles, e.g. poliomyelitis, motor neuron disease.
5. Endocrine atrophy: Loss of endocrine regulatory mechanism results in reduced metabolic activity of tissues, e.g. hypopituitarism may lead to atrophy of thyroid, adrenal and gonads.
6. Pressure atrophy: Prolonged pressure from benign tumors or cyst or aneurysm may cause atrophy of

tissues, e.g. erosion of spine by tumour in nerve root.

7. **Idiopathic atrophy:** In this, no obvious cause is present, e.g. myopathies, testicular atrophy.

Morphologic features: The organ is small, often shrunken. Shrinkage in cell size is due to reduction in cell organelles, chiefly mitochondria, myofilaments and endoplasmic reticulum. There is often increase in number of autophagic vacuoles containing cell debris, which may persist to form 'residual bodies' in cell cytoplasm.

II. Hypertrophy: Hypertrophy is an increase in size of parenchymal cells resulting in enlargement of organ or tissue, without any change in number of cells.

Causes

A. Physiologic hypertrophy: Enlarged size of uterus in pregnancy.

B. Pathologic hypertrophy

1. Hypertrophy of cardiac muscle in systemic hypertension.
2. Hypertrophy of smooth muscle, e.g. cardiac achalasia.
3. Hypertrophy of skeletal muscle, e.g. masseteric hypertrophy.
4. Compensatory hypertrophy in an organ when contralateral organ is removed, e.g. adrenal hyperplasia following removal of one adrenal gland.

Morphologic features: The affected organ is enlarged and heavy. There is enlargement of muscle fibres as well as of nuclei. At ultrastructural level, there is increased synthesis of DNA and RNA, increased protein synthesis and increased number of organelles.

C. Hyperplasia: Hyperplasia is an increase in number of parenchymal cells resulting in enlargement of organ or tissue. Hyperplasia occurs due to increased recruitment of cells from G0 (resting) phase of cell cycle to undergo mitosis, when stimulated. *Labile cells* (e.g. epithelial cells of skin and mucous membranes, cells of bone marrow and lymph nodes) and *stable cells* (e.g. parenchymal cells of liver, pancreas, kidney, adrenal, and thyroid) can undergo hyperplasia, while *permanent cells* (e.g. neurons, cardiac and skeletal muscle) have little or no capacity for regenerative hyperplastic growth.

Causes

A. Physiologic hyperplasia

1. Hormonal hyperplasia, e.g. hyperplasia of female breast at puberty, during pregnancy and lactation.
2. Compensatory hyperplasia, e.g. regeneration of liver following partial hepatectomy.

B. Pathologic hyperplasia: Due to excessive stimulation of hormones or growth factors, e.g. endometrial hyperplasia following oestrogen excess; In wound healing, there is formation of granulation tissue due to proliferation of fibroblasts and endothelial cells.

Morphologic features: There is enlargement of affected organ or tissue and increase in number of cells. This is due to increased rate of DNA synthesis and hence increased mitoses of the cells.

Q. 13. Write a short note on myoepithelial cells.
(NTR Uni., June 2014; UHSR, June 2018)

Ans. Myoepithelial (ME) (**basket cell**) cells are closely related to secretory and intercalated duct cells of salivary glands.

Location: These cells are located around the terminal secretory units and first portion of duct system. They lie between the basement membrane of parenchyma cells and are attached to cells by desmosomes.

Structure: They are stellate or spider-like, with a flattened nucleus; scanty, perinuclear cytoplasm and long branching processes that embrace the secretory and duct cells. In case of intercalated ducts, they have a more fusiform shape and are elongated with a few short processes.

Ultrastructural findings: ME cells contain cytokeratin intermediate filament and contractile actin filaments. Small dense bodies are frequently present between thin filaments. The usual cytoplasmic organelles are largely restricted to perinuclear cytoplasm. The plasma membrane of ME cell closely parallels the basal membrane of parenchymal cell. Numerous macropinocytotic vesicles, or **caveolae**, are located on plasma membranes of myoepithelial cells.

Functions

1. Accelerate the initial out flow of saliva from the acini.
2. Reduce luminal volume.
3. ME cells provide signals to acinar secretory cells that are needed for maintaining cell polarity and structural organization of acinus.
4. ME cells also produce a number of proteins that have tumor suppressor activity and anti-angiogenesis factors, which act as barriers against invasive epithelial neoplasms.

Q. 14. Write a note on pathologic calcification.
(TNMGR, Oct. 2003)

Ans. Deposition of calcium salts in tissues other than osteoid or enamel is called **pathologic** or **heterotopic calcification**. Two types:

I. Dystrophic calcification (*TNMGR, Oct. 2016*): Dystrophic calcification is characterized by deposition of calcium salts in dead or degenerated tissues with normal calcium metabolism and normal serum calcium levels.

A. Calcification in dead tissue: Phlebolith, dead parasites in hydatid cyst, Schistosoma eggs, cysticercosis, calcification in breast cancer, caseous necrosis in tuberculosis, etc.

B. Calcification in degenerated tissues: Dense old scars, long standing cysts, atheromas, calcinosis cutis, etc.

Pathogenesis: Denatured proteins in necrotic or degenerated tissue bind phosphate ions, which react with calcium ions to form precipitates of calcium phosphate.

II. Metastatic calcification: Metastatic calcification occurs in apparently normal tissues and is associated with deranged calcium metabolism and hypercalcemia.

A. Excessive mobilisation of calcium from bone: Hyperparathyroidism, bony destructive lesions, prolonged immobilization.

B. Excessive absorption of calcium from gut: Hypervitaminosis D, milk-alkali syndrome, hypercalcemia of infancy.

Sites of metastatic calcification: Kidneys, lungs, blood vessels, cornea, synovial joint.

Pathogenesis: Metastatic calcification occurs due to excessive binding of inorganic phosphate ions with calcium ions, which are elevated due to underlying metabolic derangement. This leads to formation of precipitates of calcium phosphate at the preferential sites.

Q. 15. Write a note on nerve injuries.

(BFUHS, May 2008)

Ans. The peripheral nerve injuries can be caused by a variety of mechanisms, broadly classified as systemic conditions or local pathologies. **Systemic conditions** (autoimmune inflammation, DM, vasculitis, or drug-induced), generally involve multiple nerves in multi-compartment or bilateral distribution and are best

diagnosed by a combination of clinical findings and electrophysiology. **Local pathologies** include blunt trauma, penetrating injury, chronic traction or acute stretch injury, local chemical injury, or freeze injury.

Nerve injury may involve axonal loss, myelin loss, or combination of both. Clinically, it may lead to sensory dysfunction and/or motor loss.

Classification of nerve injuries: Table 2.15 and Fig. 2.15.

Complications: Muscle weakness, sensory loss, neuropathic pain, autonomic problems.

Pathologic Reactions of Peripheral Nerves/Nerve Degeneration (*NTR Uni., April 2011*):

1. **Segmental demyelination:** It is loss of myelin of segment between two consecutive nodes of Ranvier,

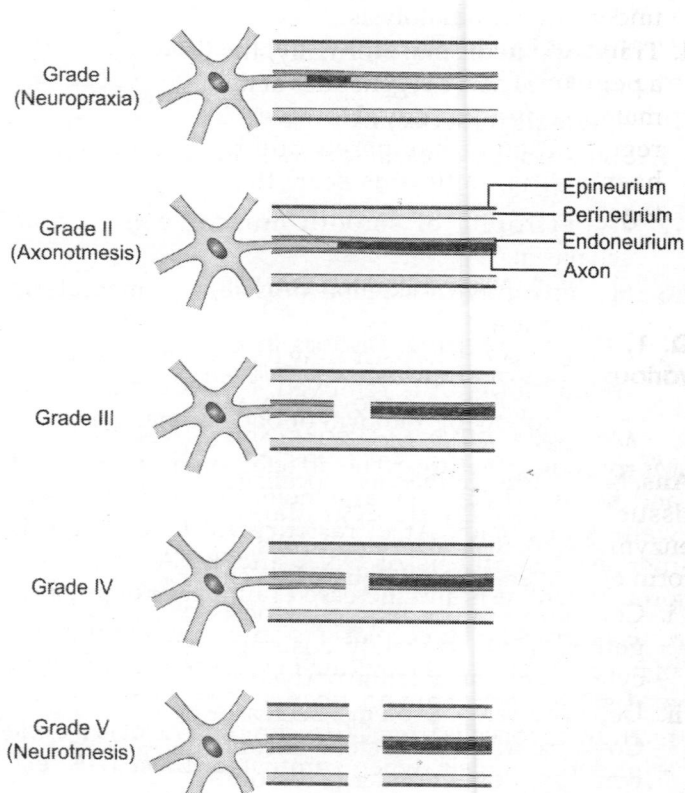

Fig. 2.15: Types of nerve injuries

Table 2.15: Classification of nerve injuries

Seddon classification (1943)	Sunderland classification (1951)	Injury
Neuropraxia	Grade I	Focal segmental demyelination
Axonotmesis	Grade II	Axon damaged with intact endoneurium
Axonotmesis	Grade III	Axon and endoneurium damaged with intact perineurium
Axonotmesis	Grade IV	Axon, endoneurium and perineurium damaged with intact epineurium
Neurotmesis	Grade V	Complete nerve transaction
	Grade VI (MacKinnon and Dellon)	Mixed nerve injury

sparing the axon. Repeated episodes of demyelination and remyelination are associated with concentric proliferation of Schwann cells around axons producing "**Onion Bulbs**" found in hypertrophic neuropathy.

2. **Wallerian degeneration (dying forward type):** Following transection, there is accumulation of organelles in proximal and distal ends of transection sites. Subsequently, axon and myelin sheath distal to transection site undergo disintegration up to next node of Ranvier, followed by phagocytosis. Process of regeneration occurs by sprouting of axons and proliferation of Schwann cells from proximal end.

3. **Axonal degeneration:** In this, degeneration of axon begins at peripheral terminal and proceeds backward towards the nerve cell body. The cell body often undergoes chromatolysis.

4. **Traumatic neuroma:** Normally, the injured axon of a peripheral nerve regenerates at the rate of approximately 1 mm per day. However, if the process of regeneration is hampered due to an interposed haematoma or fibrous scar, the axonal sprouts together.

3. NECROSIS AND GANGRENE

Q. 1. Define necrosis. Discuss in detail about the various types of necrosis. *(TNMGR, March 2008; KLE Uni., Jan. 2009; MUHS, May 2010; BFUHS, May 2011; RUHS, May 2015; NTR Uni., May 2019)*

Ans. Necrosis is defined as a localized area of death of tissue followed by its degradation by hydrolytic enzymes liberated from dead cells. It is morphologic form of irreversible cell injury. It is characterized by:

i. Cell digestion by lytic enzymes: Seen as homogeneous and intensely eosinophilic cytoplasm, cytoplasmic vacuolation or dystrophic calcification.

ii. Denaturation of proteins: Seen as nuclear changes: Condensation of nuclear chromatin (**pyknosis**) which may either undergo dissolution (**karyolysis**) or fragmentation into many granular clumps (**karyorrhexis**).

Types

1. **Coagulative necrosis:** Most common type, caused by irreversible focal injury, mostly from ischemia, and less often from bacterial and chemical agents. The organs commonly affected are heart, kidney, and spleen. *Grossly*, foci of coagulative necrosis in the early stage are pale, firm, and slightly swollen. With progression, they become more yellowish, softer, and shrunken. *Microscopically*, hallmark of coagulative necrosis is conversion of normal cells into their '*tombstones.*' The necrosed cells are swollen and appear more eosinophilic than normal. Cell digestion and liquefaction fail to occur. The necrosed focus is infiltrated by inflammatory cells and dead cells are phagocytosed, leaving granular debris and fragments of cells.

2. **Liquefaction (colliquative) necrosis** (*BBD Uni., Aug. 2017*): It occurs due to degradation of tissue by the action of powerful hydrolytic enzymes, e.g. infarct brain and abscess cavity. *Grossly*, the affected area is soft with liquefied centre containing necrotic debris. Later, a cyst wall is formed. *Microscopically*, the cystic space contains necrotic cell debris and macrophages filled with phagocytosed material. Cyst wall is formed by proliferating capillaries, inflammatory cells and proliferating glial cells in case of brain and proliferating fibroblasts in case of abscess cavity.

3. **Caseous necrosis:** Caseous necrosis is found in the centre of foci of tuberculous infections. It combines features of both coagulative and liquefactive necrosis. *Grossly*, foci of caseous necrosis resemble dry cheese and are soft, granular and yellowish. *Microscopically*, the necrosed foci are structureless, eosinophilic, and contain granular debris. The surrounding tissue shows characteristic granulomatous inflammatory reaction.

4. **Fat necrosis:** Fat necrosis is a special form of cell death occurring at two anatomically different locations but morphologically similar lesions. These are: Following acute pancreatic necrosis, and traumatic fat necrosis commonly in breasts.

In case of pancreas, there is liberation of pancreatic lipases from injured or inflamed tissue that results in necrosis of pancreas as well as of fat depots throughout the peritoneal cavity. The leaked out free fatty acids complex with calcium to form calcium soaps (**saponification**).

Grossly, fat necrosis appears as yellowish-white and firm deposits. Formation of calcium soaps imparts the necrosed foci firmer and chalky white appearance.

Microscopically, necrosed fat cells have cloudy appearance and are surrounded by an inflammatory reaction. Formation of calcium soaps is identified as amorphous, granular and basophilic material.

5. **Fibrinoid necrosis:** Fibrinoid necrosis is characterized by deposition of fibrin-like material which has the staining properties of fibrin. It is encountered in various immunologic tissue injury (e.g. immune complex vasculitis, autoimmune diseases, etc.), arterioles in hypertension, peptic ulcer, etc. *Microscopically*, fibrinoid necrosis is identified by brightly eosinophilic,

hyaline-like deposition in vessel wall. Necrotic focus is surrounded by nuclear debris of neutrophils (leuco-cytoclasis). Local hemorrhage may occur due to rupture of blood vessel.

Q. 2. Write about gangrene. *(TNMGR, March 2007; MPMS Uni., July 2017)*

Ans. Gangrene is a form of necrosis of tissue with superadded putrefaction. The type of necrosis is usually coagulative due to ischemia. **Gangrenous or necrotizing inflammation** is characterized by primarily inflammation provoked by virulent bacteria resulting in massive tissue necrosis, e.g. gangrenous appendicitis, gangrenous stomatitis (noma, cancrum oris).

1. **Dry gangrene:** This form of gangrene begins in distal part of a limb due to ischemia. Typical example is dry gangrene in toes and feet of an old patient due to arteriosclerosis. Other causes of dry gangrene foot include thromboangiitis obliterans (**Buerger's disease**), Raynaud's disease, trauma, and ergot poisoning. It is usually initiated in one of the toes which is farthest from blood supply, and then spreads slowly upwards until it reaches a point where the blood supply is adequate to keep the tissue viable. *A line of separation* is formed at this point between gangrenous part and viable part. *Grossly*, affected part is dry, shrunken and dark black (due to formation of iron sulfide), resembling foot of a mummy. *Microscopically*, there is necrosis with smudging of tissue. The line of separation consists of inflammatory granulation tissue.

2. **Wet gangrene:** Wet gangrene occurs in naturally moist tissues and organs such as mouth, bowel, lung, cervix, vulva, etc. Diabetic foot and bed sores are example of wet gangrene. Wet gangrene usually develops rapidly due to blockage of venous and less commonly, arterial blood flow from thrombosis or embolism. The affected part is stuffed with blood which favors rapid growth of putrefactive bacteria. The toxic products formed by bacteria are absorbed causing profound systemic manifestations of septicemia and finally death. *Grossly*, the affected part is soft, swollen, putrid, rotten and dark. *Microscopically*, there is coagulative necrosis with stuffing of affected part with blood.

3. **Gas gangrene:** It is a special form of wet gangrene caused by gas-forming Clostridia which gain entry into tissues through open contaminated wounds, especially in muscles, or as a complication of operation on colon. *Grossly*, the affected area is swollen, edematous, painful and crepitant due to accumulation of gas bubbles within tissues. Subsequently, affected tissue becomes dark black and foul smelling. *Microscopically*, muscle fibres undergo coagulative necrosis with liquefaction. Large number of Gram-positive bacteria can be identified.

Q. 3. Write a note on apoptosis.
(TNMGR, March 2008; RUHS, May 2015; UHSR, June 2018; NTR Uni., May 2019)

Ans. Apoptosis (**Greek:** Falling off) is a form of 'coordinated and internally programmed cell death.' Apoptosis is responsible for mediating cell death in variety of physiologic and pathologic processes.

Apoptosis in physiologic processes

1. Organized cell destruction during in sculpting of tissue development of embryo.
2. Physiologic involution of cells in hormone-dependent tissues, e.g. endometrial shedding, regression of lactating breast after withdrawal of breast-feeding.
3. Normal cell destruction followed by replacement proliferation such as in intestinal epithelium.
4. Involution of thymus in early age.

Apoptosis in pathologic processes

1. Cell death in tumors exposed to chemotherapeutic agents.
2. Cell death by cytotoxic T cells in immune mechanisms.
3. Progressive depletion of CD4+ T cells in pathogenesis of AIDS.
4. Cell death in viral infections, e.g. formation of *Councilman Bodies* in viral hepatitis.
5. Pathologic atrophy of organs and tissues on withdrawal of stimuli, e.g. atrophy of salivary gland on obstruction of ducts.
6. In degenerative diseases of CNS, e.g. Alzheimer's disease, Parkinson's disease.
7. Heart diseases, e.g. heart failure, acute myocardial infarction (20% necrosis and 80% apoptosis).

Characteristic morphologic changes: *Histologically*,

1. Involvement of single cells or small clusters of cells in the background of viable cells.
2. Apoptotic cells are round to oval shrunken masses of intensely eosinophilic cytoplasm (**mummified cell**) containing shrunken or almost-normal organelles.
3. Nuclear chromatin is condensed or fragmented (**pyknosis/karyorrehexis**).
4. Cell membrane may show convolutions or projections on the surface.
5. There may be formation of membrane-bound near spherical bodies on or around the cell (**apoptotic bodies**) containing compacted organelles.

6. Characteristically, there is no acute inflammatory reaction around apoptosis.

7. Phagocytosis of apoptotic bodies by macrophages takes place at varying speed.

Apoptotic cells can be identified and counted by:

1. Staining of chromatin condensation (haematoxylin, Feulgen, acridine orange).
2. Flow cytometry to visualize rapid cell shrinkage.
3. DNA changes detected by *in situ* techniques or by gel electrophoresis.
4. Annexin V as marker for apoptotic cell membrane.

Biochemical changes

1. Proteolysis of cytoskeletal proteins.
2. Protein-protein crosslinking.
3. Fragmentation of nuclear chromatin by activation of nuclease.
4. Appearance of phosphatidylserine (thrombospondin in some form) on outer surface of cell membrane. This facilitates early recognition by macrophages for phagocytosis prior to appearance of inflammatory cells.

Molecular mechanisms of apoptosis

1. **Initiators of apoptosis**
   i. Withdrawal of signals required for normal cell survival.
   ii. Extracellular signals triggering of programmed cell death.
   iii. Intracellular stimuli, e.g. heat, radiation, hypoxia, etc.

2. **Process of programmed cell death**
   i. Activation of caspases.
   ii. Activation of death receptors.
   iii. Activation of growth controlling genes (BCL-2 and p53).
   iv. Cell death.

3. **Phagocytosis:** Dead apoptotic cells develop membrane changes which promote their phagocytosis.

Q. 4. Write a short note on cell cycle checkpoints.
(UHSR, June 2018)

Ans. Cell cycle checkpoints are surveillance mechanisms that monitor the order, integrity, and fidelity of major events of cell cycle such as growth to appropriate size, replication and integrity of chromosomes, and their accurate segregation at mitosis. The central machines that drive cell cycle progression are the cyclin-dependent kinases (CDKs).

1. **Cell size control:** Control of cell size is critical for regulating nutrient distribution for cell, for regulating organ size and function in multicellular organisms. The existence of cell size checkpoints has been proposed for allowing cells to coordinate cell size with cell cycle progression. Cell size checkpoints have been observed in G1 and G2. Large daughter cells speed up progression through G1 and/or G2, and small daughter cells delay exit from these growth phases.

2. **DNA damage responses:** Throughout interphase, DNA damage elicits a cell cycle arrest that allows time for repair pathways to operate prior to commitment to subsequent phases of cell cycle. While there are many lesion-specific responses for DNA repair, different lesions in genomic DNA activate common checkpoint pathways whose goal is to maintain CDKs in an inactive state until the lesion is removed.

3. **Monitoring DNA replication:** S phase marks a particularly vulnerable time for cells to cope with DNA damage. DNA replication is initiated at specific sites, the replication origins. These are epigenetically defined by a number of proteins that ensure they fire (start replicating) once. Replication origin firing is controlled by the phosphorylation of two proteins, Cdt1 and Cdc6, which is catalyzed by both CDKs and the Dbf4-dependent protein kinase (DDK) Cdc7.

Checkpoint dysfunction can result in outcomes ranging from cell death to cell cycle reprogramming, which can lead to cancer.

Q. 5. Write a short note on cell adhesion molecules.

Ans. Cell adhesion molecules (CAMs) are proteins located on the cell surface involved in binding with other cells or with extracellular matrix (ECM) in the process called cell adhesion.

Types: Adhesion molecules are generally divided into five groups: Integrins; Selectins; Cadherins; Immunoglobulin superfamily (IgSF) including nectins; Others: Mucins; enzymes (vascular adhesion protein-1).

Functions

1. Cell adhesion molecules are critical to many normal physiological processes, e.g. during embryogenesis, differential expression of CAMs is responsible for selective association of embryonic cells into specific tissues.

2. In immune system, they mediate migration and homing of lymphocytes to specific tissues.

3. CAMs have also been implicated in many diverse pathological processes such as inflammation and wound healing, septic shock, transplant rejection, cancer, and atherosclerosis.

4. Cell adhesion molecules also used as either diagnostic or prognostic markers, or as potential targets for therapeutic intervention.

Q. 6. Write a short note on vascular endothelial growth factor. *(UOK, July 2017)*

Ans. Vascular endothelial growth factor (VEGF)/vascular permeability factor, was originally described as an endothelial cell-specific mitogen. VEGF is produced by many cell types including tumor cells, macrophages, platelets, keratinocytes, and renal mesangial cells. VEGF is the prototypic member of a family of structurally related dimeric proteins including VEGF-B, VEGF-C, VEGF-D, and VEGF-E, as well as placental-growth factor (PlGF)-1, -2.

Functions
- VEGF is essential for development because deletion of VEGF gene is embryonically lethal.
- VEGFs are important in physiological angiogenic processes, e.g. wound healing; ovulation, and pregnancy.
- They are important role in pathological conditions such as cancer.

Mechanism of action: VEGF ligands activate angiogenic programs through binding of several receptors. VEGFR-1 (Flt-1) binds VEGF, VEGF-B, and PlGF-1, -2 and promotes recruitment of endothelial progenitors and monocyte migration. Signal transduction through VEGFR2 regulates endothelial cell proliferation, migration, and survival. Expression of VEGFR-3 is limited to lymphatic endothelium. Neuropilin (NRP)-1, -2 bind VEGF ligands and enhance their affinity to other VEGFRs.

Approaches to inhibit VEGF pathway (anti-VEGF): Several different types of agents have been developed to target VEGF pathway.
- Monoclonal antibodies against VEGF (bevacizumab).
- Proteins that bind VEGF such as VEGF Trap.
- Antibodies that block the receptor (IMC-1121b).
- Small-molecule inhibitors of receptor tyrosine kinase such as sunitinib, sorafenib, and ZD6474.
- Others: COX-2 inhibitors, thalidomide, and EGFR inhibitors.

Clinical uses of VEGF pathway inhibitors: Addition of VEGF inhibitors (bevacizumab, sorafenib, sunitinib) to chemotherapy has provided benefit in almost all the tumor types, by increasing patients survival.

Limitations/Disadvantages: Need of developing biomarkers to predict which patients are most likely to respond to treatment; associated toxicities and complications of hemoptysis and thromboembolism and therapeutic resistance.

4. CIRCULATORY DISTURBANCES

Q. 1. Write a short note on shock and its types.
(BFUHS, May 2004; TNMGR, Aug. 2004, March 2010; RGUHS, Nov. 2011; BBD Uni., April 2015; UHSR, June 2018; NTR Uni., May 2019)

Ans. Shock is a life-threatening clinical syndrome of cardiovascular collapse characterized by acute reduction of effective circulating blood volume (hypotension) and inadequate perfusion of cells and tissues (hypoperfusion).

Classification
1. **Primary (initial shock):** Transient and usually benign vasovagal attack due to sudden reduction of venous return caused by neurogenic vasodilatation and consequent peripheral pooling of blood.
2. **Secondary (true shock):** Circulatory imbalance between oxygen supply and oxygen requirements at cellular level. In clinical practice, simple shock refers to this type.
3. **Anaphylactic (type I immunologic reaction)**

Etiologic classification
1. **Hypovolaemic shock** *(UOK, July 2016; RUHS, June 2017):* This result from inadequate circulatory blood volume by various etiologic factors that may be either from the loss of red cell mass and plasma from haemorrhage, or from the loss of plasma volume alone, e.g. acute hemorrhage, dehydration from vomiting, diarrhoea, burns, excessive use of diuretics, acute pancreatitis. The major effects of hypovolaemic shock are due to decreased cardiac output and low intra-cardiac pressure. Clinical features are tachycardia, hypotension, oliguria/anuria) and alteration in mental state (agitated to confused to lethargic).
   Classification of hypovolemic shock: Hemorrhagic *(UHSR, June 2018);* Non-hemmorrhagic.
2. **Cardiogenic shock** *(HNBG Uni., June 2015):* Acute circulatory failure with sudden fall in cardiac output from acute diseases of heart without actual reduction of blood volume (normovolaemia) results in cardiogenic shock. This occurs due to deficient emptying (e.g. MI, cardiomyopathies, cardiac arrhythmias); Deficient filling (e.g. cardiac tamponade from haemopericardium); Obstruction to outflow (e.g. pulmonary embolism, dissecting aortic aneurysm).
3. **Septic/Toxaemic shock:** Severe bacterial infections or septicaemia induce septic shock. It may be the result of:

i. Gram-negative septicemia (**endotoxic shock**), e.g. infection with *E. coli*, proteus, Klebsiella, Pseudomonas and bacteroides.

ii. Gram-positive septicemia (**exotoxic shock**), e.g. infection with streptococci, pneumococci.

Mechanism: In septic shock, there is immune system activation and severe systemic inflammatory response by: Activation of macrophages and monocytes (by altering endothelial cell adhesiveness and promoting nitric oxide synthase); Activation of other inflammatory responses (complement pathway, mast cells, coagulation system, and kinin system). The net result of all these is vasodilatation and increased vascular permeability. Increased vascular permeability causes development of inflammatory edema. DIC is prone to develop in septic shock due to endothelial cell injury by toxins. Reduced blood flow produces hypotension, inadequate perfusion of cells and tissues, finally leading to organ dysfunction.

4. **Other types**

i. **Traumatic shock:** Shock resulting from trauma is initially due to hypovolaemia, and later due to loss of plasma volume into the interstitium of injured tissue, e.g. severe injuries, obstetrical trauma.

ii. **Neurogenic shock:** Neurogenic shock results from causes of interruption of sympathetic vasomotor supply, e.g. high cervical spinal cord injury, head injury.

iii. **Hypoadrenal shock:** Hypoadrenal shock occurs from unknown adrenal insufficiency in which the patient fails to respond normally to stress of trauma, surgery or illness, administration of high doses of glucocorticoids, secondary adrenal insufficiency.

Pathogenesis: In general, all forms of shock involve following 3 derangements:

1. **Reduced effective circulating blood volume:** It may result by: Actual loss of blood volume as occurs in hypovolaemic shock or decreased cardiac output without actual loss of blood as occurs in cardiogenic shock and septic shock.

2. **Impaired tissue oxygenation:** Following reduction in effective circulating blood volume, there is decreased venous return to heart resulting in decreased cardiac output. This consequently causes reduced supply of oxygen to organs and tissues and hence tissue anoxia, which sets in cellular injury.

3. **Release of inflammatory mediators:** In response to cellular injury, innate immunity of body gets activated and release inflammatory mediators. Endotoxins in bacterial wall in septic shock stimulate massive release of pro-inflammatory mediators (cytokines). The most important being the TNF-α and IL-1.

Pathophysiology: Stages of shock (Table 4.1).

Q. 2. Discuss the pathogenesis of edema.

(TNMGR, April 1998, Oct. 2000, Aug. 2004)

Ans. Edema may be defined as abnormal and excessive accumulation of "free fluid" in the interstitial tissue spaces and serous cavities.

Classification

A. Based on extent

1. **Localized:** When limited to an organ or limb, e.g. lymphatic edema.

2. **Generalized (anasarca or dropsy):** When it is systemic in distribution, particularly noticeable in subcutaneous tissues, e.g. nutritional edema.

B. Depending upon fluid composition, edema fluid may be (Table 4.2):

A. Based on compressibility

1. **Pitting edema/cutaneous edema:** When pressure is applied to small area, the indentation persists even after the release of pressure.

Table 4.1: Stages of shock: Mechanism and effects

Stages of shock	Pathogenesis	Effects
Compensated shock (initial)	Widespread vasoconstriction, fluid conservation by kidney, stimulation of adrenal medulla	Tachycardia, cool, clammy skin
Progressive decompensated shock	Pulmonary hypoperfusion, Tissue ischemia	↓ Cardiac output, mental confusion, ↓ Urinary output, tachypnoea
Irreversible decompensated shock	Progressive vasodilation, ↑ vascular permeability, myocardial depressant factor, pulmonary hypoperfusion, anoxic damage, hypercoagulability	i. Brain: Hypoxic encephalopathy ii. Heart: Focal myocardial necrosis iii. Lungs: ARDS (adult respiratory distress syndrome) iv. Adrenals and liver: Necrosis v. GIT: Hemorrhagic gastroenteropathy vi. Blood: DIC

Table 4.2: Difference between transudate and exudate

Feature	Transudate	Exudate
Definition	Filtrate of blood plasma without changes in endothelial permeability	Edema of inflamed tissue associated with increased vascular permeability
Character	Non-inflammatory edema	Inflammatory edema
Protein content	Low	High
Glucose content	Same as in plasma	Low
Specific gravity	Less than 1.015	More than 1.018
pH	>7.3	<7.3
LDH	Low	High
Effusion LDH/serum LDH (Light's criteria)	<0.6	>0.6
Cells	Few cells, mainly mesothelial and cellular debris.	Many cells, inflammatory as well parenchymal
Examples	Edema of cardiac and renal disease	Inflammatory edema, e.g. purulent exudate

2. **Non-pitting edema:** The type of edema in which the indentation made by a pressure on the affected area does not persist.

Pathogenesis of edema: Mechanisms involved are:

1. **Decreased plasma oncotic pressure:** As in hypoprotenemia, decreased oncotic pressure results in increased outward movement of fluid from the capillary wall and decreased inward movement of fluid from the interstitial space causing edema, e.g. edema of renal disease in nephrotic syndrome.

2. **Increased capillary hydrostatic pressure:** A rise in hydrostatic pressure at venular end of capillary which is normally low (12 mmHg) to a level more than the plasma oncotic pressure results in minimal or no reabsorption of fluid at venular end, consequently leading to edema, e.g. edema of cardiac disease as in congestive cardiac failure, ascites in cirrhosis of the liver.

3. **Lymphatic obstruction:** Normally, the interstitial fluid in tissue spaces escapes by way of lymphatics. Obstruction to outflow of these channels causes localized edema, known as lymphoedema, e.g.
   i. Inflammation of lymphatics as seen in filariasis results in chronic lymphoedema of scrotum and legs known as **elephantiasis**.
   ii. **Milroy's disease or hereditary lymphoedema** is due to abnormal development of lymphatic channels.

4. **Tissue factors:** The two forces acting in the interstitial space—oncotic pressure of interstitial space and tissue tension, are normally quite small and insignificant to counteract effects of plasma oncotic pressure and capillary hydrostatic pressure respectively. However, in some situations, the tissue factors can cause edema, e.g.

   i. Elevation of oncotic pressure of interstitial fluid as occurs due to increased vascular permeability and inadequate removal of proteins by lymphatics.
   ii. Lowered tissue tension as seen in loose subcutaneous tissues of eyelids and external genitalia.

5. **Increased capillary permeability:** When capillary endothelium is injured by various 'capillary poisons', capillary permeability to plasma proteins is enhanced due to development of gaps between endothelial cells, leading to leakage of plasma proteins into interstitial fluid. This causes reduced plasma oncotic pressure and elevated oncotic pressure of interstitial fluid which leads to edema, e.g.
   i. Generalized edema occurring in systemic infections, anaphylactic reactions and anoxia.
   ii. Localized edema, e.g. inflammatory edema as seen in infections; angioneurotic edema.

6. **Sodium and water retention:** Normally, 80% of sodium is reabsorbed by proximal convoluted tubule under the influence of either intrinsic renal mechanism or extra-renal mechanism while retention of water is affected by release of ADH. The possible factors responsible for causation of edema by this mechanism are:
   i. Reduced glomerular filtration rate in response to hypovolaemia.
   ii. Enhanced tubular reabsorption of sodium and consequently its decreased renal excretion.
   iii. Increased filtration factor, i.e. increased filtration of plasma from the glomerulus.
   iv. Decreased capillary hydrostatic pressure associated with increased renal vascular resistance.

Examples of edema by this mechanism are: Edema of cardiac disease, ascites of liver disease.

Q. 3. Define thrombosis. Discuss the pathogenesis of thrombosis formation.

(TNMGR, April 2001; NTR Uni., Nov. 2017)

Ans. Thrombosis is process of formation of solid mass in circulation from the constituents of flowing blood; the mass itself is called a **thrombus. Blood clot** is mass of coagulated blood formed *in vitro*, e.g. in a test tube. **Hematoma** is the extravascular accumulation of blood clot. **Haemostatic plugs** are blood clots formed in healthy individuals at the site of bleeding. Thrombi may be life-threatening by causing one of the following harmful effects: 1. Ischemic injury. 2. Thrombo-embolism.

Pathophysiology: Virchow described three primary events which predispose to thrombus formation (**Virchow's triad**) *(TNMGR, March 2007)*: Endothelial injury; Altered blood flow; and Hypercoagulability of blood followed by activation of platelets and of clotting system.

1. **Endothelial injury:** The integrity of blood vessel wall is important for maintaining normal blood flow. Vascular injury exposes the subendothelial connective tissue which are thrombogenic and thus plays important role in initiating haemostasis as well as thrombosis. Endothelial injury is of major significance in the formation of arterial thrombi and thrombi of heart.

2. **Role of platelets:** Following endothelial cell injury, sequence of events is:
   i. Platelet adhesion: Platelets in circulation recognize the site of endothelial injury and with the help of von Willebrand's factor, adhere to exposed subendothelial collagen (**primary aggregation**).
   ii. Platelet release reaction:
      a. α-granules: Fibrinogen, fibronectin, PDGF, platelet factor 4.
      b. Dense bodies: ADP, Ca^{2+}, 5-HT, histamine and epinephrine.
   iii. Platelet aggregation: Following release of ADP, aggregation of additional platelets takes place (**secondary aggregation**). This results in formation of temporary haemostatic plug.

3. **Role of coagulation system:** Coagulation mechanism is conversion of plasma fibrinogen into solid mass of fibrin. This is involved in both haemostatic process and thrombus formation.
   • **Regulation of coagulation system:** Normally, blood is kept in fluid state and coagulation system kept in check by:
      a. Protease inhibitors: They act on coagulation factors to oppose formation of thrombin, e.g. antithrombin III, protein C, C1 inactivator, α_1-antitrypsin, α_2-macroglobulin.
      b. Fibrinolytic system: Plasmin acts on fibrin to destroy the clot and produces FSPs.

4. **Alteration of blood flow:** While stasis (slowing) allows a higher release of oxygen from blood, turbulence (unequal flow) may actually injure the endothelium resulting in deposition of platelets and fibrin. Formation of arterial and cardiac thrombi is facilitated by turbulence in blood flow, while stasis initiates venous thrombi.

5. **Hypercoagulability of blood:** Hypercoagulability occurs by:
   i. Increase in coagulation factors, e.g. fibrinogen, prothrombin, factors VIIa, VIIIa and Xa.
   ii. Increase in platelet count and their adhesiveness.
   iii. Decreased levels of coagulation inhibitors, e.g. antithrombin III, FSPs.

Predisposing factors
• **Primary (genetic) factors:** Deficiency of antithrombin, protein C or S, defects in fibrinolysis, mutation in factor V.
• **Secondary (acquired) factors**
   – Risk factors: Advanced age, prolonged bed-rest, immobilization, cigarette smoking.
   – Clinical conditions: Heart diseases, vascular diseases, hypercoagulable conditions, shock, tissue damage, late pregnancy, certain drugs (anaesthetic agents, oral contraceptives).

Morphologic features: Thrombosis may occur in heart, arteries, veins and capillaries. **Arterial thrombi** produce ischemia and infarction, whereas **cardiac** and **venous thrombi** cause embolism. *Grossly*, thrombi may be of various shapes, sizes and composition depending upon the site of origin. **Arterial thrombi** tend to be white and mural while the **venous thrombi** are red and occlusive. **Mixed or laminated thrombi** are consisting of alternate white and red layers called **lines of Zahn**. **Red thrombi** are soft, red and gelatinous, whereas **white thrombi** are firm and pale. *Microscopically*, composition of thrombus is determined by rate of flow of blood, i.e. whether it is formed in rapid arterial and cardiac circulation, or in slow moving flow in veins. **Lines of Zahn** are formed by alternate layers of light-staining aggregated platelets admixed with fibrin meshwork and dark-staining layer of red cells. **Red (venous) thrombi** have more abundant red cells, leucocytes and platelets entrapped in fibrin meshwork.

Fate of thrombus
1. **Resolution:** Thrombus activates fibrinolytic system with consequent release of plasmin which may dissolve the thrombus.

2. **Organization:** If the thrombus is not removed, phagocytic cells appear and begin to phagocytose fibrin and cell debris.
3. **Propagation:** Thrombus may enlarge in size due to more and more deposition from the constituents of blood.
4. **Thromboembolism:** Thrombi in early stage and infected thrombi are quite friable and may get detached from vessel wall as emboli.

Clinical effects
1. **Cardiac thrombi:** Sudden death by mechanical obstruction of blood flow or through thromboembolism to vital organs.
2. **Arterial thrombi:** Sudden death may occur following thrombosis of coronary artery.
3. **Venous thrombi (phlebothrombosis):** Thromboembolism, edema of area drained, poor wound healing, skin ulcer, thrombophlebitis, painful white leg (**phlegmasia alba dolens**) due to ileofemoral venous thrombosis in postpartum cases.
4. **Capillary thrombi:** DIC.

Q. 4. Define and classify embolus. *(TNMGR, March 2002; NTR Uni., Nov. 2006; RGUHS, Oct. 2010)*

Ans. Embolism is process of partial or complete obstruction of some part of the cardiovascular system by any mass carried in the circulation; the transported intravascular mass detached from its site of origin is called an **embolus**. Most usual forms of emboli (90%) are thromboemboli.

Classification of emboli
A. **Depending on the matter in emboli:** Solid (thromboemboli, tumor cell clumps); liquid (fat globules, amniotic fluid); gaseous (air, other gases).
B. **Depending on whether infected or not:** Bland (sterile) and septic (infected).
C. **Depending on the source of emboli**
   i. Cardiac emboli from left side of heart.
   ii. Arterial emboli, e.g. in systemic arteries in brain, spleen, etc.
   iii. Venous emboli, e.g. in pulmonary arteries.
   iv. Lymphatic emboli.
D. **Depending on the flow of blood**
   i. **Paradoxical/crossed embolus:** An embolus which is carried from venous side of circulation to arterial side or vice versa.
   ii. **Retrograde embolus:** An embolus which travels against the flow of blood.

Thromboembolism: It may arise in arterial or venous circulation:

1. **Arterial (systemic) thromboembolism:** Arterial emboli may be derived from within the heart (80–85%), or from within the arteries. Effects of arterial emboli are: Infarction of organ or its part, Necrosis and gangrene, arteritis and mycotic aneurysm formation, sudden death.
2. **Venous thromboembolism:** Venous emboli may arise from thrombi in veins of lower legs (most common), thrombi in pelvic veins, thrombi in veins of upper limb, CST, thrombi in right side of heart. It leads to pulmonary embolism. Consequences: Sudden death, acute cor pulmonale, pulmonary infarction, pulmonary hemorrhage, resolution, pulmonary hypertension, chronic cor pulmonale and pulmonary arteriosclerosis.
3. **Systemic embolism:** This is the type of arterial embolism originates commonly from thrombi in the diseased heart, especially in left ventricle. These arterial emboli invariably cause infarction at the sites of lodgment (lower extremity, brain, and internal visceral organs).
4. **Fat embolism** *(TNMGR, Nov. 2001)*: Obstruction of arterioles and capillaries by fat globules constitutes fat embolism. If the obstruction in the circulation is by fragments of adipose tissue, it is called **fat-tissue embolism**.
   Causes
   i. **Traumatic:** Trauma to bones (most common), trauma to soft tissue.
   ii. **Non-traumatic:** Extensive burns, DM, fatty liver, pancreatitis, decompression sickness, inflammation of bones and soft tissues, extrinsic fat or oils introduced into the body.
   Pathogenesis
   i. **Mechanical theory:** Trauma to bone and soft tissue leads to release of fat globules into the circulation.
   ii. **Emulsion instability theory:** Fat emboli are formed by aggregation of plasma lipids (chylomicrons and fatty acids) due to disturbance in natural emulsification of fat.
   iii. **Intravascular coagulation theory:** In stress, release of some factor activates DIC and aggregation of fat emboli.
   iv. **Toxic injury theory:** Small blood vessels of lungs are chemically injured by high plasma levels of free fatty acid, resulting in increased vascular permeability and consequent pulmonary edema.
   Consequences: Its consequences are:
   • Pulmonary fat embolism.
   • Systemic fat embolism: a. Brain—petechial hemorrhages. b. Kidney—tubular damage and renal insufficiency.

5. **Gas embolism** Air, nitrogen and other gases can produce bubbles within the circulation and obstruct the blood vessels causing damage to tissue. Two main forms of gas embolism are—air embolism and decompression sickness.

Q. 5. Write a short note on disseminated intravascular coagulation *(HP Uni., April 2019)*

Ans. Disseminated intravascular coagulation (DIC)/ **defibrination syndrome/consumption coagulopathy,** is a complex thrombo-hemorrhagic disorder occurring as a secondary complication in some systemic diseases.

Etiology

1. **Massive tissue injury:** In obstetrical syndromes, metastatic malignancies.
2. **Infections:** Endotoxaemia, septicemia, certain viral infections, malaria, etc.
3. **Widespread endothelial damage:** In severe burns, acute glomerulonephritis.
4. **Miscellaneous:** Snake bite, shock, acute intravascular haemolysis, heat stroke.

Pathogenesis

1. **Activation of coagulation:** Etiologic factors initiate widespread activation of coagulation pathway by release of tissue factor.
2. **Thrombotic phase:** Endothelial damage from various thrombogenic stimuli causes generalized platelet aggregation and adhesion with resultant deposition of small thrombi and emboli throughout microvasculature.
3. **Consumption phase:** Early thrombotic phase is followed by phase of consumption of coagulation factors and platelets.
4. **Secondary fibrinolysis:** As a protective mechanism, fibrinolytic system is secondarily activated at the site of intravascular coagulation, resulting formation of FSPs in circulation.

Clinical features: Bleeding (most common), organ damage, haemolytic anemia, thrombosis in larger arteries and veins.

Laboratory investigations

1. Platelet count is low.
2. Blood film: Features of microangiopathic hemolytic anaemia, schistocytes, fragmented RBCs.
3. Prothrombin time, thrombin time and activated partial thromboplastin time, are prolonged.
4. Plasma fibrinogen levels are reduced and FSPs are raised.

5. NEOPLASM

Q. 1. Define neoplasia. How does benign neoplasia differ from malignant neoplasia? Discuss in detail the various carcinogens with special reference to oral carcinoma.

(Bangalore Uni., Jan. 1992; TNMGR, Sept. 2010)

Ans. Neoplasia means "new growth," and a new growth is called a neoplasm. "A neoplasm is an abnormal mass of tissue, the growth of which exceeds and is uncoordinated with that of the normal tissues and persists in the same excessive manner after cessation of the stimuli which evoked the change" (by Willis).

All tumors have two basic components: Neoplastic cells that constitute the tumor parenchyma and reactive stroma made up of connective tissue, blood vessels, and variable numbers of cells of adaptive and innate immune system.

- **Benign tumors:** A tumor is said to be benign when its gross and microscopic appearances are considered relatively innocent, implying that it will remain localized, will not spread to other sites, and is amenable to local surgical removal.
- **Malignant tumors:** Malignant tumors can invade and destroy adjacent structures and spread to distant sites (metastasize) to cause death. Malignant tumors arising in mesenchymal tissues are usually called **sarcomas,** whereas those arising from blood-forming cells are designated **leukemias** or **lymphomas.** Malignant neoplasms of epithelial cell origin are called **carcinomas.**
- **Teratoma:** These tumors are made up of a mixture of various tissue types arising from totipotent cells derived from the three germ cell layers.
- **Blastomas (embryomas):** Group of malignant tumors which arise from embryonal or partially differentiated cells which would normally form blastoma of organs and tissue during embryogenesis.
- **Hamartoma:** Hamartoma is benign tumour which is made of mature but disorganized cells of tissues indigenous to particular organ.
- **Choristoma:** Choristoma is the ectopic islands of normal tissue.

Characteristics of tumors

I. Rate of growth: Tumour cells generally proliferate more rapidly than normal cells. It depends on:

- **Rate of cell production, growth fraction** (number of cells remaining in proliferative pool) and rate of loss of tumour cells by cell shedding.
- Rate of growth of malignant tumour is directly proportionate to degree of differentiation. Poorly

differentiated tumors show aggressive growth pattern as compared to better differentiated tumors.

II. Cancer phenotype and stem cells: Normal cells are socially desirable. However, cancer cells exhibit antisocial behavior as under:

i. Cancer cells disobey growth controlling signals in the body and thus proliferate rapidly.

ii. Cancer cells escape death signals and achieve immortality.

iii. Cancer cells lose properties of differentiation and thus perform little or no function.

iv. Cancer cells overrun their neighboring tissue and invade locally.

v. Cancer cells have the ability to travel from site of origin to other sites in the body.

Cancer cells arise from the stem cells normally present in the tissues in small number and are not readily identifiable. These stem cells have the properties of prolonged self-renewal, asymmetric replication and transdifferentiation (tumour-initiating cells).

III. Clinical and gross features (*TNMGR, Nov. 1995*): **Clinically,** benign tumors are generally slow growing, may remain asymptomatic or may produce serious symptoms. Malignant tumors grow rapidly, may ulcerate on the surface, invade locally into deeper tissues, may spread to distant sites, and also produce systemic features. In fact, two of the cardinal clinical features of malignant tumors are: Invasiveness and metastasis.

Gross appearance of almost all tumors compared to neighboring normal tissue of origin—they have a different colour, texture and consistency. Sarcomas typically have fish-flesh like consistency while carcinomas are generally firm.

IV. Microscopic features

1. Microscopic pattern: Tumour cells may be arranged in a variety of different patterns as:
   - Epithelial tumors generally consist of acini, sheets, columns or cords of epithelial cells arranged in solid or papillary pattern.
   - Mesenchymal tumors have mesenchymal tumour cells arranged as interlacing bundles, fasicles or whorls, lying separated from each other by intercellular matrix substance.
   - Hematopoietic tumors have no or little stromal support.
   - Generally, most benign tumors and low grade malignant tumors reduplicate the normal structure of origin more closely, however, anaplastic tumors differ greatly from the arrangement in normal tissue of origin of tumour.

2. **Cytomorphology of neoplastic cells:** The neoplastic cell is characterized by morphologic and functional alterations such as:

   - **Differentiation** is defined as the extent to which neoplastic parenchymal cells resemble the corresponding normal parenchymal cells, both morphologically and functionally. If the deviation of neoplastic cell in structure and function is minimal as compared to normal cell, tumour is described as 'well-differentiated'. 'Poorly differentiated', 'undifferentiated' or 'dedifferentiated' are synonymous terms for poor structural and functional resemblance to corresponding normal cell.

   - **Anaplasia** is lack of differentiation and is a characteristic feature of most malignant tumors. Depending upon the degree of differentiation, the extent of anaplasia is also variable, i.e. poorly differentiated malignant tumors have high degree of anaplasia.

   In general, benign tumors are well differentiated. In contrast, malignant neoplasms exhibit a wide range of parenchymal cell differentiation. Malignant neoplasms that are composed of poorly differentiated cells are said to be **anaplastic**. Lack of differentiation or anaplasia (**hallmark of malignancy**) is associated with many other morphologic changes. These are:

   i. **Loss of polarity:** Normally, nuclei of epithelial cells are oriented along the basement membrane (basal polarity). Early in malignancy, tumour cells lose their basal polarity.

   ii. Pleomorphism: Extent of cellular pleomorphism generally correlates with degree of anaplasia.

   iii. N : C ratio: Nucleocytoplasmic ratio is increased from normal 1:5 to 1:1 in malignant cells.

   iv. Anisonucleosis: Variation in size and shape of nuclei in malignant tumour cells.

   v. Hyperchromatism: Nuclear chromatin of malignant cell is increased and coarsely clumped, resulting in hyperchromatism.

   vi. Nucleolar changes: Malignant cells frequently have a prominent nucleolus or nucleoli in the nucleus reflecting increased nucleoprotein synthesis. This may be demonstrated as Nucleolar Organiser Region (NOR) by silver (Ag) staining.

   vii. Mitotic figures: Parenchymal cells of poorly differentiated tumors often show large number of mitoses as atypical mitotic figures (tripolar, quadripolar and multipolar spindles).

viii. Tumour giant cells: Multinucleate tumour giant cells or giant cells containing a single large and bizarre nucleus, possessing nuclear characters of adjacent tumour cells are important feature of anaplasia.

ix. Functional (cytoplasmic) changes: Functional anaplasia in neoplasms may be quantitative, qualitative, or both, e.g. absence of keratin in anaplastic squamous cell carcinoma.

x. Chromosomal abnormalities: All tumour cells have abnormal genetic composition and on division they transmit genetic abnormality to their progeny, e.g. presence of Philadelphia chromosome in CML.

3. **Tumour angiogenesis and stroma**

- In order to provide nourishment to growing tumour, new blood vessels are formed from pre-existing ones (**tumor angiogenesis**), under the influence of angiogenic factors elaborated by tumour cells, e.g. VEGF.
- Growth of fibrous tissue in tumour is stimulated by basic fibroblast growth factor (bFGF) elaborated by tumour cells.
- If collagenous tissue in tumour stroma is scanty, then the tumour is soft and fleshy.
- If collagenous tissue in tumour stroma is excessive, then the tumour is hard and gritty.
- If the epithelial tumour is almost entirely composed of parenchymal cells, it is called medullary.
- If there is excessive connective tissue stroma in the epithelial tumour, it is called **desmoplasia** and the tumour is hard or scirrhous.

4. **Inflammatory reaction:** Prominent inflammatory reaction may be present in and around the tumors, which may be acute, chronic or granulomatous.

V. Local invasion (direct spread)

- **Benign tumors:** Most benign tumors expand and push aside the surrounding normal tissues without actually invading, infiltrating or metastasizing.
- **Malignant tumors:** Malignant tumors are characterized by invasion, infiltration and destruction of surrounding tissue.

VI. Metastasis (distant spread):
Metastasis is defined as spread of tumour by invasion in such a way that discontinuous secondary tumour mass/masses are formed at the site of lodgment. Benign tumors do not metastasize while all malignant tumors (exception: gliomas of CNS, basal cell carcinoma of skin) can metastasize.

Routes of metastasis/spread of tumors (BFUHS, May 2008; HNBG Uni., June 2016; BBD Uni., April 2018; NTR Uni., May 2019):

1. **Lymphatic spread:** In general, carcinomas metastasize by lymphatic route while sarcomas metastasize by hematogenous route. The involvement of lymph nodes by malignant cells may be of two forms:

   i. Lymphatic permeation: The walls of lymphatics are readily invaded by cancer cells and may form a continuous growth in the lymphatic channels.

   ii. Lymphatic emboli: Alternatively, malignant cells may detach to form tumour emboli so as to be carried along the lymph to next draining lymph node. The tumour emboli enter lymph node at its convex surface and are lodged in the subcapsular sinus where they start growing. Generally, regional lymph nodes draining the tumour are invariably involved producing regional nodal metastasis.

   Skip metastasis: It is escape of neighboring/nearest lymph nodes of tumour from lymphatic metastases because of venous-lymphatic anastomoses or due to obliteration of lymphatics by inflammation or radiation. **Retrograde metastasis:** Spread of tumor cells against the flow of lymph due to disturbance in lymph flow caused by obstruction of lymphatics by tumour cells, resulting in metastases at unusual sites, e.g. metastasis of carcinoma prostate to supraclavicular lymph nodes.

   Virchow's lymph node is nodal metastasis preferentially to supraclavicular lymph node from cancers of abdominal organs, e.g. cancer stomach, colon, and gall bladder.

2. **Hematogenous spread:** Blood-borne metastasis is the common route for sarcomas but certain carcinomas also frequently metastasize. The sites where blood-borne metastasis commonly occurs are: Liver, lungs, brain, bones, kidney and adrenals, all of which provide 'good soil' for the growth of 'good seeds' (**seed-soil theory**). In general, only a proportion of cancer cells are capable of clonal proliferation in the proper environment; others die without establishing a metastasis. Arterial spread of tumors is less likely because they are thick-walled and contain elastic tissue which is resistant to invasion.

3. **Other routes of spread**

   i. **Transcoelomic spread:** This is spread of tumor cells through serosal wall of coelomic cavity along with coelomic fluid; peritoneal cavity is involved most commonly, e.g. carcinoma of stomach seeding to both ovaries (**Krukenberg tumour**).

ii. **Spread along epithelium-lined surfaces:** In some exception cases, malignant tumour spread along the epithelium-lined surfaces, e.g. through bronchus into alveoli.

iii. **Spread via CSF:** Malignant tumour of ependyma and leptomeninges.

iv. **Implantation:** By surgeon's scalpel, needles, sutures, or may be implanted by direct contact.

Differences between benign and malignant tumors (Table 5.1).

Q. 2. Write a short note on carcinogenesis.
(TNMGR, March 2010; RGUHS, Oct. 2010; UHSR, April 2015; NTR Uni., May 2019)

Q. List the steps from tumor inception to macrometastases.
(TNMGR, 2011)

Ans. Carcinogenesis/oncogenesis/tumorigenesis is a complex, multi-step process in which genetic events within signal transduction pathways are subverted/altered resulting enhance to cell's ability for proliferation, uncontrolled apoptosis or grow by invading locally or metastasizing to distant sites. It means mechanism of induction of tumors; agents which can induce tumors are called carcinogens. The etiology and pathogenesis of cancer includes:

A. Molecular pathogenesis of cancer (genetic mechanisms of cancer) (Fig. 5.2): The general concept of molecular mechanisms of cancer:

1. **Monoclonality of tumors:** There is strong evidence to support that most human cancers arise from a single clone of cells by genetic transformation or mutation, e.g. in multiple myeloma there is production of a single type of Ig or its chain.

2. **Field theory of cancer:** In an organ developing cancer, only limited number of cells grows into cancer after undergoing sequence of changes under the influence of etiologic agents. This is termed 'field effect' and the concept called **Field Theory of Cancer.**

3. **Multi-step process of cancer growth and progression** (Flowchart 5.2): Carcinogenesis is a gradual multi-step process involving many generations of cells. The various causes may act on the cell one after another (**multi-hit process**). The same process is also involved in further progression of tumour. Ultimately, the cells so formed are genetically and phenotypically transformed cells having phenotypic features of malignancy.

4. **Genetic theory of cancer:** In cancer, there are either genetic abnormalities in cell, or there are normal genes with abnormal expression. The abnormalities in genetic composition may be from inherited or induced mutations. The mutated cells transmit their

Table 5.1: Differences between benign and malignant tumors

Features	Benign	Malignant
I. Clinical and gross features		
Boundaries	Well-circumscribed	Poorly circumscribed
Surrounding tissue	Often compressed	Usually invaded
Size	Usually small	Often larger
Secondary changes	Less often	More often
II. Microscopic features		
Pattern	Usually resembles the tissue of origin closely	Poor resemblance to tissue of origin
Basal polarity	Retained	Often lost
Pleomorphism	Usually not present	Often present
Nucleo-cytoplasmic ratio	Normal	Increased
Anisonucleosis	Absent	Present
Hyperchromatism	Absent	Present
Mitoses	May be present but are always typical mitoses	Increased mitotic figure, atypical and abnormal
Tumour giant cells	May be present but without nuclear atypia	Present with nuclear atypia
Chromosomal abnormalities	Infrequent	Present
Function	Usually well maintained	May be retained, lost or become abnormal
III. Growth rate	Usually slow	Usually rapid
IV. Local invasion	Often compresses the surrounding tissues without invading or infiltrating them	Infiltrates and invades the adjacent tissues
V. Metastasis	Absent	Present
VI. Prognosis	Local complications	Death by local and metastatic complications

characters to next progeny of cells and result in cancer.

5. **Genetic regulators of normal and abnormal mitosis: In normal cell growth**, there are 4 regulatory genes:
   - **Proto-oncogenes** are growth-promoting genes, i.e. they encode for cell proliferation pathway.
   - **Anti-oncogenes** are growth-inhibiting or growth suppressor genes.
   - **Apoptosis** regulatory genes control programmed cell death.
   - **DNA repair genes** regulate the repair of DNA damage that has occurred during mitosis and also control the damage to proto-oncogenes and anti-oncogenes.

   In cancer, the transformed cells are produced by abnormal cell growth due to genetic damage to these normal controlling genes. Thus, corresponding abnormalities in these 4 cell regulatory genes are:
   - Activation of growth-promoting oncogenes causing transformation of cell. Mutant form of normal proto-oncogene in cancer is termed **oncogene**.
   - Inactivation of cancer-suppressor genes.
   - Abnormal apoptosis regulatory genes which may act as oncogenes or anti-oncogenes.
   - Failure of DNA repairs genes results in mutations (Flowchart 5.2).

B. Chemical carcinogenesis and carcinogens *(Nagpur Uni., Oct. 2004)*: Basic mechanism of chemical carcinogenesis is by induction of mutation in the proto-oncogenes and antioncogenes.

Stages in chemical carcinogenesis

1. **Initiation of carcinogenesis:** Initiation of carcinogenesis is done by initiator chemical carcinogens, either by a single dose of initiating agent for a short time or larger dose for longer duration (more effective). The change so induced is sudden, irreversible and permanent. It involves:

   a. **Metabolic activation:** Indirect-acting carcinogens are activated in liver by mono-oxygenases of cytochrome P-450 system in endoplasmic reticulum. In some circumstances, pro-carcinogen may be detoxified and rendered inactive metabolically.

   b. **Reactive electrophiles:** While direct-acting carcinogens are intrinsically electrophilic, indirect-acting substances become electron-deficient after metabolic activation, i.e. they become reactive electrophiles, which binds to DNA, RNA and other proteins.

   c. **Target molecules:** The primary target of electrophiles is DNA, producing mutagenesis. The change in DNA may lead to 'initiated cell' or some form of cellular enzymes may be able to repair the damage in DNA.

   d. **The initiated cell:** The unrepaired damage produced in DNA of the cell becomes permanent and fixed only if the altered cell undergoes at least one cycle of proliferation. This results in transferring the change to next progeny of cells so that the DNA damage becomes permanent and irreversible, which are the characteristics of initiated

Flowchart 5.2: Mechanism of molecular carcinogenesis

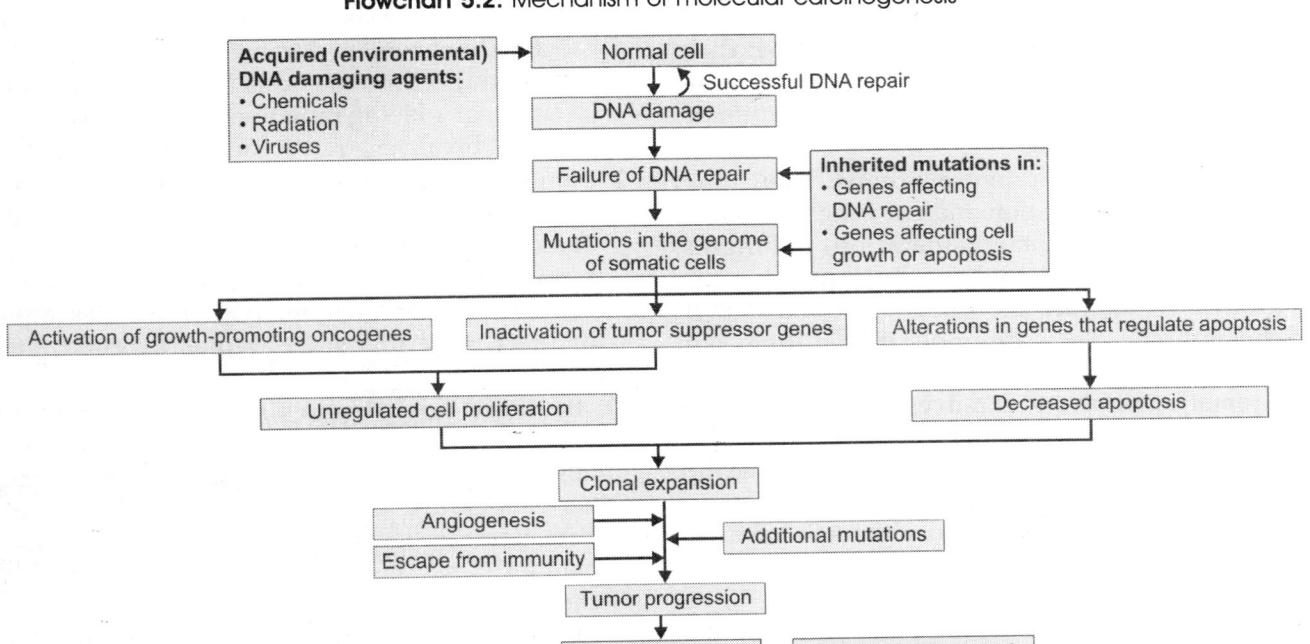

cell, vulnerable to the action of promoters of carcinogenesis.

2. **Promotion of carcinogenesis:** Promoters of carcinogenesis do not damage the DNA *per se* but instead enhance the effect of direct-acting carcinogens or procarcinogens. They do not produce sudden change and require application for sufficient time and in sufficient dose. Tumour promoters act by further clonal proliferation and expansion of initiated (mutated) cells, and have reduced requirement of growth factor.

3. **Progression of carcinogenesis:** Progression of cancer is the stage when mutated proliferated cell shows phenotypic features of malignancy, when the initiated cell starts to proliferate rapidly and acquires more and more mutations.

   • **Carcinogenic chemicals in humans:** Depending upon the mode of action of carcinogenic chemicals, they are:

I. Initiator carcinogens: Chemical carcinogens which can initiate the process of neoplastic transformation:

1. **Direct acting carcinogens:** These are chemical substances which can induce cellular transformation without undergoing any prior metabolic activation. Examples:

   a. **Alkylating agents:** This group includes mainly various anti-cancer drugs (e.g. cyclophosphamide, chlorambucil, etc). They are weakly carcinogenic and are implicated in the etiology of lymphomas and leukemias.

   b. **Acylating agents:** Acetyl imidazole and dimethyl carbamyl chloride.

2. **Indirect acting carcinogens (pro-carcinogens):** These are chemical substances which require prior metabolic activation before becoming potent 'ultimate' carcinogens. It includes:

   a. **Polycyclic aromatic hydrocarbons:** Their main sources are combustion and chewing of tobacco, smoke, fossil fuel, tar, mineral oil, pollutants. Important chemical compounds included in this group are: Anthracenes, benzapyrene and methylcholanthrene. They are implicated in lung, skin cancer and cancer of upper aerodigestive tract.

   b. **Aromatic amines and azo-dyes:** β-naphthylamine, aniline dye and rubber industry workers, benzidine (bladder cancer); Azo-dyes used for colouring foods (hepatocellular cancer).

   c. **Naturally-occurring products:** Aflatoxin B_1 (hepatocellular carcinoma), actinomycin D, mitomycin C, and betel nuts.

   d. **Miscellaneous:** Nitrosamines and nitrosamides (gastric carcinoma), vinyl chloride monomer (hemangisarcoma of liver), asbestos (bronchogenic carcinoma), metals like nickel, lead (lung cancer), insecticides and fungicides, saccharin and cyclomates.

II. Promoter carcinogens: Promoters are chemical substances which lack the intrinsic carcinogenic potential but their application subsequent to initiator exposure helps the initiated cell to proliferate further. These substances include phorbol esters, phenols, certain hormones and drugs, miscellaneous (dietary fat, cigarette smoke, viral infections, etc.)

C. Physical carcinogenesis: Physical agents in carcinogenesis are divided into 2 groups:

1. **Radiation carcinogenesis:** Ultraviolet (UV) light and ionizing radiations are two main forms of radiation carcinogens which can induce cancer. In both, appearance of mutations is followed by a long period of latency (10–20 years or more) after initial exposure. Also, radiation carcinogens may act to enhance the effect of another carcinogen (co-carcinogens) and may have sequential stages of initiation, promotion and progression in their evolution.

   • Most important biochemical effect of UV radiation is formation of pyrimidine dimers in DNA. Such UV-induced DNA damage in normal individuals is repaired, while in predisposed persons such damage remain unrepaired UV radiation also induces mutated forms of oncogenes and anti-oncogenes.

   • Ionising radiation of all kinds like X-rays, α-, β- and γ-rays, radioactive isotopes, protons and neutrons can cause cancer in animals and in man. The risk is increased by higher dose and with high LET (linear energy transfer). Damage to DNA resulting in mutagenesis is the most important action of ionizing radiation. It may cause chromosomal breakage, translocation, or point mutation.

2. **Non-radiation physical carcinogenesis:** Mechanical injury to tissues such as from stones in gallbladder, stones in urinary tract, and healed scars following burns or trauma, has been suggested as the cause of increased risk of carcinoma. Other includes implants of inert materials such as plastic, glass, etc. in prostheses.

D. Biologic carcinogenesis: The epidemiological studies indicate the involvement of transmissible biologic agents in their development, chiefly viruses. Other biologic agents implicated in carcinogenesis are:

• **Parasites:** *Schistosoma haematobium* → SCC of urinary bladder; *Clonorchis sinensis* (liver fluke) → cholangiocarcinoma.

• **Fungus:** *Aspergillus flavus* → hepatocellular carcinoma.

- Bacteria: *Helicobacter pylori* → gastric lymphoma and carcinoma,
- Viruses and human cancer *(TNMGR, April 2012)*: Based on their nucleic acid content, oncogenic viruses can be: DNA oncogenic viruses and RNA oncogenic viruses or retroviruses. Both types of oncogenic viruses usually have 3 genes:
  i. Gag gene: Codes for group antigen.
  ii. Pol gene: Codes for polymerase enzyme.
  iii. Env gene: Codes for envelope protein.

1. **Mode of DNA viral oncogenesis:** Host cells infected by DNA oncogenic viruses may have following results:
  i. Replication: Virus may replicate in host cell with consequent lysis of infected cell and release of virions. This causes cell death only.
  ii. Integration: Viral DNA may integrate into host cell DNA. This results in inducing mutation and neoplastic transformation of host cell.

■ Specific DNA oncogenic viruses
A. Papovaviruses
- **Papilloma virus:** Human wart (papilloma)—HPV 1, 2, 4, 7; Genital warts (condyloma acuminata)—HPV 6, 11; Invasive cervical cancer/oral cancer—HPV 16, 18, 31, 45.
- **Polyomavirus:** Various cancers in animals, no cancer in human.
- **SV-40 virus:** Sarcoma in hamsters.

B. Herpesviruses: EBV—Burkitt's lymphoma, nasopharyngeal carcinoma, post-transplant lymphoproliferative disease, Hodgkin's lymphoma; HHV 8—Kaposi's sarcoma.

C. Adenoviruses: Sarcomas in hamsters.

D. Poxviruses: Molluscum contagiosum and squamous cell papilloma.

E. Hepadnaviruses: HBV—Hepatocellular carcinoma

2. **Mode of RNA viral oncogenesis:** RNA viruses contain two identical strands of RNA and reverse transcriptase:
  i. Reverse transcriptase is RNA-dependent DNA synthetase that acts as a template to synthesize a single strand of matching viral DNA.
  ii. Single strand of viral DNA is then copied by DNA dependent DNA synthetase to form another strand of complementary DNA resulting in double-stranded viral DNA or provirus.
  iii. Provirus is then integrated into DNA of host cell genome and may induce mutation and thus transform the cell into neoplastic cell.

■ Specific RNA oncogenic viruses
A. Acute transforming viruses: This group includes retroviruses which transform cells infected by them into malignant cells rapidly.

B. Slow transforming viruses: These oncogenic retroviruses cause development of leukemias and lymphomas in different species of animals.

C. Human T cell lymphotropic viruses (HTLV): HTLV is a form of slow transforming virus. This is the only retrovirus implicated in human cancer. Four types of HTLVs are recognized—HTLV-I, HTLV-II, HTLV-III and HTLV-IV. HTLV-I: Cutaneous adult-T cell leukemia-lymphoma (ATLL); HTLV-II: T cell variant of hairy cell leukemia.

D. HCV: Hepatocellular carcinoma.

Q. 3. Write a short note on proto-oncogenes.
(TNMGR, March 2010)

Ans. Proto-oncogenes are growth-promoting genes, i.e. they encode for cell proliferation pathway. In cancer, the transformed cells are produced by abnormal cell growth due to genetic damage to these normal controlling genes. Mutated form of normal proto-oncogene in cancer is called **oncogenes**. Proto-oncogene becomes activated oncogenes by:
  i. By mutation in proto-oncogene which alters its structure and function.
  ii. By retroviral insertion in host cell.
  iii. By damage to DNA sequence that normally regulates growth-promoting signals of proto-oncogene resulting in its abnormal activation.
  iv. Over activity of oncogenes enhances cell proliferation and promotes development of human cancer.

  Transformation of proto-oncogene to oncogenes may occur by:
  i. Point mutations, i.e. an alteration of a single base in DNA chain.
  ii. Chromosomal translocations, i.e. transfer of a portion of one chromosome carrying proto-oncogene to another chromosome and making it independent of growth controls.
  iii. Gene amplification, i.e. increasing the number of copies of DNA sequence in protooncogene leading to increased mDNA and thus increased or over-expressed gene product.

Classification of oncogenes (proto-oncogenes in bracket) with associated human tumors
A. Growth factors
  i. PDGF-β (SIS): Gliomas, sarcomas.
  ii. TGF-α (RAS): Carcinomas, sarcomas.

iii. FGF (HST-1): Bowel cancer; INT-2: Breast cancer.

iv. HGF (HGF): Follicular carcinoma of thyroid.

B. Receptors for growth factors

i. EGF receptors (ERB B1): SCC of lung; (ERB B2): Carcinoma of breast, ovary.

ii. c-KIT receptor (c-KIT): Gastrointestinal stromal tumour.

iii. RET receptor (RET): MEN type 2A, 2B, medullary carcinoma of thyroid.

C. Cytoplasmic signal transduction proteins

i. GTP-bound (RAS): Carcinoma of lungs, colon, pancreas.

ii. Non-receptor tyrosine kinase (BCR-ABL): CML, acute leukemias.

D. Nuclear transcription factors

i. C-MYC (MYC): Burkitt's lymphoma.

ii. N-MYC (MYC): Neuroblastoma, small cell carcinoma of lung.

iii. L-MYC (MYC): Small cell carcinoma of lung.

E. Cell cycle regulatory proteins

i. Cyclins (Cyclin D): Carcinoma breast, liver, mantle cell lymphoma; (Cyclin E): Carcinoma breast.

ii. CDKs (CDK4): Glioblastoma, sarcomas.

Q. 4. Write a note on cancer suppressor genes.
(TNMGR, March 2007, 2008)

Ans. The mutation of normal growth suppressor anti-oncogenes results in removal of the brakes for growth; thus the inhibitory effect to cell growth is removed and the abnormal growth continues unchecked. In other words, mutated antioncogenes behave like growth-promoting oncogenes. The mechanisms of loss of tumour suppressor actions of genes are due to chromosomal deletions, point mutations and loss of portions of chromosomes.

Major anti-oncogenes/tumour suppressor genes implicated in human cancers are:

1. RB: Retinoblastoma, osteosarcoma.
2. P53 (TP53): Most human cancers, carcinoma of lung, head and neck, colon, breast.
3. TGF-β and its receptor: Carcinoma pancreas, colon, stomach.
4. APC and β-catenin proteins: Carcinoma colon.
5. Others:
   i. BRCA 1 and 2: Carcinoma breast, ovary.
   ii. VHL: Renal cell carcinoma.
   iii. WT 1 and 2: Wilms' tumor.
   iv. NF 1 and 2: Neurofibromatosis type 1 and 2.

Q. 5. Write a short note on tumour markers.
(MUHS, May 2015, AHSUC, May 2018)

Ans. Tumour markers are biochemical assays of products elaborated by tumour cells in blood or other body fluids. Ideally, it should be highly specific and sensitive and should provide a lead time over clinical diagnosis.

Uses

- Screening and estimating risk of developing cancer
- Differential diagnosis and determining prognosis of disease
- Predict response to therapy or progression in metastatic disease.
- Monitor for disease recurrence.

Methods of detection: Serology (enzyme assays); Immunological (immunohistochemistry, ELISA); Flow cytometry cytogenetic analysis (fluorescent *in situ* hybridization, spectral karyotyping, comparative genomic hybridization); Genetic analysis sequencing (reverse transcription gel electrophoresis, DNA microarray analysis); Proteomics (surface-enhanced laser desorption/ionization).

Classification: Tumour markers include:

1. Cell surface antigens/oncofoetal antigens:
   i. Alpha-fetoprotein (AFP): Hepatocellular carcinoma.
   ii. Carcinoembryonic antigen (CEA): Cancer of bowel, pancreas, breast.
2. Enzymes:
   i. Prostate acid phosphatase: Prostatic carcinoma.
   ii. Neuron-specific enolase: Neuroblastoma.
   iii. Lactic dehydrogenase (LDH): Lymphoma, Ewing's sarcoma.
3. Hormones:
   i. Human chorionic gonadotropin: Trophoblastic tumors.
   ii. Calcitonin: Medullary carcinoma thyroid.
   iii. Catecholamines and vanillylmandelic acid: Neuroblastoma, pheochromocytoma.
   iv. Ectopic hormone production: Paraneoplastic syndromes.
4. Cancer associated proteins:
   i. CA-125: Ovary.
   ii. CA 15-3: Breast.
   iii. CA 19-9: Colon, pancreas, breast.
   iv. CD30: Hodgkin's disease.
   v. CD25: Hairy cell leukaemia, adult T cell leukaemia/lymphoma.
   vi. Monoclonal immunoglobulins: Multiple myeloma, other gammopathies.
   vii. Prostate-specific antigen: Prostate carcinoma.

Q. 6. Write a note on grading and staging of tumors.
(TNMGR, March 2011;
PAHER, April, 2013; HP Uni., April 2019)

Ans. Grading is defined as the gross and microscopic degree of differentiation of tumour, while **staging** means extent of spread of the tumour within the patient. Thus, grading is histologic while staging is clinical.

Grading: Cancers may be graded grossly and microscopically. Gross features like exophytic or fungating appearance are indicative of less malignant growth than diffusely infiltrating tumors. However, grading is largely based on 2 important histologic features: Degree of anaplasia, and rate of growth. Based on these features, cancers are categorized from grade I as the most differentiated, to grade III or IV as the most undifferentiated or anaplastic. Broders' grading is as under:

Grade I: Well-differentiated (<25% anaplastic cells, low grade).

Grade II: Moderately-differentiated (25–50% anaplastic cells, intermediate grade).

Grade III: Moderately-differentiated (50–75% anaplastic cells, intermediate grade).

Grade IV: Poorly-differentiated or anaplastic (>75% anaplastic cells, high grade).

This is reported as: Gx: Grade cannot be assessed; G1: Well-differentiated; G2: Moderately-differentiated; G3: Poorly-differentiated; G4: Undifferentiated.

Drawback

1. It is subjective.
2. The degree of differentiation may vary from one area of tumour to other. Because of this focal variation in the degree of differentiation, the grade assigned to a small biopsy of a tumor may not always be representative of the whole neoplasm.
3. Grading has no prognostic value in some cancers.
4. Grading of salivary gland malignancies is not standardized.

Staging: The extent of spread of cancers can be assessed by 3 ways—by clinical examination, by investigations, and by pathologic examination of the tissue removed.

Clinical staging: It is based on physical examination, radiographs, and other imaging procedures.

Pathological staging: It takes into account information obtained during a surgical procedure. It includes histologic examination of all tissues removed during surgery.

Two important staging systems currently followed are: TNM staging and AJC staging.

TNM staging *(RUHS, May 2018):* (T for primary tumour, N for regional nodal involvement, and M for distant metastases) was developed by the AJCC/UICC (Americal Joint Committee on cancer/Union Internationale Centre Cancer, Geneva). For each of the 3 components, namely T, N and M, numbers are added to indicate the extent of involvement, as under *(AJCC 8th Edition, 2017)*:

T: Primary tumor
Tx: Primary tumour cannot be assessed.
T0: No evidence of primary tumour.
Tis: Carcinoma in situ.
T1: Tumor size $\leq$2 cm, depth of invasion (DOI) $\leq$5 mm.
T2: Tumor size $\leq$2 cm, DOI >5 mm, and $\geq$10 mm or tumor size >2 cm but $\leq$4 cm and DOI $\leq$10 mm.
T3: Tumor size >4 cm or DOI >10 mm, but $\leq$20 mm.
T4a: Moderately advanced local disease: (Lip) Tumor invades through cortical bone or involves inferior alveolar nerve, floor of mouth, or skin of face (oral cavity). Tumor involves adjacent structures such as cortical bone of maxilla or mandible, maxillary sinus or skin of face, or extensive tumors with bilatarel tongue involvement and/or DOI >20 mm.
T4b: Very advanced local disease; tumor invades masticator space, pterygoid plates, skull base, and/or encases the internal carotid artery.

N: Regional lymph nodes
Nx: Regional lymph nodes cannot be assessed.
N0: No Regional lymph nodes.
N1: Metastases to single lymph node, 3 cm or less in greatest diameter; node must be extranodal extension negative.
N2a: Metastases to single ipsilateral node >3 cm but not >6 cm; Node must be extranodal extension negative or single ipsilateral or node 3 cm or smaller with extranodal extension.
N2b: Metastases to multiple ipsilateral nodes >3 cm but not >6 cm; Nodes must be extranodal extension negative.
N2c: Metastases to bilateral nodes or contralateral nodes none >6 cm; Nodes must be extranodal extension negative.
N3a: Metastases to nodes >6 cm but extranodal extension negative.
N3b: Single ipsilateral node >3 cm in greatest dimension with extranodal extension, Or multiple ipsilateral, contralateral, or bilateral nodes, any with extranodal extension, Or single contralateral node 3 cm or smaller and with extranodal extension.

M: Distant metastasis
Mx: Distant metastasis cannot be assessed.
M0: No distant metastasis.
M1: Distant metastasis.

Stage grouping
Stage 0: Tis N0 M0
Stage I: T1 N0 M0

Table 5.7: Mechanisms of immune surveillance

Target gene	Target/effector cell	Tumour formation
TCR J alpha 281	NKT	MCA-induced sarcoma
TCR delta	Gamma delta T	MCA-induced sarcoma
		DMBA-induced skin tumour
TCR beta	Alpha beta T	MCA-induced sarcoma
TCR beta/TCR delta	T/gamma delta T	Reduced latency
IFN-gamma	IFN-gamma	MCA-induced sarcoma
		Spontaneous lymphoma
		Lung adenocarcinoma
Stat 1	IFK-gamma R-signalling	MCA-induced sarcoma
Perforin	CTL/NK	MCA-induced sarcoma
		Spontaneous lymphoma
		TPA/DMBA-induced sarcoma
RAG-2/Stat 1	T/B/NKT/IFN-signalling	MCA-induced sarcoma
IFNGR1 or Stat 1/p53	IFN-gamma R-signalling/tumour susceptibility	More rapid tumour formation/wider tumour spectrum
Perforin/p53 lymphoma	CTL/NK/tumour susceptibility	Enhances susceptibility to lymphoma

TCR: T cell receptor; IFN: Interferon; Stat 1: Signal transducers and activators of transcription 1; NKT: Natural killer T cell; IFNGR: Interferon gamma receptor; CTL: Cytotoxic T lymphocyte; NK: Natural killer; MCA: Methylcholanthrene; TPA: 12-O-tetradecanoylphorbol-13-acetate; DMBA: 7, 12-dimethylbenzanthracene.

Stage II: T2 N0 M0

Stage III: T1, T2 N1 M0; T3 N0, N1 M0

Stage IVA: T1, T2, T3 N2 M0; T4a N0, N1, N2, M0

Stage IVB: Any T N3 M0; T4b any N M0

Stage IVC: Any T any N M1

AJC staging: American Joint Committee staging divides all cancers into stage 0 to IV, and takes into account all the 3 components of preceding system (primary tumour, nodal involvement and distant metastases) in each stage. TNM and AJC staging systems can be applied for staging most malignant tumors.

Significance of staging: 1. Tumor burden increases and curability decreases with increasing stage, 2. Staging serves to estimate chances of survival in individual patient, 3. It helps to compare results of treatment in different institutions.

Drawback of staging: Certain tumors cannot be grouped on the basis of anatomic considerations. For example, hematopoietic tumors such as leukemia, myeloma, and lymphoma are often disseminated at presentation and do not spread like solid tumors.

Q. 7. Write about immune surveillance against cancer. *(TNMGR, Oct. 1996)*

Ans. Cancer immune surveillance is considered to be an important host protection process to inhibit carcinogenesis and to maintain cellular homeostasis. In the interaction of host and tumour cells, three essential phases have been proposed: Elimination, equilibrium and escape ('3E'). Several immune effector cells and secreted cytokines play a critical role in pursuing each process. Nascent transformed cells can initially be eliminated by an innate immune response such as by natural killer cells. During tumour progression, even though an adaptive immune response can be provoked by antigen-specific T cells, immune selection produces tumour cell variants that lose MHC I and II antigens and decreases amounts of tumour antigens in the equilibrium phase. Furthermore, tumour-derived soluble factors facilitate the escape from immune attack, allowing progression and metastasis.

Mechanisms of immune surveillance

Mechanisms of immune surveillance is given in Table 5.7.

6. DISEASES OF ORAL CAVITY

Q. 1. Write a note on histopathology of dental caries. *(BBD Uni., April 2015)*

Ans. Dental caries is an irreversible microbial disease of calcified tissues of teeth, characterized by demineralization of inorganic portion and destruction of organic substance of tooth, which often leads to cavitations.

Histopathology of dental caries:

A. Caries of enamel: The initial lesion has been divided into different zones based upon its histological appearance when longitudinal ground sections are examined with light microscope, starting from the inner advancing front of the lesion. These are the:

- **Zone 1: Translucent zone:** This lies at the advancing front of enamel lesion and is the first recognizable zone of alteration from normal enamel. It is observable when a longitudinal ground section is examined in a clearing agent having a refractive index identical to that of enamel.

- **Zone 2: Dark zone/positive zone:** This lies adjacent and superficial to translucent zone. This zone is formed as a result of demineralization and appears dark brown in ground sections examined by transmitted light.
- **Zone 3: Body of lesion:** This zone lies between the relatively unaffected surface layer and dark zone. It is the area of greatest demineralization. When a longitudinal ground section is examined in transmitted light, it appears relatively translucent and when examined with polarized light, it shows as a region of positive birefringence.
- **Zone 4: Surface zone:** The quantitative studies of the surface zone indicate a partial demineralization of about 1–4% along with a pore volume of less than 5% of spaces. After imbibing with water, the surface zone retains a negative birefringence.

B. Caries of dentin: Caries of dentin begins with the natural spread of disease process along DEJ and the rapid involvement of great numbers of dentinal tubules, each of which acts as a potential pathway leading to dental pulp along which microorganisms may travel at a variable rate of speed, depending upon a number of factors.

1. **Early dentinal changes:** The initial penetration of dentin by caries may result in alterations in dentin known as dentinal sclerosis. Close examination of dentin behind a zone of sclerosis formed reveals decalcification of dentin, which appears to occur slightly in advance of bacterial invasion of tubules.

2. **Advanced dentinal changes:** Decalcification of walls of individual tubules leads to their confluence, along with thickening and swelling of sheath of Neumann and increase in diameter of dentinal tubules due to packing by microorganisms. Tiny 'liquefaction foci' are formed by focal coalescence and breakdown of a few dentinal tubules. Beginning pulpally at the advancing edge of the lesion adjacent to normal dentin, these zones are as follows:

Zone 1: Zone of fatty degeneration of odontoblast process.

Zone 2: Zone of dentinal sclerosis characterized by deposition of calcium salts in dentinal tubules.

Zone 3: Zone of decalcification of dentin, a narrow zone, preceding bacterial invasion.

Zone 4: Zone of bacterial invasion of decalcified but intact dentin.

Zone 5: Zone of decomposed dentin.

Q. 2. Discuss recent advances in diagnosis and prevention of dental caries.

(MUHS, Dec. 2017; UOD, June 2019)

Ans.

1. Caries diagnosis: Traditionally, dental caries were detected by visible color and texture change, tactile sensation using a dental explorer, and radiographs. However, radiographs are not useful for detecting early enamel caries. Recently, several new technologies have emerged to help diagnosis are:

- DIAGNOdent uses laser fluorescence technology to measure bacterial products in caries lesions, and it may be sensitive enough to detect early demineralization.
- Digital imaging fiber-optic transillumination (DIFOTI) uses fiber-optic light to produce an image, which may be useful for detecting initial areas of demineralization.
- Quantitative light-induced fluorescence (QLF) shows reduced fluorescence of demineralized enamel.
- Electronic caries monitor (ECM) measures the changes in electrical impedance between sound enamel and demineralized tooth structure, as normal teeth have lower electrical conductivity.

2. Caries risk assessment: Past caries experience, current caries index, oral hygiene measures such as the use of fluoride toothpaste and mouth rinse, calculus deposit, deep pits and fissures, MS level, snacking habits, and salivary flow may all help assess individual caries risk and predict dental caries progression.

3. Prevention methods

- Oral hygiene: Daily plaque removal by brushing, flossing, and rinsing.
- Fluoride application: Methods of fluoride application include water fluoridation, fluoride toothpaste, fluoride mouth rinse, dietary fluoride supplements, and professionally applied fluoride compounds such as gels and varnishes.
- Pit and fissure sealants.
- Sugar substitute: Xylitol.
- Caries vaccine.
- Role of the primary caregiver in children: Maintaining oral hygiene and dental treatment in primary caregiver are also important for prevention of dental caries in young children.

Q. 3. Write about pathophysiology of periapical inflammation and associated bone resorption.

(UHSR, May 2016)

Ans. Apical periodontitis is inflammation of periodontal ligament around the root apex. The common causes of apical periodontitis include spread of infection following pulp necrosis, occlusal trauma from a high restoration or biting suddenly on a hard object, inadvertent endodontic procedures. Though the inflammatory process is similar to that occurring elsewhere, there may be resorption of periapical bone and sometimes the root apex. This process may be acute or chronic depending upon the virulence of microorganisms involved, type and severity of physical or chemical irritants, and host resistance.

Periodontal ligament shows signs of inflammation characterized by vascular dilatation and infiltration with polymorphonuclear leukocytes. Initially, these changes are localized around the root apex, as this area is richly vascular.

The inflammation is transient if it is caused by acute trauma. If the irritant is not removed, it progresses with resorption of the surrounding bone. Abscess formation may occur if it is associated with bacterial infection and is known as acute periapical abscess or alveolar abscess. Periapical granuloma that arises as a chronic process begins as a hyperaemia and edema of periodontal ligament with infiltration of chronic inflammatory cells. The inflammation and locally increased vascularity of tissue are associated with resorption of supporting bone. As the bone is resorbed, there is proliferation of fibroblasts and endothelial cells and formation of more tiny vascular channels as well as numerous delicate connective tissue fibrils. The new capillaries are usually lined by swollen endothelial cells. It is a relatively homogeneous lesion composed predominantly of macrophages, lymphocytes, and plasma cells and less frequently with mast cells and eosinophils and surrounded by a connective tissue 'capsule'. Since T cells also produce various cytotoxic lymphokines, collagenase and other enzymes, and destructive lymphokines, they may be responsible for much of the destructive potential of the periapical lesion.

Q. 4. Describe the fungal infections affecting the oral cavity. (RGUHS, May 2011; UHSR, April 2013)

Ans. Fungal infections of oral cavity can be superficial or more serious systemic illness.

Classification of fungal infections

A. Superficial mycoses

1. Candidiasis
i. Acute: Pseudomembranous type (oral thrush), atrophic type.
ii. Chronic:
    a. Chronic hyperplastic candidiasis.
    b. Chronic mucocutaneous candidiasis (CMC).
    c. Chronic atrophic candidiasis.

B. Deep mycoses (HP Uni., June 2016): Sporotrichosis, entomophthoromycosis, lobomycosis, chromomycosis, rhinosporidiosis.

C. Deep systemic mycosis

1. **Histoplasmosis (Darling's disease):** It is caused by *Histoplasma capsulatum*. Transmission and infection is through aerosolization and inhalation of spores into the lungs. It can mimic SCC with a firm base, necrotic center, and rolled borders. Most common locations intraorally are tongue, buccal mucosa, and palate.

2. **North American blastomycosis (Gilchrist's disease):** It is caused by *Blastomyces dermatitidis*. Most oral lesions are ulcerative, but there may be verrucous lesions, granulomas, sessile-based projections, abscess in the mandible with radiographic bone loss, and mobile teeth.

3. **South American blastomycosis (Lutz's disease):** It is caused by *Blastomyces brasiliensis*.

4. **Coccidioidomycosis (valley fever/great imitator):** It is caused by *Coccidioides immitis*. Usual acquisition of coccidioidomycosis is via inhalation of soil dust containing infectious spores. Cutaneous involvement is the most frequent extrapulmonary manifestation, especially of face and extremities. Tongue and lip ulcers with underlying skeletal and bone involvement can also occur.

5. **Paracoccidioidomycosis.**

6. **Cryptococcosis:** It is caused by *Cryptococcus neoformans*. Oral cryptococcosis can manifest as superficial ulcers, violaceous nodules, granuloma, cancerous looking lesions, or draining sinuses.

A. Deep opportunistic mycoses

1. **Aspergillosis:** Aspergillosis is caused by *Aspergillus* species (*Aspergillus fumigatus*), which is a mold with hyaline hyphae. Most common portal of entry is by inhalation of fungal spores into sinuses and respiratory tract. In oral and maxillary region it can cause rhinosinusitis, necrotic ulcers and orofacial osteomyelitis.

2. **Mucormycosis (zygomycosis/phycomycosis):** It is considered as the third most common opportunistic fungal infection after candidiasis and aspergillosis. The common genera (Mucorales) causing disease are Rhizopus (90%), Rhizomucor and Absidia. The infection usually results from inhalation of fungal spores, contamination of traumatized tissue, ingestion or direct inoculation. An area of ulceration or an extraction socket in the mouth can be a port of entry for mucormycosis into maxillofacial region, chiefly when the patient is immunocompromised.

Risk factors: Low immunity, uncontrolled DM.

Pathogenesis: Mucorales have the ability to damage and penetrate endothelial lining of blood vessels causing characteristics widespread angioinvasion resulting in thrombosis and tissue necrosis.

Classification: Eisenberg et al (1977) described six clinical variants: Rhinocerebral (rhinomaxillary), pulmonary, cutaneous, gastrointestinal, central nervous system and disseminated type.

I. Rhinocerebral form: Most common clinical variant, two subtypes:

- **Rhino-orbito-cerebral form:** Highly fatal, very invasive involving the ophthalmic and internal carotid arteries.
- **Rhino-maxillary form:** Less fatal, involves sphenopalatine and greater palatine arteries, resulting in thrombosis of turbinate and necrosis of palate.

Clinical features

- Malaise, headache, facial pain, swelling, an irregular black eschar, exudation of pus from eye and nose and low-grade fever.
- The disease usually starts in the nasal mucosa or palate and spread through the surrounding vessels to paranasal sinuses, frequently involving maxillary and ethmoid sinuses.
- It can involve retro-orbital region by direct extension.
- Orbital involvement can result in proptosis, ptosis, pupillary dilatation, orbital cellulitis and loss of vision.
- Direct penetration and growth of fungi through blood vessels can result in thrombosis and extensive tissue necrosis.
- Hematogenous spread to cavernous sinus can lead to fatal CST.
- Rhinocerebral mucormycosis can also spread by perineural invasion.

3. **Geotrichosis:** It is caused by *Geotrichum candidum*. Oral geotrichosis clinically resembles oral candidiasis (pseudomembranous > hyperplastic) and palatine ulcer. It mainly involves the tongue along with buccal mucosa, soft palate, and pharynx.

4. **Others:** Trichosporon, Penicilliosis, Basidiomycosis, Cephalosporiomycosis, Paecilomycosis, Alternariosis, Cercosporomycosis, Fusariomycosis.

Q. 5. Write a short note on candidiasis.

(TNMGR, March 2007)

Ans. Candidiasis is an opportunistic fungal infection caused most commonly by *Candida albicans* and occasionally by *Candida tropicalis*. In human beings, *Candida* species are present as normal flora of skin and mucocutaneous areas, intestines and vagina. The organism becomes pathogenic when the balance between the host and the organism is disturbed.

Predisposing factors: Impaired immunity, prolonged use of oral contraceptives, long-term antibiotic therapy, corticosteroid therapy, diabetes mellitus, obesity, pregnancy, etc.

Morphologic features

1. **Oral thrush:** This is the commonest form of mucocutaneous candidiasis seen especially in early life. Fully fledged lesions consist of creamy white pseudomembrane composed of fungi covering tongue, soft palate, and buccal mucosa. In severe cases, ulceration may be seen.

2. **Candidal vaginitis:** Vaginal candidiasis is characterized clinically by thick, yellow, curdy discharge. The lesions form pseudomembrane of fungi on vaginal mucosa. They are quite pruritic and may extend to involve vulva (vulvovaginitis) and perineum.

3. **Cutaneous candidiasis:** Candidal involvement of nailfolds producing change in the shape of nail plate (paronychia) and colonization in the intertriginous areas of skin, axilla, groin, infra- and inter-mammary, intergluteal folds and interdigital spaces are some of common forms of cutaneous lesions.

4. **Systemic candidiasis:** Invasive candidiasis is rare and is usually a terminal event of an underlying disorder associated with impaired immune system. The organisms gain entry into body through an ulcerative lesion on skin and mucosa or may be introduced by iatrogenic means. The lesions of systemic candidiasis are most commonly encountered in kidneys as ascending pyelonephritis and in heart as candidal endocarditis.

Q. 6. Write a short note on denture stomatitis.

(BFUHS, Nov. 2008)

Ans. Denture stomatitis refers to a visible chronic inflammation with a characteristic redness of mucosa in the oral cavity that is covered by a complete or partial removable dental appliance.

Etiology: Night wearing of dentures, ill fitting denture, inadequate denture curing, poor oral hygiene, bacterial and yeast (Candida) infection of denture.

Clinical features: Usually asymptomatic, denture bearing mucosa becomes smooth and red, in severe cases, discomfort, altered taste, burning sensation and dysphagia.

Classification (by Newton)

1. Type I: Localized redness confined to denture bearing palatal mucosa.
2. Type II: Diffuse redness of the mucosa.
3. Type III: Redness with nodular, papillary growth.

Management

1. Correction of irregularities of denture.
2. Rebasing of denture.
3. Construction of dentures.
4. Antifungal therapy.
5. Oral hygiene maintenance.

Q. 7. Write a short note on actinomycosis.
(TNMGR, Nov. 2001)

Ans. Actinomycosis is a chronic suppurative disease caused by anaerobic bacteria, *Actinomycetes israelii*. The organisms are commensals in oral cavity, alimentary tract and vagina. The infection is always endogenous in origin and not by person-to-person contact.

Morphologic features (*Cope, 1938*): 4 types:

1. **Cervicofacial actinomycosis** (*HP Uni., June 2016*): This is the commonest form (60%) and has the best prognosis. The infection enters from tonsils, carious teeth, periodontal disease or trauma following tooth extraction. Initially, a firm swelling develops in the lower jaw ('**Lumpy jaw**'), becoming progressively larger within weeks or month. Pain is rare, slight fever and sensation of superficial tension around the mass. Initially, mass may be surrounded by induration or erythema; later, it may become tender to palpation. In time, mass breaks down and abscesses and multiple sinuses are formed. The discharging pus contains typical tiny yellow BI. The infection may extend into adjoining soft tissues as well as may destroy the bone. Actinomyces rarely involves the lymph nodes.

   Treatment: Surgery with 2–4 weeks of high-dose intravenous penicillin.

2. **Thoracic actinomycosis:** Due to aspiration of organism from oral cavity or extension of infection from abdominal or hepatic lesions. Initially, the disease resembles pneumonia but subsequently the infection spreads to whole of lung, pleura, ribs and vertebrae.

3. **Abdominal actinomycosis:** This type is common in appendix, caecum and liver. The abdominal infection results from swallowing of organisms from oral cavity or extension from thoracic cavity.

4. **Pelvic actinomycosis:** Infection in pelvis occurs as a complication of intrauterine contraceptive devices (IUCDs).

Microscopically

i. The inflammatory reaction is a granuloma with central suppuration. There is formation of abscesses in the centre of lesions and at periphery, chronic inflammatory cells, giant cells and fibroblasts are seen.

ii. Centre of each abscess contains bacterial colony, '**sulphur granule**', characterized by radiating filaments (**ray fungus**) with hyaline, eosinophilic, club-like ends representative of secreted immunoglobulins.

iii. Bacterial stains reveal the organisms as gram-positive filaments, nonacid-fast, which stain positively with Gomori's methenamine silver staining.

Q. 8. Classify ulcerative lesions of the oral cavity and describe the clinical features.
(Bombay Uni., Oct. 1985; TNMGR, April, 2013)

Ans. Ulcerations are characterized by defects in the epithelium, underlying connective tissue, or both.

Classification of oral ulcers

A. Acute ulcers

I. **Acute solitary ulcers:** Traumatic ulcer, necrotizing sialometaplasia.

II. **Acute multiple ulcers:** Primary herpetic gingivostomatitis, varicella-zoster virus infection, herpangina, hand-foot-mouth disease, erythema multiforme (EM), necrotizing ulcerative gingivitis (NUG), oral hypersensitivity reactions, plasma cell stomatitis, chemotherapy related ulcers.

B. Chronic ulcers

I. **Chronic solitary ulcers:** Long-standing traumatic ulcers, necrotizing sialometaplasia, eosinophilic ulcer, ulcerative squamous cell carcinoma, cytomegalovirus associated ulceration, tuberculous ulcer, syphilitic ulceration (chancre), deep fungal ulceration (histoplasmosis, blastomycosis, mucormycosis).

II. **Chronic multiple ulcers:** Pemphigus vulgaris, Mucous membrane pemphigoid, bullous pemphigoid, lichen planus, linear IgA disease.

C. Recurrent ulcers (single/multiple): Recurrent aphthous stomatitis, recurrent herpes stomatitis, herpes associated EM, cyclic neutropenia, Behcet's disease.

Q. 9. Classify parotid tumors.
(TNMGR, April 1995)

Ans. Salivary gland neoplasms incidence is 0.4–2.5 in 100,000. Majority (80%) are parotid gland tumors. They account for 3% of head and neck tumors.

Classification

A. **Primary benign epithelial/adenomas:** Pleomorphic adenoma, Warthin's tumor, cystadenoma, myoepithelial adenoma, oncocytoma, sebaceous adenoma, lymphadenoma, ductal papilloma, canalicular adenoma, basal cell adenoma.

B. **Primary malignant epithelial/carcinomas:** Muco-epidermoid carcinoma, adenoid cystic carcinoma, acinic cell carcinoma, myoepithelial carcinoma, clear cell carcinoma (NOS), basal cell adenocarcinoma, Salivary duct carcinoma (high grade), oncocytic carcinoma (high grade), squamous cell carcinoma (SCC), polymorphous low grade adenocarcinoma, carcinoma ex pleomorphic adenoma, metastasizing pleomorphic adenoma.

C. **Soft tissue tumors:** Hemangioma.

D. **Malignant lymphomas:** Diffuse B cell lymphoma, Hodgkin lymphoma.

E. **Secondary tumors:** SCC, melanoma, lung carcinoma, angiosarcoma.

F. **Unclassified tumors:** Hemangiopericytoma, neuroendocrine tumour.

G. **Tumour-like lesions:** Sialadenosis, oncocytosis, benign lymphoepithelial lesion, salivary gland cysts, Kuttner's tumor, cystic lymphoid hyperplasia in AIDS.

■ **Pleomorphic adenoma (mixed salivary tumour)** *(NTR Uni., Oct., 2012)* is the most common tumour of major (60–75%) and minor (50%) salivary glands. The tumour is commoner in women and is seen more frequently in 3rd–5th decades of life. The tumour is solitary, smooth-surfaced but sometimes nodular, painless and slow-growing. It is often located below and in front of ear.

• **Histopathological feature:** *Grossly,* pleomorphic adenoma is a circumscribed, pseudoencapsulated, rounded, multilobulated, firm mass, 2–5 cm in diameter, with bosselated surface. The cut surface is grey-white and bluish, variegated, semi-translucent, usually solid but may show small cystic spaces. The consistency is soft and mucoid. *Microscopically,* it is characterized by pleomorphic or 'mixed' appearance: **Epithelial component** may form various patterns like ducts, acini, tubules, sheets and strands of cells of ductal or myoepithelial origin. Focal areas of squamous metaplasia and keratinisation may be present. **Mesenchymal elements** are present as loose connective tissue, and as myxoid, mucoid and chondroid matrix, which simulates cartilage (pseudocartilage) but is actually connective tissue mucin.

Prognosis: Pleomorphic adenoma is notorious for recurrences, due to incomplete surgical removal, multiple foci of tumour, pseudoencapsulation, and implantation in the surgical field.

Q. 10. Write a short note on mucocele.

(RGUHS, May 2011)

Ans. Mucocele is a common lesion of the oral mucosa that results from an alteration of minor salivary glands due to mucus accumulation causing limited swelling.

Two types

• **Extravasation mucocele:** It results from a broken salivary gland duct and consequent spillage into soft tissue around this gland. It has no epithelial lining.

• **Retention mucocele:** It appears due to decrease/absence of glandular secretion produced by blockage of salivary gland ducts. Retention cyst has an epithelial lining.

Clinical variants

• *Superficial mucocele* that is located directly under the mucosa.

• *Classic variant* located in upper submucosa.

• *Deep mucocele* located in lower corneum.

Clinical features

1. Most commonly found on lower lip, usually lateral to midline. Other sites are buccal mucosa, anterior ventral tongue, floor of mouth **(ranula)**.

2. Commonly seen in all ages; Superficial mucocele in individuals >30 years; Ranula in children and young adults; Mucus retention cysts occur in older individuals.

3. Clinically, it appears as raised, dome shaped, fluctuant vesicle, with history of rupture, collapse and refilling.

4. Superficial lesions are bluish, translucent, deeper lesions are of normal in colour; deep lesions have normal mucosal coloration and bleeding into the swelling may impart a bright red and vascular appearance.

5. Differential diagnose includes Blandin and Nuhn mucocele, hemangioma, lymphangioma, lipoma, and soft tissue abscess.

6. Diagnosis is by history and clinical examination with ultrasonography demonstrates the internal structures more clearly.

Treatment: Surgical excision with removal of accessory salivary glands, marsupialization, laser ablation, cryosurgery, and electrocautery.

Q. 11. Write a short note on salivary calculi.

(TNMGR, April 1995; BBD Uni., April 2015)

Ans. Salivary calculi (sialolithiasis) are the occurrence of calcareous concretions in salivary ducts or glands.

Sialolithiasis is the most common cause of salivary gland swelling with a reported incidence of 1 in 10000 to 1 in 30000.

Etiology: Anatomical factors (duct stenosis/inflammation); Composition factors (increased calcium content or altered enzyme function); Decreased fluid intake; Use of diuretic; Tobacco smoking.

Clinical features
1. Primary age at diagnosis is between 30 and 60 years.
2. Higher incidence in males.
3. Approximately 85% of stones occur within the submandibular gland (due to ascending position of its duct, more mucinous, viscous and alkaline saliva). Approximately 15% of salivary stones occur within parotid gland, and <5% occur within sublingual and minor salivary glands.
4. Unilateral salivary gland swelling with decreased saliva production.
5. Acute onset of pain that worsens with meals (cyclical postprandial).

Composition: Calcium phosphate, calcium carbonate, soluble salts, organic matter, water.

Treatment: Small stones can be removed by manipulation. Large stones require surgical removal.

Q. 12. Write a short note on sialadenitis.
(TNMGR, Oct. 2011)

Ans. Sialadenitis is a condition characterized by inflammation and enlargement of one or more of salivary glands.

A. **Allergic sialadenitis:** Sialadenitis due to exposure to various pharmaceutical agents and allergens, characterized by acute salivary gland enlargement, accompanied by itching over the gland. Allergic sialadenitis is self-limiting.

B. **Bacterial sialadenitis:** Bacterial infections of salivary glands are most commonly seen in patients with reduced salivary gland function. This condition was formerly referred to as "**Surgical Parotitis**" because post-surgery patients often experienced gland enlargement from ascending bacterial infection as a result of administered anticholinergic drugs and relative dehydration due to restricted fluids. Clinical features include:
- Sudden onset of unilateral or bilateral salivary gland enlargement.
- The involved gland is painful, indurated, and tender to palpation and overlying skin may be erythematous.
- Purulent discharge may be expressed from duct orifice and most commonly cultured organisms

include *Staph. aureus*, *Strept. viridans*, *Strept. pneumoniae*, *E. coli*, and *H. influenzae*.

Treatment
- Empiric intravenous administration of penicillinase resistant anti-staphylococcal antibiotic.
- Milking of involved gland, increased hydration and improve oral hygiene.
- Incision and drainage, if significant improvement is not seen after 24–48 hours.

C. **Viral sialadenitis:** It occurs in mumps. This produces pain on mastication, followed by firm, rubbery swelling of salivary glands. Treatment is conservative with maintenance of hydration, analgesics and complete rest.

D. **Sialadenitis due to mechanical obstruction:** It may occur due to sialolith in the duct or gland itself. Symptoms depend upon the site of obstruction, chronicity and size of sialolith. Treatment is removal of sialolith.

Q. 13. Write a short note on xerostomia.
(RGUHS, Oct. 2010, Nov. 2011; MUHS, June 2017; UHSR, June 2018)

Ans. Xerostomia is defined as the subjective complaint of dry mouth. A diagnosis of hyposalivation is made when stimulated salivary flow rate is ≤ 0.5–0.7 ml/min. (N=1.5–2.0 ml/min) and unstimulated salivary flow rate is ≤ 0.1 ml/min (N=0.3–0.4 ml/min).

Etiology
A. **Temporary causes:** Psychological (anxiety, depression), sialolith, sialadenitis, drugs (anticholinergic, sympathomimetic, etc.)
B. **Permanent causes:** Salivary gland disorders (aplasia, Sjögren syndrome), systemic disorders (diabetes, Parkinson's disease, cystic fibrosis, etc.), Radiotherapy, surgical desalivation.

Clinical features
1. Pain and swelling of the glands.
2. Dryness of mouth.
3. Difficulty in speech, swallowing.
4. More chances of caries development.
5. Dry, atrophic, pale oral mucosa.
6. Soreness and burning.

Diagnosis: Clinical signs pathognomonic for hyposalivation as proposed by Osailan et al:
1. Sticking of an intraoral mirror to buccal mucosa/tongue.
2. Frothy saliva.
3. No saliva pooling in floor of mouth.
4. Loss of papillae of tongue dorsum.

5. Altered/smooth gingival architecture.
6. Glassy appearance of oral mucosa (especially palate).
7. Lobulated/deeply fissured tongue.
8. Cervical caries (>2 teeth).
9. Mucosal debris on palate (except under dentures).

Dental management of patient with decreased salivation (RGUHS, November, 2011)

1. **Preventive therapy:** Supplemental fluoride, meticulous oral hygiene, frequent dental visit, brushing after meals, remineralizing solutions, non-cariogenic diet.
2. **Symptomatic treatment:** Frequent use of water and other fluids, increased humidification, mucosal lubricants, saliva substitutes, minimize caffeine and alcohol.
3. **Local salivary stimulation:** Sugar-free gums to promote chewing, electrical stimulation with low voltage current to tongue and palate, use of acupuncture needles in perioral region.
4. **Systemic salivary stimulation:** Pilocarpine (5 mg), Cevimeline (30 mg).
5. **Treatment of underlying systemic disorder**
   • Hypersalivation/sialorrhoea/ptyalism (NTR Uni., May 2008): Increased flow of saliva, occurs commonly due to: Stomatitis, teething, mentally retarded state, schizophrenia, neurological disturbances, increased gastric secretion and sialosis.

Q. 14. Write about maxillary sinus diseases.
(TNMGR, April 2012)

Ans. A broad spectrum of disease processes can involve maxillary sinus arising either from within the lining of sinus, adjacent paranasal sinuses, nasal space, dental and oral tissues, or in the adjacent bone with expansion into sinus.

A. Congenital abnormalities

1. Development variations: Aplasia, hypoplasia.
2. Facial clefts and syndromes: Cleft lip/cleft face syndrome, Crouzan syndrome, etc.
3. Choanal atresia.
4. Osteo-meatal variations: Anomalies of turbinate, uncinate process, etc.

B. Inflammatory diseases and infection

1. Sinusitis: Acute/chronic; bacterial/viral/fungal.
2. Allergic: Sino-nasal polyps, antro-choanal polyp.
3. Mucus retention cyst (mucocele).
4. Granulomatous diseases: Wegner's granulomatous disease, Churg-Strauss syndrome.

C. Trauma: Isolated fractures, complex facial fractures, transfacial fractures.

D. Neoplasm

1. **Benign:** Inverted papilloma, neurofibroma, angiofibroma, cylindrinoma.
2. **Malignant epithelial neoplasm:** SCC and its types, Adenocarcinoma, adenoid cystic carcinoma, acinic cell carcinoma, mucosal melanoma.
3. **Malignant mesenchymal neoplasms:** Soft tissue sarcoma, neurogenic sarcoma, angiosarcoma, leiomyosarcoma, rhabdomyosarcoma, fibrosarcoma, chondrosarcoma, osteosarcoma.
4. **Malignant lympho-reticular:** Lymphoma, plasmacytoma.
5. **Metastatic.**

E. Odontogenic

1. **Infections:** Pulpal/periapical, periodontal, oro-antral fistula.
2. **Cysts:** Dentigerous, radicular, OKC, calcifying odontogenic cyst.
3. **Benign tumors:** Ameloblastoma, odontoma, cementoma, adenomatoid odontogenic tumour.
4. **Fibro-osseous lesions:** Fibrous dysplasia, ossifying fibroma, cherubism.
5. **Foreign body:** Teeth, implants, restorative materials.

F. Miscellaneous lesions: Thalassaemia, giant cell reparative granuloma.

Q. 15. Write a short note on oro-antral communication.
(BBD Uni., May 2009)

Ans. Oro-antral communication (OAC) is a pathological connection between the oral cavity and maxillary sinus due to loss of soft and hard tissues that normally separates these compartments. **An oro-antral fistula** (OAF) is an epithelialized pathological unnatural communication between oral cavity and maxillary sinus.

Etiology: Extraction of maxillary posterior teeth > Pathological lesions in sinus > implant dislodgement > trauma > periodontal infections > ORN > flap necrosis.

Clinical features: Nasal regurgitation; Altered nasal resonance, difficulty in sucking through straw, unilateral nasal discharge, bad taste; Whistling sound while speaking and pain at malar region.

Diagnosis: Clinically, large fistula is easily seen on inspection. Diagnosis of small defect can be made by nose blow test. A mouth mirror placed at OAC causes fogging of the mirror. Panoramic radiograph gives an accurate estimation of dimension of bony defect of fistula and also reveals about the presence and location of dental roots/implants/foreign body. Computed tomography can be done to rule out the presence of maxillary sinusitis.

Management

I. **Perioperative:** Affected maxillary sinus should be irrigated through fistulous opening with normal saline followed by iodine-containing solution diluted with normal saline to eradicate infection. Surgical procedures for closure of OAC/OAF include local flaps, distant flaps and grafting.

II. **Postoperative:** Patients should eat soft food items and drink fluid from opposite side to avoid trauma to operated site. Strenuous physical activities should be avoided until healing occurs. The wound should be kept clean with warm saline mouth rinses. Use of straw or smoking is prohibited. Use of steam inhalations moistens the airway and stimulates serous gland activity preventing crusting of blood and mucous. All patients should receive amoxicillin plus clavulanic acid or clindamycin for at least 5 days, decongestant nasal drops and NSAIDs.

Q. 16. Write a short note on differential diagnosis of neck swellings. *(HP Uni., May 2012)*

Ans. Neck swelling is any abnormal enlargement, swelling or growth from the level of base of skull to clavicles.

Differential Diagnosis (Table 6.16)

Q. 17. Write a short note on Ludwig's angina. *(TNMGR, Oct. 2013)*

Ans. Ludwig's angina (*Wilhelm Frederick von Ludwig, 1836*) is described as a rapidly and frequently fatal progressive gangrenous cellulitis and edema of soft tissues of neck and floor of mouth, resulting in airway obstruction. It is a firm, brawny cellulitis involving submandibular, sublingual and submental spaces, bilaterally.

Etiology

1. Odontogenic infection (mainly from mandibular 2nd and 3rd molars).
2. Peritonsillar/parapharyngeal abscess.
3. Mandibular fractures, osteomyelitis.
4. Oral lacerations/piercing.

5. Submandibular sialadenitis.
6. Oral malignancy.
7. Iatrogenic—use of contaminated needle during local anesthesia.

Clinical features

1. Patient is febrile, dehydrated.
2. Marked dysphagia, impaired speech.
3. Hard brawny swelling of submandibular region, floor of mouth and neck.
4. Severe trismus, pain and malaise.
5. Airway obstruction (elevation and posterior displacement of tongue and edema of glottis).
6. Inability to swallow saliva and stridor.

Management: Early diagnosis, maintenance of patent airways, intense and prolonged antibiotic therapy (intravenous penicillin G, clindamycin or metronidazole, gentamicin), extraction of offending tooth, and surgical drainage or decompression of fascial spaces.

Q. 18. Write a short note on cancrum oris. *(TNMGR, April 1995)*

Ans. Cancrum oris (Greek: "to *devour*")/noma/gangrenous stomatitis/necrotizing ulcerative stomatitis/orofacial gangrene is a rapidly spreading mutilating, gangrenous stomatitis that occurs usually in debilitated or nutritionally deficient persons. It usually occurs in children aged 2–9 years.

Types

- **Acute noma:** Acute inflammatory phase with ulceration.
- **Chronic noma:** Healed phase in which the ulcer is healed leaving behind varying sizes of orofacial defect.

Predisposing factors: Malnutrition, poor oral hygiene, debilitating infections, blood dyscrasias, poor or lack of maternal care, HIV, and low socioeconomic groups.

Causative organism: Vincent's organism (*Borrelia vincenti*, Fusobacteria).

Clinical features

1. Usually begins as small ulcer of mucosa, which spreads rapidly and involves surrounding tissue of jaw, lips, and cheeks by gangrenous necrosis.

Table 6.16: Differential diagnosis

	Midline	Lateral
Neoplastic	Thyroid, parathyroid, pharyngeal/laryngeal	Most tumors
Congenital	Thyroglossal duct cyst, laryngocele	Cystic hygroma, branchial cleft cyst
Infectious	Ludwig's angina	Most infections (cat-scratch, mononucleosis, sialadenitis)
Inflammatory	Submental lymphadenopathy, thyroiditis	Cervical lymphadenopathy

2. Overlying skin becomes inflamed, edematous and finally necrotic.
3. Line of demarcation develops between healthy and dead tissue.
4. The large masses of tissue slough out, leaving the jaw exposed.
5. Extremely foul odor from gangrenous tissue with high grade fever.
6. Death may occur from toxemia or pneumonia.

Treatment
- Supportive care, pain control, use of oxidizing mouthwash.
- Treatment of predisposing factors.
- Local wound care: Paraffin gauze dressing soaked with betadine, and hydrogen peroxide throughout treatment.
- Intravenous administration of crystalline penicillin 10,00,000 IU q6h.

Q. 19. Describe the fibro-osseous lesion affecting the jaws. (RGUHS, May 2011)

Ans. Fibro-osseous lesions (FOLs) are a poorly defined group of lesions affecting the jaws and craniofacial bones, characterized by replacement of bone by cellular fibrous tissue containing foci of mineralization that vary in amount and appearance.

WHO classification of FOLs (2005)
1. Ossifying fibroma (OF)
2. Fibrous dysplasia
3. Osseous dysplasia: Periapical/focal/florid osseous dysplasia; Familial gigantiform cementoma
4. Central giant cell granuloma (CGCG)
5. Cherubism
6. Aneurysmal bone cyst
7. Solitary bone cyst.

Q. 20. Write about fibrous dysplasia of bone. (TNMGR, March 2008)

Ans. Reed's definition states that fibrous dysplasia (FD) is an arrest of bone maturation and presence of woven bone with ossification resulting from metaplasia of a nonspecific fibro-osseous type.

Etiology: Mutation in GNAS1 gene.

Clinical features
1. **Monostotic form** (70–80%): Involvement of single bone, may present with pain and pathological fracture in aged patient.
2. **Polyostotic form** (20–30%): FD involves > one bone. Usually patient has pain in limb followed by limp.
   i. **Jaffe's type:** FD of bones with pigmented lesions of skin or café au lait spots.

   ii. **Albright's syndrome:** FD involving nearly all bones of skeleton with endocrinal disturbances.
3. **Craniofacial form:** This form occurs in 10–25% cases of monostotic and 50% case of polyostotic form. The site most common involved is frontal, sphenoid, maxillary and ethmoidal bones. The other features include hypertelorism, cranial asymmetry, facial deformity, visual impairment, exophthalmos and blindness, vestibular dysfunction, tinnitus, hearing loss, anosmia, depending upon the bone involvement.

Radiographic features: Typically **ground-glass** appearance, **fingerprint** bone pattern, **orange peel** appearance, and superior displacement of mandibular canal in mandibular lesion. Skeletal radiographic features include "**Shepherd's crook**" deformity of femoral neck and "**bowing deformities**" in weight-bearing long bones.

Differential diagnosis: Simple bone cyst, non-ossifying fibroma, osteofibrous dysplasia, low-grade intramedullary osteosarcoma, and Paget's disease.

Treatment: Treatment protocols for FD include:
- Clinical observation for lesions that have no risk of pathologic fracture or deformity.
- Medical treatment with bisphosphonates.
- Surgery is indicated for confirmatory biopsy, correction of deformity, prevention of pathologic fracture, and/or elimination of symptomatic lesions.

Q. 21. Write a note on central giant cell granuloma. (NTR Uni., Oct 2012)

Ans. Central giant cell granuloma (CGCG) is an uncommon, benign, proliferative, intraosseous lesion representing < 7% of all benign jaw lesions. The etiology is unknown, but is thought to be a reactive process, possibly secondary to trauma or inflammation; however, some believe it is a benign neoplasm. CGCG of jaw may be divided into two categories, aggressive and nonaggressive.

Clinical features
- Most of the CGCG cases occur before age of 30, with female predilection (F:M = 2:1).
- CGCG is more prevalent in anterior than posterior jaws, often crossing midline.
- Mandible is more commonly affected than maxilla and confined to tooth-bearing areas of jaws.
- In most of cases, the lesion presents as a painless, slow-growing swelling of the jaw.
- Intraorally, swelling with bluish brown discoloration can be observed.
- Most common complaint is pain, paresthesia, and displacement of teeth.

- **Radiographically**, the lesion commonly presents as a solitary radiolucency with a multilocular appearance or, less commonly, a unilocular appearance. Lesions in mandible have an epicenter anterior to first molar, whereas in maxilla, its anterior to canine. The internal structure may show **granular pattern of calcification** which is organized into ill-defined, **wispy septa** which emanate at right angles to periphery of lesion. Displacement and resorption of teeth are also evident.
- Histologically, there is highly cellular, fibroblastic stroma with plump, spindle-shaped cells with high-mitotic rate with prominent multinucleated giant cells.
- **Differential diagnosis:** OKC, unicystic ameloblastoma, aneurysmal bone cyst, Ewing sarcoma, odontogenic myxoma, brown tumor of hyperparathyroidism, osteosarcoma, cherubism.

Treatment

A. Non-surgical treatment

- Triamcinolone hexacetonide 20 mg/ml twice weekly for 6 weeks.
- Salmon calcitonin nasal spray 200 IU/day.
- INF-α (3×10^6 IU/day) injection.

B. Surgical treatment: Simple curettage, curettage with peripheral ostectomy, enucleation, and *en bloc* resection.

Q. 22. Write a note on Paget's disease.

(NTR Uni., April 2009)

Ans. Paget's disease (PD) of bone (*Sir James Paget, 1877 as "osteitis deformans"*) is characterized by rapid bone resorption and deposition, resulting in numerous reversal line formations which give mosaic pattern to lamellar bone with profuse local vascularity and fibrous tissue in marrow.

Etiology: Genetic (chromosome 18q), environmental factors; Slow virus infections by paramyxovirus, canine distemper virus.

Clinical features

- PD is a geriatric disease reported above 5th–6th decades of life, with male predilection (3:2).
- Pain, deformity, and fracture of affected bone.
- Enlargement of skull or frontal bossing, facial disfigurement and bowing of long bones.
- *Painful fissure* fractures may occur.
- Enlarged and deformed bones may compress surrounding nerves and vessels causing neurological symptoms.
- Osteosarcomas or other sarcomas are the most serious complications of PDB.

- **Radiographic features:** Earliest lesions are lytic; Advancing lytic lesion: "**Blade of grass**" or 'V-shaped lesion' in long bones; Skull involvement typically begins with radiolucent areas (**osteoporosis circumscripta**) followed by osteoblastic activity resulting in enlargement of skull and a classic "**Cotton wool appearance.**" Others: Well-circumscribed radiolucency, loss of lamina dura, pulpal radio-opacity, root resorption, and hypercementosis.
- Histopathologically, areas of osteoclastic resorption; "**mosaic pattern or jigsaw puzzle appearance**" of osteoid seams or cement lines; space between the trabeculae and cortex is filled with collagen which gradually becomes less vascular.
- Laboratory findings: Elevated ALP, and other markers of bone formation and bone resorption; Hypercalcemia, hypercalciuria, hyperparathyroidism.
- Treatment:
  I. **Nonspecific therapy:** NSAIDs, compensatory shoe lifts or orthotics, ambulation aids, physical therapy.
  II. **Specific antipagetic drug treatment:** Specific antipagetic drugs inhibit osteoclastic activity.
  1. Salmon calcitonin (100 IU) SC, daily. Maintenance dose: 50–100 IU three times weekly.
  2. Bisphosphonates: Etidronate (400 mg); Tiludronate (400 mg); Alendronate (40 mg); Risedronate (30 mg); Pamidronate (30 mg) IV Zoledronic acid (5 mg) IV
  3. Other drugs: Gallium nitrate and plicamycin (mithramycin), denosumab (monoclonal antibody to RANKL).
  4. Surgery: Fracture stabilization, corrective osteotomy and total joint arthroplasty.

Extra-bony Paget's disease

Paget's disease of vulva is a rare condition in which the affected skin, most often on the labia majora, appears as map-like, red, scaly, elevated and indurated area.

Paget's disease of nipple: Paget's disease of nipple is an eczematoid lesion of nipple, often associated with an invasive or non-invasive ductal carcinoma of the underlying breast.

Q. 23. Write briefly about the different types of benign tumors of the jaws. *(TNMGR, Oct. 2013)*

Ans. New WHO-2017 classification of odontogenic tumors

A. Benign odontogenic tumors

I. **Epithelial origin:** 1. Ameloblastoma (conventional, unicystic, extraosseous/peripheral, metastasizing (malignant), 2. Adenomatoid odontogenic tumour, 3. Calicifying epithelial odontogenic tumors, 4. Squamous odontogenic tumor.

II. **Mixed (epithelial-mesenchymal) origin:** 1. Ameloblastic fibroma, 2. Primordial odontogenic tumor, 3. Odontoma: Compound and complex type, 4. Dentinogenic ghost cell tumor.

III. **Mesenchymal origin:** 1. Odontogenic myxoma/myxofibroma, 2. Odontogenic fibroma, 3. Cementoblastoma, 4. Cemento-ossifying fibroma.

B. Non-odontogenic tumors: 1. Central fibroma, 2. Osteoma, 3. Osteoblastoma, 4. Chondroma, 5. Giant cell granuloma, 6. Central hemangioma, 7. Benign tumors of neural tissues.

C. Fibro-osseous lesions.

Q. 24. Write a short note on brown tumour.
(RGUHS, May 2011)

Ans. Brown tumors (osteitis fibrosa cystica generalisata/von Recklinghausen's disease of bone) are giant cell focal lesion that arises as a result of abnormal bone metabolism in patients with hyperparathyroidism (HPT). It represents reparative granuloma rather than a true neoplastic process.

Clinical features

1. Prevalence of brown tumor is 0.1% and can occur in mandible, maxilla, clavicle, ribs and pelvic bones.
2. Frequency of occurrence is more among persons >50 years of age with a male to female ratio of 1:3.
3. Clinically, brown tumors may present as small, asymptomatic swelling in jaw bone or as a painful exophytic mass. Pathological fracture may be the first symptom.
4. Radiographic appearance is usually a well-demarcated unilocular or multilocular osteolytic lesion, associated with root resorption and loss of lamina dura.
5. Histologically, brown tumors are characterized by vascular fibroblastic stroma and several osteoclast-like multinucleated giant cells often interspersed with hemorrhagic infiltrates and haemosiderin deposits (that is why known as **brown tumour**).
6. **Diagnosis** is confirmed by hypocalcaemia, hypophosphatemia, and elevated levels of ALP.
7. Management involves control of HPT and a partial parathyroidectomy (small lesions) along with surgical excision (large symptomatic lesion).

Q. 25. Write a short note on ameloblastoma.
(RGUHS, Oct. 2010)

Ans. Ameloblastoma is a true neoplasm of enamel organ type tissue which does not undergo differentiation to the point of enamel formation. It was described by Robinson (1937), as a benign tumor that is "Usually unicentric, nonfunctional, intermittent in growth, anatomically benign and clinically persistent."

Pathogenesis: The tumor may be derived from: Cell rests of enamel organ; Epithelium of odontogenic cysts; Disturbance of developing enamel organ; Basal cells of surface epithelium of jaws; Heterotopic epithelium in other parts of body.

Classification: Ameloblastoma is classified, according to **WHO (2017)** classification, as a benign tumor with odontogenic epithelium, mature fibrous stroma and without odontogenic ectomesenchyme. Ameloblastoma is further classified into:

A. Conventional type

- About 80% of ameloblastoma occurs in mandible, frequently in posterior region.
- The lesions more often progresses slowly, but are locally invasive and infiltrates through medullary spaces and erodes cortical bone. If left untreated, they resorb cortical plate and extend into adjacent tissue.
- **"Crepitation or eggshell crackling"** might be elicited.
- **Radiographically,** lesion shows an expansile, radiolucent, multilocular cystic lesion, with a characteristic **"Soap bubble-like"** or **"Honeycomb"** appearance. Other findings include thinning and expansion of cortical plate with erosion, associated unerupted tooth displaced and resorption of roots of adjacent teeth.
- **Histopathologically,** classical histological pattern of ameloblastoma described by Vickers and Gorlin is characterized by peripheral layer of tall columnar cells with hyperchromasia, reverse polarity of the nuclei and sub-nuclear vacuole formation.

Histological subtypes *(BFUHS, Nov. 2009; UHSR, June 2018)* include:

a. **Follicular type** is composed of many small islands of peripheral layer of cuboidal or columnar cells with reversely polarized nucleus. Cyst formation is common. This type has the highest recurrence rate.
b. **Plexiform** is composed of anastomosing islands of odontogenic epithelium, with double rows of columnar cells in back to back arrangement.
c. In **acanthomatous type**, the cells occupying the position of stellate reticulum undergo squamous metaplasia, with keratin pearl formation in the center of tumor islands. This type has the least recurrence rate.
d. In **granular cell ameloblastoma**, cytoplasm of stellate reticulum-like cells appear coarse granular and eosinophilic.
e. In **basal cell type**, the epithelial tumor cells are less columnar and arranged in sheets.

f. **Desmoplastic variant** is composed of dense collagen stroma, which appears hypocellular and hyalinized.

g. Other histological types are **papilliferous-keratotic type**, clear cell type, and mucous cell differentiation type.

- **Treatment:** Surgery with wide resection.

B. Extraosseous/peripheral type: Peripheral ameloblastoma is confined to gingival or alveolar mucosa.

- It arises from remnants of dental lamina ("**Glands of Serres**,"), odontogenic remnants of vestibular lamina, pluripotent cells in basal cell layer of mucosal epithelium and pluripotent cells from minor salivary glands.
- In majority of cases, there is no radiological evidence of bone involvement, but superficial bone erosion (**cupping or saucerization**) may be detected at surgery.
- Overall average age is 52.1 years; M:F=1.9:1.
- Mandibular premolar region is the commonest site of occurrence.
- Treatment: Wide local excision.

C. Unicystic type: Unicystic ameloblastoma (UA) represents an ameloblastoma variant, that shows clinical and radiologic characteristics of an odontogenic cyst.

- 5–15% of all ameloblastomas are of unicystic type.
- Mean age is considerably lower (16 years) with no gender predilection.
- Three pathogenic mechanisms for its evolution are: Reduced enamel epithelium, dentigerous cyst and due to cystic degeneration of conventional ameloblastoma.
- **Radiographically**, it is well-defined unilocular to multilocular radiolucency with impacted tooth.
- Histopathological types are: Mural, luminal and intraluminal (**WHO classification, 2017**).
- **Treatment:** Radical and conservative surgical excision, curettage, chemical and electrocautery, radiation therapy or combination of surgery and radiation.

Q. 26. Describe the cysts of jaw. *(TNMGR, Oct. 2012)*

Ans. Cyst is defined as a pathological cavity filled with fluid which is solid, semisolid or gaseous form which may or may not be lined by epithelium.

A. Odontogenic cysts (WHO classification, 2017)
 i. **Developmental**
   1. Dentigerous cyst.
   2. Odontogenic keratocyst.

   3. Lateral periodontal and botryoid odontogenic cyst.
   4. Gingival cyst.
   5. Glandular odontogenic cyst.
   6. Calcifying odontogenic cyst.
   7. Orthokeartinized odontogenic cyst.
 ii. **Inflammatory:** Radicular cyst and collateral inflammatory cyst.

B. Non-odontogenic cysts
 1. Globulomaxillary cyst.
 2. Median mandibular cyst.
 3. Nasoalveolar cyst/nasolabial cyst.
 4. Palatal and alveolar cysts of newborns.
 5. Thyroglossal tract cyst.
 6. Epidermal inclusion cyst.
 7. Dermoid cyst.
 8. Heterotopic oral gastrointestinal cyst.

Q. 27. Write a short note on odontogenic keratocyst.
(RGUHS, Oct. 2010; NTR Uni., Oct. 2011)

Ans. Odontogenic keratocyst (OKC) is a developmental, non-inflammatory chronic cyst derived from remnants of dental lamina, with biological behavior like a neoplasm.

Clinical features
1. It may occur in any age (10–90 years). Peak incidence in 2–3 decades.
2. M:F=1.3:1; Mandible is affected > maxilla; In mandible, molar ramus-angle area is most commonly involved; In maxilla, molar area is most commonly involved.
3. Pain, soft tissue swelling, neurologic manifestations.
4. Radiographically, unilocular/multilocular radiolucency with well defined scalloped border. OKCs tend to grow in an anteroposterior direction within the medullary cavity of bone without causing obvious bone expansion.
5. Displacement of teeth adjacent to the cyst occurs more frequently than resorption.
6. **Aspiration (cyst content):** OKCs contain a dirty white, viscoid suspension of keratin. Electrophoresis reveals low protein content (below 4 g/100 ml).
7. **Histologic features** include a thin epithelial lining, usually consisting of <6 cell layers in a corrugated tissue composed of thin, irregular bundles of collagen, and often contain islands of epithelium that may represent "**Daughter Cysts**".

Management: Enucleation along with chemical cauterizing agent (**Carnoy's solution**) and excision of overlying mucosa, to reduce recurrence.

Q. 28. Write a short note on periapical cyst.
(TNMGR, April 2013, Oct. 2014, May 2019)

Ans. A periapical (radicular) cyst is the most common odontogenic cyst (6–55%). It is a true cyst, derived from respiratory epithelium of maxillary sinus, oral epithelium of fistulous tract.

Pathogenesis
1. Proliferation of epithelial rests in the periapical area involved by granuloma.
2. Central cell becomes separated from the source of nutrition, eventually degenerate and liquefies, to form epithelium lined cavity filled with fluid.
3. The cyst further increases in size by osmosis, local fibrinolysis, and continuous epithelial proliferations.

Clinical features
1. Most of the cysts are asymptomatic and occur between 20 and 60 years.
2. The most commonly involved teeth are maxillary anterior and non-vital.
3. Expansion of the cortical plates is uncommon.
4. Radiographically, it appears as well defined radiolucency, surrounded by well defined radiopaque corticated border.

Treatment: Extraction with removal of periapical tissue/RCT with apicoectomy.

Q. 29. Mention the white lesions of oral cavity with their clinical features. *(TNMGR, Oct. 2013)*

Ans. Oral white lesion appears white due to: Hyperkeratosis; Acanthosis; Intra- and extracellular accumulation of fluid in the epithelium; Necrosis of oral epithelium; Microbes produce whitish pseudomembranes; Reduced vascularity in the underlying lamina propria.

Classification of oral white lesions

A. Congenital/genetic lesions: Leukoedema, white sponge nevus, dyskeratosis congenital, hereditary benign intraepithelial dyskeratosis.

B. Acquired lesions
I. **Scrapable:** Superficial oral burn, pseudomembranous candidiasis, pseudomembrane of oral ulcers and materia alba, Morsicatio.
II. **Non-scrapable**
  1. **Lesions with specific pattern**
    a. **Oral lichenoid reactions:** Oral lichen planus; Oral lichen planus associated with thyroid disease, dyslipidemia, DM, HCV; Lichenoid contact reactions (LCR); Drug-induced lichenoid reactions (DILR); Graft-versus-host disease (GVHD).
    b. **Lupus erythematosus.**

2. **Lesion with non-specific pattern:** Frictional keratosis, oral leukoplakia, oral hairy leukoplakia, proliferative verrucous leukoplakia, OSCC, verrucous carcinoma, nicotinic stomatitis, actinic cheilitis, chronic mucocutaneous candidiasis, chronic hyperplastic candidiasis (candidal leukoplakia).

Q. 30. Write a short note on pre-neoplastic conditions.
(Bangalore Uni., Jan. 1992; TNMGR, Sept. 2010; NTR Uni., Nov. 2007)

Ans. Precancerous lesions are defined as a morphologically altered tissue in which cancer is more likely to occur than its apparently normal counterpart, e.g. leukoplakia, erythroplakia, proliferative verrucous leukoplakia (PVL), intraepithelial carcinoma (carcinoma *in situ*), actinic cheilitis, palatal changes with reverse smoking **(WHO, 1978)**.

Premalignant condition is defined as a generalized state associated with increased risk of cancer, e.g. OSMF, syphilis, Sideropenic dysphagia (Plummer-Vinson syndrome/Paterson-Kelly syndrome), oral lichen planus (erosive), discoid lupus erythematosus (DLE), dyskeratosis congenital, xeroderma pigmentosum, syphilis, epidermolysis bullosa **(WHO, 1978)**.

- **Leukoplakia** *(TNMGR, Oct. 2000):* Leukoplakia is defined as "a predominantly white lesion of oral mucosa that cannot be characterized as any other definable lesion" **(WHO, 2012)**.

■ **Classification**
A. According to clinical description
1. Homogenous
2. Non-homogenous.
B. According to etiology
1. Tobacco induced
2. Idiopathic.
C. According to risk of future development of oral cancer
1. High risk sites: Floor of mouth, lateral or ventral surface of tongue, soft palate.
2. Low risks: Dorsum of tongue, hard palate.
3. Intermediate group: All other sites
D. According to histology
1. Dysplastic
2. Non-dysplastic.
E. According to extend
1. Localized
2. Diffused.

■ **Staging of leukoplakia:** In this staging three parameters are used.
- **Size (L):** L1—size is <2 cm; L2–size is in range of 2–4 cm; L3—size is >4 cm; L4–size is not specified.

- **Clinical aspect (C):** C1—homogenous; C2-non-homogenous; Cx—not specified.
- **Pathological features (P):** P1: No dysplasia; P2: Mild dysplasia; P3: Moderate dysplasia; P4: Severe dysplasia; Px: Not specified.

■ Etiopathogenesis

1. **Local factor:** Tobacco (smokeless and smoking), alcohol, chronic irritation, candidiasis, electromagnetic reaction.
2. **Systemic factors:** Syphilis, vitamin deficiency, nutritional deficiency, hormones, drugs, virus.
   - **Pathogenesis:** Tobacco (chemical constituents and combustion products such as tars and resins) along with additional effect of heat from burning of tobacco causes irritation of oral mucosa producing leukoplakic changes.

■ Clinical features

a. Age—average 60 years with M:F = 3:2.
b. It can occur anywhere in oral cavity; Lip lesions are more common in men and tongue lesions are more common in women.
c. Small, well localized, irregular patches to diffused lesions involving oral mucosa.
d. Surface of lesion is often finely wrinkled, may feel rough on palpation.
e. Color may be white or yellowish white, but with heavy use of tobacco may assume brownish color.

■ Treatment

1. Tobacco cessation counseling (TCC).
2. Topical antifungal for 2 weeks.
3. Chemoprevention: Isotretinoin/13-*cis*-retinoic acid; Beta carotene: 5000 IU/day; Topical bleomycin (0.5–1% solution/2 weeks); 5-FU and cisplatin.
4. Surgical excision: Excisional biopsy if size is > 1 cm. Modalities used are: Scalpel (surgical stripping); Cryosurgery; Electrocautery; Laser ablation.
   - **Erythroplakia:** It is defined as "any lesion of the oral mucosa that presents as a bright red velvety plaque which cannot be characterized clinically or pathologically as any other recognizable condition" **(WHO, 1978).**

■ Etiology:
Tobacco and alcohol, reverse chutta smoking, HPV, Candida infection.

■ Clinical presentation:
It appears as a red macule or plaque with well-demarcated borders. The texture is characterized as soft and velvety. An adjacent area of leukoplakia may be found along with the erythroplakia. Occurs most frequently in older men. Most common sites for involvement are floor of mouth, lateral tongue, retromolar pad, and soft palate.

■ Histopathological diagnosis:
"Epithelial dysplasia" is an entity with histologic abnormalities suggesting that the lesion has a greater probability of undergoing malignant change than does normal tissue. Hyperkeratosis is an increased thickness of parakeratin or orthokeratin layer of epithelium.

■ Treatment:
Surgical excision of lesions with scalpel or CO_2 laser and regular follow-up.

Q. 31. Write a short note on submucous fibrosis.
(BFUHS, Nov. 2009, TNMGR, April 2013)

Ans. Oral submucous fibrosis (OSMF) is defined as chronic, insidious disease affecting any part of the oral cavity and sometimes the pharynx, occasionally preceded by and/or associated with vesicle formation, it is always associated with juxtaepithelial inflammatory reaction followed by a fibro-elastic change of lamina propria with epithelial atrophy, leading to stiffness of oral mucosa, causing trismus and inability to eat.

Etiology: Areca nut (most common); Predisposing factors: Nutritional deficiencies, malnutrition increase frequency of HLA-A10, HLA-B7, and HLA-DR3.

Immunopathogenesis of OSMF *(IIHSR, June 2018):*
- Clonal selection of fibroblasts with a high amount of collagen production during long-term exposure to areca quid ingredients.
- By decreased secretion of collagenase.
- Deficiency in collagen phagocytosis by OSMF fibroblasts.
- By production of collagen with a more stable structure (collagen type I trimer) by OSMF fibroblasts.
- By increase in collagen cross-linkage as caused by upregulation of lysyl oxidase by OSF fibroblasts.

There is evidence to suggest that collagen-related genes are altered due to ingredients in the quid. The genes CoL1A2, CoL3A1, CoL6A1, CoL6A3 and COL7A1 have been identified as definite TGF-β targets and induced in fibroblasts at early stages of the disease. Genetic susceptibility may also be associated because of raised frequencies of HLA-A10, -B7 and -DR3 are found in OSMF patients compared to normal subjects. Further HLA-typing done by use of PCR also demonstrates significantly increased frequencies of HLA-A24, DRB1-11 and DRB3-0202/3 antigens.

Clinical features

1. Burning sensation on eating spicy food.
2. Appearance of blisters on palate.
3. Excessive salivation with altered taste sensation.
4. Blanched oral mucosa.
5. Appearance of fibrotic bands, which are palpable.

6. Progressive reduced mouth opening with restricted tongue movements.

Grading

- **Grading of trismus**
  1. Severe: <20 mm
  2. Moderate: 20–40 mm
  3. Mild: >40 mm.
- **Grading of OSMF**
  1. Grade I: Only blanching of oral mucosa.
  2. Grade II: Burning sensation, dryness of mouth, vesicles and ulcers.
  3. Grade III: Grade II + restricted mouth opening.
  4. Grade IV: Grade III + palpable fibrotic bands all over the mouth without involvement of tongue.
  5. Grade V: Grade IV + involvement of tongue.
  6. Grade VI: OSMF with histologically proven oral cancer.

Investigations: Increase ESR, low hemoglobin, eosinophilia, decreased serum iron, increase in total iron binding capacity.

Management

1. Cessation of habit.
2. Nutritional support: High protein diet with multivitamins/antioxidants.
3. Immunomodulatory drugs: Glucocorticoids, placental extracts.
4. Physiotherapy: Forceful mouth opening, heat therapy.
5. Local drug delivery: Inj. of corticosteroids, Placental extract, hyaluronidase, collagenase.
6. Microwave diathermy: Acts by physio-fibrinolysis of fibrous bands.
7. Ultrasound: Its selectivity raises the temperature in accumulated areas.
8. CO_2 laser: It involves multiple small incisions.
9. Cryosurgery: It is the method of locally destroying abnormal tissue by applying liquid nitrogen or argon gas.
10. Combined therapy.
11. Surgical management.

Q. 32. Write a note on squamous cell carcinoma.
(Sumandeeep April 2014; BBD Uni., June 2019)

Ans. Oral cancer includes a group of neoplasms affecting any region of oral cavity, pharyngeal regions and salivary glands. It is estimated that >90% of all oral cancer are oral squamous cell carcinoma (OSCC). It is 6th most common cancer worldwide.

Etiology and major risk factors

1. **Chemical factors:** Tobacco (smoking, chewing, in betel quid, etc.), alcohol.
2. **Biological factors:** Viruses, syphilis, Candida.
3. **Dental factors:** Poor oral hygiene, sharp teeth, dental sepsis.
4. **Nutritional factors:** Dietary deficiencies.

Clinical features

1. More frequent in men than women.
2. In initial stages, it is painless but may develop a burning sensation or pain when it is advanced.
3. Common sites for OSCC to develop are on tongue, lips and floor of mouth, buccal mucosa, retromolar region, gingivobuccal sulcus.
4. *Grossly*, squamous cell carcinoma of oral cavity may have the following types: **Ulcerative type (most common)**-indurated ulcer and firm everted or rolled edges; **Papillary or verrucous type** is soft and wart-like growth; **Nodular type** appears as a firm, slow growing submucosal nodule; **Scirrhous type** is characterised by infiltration into deeper structures.
5. It may also present as a lump, as a red lesion, as a white or mixed white and red lesion, as a non-healing extraction socket or as a cervical lymph node enlargement, characterized by hardness or fixation.
6. **Histologically, SCC** ranges from well-differentiated keratinizing carcinoma to highly undifferentiated neoplasm. Changes of epithelial dysplasia are often present in the surrounding areas of lesion.

■ **Carcinoma of cheek** *(TNMGR, April 2000)*: Buccal mucosa cancer primarily occurs along the occlusal plane and is characterized by pain and ulceration, which are usually accompanied by a buccal mass. The buccal mucosa is anatomically connected to vestibule of the maxilla and mandible, retromolar trigone, and masseter muscle. Thus, buccal mucosa cancer can invade adjacent structures, such as upper and lower jaws, masticatory muscles, and cheeks, often rendering surgical resection and reconstruction more challenging.

Pathogenesis: Molecular pathogenesis: OSCC arises as a consequence of multiple molecular events that develop from combined effects of an individual's genetic predisposition and exposure to environmental carcinogens. Genetic damages may activate mutations or amplification of oncogenes that promote cell survival and proliferation. Mutations include DNA general hypomethylation, hyper- or hypomethylation of certain genes such as cyclin D, and alterations of chromatin. Genetic damages may also inactivate tumor suppressor genes involved in the inhibition of cell proliferation. All these events may lead to cell dysregulation to the extent that growth becomes autonomous and invasive mechanisms develop.

- **Field cancerization theory:** According to this theory since the oral epithelium is exposed to carcinogenic factors, the entire area is at increased risk for development of malignant lesions from accumulation of genetic alterations of oncogenes and tumor suppressor genes. In cancerization field, multiple oral cancers may develop from independent cell clones.

- **Patch field carcinoma model:** According to this model, a stem cell located in oral epithelium acquires a genetic alteration and generates daughter cells, all of which share the genetic alteration. This patch of cells expands to a size of several centimeters to surrounding oral mucosa and macroscopically is often undetectable. In some instances it may appear with distinct morphological characteristics, like leukoplakia or erythroplakia.

■ **Staging of OSCC:** Staging of OSCC is performed using the TNM system. cTNM is the stage given after clinical examination of patient, while pTNM is the stage after histopathological examination of surgical specimen.

■ **Therapeutic approaches:** In primary (I and II) stages: Surgery and/or radiotherapy; in III, IV stages: Combination of surgery, radiotherapy or chemotherapy (cisplatin and 5-FU). Recent advances: Fractionated radiotherapy or concomitant chemo-radiotherapy (CT-RT); Targeted molecular therapy (monoclonal antibodies and gene therapy).

Screening of oral cancer (NTR Uni., April 2014): Classification of diagnostic aids:

1. Clinical methods: Vital staining: Toluidine blue, Lugol's iodine, rose bengal staining
2. Light-based detection methods: Chemiluminescence; Autofluorescence.
3. Histopathological methods: Exfoliative cytology, brush biopsy (oral CDx), scalpel biopsy.
4. Molecular methods: Quantification of nuclear DNA content; tumour markers; microsatellite markers.
5. Miscellaneous: Optical coherence tomography, colposcopy, elastography.

Q. 33. Write a short note on theory of focal infection.
(BFUHS, May 2008; HP, May 2015)

Ans. Focal infection is a localized or generalized infection caused by dissemination of microorganisms or toxic products from a focus of infection. **Focus of infection** refers to a circumscribed area of tissue, which is infected with exogenous pathogenic microorganisms and is usually located near a mucous or cutaneous surface.

Mechanism of focal infection: Microorganism, thier toxins or toxic products may be carried through the blood stream or lymphatic channels from a focus to a distant site where they may incite a hypersensitive reaction.

- **Focal infection theory:** This theory (William Hunter, 1910) stated that "foci" of sepsis were responsible for initiation and progression of variety of inflammatory diseases such as arthritis, peptic ulcers, and appendicitis. In the oral cavity, therapeutic edentulation was common as a result of popularity of focal infection theory. It has become increasingly clear that oral cavity can act as the site of origin for dissemination of pathogenic organisms to distant body sites, especially in immunocompromised hosts.

Pathways of focal infection (RGUHS, May 2013): These are:

1. **Metastatic infection:** Oral infections and dental procedures can cause transient bacteremia, which can cause metastatic infections, e.g. subacute bacterial endocarditis (SABE); CST; Ludwig's angina; Orbital cellulitis.
2. **Metastatic injury:** Metastatic injury from circulation of oral microbial toxins (exotoxins and endotoxins), e.g. acute myocardial infarction; Persistent pyrexia; idiopathic trigeminal neuralgia; Toxic shock syndrome.
3. **Metastatic inflammation:** It is caused by immunological injury from oral organisms, e.g. Behcet's syndrome; Chronic uveitis; Inflammatory bowel disease; Crohn's disease.

Significance of oral foci of infection: There has evidence that shows that oral foci of infection either cause or aggravate many systemic conditions:

1. Arthritis, rheumatoid and rheumatic fever type.
2. Valvular heart disease, subacute bacterial endocarditis.
3. Gastrointestinal diseases.
4. Ocular diseases and skin diseases.
5. Renal diseases and bacterial pneumonia.
6. Diabetes mellitus and low birth weight.

Q. 34. Write a short note on enamel hypoplasia.
(TNMGR, Sept. 2008; RGUHS, Nov. 2011; NTR Uni., May 2019)

Ans. Enamel hypoplasia is defined as an incomplete formation of organic enamel matrix of teeth.

Types

A. Hereditary: Amelogenesis imperfecta: Hypoplastic, hypocalcified, hypomaturation.

B. Environmental

1. Nutritional deficiency: Vitamins A, C, D and hypocalcaemia.

2. Exanthematous diseases: Measles, chickenpox, scarlet fever.

3. Congenital syphilis (Hutchinson's incisors, Mullberry/Moon's/Fournier's molars)

4. Birth injury: Prematurity, Rh hemolytic disease.

5. Local infection/trauma: Turner hypoplasia (Turner's tooth).

6. Ingestion of chemicals: Fluorides, Tetracycline hypoplasia.

7. Idiopathic causes.

Clinically features

- Mild: It appears as small grooves, pits or fissures on the enamel surface.
- Moderate: Enamel may exhibit rows of deep pits arranged horizontally across the tooth surface.
- Severe: A considerable portion of enamel is absent.

Management: Bleaching (30% H_2O_2), laminate and veneering and capping in severe cases, microabrasion.

Q. 35. Write a short note on dry socket.
(NTR Uni., June 2014)

Ans. Dry socket (**fibrinolytic osteitis/alveolar osteitis**) is a post-extraction socket that exhibits exposed bone that is not covered by a blood clot or healing epithelium and exists inside or around the perimeter of socket or alveolus for days after the extraction procedure.

Causes: Bacteria, inflammation, fibrinolysis, traumatic extractions, smoking, oral contraceptives.

Pathogenesis: Food particles that collect inside the socket may dislodge a blood clot. Bacterial biofilm and food particles inside a socket may also hinder reformation of dislodged blood clot by obstructing contact of a reforming blood clot with the exposed bone. Food particles that collect inside a dry socket can also ferment due to bacteria. This fermentation may result in the formation of toxins or antigens that may irritate the exposed bone, produce an unpleasant taste or halitosis, and cause pain throughout the jaw.

- **Birn hypothesis:** Trauma during an extraction or presence of a bacterial infection facilitates release of plasminogen tissue activators in post-extraction socket, resulting in plasmin induction of fibrinolysis that dislodges blood clot that formed after extraction.

Clinical features: Exposed bone, acutely painful to touch, foul smell. Mostly, dry socket lesions occur in mandibular third molar extractions.

Treatment: Pharmacological measures: Antibacterial agents; Antiseptic agents and lavage; Antifibrinolytic agents; Steroid anti-inflammatory agents; Obtundent dressings; Clot supporting agents.

Q. 36. What is osteomyelitis. Mention the management of osteomyelitis of body of mandible.
(BFUHS, May 2004; TNMGR, Oct. 2013)

Ans. Osteomyelitis is defined as an inflammatory condition of the bone, beginning in the medullar cavity and havarian systems and extending to involve the periosteum of affected area. The infection becomes established in calcified portion of the bone when pus and edema in the medullary cavity and beneath the periosteum compromises or obstructs the local blood supply. Following ischemia, infected bone becomes necrotic and leads to **sequestrum** formation, which is considered a classical sign of osteomyelitis (*Topazian 1994, 2002*). The surrounding viable, reactive bone is called **involucrum** (Fig. 6.36).

Predisposing factors: Fracture due to trauma, gunshot wounds, radiation damage, Paget's disease, osteopetrosis, systemic conditions (malnutrition, acute leukemia, uncontrolled diabetes).

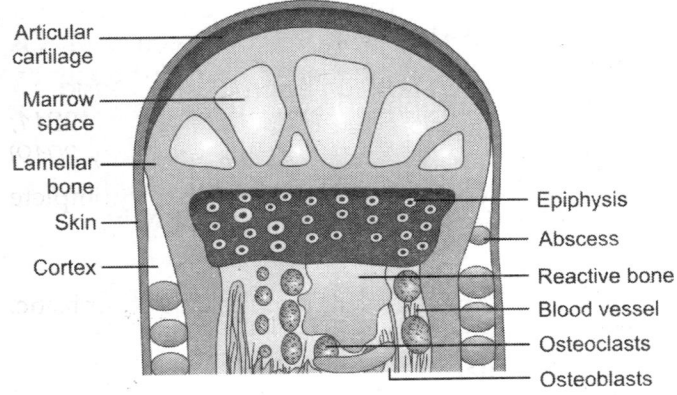
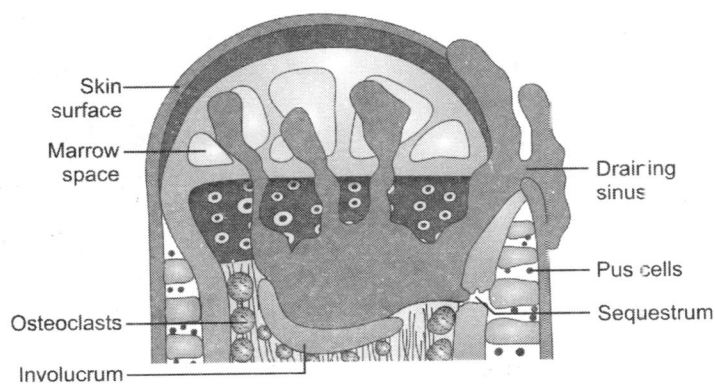

Fig. 6.36: Pathogenesis of osteomyelitis

Classification

a. **Acute:** Acute suppurative osteomyelitis.

b. **Chronic**

i. Chronic suppurative osteomyelitis.

ii. Chronic focal sclerosing osteomyelitis (condensing osteomyelitis).

iii. Chronic diffuse sclerosing osteomyelitis and SAPHO syndrome (synovitis, acne, pustulosis, hyperostosis, and osteitis)

iv. Garre's osteomyelitis (chronic osteomyelitis with proliferative periostitis, ossifying periostitis).

c. **Specific types:** Tuberculous osteomyelitis, syphilitic osteomyelitis, actinomycotic osteomyelitis.

Etiopathogenesis *(NTR Uni., April 2013)*: (Flowchart 6.36).

Management

1. General principles of management include debridement, drainage and antimicrobial therapy.

2. If sequestrum is large, surgical excision. Drainage, curettage, sequestrectomy, saucerization, decortications and resection.

Q. 37. Write a short note on Garre's osteomyelitis.
(TNMGR, March 2007)

Ans. Garre's osteomyelitis, which was first described by Carl Garre in 1893 as a focal gross thickening of periosteum with peripheral reactive bone formation resulting from infection, is a chronic non-suppurative sclerotic type of osteomyelitis.

Flowchart 6.36: Pathogenesis of osteomyelitis *(Topazian, 2002)* A. Acute , B. secondary chronic osteomyelitis

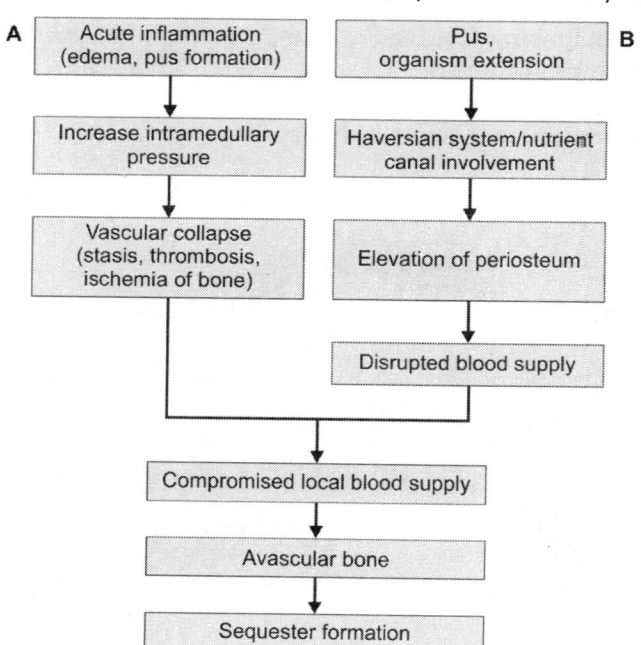

Clinical features

1. Occur commonly in younger age (<30); M>F.

2. Mandible is affected > Maxilla, mostly at inferior border of mandible, in first molar region.

3. It is presented as hard non-tender swelling with medial and lateral expansion of jaw.

4. It may become secondarily affected to cause discomfort.

5. Histopathological examination may show micro-abscess and micro-sequesters.

6. Radiographically, appearance is "**Onion Skin**".

Differential diagnosis: Ewing's sarcoma, Caffey disease, fibrous dysplasia, Paget's disease, osteosarcoma.

Treatment: Endodontically treated or removal of carious tooth with no surgical intervention for periosteal lesion.

Q. 38. Write a short note on osteoradionecrosis.
(TNMGR, March 2008; Oct. 2019)

Ans. Osteoradionecrosis (ORN) is a radiation-induced pathologic process characterized by a chronic and painful infection and necrosis accompanied by late sequestration and sometimes, permanent deformity.

Etiopathogenesis: Flowchart 6.38.

Theories of pathophysiology of ORN

1. **Meyer's theory or radiation, trauma and infection theory:** He suggested that injury provided the opening for invasion of oral microbiological flora into the underlying irradiated bone.

2. **Marx theory or hypoxic-hypocellular-hypovascular theory:** The pathophysiological sequence suggested by Marx is: Irradiation; formation of **Hypoxic-Hypocellular, Hypovascular tissue (3H)**; and breakdown of tissue driven by persistent hypoxia that can cause a chronic non-healing wound.

3. **Radiation-induced fibroatrophic theory (2004):** It suggests that the key event in progression of ORN is activation and dysregulation of fibroblastic activity that leads to atrophic tissue within a previously irradiated area.

Classification/staging of ORN: Notani classification: Based on clinical examination and OPG findings.

1. Class I: ORN confined to dentoalveolar bone.

2. Class II: ORN limited to dentoalveolar bone or mandible above inferior alveolar canal or both.

3. Class III: ORN involving mandible below inferior dental canal, or pathological fracture or skin fistula.

Flowchart 6.38: Etiopathogenesis of osteoradionecrosis

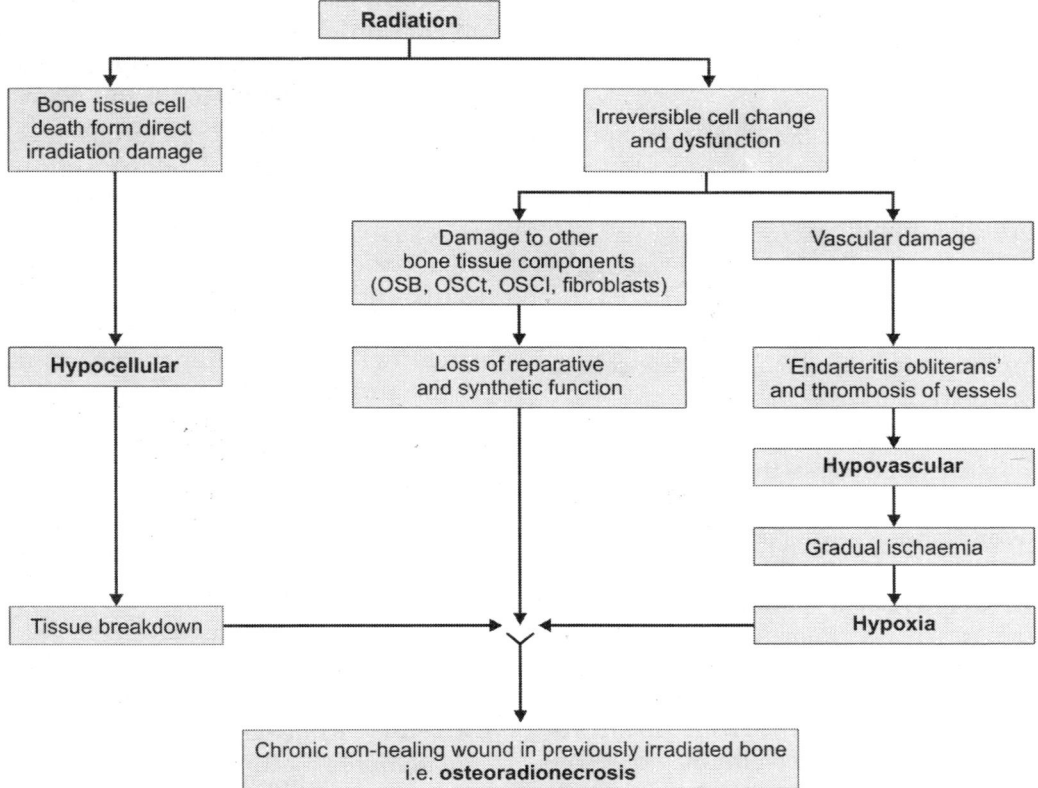

Clinical features

1. Early ORN may be asymptomatic, exposed devitalized bone through ulcerated mucosa or skin can be seen clearly.
2. Pain is a common symptom; Other symptoms include dysaesthesia, halitosis, dysgeusia and food impaction in the area of exposed sequestra.
3. In severe cases, patients can present with fistulation from oral mucosa or skin, complete devitalisation of bone and pathological fractures.
4. ORN usually develops during the first 6–12 months after radiotherapy.

Prevention: Before treatment, a thorough dental exploration is indicated, evaluating those teeth with a poor prognosis due to caries, periodontal disease, or with latent infections. In these cases extractions should be made at least 2–3 weeks before treatment. After treatment for lessening the risk of ORN is good fitting, support and stability of removable dentures, avoiding points of excessive pressure that may give rise to pressure ulcers. All patients should be instructed on meticulous oral hygiene and fluoride should be applied to dentition daily via custom molded trays and "close follow-up" schedule. Those who require dental extractions >4 months after radiation therapy should be treated with HBO (Marx protocol: 20 dives, 2.4 atmospheres for 90 min/dive before extraction and 10 dives after extraction).

Management

A. Conservative treatment: Local irrigation (saline solution, NaHCO$_3$, or chlorhexidine 0.2%), systemic antibiotics in acute infectious episodes, avoidance of irritants, oral hygiene instruction, gentle removal of sequestrum and PENTO regimen [pentoxifylline (400 mg) BD + tocopherol (1000 IU) OD].

B. Definitive treatment

1. **Hyperbaric oxygen therapy (HBO):** The rationale for use of HBO in radiation tissue damage is to revascularize irradiated tissues and to improve fibroblastic cellular density, thus limiting the amount of non-viable tissue to be surgically removed; enhancing wound healing and preparing the tissues for reconstruction when indicated. "**Wilfred-Hall Protocol**" to treat established osteonecrosis of jaws (by Marx and Ames):
   - **Stage I:** 30 consecutive treatments. If the wound shows no definitive clinical improvement, a further 10 exposures are given. If there is failure to heal after 3 months, the condition is advanced to stage II.

- **Stage II:** Exposed bone is removed by alveolar sequestrectomy and further 20 HBO treatments are given, to a total of 60 exposures. If wound dehiscence or failure to heal occurs, patient is advanced to stage III.
- **Stage III:** The criteria for this category are failure of stage II, pathological fracture, orocutaneous fistula, or radiographic evidence of résorption to inferior border of mandible.

2. **Ultrasound:** Therapeutic US can result in healing by induction of angiogenesis.
3. **Surgery:** Reconstruction surgery (fibular flap, iliac crest flap, scapular-parascapular flaps); Cancellous bone grafting (distraction osteogenesis).

■ **Osteochemonecrosis:** Many drugs/chemicals can facilitates or induce osteonecrosis of the jaws. Examples:
1. **Phossy jaw/phosphorous necrosis of jaw:** Due to exposure to white phosphorous among workers in match-stick industry.
2. **Bisphosphonates associates osteonecrosis of jaws:** Osteonecrosis of jaws in patient receiving bisphosphonate therapy. The mandible is more commonly affected than the maxilla, and 60% of cases are preceded by a dental surgical procedure. All sites of potential jaw infection should be eliminated before bisphosphonate therapy is initiated in these patients to reduce the necessity of subsequent dentoalveolar surgery. Conservative debridement of necrotic bone, pain control, infection management, use of antimicrobial oral rinses and withdrawal of bisphosphonates are preferable to aggressive surgical measures for treating this condition.

Q. 39. Discuss the pathophysiology of residual ridge resorption. *(TNMGR, March 2009)*

Ans. Residual ridge resorption (RRR) is defined as diminishing quantity and quality of residual ridge after teeth are lost. It is primarily localized loss of bone structure.

Etiology: Atwood postulated four main factors that are responsible for RRR *(Atwood, 1957, 1962):*
1. **Anatomic factor:** Rate of resorption of alveolar bone depends on anatomic factors include size, shape, cortical, cancellous and density of ridges, thickness and character of mucosal covering, ridge relationships, number and depth of sockets.
2. **Metabolic factors:** These are multiple nutritional and hormonal factors which influence the cellular activity of bone forming cells. 1. Osteoporosis, 2. Calcium and vitamin D.
3. **Functional factors:** Intensity, duration and direction of force applied are translated into biologic cell activity resulting in either bone formation or bone resorption.
4. **Prosthetic factor:** Includes various techniques, materials, concepts, principles incorporated in the prosthesis, tooth material and form.

Pathophysiology: RRR is a localized pathologic loss of bone that is not built back by simply removing the causative factors. Immediately following the extraction, any sharp edges remaining are rounded off by external osteoclastic resorption, leaving a high well rounded residual ridge. As resorption continues from the labial and lingual aspects, the crest of the ridge becomes increasingly narrow ultimately becoming knife-edged. As the process continues, the knife-edge becomes shorter and even eventually disappears, leaving a low well rounded or flat ridge. Eventually, this too resorbs, leaving a depressed ridge.

Residual ridge form: Classification by Cawood and Howell as:
1. Class I: Dentate.
2. Class II: Post-extraction.
3. Class III: Convex ridge form, with adequate height and width of alveolar process.
4. Class IV: Knife edge form with adequate height but inadequate width of alveolar process.
5. Class V: Flat ridge form with loss of alveolar process.
6. Class VI: Loss of basal bone that may be extensive but follows no predictable pattern.

Assessment of RRR: Mandibular RRR was assessed by using the mental foramen and the inferior border of the mandible, as they appear in OPGs, as reference points, using Wical and Swoope analysis method; in which the original height of mandible is assumed to be three times the distance between inferior border of mandible to lower border of mental foramen. The amount of resorption was calculated according to formula: $R = 3 \times -L$ (R: Amount of mandibular RRR; ×: Distance from inferior border of mandible to lower border of mental foramen; L: Height of mandibular residual alveolar ridge).

Q. 40. Write about oral manifestations of systemic conditions of dental relevance. *(TNMGR, Sept. 2008; TNMGR, April 2015; MUHS June 2017)*

Ans. The mouth has been called a "Mirror of the body". The oral cavity provides many diagnostic clues to systemic disease and may be the first indication of a systemic condition.
A. **Blood dyscrasias:** The mouth may be the site of the earliest signs of blood dyscrasias. Manifestations may include hemorrhage, infection, and cellular infiltration of tissues. Diffuse gingival hypertrophy

may be present in leukemia. Gingival bleeding or accumulation of blood in tissues may occur secondary to a platelet deficiency. Patients are predisposed to fungal infections and certain viral infections which may be the initial complaint in a blood dyscrasia. Also, medical management of leukemias may occasion secondary complications in oral cavity. These may include secondary microbial infections, stomatitis, and secondary bone marrow depression and related changes. Gingival hemorrhage and oozing may be evidence of thrombocytopenia. Anemia may manifest as fatigue, shortness of breath, and pallor, together with oral manifestations like pallor of oral mucosa, pain and burning in tongue with loss of papillae.

B. **Metabolic disease:** Oral manifestations may result from abnormal hormonal regulation. Manifestations of diabetes frequently occur in the oral cavity. These may include dry mouth, symptoms of burning, tenderness of the mucosa, and heightened reactivity to local irritation of bacterial plaque. Sex hormone imbalance can result in marked reaction to local irritations of oral tissues. This may occur during puberty, pregnancy, and with use of oral contraceptives. Also hyperplastic tissue responses are commonly seen, resulting in soft tissue growths on the gum tissue. Hypofunction of the adrenal cortex, resulting in Addison's disease, may present accumulation of brownish melanotic pigment in a general fashion, or as blotches in the oral soft tissue.

C. **Dermatological disease:** Lichen planus is a common dermatologic condition occurring in the oral cavity. Clinically, the condition presents diagnostic white striations (Wickham's striae) and plaque-like white areas on the tissue. Benign mucous membrane pemphigoid (BMMP) is a dermatologic condition principally affecting the gum tissues. Bullae and ulceration may occur in the oral tissues, or the condition may be relatively asymptomatic. In pemphigus, oral lesions may be the initial, and possibly the only manifestation of the condition. The sites most commonly affected are the lips, cheeks, and floor of the mouth. The mucosal surfaces are friable and will slough when subjected to minor physical irritation.

D. **Connective tissue disease:** Sjögren's syndrome is characterized by dry mouth, keratoconjunctivitis sicca, and other collagen diseases—often rheumatoid arthritis. Rheumatoid arthritis may affect the temporomandibular joint. Signs and symptoms include pain, clicking and grinding in the joint, limitation of jaw function, and a changing occlusion of teeth. Radiographic evidence of rheumatoid arthritis may be present.

E. **Nutritional deficiencies:** Due to rapid cell turnover of oral mucosa, nutritional deficiencies may present first with oral manifestations. Changes may occur in tongue papillae, mucosal color and integrity, and in oral sensation. The most common oral changes are: Inflammation and loss of tongue papillae (glossitis), a burning sensation and pain in the corners of mouth.

Q. 41. Write a note on syndromes related to maxillofacial region. *(TNMGR, March 2010)*

Ans. Syndrome is defined as a pattern of multiple anomalies pathogenetically related but not representing a single sequence or developmental field.

Syndrome related to maxillofacial region

1. **Syndrome of developmental disturbances during growth:** Cleft lip/palate, Parry Romberg syndrome, Vander Woude's syndrome, Ascher's syndrome, orofacial digital syndrome, median cleft face syndrome, Meischer's syndrome, Melkerson-Rosenthal syndrome, branchial arch syndrome, Peutz-Jeghers syndrome, Rubinstein-Taybi syndrome, Klinefelter's syndrome, Gardner's syndrome.

2. **Syndrome related to benign and malignant tumors:** Cowden's syndrome, B-K mole syndrome, multiple endocrine neoplasia syndromes, Sipple syndrome.

3. **Syndrome related to salivary gland:** Sjögren's syndrome.

4. **Syndrome of odontogenic cysts and tumors:** Gorlin-Goltz syndrome.

5. **Syndrome related to infections:** Heerfordt's syndrome, Behcet's syndrome, Reiter's syndrome, Ramsay Hunt's syndrome.

6. **Syndromes related to bone and joints:** Albright's syndrome, Crouzan syndrome, Apert syndrome, Treacher Collins syndrome, Pierre-Robin syndrome, Marfan syndrome, Down syndrome (trisomy 21), van Buchem syndrome, Gorham syndrome, Albright syndrome, Caffey-Silverman syndrome, Costen syndrome, myofascial pain dysfunction syndrome, Maffucci's syndrome.

7. **Syndrome related to blood:** Fanconi syndrome, Plummer-Vinson syndrome, Aldrich syndrome, Chédiak-Higashi syndrome, Kostmann syndrome.

8. **Syndrome related to skin diseases:** Steven-Johnson syndrome, CREST syndrome, Ehlers-Danlos syndrome, Papillon-Lefèvre syndrome.

9. **Syndromes related to neuromuscular system:** Reader's syndrome, Frey's syndrome, Horner's syndrome, jaw-winking syndrome, Trotter's syndrome, Eagle's syndrome, floppy infant syndrome, mobius syndrome, Horton's syndrome.

10. **Syndrome related to metabolic disorders:** Cushing's syndrome, Hurler's syndrome, Hunter's syndrome, Waterhouse-Friederichsen syndrome.

Q. 42. Write a short note on trisomy 21.
(TNMGR, March 2009; NTR Uni., May 2019)

Ans. Trisomy 21 or Down syndrome is a common form of mental retardation associated with mongolism and other somatic abnormalities. It is the most common autosomal abnormality, occurring 1/700 live births. Both genders are affected equally.

Types of Down syndrome

- **Trisomy 21:** About 95% of people with Down syndrome have Trisomy 21. In this type, each cell in the body has 3 separate copies of chromosome 21.
- **Translocation Down syndrome (3%):** This occurs when an extra part or a whole extra chromosome 21 is present, but it is attached or "trans-located" to a different chromosome.
- **Mosaic Down syndrome (2%):** For children with mosaic Down syndrome, some of their cells have 3 copies; other cells have 2 copies of chromosome 21.

Clinical features: Mental retardation; Brachycephaly; Hypertelorism; Depressed nasal bridge; Flat occiput; Broad short neck; Mongoloid face; Medial epicanthal fold; Strabismus; Ocular anomalies; Short stature, feet and hands; Clinodactyly; Wide gap between first and second toes.

Oral manifestations: Microstomia, macroglossia, scrotal tongue, hypoplasia of maxilla, delayed tooth eruption, partial anodontia, enamel hypoplasia, juvenile periodontitis, cleft lip/palate, angular cheilitis, geographic tongue.

Diagnosis

1. **Screening tests:** Measuring the amount of various substances in mother's blood (e.g. MS-AFP, triple screen, quad-screen), and ultrasound.
2. **Diagnostic tests:** Chorionic villus sampling (CVS); Amniocentesis; Percutaneous umbilical blood sampling (PUBS).

Q. 43. Write about Treacher Collins syndrome.
(TNMGR, Sept. 2007)

Ans. Treacher Collins syndrome (mandibulofacial dysostosis/Franceschetti-Klein syndrome) is a congenital disorder of craniofacial development characterized by bilateral symmetrical oto-mandibular dysplasia without abnormalities of extremities, and associated with several head and neck defects. Inheritance is autosomal dominant, with males and females are equally affected.

Etiology: Mutations in: *TCOF1* gene (5q32); or *POLR1C* (6p21.1) or *POLR1D* (13q12.2).

Clinical features

1. Anti-mongoloid palpebral fissures with coloboma of outer portion of lower lids and deficiency of eyelashes.
2. Hypoplasia of facial bones, malformation of external ears and macrostomia.
3. High palate and Malocclusion of teeth.
4. Blind fistula between angle of ears and angle of mouth.
5. Tongue-shaped process of hairline extending towards the cheeks.
6. Facial clefts and skeletal deformities.
7. Characteristic **bird-like** or **fish-like** face.

Differential diagnosis: Nager syndrome, Miller syndrome, Goldenhar syndrome.

Antenatal diagnosis: Molecular analysis of chorionic villus samples (CVS); Antenatal ultrasound may show typical facial dysmorphism and bilateral ear abnormalities.

Management and treatment: In cases with postnatal respiratory distress, tracheostomy, non-invasive ventilation or mandibular distraction should be done. Maxillofacial and plastic surgery can correct the soft tissue hypoplasia (facial recontouring with lipostructure), bone hypoplasia (surgical bone distraction, bone grafts), eyelid coloboma and cleft palate (surgical repair). Specialist ENT surgery is required for abnormalities of middle ear and external ear. Management of hearing impairment includes hearing aids and functional surgery.

Q. 44. Write a short note on long face syndrome.
(TNMGR, Oct. 2013)

Ans. "Long face syndrome" includes multiple anomalies like open bite, hyper divergent face, maxillary alveolar hyperplasia, maxillary vertical excess, anterior vertical excess of the lower face level, high angle facial type. Long face morphology is a relatively common presentation among orthodontic patients. Etiological factors such as enlarged adenoids, nasal allergies, weak masticatory muscles, oral habits, and genetic factors have all been implicated in the development of the long face morphology.

Clinical features: Longer lower third of face, facial retrognathism, depressed nasolabial areas, excessive exposure of maxillary teeth and gingiva, lip incompetence, narrow palate, posterior cross-bites, anterior open-bite.

Treatment: The clinician must address the three-dimensional dentoalveolar and skeletal problems that present in long face syndrome. Two traditional methods for impeding excessive vertical growth are: High-pull headgear with maxillary fixed appliance and functional appliance with bite blocks.

Q. 45. Write a short note on Ehlers-Danlos syndrome.

Ans. "Ehlers-Danlos syndrome (EDS)/elastic man" or "India rubber man" is a hereditary collagen characterized by hyperelasticity of skin and strong tendency to bruising.

Diagnosis: By clinical findings and family history.

Clinical features: Joint hypermobility; Skin hyperelasticity; Presence of dystrophic scars; and a tendency to excessive bleeding manifested by bruises, ecchymoses and hematomas. Types:

Type I: Hyperelastic skin, bony prominences, pigmented and atrophic scars ("**Cigarette Paper Scar**"), fibrous nodules, abnormal bleeding tendency, mitral valve prolapse.

Type II: Similar to type I, but less severe clinically.

Type III: Tall and thin, joint hypermobility and hyperelastic and velvety skin.

Type IV: Marked fragility of vascular system, short stature, acrogeria, hypertelorism, narrow nose, atrophied ear lobes, aneurysms, joint hypermobility, mitral valve prolapse.

Type V: Women are carriers; similar to types I and II.

Type VI: Type I + ocular involvement.

Type VII: Joint hypermobility, bilateral dislocation of hips, small stature.

Type VIII: Generalized early-onset periodontitis, large patches of scar tissue on shins, premature loss of teeth before age 30, skin hyperelasticity, hypermobility of joints, hypertelorism, narrow curved nose, narrow face and scarring on forehead and chin.

Oral manifestations of EDS

A. **Extraoral:** Presence of scarring on chin and forehead, a history of repeated luxation of TMJ, epicanthus, hypertelorism, narrow curved nose, sparse hair and hyperelasticity of skin.

B. **Intraoral**
   - **Mucosa:** Fragile mucosa/gingiva, early-onset generalized periodontitis, premature loss of deci-

duous and permanent teeth, and **supple tongue** with positive "**Gorlin's sign**".
   - **Teeth:** Enamel hypoplasia, fragile teeth, microdontia, pulp stones, short roots, multiple supernumerary teeth, high arched palate.

Differential diagnosis: Marfan's syndrome, generalized familial joint hypermobility syndrome, cutis laxa, pseudoxanthoma elasticum and Larsen's syndrome.

Q. 46. Write a short note on fragile X syndrome.

Ans. Fragile X syndrome (Martin-Bell syndrome) is the most common cause of inherited mental retardation and it is transmitted as dominant linked to X chromosome. The gene responsible for fragile X syndrome is FMR1 gene of X chromosome.

Characteristic features

- **Primary features:** Elongated and narrow face; large forehead and prominent chin; large and anteverted ears, joint hyperlaxity, macroorchidism.
- **Secondary features:** Tallness, soft and silky skin, widened fingertips and flat feet, cardiac anomalies.
- **Oral and maxillofacial features:** Macrocephalia, prominent frontal bone, hypotelorism, strabismus, hypoplasia of middle 3rd of face, mandibular protrusion, micrognathia, glossoptosis and cleft palate, high arched palate, mesiodens, dental hypomineralization, abraded occlusal surfaces.
- **Beahivioural features:** Low IQ score, attention disorders, behavioral disturbances, extremely shy, poor tolerance of frustration.

Q. 47. Write a short note on Marfan syndrome.

Ans. Marfan syndrome is an autosomal-dominant genetic disorder of connective tissue with genetic defect in fibrillin which is a connective tissue protein required for elastic tissue formation. This alteration was caused by mutation of FBN1 gene, located on long arm of chromosome 15 and mutation of TGFBR2 gene.

Diagnosis: By Ghent's 1996 nosology, which is based on the combination of "major manifestations" and "minor manifestations." The diagnosis of Marfan syndrome is made with the presence of 1 major criterion in the family history and 1 major criterion in an organ system plus involvement of a second organ system.

Clinical features

- Dilatation of ascending aorta, mitral valve prolapse, dilatation of main pulmonary artery, and calcification of mitral annulus.
- Disproportionate growth of long bones, pectus excavatum (hollowed chest) or pectus carinatum (overgrowth of ribs), acetabular protrusion, scoliosis.

- Dolichocephaly, retrognathia, micrognathia, deep palate, and a convex profile.
- More dental caries, hypoplastic enamel, root deformity, abnormal pulp shape, pulp calcifications, gingival inflammation, supernumerary teeth, dental crowding, TMJ subluxation and disorder.
- Ectopia lentis, abnormally flat cornea, increased axial length of globe, myopia, strabismus.
- Others: Spontaneous pneumothorax, apical blebs, and recurrent or incisional hernias, nephritic syndrome, hematologic abnormalities, primary hypogonadism, and alopecia.

Differential diagnoses: Lujan-Fryns syndrome, Beals syndrome, MASS phenotype (mitral valve prolapse, aortic enlargement, skin and skeletal findings), Stickler syndrome, Ehlers-Danlos syndrome.

Q. 48. Write a note on Sjögren's syndrome.
(NTR Uni., April 2013)

Ans. Sjögren's syndrome (Gougerot-Houwer-Sjögren syndrome/keratoconjunctivitis sicca/secreto-inhibitor-xerodermostenosis/sicca syndrome) is a chronic inflammatory autoimmune disease of unknown origin, affecting in particular the tear and salivary glands. Sicca symptoms are the hallmarks of Sjögren's syndrome. Types:

- **Primary Sjögren's syndrome (PSS):** Idiopathic, comprises the "sicca syndrome" without any associated autoimmune disease. Exocrine function are more severely impaired than in secondary type and are frequently associated with extraglandular manifestations.
- **Secondary Sjögren's syndrome (SSS):** It consists of "Sicca complex" which may be relatively mild and associated with autoimmune diseases.

Clinical features
1. **Ocular involvement:** Dry, sore and gritty eyes, corneal ulceration, uveitis, cataract and glaucoma, keratoconjunctivitis, foreign body sensation, burning, photophobia, irregularity of the corneal image, discharge.

Table 6.48: ACR/EULAR-2017 classification criteria for Primary Sjögren's syndrome

Items	Score
Labial salivary gland with focus score of >1 foci/4 mm³	3
Anti-SSA/Ro60 antibodies	3
SICCA ocular staining score >5	1
Schirmer's test <5 mm/5 min. in at least 1 eye	1
Unstimulated whole saliva flow rate <0.1 ml/min	1

2. **Oral involvement:** Dryness of mouth, lip cracking, difficulty in mastication, dysphagia, angular stomatitis, fissuring and ulceration of tongue, dental caries and candidiasis.
3. **Others:** Arthralgia, annular erythema, skin dryness, Raynaud's phenomenon, dry cough, dyspnoea, interstitial lung disease, esophageal dryness, dysphagia, atrophic gastritis, renal tubular acidosis, hypothyroidism.
4. **Complication:** Patients with Sjögren's syndrome have 44 times increased risk of developing lymphoma.

Diagnostic criteria: PSS is diagnosed in any individual who has a score of >4 when the classification criteria of American College of Rheumatology (ACR)/European League Against Rheumatism (EULAR) given in 2017 is applied (Table 6.48).

Inclusion criteria: Any patient with at least 1 symptom of ocular or oral dryness or the presence of systemic manifestations suggestive of PSS.

Exclusion criteria: History of head and neck radiation treatment; active HCV infection on PCR assay; receipt of anticholinergic drugs; Sarcoidosis; graft-versus-host disease; IgG4-related disease.

Treatment: Symptomatic relief, achieved by keeping the mucosal surfaces moist.

- For dry eyes: Artificial tears, hydroxyethylcellulose, acetylcysteine, dispersants like dextran, polyethylene glycol.
- Regular and proper oral hygiene and frequent dental assessment is required.
- Topical oral treatment with fluoride may slow down damage to teeth.
- Bromhexine (48 mg/day), pilocarpine (5 mg TDS) may help in sicca symptoms.
- Lubricant jellies are used to treat vaginal dryness.
- Dry skin is treated with moisturizing creams.
- Arthralgia or joint symptoms are treated with NSAIDs. Hydroxychloroquine (200 mg a day) helps both arthralgia and fatigue of Sjögren's syndrome. It also reduces hypergammaglobulinaemia, decreases titre of IgG antibodies to La/SS-B, and increases haemoglobin.
- Corticosteroids (0.5–1.0 mg/kg/day) are used in patients with severe extraglandular disease including interstitial pneumonitis, glomerulonephritis, vasculitis, and peripheral neuropathy.
- Other drugs: Cyclosporin; IFN-α; High dose IV immunoglobulin; plasma exchange; Anti-CD4 monoclonal antibodies.

Q. 49. Write a short note on burning sensation in tongue. *(NTR Uni., Nov. 2008)*

Ans. Burning mouth syndrome (BMS) has been defined as "A pain of at least 4–6 months duration located on tongue or other oral mucosal membranes associated with normal clinical or laboratory findings" (IASP).

Synonyms: Stomatodynia, stomatopyrosis, oral dysesthesia, sore mouth and sore tongue/glossodynia (painful tongue)/glossopyrosis (burning tongue)/glossalgia.

Etiological factors

A. **Local conditions:** Xerostomia, ill fitting denture, allergic reactions (lichenoid, stomatitis), infections, oral mucosal lesions, chemical burn.

B. **Systemic factors:** Nutritional deficiency, endocrine disorders, anaemia, GIT disorders, peripheral neuropathies.

C. **Psychological factors:** Anxiety, depression, cancer phobia, compulsive disorder.

Clinical features

- Female/male ratio of occurrence of BMS is 7:1.
- Prevalence of BMS increases with age in both genders.
- It mainly affects middle aged females in 5th–7th decades of life.
- The condition affects multiple sites in oral cavity (tip of tongue > lips > lateral border of tongue > palate).
- Patients usually complains of classic triad of chronic oral mucosal burning pain associated with dysgeusia and xerostomia with no visible disease in oral mucosa for 4–6 months duration.
- Some patient may report with dry mouth, bitter/metallic taste, and altered taste perception.

Classification

I. Scala classification

1. Primary BMS/idiopathic BMS: No organic local/systemic causes are identified.
2. Secondary BMS: Due to local/systemic pathological conditions.

II. Lamey and Lamb (1994) classification

1. Type 1: Progressive burning pain, which increases gradually throughout the day.
2. Type 2: Symptoms are constant throughout the day and patients find it difficult to get sleep.
3. Type 3: Symptoms are intermittent, with atypical location and pain.

Diagnostic criteria: Scala's diagnostic criteria:

I. Fundamental criteria

- Daily deep burning sensation of bilateral oral mucosa.
- Burning sensation for at least 4–6 months.
- Constant intensity or increasing intensity during the day.
- No worsening on eating or drinking rather it may reduce.
- No interference with sleep.

II. Additional criteria: Dysgeusia and/or xerostomia; Sensory or chemosensory alterations; Mood changes or psychopathological alterations.

Management: The initial step in management is to identify primary versus secondary BMS. The objective of management for secondary BMS should initially be directed at treating the causative local or systemic disease and withdrawing the use of offending medications (such as ACE inhibitors).

1. **Psychological therapy:** Cognitive behavioral therapy, electroconvulsive therapy, yoga meditation, relaxation therapy.
2. **Topical medication:** Benzodiazepine (clonazepam 0.25 mg), local anesthetics, capsaicin, benzydamine rinse, srtificial saliva.
3. **Systemic medication:** Low dose benzodiazepine and antidepressants, antioxidants, salivary stimulants.

Q. 50. Write a short note on lower lip paresthesia. *(NTR Uni., Nov. 2008; BBD Uni., April 2015)*

Ans. Lower lip paresthesia is a common symptom, usually described by patient as a unilateral loss of sensitivity of lower lip and gums, numbness, tingling sensation, and dryness of affected mucosa. It is often preceded by intense pain and burning sensation in affected area.

Causes

- Local factors: Anesthetic injections, surgical interventions, compressive phenomena or local infections, and endodontic treatment.
- Systemic factors: Multiple sclerosis, viral and bacterial infections, leukemia and lymphoma.

Diagnosis: Examination of area by thermal, mechanical, electrical, or chemical tests, electrophysiologic analysis of nerve, radiographic and neurophysiologic screening.

Treatment: Removal of cause and conservative (promotion of nerve regeneration) or surgical (nerve repair) procedures along with antibiotics, NSAIDs, corticosteroids, proteolytic enzymes, and vit. B.

Q. 51. Write a short note on desquamative gingivitis. *(RGUHS, May 2011)*

Ans. Desquamative gingivitis (DG) is characterized by erythematous gingiva, desquamation and erosion of gingival epithelium with blister formation. It is a common clinical manifestation in several diseases.

Classification/etiology

A. **Dermatological diseases:** Cicatricial pemphigoid, lichen planus, pemphigus, bullous pemphigoid, psoriasis, epidermolysis bullosa acquisita, contact stomatitis.

B. **Endocrine disturbances:** Estrogen deficiencies, testosterone imbalance, hypothyroidism.

C. **Aging**

D. **Abnormal response to bacterial plaque**

E. **Idiopathic**

F. **Chronic infections:** Tuberculosis, chronic candidiasis, histoplasmosis.

Clinical features

1. Predominantly occurs in women of age group 40–55 years.

2. Gingiva is red, swollen and glossy, with loss of stippling.

3. Multiple vesicles with superficial denuded areas, with bleeding on provocation.

4. The normal mucosa is peeled off on rubbing, leaving a raw, bleeding surface.

5. Patient is unable to eat hot, cold and spicy due to sensitive gingiva.

Diagnosis: Definitive diagnosis can be made by histopathological, direct (DIF) and indirect immune fluorescent (IIF) and autoantibodies in circulation.

Treatment: If there are previously determined etiologic factors (allergen materials, etc.) that cause DG, those should be eliminated and oral hygiene practices should be improved. Besides, patients should be warned about mechanical and chemical trauma. Intraoral restorations or prosthesis should be removed. Systemic and topical corticosteroids are used for the medical treatment of DG.

Q. 52. Write a short note on inflammatory enlargement of gingiva. *(NTR Uni., Nov. 2008)*

Ans. Gingival enlargement, also known as gingival hyperplasia or hypertrophy, is an abnormal overgrowth of gingival tissues. Causes are:

1. **Inflammatory gingival enlargement:** The most common form of enlargement, which is due to plaque induced inflammation of gingival tissues. It can be localized or generalized, or can be exaggerated by hormonal effects, as seen in puberty or pregnancy, or may be complicated by certain systemic medications. Gingival overgrowth varies from mild enlargement of isolated interdental papillae to uniform marked enlargement affecting either one or both the jaws. This is caused due to tissue edema and infective cellular infiltration as a result of long standing bacterial plaque, which are treated with conventional periodontal therapy, such as scaling and root planing. The most widely employed surgical approaches for the treatment of gingival enlargements is gingivectomy, flap technique by laser, electrocautery or conventional means.

2. **Medication-induced gingival enlargement:** Patients who take certain medications may develop gingival enlargement. In this, gum tissues are typically firm, non-tender, pale pink in color, and do not bleed easily. In severe cases, the gingiva may completely cover the crowns of teeth causing periodontal disease as well as problems with tooth eruption and alignment. Medication-induced gingival enlargement may resolve either partially or completely when the medication is discontinued. If the medication cannot be discontinued, surgical removal of the excess gingiva (gingivectomy) may be performed but the condition will likely recur. As this condition is somewhat worsen by the level of plaque accumulation on the teeth, effective oral hygiene measures will reduce the severity. For example Anticonvulsants (phenytoin), calcium channel blockers (verapamil, nifedipine), immunosuppressants (cyclosporine).

3. **Hereditary gingival fibromatosis:** This is a rare hereditary condition that usually develops during childhood, although some cases may not become evident until adulthood. The condition presents as a slow growing generalized or occasionally localized non-tender, firm, pale pink enlargement of gingiva. Repeated surgical removals may be required because of the recurrent nature of this condition.

4. **Systemic causes of gingival enlargement:** There are numerous physiologic and systemic conditions that may promote localized and/or generalized gingival enlargement such as pregnancy, hormonal imbalances, and leukemia. Gingival enlargement associated with systemic conditions usually resolves when the underlying condition is treated. Effective oral hygiene measures will reduce the risk of developing gingival enlargement.

- **Leukemic gingival enlargement** *(BBD Uni., June 2016):* Gingival enlargement in leukemia occurs due to infiltration of premature leukocytes. This is a common symptom that aids in the diagnosis of leukemia and warrants dental consultation. Acute monocytic leukemia (AML) has the greatest incidence of gingival infiltrates (M5) followed by acute myelomonocytic leukemia (M4) and acute myeloblastic leukemia (M1, M2). Gingival overgrowth may vary in severity, from minimal to complete tooth coverage and hinders with the function and aesthetics. Leukemic gingival infiltration is not seen in edentulous individuals, thus, suggesting a potential role of tooth-associated local factors in its pathogenesis. The diagnosis is suggested by a complete blood cell count showing pancytopenia and blast cells and is confirmed by examination of bone marrow. Treatment options in acute leukemias include aggressive multidrug chemotherapy and allogenic bone marrow transplantation. Periodontal and dental treatment for leukemic patients should always be planned after medical evaluation and physicians consent and under prophylactic antibiotics. Patients are advised 0.12% chlorhexidine mouth rinses postoperative oral hygiene procedures.

Q. 53. Write a short note on gingival pigmentation.
(NTR Uni., Oct. 2013; BBD Uni., June 2019)

Ans. Gingival pigmentation is presented as a diffuse deep purplish discoloration or as irregularly shaped brown and light brown or black patches, striae or strands. Gingival color depends primarily upon: Number and size of vasculature; Epithelial thickness; Degree of keratinization; Pigments within the gingival epithelium.

Classification (Table 6.53)

Q. 54. Discuss the bite mark analysis.
(RGUHS, May 2011)

Ans. Bite mark refers to a mark caused by the teeth either alone or in combination with other mouth parts (MacDonald).

Classification

A. Cameron and Sims classification
1. Agents: Human, animal.
2. Materials: Skin, body tissues, foodstuff, other materials.

B. MacDonald's classification
1. Tooth pressure marks.
2. Tongue pressure marks.
3. Teeth scrape marks.

C. Webster's classification
1. Type I: Fractured food items with limited depth of penetration.
2. Type II: Fractured food items with considerable depth of penetration.
3. Type III: Complete penetration with slide marks.

Bite mark appearance

Type of injury: Identifying the injury as a bite mark
a. Gross features: Circular or elliptical with central area of ecchymosis.
b. Class features: Incisor → rectangular; Canines → triangular or rectangular; Premolars and molars → spherical or point shaped
c. Individual features: Characteristics such as fractures, rotation, etc.
   - Site of bite marks: Females → on breast, legs (inner part of thigh)—sexual assault; Male children → genitals—child abuse; Adult Males → finger, arms and shoulders—fight.

Bite marks investigations
1. Preliminary relevant questions.
2. Evidence collection from the victim.
3. Visual examination.

Table 6.53: Classification of gingival pigmentation (Peeran et al, 2014)

Class	Criteria of classifications
I	Coral pink/salmon pink colored gingiva
II	Localized/isolated spots/areas of gingival melanin pigmentation which does not involve all parts of gingiva
	Mild, moderate, sever pigmentation
III	Localized/isolated unit/s of melanin pigmentation which involves all parts of gingiva
	Mild, moderate and severe pigmentation
IV	Generalized diffuse pigmentation which involves all parts of gingiva
	Mild, moderate and severe pigmentation
V	Tobacco associated pigmentation
VI	Gingival pigmentation due to exogenous pigments
VII	Gingival pigmentation due to endogenous pigments
VIII	Drug-induced gingival pigmentation
IX	Gingival pigmentation associated with systemic diseases and syndromes
X	Pigmented benign and malignant lesions involving the gingiva

4. Photography.
5. Saliva swab: WBCs, sloughed epithelial cells (potential source of DNA).
6. Impressions: Vinyl polysiloxane.
7. Evidence collection from the suspect.

7. DISEASES OF BLOOD, NUTRITIONAL DISEASES AND MISCELLANEOUS

Q. 1. Write a short note on scurvy.

(TNMGR, Sept. 2007)

Ans. Vitamin C deficiency in the food or as a conditioned deficiency results in scurvy. The lesions and clinical manifestations of scurvy are seen more commonly at two peak ages: In early childhood and in the very aged. These are:

1. **Hemorrhagic diathesis:** A marked tendency of bleeding is characteristic of scurvy. This may be due to deficiency of intercellular cement which holds together the cells of capillary endothelium. There may be hemorrhages in skin, mucous membranes, gums, muscles, joints and underneath the periosteum.

2. **Skeletal lesions:** These changes are more pronounced in growing children. The most prominent change is deranged formation of osteoid matrix and not derranged mineralization. The epiphyseal ends of growing long bones have cartilage cells in rows which normally undergo provisional mineralization. But, due to vitamin C deficiency, the next step of lying down of osteoid matrix by osteoblasts is poor and results in failure of resorption of cartilage. Consequently, mineralized cartilage under the widened and irregular epiphyseal plate's project as "**Scorbutic Rosary**".

3. **Delayed wound healing:** Due to: Derranged collagen synthesis; poor preservation and maturation of fibroblasts; and localization of infections in wounds.

4. **Anemia:** It may be result of hemorrhage, interference with formation of folic acid or deranged iron metabolism.

5. **Lesions in teeth and gums:** Scurvy may interfere with development of dentin. The gums are soft and swollen, may bleed readily and get infected commonly.

6. **Skin rash:** Hyperkeratotic and follicular rash may occur in scurvy.

Q. 2. Write a short note on bleeding time and clotting time.

(TNMGR, April 1998; NTR Uni., Nov. 2007)

Ans. Bleeding time (BT) is the time interval from oozing of blood after a cut or injury till arrest of bleeding. Usually, it is determined by Duke method using blotting paper or filter paper method. Its normal duration is 3 to 6 minutes. It is prolonged in purpura. BT is increased in females due to presence of estrogens which, in turn, reduce the functions of platelets. BT is decreased in males due to increased activation and aggregation of platelets.

Clotting time (CT) is the time interval from oozing of blood after a cut or injury till the formation of clot. It is usually determined by capillary tube method. Its normal duration is 3 to 8 minutes. It is prolonged in hemophilia. CT is higher in females as compared to males. This is because of increased estrogen in females which prolongs CT and decreases plasma fibrinogen level.

Q. 3. Write a note on bleeding disorders.

(TNMGR, March 2008)

Ans. Bleeding disorders/hemorrhagic diatheses are a group of disorders characterized by defective haemostasis with abnormal bleeding. The tendency to bleeding may be spontaneous in the form of small hemorrhages (e.g. petechiae, purpura, ecchymoses), or there may be excessive external or internal bleeding (e.g. hematoma, haemarthroses, etc.).

Causes

I. Hemorrhagic diathesis due to vascular abnormalities.
II. Hemorrhagic diathesis related to platelet abnormalities.
III. Disorders of coagulation factors.
IV. Hemorrhagic diathesis due to fibrinolytic defects.
V. Combination of all these.

Investigations of haemostatic function

A. Comprehensive clinical evaluation, including patient's history, family history and details of site, frequency and character of haemostatic defect.
B. Screening tests and specific tests.

I. Investigation of disordered vascular haemostasis

1. **Bleeding time:** A prolonged bleeding time may be due to: Thrombocytopenia, disorders of platelet function, von Willebrand's disease, vascular abnormalities, severe deficiency of factors V and XI.
2. **Platelet count:** Thrombocytopenia.
3. **Prothrombin time:** It is prolonged in: Oral anticoagulant therapy, DIC, liver disease.
4. **Partial thromboplastin time:** Parenteral heparin therapy, DIC, liver disease.
5. **Thrombin time:** Evaluation of common pathway. It is prolonged in afibrinogenaemia, DIC, and parenteral heparin therapy.

II. Hemorrhagic diatheses due to platelet disorders

a. **Thrombocytopenia.**

b. **Thrombocytosis.**

c. **Disorders of platelet functions**
  i. **Hereditary disorders:** Bernard-Soulier syndrome, von Willebrand's disease, Glanzmann's disease.
  ii. **Acquired disorders:** Aspirin therapy, uremia, liver disease, multiple myeloma, Waldenström's macroglobulinaemia and various myeloproliferative disorders.

III. Hemorrhagic diatheses due to vascular disorders:

They are characterized by petechiae, purpura or ecchymoses. Vascular bleeding disorders may be inherited or acquired.

a. **Inherited:** Hereditary hemorrhagic telangiectasia (Osler-Weber-Rendu disease); Marfan's syndrome; Ehlers-Danlos syndrome and pseudoxanthoma elasticum.

b. **Acquired vascular bleeding disorders:** Henoch-Schönlein purpura, haemolytic-uraemic syndrome, **Devil's pinches:** Easy bruising of unknown cause, infection and drug reactions, steroid purpura and senile purpura, scurvy.

Q. 4. Write a short note on iron deficiency anemia.
(TNMGR, March 2008, 2011; RGUHS, Oct. 2010; NTR Uni., May 2018)

Ans. The commonest nutritional deficiency disorder present throughout the world is iron deficiency. Iron deficiency anaemia (IDA) is always secondary to an underlying disorder.

Etiology

I. **Increased blood loss:** Uterine (excessive menstruation, repeated miscarriages, etc.); Gastrointestinal (peptic ulcer, hemorrhoids, hookworm infestation, etc.); Renal tract (haematuria, haemoglobinuria); Nose (repeated epistaxis); Lungs (haemoptysis).

II. **Increased requirements:** Spurts of growth in infancy, childhood and adolescence; Prematurity; Pregnancy and lactation.

III. **Inadequate dietary intake:** Poor economic status, anorexia (e.g. in pregnancy), elderly individuals due to poor dentition, apathy and financial constraints.

IV. **Decreased absorption:** Partial or total gastrectomy; Achlorhydria; Intestinal malabsorption such as in celiac disease.

Clinical features

1. IDA is much more common in women between age of 20 and 45 years; at periods of active growth in infancy, childhood and adolescence.

2. The usual symptoms are weakness, fatigue, and dyspnoea on exertion, palpitations and pallor of skin, mucous membranes and sclera.

3. Older patients may develop angina and congestive cardiac failure.

4. Patients may have unusual dietary cravings such as pica.

5. Menorrhagia is a common symptom in iron deficient women.

6. Long-standing chronic IDA causes epithelial tissue changes in some patients. The changes occur in nails (**koilonychias:** Spoon-shaped nails), tongue (**atrophic glossitis**), mouth (**angular stomatitis**), and esophagus causing dysphagia from development of thin, membranous webs at postcricoid area (**Plummer-Vinson syndrome**).

Treatment

Correction of the underlying disorder: Correction of iron deficiency: Oral therapy (iron salts such as ferrous sulfate, ferrous fumarate, ferrous gluconate and polysaccharide iron) and parenteral therapy (iron dextran, sodium ferric gluconate and iron sucrose; dose is calculated by multiplying the grams of hemoglobin below normal with 250, plus an additional 500 mg).

Q. 5. Write a short note on megaloblastic anemia.
(TNMGR, Sept. 2009; NTR Uni., May 2018)

Ans. Megaloblastic anaemias are disorders caused by impaired DNA synthesis and are characterized by delayed maturation of nucleus than cytoplasm in the hematopoietic precursors in bone marrow. The underlying defect for asynchronous maturation of nucleus is defective DNA synthesis due to deficiency of vitamin B_{12} and/or folic acid. Other causes include drugs which interfere with DNA synthesis, acquired defects of hematopoietic stem cells.

Clinical features

1. **Anaemia:** Macrocytic megaloblastic anaemia.

2. **Glossitis:** Smooth, beefy, red tongue.

3. **Neurologic manifestations:** Numbness, parasthesia, weakness, ataxia, poor finger coordination and diminished reflexes.

4. **Others:** Mild jaundice, angular stomatitis, purpura, melanin pigmentation, symptoms of malabsorption, weight loss and anorexia.

Laboratory findings

A. Lab investigations for anaemia

1. **Blood**
  i. Hemoglobin: Hemoglobin values are below the normal range.
  ii. Red cells: Macrocytosis, anisocytosis, poikilocytosis and presence of macro-ovalocytes.

iii. Reticulocyte count: Reticulocyte count is generally low.

iv. Absolute values: Red cell indices reveal an elevated MCV, elevated MCH and normal or reduced MCHC.

v. Leucocytes: Hyper-segmented neutrophils in blood film.

vi. Platelets: Platelet count may be moderately reduced.

2. **Bone marrow findings:** Hypercellular, decreased myeloid–erythroid ratio, erythroid hyperplasia. Megaloblasts are abnormal, large, having nuclear-cytoplasmic asynchrony. The nuclei are large, having fine, reticular and open chromatin that stains lightly. Increase in the number and size of iron granules in erythroid precursors and chromosomal abnormalities.

3. **Biochemical findings:** Rise in serum unconjugated bilirubin and LDH, serum iron and ferretin may be normal or elevated.

B. Special tests for cause of specific deficiency

1. Tests for vitamin B_{12} deficiency: Serum vitamin B_{12} assay, Schilling test and serum enzyme levels.

2. Tests for folate deficiency: Urinary excretion of FIGLU, serum and red cell folate assay.

Treatment: Hydroxycobalamin (1000 µg) as IM injection for 3 weeks and Tab. Folic acid (5 mg) OD for 4 months.

Q. 6. Write a short note on Schilling tests.
(HNBG Uni., June 2016)

Ans. Schilling test (Dr. Robert F. Schilling) is very helpful in detecting the absorption rate of an administered load of vitamin B_{12} in a patient.

Procedures

Stage 1: The patient is given radio labeled vitamin B_{12} orally, following an IM dose of unlabeled vitamin B_{12} one hour later. The injection is given to ensure that none of the radioactive B_{12} binds to any vitamin B_{12} depleted tissues. A 24-hour urine collection monitors the absorption and excretion.

Stage 2: If the previous stage provides an abnormal result, stage 2 can be done to assess whether there is a deficiency of intrinsic factor. Stage 1 is repeated along with an oral dose of intrinsic factor. A 24-hour urine collection is carried out to assess the level of vitamin B_{12}.

Potential diagnosis: During stage 1, a healthy person will be able to absorb the administered radioactive B_{12} in their terminal ileum. It will then be excreted in urine. If there are any defects with the cubam receptor at the terminal ileum, the result will show a low level of labeled cobalamin in urine as it will remain in intestines and is likely to be excreted in feces. A defect associated with low levels of an intrinsic factor will also produce a similar abnormal result.

If stage 2 shows a normal level of excreted vitamin B_{12}, it means that the patient has low levels of intrinsic factor and one possible cause is pernicious anemia. If the test still indicates a low level of vitamin B_{12} in the urine, it means that the patient has a poor intestinal absorption of cobalamin.

Q. 7. Write a short note on polymorphonuclear neutrophil (PMN) defects.
(Sumandeep Vidyapeeth, April 2011; TNMGR, April 2014; NTR Uni., May 2019)

Ans. A polymorphonuclear neutrophil (PMN), commonly called polymorph or neutrophil, is 12–15 µm in diameter. It consists of a characteristic dense nucleus, having 2–5 lobes and pale cytoplasm containing numerous fine violet-pink granules.

Pathologic variations

A. Neutrophil leucocytosis

1. Acute infections, e.g. actinomycosis, poliomyelitis, abscess, furuncle, carbuncle, tonsillitis, otitis media, osteomyelitis, etc.

2. Other inflammations, e.g. burn, operations, collagen-vascular diseases, hypersensitivity reactions, etc.

3. Intoxication, e.g. uremia, poisonings.

4. Acute hemorrhage/haemolysis.

5. Disseminated malignancies.

6. Myeloproliferative disorders, e.g. myeloid leukemia, polycythemia vera.

7. Miscellaneous, e.g. corticosteroid therapy, idiopathic neutrophilia.

B. Neutropenia

1. Certain infections, e.g. typhoid, paratyphoid, measles, viral hepatitis, malaria, etc.

2. Overwhelming bacterial infections, e.g. miliary tuberculosis, septicemia.

3. Drugs, chemicals and physical agents causing aplasia of bone marrow, e.g. antimetabolite and antihistaminic.

4. Certain hematological and other diseases, e.g. pernicious anaemia, cirrhosis of liver with splenomegaly, SLE, Gaucher's disease.

5. Cachexia and debility.

6. Anaphylactoid shock.

7. Certain rare hereditary, congenital or familial disorders, e.g. cyclic neutropenia.

C. Defective functions

1. Defective chemotaxis, e.g. lazy-leukocyte syndrome; following corticosteroid therapy, aspirin ingestion, alcoholism, myeloid leukemia.
2. Defective phagocytosis, e.g. hypogammaglobulinaemia, hypocomplementaemia, after splenectomy, sickle cell disease.
3. Defective killing, e.g. chronic granulomatous disease, Chédiak-Higashi syndrome, myeloid leukemia.

Q. 8. Write a short note on thrombocytopenia.

(TNMGR, Oct. 1999; RUHS, July 2016)

Ans. Thrombocytopenia is defined as a reduction in peripheral blood platelet count below the lower limit of normal, i.e. below 150,000/µl. Thrombocytopenia may result from: Impaired platelet production; Accelerated platelet destruction; Splenic sequestration; Dilutional loss.

Types of thrombocytopenia

I. Drug-induced thrombocytopenia: Chemotherapeutic agents, antibiotics (sulfonamides, penicillins), other drugs (digitoxin, thiazide diuretics) and excessive consumption of ethanol. Clinically, the patient presents with acute purpura. The platelet count is markedly lowered, often below 10,000/ml and bone marrow shows normal or increased number of megakaryocyte. Immediate treatment is to stop or replace the suspected drug. Occasional patients may require temporary support with glucocorticoids, plasmapheresis or platelet transfusions.

II. Immune thrombocytopenic purpura (ITP) *(HP Uni., April 2019)*: Characterized by immunologic destruction of platelets and normal or increased megakaryocyte in bone marrow.

Pathogenesis

- **Acute ITP:** This is a self-limited disorder, seen mostly in children following recovery from a viral illness. Mechanism is by formation of immune complexes containing viral antigens, and by formation of antibodies against viral antigens which cross react with platelets and lead to their destruction.
- **Chronic ITP:** It is more commonly in adults, particularly in women of child-bearing age. Pathogenesis of chronic ITP is explained by formation of antiplatelet autoantibodies. These antibodies are directed against target antigens (platelet glycoproteins).

The usual manifestations are petechial hemorrhages, easy bruising, and mucosal bleeding such as menorrhagia in women, nasal bleeding, bleeding from gums, melaena and haematuria. Intracranial hemorrhage is, however, rare. Splenomegaly and hepatomegaly may occur.

Laboratory findings

1. Platelet count is markedly reduced.
2. Blood film shows occasional platelets.
3. Bone marrow shows increased number of megakaryocyte.

Treatment: Corticosteroid therapy; Immunosuppressive drugs; Splenectomy; Platelet transfusions.

III. Thrombotic thrombocytopenic purpura (TTP): Triad of thrombocytopenia, microangiopathic hemolytic anaemia and formation of microthrombi.

Pathogenesis: TTP is initiated by endothelial injury followed by release of von Willebrand factor and other procoagulant material from endothelial cells, leading to the formation of microthrombi.

Laboratory findings

1. Thrombocytopenia.
2. Microangiopathic hemolytic anaemia with negative Coombs' test.
3. Leucocytosis, sometimes with leukaemoid reaction.
4. Bone marrow examination reveals normal or slightly increased megakaryocyte.
5. Diagnosis is established by examination of biopsy (e.g. from gingiva).

Q. 9. Write a short note on transfusion reactions.

(TNMGR, March 2002; KLE Uni. Jan.2009)

Ans. Transfusion reactions are defined as adverse events associated with transfusion of whole blood or one of its components. These may range in severity from minor to life-threatening. Reactions can occur during the transfusion (**acute**) or days to weeks later (**delayed**). Transfusion reactions are generally classified into two types:

I. Immunologic transfusion reactions may be against RBCs (**hemolytic reactions**), leucocytes, platelets or immunoglobulins. These are as under:

1. **Hemolytic transfusion reactions**
   a. **Intravascular haemolysis:** Due to ABO incompatibility. Symptoms include restlessness, anxiety, flushing, chest or lumbar pain, tachypnoea, tachycardia and nausea, followed by shock and renal failure.
   b. **Extravascular haemolysis:** Due to immune antibodies of Rh system, symptoms are malaise and fever but shock and renal failure may rarely occur. Some patients develop delayed reactions because of previous transfusion or pregnancy, in which the patient develops anaemia due to destruction of red cells in the RE system about a week after transfusion (**anamnestic reaction**).
2. **Transfusion-related acute lung injury (TRALI):** An uncommon reaction resulting from transfusion of

donor plasma containing high levels of anti-HLA antibodies which bind to leucocytes of recipient.

3. **Other allergic reactions**
   i. Febrile reaction: Immunologic reaction against WBCs, platelets, or IgA.
   ii. Anaphylactic shock.
   iii. Allergic reactions: Urticaria.
   iv. Transfusion-related graft-versus-host disease.

II. Non-immune transfusion reactions: Transfusion associated circulatory overload (TACO); Massive transfusion; Transmission of infection; Air embolism; Thrombophlebitis; Transfusion haemosiderosis.

Differential diagnosis: Anaphylaxis, DIC, hemolytic anemia, septic shock.

Treatment
- Immediately stop the transfusion and start intravenous fluids (usually 0.9% saline).
- Monitoring of patient's vital signs at every 15 min. intervals.
- Treatment of specific transfusion reactions is most often supportive.

Q. 10. Define hemorrhage. Classify it. Describe the management of secondary hemorrhage from extraction socket. *(BFUHS, Oct. 2010)*

Ans. Hemorrhage is the escape of blood from a blood vessel. **Lockhart (2003)** has provided four criteria to define post-extraction bleeding (**PEB**): Continues for >12 hours; causes patient to call or return to dentist, or go to emergency department; results in development of large hematoma or ecchymosis within oral soft tissues; or requires a blood transfusion and/or hospitalization.

Classification

A. Based on the type of blood vessel involved
1. **Arterial hemorrhage:** Bleeding from ruptured artery. It is pulsatile, brisk and bright red in colour.
2. **Venous hemorrhage:** Bleeding from veins. Non-pulsatile, dark in color.
3. **Capillary hemorrhage:** Oozing from the capillaries. The blood is bluish red in color.

B. Based on the duration
1. **Primary hemorrhage:** Bleeding occurs during and immediately after extraction, usually due to infection/trauma to blood vessels.
2. **Secondary hemorrhage:** Bleeding begins 7–10 days after post-extraction. It is mainly due to secondary infection.
3. **Intermediate/reactionary hemorrhage:** Bleeding occurs within 2–3 hours, usually due to underlying systemic conditions.

Management of secondary bleeding *(NTR Uni., May 2019):*

Causes: Dislodgement of clot, secondary trauma to wound, infection, elevation of blood pressure.

Management: Local and systemic haemostatic measures:
1. **Mechanical methods:** Local pressure with gauze, use of hemostat, suture and ligation, embolization of the vessels, acrylic/surgical splints.
2. **Thermal agents:** Cautery, electrosurgery, cryosurgery, argon-beam coagulator.
3. **Chemical methods:** Astringents and styptics, bone wax, adrenaline, whole blood, platelet rich plasma, fresh frozen plasma, cryoprecipitate, oxidized cellulose, gel foam, thrombin, collagen fleeces, cyanoacrylate glue, local antifibrinolytic solutions such as tranexamic acid mouthwash, fibrin glue/adhesive, resorbable gelatin sponge, collagen sponge, gauze soaked with tranexamic acid, chlorhexidine bio-adhesive gel, calcium alginate, haemocoagulase, ankaferd blood stopper, green tea extract, chitosan-based dressings.

Q. 11. Write in detail about HIV/AIDS.
(NTR Uni. Nov. 2008; TNMGR, March 2010; MUHS, June 2018)

Ans. Acquired immune deficiency syndrome (AIDS) is defined by a loss of CD4 T lymphocytes or the occurrence of opportunistic infections or cancers.

Etiologic agent: AIDS is caused by a RNA retrovirus called human immunodeficiency virus (HIV) which is a type of human T cell leukemia-lymphoma virus (HTLV). HIV has tropism for CD4 molecules present on subpopulation of T cells which are the particular targets of attack by HIV. HIV is cytolytic for T cells causing immunodeficiency. Two forms: HIV1 is the etiologic agent for AIDS in US and Central Africa; HIV2 causes a similar disease in West Africa and parts of India.

Routes of transmission: Transmission of HIV infection occurs by:
1. **Sexual transmission.**
2. **Transmission via blood and blood products:** (i) Intravenous drug abusers; (ii) Haemophilics; (iii) Recipients of HIV-infected blood and blood products.
3. **Perinatal transmission.**
4. **Occupational transmission.**
5. **Transmission by other body fluids:** Saliva, tears, sweat, urine, semen, vaginal secretions, cervical secretions, breast milk, CSF, synovial, pleural, peritoneal and pericardial fluids.

Pathogenesis: The pathogenesis of HIV infection is largely related to depletion of CD4+ T cells (helper T cells) resulting in profound immunosuppression.

1. **Selective tropism for CD4 molecule receptor:** gp120 envelope glycoprotein of HIV has selective tropism for cells containing CD4 molecule receptor on their surface, e.g. CD4+ T cells (T helper cells); Monocyte-macrophages; microglial cells, epithelial cells of cervix, Langerhans cells of skin and follicular dendritic cells.

2. **Internalization:** gp120 of virion combines with CD4 receptor, but for fusion of virion with the host cell membrane, a chemokine coreceptor (CCR) is necessary. Once HIV has combined with CD4 receptor and CCR, gp41 glycoprotein of envelope is internalized in CD4+ T cell membrane.

3. **Uncoating and viral DNA formation:** Once the virion has entered T cell cytoplasm, reverse trans-criptase of viral RNA forms a single-stranded DNA. Using the single-stranded DNA as a template, DNA polymerase copies it to make it double-stranded DNA, while destroying the original RNA strands.

4. **Viral integration:** Viral integrase protein inserts the viral DNA into nucleus of host T cell and integrates in the host cell DNA. At this stage, viral particle is termed **HIV provirus.**

5. **Viral replication:** HIV provirus having become part of host cell DNA, host cell DNA transcripts for viral RNA with presence of tat gene. Multiplication of viral particles is further facilitated by release of cytokines from T helper cells (CD4+ T cells). RNA viral particles thus fill the cytoplasm of host T cell from where they acquire protein coating.

6. **Latent period and immune attack:** In an inactive infected T cell, the infection may remain in latent phase for a long time, accounting for long incubation period.

7. **CD4+ T cell destruction:** Viral particles replicated in CD4+ T cells start forming buds from the cell wall of host cell. As these particles detach from the infected host cell, they damage part of the cell membrane of host cell and cause death of host CD4+ T cells by apoptosis.

8. **Viral dissemination:** Release of viral particles from infected host cell spreads the infection to more CD4+ host cells and produces viraemia. Through circu-lation, virus gains entry to lymphoid tissues where it multiplies further (virus reservoir).

Natural history generally, the biologic course passes through 3 phases:

1. Acute HIV syndrome (3–12 weeks)
  i. High levels of plasma viraemia due to replication of virus.
  ii. Virus-specific immune response by formation of anti-HIV antibodies (seroconversion) after 3 weeks of initial exposure to HIV.
  iii. Initially, sudden marked reduction in CD4+ T cells (helper T cells) followed by return to normal levels.
  iv. Rise in CD8+ T cells (cytotoxic T cells).
  v. Appearance of self-limited non-specific acute viral illness in 50–70% of adults within 3–6 weeks of initial infection. Manifestations include: Sore throat, fever, myalgia, skin rash, and sometimes, aseptic meningitis. These symptoms resolve spontaneously in 2–3 weeks.

2. Middle chronic phase (10–12 years)
  i. With passage of time viral load increases due to crumbling host defenses.
  ii. Chronic stage, depending upon host immune system, may continue as long as 10 years.
  iii. CD4+ T cells continue to proliferate but net result is moderate fall in CD4+ T cell counts.
  iv. Cytotoxic CD8+ T cell count remains high.
  v. Clinically, it may be a stage of latency and patient may be asymptomatic, or may develop mild constitutional symptoms and persistent genera-lized lymphadenopathy.

3. Final crisis phase: Full-blown AIDS
  i. Marked increase in viraemia.
  ii. Time period from HIV infection through chronic phase into full-blown AIDS may last 7–10 years and culminate in death.
  iii. CD4+ T cells are markedly reduced (<200/μl). Avg. survival after the onset of full-blown AIDS is 2 years.

Revised CDC HIV classification system: Centers for Disease Control and Prevention (CDC), US in 1993 revised the classification system for HIV infection in adults and children based on 2 parameters: Clinical manifestations and CD4+ T cell counts. According to this classification, HIV/AIDS has 3 categories: A, B and C.

Category A: Includes a variety of conditions: Asympto-matic case, persistent generalized lymphadenopathy (PGL), and acute HIV syndrome. CD4+ T cell counts >500/μl.

Category B: Symptomatic cases and includes conditions secondary to impaired cell-mediated immunity, e.g. bacillary dysentery, mucosal candidiasis, fever, oral hairy leukoplakia, ITP, pelvic inflammatory disease, peripheral neuropathy, cervical dysplasia and carci-noma *in situ* cervix etc. CD4+ T cell counts is 200–499/μl.

Category C: This category includes conditions listed for AIDS surveillance case definition, e.g. mucosal candidiasis, cancer uterine cervix, bacterial infections (e.g. tuberculosis), fungal infections (e.g. histoplasmosis), parasitic infections (e.g. *Pneumocystis carinii*, pneumonia), malnutrition, wasting of muscles, etc. CD4+ T cell counts are <200/µl.

Pathological lesions and clinical manifestations of HIV/AIDS

1. **Wasting syndrome:** It is defined as 'involuntary loss of body weight by >10%'. It occurs due to malnutrition, increased metabolic rate, malabsorption, anorexia, and ill-effects of multiple opportunistic infections.

2. **Persistent generalized lymphadenopathy (PGL):** PGL is defined as presence of enlarged lymph nodes >1 cm at two or more extra inguinal sites for >3 months without an obvious cause.

3. **Gastrointestinal manifestations:** Chronic watery/bloody diarrhoea, oral, oropharyngeal and esophageal candidiasis, anorexia, nausea, vomiting, mucosal ulcers, abdominal pain. Advance cases may develop secondary tumors occurring in GIT.

4. **Pulmonary manifestations:** Pneumonia, lung abscess, ARDS and secondary tumors.

5. **Mucocutaneous manifestations:** Mucocutaneous viral exanthem (erythematous rash), allergic (e.g. drug reaction, seborrhoeic dermatitis), infectious (viral infections such as herpes, varicella zoster, EB virus, HPV; bacterial infections such as *M. avium*, *Staph. aureus*; fungal infections such as Candida, Cryptococcus, Histoplasma), and neoplasia (e.g. Kaposi's sarcoma, SCC, basal cell carcinoma, cutaneous lymphoma).

6. **Hematologic manifestations:** Anaemia, leucopenia, and thrombocytopenia.

7. **CNS manifestations:** HIV encephalopathy/AIDS associated dementia complex, meningitis, demyelinating lesions of spinal cord, peripheral neuropathy and lymphoma of brain.

8. **Gynecologic manifestations:** Monilial (candidal) vaginitis, cervical dysplasia, carcinoma cervix, and pelvic inflammatory disease.

9. **Renal manifestations:** Nephropathy, genitourinary tract infections and pyelonephritis.

10. **Hepatobiliary manifestations:** Drug-induced hepatic injury, steatosis, granulomatous hepatitis and opportunistic infections.

11. **Cardiovascular manifestations:** HIV-associated cardiomyopathy, pericardial effusion, lymphoma and Kaposi's sarcoma.

12. **Ophthalmic lesions:** Opportunistic infections (e.g. CMV retinitis), HIV retinopathy, and secondary tumors.

13. **Musculoskeletal lesions:** Osteoporosis, osteopenia, septic arthritis, osteomyelitis and polymyositis.

14. **Endocrine lesions:** Due to dyslipidaemia, hyperinsulinaemia and hyperglycemia.

Oral manifestations of AIDS (*TNMGR, April 1995; UHSR, April 2009; Sumandeep Uni., April 2013*): Oral manifestations of HIV/AIDS infection occur in 30–80% of the affected patient.

Group 1: Lesions strongly associated with HIV infection

1. Candidiasis: Pseudomembranous, erythematous, angular cheilitis.
2. Periodontal diseases: Linear gingival erythema, necrotizing ulcerative gingivitis/periodontitis.
3. Non-Hodgkin's lymphoma.
4. Hairy leukoplakia.
5. Kaposi's sarcoma.

Group 2: Lesions less commonly associated with HIV infection

1. Bacterial infections: *Mycobacterium avium-intracellulare*, *Mycobacterium tuberculosis*.
2. Melanotic hyperpigmentation.
3. Necrotizing ulcerative stomatitis.
4. Salivary gland disease: Hyposalivation, swelling of gland.
5. Thrombocytopenic purpura.
6. Ulceration (not otherwise specified)
7. Viral infections: HSV, HPV, condyloma acuminatum, focal epithelial hyperplasia, verruca vulgaris, VZV, herpes zoster.

Group 3: Lesions seen in HIV infection

1. Bacterial infections: *Actinomyces israelii*, *E. coli*, *Klebsiella pneumoniae*.
2. Fungal infection other than candidiasis: Cryptococosis, histoplasmosis, aspergillosis, mucormycosis.
3. Recurrent aphthous stomatitis.
4. Cat-scratch disease.
5. Drug reactions: Ulcerative lesion, Erythema multiforme, lichenoid reaction, toxic epidermolysis.
6. Bacillary epithelioid angiomatosis.
7. Neurological disturbances: Trigeminal neuralgia, facial palsy.
8. Viral infections: Molluscum contagiosum, CMV infection.

Diagnosis of HIV/AIDS (*UHSR, May 2016*):

1. Tests for establishing HIV infection

  i. Antibody tests:

    a. ELISA: Initial screening is done for antibodies against gag and env proteins by ELISA.

b. Western blot: If ELISA is positive, confirmation is done by Western blot for presence of specific antibodies against all three HIV antigens—gag, pol and env.

ii. Direct detection of HIV:

a. p24 antigen capture assay.

b. HIV RNA assay methods by reverse transcriptase (RT) PCR branched DNA, nucleic acid sequence-based amplification (NucliSens).

c. DNA-PCR by amplification of proviral DNA.

d. Culture of HIV from blood monocytes and CD4+ T cells.

2. **Tests for defects in immunity:** These tests are used for diagnosis as well as for monitoring treatment of cases.

i. CD4+ T cell counts: Progressive fall.

ii. Rise in CD8+ T cells.

iii. Reversal of CD4+ to CD8+ T cell ratio.

iv. Lymphopenia.

v. Polyclonal hypergammaglobulinaemia.

vi. Increased β_2 microglobulin levels.

vii. Platelet counts: Thrombocytopenia.

3. **Tests for detection of opportunistic infections and secondary tumors:** By aspiration or biopsy.

Prevention: Individuals can reduce the risk of HIV infection by limiting exposure to risk factors. Key approaches for HIV prevention by WHO are:

1. Use of condoms for all forms of sexual intercourse.

2. Use of clean needles and syringes.

3. Testing of individuals in high risk groups.

4. Antiretroviral treatment for HIV positive women during pregnancy.

5. Offering HIV positive pregnant women caesarean section deliveries.

6. Advising all HIV positive women not to breastfeed.

Q. 12. Write a note on addiction and dental diseases.
(TNMGR, April 2013)

Ans. Drug abuse: When drugs are used in a manner or amount inconsistent with the medical or social pattern or culture it is called drug abuse.

Drug dependence: Most controlled substances are capable of producing dependence either physical, psychological or both after repeated use of the drug that necessitates continued administration of drug to prevent withdrawal symptoms.

Drug addiction: It is defined as physical and psychological dependence on psychotic substances, which cross the blood–brain barrier once ingested, temporarily altering the chemical milieu of the brain.

Oral manifestations of substance abuse

1. **Opiates:** Tooth loss, generalized tooth decay especially on smooth and cervical surfaces, salivary hypofunction, burning mouth, taste impairment, eating difficulties, mucosal infections, periodontal diseases. Heroin users show poor oral health in terms of caries and periodontal diseases. Caries in these patients is darker and usually limited to buccal and labial surfaces.

2. **Cannabis:** Cannabis abuse, mainly hashish and marijuana, leads to increased risk of oral cancer, dry mouth, and periodontitis, xerostomia, leukoedema, high prevalence of *Candida albicans* but not candidiasis, and higher DMF scores.

3. **Stimulants:** Stimulants includes amphetamine, methamphetamine, cocaine, and crack-cocaine. **Cocaine snorting** is associated with nasal septum perforation, changes in sense of smell, chronic sinusitis, and perforation of palate. Oral administration of cocaine may result in gingival lesions, bruxism, dental attrition. Crack-cocaine smoking produces burns and sores on lips, face, and inside of mouth. Cocaine can result in movement disorder and manifest itself as **transient chorea and buccolingual dyskinesia ("crack dancing" or boca torcida-twisted mouth)**. Methamphetamine abusers show bruxism, excessive tooth wear, xerostomia, rampant caries and gum problem **(meth mouth)**.

4. **Hallucinogens:** Hallucinogens such as ecstasy and LSD (lysergic acid diethylamide) results in dry mouth, bruxism, and problems associated with malnutrition caused by drug-induced anorexia, chewing, grinding, and temporomandibular joint (TMJ) tenderness.

5. **Club drugs:** Club drugs including methylenedioxymethamphetamine (MDMA), ketamine, gamma-hydroxybutyrate (GHB), and flunitrazepam are chemical substances used mainly by young people in recreational settings such as dance clubs and rave parties. These drugs are associated with dry mouth, bruxism, increased risk of dental erosion, ulcers, vestibular swelling, edema, and necrosis.

6. **Indirect effects of drugs on oral health:** It is difficult to identify and isolate the root causes of oral diseases among addicts, since they show a variety of unhealthy behaviors. Poor oral hygiene, increased sugar intake, and inappropriate nutrition are examples.

- **Oral health and HIV transmission:** Illicit drugs such as methamphetamines may lead to an increase in risky sexual behaviors resulting in the spread of infectious diseases such as HIV and AIDS.

Barriers against oral health promotion among drug addicts

1. It is difficult to access drug addicts as a target population.
2. In addition to problems with drug abusers' cooperation with and compliance in oral health studies, problems with their long-term follow-up are common.
3. Finally, lack of appropriate policies to improve access to oral health services.
4. Poor collaboration between dental and general health care sectors serving drug addicts.

Q. 13. Effects of radiations on oral and paraoral structures. *(RUHS, June 2017)*

Ans. Radiotherapy is a curative medical intervention in cancer therapeutics. High doses of radiation used to destroy cancer cells can cause side effects because radiation can damage healthy cells and tissues near the zone of radiation.

Rationale of radiotherapy of oral cavity: Radiation therapy is part of oral cancer treatment, either as a primary mode of treatment, pre-surgery/post-surgery, part of radiochemotherapy, or as palliative therapy. Radiation therapy is indicated when the lesion is radiosensitive, advanced or deeply invasive, and cannot be approached surgically.

I. Acute effects

1. **Mucositis:** Earliest signs and symptoms of oral mucositis include erythema and edema, burning sensation and increased sensitivity to hot and spicy food followed by redness, inflammation, with formation of white to yellow pseudomembrane. For grading (Table 7.13).
2. **Effect on salivary gland:** Initial effects include degeneration or destruction of acinar tissue with subsequent inflammation and marked loss of salivary secretion in first few weeks. Late effects after months are progressive fibrosis, adiposis, loss of fine vasculature, and concomitant parenchymal degeneration. These all leads to hyposalivation; Alterations in composition of saliva; Taste dysfunction; Infections.

II. Late effects

1. **Dental alterations:** Dental hypersensitivity, taste variations.
2. **Effects on teeth:** Before calcification, radiation leads to destruction of tooth bud while irradiation after calcification causes inhibition of cellular differentiation, causing malformations and arrest in general growth.
3. **Effects on odontogenesis:** Maturing ameloblasts may be permanently damaged with as little as 10 Gy, and ameloblastic activity ceases after exposure to 30 Gy.
4. **Radiation caries:** Radiation caries is rampant form of caries that may occur in individuals who receive a course of radiotherapy that includes exposure to salivary glands. They are as follows:
   - Widespread superficial lesions attacking buccal, occlusal, incisal, and palatal surfaces.
   - Lesions involving primarily cementum and dentin in cervical region, may progress around the teeth circumferentially and result in loss of the crown.
   - Dark pigmentation of entire crown and wearing away of the incisal edges.
5. **Periodontal problems:** Decrease in vascularity and acellularity of PDL; Disorientation and rupture of Sharpey's fibers; thickening and widening of periodontal space. Cementum gets acellular, and its repair and regeneration capacity is severely reduced.
6. **Pulpal defects:** Pulpal tissue will demonstrate long-term fibroatrophy after irradiation. Patients may exhibit hypersensitivity, pulpal pain, and necrosis.
7. **Osteoradionecrosis.**
8. **Trismus:** Trismus develops in most patients within 3–6 months after radiotherapy and frequently becomes a long lasting problem.
9. **Soft tissue necrosis:** Due to excessive dose delivered to tissues via interstitial implants or secondary to soft tissue irritation from an inadequate fitting prosthesis.

Q. 14. Write a short note on amalgam tattoo. *(RGUHS, May 2014)*

Ans. An amalgam tattoo (focal argyrosis) is the most common localized pigmented lesion in the mouth. It develops when a piece of amalgam filling material becomes inadvertently lodged in the oral mucosa. This can happen whilst the fillings are being placed or

Table 7.13: Scoring system for radiation mucositis

Score	National cancer institute rating	WHO rating
0	None	No symptoms
1	Painless ulcers, erythema, or mild soreness	Sore mouth, no ulcer
2	Painful erythema, edema, or ulcers; however, patient can eat solid food	Sore mouth with ulcers but able to eat normally
3	Painful erythema, edema, or ulcers; patient cannot eat solid food	Liquid diet only
4	Requires parenteral or enteral support (such as gastric feeding tube) to provide nutrition	Unable to eat or drink

polished, or during the removal of a filling following the use of dental drills.

Clinical features
1. Amalgam tattoo presents as a dark gray or blue, flat macule located adjacent to a restored tooth.
2. Most are located on the gingiva and alveolar mucosa followed by the buccal mucosa and floor of mouth.
3. *Microscopically*, amalgam is seen two forms: As irregular dark, solid fragments of metal or as numerous, discrete fine, brown or black granules dispersed along collagen bundles and around small blood vessels and nerves.
4. Large fragments become surrounded by dense fibrous connective tissue. Smaller particles are associated with mild to moderate chronic inflammatory response with individual macrophages engulfing small amalgam particles.

Diagnosis: Usually obvious from the location and clinical appearance. A radiograph is recommended to confirm the presence of metallic particles. When there is no radiographic evidence or an adjacent restored tooth, biopsy is recommended.

Treatment: Surgical excision; Q-switched ruby laser; Q-switched alexandrite laser.

Q. 15. Write a short note on tracheostomy.
(HP Uni., May 2018; UHSR, June 2018)

Ans. A tracheostomy is a surgically created opening in the neck leading directly to trachea, and is maintained open with a hollow tube called tracheostomy tube.

Indications
1. To bypass an obstructed upper airway.
2. To clean and remove secretions from the airway.
3. To prolong mechanical ventilation.
4. To more easily and usually more safely, deliver oxygen to lungs.

Complications: Airway obstruction and aspiration of secretions; Bleeding; Damage to larynx; Infection; Air trapping in surrounding tissues/chest; Scarring of airway; Erosion of tube into surrounding structures; Impaired swallowing and vocal function; Scarring of neck.

During a tracheostomy procedure, surgery is performed in intensive care unit or in operating room. In either location, patient is continuously monitored by pulse oximeter and cardiac rhythm. The anesthesiologists usually use a mixture of an intravenous medication and a local anesthetic in order to make the procedure comfortable for patient. The surgeon makes an incision low in the neck. The trachea is identified in the middle and an opening is created to allow for the new breathing passage (tracheostomy tube) to be inserted below the larynx.

Q. 16. Write a short note on hemothorax.
(HP Uni., Nov. 2018).

Ans. Hemothorax is a collection of blood in the pleural space, a potential space between the visceral and parietal pleura. The most common mechanism of trauma is a blunt or penetrating injury to intrathoracic or extrathoracic structures that result in bleeding into thorax.

Clinical features: Respiratory distress, tachypnea, decreased or absent breath sounds, dullness to percussion, chest wall asymmetry, tracheal deviation, hypoxia, narrow pulse pressure, and hypotension.

CT scan is the preferred method of evaluation for intrathoracic injuries.

Physical findings
- Distended neck veins → pericardial tamponade, tension pneumothorax, cardiogenic failure, air embolism.
- "Seat belt sign" → deceleration or vascular injury; chest wall contusion/abrasion
- Paradoxical chest wall movement → flail chest
- Facial/neck swelling or cyanosis → superior mediastinum injury with occlusion or compression of superior vena cava.
- Subcutaneous emphysema → torn bronchus or lung parenchyma laceration.
- Scaphoid abdomen → diaphragmatic injury with herniation of abdominal content into the chest.
- Excessive abdominal movement with breathing → chest wall injury.

Differential diagnosis: Visceral injuries; skeletal injuries; Cardiovascular injuries.

Management: Perform initial resuscitation and management of a trauma patient according to the ATLS protocol. Every patient should have two large bore IVs access, be placed on a cardiac and oxygen monitor, and have a 12-lead EKG. Immediate life-threatening injuries require prompt intervention, such as decompression needle thoracostomy, and/or emergent tube thoracostomy for large pneumothorax, and initial management of hemothorax.

Q. 17. Write a short note on velopharyngeal incompetence. *(NTR Uni., Oct. 2011)*

Ans. When velum (soft palate) fails to close tightly against the posterior wall or pharyngeal wall of throat, during speech, allowing the air to come out of the nose and making the speech difficult to understand due to hypernasality and/or nasal air emission is called velopharyngeal insufficiency (VPI).

Symptoms of VPI: Hypernasality (nasal speech) and nasal air escape (sounds)/nasal air emission.

Causes: Structural causes (cleft palate); Neuromuscular causes (velocardiofacial syndrome); Functional causes (splinting of palate after tonsillectomy surgery); Abnormal anatomy, abnormal neurophysiology; Particular articulation errors (velopharyngeal mislearning).

Diagnosis of velopharyngeal insufficiency: Speech analysis, nasometry, nasopharyngoscopy, videofluoroscopy, MRI.

Treatment of velopharyngeal insufficiency: Speech therapy; Nasal continuous positive airway pressure therapy (CPAP); Surgical techniques (pharyngeal flap, sphincter palatoplasty, posterior wall augmentation); Non-surgical techniques (prosthesis).

Q. 18. Write a short note on subacute bacterial endocarditis. *(NTR Uni., April 2011)*

Ans. Infective or bacterial endocarditis (IE or BE) is serious infection of valvular and mural endocardium caused by different forms of microorganisms and is characterized by typical infected and friable vegetations.

Predisposing/risk factors: Structural heart disease, prosthetic heart valves, indwelling cardiovascular device, an intravascular catheter, history of infective endocarditis. Other risk factors include male >60 years, intravenous (IV) drug use, poor dentition, or dental infection.

Types

- **Acute bacterial endocarditis (ABE):** It presents as fulminant and destructive acute infection of endocardium by highly virulent bacteria (*Staph. aureus*) in a previously normal heart and almost invariably runs a rapidly fatal course in a period of 2–6 weeks.
- **Sub-acute bacterial endocarditis (SABE) or endocarditis lenta:** It is caused by less virulent bacteria (*Strept. viridans*) in a previously diseased heart and has a gradual downhill course in a period of 6 weeks to a few months and sometimes years.

Pathogenesis: Bacteria causing BE on entering the bloodstream are implanted on the cardiac valves or mural endocardium because they have surface adhesion molecules which mediate their adherence to injured endocardium.

Complications and sequelae: Acute form: High grade fever, chills, weakness and malaise. SABE: Slight fever, fatigue, loss of weight and flu-like symptoms.

A. **Cardiac complications:** Valvular stenosis/insufficiency; Perforation, rupture, and aneurysm of valve leaflets; Abscess in valve ring; Myocardial abscess; Suppurative pericarditis; Cardiac failure.

B. **Extra-cardiac complications:** Vegetations are typically friable and tend to get dislodged due to rapid stream of blood and give rise to embolism, which is responsible for extra-cardiac complications, e.g. infarcts, abscesses and mycotic aneurysms, petechiae. In SABE, there are painful, tender nodules on finger tips of hands and feet (*Osler's nodes*), and focal necrotising glomerulonephritis. In ABE, there is appearance of painless, non-tender subcutaneous maculopapular lesions on the pulp of fingers (*Janeway's spots*).

Treatment: High dose antibiotics (pencillin).

Q. 19. Write a short note on tetralogy of Fallot (TOF).

Ans. Tetralogy of Fallot is the most common cyanotic congenital heart disease, found in about 10% of children with anomalies of heart.

Etiology: Untreated maternal diabetes, maternal intake of retinoic acid, phenylketonuria, chromosomal anomalies (trisomies 21, 18, 13), micro-deletions of chromosome 22q11.2, Alagille syndrome, methylene-tetrahydrofolate reductase polymorphism, and mutations in TBX1 and ZFPM2.

Morphologic features: Four features of tetralogy are:
  i. Ventricular septal defect (VSD) ('shunt').
  ii. Displacement of aorta to right so that it overrides VSD.
  iii. Pulmonary stenosis ('obstruction').
  iv. Right ventricular hypertrophy.

Types

a. **Cyanotic tetralogy:** Pulmonary stenosis is greater and VSD is mild so that there is more resistance to outflow of blood from right ventricle resulting in right-to-left shunt at ventricular level and cyanosis.

b. **Acyanotic tetralogy:** VSD is larger and pulmonary stenosis is mild so that there is mainly left-to-right shunt with increased pulmonary flow and increased volume in left heart but no cyanosis.

Clinical features

- More commonly present in neonates with a certain degree of cyanosis and clubbing.
- Prominent murmur (crescendo-decrescendo) with harsh systolic ejection quality.
- Systolic click may be auscultated along left sternal border.
- Prominent ventricular impulse and systolic thrill.

- Others: Right aortic arch, abnormal coronary arteries, significant aorticopulmonary collaterals, patent ductus arteriosus, multiple septal defects, and aortic valve regurgitation.
- "**Tet spells**" or hypercyanotic episodes are present during infancy and decrease after 4–5 years of age.

Diagnosis: Fetal echocardiography. After birth—chest radiograph, electrocardiogram, and echocardiogram. Chest radiographs usually show a normal-size heart silhouette ("**Boot-shaped**").

Treatment: Prostaglandin therapy, surgical repair.

Q. 20. Write a short note on cardiomyopathy.
(RUHS, June 2017)

Ans. Cardiomyopathy literally means disease of the heart muscle.

Classification

A. Primary cardiomyopathy: Myocardial disease with no known underlying cause. It is subdivided into 3 pathophysiologic categories:

1. Idiopathic dilated (congestive) cardiomyopathy.
2. Idiopathic hypertrophic cardiomyopathy: Obstructive and non-obstructive.
3. Idiopathic restrictive or obliterative or infiltrative cardiomyopathy: Cardiac amyloidosis, Loeffler's endocarditis (fibroplastic parietal endocarditis with peripheral blood eosinophilia), other forms of restrictive cardiomyopathy (haemochromatosis, myocardial sarcoidosis, carcinoid syndrome, scleroderma, neoplastic infiltration in heart).

B. Secondary cardiomyopathy: Myocardial disease with known underlying cause, e.g. nutritional disorders (thiamine deficiency), toxic chemicals (cobalt), drugs (cyclophosphamide), metabolic diseases (glycogen storage diseases), neuromuscular diseases (muscular dystrophies), infiltrations (leukemia), connective tissue diseases.

Morphologic features: *Grossly*, the heart is enlarged and increased in weight. Most characteristic feature is prominent dilatation of all the four chambers giving the heart typical "**Globular appearance**". The endocardium is thickened and mural thrombi are often found in ventricles and atria. *Microscopically*, endomyocardial biopsies or autopsy examination of heart reveal non-specific and variable changes.

Q. 21. Write a note on giant cell tumor.
(NTR Uni., May 2019).

Ans. Giant cell tumors (GCTs) are benign bone tumors arising from bone marrow, which account for about 5% of all biopsied primary bone tumors. GCTs arising in the head and neck region constitute approximately 2% of all GCTs, with the majority occurring in sphenoid, ethmoid, or temporal bones.

GCT is a true neoplastic process originating from the undifferentiated mesenchymal cells of the bone marrow. It is generally considered as benign but severe bony destruction may result occasionally depending on the location and clinical presentation of tumor.

Patients with head and neck GCT may present with swelling, pain, epistaxis, neurological deficits, proptosis, visual defects, tinnitus, and hearing loss.

Radiologic examination of GCT usually reveals a well-circumscribed lytic lesion surrounded by little or no sclerosis. The tumors may break through cortex and invade soft tissue or articular space.

Histologically, GCTs are composed of multinucleated giant cells in a vascular stroma of epithelioid or spindle-shaped mononuclear cells. Pathologic differential diagnosis of GCT is also extensive, including giant cell reparative granuloma, brown tumor of hyperparathyroidism, osteoblastoma, chondroblastoma, aneurysmal bone cyst, non-ossifying fibroma, foreign body reaction, and osteosarcoma with abundant giant cells.

Treatment: Surgical excision.

Q. 22. Write a short note on Bence Jones protein.
(NTR Uni., June 2014)

Ans. Bence Jones protein (BJP) is characterized by precipitation of urine at 40–60°C and re-dissolving of the precipitate at 100°C. They are known as light chain of immunoglobulins without accompanying heavy chain.

BJP, or free light chains, are found in urine as low molecular weight monomers, dimers, or high molecular weight polymers and as tetramers in serum. Their molecular weight is 22000, and the kidney metabolizes them. Bence Jones proteins spill into the urine once capacity for tubular absorption becomes saturated.

Specimen collection: A 24-hour urine catch is desirable to accurately quantify the amount of BJP excreted. Methods for detection include conventional high-resolution electrophoresis or capillary zone electrophoresis followed by confirmation through immunofixation electrophoresis or immunoelectrophoresis.

Clinical significance: Testing for Bence Jones proteinuria is indicated when plasma cell disorders such as multiple myeloma are suspected. Patient signs and symptoms that may prompt testing include anemia, hypercalcemia, and renal impairment. Excessive secretion of Bence Jones proteins causes acute kidney injury from tubular obstruction and tubular nephropathy. Tubular damage results in Fanconi syndrome with glycosuria, aminoaciduria, phosphaturia, and renal tubular acidosis type 2.

Q. 23. Write a short note on basal cell carcinoma.

(NTR Uni., Oct. 2013)

Ans. Basal cell carcinoma (BCC) or **basal cell epithelioma** is the most common cancer in humans, mostly arises on sun-damaged skin and rarely develops on mucous membranes or palms and soles. Basal cell carcinoma is usually a slow-growing tumor for which metastases are rare.

Subtypes of BCC: Nodular, superficial, morpheaform, and fibroepithelial (**fibroepithelioma of Pinkus**).

Etiology: Exposure to UV light (UVB > UVA wavelengths), ionizing radiation exposure, arsenic exposure, immunosuppression, and genetic predisposition (xeroderma pigmentosum, basal cell nevus syndrome (Gorlin syndrome), Bazex-Dupre-Christol syndrome, and Rombo syndrome).

Pathophysiology: Mechanism via ultraviolet radiation is by direct DNA damage, indirect DNA damage through reactive oxygen species, and immune suppression. Ultraviolet exposure also causes dose-dependent suppression of the cutaneous immune system, impairing immune surveillance of skin cancer.

Clinical features

- Men generally have higher rates of BCC than women.
- BCC is more frequent in geographic locations with greater UV exposure.
- Incidence rates for BCC also increase with age, with the median age of diagnosis being 68 years.
- BCC typically presents as a shiny, pink- or flesh-colored papule or nodule with surface telangiectasia.
- Tumor may enlarge and ulcerate, giving the borders a **rolled/rodent ulcer** appearance.
- Most common sites for nodular basal cells are nose, cheeks, forehead, nasolabial folds, and eyelids.
- **Histopathology:** Characteristic features are islands or nests of basaloid cells, with cells palisading at periphery in a haphazard arrangement in the centers of islands. Each of these small pleomorphic cells is composed of a basophilic nucleus without a discernible nucleolus and scanty cytoplasm. Mucin deposition may be present within the tumor and in the stroma around tumor. Mitotic figures also may be present.

Diagnosis: Skin biopsy; Dermoscopy: Presence of well-focused *arborizing vessels* (hallmark), multiple blue-gray globules, leaf-like structures, large blue-gray ovoid nests, and spoke-wheel areas.

Treatment/management: Mohs micrographic surgery (MMS), standard surgical excision, EDC, radiation, photodynamic therapy, cryosurgery, topical therapy (5-FU, imiquimod 5% cream), and systemic medications such as vismodegib.

Q. 24. Write a note on condrosarcoma.

(NTR Uni., April 2009)

Ans. Chondrosarcoma is a malignant tumour of chondroblasts. Chondrosarcomas of the head and neck regions are rare malignancies. Two types:

- **Central chondrosarcoma** is more common and arises within the medullary cavity of bone and occurs *de novo*.
- **Peripheral chondrosarcoma** arises in the cortex or periosteum of bone. It may be primary or secondary occurring on a pre-existing benign cartilaginous tumour.

Clinical features

- Chondrosarcomas generally occurs in 3rd–6th decades of life with M:F = 2:1; Maxilla > mandible.
- Tumour is slow-growing with gradual enlargement over years.
- Mucosa is often intact, with painless swelling.
- Tumors located in skull base can cause neurological symptoms.
- High grades cause metastatic dissemination, commonly to lungs, liver, kidney and brain.
- **Radiographically,** lytic lesions, intralesional calcifications (**popcorn calcification or rings and arcs calcification**), endosteal scalloping, permeative appearance/moth-eaten appearance in high-grade chondrosarcomas, cortical remodeling, thickening, and periosteal reaction.
- *Histologically,* hallmarks of chondrosarcoma are invasive character and formation of lobules of anaplastic cartilage cells. These tumour cells show cytologic features of malignancy such as hyperchromatism, pleomorphism, two or more cells in the lacunae and tumour giant cells.
- **Differential diagnosis:** Chondromyxoid fibroma, enchondroma, chondroblastic osteosarcoma, fracture callus.

Treatment

1. **Surgery:** Intralesional curettage, burring and surgical adjuvant application such as hydrogen peroxide, wide surgical excision, wide en bloc excision.
2. **Chemotherapy:** For dedifferentiated chondrosarcomas containing high-grade spindle cell component.
3. **Radiation therapy:** For locally recurrent tumors, intermediate to high-grade tumors, and tumors in locations where surgical resection is challenging or limited.

Q. 25. Write a short note on paraneoplastic syndrome.

Ans. Paraneoplastic syndromes (PNS) represent a clinical spectrum of manifestations of the indirect and remote effects produced by tumor metabolites or other products and exclude metastasis or any other normal events associated with tumor progression. Their clinical presentation could be the first or prominent clinical manifestation so it can raise suspicion of a deep-seated tumor.

Pathogenesis: Tumor cells can produce hormones, enzymes or fetal proteins, cytokines, stimulate antibody production and metabolize steroids. Any of these tumor products can produce manifestations of PNS.

PNS associated with oral SCC

1. **Endocrine manifestations:** Syndrome of inappropriate antidiuretic hormone (SIADH) humoral hypercalcemia of malignancy (HHM), ectopic ACTH-producing tumors, chemical hyperadrenocorticism, paraneoplastic gynaecomastia.
2. **Neuromuscular manifestations:** Subacute cerebellar degeneration, Eaton-Lambart myasthenic syndrome, Paraneoplastic encephalomyelitis.
3. **Ocular manifestations:** Carcinoma-associated retinopathy.
4. **Rheumatological manifestations:** Polyarthritis, pseudo-stills disease, hypertrophy osteoarthropathy.
5. **Dermal manifestations:** Paraneoplastic pruritus, herpes zoster, alopecia, acanthosis nigricans, acrokeratosis paraneoplastica (Bazex syndrome), sweets syndrome, yellow nail syndrome, paraneoplastic pemphigus.
6. **Hematological manifestations:** Trousseaus's syndrome, paraneoplastic polyvasculitis, leukocytosis, erythrocytosis or anemia, thrombocytosis, DIC, leukaemoid reactions, and hypereosinophilia.

Q. 26. Write a short note on myeloid leukemia.
(NTR Uni., May 2005)

Ans. Leukemia is a hematological disorder which is caused by proliferating white blood cell-forming tissues resulting in a marked increase in circulating immature or abnormal WBCs.

Causes: Ionizing radiation, certain chemicals (benzene), and infection with specific oncogenic viruses, cigarette smoking, exposure to electromagnetic fields.

Classification: Leukemia is classified based on clinical behavior (acute or chronic) and the primary hematopoietic cell line affected (myeloid or lymphoid): Acute myelogenous leukemia (AML); Acute lymphocytic leukemia (ALL); Chronic myelogenous leukemia (CML); Chronic lymphocytic leukemia (CLL).

I. Acute myeloid leukaemia: AML is a heterogeneous disease characterized by infiltration of malignant myeloid cells into the blood, bone marrow and other tissues. AML is mainly a disease of adults, while children and older individuals may also develop it. AML develops due to inhibition of maturation of myeloid stem cells due to mutations.

Classification

a. **FAB classification:** According to this, a leukaemia is acute if bone marrow consists of >30% blasts. FAB divides AML into 8 subtypes (M0 to M7).
b. **WHO classification (2002):** WHO classification for AML is more clinical and has lowered the cut off percentage of marrow blasts to 20% from 30% in FAB classification.

Clinical features: Anemia, bleeding disorders, infections, fever, pain and tenderness of bones, lymphadenopathy, enlarged tonsils, splenomegaly, hepatomegaly, gum hypertrophy, chloroma, meningeal involvement.

Laboratory findings

a. **Blood picture:** Anaemia, reticulocytosis, thrombocytopenia, leukocytosis.
b. **Bone marrow examination**
   - Hypercellular, or 'dry tap', leukemic blast cells, reduced erythropoietic cells, dyserythropoiesis, megaloblastic features and ring sideroblasts, reduced megakaryocytes.
   - Chromosomal analysis: M3 have t(15;17)(q22;q12); M4E0 have inv(16)(p13q22).

Treatment: Fresh blood transfusions and platelet and leukocyte concentrates; Systemic antibiotics; Cytotoxic therapy (cytosine arabinoside, anthracyclines, 6-thioguanine, amsacrine); Bone marrow transplantation.

II. Chronic myeloid leukaemia (CML): By WHO definition, CML is established by identification of clone of haematopoietic stem cell that possesses reciprocal translocation between chromosomes 9 and 22, forming **Philadelphia chromosome**.

Clinical features: CML comprises 20% of all leukemias and its peak incidence is seen in 3rd–4th decades of life. Both sexes are affected equally. Common manifestations are: Anaemia, hypermetabolism, splenomegaly, bleeding tendencies, gout, visual disturbance, neurologic manifestations and priapism.

Laboratory findings

a. **Blood picture:** Anaemia, marked leucocytosis, platelet count normal or elevated.
b. **Bone marrow examination:** Hypercellular, increased myeloid-erythroid ratio; reduction in erythropoietic

cells; smaller megakaryocytes. Cytogenetic studies show characteristic Philadelphia (Ph) chromosome.

Treatment: Imatinib oral therapy; Bone marrow transplantation; IFN-α; Chemotherapeutic agents (busulfan, cyclophosphamide, hydroxyurea); Others (splenic irradiation, splenectomy, leucopheresis).

Oral manifestations: Gingival bleeding, petechiae, ecchymoses, thrombocytopenia, gingival enlargement (more common in acute than chronic leukemia), gingival ulceration, oral infection, pale oral mucosa.

Q. 27. Write a note on oral manifestations of diabetes mellitus. *(NTR Uni., April 2014)*

Ans. Diabetes mellitus (DM) is defined as a heterogeneous metabolic disorder characterized by chronic hyperglycemia with disturbance of carbohydrate, fat and protein metabolism (WHO).

Complications of diabetes

I. Acute metabolic complications: Diabetic ketoacidosis, hyperosmolar nonketotic coma, and hypoglycemia.

II. Late systemic complications: Atherosclerosis, diabetic microangiopathy, diabetic nephropathy, diabetic neuropathy, diabetic retinopathy and infections.

Oral manifestations

i. **Diabetes and periodontal disease:** Main oral complication of DM is periodontal disease, considered as 6th complication of DM. Simple chewing can cause systemic dissemination of periodontal pathogens and their metabolic products in patients, causing endotoxemia or bacteremia, which results in an increase in serum levels of inflammatory mediators (IL-6, fibrinogen, and C-reactive protein). Furthermore, systemic inflammation can exacerbate insulin resistance.

ii. **Diabetes and periapical pathology:** Patients with DM2 have increased incidence of periapical lesions and a lower success rate in primary root canal treatment. Patients with diabetes are at increased risk of need for tooth extraction following endodontic treatment. The dental pulp of diabetic patients may have limited dental collateral circulation, impaired immune response, and increased risk of infection/pulp necrosis.

iii. **Diabetes and dental caries:** Patients with DM may have fewer cavities due to content of their diet which usually contains more protein and fewer fermentable carbohydrates. Meanwhile, other studies have found a higher incidence of dental caries, which could be explained by decrease salivary secretion in diabetics.

iv. **Diabetes and oral mucosa:** DM patients may have a higher prevalence of mucosal disorders possibly associated with chronic immunosuppression, delayed healing, and/or salivary hypofunction. These alterations include: Oral fungal infections; fissured tongue, irritation fibroma, traumatic ulcers and lichen planus.

v. **Diabetes and xerostomia:** DM can cause xerostomia. In addition, increased salivary glucose promotes proliferation and colonization of bacteria in oral cavity.

vi. **Diabetes and taste disturbance:** Taste detection follows a hereditary pattern, but can be influenced by appearance of neuropathies. When this sensory dysfunction occurs, it can inhibit the ability to maintain a proper diet and can lead to poor glycemic control. Taste alteration has been associated with diabetes and development of obesity.

vii. **Diabetes and BMS:** Patients with diabetes often have burning mouth syndrome.

Q. 28. Write a short note on syncope.
(NTR Uni., April 2013; RGUHS, July 2017)

Ans. Syncope is a short-term, temporary loss of consciousness, after which the patient regains consciousness spontaneously.

Types:
1. Cerebral (neurogenic)
2. Cardiac (cardiogenic)
3. Neuro-cardiogenic
4. Vascular
5. Metabolic
6. Drug-induced

In dental practice, most common type is neurocardiogenic syncope (syncope caused by reflexive reaction of autonomous nervous system), which can be:

1. **Vasovagal syndrome:** It is reflective bradycardia and hypotension caused by erect position. This leads to a drop in blood pressure, lower heart ejection fraction resulting in cerebral hypoxia with subsequent loss of consciousness. It may be preceded by nausea, vomiting, heat sensation and vertigo.

2. **Postural syncope:** It occurs when one quickly changes body position to standing after being in a recumbent or sitting position for a long time. This causes a sudden drop in hydrostatic blood pressure in brain as a result of absence or insufficient activity of neurohumoral mechanisms. Patients at risk for postural syncope include those taking antihypertensive drugs, antidepressants, sedatives, hypnotics.

3. **Carotid sinus hypersensitivity:** It is characterized by reflexive bradycardia or drop in blood pressure due to hypersensitivity of carotid sinus baroreceptors. It is caused by tight collar or tie or after a suddenly turning the head to the side.

4. **Hyperventilation-induced syncope:** It usually occurs in minors, who are generally healthy, and is caused by hysterical fear. Often the first symptom of hyperventilation is inability to take a deep and slow breath. Apart from anxiety, patient may present with an increased respiration rate and deeper respiration leading to respiratory alkalosis, vertigo, xerostomia, tingling and numb sensations in lips and fingers, palpitations, tachycardia, muscle tremor and pains.

Management of syncope

1. Discontinue treatment, unfold the dental chair, lift the lower limbs.
2. Administer oxygen (2–5 L/min.).
3. Loosen tight clothing, take the glasses off.
4. Assess the pulse, arterial blood pressure, state of consciousness.
5. If the patient does not regain consciousness: Apply basic resuscitation procedures; call an ambulance.

Q. 29. Write a short note on autoimmune disease.
(RGUHS, May 2013)

Ans. Autoimmunity *(UHSR, April 2015)*: Autoimmunity is the failure of an organism in recognizing its own constituent parts as non-self, which allows an immune response against its own cells and tissues. Autoimmune disease is any disease that results from an immune response against self. **Autoimmune disease** may be primarily due to either antibodies (autoantibodies) or immune cells, but a common characteristic is presence of a lymphocytic infiltration in target organ. Autoimmunity is the opposite of **immune tolerance.** Immune tolerance is defined as the ability of an individual to recognize self tissue and antigens.

Mechanisms of autoimmunity *(BFUHS, May 2015)*: Autoimmunity results from a failure of the mechanisms of self-tolerance in T or B cells, which may lead to an imbalance between lymphocyte activation and control mechanisms.

- Defects in deletion (negative selection) of T or B cells or receptor editing in B cells during maturation in respective lymphoid organs.
- Defective numbers and functions of regulatory T lymphocytes.
- Defective apoptosis of mature self-reactive lymphocytes.

- Inadequate function of inhibitory receptors.
- Activation of sntigen presenting cells (APCs), which results in excessive T cell activation.

Classification of autoimmune diseases

A. Organ non-specific (systemic): In these, autoantibodies formed reacts with antigens in many tissues and thus cause systemic lesions. Examples: Systemic lupus erythematosus (SLE), rheumatoid arthritis, scleroderma (progressive systemic sclerosis), polymyositis, dermatomyositis, polyarteritis nodosa (PAN), Sjögren's syndrome, Reiter's syndrome, Wegener's granulomatosis.

B. Organ specific (localized): In these, autoantibodies formed react specifically against an organ or target tissue component and cause its chronic inflammatory destruction. Examples:

1. **Endocrine glands:** Hashimoto's (autoimmune) thyroiditis, Graves' disease, type 1 diabetes mellitus, idiopathic Addison's disease.
2. **Alimentary tract:** Autoimmune atrophic gastritis, ulcerative colitis, Crohn's disease.
3. **Blood cells:** Autoimmune haemolytic anaemia, autoimmune thrombocytopenia, pernicious anaemia.
4. **Others:** Myasthenia gravis, autoimmune orchitis, autoimmune encephalomyelitis, Goodpasture's syndrome, primary biliary cirrhosis, lupoid hepatitis, membranous glomerulonephritis, autoimmune skin diseases.

Treatment: Anti-inflammatory drugs, corticosteroids, immunosuppressant drugs, methotrexate, radiation, plasmapheresis, monoclonal antibodies, thymectomy, plasmapheresis.

Q. 30. Discuss immunodeficiency disorders and management of immune deficiency patients who require surgical procedures.

Ans. Immunodeficiency relates to body's immune system being unable to perform its normal functions in protecting the host. Broadly it can be classified as:

A. **Primary immunodeficiency:** Genetically determined, typically manifesting during infancy or childhood.

B. **Secondary immunodeficiency:** Acquired type. Individuals are born with normal immunity but some conditions or external factor results in an immunocompromised state, e.g. AIDS, malnutrtion, immunosuppressive treatment, malignancies, uncontrolled diabetes, autoimmune disorders, toxic exposures, stress, aging.

Clinical manifestations of immunodeficiency: Recurrent infections; Chronic diarrhea; Failure to thrive; Skin lesions, oral or esophageal thrush, oral ulcers, and periodontitis, severe viral infection, CNS problems, and autoimmune disorder.

Diagnosis

- Onset <6 month: T cell defect.
- Onset between age of 6 and 12 months: Combined B and T cell defects or a B cell defect.
- Onset >12 months: B cell defect or secondary immunodeficiency.

Classification of primary immunodeficiency: International Union of Immunological Societies (IUIS) 2014 classification

1. Combined immunodeficiency (CID): These disorders are characterized by decreased numbers of T cells and often reduction in B cell count.

a. **Severe combined immunodeficiency (SCID):** This group is represented by little or no T and B cells and defective antibody responses. This disease is fatal within first two years of life. Diarrhea, failure to thrive, life-threatening infections, maculopapular rash, splenomegaly, candidiasis, viral infections, and ulcerative stomatitis.

b. **MHC class I and II deficiency** (bare lymphocyte syndrome).

2. Combined immunodeficiencies (CID) with associated or syndromic features: CID with syndromic features predominantly affects T cells.

a. **DiGeorge anomaly (deletion 22 syndrome):** This disorder can be inherited or as a consequence of *de novo* defect. Most cases have a thymic deficiency, hypoparathyroidism, hypocalcaemic tetany, cardiac defects, opportunistic infections, distinguishing maxillofacial/head and neck defects, include laryngeal, pharyngeal, esophageal, tracheal, cleft palatal deformities, malformations in dental anatomy, enamel hypoplasia, missing teeth, dental eruption patterns, and caries.

b. **Ataxia:** Telangiectasia.

c. **Wiskott-Aldrich syndrome (WAS):** WAS is a rare X-linked disorder arising from an alteration in WAS protein gene, which affects immune response, cell motility, and protection against autoimmune diseases. T cells are decreased and IgM production is decreased. Clinical features associated with WAS are microthrombocytopenia, eczema, lymphoma, recurrent bacterial and viral infections, IgA nephropathy, and a high incidence of autoimmunity, gingival ulceration with bleeding tendency.

d. **Hyper IgE syndromes** (Job's syndrome).

e. **Dyskeratosis congenita** (DKC).

f. **Schimke syndrome** (SIOD).

3. Predominantly antibody deficiencies

a. BTK deficiency (X-linked agammaglobulinemia or Bruton's agammaglobulinemia).

b. Common variable immunodeficiency disorders (CVID).

c. CD40L/CD40 deficiencies (hyper-IgM syndrome).

d. Selective IgA deficiency.

e. Isolated IgG subclass deficiency (selective IgG deficiency).

f. **Thymoma with immunodeficiency** (good syndrome).

4. Diseases of immune dysregulation: This group is characterized by difficulties in regulating immunity.

a. **Chédiak-Higashi syndrome (CHS):** CHS is a rare AR disorder wherein the genetic defect is mutations throughout lysosomal trafficking (LYST) genes. Disease characteristics of CHS include partial albinism, hepatosplenomegaly, neutropenia, severe recurrent bacterial infections, platelet abnormalities, lymphoma-like disease, and neurologic problems. Oral manifestations described are recurrent ulcers, candidiasis, and early-onset aggressive periodontitis.

b. **APECED (APS-1)** (autoimmune polyendocrinopathy with candidiasis and ectodermal dystrophy).

c. **SAMHD1** deficiency.

5. Congenital defects of phagocyte number, function, or both

I. **Defects of neutrophil differentiation**

   a. **Severe congenital neutropenia** (SCN).

   b. **Cyclic neutropenia (CyN):** CyN is characterized by severe fluctuating neutropenia every 21 days. It is an autosomal dominant defect in ELANE. Patients are susceptible to bacterial and fungal infections, fever, septic shock, periodic aphthous stomatitis and severe periodontal disease.

   c. **Glycogen storage disease type 1b** (GSD1).

II. **Defects of motility**

   a. **Leukocyte adhesion deficiency type 1 (LAD1)/Lazy leukocyte syndrome:** LAD syndromes are rare Autosomal recessive disorders that transpire as a result of defective recruitment of leukocytes from the intravascular compartment. There is a defect in β_2 integrin gene (ITGB2) subunit of leukocyte cell adhesion protein. Clinical features are recurrent infections without pus formation, delayed umbilical cord separation, leukocytosis, skin ulcers, and severe aggressive periodontitis that may affect primary and permanent dentition.

b. **Papillon-Lefèvre syndrome (PLS):** PLS (AR) disorder is characterized by palmoplantar hyperkeratosis (PPK) and severe periodontitis. Haim-Munk syndrome (HMS) is a phenotypic variant of PLS. The genetic mutation in PLS is within cathepsin C (CTSC), an enzyme which coordinates activation of serine proteases necessary for immune cell function. This results in a chemotactic defect in neutrophils and monocytes-macrophages. Severe destructive periodontitis, early loss of primary and permanent teeth, increased incidence of liver, brain, and kidney abscesses, chronic granulomatous infection malignant melanoma.

III. **Defects of respiratory burst:** Chronic granulomatous disease.

6. Defects in innate immunity: These disorders have defects in innate system, e.g. chronic mucocutaneous candidiasis (CMC).

7. Autoinflammatory disorders: These disorders are also known as "periodic fever syndromes."

a. **Periodic fever, aphthous, pharyngitis, adenitis syndrome (PFAPA):** PFAPA Syndrome **(Marshall's syndrome)**, is characterized by recurring high fever, aphthous stomatitis, pharyngitis, cervical adenitis, and sometimes genital ulcers. It is linked to IL-1 pathway.

b. **Familial Mediterranean fever** (FMF).

c. **Hyper IgD syndrome** (HIDS).

d. **Cherubism:** Cherubism is a rare fibro-osseous condition of maxillofacial region where bone is resorbed and replaced by fibrous tissue, resulting in disfigurement. The genetic defect is a neomorphic mutation of SH3BP2 protein, which leads to increased TNF-α.

e. **Chronic atypical neutrophilic dermatitis with lipodystrophy syndrome** (CANDLE syndrome/elevated temperature syndrome).

8. Complement (C) deficiencies.

9. Phenocopies of PID: This group contains conditions present as inherited immunodeficiencies, but is result of acquired changes instead of hereditary (germline) mutations.

Laboratory investigations

- Complete blood count (CBC) with manual differential: Neutropenia, lymphopenia, leukocytosis, thrombocytopenia, anemia, peripheral blood smear.
- Quantitative immunoglobulin (Ig) measurements and antibody titers.
- Skin testing for delayed hypersensitivity.
- Chest X-ray: Absent thymic shadow suggests a T cell disorder.

Treatment: Treatment of immunodeficiency disorders generally involves:

1. **Infection prevention:** By avoiding environmental exposures and not giving live-virus vaccines and using prophylactic antibiotics.
2. **Management of acute infection:** Antibiotics, antiviral, surgery.
3. **Replacement of missing immune components**
   - **IV immune globulin** (400 mg/kg once a month); Subcutaneous immune globulin (100–150 mg/kg once a week).
   - **Hematopoietic stem cell transplantation.**

Q. 31. Write a short note on acoustic neuroma.

Ans. Vestibular schwannoma (acoustic neuroma/acoustic neurinoma/acoustic neurilemoma) is a benign tumour of Schwann cells of the 8th cranial nerve. It may manifest as isolated case or part of neurofibromatosis. It usually occurs after 3rd decade and more frequently in females.

Clinical features: Hearing loss, sensory disturbances of face, vertigo, ataxia, cerebellar signs in limbs, hydrocephalus, facial palsy after removal of tumor.

Investigations: MRI, CT, electro-nystagmography (to evaluate balance), and brainstem auditory evoked response (**BAER**).

Differntial diagnosis: Meniere's disease, Bell's palsy, meningioma.

Treatment: Treatment of acoustic neuroma may involve observation (if the tumor is small and does not cause symptoms), surgical removal (microsurgery or excision) or use of radiation.

Q. 32. Write a short note on thyroglossal duct cyst.

Ans. Thyroglossal duct cysts are the most frequently occurring congenital cervical anomalies, and can form anywhere along thyroid's route of migration from tongue base to inferior neck.

Etiology: A thyroglossal duct cyst is an embryologic remnant that forms due to failure of closure of thyroglossal duct extending from the foramen cecum in the tongue to thyroid's location in the neck.

Clinical features

1. Thyroglossal duct cysts typically present as mobile midline neck masses near the hyoid bone.
2. They often are asymptomatic, however, they can present as an abscess or intermittently draining sinus.
3. The mass will elevate with tongue protrusion or swallowing.
4. Ultrasound is the ideal initial imaging choice.

Histopathological features: They are lined by pseudo-stratified columnar epithelium which may be ciliated or stratified squamous epithelium. Connective tissue wall of cyst contains small patches of lymphoid tissue, thyroid tissue and mucous gland.

Differential diagnosis: Midline neck masses, cystic neck masses, cystic metastatic lymph nodes, dermoid or epidermoid cysts, and second branchial cleft cysts.

Treatment: Sistrunk operation.

Q. 33. Write a note on obstructive sleep apnea.
(RGUHS, May 2012; KUHS, Jan., 2014; HP Uni., April 2019)

Ans. Obstructive sleep apnea (OSA) is characterized by repetitive episodes of complete or partial collapse of the upper airway during sleep, with a consequent cessation/reduction of airflow. The obstructive events (apnoeas or hypopnoeas) cause a progressive asphyxia that increasingly stimulates breathing efforts against the collapsed airway, typically until the person is awakened.

Symptoms of OSA

- Nocturnal: Snoring, witnesses apnoes, choking at night, nocturia, insomnia.
- Diurnal: Excessive sleepiness, morning headaches, depression/irritability, memory loss, decreased libido.

Diagnosis: Nocturnal monitoring of respiratory, sleep and cardiac parameters (polisomnography or nocturnal cardiorespiratory poligraphy); Changes in blood oxygen saturation (SaO_2). A common measurement of sleep apnea is the *apnea-hypopnea index* (AHI) which is an average that represents the combined number of apneas and hypopneas/hour of sleep.

1. **Mild OSA:** AHI of 5–15: Involuntary sleepiness during activities that require little attention, such as watching TV or reading.
2. **Moderate OSA:** AHI of 15–30: Involuntary sleepiness during activities that require some attention, such as meetings or presentations.
3. **Severe OSA:** AHI of more than 30: Involuntary sleepiness during activities that require more active attention, such as talking or driving.

Risk groups: People who are **overweight** and **obese**; With **large neck sizes**; **Middle-aged** and **older men**, and **post-menopausal** women; **Ethnic** minorities; People with **abnormalities** of the bony and soft tissue structure of the head and neck; Adults and children with **Down syndrome**; Children with **large tonsils** and **adenoids**; Anyone who has a **family member** with OSA; People with endocrine disorders such as **acromegaly** and **hypothyroidism**; **Smokers**; Those suffering from nocturnal nasal congestion due to **abnormal morphology, rhinitis** or both.

Effects

1. Fluctuating oxygen levels and increased heart rate.
2. Chronic elevation in daytime blood pressure and increased risk of stroke.
3. Higher rate of death due to heart disease.
4. Impaired glucose tolerance and insulin resistance.
5. Impaired concentration and mood changes.
6. Increased risk of being involved in a deadly motor vehicle accident.
7. Disturbed sleep of the bed partner.

Treatment

1. **Continuous positive airway pressure (CPAP):** CPAP is the standard treatment option for moderate to severe cases of OSA and a good option for mild sleep apnea. CPAP provides a steady stream of pressurized air to patients through a mask that they wear during sleep. This airflow keeps the airway open, preventing pauses in breathing and restoring normal oxygen levels.
2. **Oral appliances:** An oral appliance is an effective treatment option for people with mild to moderate OSA who either prefer it to CPAP or are unable to successfully comply with CPAP therapy. The most commonly used oral appliances are mandibular advanced splints (MAS). These devices attach to both the upper and lower dental arches in order to advance and retain the mandible in a forward position. This will relocate laterally the pharyngeal fat pads from the airway and the tongue base will move forward. Consequently, the upper airway will be widened, particularly in its lateral dimension, and the function of upper airway dilator muscles, particularly the genioglossus, will improve
3. **Surgery:** Surgery is indicated when non-invasive treatments have been unsuccessful.
4. **Behavioral changes:** Weight loss benefits many people with sleep apnea, and changing from back-sleeping to side-sleeping may help those with mild cases of OSA.
5. **Over-the-counter remedies:** External nasal dilator strips, internal nasal dilators, and lubricant sprays may reduce snoring.
6. **Position therapy:** A treatment used for patients suffering from mild OSA. Patients are advised to stay off of the back while sleeping and raise the head of the bed to reduce symptoms.
7. **Emerging therapeutic options:** Stimulation of upper airway muscles, nasal expiratory PAP (nEPAP), oral negative.

Q. 34. Discuss about prions in dentistry.

(TNMGR, April 2012)

Ans. Spongiform encephalopathy, also called **Creutzfeldt-Jakob disease** (CJD) or **mad-cow disease,** is caused by accumulation of prion proteins. Prion proteins are a modified form of normal structural proteins present in the mammalian CNS and are peculiar in two respects: They lack nucleic acid, and they can be transmitted as an infectious proteinaceous particles. Method of transmission are by iatrogenic route (e.g. by tissue transplantation from an infected individual) and by human consumption of BSE (bovine spongiform encephalopathy)-infected beef. Clinically, CJD is characterized by rapidly progressive dementia with prominent association of myoclonus. CJD is invariably fatal.

Oral manifestations: Oral manifestations are rarely seen in prion diseases.

1. Dysphagia (difficulty in swallowing) and dysarthria (poor articulation of speech).
2. Paraesthesia (tingling, pricking or numbness).
3. Orofacial dysesthesia (abnormal sensations in the absence of stimulation).
4. Loss of taste and smell.

There are two possible mechanisms assessed for the transfer of CJD via dental instruments:

a. Accidental abrasion of lingual tonsil during dental procedures. Such a chance is extremely low.
b. Contact of dental instruments with pulp tissue. As dental pulp originates from richly innervated neural crest cells, it is theoretically possible that the dental pulp of individuals infected with CJD may be infectious.

Guidelines for dental management of patients with prion disease: In general, the suggested infection control procedures for the dental management of patients with known prion disease are similar to those of all other patients, with certain important modifications. At present, oral tissues are considered to be of low infectivity, so persons liable to iatrogenic CJD are considered at low risk of prion transmission, hence no additional infection control measures are recommended other than those employed in universal cross-infection control. Brief recommendations are:

1. All health care instruments employed in treatment of patient with known prion disease should be discarded.
2. Single-use instruments are preferred.
3. Dental unit waterlines must not be activated.
4. An independent suction and spittoon other than those of dental unit should be used.
5. Non-disposable instruments should be mechanically cleaned and passed thorough stringent decontamination protocols before reuse, as recommended by WHO.
6. Source of refrigeration and aspiration system should be external to the equipment.
7. Histological samples of high-risk patients must be immediately immersed in 98% formic acid for 1 hour prior to paraffin embedding and labeled as biohazardous.
8. In patients with suspicion of CJD, all the instruments must be stored separately in a rigid container labeled with data of the patient, type of treatment provided and details of the attending clinician until a definitive diagnosis is arrived.
9. The instruments are incinerated if the diagnosis is confirmed or sterilized by conventional methods like autoclaving if diagnosis is ruled out.

Pharmacology

1. PHARMACODYNAMIC AND PHARMACOKINETIC OF DRUGS

Q. 1. Describe various routes of drug administration.
(MAHE, July 2001; RGUHS, September, 2007; TNMGR, March, 2010; BBD Uni., June 2016; AHSUC, May 2017; RUHS, May 2018; HP Uni., April 2019)

Ans. A route of administration is the path by which a drug, fluid, poison or other substance is brought into contact with the body.

Factors governing choice of route

1. Physical and chemical properties of the drug-solid/liquid/gas; Solubility, stability, pH, irritancy.
2. Site of desired action: Localized and approachable or generalized and not approachable.
3. Rate and extent of absorption of drug from different routes.
4. Effect of digestive juices and first pass metabolism on the drug.
5. Rapidity with which the response is desired: Routine treatment or emergency.
6. Accuracy of dosage required: IV and inhalational can provide fine tuning.
7. Condition of the patient.

Routes of drug administration

A. Local routes

1. **Topical:** External application of drug to the surface for localized action. Drugs can be efficiently delivered to the localized lesions on skin, oropharyngeal/nasal mucosa, eyes, ear canal, anal canal or vagina.

a. **Skin**
   i. **Dermal:** Cream, ointment (local action)
   ii. **Transdermal:** This is absorption of drug through skin (systemic action). It is used for highly lipid soluble drugs can be applied over the skin.

Advantages: Prolonged action; Constant plasma drug levels (controlled drug delivery system); Good patient compliance.

Types

- *Adhesive units* (transdermal therapeutic systems) (Fig. 1.1) are adhesive patches of different sizes and shapes made to suit the area of application. Drug is held in a reservoir between an outer layer and a porous membrane and membrane is smeared with adhesive on the area of application. The drug slowly diffuses through the membrane and percutaneous absorption takes place. Sites of application: Chest, abdomen, upper arm, back mastoid region, and scrotum, e.g. highly potent drugs and short acting drugs, hyoscine, GTN, fentanyl transdermal patches.
- *Inunction:* In this, drug is rubbed on the skin, which gets absorbed to produce systemic effects.
- *Iontophoresis:* In this, galvanic current is used for penetration of lipid insoluble drugs into deeper tissues, e.g. fluoride iontophoresis for dental hypersensitivity.
- *Jet injection:* As absorption of drug occurs across the layers of skin, dermojet may also be considered as a form of this route.

b. **Mucous membrane:** Eye/ear drops; Intranasal route.

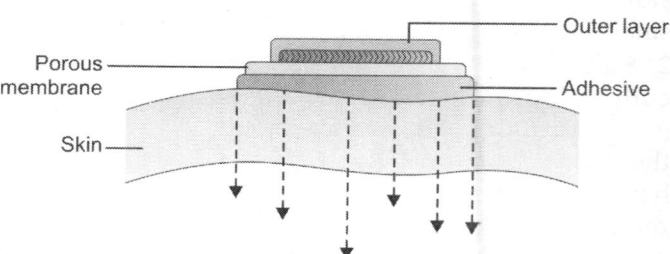

Fig. 1.1: Structure of transdermal therapeutic systems

2. **Deeper tissues:** Certain deep areas can be approached by using a syringe and needle, but the drug should be such that systemic absorption is slow, e.g. intra-articular injection, infiltration around a nerve or intrathecal injection, retro-bulbar injection.

3. **Arterial supply:** Close intra-arterial injection is used for contrast media in angiography; anticancer drugs can be infused in femoral or brachial artery to localize the effect for limb malignancies.

B. Systemic routes

1. **Oral/enteral route:** Oral ingestion is the oldest and commonest mode of drug administration.

Advantages: It is safer, more convenient, does not need assistance, non-invasive, often painless, the medicament need not be sterile and so is cheaper. Both solid dosage forms (powders, tablets, capsules, spansules, and gastrointestinal therapeutic systems) and liquid dosage forms (elixirs, syrups, emulsions, and mixtures) can be given orally.

Limitations

- Action of drugs is slower and thus not suitable for emergencies.
- Unpalatable drugs are difficult to administer.
- May cause nausea and vomiting.
- Cannot be used for uncooperative/unconscious/vomiting patient.
- Absorption of drugs may be variable and erratic.
- Drugs may be destroyed by digestive juices, e.g. insulin.
  - Some drugs may undergo extensive first pass metabolism in the liver.

■ **First pass metabolism/effect:** It is hepatic metabolism of pharmacological agents when it is absorbed from the gut and delivered to the liver via portal circulation. The greater the effect, lower is the bioavailability of the drug.

■ **Enteric coated tablets:** Some tablets are coated with substances like cellulose-acetate, phthalate, gluten, etc. which are not digested by gastric acid but get disintegrated in alkaline juices of intestine. This will: Prevent gastric irritation; avoid destruction of drug by stomach; Provide higher concentration of drug in the small intestine.

2. **Sublingual (s.l.) or buccal:** The tablet or pellet containing the drug is placed under the tongue (sublingual) or crushed in the mouth and spread over the buccal mucosa (buccal). Buccal tablets are often harder, designed to dissolve slowly. Absorption is relatively rapid; action can be produced in minutes. The chief advantage is that liver is bypassed and drugs with high first pass metabolism can be absorbed directly into systemic circulation. Drug is more stable due to relative neutral pH of mouth, e.g. glycerotrinitrate (GTN), buprenorphine.

Disadvantages: Inconvenient; Unpleasant taste of some drugs.

3. **Rectal:** Certain irritant and unpleasant drugs can be put into rectum as suppositories or retention enema for systemic effect. This route can also be used when the patient is having recurrent vomiting or is unconscious or with younger patients. Liver is bypassed. However, absorption is slower, irregular and often unpredictable.

4. **Cutaneous:** Highly lipid soluble drugs can be applied over the skin for slow and prolonged absorption. The liver is also bypassed. Absorption of the drug can be enhanced by rubbing the preparation, by using an oily base and by an occlusive dressing. **Transdermal therapeutic systems** are devices in the form of adhesive patches of various shapes and sizes (5–20 cm^2) which deliver the contained drug at a constant rate into systemic circulation.

5. **Inhalation:** Volatile liquids and gases are given by inhalation for systemic action, e.g. general anesthetics. Advantage: Rapid onset of action; More effective and less harmful; First pass metabolism is avoided; Blood levels of volatile anesthetics can be conveniently controlled.

Disadvantages: Most addictive route; Difficulties in regulating the exact amount of dosage.

6. **Nasal:** The mucous membrane of the nose can readily absorb many drugs; Digestive juices and liver are bypassed.

7. **Parenteral (Par—beyond, enteral—intestinal):** It refers to administration by injection which takes the drug directly into the tissue fluid or blood without having to cross the intestinal mucosa.

Advantages

1. Drug action is faster and predictable.
2. Gastric irritation and vomiting are not provoked.
3. Can be used in unconscious, uncooperative or vomiting patients.
4. No chances of interference by food or digestive juices.
5. No first pass metabolism.

Disadvantages

1. Only sterilized preparation can be used.
2. Expensive, invasive and painful.
3. Assistance required.
4. Chances of local tissue injury; More risky.

Various parenteral routes are:

i. Subcutaneous (SC): Drug is deposited in loose subcutaneous tissue which is richly supplied by nerves but is less vascular (under the skin), e.g. insulin. Self-injection is possible. Absorption can be enhanced by addition of enzyme hyaluronidase. Only small volumes can be injected. Irritant drugs cannot be injected. In shock, absorption is not dependable. Repeated injections at same site can cause lipoatrophy. Some special forms are:

a. **Dermojet:** A high velocity jet of drug solution is projected from a microfine orifice using a gun. It is essentially painless and suited for vaccines.

b. **Pellet implantation:** Drug in the form of small pellets is introduced with a trochar and cannula, e.g. DOCA, testosterone.

c. **Nonbiodegradable (sialistic)** and biodegradable implants: Crystalline drug is packed in tubes or capsules made of suitable materials and implanted under the skin, e.g. hormones, contraceptives (e.g. NORPLANT).

ii. Intramuscular (IM): Drug is injected in one of the large skeletal muscles—deltoid, triceps, gluteus maximus, rectus femoris. Muscle is less richly supplied with sensory nerves and is more vascular (absorption of drugs is faster and reliable). Advantage is that it is suitable for drug in aqueous solution, in suspension or emulsion. Self injection is often impracticable. It may be painful, may even result in an abscess. Irritant solutions can damage the nerve. It should be avoided in anticoagulant treated patients.

iii. Intravenous (IV): Drug is injected into one of the superficial veins so that it directly reaches the circulation and is immediately available for action. Drugs can be given as *bolus; Slow injection; or Slow infusion.* **Advantages:** Most useful route in emergencies, as drug is immediately available for action; Provides predictable blood concentrations with 100% bioavailability; Large volumes of solutions can be given; Irritants can be given by this route; Rapid dose adjustments are possible. **Disadvantages:** Once injected, drug cannot be withdrawn; Irritation of veins may cause thrombophlebitis; Extravasation of drugs may cause severe irritation and sloughing; Only aqueous solutions can be given; Self medication is difficult.

iv. Intradermal injection: Drug is injected into the skin raising a bleb (e.g. BCG vaccine, allergy testing) or scarring/multiple puncture of epidermis through a drop of drug is done. Only a small quantity can be administered by this route and it may be painful.

v. Intrathecal/intraventricular: Into the spine/CSF, most commonly used for spinal anesthesia.

vi. Intraperitoneal: Infusion or injection into peritoneum, e.g. peritoneal dialysis in renal insufficiency.

C. Special drug delivery systems

1. **Ocusert system:** These are thin elliptical units that contain drug in a reservoir which slowly releases it through a membrane by diffusion at a steady rate, e.g. pilocarpine ocusert used in glaucoma.

2. **Progestasert:** It is inserted into uterus, to deliver progesterone constantly for a period.

3. **Transdermal adhesive units.**

4. **Prodrug:** It is an inactive form of drug which gets metabolized to active derivative in body, e.g. Levodopa/dopamine; Bacampicillin/ampicillin; Aspirin/salicylic.

5. **Osmotic pumps/gastrointestinal therapeutic system (GITS):** They are small tablet-shaped units containing drug and an osmotic substance in two different chambers. The tablet is coated with a semipermeable membrane in which a minute laser-drilled hole is made. When tablet is swallowed and reaches the gut, water enters into the tablet through semipermeable membrane. The osmotic layer swells and pushes the drug slowly out of the laser-drilled orifice. This allows slow and constant delivery of the drug over a long period of time, e.g. iron, prazosin.

6. **Computerised miniature pumps:** These are programmed to release drugs at a definite rate either continuously or intermittently in pulses.

7. **Liposomes** are phospholipids suspended in aqueous vehicles to form minute vesicles. Drugs encapsulated in liposomes are taken up mainly by reticuloendothelial cells of liver and are also concentrated in malignant tumors.

Q. 2. Write a short note on saturation kinetics.

(TNMGR, April 1998)

Ans. Pharmacokinetics is the quantitative study of drug movement in, through and out of the body. It involves absorption, distribution, metabolism and excretion.

1. **Absorption:** Absorption is movement of drug from its site of administration into the circulation. Except for IV route, for absorption, drug must pass through various biological membranes. Factors affecting are: Disintegration and dissolution time, formulation, particle size, lipid solubility, pH and ionization, area and vascularity of absorbing surface, gastrointestinal motility, presence of food, metabolism and diseases of gut.

2. **Distribution:** Once a drug has gained access to blood stream, it gets distributed to other tissues that initially had no drug, concentration gradient being in the direction of plasma to tissues. The extent of

distribution of a drug depends on its lipid solubility, ionization at physiological pH (a function of its pKa), extent of binding to plasma and tissue proteins, presence of tissue-specific transporters and differences in regional blood flow.

3. **Biotransformation (metabolism):** Biotransformation means chemical alteration of the drug in the body. It is needed to render non-polar (lipid-soluble) compounds polar (lipid insoluble) so that they are not reabsorbed in renal tubules and are excreted. Most hydrophilic drugs, e.g. streptomycin, neostigmine, pancuronium, etc. are little biotransformed and are largely excreted unchanged. Primary site for drug metabolism is liver; Others are—kidney, intestine, lungs, mucosa/skin and plasma. Biotransformation of drugs may lead to:

   i. Active drug to inactive metabolite, e.g. morphine, chloramphenicol, etc.
   ii. Active drug to active metabolite, e.g. primidone → phenobarbitone.
   iii. Inactive drug to active metabolite (prodrug), e.g levodopa → dopamine.

Factors influencing biotransformation: Genetic variation; Environmental pollutants; Age; Diseases of liver.

Biotransformation reactions can be classified into:

a. **Nonsynthetic/phase I/functionalization reactions:** These convert the drug to a more polar metabolite by oxidation (phenytoin), reduction (chloramphenicol) or hydrolysis (procaine).

b. **Synthetic/conjugation/phase II reactions:** In phase II reactions, endogenous water-soluble substances like glucuronic acid, sulfuric acid, glutathione or an amino acid combine with the drug or its phase I metabolite to form a highly polar conjugate which is inactive and gets readily excreted by kidneys. Large molecules are excreted through bile. Examples: Glucuronide conjugation (chloramphenicol, morphine); Acetylation (sulfonamides, isoniazid); Methylation (adrenaline, histamine); Glutathione conjugation (paracetamol).

4. **Excretion:** Excretion is the passage out of systemically absorbed drug. Drugs and their metabolites are excreted in: 1. Urine, 2. Faeces, 3. Exhaled air, 4. Saliva and sweat, 5. Milk.

Kinetics of elimination: There are three fundamental pharmacokinetic parameters:

1. **Bioavailability:** Bioavailability is the fraction of the drug that reaches the systemic circulation following administration by any route.

2. **Volume of distribution (Vd):** It is defined as the volume necessary to accommodate the entire amount of drug administered, if the concentration throughout the body were equal to that in plasma. It relates the amount of drug in body to the concentration of drug in plasma. It is calculated as: Amount of drug in the body/plasma concentration.

3. **Clearance (CL):** It is the volume of plasma freed completely of the drug in unit time. It is calculated by:

CL = Rate of elimination/plasma concentration (C).

Drugs are metabolized/eliminated from the body by:

1. **First order (exponential) kinetics:** Rate of elimination is directly proportional to the drug concentration, CL remains constant.

2. **Zero order (linear/saturation) kinetics:** Rate of elimination remains constant irrespective of drug concentration, CL decreases with increase in concentration, e.g. ethyl alcohol, aspirin. The elimination of some drugs approaches saturation over the therapeutic range, kinetics changes from first order to zero order at higher doses. As a result plasma concentration increases disproportionately with increase in dose, e.g. phenytoin, theophylline.

   • Plasma half-life: Plasma half-life ($t\frac{1}{2}$) of a drug is the time taken for its plasma concentration to be reduced to half of its original value. It helps in calculating loading and maintenance doses of a drug. It also indicates duration of action of a drug. As such, half-life is a derived parameter from two variables Vd and CL both of which may change independently, i.e. after

   1. $t\frac{1}{2}$: 50% drug is eliminated.
   2. $t\frac{1}{2}$: 75% (50 + 25) drug is eliminated.
   3. $t\frac{1}{2}$: 87.5% (50 + 25 + 12.5) drug is eliminated.
   4. $t\frac{1}{2}$: 93.75% (50 + 25 + 12.5 + 6.25) drug is eliminated.

Thus, nearly complete drug elimination occurs in 4–5 half lives.

For first order kinetics: $t\frac{1}{2}$ remains constant; For zero order kinetics: $t\frac{1}{2}$ increases with dose.

   • **Plateau principle:** If a drug is administered repeatedly at short intervals before complete elimination, the drug accumulates in the body and reaches a 'state' at which the rate of elimination equals the rate of administration. This is known as the 'Steady-state' or **plateau level**. After attaining this level, the plasma concentration fluctuates around an average steady level. This is known as the plateau principle of drug accumulation. It takes 4–5 half-lives for the plasma concentration to reach the plateau level.

Q. 3. Write about mechanism of action of drug.
(TNMGR, March 2008)

Ans. Pharmacodynamic is the study of actions of drugs on the body and their mechanisms of action, i.e. to know what drugs do and how they do it.

Principles of drug action: Basic types of drug action are:

1. **Stimulation:** It is selective enhancement of level of activity of specialized cells, e.g. adrenaline (Adr) stimulates heart.

2. **Depression:** It is selective diminution of activity of specialized cells, e.g. quinidine depresses heart.

3. **Irritation:** This connotes a nonselective, often noxious effect and is particularly applied to less specialized cells. Mild irritation may stimulate associated function, e.g. bitters increase salivary secretion. But strong irritation results in inflammation, corrosion, necrosis and morphological damage, e.g. astringent and counterirritant.

4. **Replacement:** This refers to use of natural metabolites, hormones or their congeners in deficiency states, e.g. levodopa in parkinsonism, insulin in DM.

5. **Anti-infective and cytotoxic action:** Drugs may act by specifically destroying infective organisms, e.g. penicillins, or by cytotoxic effect on cancer cells, e.g. anticancer drugs.

6. **Modification of immune status:** Vaccines and sera act by improving immunity while immunosuppressant acts by depressing immunity, e.g. glucocorticoids.

Mechanism of drug action: Basic mechanisms of drug action are:

I. Through receptors: Drugs may act by interacting with specific receptors in the body. Receptor has two functional domains (areas): A ligand binding domain (site to bind drug molecule); an effector domain (undergoes change to propagate the message).

Functions of receptors

- To propagate regulatory signals from outside to within the effector cell when the molecular species carrying signal cannot itself penetrate the cell membrane.
- To amplify the signal.
- To integrate various extracellular and intracellular regulatory signals.
- To adapt to short-term and long-term changes in the regulatory melieu and maintain homeostasis.

Types of receptors (Fig. 1.3):

1. **G-protein coupled receptors (GPCR):** These are a large family of cell membrane receptors which are linked to effector through one or more GTP-activated proteins (G-proteins). G-proteins consist of three subunits, viz. α, β and γ. In inactive state GDP is bound to their exposed domain; activation through the receptor leads to displacement of GDP by GTP. G-proteins are of different classes like G_s, G_i, G_o, and Gq-GS is stimulatory and Gi is inhibitory. One receptor can utilize more than one G-protein (**agonist pleiotropy**). There are three major effector pathways (Second messenger) through which GPCRs function.

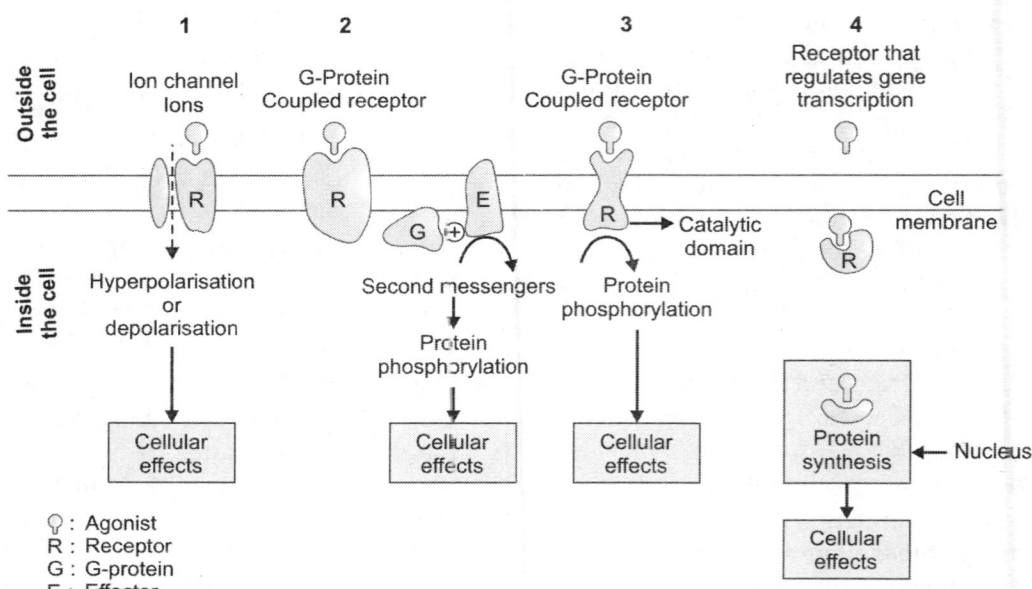

Fig. 1.3: Types of receptors involved in drug action

a. **Adenylyl cyclase/cAMP pathway:** Activation of adenylylcyclase results in the formation and accumulation of cAMP within the cell. This cAMP acts through protein kinases which phosphorylate various proteins to regulate the cell function.

b. **Phospholipase C/IP$_3$-DAG pathway:** Activation of phospholipase C (PLc) hydrolyses the membrane phospholipid, phosphatidylinositol 4, 5-bisphosphate (PIP$_2$) to generate second messengers, inositol 1, 4, 5-trisphosphate (IP$_3$) and diacylglycerol (DAG). IP3 mobilises Ca^{2+} from intracellular depots and this mediates responses like secretion, contraction, metabolism and hyperpolarisation. DAG enhances protein kinase C (PKc), which regulates cell function.

c. **Ion channel regulation:** Activated G-proteins can also open or close ionic channels specific for Ca^{2+}, K$^+$ or Na$^+$, without intervention of any second messenger and bring about hyperpolarization/depolarization/changes in intracellular Ca^{2+}.

2. Receptors with intrinsic ion channel (inotropic receptors): These cell surface receptors, also called ligand-gated ion channels, enclose ion selective channels (for Na$^+$, K$^+$, Ca^{2+} or Cl$^-$) within their molecules. Agonist binding opens the channel and causes depolarization/hyperpolarization/changes in cytosolic ionic composition, depending on the ion that flows through, e.g. nicotinic cholinergic receptor channel permits passage of Na$^+$ ions resulting in depolarization.

3. Enzymatic receptors/kinase linked receptors: These are transmembrane proteins with an extracellular site for ligand binding and intracellular domain to carry out the catalytic activity. Binding of agonist to ligand binding domain results in auto-phosphorylation of intracellular domain, which triggers phosphorylation of various intracellular proteins resulting in the responses, e.g. receptors of insulin, and growth factors.

4. Receptors regulating gene expression (transcription factors/nuclear receptors): They are intracellular proteins which are in an inactive state. Binding of agonist activates the receptor. Agonist-receptor complex moves to nucleus where it interacts with DNA, regulates gene transcription and thereby directs synthesis of specific proteins to regulate the activity of target cells, e.g. receptors for steroidal hormones, thyroid hormones.

II. Through enzymes: Drugs can either increase or decrease the rate of enzymatically mediated reactions.

1. Enzyme stimulation: It is relevant to some natural metabolites only, e.g. pyridoxine acts as a cofactor and increases decarboxylase activity. Several enzymes are stimulated through receptors and second messengers, e.g. Adr. stimulates hepatic glycogen phosphorylase through β receptors and cyclic AMP. Apparent increase in enzyme activity can also occur by enzyme induction.

2. Enzyme inhibition: It is a common mode of drug action.

a. **Nonspecific inhibition:** Many chemicals alter the tertiary structure of any enzyme with which they come in contact and thus inhibit it nonspecifically, e.g. heavy metal salts, strong acids.

b. **Specific inhibition:** Many drugs inhibit a particular enzyme without affecting others. Such inhibition is:

    i. **Competitive (equilibrium type):** Drug being structurally similar competes with the normal substrate for catalytic binding site of enzyme so either the product is not formed or a nonfunctional product is formed, e.g. physostigmine and neostigmine compete with acetylcholine for cholinesterase.

    Nonequilibrium type of enzyme inhibition: Drugs which react with the same catalytic site of enzyme but form strong covalent bonds so that the normal substrate is not able to displace the inhibitor, e.g. organophosphates react covalently with esteretic site of enzyme cholinesterase.

    ii. **Noncompetitive:** Inhibitor reacts with an adjacent site and not with the catalytic site, but alters the enzyme in such a way that it loses its catalytic property, e.g. H$^+$ K$^+$ ATPase inhibition by Omeprazole.

III. Through ion channels: Drugs may interfere with the movement of ions across specific channels, e.g. calcium channel blockers, sodium channel blockers.

IV. Transporters/pumps: Many drugs produce their action by directly interacting with the solute carrier class of transporter proteins to inhibit physiological transport of metabolite/ion, e.g. amphetamines selectively block dopamine reuptake in brain neurons by dopamine transporter (DAT).

V. Physical action: The action of a drug can be because of its physical properties, e.g. adsorption-activated charcoal in poisoning; Mass of drug—bulk laxatives; Osmotic property—osmotic diuretics; Radioactivity—^{131}I; Radio-opacity—barium sulphate.

VI. Chemical interaction: Drugs may act by chemical reaction, e.g. antacids neutralize gastric acids; Chelating agents bind heavy metals.

VII. Altering metabolic processes: Drugs may alter metabolic pathway in microorganisms resulting in its destruction, e.g. sulfonamides interfere with bacterial folic acid synthesis.

Q. 4. Discuss the role of receptors in the mechanism of drug action. (TNMGR, Oct. 2012)

Ans. Receptor is defined as a macromolecule or binding site located on the surface or inside the effector cell that serves to recognize the signal molecule/drug and initiate the response to it, but itself has no other function.

Drug action through receptors: Also refer Q. 3

1. **Receptor occupation theory:** The drug action is based on occupation of receptors by specific drugs and the pace of a cellular function can be altered by interaction of these receptors with drugs.

2. **The two-state receptor model:** The receptor is believed to exist in two interchangeable states: Ra (active) and Ri (inactive) which are in equilibrium. In case, Ri state is favored at equilibrium—no/very weak signal is generated in absence of agonist, the receptor exhibits no constitutive activation. The agonist (A) binds preferentially to Ra conformation and shifts the equilibrium → Ra predominates and a response is generated depending on the concentration of A.

Nature of receptors

1. Physiological receptors: Mediate responses to transmitters, hormones, autacoids and other endogenous signal molecules, e.g. cholinergic, adrenergic, histaminergic, steroid.

2. **Drug receptors:** No known physiological ligands, e.g. benzodiazepine receptor, sulfonylurea receptor.

Receptor subtypes: The following criteria have been utilized in classifying receptors:

a. **Pharmacological criteria:** It is based on relative potencies of selective agonists and antagonists, e.g. α- and β-adrenergic receptors.

b. **Tissue distribution:** The relative organ/tissue distribution is the basis for designating the subtype.

c. **Ligand binding:** Measurement of specific binding of high affinity radio-labeled ligand to cellular fragments *in vitro*, and its displacement by various selective agonists/antagonists is used to delineate receptor subtypes, e.g. subtypes of 5-HT receptors.

d. **Transducer pathway:** Receptor subtypes may be distinguished by the mechanism through which their activation is linked to the response, e.g. M cholinergic receptor acts through G-proteins, while N cholinergic receptor gates influx of Na^+ ions.

e. **Molecular cloning:** The receptor protein is cloned and its detailed amino acid sequence as well as three dimensional structures is worked out. Subtypes are designated on the basis of sequence homology.

f. **Silent receptors:** These are sites which bind specific drugs but no pharmacological response is elicited. They are better called *drug acceptors* or *sites of loss*, e.g. plasma proteins which have binding sites for many drugs.

Q. 5. Write about local drug delivery systems in the oral cavity.
(TNMGR, March 2007; RGUHS, April 2007)

Ans. Oral cavity has been proposed as a potential topical delivery site for the local and systemic delivery of therapeutic agents. The target sites for local drug delivery in the oral cavity include the buccal, sublingual and periodontal region. Delivery of drugs via the membranes of the oral cavity is classified into three Categories: Buccal delivery; Sublingual delivery; Local drug delivery (LDD).

LDD: Drug delivery to periodontal, gingival, delivery for the local treatment of ulcers, bacterial and fungal infections and periodontal disease.

Advantages: Accessible, self-administrable, rapid repair of mucosa, different areas of oral cavity has different permeability characteristics, highly hydrated environment to dissolve drug, sustained delivery possible, potential reduction of systemic side effects.

Disadvantages: Permeability barrier of oral mucosa, dilution by saliva, jaw movements may dislodge delivery device, taste consideration, highly enzymatic environment, relatively small surface area, risk of aspiration of delivery device.

These include:

A. **Oral rinses:** It requires patient compliance; Easy to use, high concentration of the agent can be delivered.

B. **Oral irrigation:** Easy to use, high concentration of the agent can be delivered; Subgingival areas can be irrigated safely.

C. **Controlled release devices:** It is reproducible and drug can be delivered at constant rate. It requires less frequent administration and has greater patient compliance, with reduced side effects.

Types

1. Reservoirs without rate controlling system: Hollow fibers filled with agent.

2. Reservoirs with rate controlling system: Microcapsules filled with agent.

3. Monolithic system: Agent dispersed in inert polymeric matrix.

4. Laminated system: Multiple layers of polymers with different diffusion capacity.

Most common oromucosal lesions and suitable drug formulations

1. Recurrent apthous stomatitis: Amlexanox (muco-adhesive tablets, patches)
2. Hydroxyapetite (mucoadhesive gel): Doxycycline (mucoadhesive gel)
3. Oral lichen planus: Tacrolimus (oral rinse), cyclosporine (mucoadhesive gel); Clobetasol (mucoadhesive gel)
4. Xerostomia: Physostigmine (mucoadhesive gel); Interferon alpha (mucoadhesive tablets)
5. Oral mucositis: Gelclair, MuGaurd (mucoadhesive covering agents); TGF-β3 (mucoadhesive gel)
6. Oral infections: Metronidazole (mucoadhesive tablets), tetracycline (mucoadhesive patch)

Q. 6. Write a short note on drug antagonism.
(TNMGR, March 2007)

Ans. When two or more drugs are given concurrently, the effect may be:

1. **Additive:** The total effects two-drug is equal to the sum of their individual actions. Effect of drug A + B = Effect of drug A + effect of drug B, e.g. nitrous oxide and ether as general anesthetics.
2. **Synergism:** When the action of one drug is enhanced or facilitated by another drug, the combination is synergistic. It is also called '**Potentiation**' or '**Supra-additive**' effect. Effect of drug A + B > Effect of drug A + Effect of drug B, e.g. acetylcholine + physostigmine.
3. **Antagonism:** When one drug decreases or abolishes the action of another, they are said to be antagonistic. Effect of drug A + B < effect of drug A + effect of drug B.

Types: Based on mechanism of antagonism

1. **Physical antagonism:** Based on the physical property of drugs, e.g. charcoal adsorbs alkaloid.
2. **Chemical antagonism:** Drug reacts chemically and form inactive product, e.g. $KMnO_4$ + alkaloids → inactive product.
3. **Physiological/functional antagonism:** Two-drug acts on different receptors or by different mechanism to produce opposite effect on same physiological function, e.g. glucagon + insulin → effects on blood sugar level.
4. **Pharmacokinetic antagonism:** By reducing the concentration of active drug at its site of action by: Increase in metabolism; Increase in its excretion; Decreses in its absorption.
5. **Pharmacodynamic/receptor antagonism:** One drug (antagonist) blocks the receptor action of other (agonist). Receptor antagonism can be competitive or noncompetitive.
   - Competitive antagonism: Equilibrium (reversible) and nonequilibrium (irreversible).
   - Non-competitive.

Q. 7. Discuss the various factors modifying the actions of a drug in the human body. *(TNMGR, Sept. 2009)*

Q. Write a short note on determinants of drug dosage. *(RUHS, July 2016)*

Ans. The various factors are discussed below:

1. **Body size:** It influences the concentration of drug attained at the site of action. The average adult dose refers to individuals of medium built. For exceptionally obese or lean individuals and for children dose may be calculated on body weight (BW) basis:
   - Individual dose = BW (kg)/70 × average adult dose
   - Individual dose = BSA (m²)/1.7 × average adult dose; BSA (body surface area).
2. **Age:** In newborn, liver and kidneys are not fully mature; blood–brain barrier is not well-formed; Gastric acidity is low, intestinal motility is slow. Dose of drug for children is calculated from the adult dose as:
   - Child dose = Age (in years)/age + 12 × adult dose (Young's formula)
   - Child dose = Age (in years)/20 × adult dose (Dilling's formula)

   In elderly, renal function progressively declines so the GFR is ~75% at 50 years and ~50% at 75 years age compared to young adults. Drug doses have to be reduced.
3. **Sex:** Females have smaller body size and require doses that are on the lower side of range. Special care is necessary while prescribing for pregnant and lactating women and during menstruation.
4. **Species and race:** Response to drugs may vary with species and race, e.g. Indians tolerate thiacetazone better than Whites. Blacks need higher doses of atropine to produce mydriasis.
5. **Genetics:** All key determinants of drug response are controlled genetically. Hence, a great deal of individual variability can be traced to the genetic composition of subject. The study of genetic basis for variability in drug response is called 'Pharmacogenetics', e.g. in G6PD deficiency, primaquine, sulphones and quinolones can cause hemolysis in such people.
6. **Route of administration:** A drug may have entirely different uses through different routes, e.g. magnesium sulfate given orally causes purgation, applied

on sprained joints—decreases swelling, while IV, it produces CNS depression and hypotension.

7. **Environmental factors and time of administration:** Food interferes with the absorption of many drugs, e.g. tetracyclines form complexes with calcium present in food. Polycyclic hydrocarbons present in cigarette smoke may induce microsomal enzymes resulting in enhanced metabolism of some drugs.

8. **Psychological factor:** Efficacy of a drug can be affected by patient's beliefs, attitudes and expectations. This is particularly applicable to centrally acting drugs.

   Placebo (*NTR Uni., April 2011*) is an inert substance which is given in the garb of a medicine. It works by psychological rather than pharmacological means and often produces responses equivalent to the active drug. It is the inert dosage form with no specific biological activity but only resembles the actual preparation in appearance (dummy medication). Placebo means 'I shall be pleasing' (in Latin).

   Placebo medicines are used in: 1. Clinical trials as a control to compare and assess whether the new compound is significantly better than the placebo. 2. To benefit or please a patient psychologically when he does not actually require an active drug as in mild psychosomatic disorders and in chronic incurable diseases. In fact, all forms of treatment including physiotherapy and surgery have some placebo effect. Substances used as placebo include lactose, some vitamins, minerals and distilled water injections. **Nocebo** is the converse of placebo, and refers to negative psychodynamic effect evoked by loss of faith in medication and/or the physician. Nocebo effect can oppose the therapeutic effect of active medication.

9. **Pathological states:** Several diseases can influence drug disposition and drug action, e.g. in malabsorption, drugs are poorly absorbed; In liver diseases, rate of drug metabolism is reduced due to dysfunction of hepatocytes.

10. **Other drugs:** Drugs can modify the response to each other by pharmacokinetic or pharmacodynamic interaction between them.

11. **Dose:** It is observed that the response to a drug may be modified by the dose administered. Generally as the dose is increased, the magnitude of response increases proportionately; further increases in doses may produce effects opposite to their lower-dose effect, e.g. physiological doses of vitamin D promotes calcification while hypervitaminosis D leads to decalcification.

12. **Repeated dosing:** It can result in:
    - **Cumulation:** Drugs like digoxin which are slowly eliminated may cumulate resulting in toxicity.
    - **Tolerance:** It is requirement of higher doses of a drug to produce a given response. Tolerance may be natural or acquired. Tolerance may develop to some actions of drug and not to others, e.g. barbiturates—tolerance develops to sedative but not antiepileptic effects of barbiturates. Mechanisms of development of tolerance could be: Pharmacokinetic (**dispositional tolerance**); Pharmacodynamic (**functional tolerance**). **Cross tolerance** is the development of tolerance to pharmacologically related drugs, e.g. alcoholics are relatively tolerant to barbiturates and general anesthetics.
    - **Tachyphylaxis/acute tolerance** is rapid development of tolerance when doses of a drug repeated in quick succession result in marked reduction in response.

Q. 8. Write in detail about adverse drug reactions.
(TNMGR, April 1995)

Q. Write a short note on drug allergy.
(TNMGR, Oct. 2013)

Ans. Adverse drug reactions (ADRs) can be defined as 'A response to a drug which is noxious and unintended, and which occurs at doses normally used in man for the prophylaxis, diagnosis, or therapy of disease, or for the modifications of physiological function' (**WHO, 1972**).

A. According to predictability of adverse effects

1. **Predictable (type A or augmented) reactions:** These are based on the pharmacological properties of drug, which means that they are augmented, but qualitatively normal response to the drug; include side effects, toxic effects and consequences of drug withdrawal. They are more common, dose related and mostly preventable and reversible.

2. **Unpredictable (type B or bizarre) reactions:** These are based on peculiarities of the patient and not on drug's known actions; include allergy and idiosyncrasy. They are less common, often non-dose related, generally more serious and require withdrawal of the drug.

B. According to severity of adverse effects

1. **Minor:** No therapy, antidote or prolongation of hospitalization is required.

2. **Moderate:** Requires change in drug therapy, specific treatment or prolongs hospital stay.

3. **Severe:** Potentially life-threatening, causes permanent damage or requires intensive medical treatment.
4. **Lethal:** Directly or indirectly contributes to death of patient.

C. Adverse drug effects may be categorized into:

1. **Side effects:** These are unwanted effects of a drug that are extension of pharmacological effects and are seen with the therapeutic dose of drug. They are predictable, common and can occur in all people, e.g. hypoglycemia due to insulin.
2. **Secondary effects:** These are indirect consequences of a primary action of drug, e.g. super infections due to suppression of bacterial flora by tetracyclines.
3. **Toxic effects:** These are the result of excessive pharmacological action of the drug due to over dosage or prolonged use, e.g. morphine (analgesic) causes respiratory depression in over dosage.
4. **Intolerance:** Drug intolerance is the inability of a person to tolerate a drug and is unpredictable. Patients show exaggerated response to even small doses of drug, e.g. vestibular dysfunction after a single dose of streptomycin in some patients. Intolerance could also be qualitative, e.g. idiosyncrasy and allergic reactions.
5. **Idiosyncrasy:** It is genetically determined abnormal reactivity to a chemical. The drug interacts with some unique feature of the individual, and produces the uncharacteristic reaction, e.g. barbiturates cause excitement and mental confusion in some individuals. In some cases, the person may be highly sensitive even to low doses of a drug or highly insensitive even to high doses of the drug.
6. **Drug allergy:** It is an immunologically mediated reaction producing stereotype symptoms which are unrelated to the pharmacodynamic profile of drug, generally occur even with much smaller doses and have a different time course of onset and duration. This is also called drug hypersensitivity; but does not refer to increased response which is called super sensitivity. Prior sensitization is needed and a latent period of at least 1–2 weeks is required after the first exposure. The drug or its metabolite acts as antigen (Ag) or more commonly hapten and induce production of antibody (Ab)/sensitized lymphocytes.

   Mechanism and types of allergic reactions

   A. **Humoral mediated:** Type I: Anaphylactic reactions (IgE mediated); Type II: Cytolytic reactions (complement); Type III: Retarded, arthus reactions (immune complex).

   B. **Cell mediated:** Type IV: Delayed hypersensitivity reactions (contact dermatitis, some rashes, fever, photosensitization).

7. **Photosensitivity:** It is a cutaneous reaction resulting from drug-induced sensitization of the skin to UV radiation. The reactions are of two types:

   a. **Phototoxic:** Drug or its metabolite accumulates in the skin, absorbs light and undergoes a photochemical reaction followed by a photo-biological reaction resulting in local tissue damage (sunburn-like), i.e. erythema, edema, blistering followed by hyperpigmentation and desquamation. The shorter wavelengths (290–320 nm, UVB) are responsible and this is more common than photo-allergic reaction.
   - Acute phototoxic reactions: Tetracyclines (especially demeclocycline) and tar products.
   - Chronic phototoxic reactions: Nalidixic acid, fluoroquinolones, sulfonamides, phenothiazines, thiazides.

   b. **Photo-allergic:** Drug or its metabolite induces a cell-mediated immune response which on exposure to light of longer wavelengths (320–400 nm, UV-A) produces a papular or eczematous contact dermatitis. Drugs involved are sulfonamides, sulfonylureas, griseofulvin, chloroquine, and chlorpromazine.

8. **Drug dependence:** Drug dependence is a state in which use of drugs for personal satisfaction is accorded a higher priority than other basic needs, often in the face of known risks to health.

   a. **Psychological dependence:** It is compulsive drug-seeking behaviour to obtain its pleasurable effects, e.g. smoking.
   b. Physical dependence: It is an altered physiological state produced by repeated administration of a drug which necessitates the continued presence of the drug to maintain physiological equilibrium. Stopping of drug results in 'Withdrawal syndrome.' e.g. opioid, alcohol.
   c. **Drug abuse:** It is the use of a drug by self-medication in a manner and amount that deviates from the approved medical and social patterns in a given culture at a given time.
   d. **Drug addiction:** It is a pattern of compulsive drug use characterized by overwhelming involvement with the use of a drug, e.g. amphetamines, cocaine.
   e. **Drug habituation:** It denotes less intensive involvement with the drug, so that its withdrawal produces only mild discomfort, e.g. consumption of tea, coffee.

9. **Drug withdrawal reactions:** Sudden interruption of drug therapy may result in adverse consequences, e.g. acute adrenal insufficiency may be precipitated by abrupt cessation of corticosteroid therapy.

10. **Teratogenicity:** It refers to capacity of a drug to cause fetal abnormalities when administered to the pregnant mother. The placenta does not strictly constitute a barrier and any drug can cross it to a greater or lesser extent. The embryo is one of the most dynamic biological systems and in contrast to adults, drug effects are often irreversible. *Thalidomide disaster* (1958–1961) resulting in thousands of babies born with **phocomelia** (seal-like limbs) and other defects focused attention to this type of adverse effect. Drugs can affect the fetus at 3 stages:

    i. Fertilization and implantation (conception to 17 days): Failure of pregnancy which often goes unnoticed.

    ii. Organogenesis (18–55 days of gestation): Most vulnerable period, deformities are produced.

    iii. Growth and development (56 days onwards): Developmental and functional abnormalities can occur.

    Therefore, in general, drugs should be avoided during pregnancy especially in first trimester. The type of malformation also depends on the drug, e.g. thalidomide causes phocomelia; Tetracyclines cause deformed teeth; Sodium valproate causes spina bifida, ACE inhibitors can cause hypoplasia of organs, NSAIDs may induce premature closure of ductus arteriosus.

11. **Mutagenicity and carcinogenicity:** It refers to capacity of a drug to cause genetic defects and cancer respectively. Drugs implicated in these adverse effects are—anticancer drugs, radioisotopes, estrogens, tobacco.

12. **Drug-induced/iatrogenic/physician-induced diseases:** These are functional disturbances (disease) caused by drugs which persist even after the offending drug has been withdrawn and largely eliminated, e.g. peptic ulcer by salicylates and corticosteroids.

Prevention of adverse effects to drugs

1. Avoid all inappropriate use of drugs.
2. Use appropriate dose, route and frequency of drug administration.
3. Elicit and take into consideration previous history of drug reactions.
4. Elicit history of allergic diseases.
5. Rule out possibility of drug interactions when more than one drug is prescribed.

6. Adopt correct drug administration technique.
7. Carry out appropriate laboratory monitoring.

Oral manifestations of drug reactions (*BFUHS, May 2017*):

1. **Saliva and salivary glands involvement:** Xerostomia, ptyalism, salivary gland enlargement, salivary gland pain, discoloration of saliva.

2. **Soft tissue (mucosal) involvement:** Lichenoid reaction, erythema multiform, pemphigoid, lupus erythematous, fixed drug eruption, angioedema, mucous membrane pigmentation, drug-induced gingival enlargement.

3. **Hard tissue involvement:** Drug-related osteonecrosis of the jaw, dental caries, dry socket, tooth discoloration.

4. **Non-specific conditions:** Taste disorders, halitosis (malodor), neuropathies, movement disturbance, infection.

Q. 9. Write a note on drug reactions and interactions.
(BFUHS, May 2010; TNMGR, Sept. 2010)

Ans. Drug interaction refers to modification of response to one drug by another when they are administered simultaneously or in quick succession. The response is either increased or decreased in intensity (quantitative), or an abnormal/different type of response is produced (qualitative).

Types of drugs most likely to be involved in clinically important drug interactions: Drugs with narrow safety margin (aminoglycoside); Drugs affecting closely regulated body functions (antihypertensive); Highly plasma protein bound drugs (NSAIDs); Drugs metabolized by saturation kinetics (phenytoin).

Site: Drug interactions can occur: (i) *In vitro*: Mixing of drugs in syringes can cause chemical or physical interactions, e.g. penicillin and gentamicin, (ii) *In vivo*, i.e. in the body after administration.

Mechanism of drug interactions

A. **Pharmacokinetic interactions:** These interactions alter the concentration of the object drug at its site of action by affecting:

   i. **Absorption:** Absorption of an orally administered drug can be affected by other concurrently ingested drugs, e.g. tetracyclines and calcium/iron salts, antacids or sucralfate.

   ii. **Distribution:** Competition for plasma protein or tissue binding results in displacement interactions, e.g. warfarin is displaced by phenylbutazone from protein binding sites.

   iii. **Metabolism:** Enzyme induction and inhibition of metabolism can both result in drug interactions, e.g. phenytoin, phenobarbitone, carbamazepine and rifampicin are enzyme inducers while chloramphenicol and cimetidine are enzyme inhibitors.

iv. **Excretion:** When drugs compete for the same renal tubular transport system, they prolong each other's duration of action, e.g. penicillin and probenecid.

B. **Pharmacodynamic interactions:** Drugs acting on the same receptors or physiological systems result in additive, synergistic or antagonistic effects, e.g. atropine opposes effects of physostigmine; naloxone antagonises morphine; Aspirin inhibits platelet aggregation; Many antihistamines produce sedation, which may be enhanced by alcohol intake.

2. DRUGS ACTING ON RESPIRATORY SYSTEM

Q. 1. Write a short note on expectorants.
(TNMGR, Sept. 2002)

Ans. Expectorants (mucokinetics) are drugs believed to increase bronchial secretion or reduce its viscosity, facilitating its removal by coughing.

Classification
A. Bronchial secretion enhancers
1. Sodium/potassium citrate: Increase bronchial secretion by salt action.
2. Potassium iodide: Secreted by bronchial mucosa and can irritate the airway mucosa.
3. Guiphenesin (glyceryl guaiacolate), balsam of tolu, Vasaka (plant products): Enhance bronchial secretion and mucocilliary function while being secreted by trachebronchial glands.
4. Ammonium chloride: They are nauseating—reflexly increases respiratory secretions.

B. Mucolytics
1. Bromhexine: It produces thin copious bronchial secretions by depolymerising mucopolysaccharides. Side effects: Rhinorrhea, lacrimation, gastric irritation. Dose: Bromhexine (8 mg) TDS, 4 mg/5 ml elixir.
2. Ambroxol: It is a metabolite of bromhexine with similar effects. Dose: 15–30 mg TDS.
3. Acetylcysteine: It opens disulfide bonds in mucoproteins present in sputum. It is given by aerosol directly into respiratory tract.
4. Carbocysteine: Action is similar to acetylcysteine, but administered orally (250–750 mg TDS).

Q. 2. Write a short note on atropine sulfate.
(TNMGR, Aug. 2004)

Ans. The prototype drug of anticholinergic drugs is highly selective for muscarinic receptors, but some of its synthetic substitutes do possess significant nicotinic blocking property.

Classification
A. According to source
1. Natural alkaloids: Atropine, hyoscine (scopclamine).
2. Semisynthetic: Homatropine, ipratropium bromide.
3. Synthetic: Tropicamide, propantheline, dicyclomine, glycopyrrolate.

B. According to selectivity
1. Non-selective muscarinic antagonist: Atropine, hyoscine
2. Selective muscarinic antagonists:
   a. Selective M1 antagonist: Pirenzepine, telenzepine, dicyclomine
   b. Selective M2 antagonist: Gallamine
   c. Selective M3 antagonist: Tolterdine

Pharmacokinetics: Atropine and hyoscine are rapidly absorbed from GIT. About 50% of atropine is metabolized in liver and rest is excreted unchanged in urine. It has a $t\frac{1}{2}$ of 3–4 hours.

Dose: Atropine sulfate: 0.6–2 mg IM, IV (children 10 µg/kg), 1–2% topically in eye.

Mechanism of action: Atropine causes reversible non-selective blockade of cholimimetic actions at muscarinic receptors.

Pharmacological actions (atropine as prototype):
1. **CNS:** CNS stimulant action due to blockade of muscarinic receptors.
2. **CVS:** Tachycardia due to blockade of M2 receptors on SA node.
3. **Eye:** Mydriasis, abolition of light reflex and cycloplegia.
4. **Smooth muscles:** Atropine causes bronchodilatation and reduces airway resistance. Atropine has relaxant action on ureter and urinary bladder; Urinary retention can occur in older males with prostatic hypertrophy.
5. **Glands:** Atropine markedly decreases sweat, salivary, tracheobronchial and lacrimal secretion (M3 blockade). Atropine decreases secretion of acid, pepsin and mucus in stomach.
6. **Body temperature:** Rise in body temperature occurs at higher doses.
7. **Local anaesthetic:** Atropine has a mild anaesthetic action on the cornea.

Therapeutic uses
1. Ophthalmic: For accurate measurements of refractive errors.

2. Antidote: For cholinesterase inhibitor insecticides and mushroom poisoning.
3. In treatment of Parkinson's disease.
4. As pre-anaesthetic medication.
5. In myocardial infarction.
6. Symptomatic relief in urinary urgency.
7. In hyperhydrosis (excessive sweating)

Adverse effects: Tachycardia, palpitation, dry mouth, constipation, urine retention, blurred vision, xerophthalmia, agitation, flushing.

3. DRUGS ACTING ON CVS

Q. 1. Write a short note on beta blockers.
(TNMGR, Oct. 2000)

Ans. These drugs inhibit adrenergic responses mediated through β-receptors.

Classification

A. Nonselective (both β_1 and β_2 blockers):
1. With intrinsic sympathomimetic activity: Pindolol.
2. Without intrinsic sympathomimetic activity: Propranolol, sotalol, timolol.
3. With additional α-blocking property: Labetalol, carvedilol, celiprolol, nebivolol.

B. Cardioselective (β_1): Metoprolol, atenolol, acebutol, bisoprolol, esmolol, etc.

Pharmacological actions
1. **CVS:** β-blockers decreases heart rate, force of contraction and cardiac output (CO). It has no direct effect on blood vessels. On prolonged administration BP gradually falls in hypertensive subjects.
2. **Respiratory tract:** Increases bronchial resistance by blocking β_2 receptors (bronchoconstriction).
3. **CNS:** Forgetfulness, increased dreaming and nightmares.
4. **Local anaesthetic:** Propranolol is a potent local anaesthetic.
5. **Metabolic:** Propranolol blocks adrenergically induced lipolysis and glycogenolysis.
6. **Skeletal muscle:** Propranolol inhibits adrenergically provoked tremor.
7. **Eye:** It reduces intraocular pressure by decreasing secretion of aqueous humor.
8. **Uterus:** Relaxation of uterus in response to β_2 agonists is blocked by propranolol.

Pharmacokinetics: Propranolol is well absorbed after oral administration, but has low bioavailability due to high first pass metabolism in liver.

Dose: Oral: 10 mg BD to 160 mg QID (average 40–160 mg/day).

Therapeutic uses
1. Cardiovascular: Hypertension, congestive heart failure (CHF), angina pectoris, myocardial infarction (MI), cardiac arrhythmias, dissecting aortic aneurysm, hypertrophic obstructive cardiomyopathy.
2. Non-cardiovascular: Hyperthyroidism, glaucoma, pheochromocytoma, migraine, anxiety, alcohol withdrawal.

Contraindications: Asthma, COPD, bradycardia, heart block.

Interactions
1. Additive depression of sinus node and AV conduction with digitalis and verapamil.
2. Propranolol delays recovery from hypoglycemia due to insulin and oral antidiabetic.
3. Phenylephrine, ephedrine and other α agonists present in cold remedies can cause marked rise in BP due to blockade of sympathetic vasodilatation.
4. Indomethacin and other NSAIDs attenuate the antihypertensive action of β blockers.
5. Cimetidine inhibits propranolol metabolism.

Q. 2. Write a short note on antihypertensive drugs.
(MUHS, June 2016)

Ans. Antihypertensive drugs comprise several classes of compound with the therapeutic intention of preventing, controlling, or treating hypertension.

American College of Cardiology (ACC) and AHA definition of hypertension (HTN) stages is:
- Normal BP: SBP <120, DBP <80.
- Elevated BP: SBP = 120–130, DBP <80.
- Stage 1 HTN: SBP = 130–139 or DBP = 80–89.
- Stage 2 HTN: SBP at least 140 or DBP at least 90.
- Hypertensive crises: SBP >180 and/or DBP >120.

ACC/AHA 2019 guidelines on primary prevention of cardiovascular disease: All patients with elevated BP are recommended to have lifestyle modifications as initial treatment, including weight loss, health heart diet, increased physical activity, low sodium diet and limitation of alcohol consumption.

Classification of drugs
1. ACE inhibitors: Captopril, enalapril, lisinopril, perindopril, ramipril.
2. Angiotensin antagonists: Losartan, irbesartan, candesartan.
3. Calcium channel blockers: Verapamil, diltiazem, nifedipine, felodipine, amlodipine, lacidipine.
4. Diuretics: Thiazide, high ceiling, K+ sparing.
5. β-Adrenergic blockers: Propranolol, metaprolol, atenolol.

6. α- + β-adrenergic blockers: Labetalol, carvedilol. Sodium.

7. α-Adrenergic blockers: Prazosin, terazosin, phentolamine.

8. Central sympatholytic: Clonidine, methyldopa.

9. Vasodilators: Hydralazine, minoxidil.

10. Renin inhibitors: Aliskiren.

Q. 3. Write about potassium sparing diuretics.

(TNMGR, Oct. 1999)

Ans. Diuretics (**water pills**) are the drugs which increase the urine output.

Classification

1. **High efficacy diuretics:** Furosemide, bumetanide, torsemide, azosemide.

2. **Moderate efficacy diuretics**
   - Thiazides: Benzothiadiazines—chlorothiazide, hydrochlorothiazide, polythiazide, cyclopenthiazide.
   - Thiazide-related agents: Chlorthalidone, clopamide, metolazone.

3. **Low efficacy diuretics**
   - Potassium sparing diuretics: Aldosterone antagonist (spironolactone, eplerenone); Inhibitors of renal epithelial Na^+ channel (triamterene, amiloride).
   - Carbonic anhydrase inhibitors: Acetazolamide, methazolamide, dorzolamide.
   - Osmotic diuretics: Mannitol, urea, glycerol.
   - Methylxanthines: Theophylline.

Mechanism of action: Aldosterone antagonist acts from the interstitial side of the tubular cell, combines with the mineralocorticoid receptor and inhibits the formation of aldosterone-induced proteins (AIPs), thus reducing Na^+ reabsorption and K^+ secretion, in a competitive manner. It increases Ca^{2+} excretion by a direct action on renal tubules. Inhibitors of renal epithelial Na^+ channel decreases K^+ excretion, particularly when it is high due to large K^+ intake or use of a diuretic that enhances K^+ loss.

Pharmacokinetics: Oral bioavailability of spironolactone is 75%. It is highly bound to plasma proteins and completely metabolized in liver; converted to active metabolites. The $t\frac{1}{2}$ of spironolactone is 1–2 hours.

Dose: 25–50 mg BD-QID.

Use

1. **Edema:** It is more useful in cirrhotic and nephritic edema.

2. To counteract K^+ loss due to thiazide and loop diuretics.

3. Hypertension.

4. CHF

Interactions

1. Given together with K^+ supplements—dangerous hyperkalaemia can occur.

2. Aspirin blocks spironolactone action.

Adverse effects: Drowsiness, confusion, abdominal upset, hirsutism, gynaecomastia, impotence and menstrual irregularities, hyperkalaemia, acidosis.

Q. 4. Write about role of diuretics in hypertension.

(TNMGR, Sept. 2002)

Ans. Thiazides are the first-line antihypertensives and are inexpensive (12.5–25 mg). They may be combined with a K^+ sparing diuretic which is the best way to avoid hypokalaemia. Proposed mechanism of antihypertensive action is:

1. Initially, they reduce plasma and ECF volume by 5–15% → decreased cardiac output.

2. Subsequently, compensatory mechanisms operate to almost regain Na^+ balance and plasma volume; Cardiac output is restored, but fall in BP is maintained.

3. The reduction in total peripheral resistance (TPR) is most probably an indirect consequence of a small persisting Na^+ and volume deficit.

They are indicated in hypertension only when it is complicated by: Coexisting refractory CHF; Resistance to combination regimens containing a thiazide, or marked fluid retention due to use of potent vasodilators.

Loop diuretics: Their antihypertensive efficacy is low. They are used only in hypertension with chronic renal failure or congestive heart failure.

Hypertension and dentistry: For major dental procedures, good control of BP should be ensured before, during and after the procedure. BP is maintained below 150/100 mm of Hg. To control postoperative bleeding ethamsylate is given. When local anaesthetic is required, for minor procedures plain lignocaine is used and adrenaline avoided. Procedures are done in multiple sittings.

Q. 5. Write a short note on furosemide.

(TNMGR, Oct. 2003)

Ans. Frusemide (furosemide) is a sulfonamide derivative. It is a powerful and most commonly used Loop/high ceiling diuretic (inhibitors of Na^+–K^+–$2Cl^-$ cotransport). Furosemide may be given as an adjunct with drugs if there is volume overload or cerebral edema, but should be avoided when patient may be hypovolaemic.

The onset of action is prompt and duration short (3–6 hours). The major site of action is the thick ascending limb of loop of Henle, where furosemide inhibits Na^+–K^+–$2Cl^-$ cotransport. It is secreted in proximal tubule by organic anion transport and reaches ascending limb of loop of Henle, where it acts from luminal side of the membrane. It abolishes the cortico-medullary osmotic gradient and blocks positive as well as negative free water clearance. K^+ excretion is increased mainly due to high Na^+ load reaching distal tubule.

Pharmacokinetics: Furosemide is rapidly absorbed orally but bioavailability is about 60%. It is highly bound to plasma proteins. It is partly conjugated with glucuronic acid and mainly excreted unchanged by glomerular filtration as well as tubular secretion. Plasma t½ averages 1–2 hours.

Dose: Usually 20–80 mg once daily in the morning.

Therapeutic uses: 1. Edema, 2. Acute pulmonary edema (acute LVF, following MI), 3. Cerebral edema, 4. Hypertension, 5. Along with blood transfusion in severe anaemia, to prevent vascular overload, 6. Hypercalcemia and renal calcium stones.

Adverse effects: Ototoxicity, hyperuricaemia, hypokalemia, hypomagnesaemia, acute hypovolumia, allergy.

Q. 6. Write a short note on calcium channel blockers.
(TNMGR, March 2009)

Ans. Calcium channel blockers (CCBs)/calcium antagonists disrupt the movement of calcium through calcium channels.

Classification

A. Dihydropyridine: Nifedipine, amlodipine, nicardipine, nimodipine, felodipine.

B. Non-dihydropyridine:
1. Phenyl alkylamine: Verapamil, gallopamil
2. Benzothiazepine: Diltiazem.

The dihydropyridines (DHPs) are the most potent Ca^{2+} channel blockers.

Mechanism of action: CCBs inhibit the entry of calcium by blocking the L-type of calcium channels. (3 types: L, N and T). This decreases calcium current and calcium entry into cardiac and vascular smooth muscle cells. The two most important actions of CCBs are: Smooth muscle (especially vascular) relaxation; Negative chronotropic, inotropic and dromotropic action on heart.

Pharmacokinetics: CCBs are well-absorbed but undergo extensive first pass metabolism. They are all highly plasma protein bound and are metabolized in liver.

Therapeutic uses: Angina pectoris; Supraventricular arrhythmias; Hypertension; Migraine; Raynaud's phenomenon; Hypertrophic cardiomyopathy; Subarchnoid hemorrhage; Preterm labor.

Adverse effects: Postural hypotension, palpitation, reflex tachycardia, AV block, hypotension, facial redness, gingival overgrowth.

Q. 7. Write a note on drugs in myocardial infarction.
(TNMGR, Sept. 2002)

Ans. Myocardial infarction (MI) is ischemic necrosis of a portion of the myocardium due to sudden occlusion of a branch of coronary artery. An acute thrombus at the site of atherosclerotic obstruction is the usual cause. The drug therapy for MI can be is directed to:

1. Pain, anxiety and apprehension: Opioid analgesics, morphine (10 mg); Pethidine (50 mg); Diazepam administered parenterally.
2. Oxygenation: By O_2 inhalation and assisted respiration, if needed.
3. Maintenance of blood volume, tissue perfusion and microcirculation: Slow IV infusion of saline/low molecular weight dextran (avoid volume overload).
4. Correction of acidosis: Due to lactic acid production: Sodium bicarbonate by IV infusion.
5. Prevention and treatment of arrhythmias: Prophylactic IV infusion of a β-blocker (atenolol, 5–10 mg over 5 minutes). Tachyarrhythmias may be treated with lidocaine, procainamide or other anti-arrhythmics. Bradycardia and heart block may be managed with atropine or electrical pacing.
6. Pump failure: The objective is to increase cardiac output and/or decrease filling pressure without unduly increasing cardiac work or reducing BP. Drugs used for this purpose are: Furosemide; Vasodilators (GTN IV or nitroprusside); Inotropic agents (dopamine or dobutamine).
7. Prevention of thrombus extension, embolism, and venous thrombosis: Aspirin (162–325 mg) should be given for chewing and swallowing as soon as MI is suspected. This is continued at 80–160 mg/day.
8. Thrombolysis and reperfusion: Fibrinolytic agents (clot busters), streptokinase 1.5 MU infusion over 1 hour. Thrombolytics should be started at the earliest possible (within 6–12 hours) as they can limit the extent of damage and reduce mortality.
9. Prevention of remodeling and subsequent CHF: ACE inhibitors/angiotensin receptor blockers (ARBs).

10. Prevention of future attacks:
    a. Platelet inhibitors: Aspirin or clopidogrel given on long-term basis are routinely prescribed.
    b. β-blockers: Reduce risk of reinfarction, CHF and mortality.
    c. Control of hyperlipidaemia: Dietary substitution with unsaturated fats, hypolipidemic drugs especially statins.

Dental implications: A majority of dental procedures can evoke anxiety in patient, that could precipitate an attack of angina or rarely even myocardial infarction. Utmost importance is given to keep the patient stress free. Adequate antianxiety agents, analgesics and anesthetics are used to avoid pain and anxiety. Patient is taken for the procedure as the first case in the morning. Adrenaline is avoided in such patients. For an acute episode of angina, nitroglycerine 0.5 mg is given sublingually immediately. If MI is suspected, injection pethidine 50 mg should be given immediately even before shifting the patient to emergency.

4. DRUGS ACTING ON CNS

Q. 1. Write a short note on anxiolytic/sedative drugs.

Ans. Sedative is a drug that produces a calming or quietening effect and reduces excitement. It may induce drowsiness. Hypnotic is a drug that induces sleep resembling natural sleep.

Classification
1. Benzodiazepines (BZDs)
   * Long-acting (24–48 hours): Diazepam, chlordiazepoxide, clonazepam, flurazepam, chlorazepate, clobazam.
   * Short-acting (12–24 hours): Temazepam, lorazepam, oxazepam, nitrazepam, alprazolam, halazepam.
   * Ultra short acting (<6 hours): Triazolam, midazolam
2. Newer agents: Zolpidem, zopiclone, zaleplon
3. Barbiturates: Phenobarbitone, mephobarbitone, secobarbitone, pentobarbitone, thiopentone, hexobarbitone,
4. Miscellaneous: Paraldehyde, chloral hydrate, glutethimide, meprobamate.

Q. 2. Explain the pharmacological basis for phenytoin sodium in grandmal epilepsy.

(TNMGR, April 2001)

Ans. Generalized grandmal epilepsy/tonic–clonic seizures is characterized by sudden loss of consciousness followed by sustained contraction of muscles throughout the body (**tonic phase**), lasting for 1 minute and then, a series of jerks, i.e. periods of muscle contraction alternating with periods of relaxation (clonic phase) lasting for 2–4 minutes follow. CNS depression then occurs and the person goes into sleep.

Phenytoin (diphenylhydantoin): Phenytoin has good anti-seizure activity and is one of the most effective drugs against generalized tonic–clonic seizures and partial seizures. It brings about its effects without causing general depression of the CNS.

Mechanism of action: Phenytoin causes blockade of voltage dependent sodium channels and stabilizes the neuronal membrane. It inhibits the generation of repetitive action potentials. Voltage dependent Na^+ channels enter an inactive stage after each action potential. Phenytoin blocks the Na^+ channels which are in an inactivated state and delay the recovery of these channels from inactivation. It decreases the number of channels which are available for the generation of action potentials.

Pharmacokinetics: Absorption of phenytoin by oral route is slow. It is widely distributed in the body and is 80–90% bound to plasma proteins. Phenytoin is metabolized in liver by hydroxylation and glucuronide conjugation. The t½ (12–24 hours) progressively increases (up to 60 hr) when plasma concentration rises above 10 μg/ml. Only 5% unchanged phenytoin is excreted in urine.

Adverse effects
* **At therapeutic levels (5H):** Gum hypertrophy; Hirsutism; Hypersensitivity reactions; Megaloblastic anaemia; Osteomalacia; Hyperglycemia; Fetal Hydantoin syndrome (hypoplastic phalanges, cleft palate, harelip and microcephaly in the offspring).
* **At high plasma levels (dose-related toxicity)**
   a. Cerebellar and vestibular manifestations.
   b. Drowsiness, behavioral alterations, mental confusion, hallucinations, disorientation and rigidity.
   c. Epigastric pain, nausea and vomiting.
   d. Intravenous injection can cause local vascular injury, hypotension, and cardiac arrhythmia.

Therapeutic uses: Phenytoin is a first line antiepileptic drug for:
1. Generalized tonic–clonic, simple and complex partial seizures. It is ineffective in absence seizures. **Dose:** 100 mg BD, maximum 400 mg/day; Children 5–8 mg/kg/day.
2. Status epilepticus.
3. Trigeminal neuralgia.
4. Digitalis-induced cardiac arrhythmias.

Q. 3. Write about clinical uses of muscle relaxants.
(TNMGR, Nov. 2001)

Q. Write a short note on muscle relaxants.

Ans. Skeletal muscle relaxants are drugs that act peripherally at NMJ/muscle fiber itself or centrally in the cerebrospinal axis to reduce muscle tone and/or cause paralysis.

Classification

1. **Drugs acting peripherally at NMJ**
   a. **Competitive blockers** (non-depolarizing agents):
      - Long acting: d-Tubocurarine, pancuronium, doxacurium, pipecuronium.
      - Intermediate acting: Vecuronium, atracurium, cisatracurium, rocuronium, rapacuronium.
      - Short acting: Mivacurium.
   b. **Depolarising blockers:** Succinylcholine (Sch), suxamethonium, decamethonium.
   c. **Others:** Botulinum toxin A
2. **Drugs acting centrally:** Diazepam, baclofen, mephenesin, tizanidine.
3. **Drugs acting directly on the muscle:** Dantrolene sodium, quinine.

A. Peripherally acting skeletal muscle relaxants

Mechanism of action: Non-depolarizing blockers bind to nicotinic receptors on the motor end plate and block the actions of acetylcholine by competitive blockade. Depolarizing blocker reacts with nicotinic receptors and depolarizes the skeletal muscle membrane.

Uses

1. Most important use of neuromuscular blockers is as adjuvant to general anesthesia.
2. Assisted ventilation: Competitive neuromuscular blocker which reduces the chest wall resistance to inflation.
3. Convulsions and trauma from electroconvulsive therapy can be avoided by use of muscle relaxants.
4. Severe cases of tetanus and status epilepticus may be paralyzed by a neuromuscular blocker.

B. Centrally acting muscle relaxants: They selectively depress spinal and supraspinal polysynaptic reflexes involved in the regulation of muscle tone without significantly affecting monosynaptically mediated stretch reflex.

Classification

i. Mephenesin congeners: Mephenesin, carisoprodol, chlorzoxazone, chlormezanone, methocarbamol.
ii. Benzodiazepines: Diazepam and others.
iii. GABA derivative: Baclofen.
iv. Central α_2 agonist: Tizanidine.

Uses

1. Acute muscle spasms.
2. Torticollis, lumbago, backache, neuralgias.
3. Anxiety and tension.
4. Spastic neurological diseases.
5. Tetanus.
6. Electroconvulsive therapy.
7. Orthopedic manipulations.

Skeletal muscle relaxants (SMRs) in dentistry *(NTR Uni., April 2013):*

1. Mephenesin, diazepam and others along with analgesics are used to relieve spasm of masticatory muscles (trismus).
2. Dislocation: Relaxing the related muscles with SMRs may be sufficient to set right the TMJ dislocation.
3. Fractures: SMRs may also be used to reduce fractures of mandible.

Q. 4. Write a note on tricyclic antidepressants (TCAs).
(TNMGR, Oct. 2012)

Ans. TCAs are first generation class of antidepressants. They inhibit axonal reuptake of noradrenaline (NA) and 5-hydroxytryptamine (5HT) in neurons and increase concentration of these neurotransmitters in brain.

Classification

A. **Predominantly 5-HT reuptake inhibitors:** Imipramine, amitriptyline, trimipramine, doxepin, dothiepin, clomipramine (potent anticholinergic, more sedative).
B. **Predominantly NA reuptake inhibitors:** Desipramine, nortriptyline, amoxapine, reboxetine (less sedative).

Pharmacological actions: Most prominent action of TCAs is their ability to inhibit norepinephrine transporter (NET) and serotonin transporter (SERT) located at neuronal/platelet membrane at low and therapeutically attained concentrations. TCAs inhibit monoamine reuptake and interact with a variety of receptors, viz. muscarinic, α-drenergic, histamine H_1, $5\text{-}HT_1$, $5\text{-}HT_1$ and occasionally dopamine D2. The actions of imipramine are described as prototype.

1. CNS

- In normal individuals: It induces clumsy feeling, tiredness, light-headedness, and sleepiness, difficulty in concentrating and thinking, unsteady gait.
- In depressed patients: Little acute effects. After 2–3 weeks of continuous treatment, the mood is gradually elevated; patients become more communicative and start taking interest in self and surroundings.

2. ANS: Most TCAs are potent anticholinergic.

3. CVS: Tachycardia, postural hypotension, T wave suppression or inversion, cardiac arrhythmias.

Pharmacokinetics: Oral absorption of TCAs is good. They are extensively metabolized in liver. Metabolites are excreted in urine over 1–2 weeks. Plasma t½ range between 16 and 24 hours.

Adverse effects

1. Anticholinergic: Dry mouth, bad taste, constipation, epigastric distress, urinary retention, blurred vision, palpitation.
2. Sedation, mental confusion and weakness.
3. Increased appetite and weight gain.
4. Dysphoric agitated state or mania.
5. Sweating and fine tremors.
6. Seizure threshold is lowered—fits may be precipitated.
7. Postural hypotension.
8. Cardiac arrhythmias.
9. Rashes and jaundice.

Q. 5. Write a note on use of diazepam in dentistry. Mention also the contradictions. *(BFUHS, Nov. 2009)*

Ans. Diazepam (VALIUM) is a long acting (t½ = 30–60 hr) lipid soluble benzodiazepine, which acts on CNS.

Mechanism of action: It binds to GABAA-receptor Cl⁻ channel complex and potentiates the inhibitory effect of GABA, which increases the frequency of opening of Cl⁻ channels. This leads to increase in chloride conductance, membrane hypopolarization leading to CNS depression.

Uses

1. For sedation and hypnosis.
2. As anticonvulsant.
3. During diagnostic and minor operative procedures.
4. In conscious sedation.
5. In preanaesthetic medication.
6. As antianxiety: 5 mg on night before dental procedure and 5 mg two hours before dental procedure.
7. Muscle relaxant.
8. To treat alcohol withdrawal symptoms.

Dose: 2–10 mg

Side-effects: Drowsiness, confusion, blurred vision, amnesia, disorientation, tolerance and drug dependence. It may cause respiratory depression and hypotonia in the newborn (**floppy baby syndrome**), if used during pregnancy.

Contraindications: Hypersensitivity to BZDs, myasthenia gravis, pediatric patients <6 months, severe respiratory/hepatic insufficiency, OSA, acute narrow-angle glaucoma.

Q. 6. Write a short note on ultra short action barbiturates. *(TNMGR, April 1998)*

Ans. Barbiturates are substituted derivatives of barbituric acid (malonyl urea). Barbiturates have variable lipid solubility; the more soluble ones are more potent and shorter acting.

Classification

1. Ultra-short acting (~30 min): Thiopentone, methohexitone.
2. Short acting (~2 hr): Butobarbitone
3. Intermediate acting (~3–5 hr): Amobarbitone, butabarbitone.
4. Long acting (~6hr): Phenobarbitone, mephobarbitone.

Only ultra-short acting barbiturates are useful as anaesthetic agent.

Mechanism of action

i. *Barbiturates act at GABA: BZD receptor — Cl⁻ channel complex* and potentiate GABAergic inhibition by increasing the lifetime of Cl⁻ channel opening induced by GABA. (Contrast to BZDs which enhance frequency of Cl⁻ channel opening.)

ii. At high concentrations, barbiturates directly increase Cl⁻ conductance (GABAmimetic action; Contrast BZDs which have only GABAfacilitatory action) and inhibit Ca²⁺ dependent release of neurotransmitters.

iii. At very high concentrations, barbiturates depress voltage sensitive Na⁺ and K⁺ channels as well.

Pharmacological actions: Barbiturates are general depressants for all excitable cells, the CNS is most sensitive.

1. **CNS:** Dose-dependent effects: Sedation → sleep → anaesthesia → coma.
   Other systems: Respiration is depressed by relatively higher doses.
2. **CVS:** Decrease in BP and heart rate, reflex tachycardia.
3. **Skeletal muscle:** Reduce muscle contraction.
4. **Smooth muscles:** Tone and motility of bowel is decreased.
5. **Kidney:** Barbiturates tend to reduce urine flow by decreasing BP and increasing ADH release.
6. **Immunologic:** Thiopentone impair neutrophil function.

Pharmacokinetics: Barbiturates are well absorbed from GIT. The rate of entry into CNS is dependent on lipid solubility. Barbiturates cross placenta and are secreted in milk; can produce effects on fetus and suckling infant.

Dose: Thiopentone (2.5%): 50–100 mg; Methohexitone (1%): 20–40 mg.

Uses

1. Induction and maintenance of anesthesia
2. Treatment of increased intracranial pressure
3. Status epilepticus and grandmal seizures.
4. Cardioversion.
5. Narcoanalysis.
6. As hypnotic and anxiolytic (rarely).
7. As adjuvant in psychosomatic disorders.
8. Congenital nonhaemolytic jaundice and kernicterus.

Side effects: Hangover; Tolerance and dependence; Mental confusion, impaired performance and traffic accidents; Idiosyncrasy; Precipitation of porphyria; Hypersensitivity rashes, swelling of eyelids, lips, etc.

Contraindications: Acute intermittent porphyria (absolute). Liver and kidney disease; Severe pulmonary insufficiency; OSA; Shock; Coronary artery disease; hypothyroidism.

Sodium thiopentone as inducing agent for general anesthesia (TNMGR, April 2001; BFUHS, Oct. 2010): Thiopentone sodium is an ultra short-acting barbiturate which when administered, IV rapidly induces hypnosis and anesthesia without analgesia. It is highly water-soluble. Extravasation of solution produces intense pain, necrosis and gangrene. On IV inj (3–5 mg/kg as a 2.5% solution) it produces unconsciousness in 20–30 sec. Duration of action is 4–7 minutes. It is highly lipid soluble and gets rapidly redistributed in the body tissues.

Advantages: Quick onset of action; Induction is smooth, rapid and pleasant.

Disadvantages: It is not a good analgesic and not a muscle relaxant. It cannot be used alone as the dose required results in delayed recovery, respiratory and circulatory depression. A short period of apnea occurs. Overdosage results in profound respiratory depression.

Uses: It is used for induction of anesthesia prior to administration of inhalational anesthetics.

Q. 7. Write about the objectives of preanaesthetic medication? (TNMGR, Nov. 1995; BFUHS, Oct. 2010; NTR Uni., Nov. 2017; Sumandeep Uni., May 2018)

Ans. Preanaesthetic medication is defined as use of drugs before anesthesia to make it more pleasant and safe. The objectives of preanaesthetic medication are:

1. Relief of anxiety and apprehension preoperatively.
2. To facilitate smooth induction.
3. Amnesia for pre- and postoperative events.
4. To supplement and potentiate the analgesic action of anesthetics, so that less anaesthetic is needed.
5. To decrease secretions vagal stimulation caused by anesthetics.
6. Antiemetic effect which extends postoperatively.
7. To decrease acidity and amount of gastric secretions so that it is less damaging, if aspirated.
8. As prophylaxis for suppression of autonomic reflex activity.

Drugs used for preanaesthetic medication

1. **Sedative-antianxiety drugs:** Benzodiazepines like diazepam (5–10 mg oral), lorazepam (2 mg or 0.05 mg/kg IM 1 hr before), midazolam (IV), and antihistaminic like promethazine (50 mg IM).
2. **Opioids:** Morphine (10 mg) or pethidine (50–100 mg) IM Because of side effects of opioids, their use is highly restricted to those having preoperative pain. Fentanyl (50–100 µg IM or IV) is preferred nowadays.
3. **Anticholinergics:** Atropine or hyoscine (0.6 mg IM/IV), glycopyrrolate (0.1–0.3 mg IM).
4. **Neuroleptics:** Chlorpromazine (25 mg), triflupromazine (10 mg), or haloperidol (2–4 mg IM).
5. **H_2 Blockers:** Ranitidine (150–300 mg), or famotidine (20–40 mg), omeprazole/pantoprazole (20 mg).
6. **Antiemetics:** Metoclopramide (10–20 mg IM), domperidone (10 mg oral), selective 5HT3 blocker odansetron (4–8 mg IV).

   - **Ketamine anaesthesia** (TNMGR, April 2012): Ketamine is a phencyclidine derivative. In anaesthetic doses it produces a transe-like state known as "Dissociative anesthesia," characterized by intense analgesia, immobility, amnesia and a feeling of dissociation from one's own body and surroundings with or without actual loss of consciousness.

     Mechanism of action: Its mechanism of action is mainly by noncompetitive antagonism of the N-methyl D-aspartic acid (NMDA) receptor. It also interacts with opioid receptors, monoamine, cholinergic, purinergic and adrenoreceptor systems as well as having local anesthetic effects.

Advantages

1. Anaesthesia persists for up to 15 min., and is characterized by profound analgesia.
2. Ketamine may be used as sole agent for diagnostic and minor surgical interventions.
3. It is less likely to induce vomiting. hypotension.
4. Its sympathomimetic effects are of particular value in patients who are shocked, severely dehydrated or severely anemic.
5. Pharyngeal and laryngeal reflexes are only slightly impaired.

6. It is of particular value in children and poor-risk patients, and in asthmatic patients.

Disadvantages

1. No muscular relaxation.
2. It tends to raise heart rate and intracranial and intraocular pressure.
3. Hallucinations.

Uses

1. Sub-anaesthetic concentrations of ketamine may be used to provide analgesia for painful procedures of short duration.
2. Ketamine may be used for induction of anesthesia prior to administration of inhalational anesthetics, or for both induction and maintenance of anesthesia for short-lasting diagnostic and surgical interventions, including dental procedures that do not require skeletal muscle relaxation.

   • **Induction of anesthesia:** Induction of anesthesia is produced by administration of ketamine by IV or IM consciousness is lost in 30–60 seconds after IV administration and 2–4 min. after IM administration. Return of consciousness usually occurs in 10–20 min. after an injected induction dose of ketamine but return of full orientation may require additional 60–90 min. Amnesia persists for about 60–90 min. after recovery of consciousness.

Dosage and administration

1. Induction: 1–2 mg/kg by slow IV injection over a period of 60 sec.; 6–8 mg/kg by deep IM injection.
2. Induction and maintenance: Serial doses of 50% of original IV dose or 25% of IM dose are administered as required.
3. As analgesic: 500 µg/kg IM or IV followed, if necessary, by a dose of 250 µg/kg.

Contraindications

• Hypersensitivity to ketamine.
• Moderate to severe hypertension, CHF, or history of cerebrovascular accident.
• Alcohol intoxication.
• Cerebral trauma, raised intracranial pressure.
• Eye injury and increased intraocular pressure.
• Psychiatric disorders such as schizophrenia and acute psychoses.

Q. 8. Write on stages of general anesthesia.
(BFUHS, May 2010)

Ans. General anesthesia (GAs) is a drug-induced loss of consciousness during which the patient is not arousable, even by painful stimuli, accompanied by complete loss of protective reflexes including the ability to independently maintain ventilator function and respond purposefully to physical stimulation or verbal command.

Stages of General Anesthesia (GA): By Arthur Ernest Guedel in 1937.

I. Stage of analgesia: Starts from beginning of anaesthetic inhalation and lasts up to the loss of consciousness. Pain is progressively abolished. Patient remains conscious, can hear and see, and feels a dream like state; Amnesia develops by the end of this stage. Reflexes and respiration remain normal. Its use is limited to short procedures.

II. Stage of delirium: From loss of consciousness to beginning of regular respiration. Apparent excitement is seen; patient may shout, struggle and hold his breath; muscle tone increases, jaws are tightly closed, breathing is jerky; Vomiting, involuntary micturition or defecation may occur. Heart rate and BP may rise and pupils dilate due to sympathetic stimulation. No stimulus or operative procedure carried out during this stage.

III. Surgical anesthesia: Extends from onset of regular respiration to cessation of spontaneous breathing. This has been divided into 4 planes:

• Plane 1: Roving eyeballs. This plane ends when eyes become fixed.
• Plane 2: Loss of corneal and laryngeal reflexes.
• Plane 3: Pupil starts dilating and light reflex is lost.
• Plane 4: Intercostal paralysis, shallow abdominal respiration, dilated pupil.

IV. Medullary/respiratory paralysis: It is seen only with overdose. It is the stage of medullary depression → cessation of breathing, circulatory failure and death may follow.

Ideal anaesthetic should be pleasant, nonirritating, provide adequate analgesia, immobility and muscle relaxation; should be non-inflammable and administration should be easy and controllable and have a wide margin of safety. Induction and recovery should be smooth and should not affect cardiovascular functions. It should be inexpensive.

Mechanism of action of GAs: Most accepted mechanisms of action are as follows:

1. Inhaled and some intravenous anesthetics bind to specific sites on GABA receptor chloride channels and activate these receptors. By this they increase the inhibitory neurotransmission and depress the CNS.
2. Inhalational anesthetics enhance the sensitivity of glycine-gated chloride channels to glycine. These glycine receptors bring about inhibitory neurotransmission in the brainstem.

3. Ketamine and nitrous oxide bind to and inhibit N-methyl-D-aspartate (NMDA) receptors.
4. Inhalational and intravenous agents act at multiple sites in the nervous system and depress the neuronal activity at many sites in the brain.

Classification

I. Inhalational *(NTR Uni., May 2018)*

A. Gases: Nitrous oxide, cyclopropane.
B. Liquids: Ether, halothane, enflurane, isoflurane, methoxyflurane, desflurane, sevoflurane.

II. Intravenous

A. Inducing agents: Thiopentone sodium, methohexitone, propofol, etomidate.
B. Dissociative anesthesia: Ketamine.
C. Neuroleptanalgesia: Fentanyl + droperidol.
D. Benzodiazepines (BZDs): Diazepam, lorazepam, midazolam.

Q. 9. Write a note on conscious sedation.
(BFUHS, May 2008; RUHS, June 2017)

Ans. Conscious sedation (moderate sedation/analgesia) is defined as a state of altered consciousness that allows the patient to retain his airway and protective reflexes and respond appropriately to physical stimulation and/or verbal command.

Agents commonly used for conscious sedation are:

A. **Inhalation agents:** Nitrous oxide and oxygen.
B. **Systemic agents**
   I. **Conventional:** Lytic cocktail; Barbiturates (phenobarbitone); Chloral hydrate; Antihistaminic (promethazine, hydroxyzine); BZDs (diazepam).
   II. **Contemporary:** Newer benzodiazepines (midazolam, triazolam); Newer antihistaminic (loratidine).

Routes of drug administration for conscious sedation: Oral, rectal, inhalational, submucosal, intramuscular, intravenous.

Indications for conscious sedation

1. Children with low coping capacity.
2. Behavior management problem.
3. Dental fear and anxiety.
4. Mental retardation.
5. General disorder, psychiatric conditions.
6. Emergency treatment.
7. Moderate to large and complicated need.

Contraindication: Children <1 year, COPD, pregnancy, prolonged surgery, psychoses.

1. **Nitrous oxide:** It is delivered by means of flow meter utilizing nasal mask or hoods. It has anxiolytic and sedative properties with varying degree of analgesia and muscle relaxation. It should be the first choice for pediatric dental patients who are unable to tolerate local anesthesia alone and have sufficient understanding to accept the procedure. It is very safe because the child remains awake, responsive, and breaths on his/her own.

   Advantages: Easy to administer; Dose can be controlled; Patient remains calm and relax; Minimum side effects; No respiratory irritation.

   Contraindications: Common cold, tonsillitis, nasal blockage, pophyria, psychotic patients, COPD.

   Concentration used during various stages
   1. Induction: Slow: 0.5–1 L/min., rapid: 2–4 L/min., 40% nitrous oxide and 60% oxygen.
   2. Maintenance: 20–30% nitrous oxide.
   3. Reversal: 100% oxygen.

   Effects on body: CNS depression; Decreased cardiac output; Increases peripheral resistance; Respiratory depression.

2. **Midazolam:** It is twice as potent as diazepam. It is water-soluble, so less thrombophlebitis, sedation occurs within 3–5 minutes. Side effects include respiratory depression, hypertension.

   Dose: Adult: 0.1–0.15 mg/kg. Pediatric: 0.05–0.1 mg/kg.

3. **Propofol:** Propofol is water-immiscible oil which is formulated as an emulsion with a soya oil base to facilitate injection. Its rapid effect and moderate amnesia makes it an ideal drug for IV sedation.

   Dose: Loading dose: 1 mg/kg; **Maintenance dose:** 0.3–4 mg/kg/hr.

4. **Sevoflurane:** Potent ether inhalational anesthetic with low blood-gas solubility resulting in fast onset and offset (induction in 1 min). Therefore, ideal for induction before infusion of a total intravenous anesthetic to maintain the sedation.

5. **Chloral hydrate:** It is a chlorinated derivative of ethyl alcohol, can be given orally or rectally. Onset of action is within 15–30 minutes. Drug can cause nausea, vomiting. It is contraindicated in patients with heart diseases, renal or hepatic impairment.

   Dose: 25–50 mg/kg.

6. **Lytic cocktail:** It is a mixture of chlorpromazine with meperidine and promethazine. Dose used is 0.5 mg/kg.

7. **Dexmedetomidine:** Dextroisomer of medetomidine (imidazole), selective α_2-adrenoceptors agonist, decreases sympathetic tone, causing sedation and analgesia.

   Dose: 2 µg/kg, 45 min. before procedure.

8. **Fentanyl:** For painful procedures. It may be administered by parenteral, transdermal, nasal, and oral

routes, oral transmucosal (**"Lollipop" delivery system**).

Dose: 1 µg/kg/dose IV; Not to exceed total dose of 4 µg/kg.

9. **Sufentanil:** It is 10 times more potent than fentanyl. Potential side effects and prolonged hospital stay after nasal sufentanil makes it an unpopular choice for premedication.

Q. 10. Describe in detail the composition and mode of action of local anaesthetic agent lignocaine hydrochloride and briefly write its complications and its management.

(TNMGR, April 1995; HP Uni., May 2017; TNMGR, June 2017; MUHS, Dec. 2017; Sumandeep Uni., May 2018)

Ans. Local anesthesia is defined as a loss of sensation in a circumscribed area of the body caused by depression of excitation in nerve endings or an inhibition of the conduction process in peripheral nerves **(Stanley F. Malamed, 1980).**

Local anesthetics are the drugs which upon topical application or local injection cause reversible loss of sensory perception, especially pain in a localized area.

Desirable properties of local anesthesia

1. It should not be irritating to tissue.
2. It should not cause any permanent alteration of nerve structure.
3. Its systemic toxicity should be low.
4. Time of onset of anesthesia should be short.
5. It should be effective regardless of its route of application.
6. The duration of action should be long enough to permit the completion of procedure.

First classification

A. Injectable anaesthetic

    I. Low potency: Procaine, chloroprocaine.

    II. Intermediate Potency: Lidocaine (lignocaine), prilocaine.

    III. High potency: Tetracaine (amethocaine), bupivacaine, ropivacaine, mepivacaine, dibucaine (cinchocaine).

B. Surface anaesthetic: Soluble (cocaine, lidocaine, tetracaine, benoxinate); and insoluble (benzocaine, butylaminobenzoate, oxethazaine).

C. Miscellaneous: Clove oil, phenol, chlorpromazine, diphenhydramine, etc.

Second classification (structure based)

1. **Esters:** Cocaine, procaine, chloroprocaine, benzocaine, tetracaine.
2. **Amides:** Lidocaine, mepivacaine, bupivacaine, prilocaine, ropivacaine.

Third classification (duration based)

1. **Ultra short:** Pulpal = <10 min; Soft tissue = 30–45 min., e.g. chlorprocaine, procaine.
2. **Short:** Pulpal = 5–10 min; Soft tissue = 60–120 min., e.g. lidocaine, prilocaine.
3. **Medium:** Pulpal = 45–90 min; Soft tissue = 120–240 min., e.g. mepivacaine, articaine.
4. **Long:** Pulpal = 90–180 min; soft tissue = 240–540 min., e.g. bupivacaine, Etidocaine.

Pharmacokinetics: Soluble surface anesthetics (lidocaine, tetracaine) are rapidly absorbed from mucous membranes and abraded areas. The absorbed LA being lipophilic is widely distributed; rapidly enters highly perfused brain, heart, liver, and kidney, followed by muscle and other viscera. Ester-linked LAs are rapidly hydrolyzed by plasma pseudocholinesterase and the remaining by esterase in liver. Amide-linked LAs are degraded only in the liver microsomes by dealkylation and hydrolysis.

Mechanism of action (Fig. 4.10): Local anesthetics (LAs) block nerve conduction by decreasing the entry of Na^+ ions during upstroke of action potential (AP). As the concentration of LA is increased, the rate of rise of AP and maximum depolarization decreases, causing slowing of conduction. Finally, local depolarization fails to reach the threshold potential and conduction block ensues. LAs interact with a receptor situated within the voltage sensitive Na^+ channel and raise the threshold of channel opening, Na^+ permeability fails to increase in response to an impulse or stimulus. The equilibrium between the unionized base form (B) and ionized cationic form (BH^+) depends on the pKa of LA. The predominant active species (cationic form of LA) is able to approach its receptor only when the channel is open at the inner face and it binds more avidly to the inactive state of the channel, prolonging the inactive state. The channel takes longer to recover and hence refractory period of the fiber is increased.

A. Local actions: The clinically used LAs block sensory nerve endings, nerve trunks, NMJ, ganglionic synapse and receptors (non-selectively). They also reduce

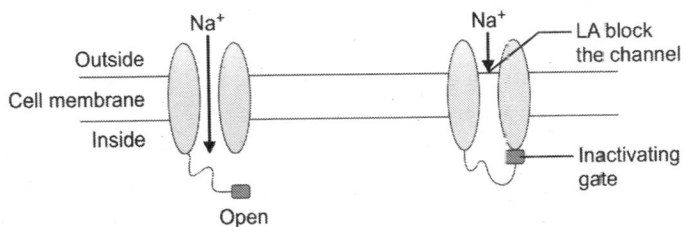

Fig. 4.10: Mechanism of action of local anesthetics

release of ACh from motor nerve endings. Sensory and motor fibres are inherently equally sensitive. Myelinated nerves are blocked earlier than nonmyelinated. Smaller fibres are more sensitive than larger fibres. Sensory fibres are more vulnerable than the motor fibres. Autonomic fibres are generally more susceptible than somatic fibres. Among the somatic afferents order of blockade is: Pain, temperature, touch, deep pressure. In general, fibres that are more susceptible to LA are the first to be blocked and the last to recover. Nerve sheaths restrict diffusion of LA into the nerve trunk so that fibres in the outer layers are blocked earlier than the inner or core fibres. As a result, the more proximal areas supplied by a nerve are affected earlier. In a mixed nerve, motor fibres are usually present circumferentially; may be blocked earlier than the sensory fibres in the core of nerve.

LA fails to afford adequate pain control in inflamed tissues (like infected tooth). The likely reasons are:

a. Inflammation lowers pH of the tissue—greater fraction of LA is in ionized form, hindering diffusion into the axolemma.

b. Blood flow to inflamed area is increased—LA is removed more rapidly from the site.

c. Effectiveness of Adr. injected with the LA is reduced at inflamed site.

d. Inflammatory products may oppose LA action.

Addition of a vasoconstrictor (*RGUHS, May 2011; NTR Uni., Oct. 2012):* e.g. Adrenaline (1:50,000 to 1:200,000):

- Prolongs duration of action of LAs by decreasing their rate of removal from the local site into circulation.
- Enhances the intensity of nerve block.
- Reduces systemic toxicity of LAs: Rate of absorption is reduced and metabolism keeps the plasma concentration lower.
- Makes the injection more painful.
- Provides a more bloodless field for surgery.
- Increases the chances of subsequent local tissue edema and necrosis as well as delays wound healing by reducing oxygen supply and enhancing oxygen consumption in the affected area.
- May raise BP and promote arrhythmia in susceptible individuals.

Maximum dose in dental practice: Healthy patient: 0.2 mg; Cardiac patient: 0.04 mg.

B. Systemic actions: Any LA injected or applied locally is ultimately absorbed and can produce systemic effects depending on the concentration attained in the plasma and tissues.

1. **CNS:** There is a sequence of stimulation followed by depression. Euphoria-excitement → mental confusion → restlessness → tremor and twitching of muscles → convulsions → unconsciousness → respiratory depression → death, in a dose-dependent manner.

2. **CVS**
   i. *Heart:* LAs at high doses or on inadvertent IV injection, decrease automaticity, excitability, contractility, conductivity and increases effective refractory period (ERP).
   ii. *Blood vessels:* LAs tend to produce fall in BP.

Adverse effects: Systemic toxicity on rapid IV injection is related to intrinsic anaesthetic potency of LA. However, toxicity after topical application or regional injection is influenced by relative rates of absorption and metabolism; those rapidly absorbed but slowly metabolized are more toxic.

- **Lidocaine (lignocaine)** (*TNMGR, April 2012; KUHS, Jan., 2014):* It is a versatile LA, good both for surface application as well as injection and is available in a variety of forms. Injected around a nerve it blocks conduction within 3 min. Also anesthesia is more intense and longer lasting. Vasodilatation occurs in the injected area. It is used for surface application, infiltration, nerve block, epidural, spinal and intravenous regional block anesthesia. In contrast to other LAs, early central effects of lidocaine are drowsiness, mental clouding, altered taste and tinnitus. Overdose causes muscle twitching, convulsions, cardiac arrhythmias, fall in BP, coma and respiratory arrest like other LAs. Lidocaine is popular antiarrhythmics.

Composition

a. Local anesthetic agent: Lignocaine 2%
b. Vasoconstrictor: Adr. 1:80,000.
c. Sodium metabisulphite: Reducing agent (antioxidant)
d. Methylparaben: Bacteriostatic agent.
e. Thymol: Fungicide.
f. Vehicle: Distilled water and NaCl → volume and isotonicity of solution.

Maximum recommended dose: Without adrenaline: 4.4 mg/kg; With adrenaline: 6.6 mg/kg

Use

a. 2% lidocaine with 1:50000 adrenaline: Hemostasis
b. 2% lidocaine with 1:100000 or 1:200000 adrenaline: Local anesthesia.

Techniques of local anesthesia

1. **Surface anesthesia (topical anesthesia):** LA is applied on the abraded skin, mucous membrane.

2. **Infiltration anesthesia:** LA is directed into tissues to be operated, it blocks small, terminal sensory nerve endings. LA is infiltrated into skin, subcutaneous tissue or deeper structures. Most frequently used LAs are lignocaine (0.5–1%), procaine (0.5–1%), bupivacaine (0.125–0.25%). It is suitable only for small areas. It can be used for drainage of an abscess, excision of small swelling, suturing of cut wounds, before root canal treatment. It is contra-indicated if there is local infection and clotting disorders.

3. **Field block anesthesia:** It is achieved by injecting LA in proximity to larger nerve branches, which anaesthetize the area distal to the injection. This principle is used in cases of minor procedures of scalp, anterior abdominal wall, extremities, and teeth.

4. **Nerve block anesthesia** (1.8–2.0 ml): LA is injected very close to or around the main nerve trunk. It produces larger areas of anesthesia than field block.

5. **Intraligamentary (0.2 ml):** LA is injected within PDL through gingival sulcus. It is indicated in patients with bleeding disorder and young handicapped.

6. **Intraseptal (0.1 ml):** Similar technique as intraligamentary. Useful in providing osseous and soft tissue anesthesia and hemostasis for periodontal curettage and surgical flap procedures.

7. **Intrapapillary:** For palatal and lingual anesthesia.

8. **Intrapulpal:** In case of pulp therapy where other techniques have failed.

9. **Spinal anesthesia:** LA is injected into the subarachnoid space to anaesthetize spinal roots. It is injected into the space between L2–3 and L3–4. Agents used are lignocaine, tetracaine, bupivacaine, etc. It is used for surgical procedures below the level of umbilicus. Advantages: No loss of consciousness, good muscle relaxation and analgesia. Complications are headache, hypotension, respiratory paralysis, septic meningitis, nerve injury.

10. **Epidural anesthesia:** LA is injected into epidural space where it acts on spinal nerve roots. It is safer but the technique is little difficult than spinal anesthesia. It is slower in onset, require much larger doses. It is mainly used in obstetric analgesia.

11. **Intravenous regional anesthesia:** It is mainly used in anaesthetizing the upper limb. LA is injected into the vein of the limb whose blood flow is occluded by a tourniquet.

Q. 11. Write a short note on topical anesthetics.

(TNMGR, Sept. 2007)

Ans. Topical anesthetics reversibly block nerve conduction near their site of administration by targeting free nerve endings in dermis or mucosa, thereby producing temporary loss of sensation in a limited area.

Methods of enhancing permeation of topical anesthetics: Iontophoresis, electroporation, sonophoresis/phonophoresis, magnetophoresis/magnetokinesis, delivery from lipid vesicles (liposomes, niosomes, and transfersomes).

Various topical anaesthetic agents used: Benzocaine (20%); Tetracaine hydrochloride (0.2–2.0%); Lidocaine hydrochloride (2%, 5% gel; 2%, 4%, 5% solution; 5% ointment, or 10% spray); Prilocaine (4% prilocaine or 4% prilocaine with 1:200,000 epinephrine); Eutectic mixtures of local anesthesia (EMLA) cream: 1:1 mixture of 2.5% prilocaine and 2.5% lidocaine; Tetracaine, adrenaline (epinephrine), and cocaine (TAC): 0.5% tetracaine, 0.05% adrenaline, and 11.8% cocaine; Lidocaine, epinephrine, and tetracaine (LET): 4% lignocaine with 0.1% epinephrine and 0.5% tetracaine; Bupivanor: 0.48% bupivacaine and 1:26000 norepinephrine; ELA-max: 4 or 5% lignocaine cream in a liposomal matrix; Betacaine-LA: Lignocaine, prilocaine and phenylephrine; 4% tetracaine; Topicaine (4% lignocaine in gel microemulsion); Lidoderm patch (5%); Proparacaine or proxymetacaine (0.5% solution); Miscellaneous agents (8–10% capsaicin, tetradotoxin, 0.8% nalbuphine, ethyl chloride spray, etc).

Clinical applications

a. For local analgesia on intact skin: EMLA, 4% tetracaine.

b. Minimize discomfort prior to injections or before intravenous and arterial line access: EMLA, 4% tetracaine.

c. For symptomatic relief of chronic pain: Heated lidocaine/tetracaine patch.

d. To relieve pruritus and pain due to minor burns, skin eruptions, stings, poison ivy, and minor cuts and scratches: EMLA, lidocaine, epinephrine, and tetracaine (LET), bupivanor, ELA max.

e. In ophthalmology: 0.5% proparacaine, 0.4% oxybuprocaine, 2% lignocaine aqueous gel and drops, 0.5% tetracaine.

f. Otorhinolaryngology: 80–90% liquefied phenol, 8% tetracaine base in 70% isopropyl alcohol.

g. For superficial dermatologic, esthetic, and laser procedures: EMLA 5%.

Indications for surface anesthesia in dentistry

1. Needle insertion for conduction or infiltration anesthesia.
2. Control of pain in a wounded area
3. Placement of orthodontic bands
4. Inhibition of vomiting (for radiographic imaging or impression)
5. Dry socket
6. Simple extraction of primary tooth
7. Rubber-dam clamp placement
8. Surgical treatment of mucosal surface, such as superficial submucosal abscess incision.
9. Inhibition of reflexes during endotracheal intubation.
10. Root planning or scaling.

Recent developments: HurriPAK Periodontal Anesthetic Kit (20% benzocaine solution); Cetacaine (14% benzocaine, 2% butamben, and 2% tetracaine hydrochloric acid); Oraqix subgingival anesthetic (2.5% lidocaine and 2.5% prilocaine).

Side effects and precautions

1. Tissue stimulation (when applied for prolonged periods), temporary altered sense of taste.
2. Ester-based agents, as PABA derivatives, are known allergens.
3. Systemic toxicity: Metallic taste, circumoral numbness, diplopia, tinnitus, dizziness, CNS excitation or depression, hypertension, tachycardia, ventricular arrhythmias, gag-reflex suppression, methemoglobinemia, skin discoloration, swelling, neuritis, tissue necrosis, sloughing, etc.

Q. 12. Write about merits and demerits of procaine.
(TNMGR, April 2000)

Ans. Procaine is low potency, short duration injectable anaesthetic agent. It is the first synthetic local anaesthetic introduced in 1905. It is not a surface anaesthetic. It is derivatives of para-aminobenzoic acid. Procaine forms poorly soluble salt with benzyl penicillin; Procaine penicillin injected IM acts for 24 hours due to slow absorption from the site of injection.

Merits

1. It is a non irritant.
2. As effective as cocaine as local anaesthetic.
3. Much less toxic.
4. Does not produce drug dependence.
5. Compatible in solutions with all vasoconstrictor.
6. It aid in breaking arteriospasm.
7. Safe in patients with hepatic dysfunction.

Demerits

1. Less potent than other.
2. Can reduce the effectiveness of sulfonamides.
3. Poor diffusion through interstitial tissue.
4. Because of extreme vasodilating property, chances of more bleeding.
5. Slow clinical onset of anesthesia.

5. ANTIBIOTICS AND OTHER CHEMOTHERAPEUTICS.

Q. 1. Write about the principle of antibiotic therapy.
(TNMGR, March 2010; BFUHS, May 2011; NTR Uni., June 2017)

Q. Discuss on selection of antimicrobial agent in orofacial infections.
(TNMGR, Sept. 2007)

Ans. An **antimicrobial** is any substance of natural, semisynthetic or synthetic origin that kills or inhibits the growth of microorganisms but causes little or no damage to the host. An **antibiotic** is a low molecular substance produced by a microorganism that at a low concentration inhibits or kills other microorganisms.

All antibiotics are antimicrobials, but not all antimicrobials are antibiotics.

Principles which govern selection of antibiotics are:

A. Drug factors

1. **Obtaining an accurate infectious disease diagnosis:** An infectious disease diagnosis is reached by determining the site of infection, defining the host, and establishing a microbiological diagnosis.
2. **Timing of initiation of antimicrobial therapy:** In critically ill patients, empiric therapy should be initiated immediately. In stable patients, antimicrobial therapy should be deliberately withheld until appropriate specimens have been collected.
3. **Empiric vs definitive antimicrobial therapy:** A common approach is to use broad-spectrum antimicrobial agents as initial empiric therapy. Once microbiology results are available, switch over to definitive therapy of narrow antibiotic spectrum.
4. **Interpretation of antimicrobial susceptibility tests:** Antimicrobial susceptibility testing measures the ability of a specific organism to grow in the presence of a particular drug *in vitro*. The goal is to predict the clinical success or failure of the antibiotic being tested against a particular organism.
5. **Bactericidal vs bacteriostatic therapy:** Bactericidal drugs, include drugs that primarily act on the cell wall (e.g. β-lactams), cell membrane (e.g. daptomycin), or bacterial DNA (e.g. fluoroquinolones). Bacteriostatic agents inhibit bacterial replication without killing the organism.

6. **Use of antimicrobial combinations:** Combination of 2 or more antimicrobial agents is recommended:
   i. When agents exhibit synergistic activity against a microorganism.
   ii. When critically ill patients require empiric therapy.
   iii. To extend the antimicrobial spectrum beyond that is achieved by use of a single agent for treatment of polymicrobial infections.
   iv. To prevent emergence of resistance.

B. Host factors

1. **Renal and hepatic function:** If there is impairment of kidney and liver function, drugs dose need to be reduced.
2. **Age:** Most pediatric drug dosing is guided by weight. In geriatric patients, the serum creatinine level, creatinine clearance should be estimated by age and weight for these patients.
3. **Genetic variation:** Genetic susceptibility to the adverse effects of antimicrobial agents is occasionally significant, before administration of certain drugs, e.g. in G6PD deficiency, certain antibiotics can cause hemolysis.
4. **Pregnancy and lactation:** Higher antimicrobial doses are not routinely recommended in third trimester of pregnancy and lactation.
5. **History of allergy or intolerance.**
6. **History of recent antimicrobial use:** Eliciting a history of exposure to antimicrobial agents in the recent past (3 months) can also help in selection of antimicrobial therapy.
7. **Oral vs intravenous therapy:** Patients hospitalized with infections are often treated with intravenous antimicrobial therapy. Patients with mild to moderate infections are treated with oral antimicrobial agents.

C. Pharmacodynamic characteristics: Drugs that exhibit time-dependent activity (β-lactams and vancomycin) have relatively slow bactericidal action, whereas drugs that exhibit concentration-dependent killing (aminoglycosides, fluoroquinolones, metronidazole, and daptomycin) have enhanced bactericidal activity as the serum concentration is increased.

D. Efficacy at the site of infection: Efficacy of antimicrobial agents depends on their capacity to achieve a concentration equal to or greater than the MIC at the site of infection and modification of activity at certain sites. Antimicrobial concentrations attained at some sites are often much lower than serum levels, e.g. first- and second-generation cephalosporins and macrolides do not cross blood–brain barrier; Fluoroquinolones achieve high concentrations in prostate. Many antibiotics (aminoglycosides) are less active in low-oxygen, low-pH, and high-protein environment of abscesses. Presence of foreign bodies at the site of infection also affects antimicrobial activity.

Considerations for continuing antibiotic therapy

1. **Duration of antimicrobial therapy:** It is important for clinicians to ensure that their patients fit the profile of the study population and carefully monitor high-risk patients for improvement.
2. **Assessment of response to treatment:** Response to treatment of an infection can be assessed using both clinical and microbiological parameters.
3. **Adverse effects:** A history of serious allergic reaction should be carefully documented to avoid inadvertent administration of same drug or another drug in same class.

Special situations in infectious disease therapy

1. **Antimicrobial therapy for foreign body associated infections:** As an alternative, for patients unable to tolerate implant removal, long-term suppressive antimicrobial therapy is sometimes used, with variable success.
2. **Use of antimicrobial agents as prophylactic or suppressive therapy:** For use of an antimicrobial agent as prophylactic treatment, the infection would occur predictably in a certain setting and would be well known to be associated with a specific organism or organisms, and an effective antimicrobial agent would be available with no or limited long-term toxicity.

Common misuses of antibiotics

1. Prolonged empiric antimicrobial treatment without clear evidence of infection.
2. Treatment of a positive clinical culture in the absence of disease.
3. Failure to narrow antimicrobial therapy when a causative organism is identified.
4. Prolonged prophylactic therapy.
5. Excessive use of certain antimicrobial agents.

Q. 2. Discuss the beneficial antimicrobial combinations and their clinical utility.

[TNMGR, Nov. 1995, April 1998
NTR Uni., June 2014; MUHS, Dec. 2018]

Ans. Antimicrobial combinations can result in: Additive (indifferent) effect; synergistic effect or antagonistic effect. The objectives of using antimicrobial combinations are:

1. **To achieve synergism:** Synergism may manifest in terms of decrease in MIC of antimicrobial agent (AMA). General guidelines are:
   a. Two bacteriostatic agents are often additive, rarely synergistic.
   b. Two bactericidal drugs are frequently additive and sometime synergistic, if the organism is sensitive to both.
   c. Combination of a bactericidal with a bacteriostatic drug may be synergistic or antagonistic depending on the organism. In general, if the organism is highly sensitive to the cidal drug-response to the combination is equal to static drug given alone. If organism has low sensitivity to cidal drug-synergism may be seen.

   Example: Bacterial endocarditis: Penicillin + streptomycin/gentamicin.
   - Pseudomonas infections: Carbenicillin + gentamicin.
   - *Pneumocystis carinii* pneumonia: Trimethoprim + sulfamethoxazole.
   - β-lactamase producing organisms like *H. influenzae:* Amoxicillin + clavulinic acid.
   - Tuberculosis: INH + rifampicin.
2. **To reduce severity or incidence of adverse effects:** This is possible only if the combination is synergistic so that doses can be reduced.
3. **To prevent emergence of resistance:** Decreased resistant *Mycobacterium tuberculosis* with combination.
4. **To broaden the spectrum of antimicrobial action:** For example, mixed aerobic and anaerobic infection.
5. **As initial therapy:** In patient where nature of infection is not clear yet; Drugs covering both gram-positive and gram-negative pathogens may be used initially till the culture report is available.

Disadvantages of antimicrobial combinations
1. They foster a casual rather than rational outlook in the diagnosis of infections and choice of AMA.
2. Increased incidence and variety of adverse effects.
3. Increased chances of superinfections (alteration of normal flora).
4. If inadequate doses of non-synergistic drugs are used, emergence of resistance may be promoted.
5. Selection of resistant strains (few resistant mutants that remain may multiply unchecked).
6. Increased cost of therapy.

Q. 3. Write a note on uses of antibiotics in dentistry.
(TNMGR, March 2007; MUHS, May 2009; MPMS, July 2017; NTR Uni., May 2019)

Ans. The use of antibiotics (Abs) in dental practice is characterized by empirical prescription based on clinical and bacteriological epidemiological factors, with use of broad-spectrum antibiotics for short periods of time, and application of a very narrow range of antibiotics.

Classification
A. According to their type of activity
   i. Bactericidal agents: Penicillins, cephalosporins, aminoglycoside, fluoroquinolones, rifampicin, metronidazole.
   ii. Bacteriostatic agents: Tetracyclines, chloramphenicol, sulphonamides, dapsone, macrolides.
B. According to spectrum of activity
   i. Narrow spectrum: Penicillins, aminoglycoside.
   ii. Broad-spectrum: Tetracyclines, chloramphenicol.
C. According to mechanism of action
   i. Inhibition of cell wall synthesis: Penicillins, cephalosporins, vancomycin, bacitracin, cycloserine.
   ii. Inhibition of cell membrane function: Amphotericin B, nystatin, polymyxins, colistin.
   iii. Inhibition of protein synthesis: Tetracyclines, aminoglycoside, macrolides, chloramphenicol.
   iv. Inhibition of DNA synthesis: Acyclovir, ganciclovir
   v. Inhibition of DNA function (DNA-dependent RNA polymerase): Rifampicin, metronidazole.
   vi. Inhibition of DNA gyrase: Fluoroquinolones.
   vii. Antimetabolite: Sulphonamides, dapsone.

Indications
1. As treatment for acute odontogenic infections: e.g. pulpitis, ANUG, periapical abscess, aggressive periodontitis, and space infections.

   Antibiotics commonly used in application to odontogenic infections.
   a. Amoxicillin: 500 mg TDS OR 1000 mg BD
   b. Amoxicillin-clavulanic acid:500–875 mg TDS OR 2000 mg BD;1000–2000 mg (IV) TDS
   c. Clindamycin 300 mg TDS; 600 mg (IV) TDS .
   d. Azithromycin: 500 mg OD for 3 days.
   e. Ciprofloxacin: 500 mg BD.
   f. Metronidazole: 500–750 mg TDS.
   g. Gentamicin: 240 mg (IM/IV) OD.
   h. Penicillin: 1.2–2.4 million IU (IM/IV) OD.

   Antibiotics are not recommended: Chronic gingivitis, periodontal abscess (non-disseminated).
2. As treatment for non-odontogenic infections, e.g. specific infections of oral cavity (tuberculosis, syphilis, leprosy), and nonspecific infections of mucosal membranes, muscles and fascias, salivary glands and bone infections.

a. Clindamycin: Used because of its high concentration on bone.

b. Fluoroquinolones: To include Gram-negative bacilli, Gram-positive aerobic cocci, and anaerobes.

c. Doxycycline: 100 mg OD

d. Mycobacterial infection: Anti-tubercular drugs.

3. As prophylaxis against focal infection in patients at risk of endocarditis and joint prostheses.

a. Infective endocarditis antibiotic prophylaxis by AHA.

4. As prophylaxis against local infection and systemic spread in oral surgery: Removal of impacted teeth, periapical surgery, bone surgery, implant surgery, bone grafting and surgery for benign tumors.

Local or systemic infection—including oncological patients, immune suppressed individuals, patients with metabolic disorders such as diabetes, and splenectomized patients, prophylactic antibiotic coverage should be provided before attempting any invasive procedure.

5. In patient where the host response is decreased by diseases like diabetes mellitus, malnutrition, etc.

■ **Antibiotic use in endodontics** (*BBD Uni., April 2014; TNMGR, June 2017*): Use of antibiotics in endodontics should be reserved for patients with signs of local infection, malaise of fever.

1. Reversible and irreversible pulpitis: No ABs.
2. Apical periodontitis: No ABs except in compromised host.
3. Periapical abscess: Incision and drainage (I and D) followed by ABs for 3–5 days.
4. Avulsed tooth: Doxycycline 200 mg loading dose followed by 100 mg for 4 days
5. Periapical pathology (cyst and granuloma): No ABs Except 1 gm preoperative followed by 500 mg thrice daily for 3 days.

■ **Antibiotics in periodontics**

1. Gingivitis and chronic periodontitis: No ABs.
2. Aggressive periodontitis: Amoxicillin + metronidazole.
3. NUG/NUP: ABs only when patient has systemic complications.
4. Periodontal abscess: Curetting of pocket; ABs is indicated in patients with signs of systemic infections.
5. Peri-implantitis: ABs are indicated when: Presence of bleeding on probing, suppuration, periodontal pocket depth >6 mm and bone loss >2 mm.
6. Periodontal surgeries.

■ **Indications for AB prophylaxis in oral surgery**

1. Exodontia and dentoalveolar surgery: No ABs, except high risk of infection; Communication with sinus or oral cavity.

2. 3rd molar surgery: No ABs except high risk of infection.
3. Dental implants: Preoperative and postoperative AB prophylaxis in high risk of infection.
4. Orthognathic surgery e/o approach: No ABs except pre-operative when anticipate oral communication.
5. Orthognathic surgery i/o approach: Preoperative and 1 day postoperative.
6. Mandibular fractures (no oral communication): No ABs.
7. Mandibular fractures (oral communication): Preoperative and postoperative 3–5 days.
8. Facial bone fractures: Preoperative.
9. Soft tissue trauma i/o or e/o: No ABs except high risk infection.
10. Soft tissue trauma with dirty e/o wound: Preoperative and postoperative 3–5 days.
11. Major head and neck surgery: Preoperative and postoperative 3–5 days.

■ **Antibiotics used in pediatric dentistry** (*TNMGR, April 2013*):

Calculation of pediatric dose: Young's rule; Dilling's rule; Clarke's rule: Weight (lb) × adult dose/150.

Commonly used antibiotics:

1. Natural penicillins: Penicillin G; **Dose:** Neonates—50 mg/kg/day; Infants and children: 100 mg/kg/day.
2. **Acid resistant penicillins:** Potassium phenoxymethyl penicillin. **Dose:** 6–12 years: 250 mg; 1–5 years: 125 mg; <1 years: 62.5 mg, in four divided doses.
3. Penicillinase resistant penicillins: Cloxacillin: 0.5–1 g/day, in 3–4 divided doses.
4. Extended spectrum penicillins: Ampicillin: Children up to: 50–100 mg/kg/day. Amoxicillin: <12 years: 20–40 mg/kg/day TDS.
5. Metronidazole: 10–50 mg/kg/day TDS.
6. Erythromycin: 30–50 mg/kg/day QID.
7. Clindamycin: <1 month: 15–20 mg/kg/day, older children: 20–40 mg/kg/day.
8. Tetracycline: 20–40 mg/kg/day in divided doses.

■ **Nystatin:** <1 year: 100000 units TDS, 1–6 years: 200000 units TDS, >6 years: 500000 units, TDS.

Precautions in using antibiotics

1. United States Food and Drug Administration (FDA) drug risk during pregnancy:
   i. (A) without demonstrated risk; No antibiotics.
   ii. (B) Without effects in animals, though with undemonstrated innocuousness in humans, e.g. azithromycin, cephalosporins, erythromycin, metronidazole and penicillins with or without β-lactamase inhibitors.

Table 5.3: Dose adjustment in patients with chronic kidney failure

Drug	Cr cl: 10–50 ml/min	Cr cl: <10 ml/min
Amoxicillin	Every 8–12 h	Every 12–14 h
Amoxicillin-clavulanate	Every 8 h	Every 12–24 h
Clindamycin	Not needed	Not needed
Doxycycline	Not needed	Not needed
Erythromycin	Not needed	Not needed
Metronidazole	Every 8–12 h	Every 12–24 h
Penicillin G	50–100% of the dose every 8–12 h	25–50% of the dose every 12 h
Azithromycin	Not needed	Not needed

iii. (C) No studies conducted in either animals or humans, or teratogenic effects recorded in animals without due evaluation in humans, e.g. clarithromycin, fluorquinolone, sulfa drugs.

iv. (D) Teratogenic effects upon the fetus—use of the drug being conditioned to obtainment of benefit that outweighs the risks, e.g. aminoglycosides and tetracyclines.

v. (X) In turn contemplates teratogenic effects that outweigh any possible benefit derived from the drug.

2. Kidney failure: Presence of impaired renal function requires reduction of drug dose. Dose adjustment in patients with chronic kidney failure: According to creatinine clearance (Cr cl) (Table 5.3).

3. Liver failure: Erythromycin, clindamycin, metronidazole and anti-tuberculosis drugs require dose adjustments in patients with liver failure. Tetracyclines should be avoided.

Q. 4. Discuss tetracyclines in detail. *(MAHE, July 1999)*

Ans. Tetracyclines (TCs) are broad-spectrum agents, exhibiting activity against a wide range of gram-positive and gram-negative bacteria, atypical organisms such as chlamydiae, mycoplasmas, and rickettsiae, and protozoan parasites. The tetracyclines include: Tetracyclines (chlortetracycline, oxytetracycline); Semisynthetic derivatives (demeclocycline, methacycline, doxycycline, minocycline).

Mechanism of action: Tetracyclines are primarily bacteriostatic; Inhibit protein synthesis by binding to 30S ribosomes in susceptible organism. Subsequent to such binding, attachment of aminoacyl-t-RNA to mRNA-ribosome complex is interfered. As a result, the peptide chain fails to grow.

Antimicrobial spectrum: All types of pathogenic microorganisms except fungi and viruses.

Resistance: In such bacteria, usually the tetracycline concentrating mechanism becomes less efficient or the bacteria acquire capacity to pump it out. Another mechanism is plasmid mediated synthesis of a 'protection' protein which protects the ribosomal binding site from tetracycline. Elaboration of tetracycline inactivating enzymes is an unimportant mechanism of tetracycline resistance.

Pharmacokinetics: Older TCs are incompletely absorbed from GIT; Absorption is better if taken in empty stomach. Doxycycline and minocycline are completely absorbed irrespective of food. TCs chelate calcium and other metals which reduce their absorption. Hence, tetracyclines should not be given with milk, iron preparations and antacids. Tetracyclines are widely distributed in the body. Most tetracyclines are primarily excreted in urine by glomerular filtration; dose has to be reduced in renal failure; Doxycycline and minocyclin are exception to this. They are partly metabolized and significant amounts enter bile—some degree of enterohepatic circulation occurs.

Dose: Chlortetracycline: 250–500 mg QID; Tetracycline: 250–500 mg QID; Doxycycline: 200 mg initially then 100 mg OD; Minocycline: 200 mg initially then 100 mg OD.

Adverse effects: Epigastric pain; Nausea; Vomiting; Diarrhoea; Esophageal ulceration; Intramuscular injection of tetracyclines is very painful; Thrombophlebitis.

Dose related toxicity
1. Liver damage.
2. Kidney damage.
3. Phototoxicity.
4. **Teeth and bones:** TCs chelate calcium; Calcium-tetracycline-orthophosphate complexes get deposited in the developing teeth and bones. The deformities depend on the time of tetracycline administration as:
   - Mid-pregnancy to 5 months of extra uterine life: Deciduous teeth are affected: Brown discoloration, enamel hypoplasia, more susceptible to caries.

- 3 months and 6 years of age: Pigmentation and discoloration of permanent dentition.
- Pregnancy and childhood up to 12 years: Depressed skeletal growth.

5. Antianabolic effect
6. Increased intracranial pressure
7. Diabetes insipidus
8. Vestibular toxicity
9. Hypersensitivity
10. Superinfection

Precautions

1. Tetracyclines should not be used during pregnancy, lactation and in children.
2. They should be avoided in patients on diuretics: blood urea may rise in such patients.
3. They should be used cautiously in renal or hepatic insufficiency.
4. Preparations should never be used beyond their expiry date.
5. Do not mix injectable tetracyclines with penicillin-inactivation occurs.
6. Do not inject tetracyclines intrathecally.

Contraindications: Pregnancy, lactation, children up to 12 years of age.

Uses

1. Empirical therapy.
2. TCs as first choice drugs in: Venereal diseases (chlamydial nonspecific urethritis/endocervicitis, lymphogranuloma venereum, granuloma inguinale); Atypical pneumonia; Cholera; Brucellosis (doxycycline 200 mg + rifampicin 600 mg daily for 6 weeks); Plague; Relapsing fever; Rickettsial infections.
3. TCs as second choice drug in: Tetanus, anthrax, actinomycosis, gonorrhoea; Leptospirosis; Patients allergic to penicillin.
4. TCs may be used in: Urinary tract infections, community-acquired pneumonia, amoebiasis, chronic obstructive lung disease.
5. **In periodontitis:** Low dose tetracyclines (250 mg QID) are used as adjuvants in periodontitis. Doxycycline (20 mg) BD for 2–4 weeks is thought to act by inhibiting crevicular bacterial collagenases (calcium dependent). By chelating Ca^{2+}, TCs suppress collagenase activity and suppress inflammation. Doxycycline polymer gel is placed into periodontial pocket so that the drug gets slowly absorbed. For systemic activity, tetracycline is combined with metronidazole or ciprofloxacin.

- **Chemically modified tetracyclines** (NTR Uni., Nov. 2007; Sumandeep Uni., June 2017): Host modulation therapy (HMT) along with conventional mechanical therapy is an ideal approach for treatment of periodontal disease. Chemically modified tetracyclines (CMTs) are derivatives of tetracycline in which antibiotic property has been removed, but retain the host modulatory, anti-collagenolytic property by eliminating dimethyl-amino group from carbon 4 position of A ring of four ringed (A, B, C, D) structure. Presently, CMT 1–8 have been evolved. Among them CMT 1, CMT 3 and CMT 8 have been used for periodontal applications.

Mechanism of action: CMTs act as HMT agents in treatment of periodontitis by inhibiting MMPs, inhibiting proinflammatory cytokines, inducible nitric oxide synthase (iNOS), inhibiting bone resorption and by increasing attachment of fibroblasts and connective tissues to tooth surface.

Advantages of CMTs

- No development of antibiotic resistant microbial flora in long-term therapy.
- No gastrointestinal toxicity on long-term therapy.
- Higher plasma concentrations can be obtained with less frequent administration regimens.

Limitations of CMTs: Photosensitivity; SLE; Altered liver function tests; Neurotoxicities. Non-dose related toxicities (anemia, anorexia, constipation, dizziness, fatigue, fever, headache, heartburn, nausea, vomiting).

Applications of CMTs

- In periodontal disease, as host-modulating therapy.
- Non-infected corneal ulcers, rheumatoid arthritis and diabetes mellitus.
- Tumor metastasis.
- Antifungal agents.
- In acne, epidermolysis bullosa and ARDS.
- Inhibition of intimal thickening after arterial injury.
- Inhibition of orthodontic tooth displacement.

Q. 5. Write a short note on doxycycline.
(UHSR, RUHS, June 2018)

Ans. Doxycycline hyclate is a water-soluble tetracycline antibiotic that kills and prevents the growth of a wide range of Gram-positive and Gram-negative bacteria.

Pharmacokinetics: Oral dose is rapidly absorbed and detectable in blood as soon as 15 minutes after administration. Peak plasma concentration is reached after 2 to

3 hours and an elimination half-life of 15–30 hours. It is metabolism mainly in duodenum. Elimination primarily occurs through GIT.

Mechanism of action: Its high lipophilicity, compared to other tetracyclines, allows it to cross multiple membranes to reach target molecules.

- **As antibacterial**
- **As immunomodulator:** It inhibits leukocyte movement during inflammation by preventing calcium-dependent microtubular assembly and lymphocytic proliferation.
- **As anti-inflammatory:** By inhibition of nitric acid synthase.

Dose

- For antibacterial: For mild to moderate infections, 100 mg, q12h on first day and then 100 mg/day onwards. For pelvic infections, 100 mg BD for one week.
- For anti-inflammation: 40 mg daily.
- For malaria prevention: 100 mg OD.

Therapeutic uses: Treatment of acne, malaria (for prophylaxis and treatment), skin infections, STDs, Lyme disease. Cholera, mycoplasma, tularemia, typhus, and rickettsia infections, rheumatoid arthritis, rosacea, bullous dermatoses, granulomatous disease. Doxycycline hyclate has a specific indication for adult periodontal disease for its anti-collagenase and anti-matrix metalloproteinase activity in GCF.

Adverse effects: Mild diarrhea, photosensitivity, nausea, vomiting, skin rash/itching, headaches, tooth discoloration.

Contraindications

- Absolute: Pregnancy or breastfeeding; Children <12 years; Allergy to tetracycline antibiotics; Use with penicillin or isotretinoin.
- Relative: Liver disease, history of yeast infections, kidney disease, diarrhea from *C. difficile*, history of lupus, porphyria, myasthenia gravis.

Q. 6. Write a short note on newer penicillins.
(TNMGR, Oct. 1999; UHSR, June2018)

Q. Write a short note on extended spectrum penicillins. *(TNMGR, March 2007)*

Ans. The β-lactam antibiotics have a β-lactam ring, e.g. penicillins, cephalosporins, monobactams and carbapenems.

Penicillins: Sir Alexander Fleming discovered penicillin in 1928. Penicillins are one of the most important groups of antibiotics. Penicillin is now obtained from the fungus *Penicillium chrysogenum*.

Mechanism of action: All β-lactam antibiotics inhibit bacterial wall synthesis, resulting in formation of cell wall deficient bacteria. Such bacteria undergo lysis. Thus, penicillins are bactericidal.

Classification

1. Narrow spectrum penicillin (β-lactamase sensitive, natural)

a. Acid labile: Penicillin G (benzyl penicillin), procaine penicillin, benzathine penicillin
b. Acid-resistant alternative to penicillin G: Phenoxymethyl penicillin (penicillin V).

2. Penicillinase (β-lactamase sensitive, antistaphylococcal) resistant penicillins.

a. Acid labile: Methicillin, nafcillin
b. Acid-resistant: Cloxacillin, dicloxacin, flucloxacillin.

3. Extended spectrum penicillins

a. Acid labile (antipseudomonal): Carboxypenicillins (carbenicillin, ticarcillin); Ureidopenicillins (piperacillin, mezlocillin, azlocillin).
b. Acid-resistant: Aminopenicillins: Ampicillin, amoxicillin, bacampicillin, talampicillin.

4. β-lactamase inhibitors *(HNBG Uni., July 2016):* Clavulanic acid, sulbactam, tazobactam.

1. **Penicillin G (benzyl penicillin):** Penicillin G (PnG) has a narrow antibacterial spectrum, is effective against Gram-positive cocci and bacilli and a few Gram-negative cocci. Many organisms like staphylococci produce a penicillinase which is a β-lactamase, which opens β-lactam ring and inactivates penicillins.

Pharmacokinetics: PnG is destroyed by gastric juice; Food interferes with its absorption. It has a short t½ of 30 min. It is excreted by kidneys. Probenecid blocks renal tubular secretion of penicillin, prolongs its duration of action.

Preparations and dose: PnG is mainly given parenterally though orally effective form—potassium PnG is also available. Procaine penicillin is given 12–24 hr; Single injection of benzathine penicillin is effective for 3–4 weeks.

Adverse effects: Hypersensitivity, local pain, thrombophlebitis, suprainfections, *Jarisch-Herxheimer reaction* (when PnG is injected in a syphilitic patient, the sudden destruction of spirochetes releases lytic products, resulting in fever, myalgia, shivering, exacerbation of syphilitic lesions and vascular collapse).

Uses: Penicillin G is antibiotic of choice for several infections unless the patient is allergic to it.

a. Orodental infections.
b. Other infections: Pneumococcal infections; Streptococcal infections; Meningococcal infections;

Syphilis; Anaerobic infections; Actinomycosis; Gas gangrene; Anthrax, trench mouth, rat bite fever and Listeria infections.

c. **Prophylactic uses:** Rheumatic fever benzathine penicillin 1.2 MU/month prevents; Gonorrhoea and syphilis; Valvular heart diseases.

Disadvantages of natural penicillins: Orally not effective; Narrow spectrum of activity; Susceptible to β-lactamase; Hypersensitivity.

To overcome this, semisynthetic penicillins have been introduced. Semisynthetic penicillins are produced by chemically combining specific side chains or by incorporating specific precursors.

2. **Acid-resistant alternative to penicillin-G (PnG).**
   (i) Phenoxymethyl penicillin (penicillin V): It is acid stable oral absorption is better. The antibacterial spectrum of penicillin V is identical to PnG.
   Dose: 250–500 mg q6h.

1. **Penicillinase-resistant penicillins:** These congeners have side chains that protect β-lactam ring from attack by staphylococcal penicillinase. These drugs are not resistant to Gram-negative β-lactamases.
   i. **Methicillin:** It is highly penicillinase resistant, must be injected. Haematuria, albuminuria and reversible interstitial nephritis are specific adverse effects of methicillin.
   ii. **Cloxacillin:** It is highly penicillinase as well as acid resistant. It is less active against PnG sensitive organisms.
   Dose: 0.25–0.5 g orally every 6 hours; 0.25–1 g IM or IV.

2. **Extended spectrum penicillins:** These semisynthetic penicillins are active against a variety of Gram-negative bacilli as well.
   1. Aminopenicillins: This group has an amino substitution in the side chain. None is resistant to penicillinase or other β-lactamases.
      i. **Ampicillin:** It is active against all organisms sensitive to PnG; in addition, many gram-negative bacilli, e.g. *H. influenzae, E. coli,* Proteus, Salmonella and Shigella. Ampicillin is not degraded by gastric acid; oral absorption is incomplete but adequate. Food interferes with absorption. It is partly excreted in bile and reabsorbed, enterohepatic circulation occurs. However, primary channel of excretion is kidney, but tubular secretion is slower than for PnG; plasma t½ is 1 hr.
      Dose: 0.5–2 g oral/IM/IV depending on severity of infection, every 6 hours; children 25–50 mg/kg/day.

Uses: Urinary tract infections, meningitis, gonorrhea (drug of choice; DOC); Respiratory tract infections; Typhoid fever; Bacillary dysentery; Cholecystitis; SABE; Oro-dental infections; Septicemias and mixed infections.
Adverse effects: Diarrhoea, rashes, hypersensitivity reactions.

ii. **Bacampicillin:** It is an ester prodrug of ampicillin which is nearly completely absorbed from GIT, and is largely hydrolyzed during absorption. Tissue penetration is better and incidence of diarrhoea is lower.
   Dose: 400–800 mg BD.

iii. **Amoxicillin** *(NTR Uni., June 2017)*: It is a close congener of ampicillin (but not a prodrug); similar to it in all respects *except:*
   • Oral absorption is better; Food does not interfere with absorption; Higher and more sustained blood levels are produced.
   • Incidence of diarrhoea is lower.
   • It is less active against Shigella and *H. influenzae.*
   Dose: 0.25–1 g TDS; Oral/IM

2. **Carboxypenicillins**
   i. **Carbenicillin:** It is active against *Pseudomonas aeruginosa* and indole positive Proteus but neither penicillinase-resistant nor acid resistant. It is inactive orally and is excreted rapidly in urine (t½–1 hr). It is used as sodium salt in a dose of 1–2 g IM or 1–5 g IV q4–6 hr. High doses have also caused bleeding by interfering with platelet function.
   ii. **Ticarcillin:** It is more potent than carbenicillin against Pseudomonas.

3. **Ureidopenicillins**
   i. **Piperacillin:** This antipseudomonal penicillin is about 8 times more active than carbenicillin. It has good activity against Klebsiella and is used mainly in neutropenic/immunocompromised patients having serious Gram-negative infections, and in burns. Elimination t½ is 1 hour. Concurrent use of gentamicin or tobramycin is advised.
   Dose: 100–150 mg/kg/d in 3 divided doses (max. 16 g/day) IM/IV.
   ii. **Mezlocillin:** It has activity similar to ticarcillin against Pseudomonas and inhibits Klebsiella as well. It is given parenterally primarily for infections caused by enteric bacilli.

4. **β-lactamase inhibitors:** β-lactamase inhibitors bind to and inactivate β-lactamases preventing destruction of β-lactam antibiotics.
   i. Clavulanic acid inhibits β-lactamases and is combined with amoxicillin for both oral and

parenteral administration. It extends the anti-bacterial spectrum of amoxicillin and the combination inhibits organisms like β-lactamase producing staphylococci, gonococci, *E. coli* and *H. influenzae*. The combination is used for mixed aerobic-anaerobic infections including orodental infections, gonorrhoea and nosocomial infections. Clavulanic acid is also combined with ticarcillin.

ii. Sulbactam is combined with ampicillin. It is given parenterally for mixed aerobic-anaerobic infections including orodental, intra-abdominal, gynaecological, surgical, pelvic and other infections.

iii. Tazobactam is combined with piperacillin for parenteral administration.

They are available in fixed combinations.

Q. 7. Write a short note on cephalosporins.
(TNMGR, Sept. 2008; HP Uni., April 2019)

Ans. Cephalosporins are a group of semi-synthetic antibiotics derived from 'cephalosporin-C' obtained from a fungus Cephalosporium. The nucleus consists of a β-lactam ring fused to a dihydrothiazine ring (7-aminocephalosporanic acid). All cephalosporins are bactericidal and have same mechanism of action as penicillin. However, they bind to different proteins than those which bind penicillins.

- **First generation cephalosporins:** These were developed in the 1960s, have high activity against Gram-positive cocci but weaker against Gram-negative bacteria.

Parenteral	Oral
Cephalothin	Cephalexin
Cefazolin	Cephradine
Cefapirin	Cefadroxil
Cephradine	

- **Second generation cephalosporins:** These were developed subsequent to the first generation compounds and are more active against Gram-negative organisms, with some members active against anaerobes, but none inhibits *P. aeruginosa*.

Parenteral	Oral
Cefuroxime	Cefprozil
Cefoxitin	Cefuroxime axetil
Cefmetazole	
Cefotetan	

- **Third generation cephalosporins:** These compounds introduced in the 1980s have highly augmented activity against Gram-negative Enterobacteriaceae; some inhibit Pseudomonas as well. All are highly resistant to β-lactamases from Gram-negative

bacteria. However, they are less active on Gram-positive cocci and anaerobes.

Parenteral	Oral
Cefotaxime	Cefixime
Ceftazidime	Cefpodoxime proxetil
Ceftriaxone	Cefdinir

- **Fourth generation cephalosporins:** Similar coverage as third generation cephalosporins but with additional coverage against Gram-negative bacteria with a mechanism of resistance.

  Parenteral: Cefepime, cefpirome.

- **Fifth generation cephalosporins:** They have coverage against methicillin-resistant staphylococci (MRSA) and penicillin-resistant pneumococci.

  Parenteral: Ceftarolin

Mechanism of action: Bacteria synthesize a cell wall by cross-linking peptidoglycan using penicillin-binding proteins (PBP, transpeptidase). The beta-lactam rings bind to the penicillin-binding protein and inhibit its normal activity. Unable to synthesize a cell wall, the bacteria die.

Adverse effects: Pain after injection, thrombophlebitis, diarrhoea, hypersensitivity reactions, nephrotoxicity, drug-induce immune hemolytic anemia (DIIHA), pseudomembranous colitis, *disulfiram-like interaction* with alcohol.

Contraindications: Patients with known allergy to cephalosporins or other beta-lactams antibiotics. Ceftriaxone is contraindicated in hyperbilirubinemic neonates and infants <28 days old if they are expected to receive any calcium product.

Uses

1. As alternatives to PnG; Particularly in allergic patients.
2. Respiratory, urinary and soft tissue infections caused by Gram-negative organisms.
3. Penicillinase producing staphylococcal infections.
4. Septicemias caused by Gram-negative organisms.
5. Surgical prophylaxis.
6. Meningitis, gonorrhea, typhoid.
7. Mixed aerobic-anaerobic infections in cancer patients.
8. Hospital acquired infections.
9. Prophylaxis and treatment of infections in neutropenic patients.

Q. 8. Write a short note on ciprofloxacin.
(TNMGR, Oct. 2000)

Ans. Ciprofloxacin is the most potent (bactericidal) first generation fluoroquinolones (FQs) active against broad range of bacteria.

Highly susceptible organism: Aerobic Gram-negative bacilli, e.g. *E.coli*, *K. pneumoniae*, *Salmonella* sp., Shigella, *N. gonorrhoeae*, *H. influenzae*, etc.

Moderately susceptible: *P. aeruginosa*, *Staph. aureus*, *Bacillus anthracis*, *M. tuberculosis*, etc.

Mechanism of action: FQs inhibit DNA replication by inhibiting the enzyme bacterial DNA gyrase, which nicks double-stranded DNA, introduces negative super coils and then reseals the nicked ends. DNA gyrase consists of two A and two B subunits: A subunit carries out nicking of DNA, B subunit introduces negative super coils and then A subunit reseals the strands. FQs bind to A subunit with high affinity and interfere with its strand cutting and resealing function.

In **Gram-positive bacteria**, major target of FQ action is a similar enzyme topoisomerase IV which nicks and separates daughter DNA strands after DNA replication. The bactericidal action probably results from digestion of DNA by exonucleases whose production is signaled by the damaged DNA.

In **mammalian cells,** possess an enzyme topoisomerase II (that also removes positive super coils) which has very low affinity for FQs—hence low toxicity to host cells.

Mechanism of resistance: Resistance is due to chromosomal mutation producing a DNA gyrase or topoisomerase IV with reduced affinity for FQs, or due to reduced permeability/increased efflux of these drugs across bacterial membranes.

The remarkable microbiological features of ciprofloxacin (also other FQs) are:

• Rapidly bactericidal activity and high potency.
• Relatively long post-antibiotic effect on Enterobacteriaceae, Pseudomonas and Staph.
• Low frequency of mutational resistance.
• Low propensity to select plasmid type resistant mutants.
• Protective intestinal streptococci and anaerobes are spared.
• Active against many β-lactam and aminoglycoside resistant bacteria.
• Less active at acidic pH.

Pharmacokinetics: Ciprofloxacin is rapidly absorbed orally, but food delays absorption, and first pass metabolism occurs. It is excreted primarily in urine; Urinary and biliary concentrations are 10–50 folds higher than plasma.

Adverse effects: Gastrointestinal: Nausea, vomiting, bad taste, anorexia; CNS: Dizziness, headache, restlessness, anxiety, insomnia, impairment of concentration and dexterity, tremor, peripheral neuropathy, seizures; Skin/hypersensitivity: Rash, pruritus, photosensitivity, urticaria, swelling of lips, drug-induced bullous pemphigoid, etc.; Tendonitis and tendon rupture.

Contraindications: Hypersensitivity, myasthenia gravis, concurrent use of tizanidine.

Uses: Gonorrhoea, typhoid (DOC); Urinary tract infections, chancroid, bacteria gastroenteritis, bone, soft tissue, gynecological and wound infections; Respiratory infections; Tuberculosis; Meningitis; Prophylaxis of infections in netropenic/cancer patients; Conjuctivitis.

Dose: Oral: 250–750 mg BD. 200–400 mg BD; IV.

Q. 9. Write a short note on aminoglycoside.
(TNMGR, Oct. 2011)

Ans. These are a group of natural and semi-synthetic antibiotics having polybasic amino groups linked glycosidically to two or more amino sugar (streptidine, 2-deoxy streptamine, garosamine) residues. All aminoglycosides are produced by soil actinomycetes.

A. **Systemic aminoglycoside:** Streptomycin, amikacin, gentamicin, sisomicin, kanamycin, netilmicin, tobramycin.

B. **Topical aminoglycoside:** Neomycin, framycetin.

C. **Newer aminoglycoside:** Plazomicin, arbekacin.

Properties

1. All are used as sulfate salts, which are highly water soluble; Solutions are stable for months.
2. They ionize in solution; Not absorbed orally; Do not penetrate brain or CSF.
3. All are excreted unchanged in urine by glomerular filtration.
4. All are bactericidal and more active at alkaline pH.
5. They act by interfering with bacterial protein synthesis.
6. All are active primarily against aerobic Gram-negative bacilli like *E. coli*, Proteus, Pseudomonas, Brucella, Salmonella, Shigella and Klebsiella.
7. There is only partial cross resistance among them.
8. They have relatively narrow margin of safety.
9. All exhibit ototoxicity and nephrotoxicity.

Pharmacokinetics: Aminoglycosides are not absorbed from gut but when instilled into body cavities or applied over large wounds, they may get rapidly absorbed. Following IM injection, peak levels are seen in 60 minutes. They are not bound to plasma proteins and do not enter cells or cross barriers.

Mechanism of action: They diffuse across the outer coat of Gram-negative bacteria through porin channels.

Inside the bacterial cell, streptomycin binds to 30S ribosome, but other aminoglycoside bind to additional sites on 50S subunit, as well as to 30–50S interface. They freeze initiation of protein synthesis, prevent polysome formation and promote their disaggregation to monosomes so that only one ribosome is attached to each strand of mRNA (protein inhibition).

Mechanism of resistance

- Acquisition of cell membrane bound inactivating enzymes (most important).
- Low affinity of ribosomes—acquired by mutation.
- Decrease in permeability to the antibiotic.

Uses

1. Serious, life-threatening Gram-negative infection.
2. Complicated skin, bone or soft tissue infection, urinary tract infection.
3. Septicemia, endocarditis and neonatal sepsis.
4. Peritonitis and other severe intra-abdominal infections.
5. Mycobacterium infection.
6. Ocular infections, otits externa (topical)

Shared toxicities

1. **Ototoxicity:** Vestibular or cochlear part may be affected. Headache is usually first to appear, followed by nausea, vomiting, dizziness, nystagmus, vertigo and ataxia.
2. **Nephrotoxicity:** It manifests as tubular damage resulting in loss of urinary concentrating power, low GFR, nitrogen retention, albuminuria and casts.
3. **Neuromuscular blockade:** All aminoglycoside reduce acetylcholine release from the motor nerve endings.

Precautions and interactions

1. Avoid aminoglycoside during pregnancy: Risk of fetal ototoxicity.
2. Avoid concurrent use of other ototoxic drugs, e.g. high ceiling diuretics, minocycline.
3. Avoid concurrent use of other nephrotoxic drugs, e.g. amphotericin B, vancomycin, cyclosporine and cisplatin.
4. Cautious use in patients past middle age and in those with kidney damage.
5. Cautious use of muscle relaxants in patients receiving an aminoglycoside.
6. Do not mix aminoglycoside with any drug in the same syringe/infusion bottle.

Q. 10. Write a short note on metronidazole.

(TNMGR, March 2008, Oct. 2012; AHSUC, July 2016)

Ans. It is the prototype nitroimidazole, and one of the mainstay drugs for the treatment of anaerobic bacterial infections, protozoal infections, and microaerophilic bacterial infections. It is cytotoxic to facultative anaerobic microorganisms.

Mechanism of action: Metronidazole is a prodrug. Susceptible microorganisms reduce the nitro group of metronidazole by a nitroreductase and convert it to a cytotoxic derivative which binds to DNA and inhibits protein synthesis. Aerobic bacteria lack this nitroreductase and are therefore not susceptible to metronidazole.

Pharmacokinetics: Metronidazole is almost completely absorbed from small intestines. It is widely distributed in body, attaining therapeutic concentration in vaginal secretion, semen, saliva and CSF. It is metabolized in liver primarily by oxidation and glucuronide conjugation, and excreted in urine. Plasma t½ is 8 hours.

Adverse effects: Anorexia, nausea, metallic taste, confusion, peripheral neuropathy, abdominal cramps, headache, stomatitis, glossitis and furry tongue.

Contraindications: Known hypersensitivity, neurological disease, blood dyscrasias, first trimester of pregnancy and chronic alcoholism.

Interactions: A disulfiram-like intolerance to alcohol. Enzyme inducers may reduce its therapeutic effect. Cimetidine can reduce metronidazole metabolism. Metronidazole enhances warfarin action by inhibiting its metabolism.

Uses

1. Amoebiasis: Metronidazole is a first line drug for all forms of amoebic infection. For invasive dysentery and liver abscess: 800 mg TDS (children 30–50 mg/kg/d) for 7–10 days. For mild intestinal disease: 400 mg TDS for 5–7 days.
2. Giardiasis: 400 mg TDS for 7 days.
3. *Trichomonas vaginitis:* It is the drug of choice; 400 mg TDS for 7 days.
4. Anaerobic bacterial infections.
5. Pseudomembranous enterocolitis due to *C. difficile* is generally associated with use of antibiotics. Oral metronidazole 800 mg TDS is effective.
6. Ulcerative Gingivitis, trench mouth/Vincent angina: 200–400 mg TDS (15–30 mg/kg/day).
7. Guinea worm infestation.
8. *Helicobacter pylori* eradication:
   - **Triple regimen:** Metronidazole (500 mg) TDS combined with clarithromycin (500 mg) BD and a standard-dose or double-dose proton pump inhibitor (PPI) BD; for 14 days.
   - **Quadruple regimen:** Metronidazole (250 mg) QID or (500 mg) TDS/QID in combination with

Bismuth subsalicylate (300–524 mg) or bismuth subsalicylate (120–300 mg) QID, tetracycline (500 mg) QID, and a standard-dose PPI, BD; for 10–14 days

- **Concomitant regimen:** Metronidazole (500 mg) BD in combination with clarithromycin (500 mg) BD, amoxicillin (1 g) BD, and a standard-dose PPI, BD; for 10–14 days.

- **Uses in oral infections** (NTR Uni., May 2019): Odontogenic infections like acute periapical abscess, periodontitis, acute ulcerative gingivitis, pericoronitis and other oral infections and salivary gland infections are treated with metronidazole (200–400 mg TDS) in combination with an antibiotic effective against aerobes like a penicillin or a macrolide. Clindamycin being effective against Gram-positive and anaerobic bacteria is an alternative.

Q. 11. Write a short essay on azithromycin.
(RUHS, July 2016)

Ans. Azithromycin belongs to macrolides antimicrobials along with erythromycin, clarithromycin, roxithromycin and spiramycin.

Mechanism of action: Inhibits protein synthesis by reversibly binding to 50S ribosomal subunit by inhibiting translocation of mRNA. It is bacteriostatic at low and cidal at high concentration.

Spectrum of activity: Narrow spectrum, effective against aerobic Gram-positive bacteria and a few gram-negative organisms. Streptococci, pneumococci, staphylococci, gonococci, *C. diphtheriae*, *C. jejuni*, Mycoplasma, Chlamydiae and some atypical mycobacteria are sensitive.

Bacterial resistance: It develops by Methylation of a guanine residue on ribosomal RNA which leads to lower affinity for macrolides.

Pharmacokinetics: Acid stable, food decreases absorption. It accumulates in neutrophils, macrophages, fibroblasts and has large volume of distribution and longest $t\frac{1}{2}$ >40 hr. Excretion is through bile as active drug.

Adverse effects: Anorexia, nausea, vomiting, ototoxicity, eosinophilia, rash, pseudomembranous colitis.

Contraindications: Prolonged QT interval, patient on antiarrhythmics, pregnancy

Dose: 500 mg OD (Day 1) → 250 mg OD (Day 2–5)

Uses: Food borne illness; Bacteremia; Meningitis; Acute bacterial infection; Sinusitis; Chancroid; Non-gonococcal infections; Atypical pneumonia; Orodental infections, as an alternative to penicillin.

Q. 12. Discuss briefly antibiotic prophylaxis recent protocol.
(TNMGR, April 2000; RGUHS, Nov. 2011; HP Uni., May 2017; NTR Uni., May 2019)

Ans. Infective endocarditis (IE), also called bacterial endocarditis (BE), is an infection caused by bacteria that enter the bloodstream and settle in the heart lining, a heart valve or a blood vessel (Table 5.12).

Antibiotics before dental procedures are only recommended for patients with highest risk of IE, those who have:

1. Prosthetic heart valve or who have had a heart valve repaired with prosthetic material.
2. History of endocarditis.
3. Heart transplant with abnormal heart valve function.
4. Certain congenital heart defects including:
   - Cyanotic congenital heart disease that has not been fully repaired, including children who have had a surgical shunts and conduits.
   - Congenital heart defect that's been completely repaired with prosthetic material or a device for the first six months after the repair procedure.
   - Repaired congenital heart disease with residual defects, such as persisting leaks or abnormal flow

Table 5.12: Guidelines to use antibiotic prophylaxis by American Heart Association (AHA), 2007

Sl. No.	Patient category	Oral medications	Non-oral medications* (IM/IV)
1.	Adults, not allergic to penicillin	Amoxicillin (2 g)	Ampicillin (2 g) or cefazolin/
2.	Adults, penicillin allergic	Clindamycin (600 mg)/cephalexin (2 g) or azithromycin/clarithromycin (500 mg)	Ceftriaxone (1 g) clindamycin (600 mg) or cefazolin (1 g)
3.	Children, not allergic to penicillin	Amoxicillin (50 mg/kg)[†]	Ampicillin (50 mg/kg) or cefazolin/ ceftriaxone (50 mg/kg)[†]
4.	Children, penicillin allergic	Clindamycin (20 mg/kg) or cephalexin/ cefadroxil (50 mg/kg) or azithromycin/ clarithromycin (15 mg/kg)	Clindamycin (20 mg/kg) or cefazolin/ceftriaxone (50 mg/kg)

*For patients who are unable to take oral medications; Oral drugs are given 1 hour before procedure; Parenteral drugs 30 min prior to procedure.

[†]The total pediatric dose calculated by weight should not exceed the adult dose.

at or adjacent to a prosthetic patch or prosthetic device.

Dental procedures: Prophylaxis is recommended for the patients identified in the previous section for all dental procedures that involve manipulation of gingival tissue or periapical region of teeth, or perforation of oral mucosa.

Q. 13. Write a note on probiotics. *(RUHS, June 2017)*

Ans. Probiotics are "live microorganisms which when administered in adequate amounts confer a health benefit to the host": Food and Agriculture Organization of United Nations (FAO) and WHO.

Prebiotics are selectively fermented ingredients that result in specific changes in the composition and/or activity of gastrointestinal microbiota, thus conferring benefit(s) upon host health. Synbiotics are products that contain both probiotics and prebiotics.

Composition: Probiotics can be bacteria, molds or yeast. Among bacteria, lactic acid bacteria are more popular, e.g. *Lactobacillus acidophilus, L. casei, L. lactis, L. salivarius, L. plantarum, L. bulgaricus, L. rhamnosus, L. reuteri, L. fermentum, Strept. thermophilus, E. faecium, E. faecalis, Bifidobacterium breve, B. longum,* and *Saccharomyces boulardii.*

Features of probiotics: Non-pathogenic, non-toxic, resistant to gastric acid, adhere to gut epithelial tissue and produce antibacterial substances.

Mechanisms of action: Modulation of host immune response leading to strengthening of resistance to pathogenic challenge and alteration of composition and metabolic activity of host micro-flora at the specific location.

Probiotics products

1. A culture concentrate added to a beverage or food (such as a fruit juice).
2. Inoculated into prebiotic fibers.
3. Inoculants into a milk-based food.
4. As concentrated and dried cells packaged as dietary supplements such as powder, capsule, gelatin tablets.

Indications: Rotavirus diarrhea, reduction of antibiotic-associated side effects, food allergies and lactose intolerance, actopic eczema, prevention of vaginitis, urogenital infections, irritable/inflammatory bowel syndrome, cystic fibrosis, Traveler's diarrhea, *H. pylori* infection, various cancers.

Probiotics and oral cavity

1. In periodontal infection: Probiotics decrease pH of oral cavity so that plaque bacteria cannot form dental plaque and calculus that causes the periodontal disease.
2. In halitosis: By fixating on the toxic gases (volatile sulfur compounds) and changing them to gases needed for metabolism.
3. In dental caries: By replacing cariogenic bacteria with non-cariogenic bacteria.
4. In oral candidiasis: Lactobacilli probiotics inhibit growth of *C. albicans* due to low pH milieu produced by them.
5. Probiotics and voice prosthesis: Probiotics reduces occurrence of pathogenic bacteria in voice prosthetic biofilms.

Side effects and risks: Mild, such as gas or bloating. More serious effects in people with underlying health conditions.

Q. 14. Write a note on antifungal agents.
(TNMGR, Oct. 2003; BFUHS, May 2011; AHSUC, May 2017)

Ans. An antifungal agent is a drug that selectively eliminates fungal pathogens from a host with minimal toxicity to the host.

Classification

1. Antibiotics

A. Polyenes: They bind with ergosterol and cause membrane disruption, loss of potassium ions and decrease in ATPase, e.g. amphotericin B (AMB), nystatin, hamycin, natamycin (pimaricin).

B. Heterocyclic benzofuran: Mitotic spindle poison, e.g. griseofulvin.

2. Antimetabolite (pyrimidine derivatives): They inhibit both DNA and RNA synthesis via the intra-cytoplasmic conversion of 5-fluorocytosine to 5-fluorouracil. e.g flucytosine (5-FC).

3. Azoles: Broad spectrum; Antibacterial, antiprotozoal, anthelminthic, and antifungal. Mechanism of Action: Inhibit the fungal cytochrome P450 enzyme, (α-demethylase) which is responsible for converting lanosterol to ergosterol (main sterol in fungal cell membrane). Inhibition of mitochondrial cytochrome oxidase leading to accumulation of peroxides that causes auto digestion of the fungus. Imidazole may alter RNA and DNA metabolism

A. **Imidazole (topical):** Clotrimazole, econazole, miconazole, oxiconazole, mebendazole, isoconaole, sertaconazole, thiabendazole, bifonazole, buto-conazole, fenticonazole, sulconazole, tiaconazole, ketoconazole.

B. **Triazoles (systemic):** Fluconazole, itraconazole, voriconazole, ravuconazole, posaconazole.

4. Allylamine: Interfere with early step of ergosterol biosynthesis, e.g. terbinafine, naftifine, butenafine, tolnaftate.

5. Morpholine: Interfere with later step of ergosterol biosynthesis, e.g. amorolfine.

6. Echinocandins: Inhibits β(1,3) glucan synthesis, blocking cell wall synthesis, e.g. caspofungin, micafungin, anidulafungin.

7. Other topical agents: Undecylenic acid, benzoic acid, quiniodochlor, ciclopiroxolamine, butenafine, sodium thiosulfate, potassium iodide.

Q. 15. Write a short note on antitubercular drugs.

(HP, May 2008)

Ans. Tuberculosis is a chronic granulomatous disease caused by *Mycobacterium tuberculosis*.

Drugs used in tuberculosis (antitubercular drugs):

First line drugs: Kills active bacteria in early stages of infection.

1. Isoniazid (H), inhibits synthesis of mycolic acid. Dose: 300–400 mg.
2. Rifampin (R), inhibits RNA synthesis. Dose: 450–600 mg.
3. Pyrazinamide (Z), inhibits cell wall synthesis by interacting gene encoding fatty acid synthesis. Dose: 1200–1500 mg.
4. Ethambutol (E), inhibits mycobacterial arabinosyl transferase. Dose: 800–1000 mg.
5. Streptomycin (S): Inhibition of protein synthesis by misreading of code on mRNA. Dose: 750–1000 mg.

Second line drugs: These drugs hinder bacterial growth have either low antitubercular efficacy or high toxicity or both; are used in special circumstances only, e.g. thiacetazone (Tzn), para-aminosalicylic acid (PAS), ethionamide (Etm), cycloserine (Cys), kanamycin (Kmc), amikacin (Am), capreomycin (Cpr). Newer drugs: Ciprofloxacin, ofloxacin, clarithromycin, azithromycin, rifabutin.

Regimen: Standard regimens

1. **Regimen 1:** Isoniazid, rifampin, pyrazinamide and ethambutol or streptomycin for 2 months followed by isoniazid and rifampin for 4 months.
2. **Regimen 2:** Isoniazid, rifampin, pyrazinamide for 2 months followed by isoniazid and rifampin for 7 months.

DOTS: Directly observed treatment short course (WHO): For noncompliant patient.

Q. 16. Write a short note on antisyphilitic drugs.

(BFUHS, May 2011)

Ans. A substance that is used in the treatment of syphilis.

1. Primary, secondary or early latent: Penicillin G benzathine (single dose of 2.4 mU IM). If allergic to penicillin: Tetracycline hydrochloride (500 mg QID) or doxycycline (100 mg BID) for 2 weeks.
2. Neurosyphilis: Aqueous PnG (18–24 mU/day IV, given as 3–4 mU, q4h, for 10–14 days).
3. Syphilis in pregnancy: According to stage.

Q. 17. Write a short note on antiviral drugs.

(NTR Uni., May 2008; PAHER, May 2014)

Ans. Antivirals (AV) are a class of medications that are used to treat viral infections.

Classification

1. **Anti-herpes virus:** Idoxuridine, acyclovir, valacyclovir, penciclovir, famciclovir, ganciclovir, valganciclovir, foscarnet.
2. **Anti-retrovirus (for HIV)** *(RGUHS, October 2010)*
   a. **Nucleoside reverse transcriptase inhibitors (NRTIs):** Zidovudine (AZT), didanosine, zalcitabine, stavudine, lamivudine, abacavir.
   b. **Non-nucleoside reverse transcriptase inhibitors (NNRTIs):** Nevirapine, efavirenz, delavirdine.
   c. **Protease inhibitors (PIs):** Ritonavir, indinavir, nelfinavir, saquinavir, amprenavir, lopinavir.
   d. **Nucleotide reverse transcriptase inhibitors (NTRTI):** Tenofovir.
3. **Anti-Influenza virus:** Amantadine, rimantadine
4. **Nonselective antiviral drugs:** Ribavirin, adefovir dipivoxil, interferon-α.

Q. 18. Write a short note on chemotherapy for oral cancer.

(TNMGR, March 2007; NTR Uni., May 2008; BFUHS, Nov. 2013)

Ans. Chemotherapy is administration of one or more cytotoxic drugs to destroy or inhibit the growth and division of malignant cells in the treatment of cancer. Chemotherapy is either used as primary treatment modality or in combination with radiation, where it is used as radiation sensitizer (primary chemoradiation)

Types

1. **Induction chemotherapy:** Given before other definitive local therapies. Objective is to promote initial tumour reduction, and provide early treatment of micrometastases. *(Docetaxel, Cisplatin, 5-FU.)*
2. **Concurrent chemotherapy:** Simultaneous with other therapy like radiotherapy is now the standard protocol treatment.
3. **Adjuvant chemotherapy:** It is given after the local therapy.

Standard chemotherapy for metastatic disease: Cisplatin or carboplatin combined with 5-FU docetaxel, paclitaxel.

Agents used for the chemotherapy of oral cancer are:

1. Methotrexate.
2. Bleomycin.

3. Taxol and derivatives.
4. Platinum derivatives (cisplatin, carboplatin).
5. 5-fluorouracil.
6. Ifosphamide
7. Newer target directed agents: EGFR, bevacizumab, erlotinib, capecitabine, interferon α-2b.
8. **Non-platinum based:** Gemcitabine paclitaxel, docetaxel, panitumumab (human monoclonal antibody), cetuximab, nivolumab, pembrolizumab, atezolizumab (programmed cell death-1 inhibitor), small molecule tyrosine kinase inhibitors (gefitinib, afatinib, sunitinib, erlotinib).

All chemotherapeutic agents act by interfering with cell division. For treating cancer, majority of the agents exploit kinetic differences between normal and malignant cells by acting preferentially on the cells that are dividing at a faster rate.

Side effects: Myelosuppression, leukopenia, thrombocytopenia, anaemia, nausea, vomiting, diarrhoea, mucositis, dermatitis, alopecia.

Q. 19. Write a short note on antimetabolites.

(TNMGR, Oct. 2013)

Ans. Antimetabolites are defined as cytotoxic agents, which interfere with the synthesis of DNA constituents. They competitively inhibit utilization of the normal substrate or get themselves incorporated forming dysfunctional macromolecules.

Classification
1. **Folate antagonist:** Methotrexate (Mtx).
2. **Purine antagonist:** 6-Mercaptopurine (6-MP), 6-thioguanine (6-TG), azathioprine, fludarabine.
3. **Pyrimidine antagonist:** 5-Fluorouracil (5-FU), cytarabine (cytosine arabinoside).

1. Folate antagonist

Methotrexate (Mtx): It binds to dihydrofolate reductase (DHFR) and prevents the formation of tetrahydrofolate (THF). This THF is a coenzyme essential in several reactions in protein synthesis. The deficiency results in inhibition of protein synthesis.

Cytotoxic actions: Methotrexate mainly affects bone marrow, skin and gastrointestinal mucosa and other rapidly dividing cells. It also has immunosuppressant and some anti-inflammatory properties.

Methotrexate toxicity can be largely prevented by administering folinic acid. This folinic acid (**leucovorin or citrovorum factor**) gets converted to a form of THF that can be utilized by the cells.

Methotrexate is absorbed orally, 50% plasma protein bound, little metabolized and largely excreted unchanged in urine.

Methotrexate is apparently curative in choriocarcinoma: 15–30 mg/day for 5 days orally or 20–40 mg/m^2 BSA IM or IV twice weekly.

It is highly effective in maintaining remission in children with acute leukemias (2.5–15 mg/day). It is also useful in other malignancies, rheumatoid arthritis, psoriasis and as immunosuppressant.

2. Purine antagonists

- **6-Mercaptopurine (6-MP) and 6-thioguanine (6-TG):** Purine antagonists enter the cells and get converted to active metabolites (triphosphates in most compounds) which are incorporated into DNA. They cause breakages in DNA strands and inhibit protein synthesis. They are especially useful in childhood acute leukemia, choriocarcinoma and have been employed in some solid tumors as well.

- **Azathioprine:** It has marked effect on T lymphocytes; suppresses cell-mediated immunity (CMI) and is used primarily as immunosuppressant in organ transplantation, rheumatoid arthritis, etc. Azathioprine and 6-MP are metabolized by xanthine oxidase; their metabolism is inhibited by allopurinol. Methylation by thiopurine methyl transferase (TPMT) is an additional pathway of 6-MP metabolism. Toxicity of azathioprine is also enhanced in TPMT deficiency.

The main toxic effect of antipurines is bone marrow depression. Mercaptopurine causes more nausea and vomiting than 6-TG. It also produces a high incidence of reversible jaundice. Hyperuricaemia occurs with both. 6-Mercaptopurine: 2.5 mg/kg/day, half dose for maintenance.

3. Pyrimidine antagonists:
Pyrimidine antagonists have varied applications as antineoplastic, antifungal and antipsoriatic agents.

- **5-Fluorouracil (5-FU):** It inhibits the enzyme thymidylate synthetase due to which it inhibits the synthesis of thymine and thereby inhibits DNA synthesis. It is used in carcinoma of the stomach, colon, rectum, breast and ovaries.

Dose: 1 g orally on alternate days (6 doses) then 1 g weekly or 12 mg/kg/day IV for 4 days to 6 mg/kg IV on alternate days.

It has been particularly used for many solid tumors—breast, colon, urinary bladder, liver, etc. Topical application in cutaneous basal cell carcinoma has yielded gratifying results.

Cytarabine: It is phosphorylated in the body to the corresponding nucleotide which inhibits DNA synthesis. It also interferes with DNA repair. Its main use is to induce remission in acute leukemia in children, also in adults. Other uses are: Hodgkin's disease and non-Hodgkin lymphoma.

Dose: 1.5–3 mg/kg IV BD for 5–10 days.

Q. 20. Write a note on immunomodulatory drugs.

Ans. Immunomodulatory drugs modify the response of immune system by increasing (immunostimulator) or decreasing (immunosuppressive) the production of serum antibodies. Immunostimulators are prescribed to enhance the immune response against infectious diseases, tumours, primary or secondary immunodeficiency, and alterations in antibody transfer, among others. Immunosuppressive drugs are used to reduce the immune response against transplanted organs and to treat autoimmune diseases such as pemphigus, lupus, or allergies.

Classification:

1. Bacterial and fungal products: BCG, muramyl dipeptide, LPS, *Propionibacterium* spp., glucan.
2. Thymic factors: Thymosins.
3. Synthetic drugs: Levamisole, isoprinosine.
4. Polyclonal antibodies: Specific antibodies.
5. Recombinant cytokines: IL-1, IL-2, IL-12, IFN-γ.
6. Monoclonal antibodies: Specific antibodies.
7. Vaccines: Antigens.

Mechanisms of action: Immunomodulators selectively inhibit or intensify the specific populations and subpopulations of immune responsive cells, i.e. lymphocytes, macrophages, neutrophils, natural killer (NK) cells, and cytotoxic T lymphocytes (CTL). Immunomodulators affect the cells producing soluble mediators such as cytokines. Thus, in immunotherapy the immune system is targeted in order to help the healing of a given disease.

Adverse effects: Increase the risk of infection/opportunistic infections.

Q. 21. Write a short note on hydroxychloroquine.

Ans. Hydroxychloroquine (HCQ) belongs to the group of antimalarial agents, with immunomodulatory effects.

Mechanisms of action

- Interference with lysosomal acidification and inhibition of proteolysis, chemotaxis, phagocytosis, and antigen presentation.
- Decreasing macrophage-mediated cytokine production, especially interleukin (IL)-1 and IL-6.
- Inhibition of phospholipase A_2 and thereby antagonizing the effects of prostaglandins.
- Absorption and blocking of UV light cutaneous reactions.
- Binding and stabilizing DNA.
- Inhibition of T and B cell receptors calcium signaling.
- Inhibition of matrix metalloproteinases.

Therapeutic indications

1. Malaria (acute): 800 mg followed by 400 mg at 6, 24, and 48 hours.
2. Rheumatoid arthritis: 400–600 mg/day.
3. SLE: 200–400 mg/day.
4. Palindromic rheumatism: 200–400 mg/day.
5. Eosinophilic fasciitis: 400 mg/day.
6. Dermatomyositis: 400 mg/day.
7. Sjögren's syndrome: 6–7 mg/kg/day.
8. Porphyria cutanea tarda: 250–500 mg/week.
9. Polymorphous light eruption: 200–400 mg/day.
10. Granuloma annulare: 2–9 mg/gk/day.
11. Lichen planus: 200–400 mg/day.
12. Lupus panniculitis: 200–400 mg/day.
13. Discoid lupus: 400 mg/day

    Antimicrobial effects: Antibacterial in *Coxiella burnetii* infections; In HIV, HCQ inhibit virus replication in T cells, by inhibiting the surface envelope glycoprotein 120. Severe acute respiratory syndrome-coronavirus-2 (**SARS-CoV-2**) has caused a pandemic of coronavirus disease (**COVID-19**) 2019–2020. HCQS has shown to inhibit replication and spread of corona virus *in vitro* and prevent infection with COVID-19.

14. Others indications: Improves lipid profile, antithrombotic effects, antineoplastic effects, kikuchi-fujimoto disease, sarcoidosis, sensory neuropathy syndrome.

Antimalarial toxicity: Hypersensitivity, retinopathy, irreversible retinopathy and ototoxicity.

Prophylaxis of COVID-19 (recent pandemic): As recommended by ICMR:

- All health care workers those who are involved in the care of suspected or confirmed cases of COVID-19: 400 mg twice a day on day 1, followed by 400 mg once weekly for next 7 weeks; to be taken with meals.
- Asymptomatic household contacts of laboratory confirmed cases may be prescribed 400 mg twice a day on day 1, followed by 400 mg once weekly for next 3 weeks; to be taken with meals.

Q. 22. Discuss the immunosuppressive drugs and their effects on oral tissue. *(RGUHS, April, 2006)*

Ans. Immunosuppressive agents are drugs that suppress the immune system and reduce the risk of rejection of foreign bodies such as transplant organs, also used as cancer chemotherapy.

I. Macrolides immunosuppressant: Cyclosporine, tacrolimus, sirolimus.

- **Effect on oral mucosa:** Increased risk of infections, cytochrome P-450 system alteration, gingival hyperplasia, may effect renal elimination of drugs, risk of neoplasm.

II. Antimetabolite drugs: Azathioprine, mycophenolate mofetil.

- **Effect on oral mucosa:** Increased risk of infections, risk of neoplasm, dental erosion due to gastric problem, petechial hemorrhages, profuse bleeding from gingiva on manipulation, increase risk of oral ulceration and periodontal breakdown.

III. Polyclonal antibody: Antithymocyte globulin, anti-lymphocyte globulin.

- **Effect on oral mucosa:** Increased risk of infections.

IV. Monoclonal antibody: Muromonab—CD3, daclizumab, basiliximab.

- **Effect on oral mucosa:** Increased risk of infections, risk of neoplasm.

V. Non-specific immunosuppressant: Corticosteroids.

- **Effect on oral mucosa:** Increased risk of osteoporosis, periodontal disease with an increased risk of tooth loss, increased risk of opportunistic infections, easy bruising of mucosa, poor wound healing, risk of neoplasm, steroid supplement needed during stressful procedure.

6. ANALGESICS AND ANTI-INFLAMMATORY

Q. 1. Write a note on NSAIDs used in dentistry.
(RGUHS, April, 2006; BFUHS, May 2009; UHSR, May 2016; Sumandeep Uni., June 2016; HP Uni., May 2017; TNMGR, May 2019)

Q. Classify analgesics. Discuss in detail newer analgesics. *(DYP Uni., May 2019)*

Ans. Analgesics: A drug that selectively relieves pain by acting on CNS or on peripheral pain mechanism, without significantly altering consciousness.

Anti-inflammatory: A drug or substance that reduces inflammation in the body.

Classification of analgesics

A. Opioid/narcotic/morphine-like analgesics: Act centrally.

1. **Natural opium alkaloids:** Morphine, codeine.
2. **Semi-synthetic:** Diacetylmorphine oxymorphone, pholcodeine.
3. **Synthetic:** Pethidine, fentanyl, methadone, dextropropoxyphene, ethoheptazine, tramadol.

B. Non-opioid/non-narcotic/aspirin-like analgesics/NSAIDs:

I. Nonselective COX inhibitors (traditional NSAIDs)
1. Salicylates: Aspirin.
2. Propionic acid derivatives: Ibuprofen, naproxen, ketoprofen, flurbiprofen.

3. Anthranilic acid derivatives: Mefenamic acid.
4. Aryl-acetic acid derivatives: Diclofenac, aceclofenac.
5. Oxicam derivatives: Piroxicam, tinoxicam.
6. Pyrrolo-pyrrole derivative: Ketorolac.
7. Indole derivatives: Indomethacin
8. Pyrazolone derivatives: Phenylbutazone, oxyphenbutazone.

II. Preferential COX-2 inhibitors: Nimesulide, meloxicam, nebumetone.

III. Selective COX-2 inhibitors: Celecoxib, etoricoxib, parecoxib.

IV. Analgesics-antipyretics with poor anti-inflammatory action

1. **Para-aminophenol derivative:** Paracetamol (acetaminophen).
2. **Pyrazolone derivatives:** Metamizole (dipyrone), propiphenazone.
3. **Benzoxazocaine derivatives:** Nefopam.

Mechanism of action of NSAIDs: Prostaglandins (PGs), prostacyclin (PGI_2) and thromboxane A_2 (TXA_2) are produced from arachidonic acid by enzyme cyclooxygenase, which exists in a constitutive (COX-1) and an inducible (COX-2) isoforms; former serves physiological 'housekeeping' functions, while the latter, normally present in minute quantities, is induced by cytokines and other signal molecules at the site of inflammation → generation of PGs locally which mediate many of the inflammatory changes. Most NSAIDs inhibit COX-1 and COX-2 nonselectively, but now some selective COX-2 inhibitors have been produced. Aspirin inhibits COX irreversibly by acetylating one of its serine residues; return of COX activity depends on synthesis of fresh enzyme. Beneficial actions due to PG synthesis inhibition are: Analgesia, antipyresis, anti-inflammatory, antithrombotic, and closure of ductus arteriosus in newborn.

Other NSAIDs are competitive and reversible inhibitors of COX, return of activity depends on their dissociation from enzyme which is governed by pharmacokinetic characteristics of compound.

Pharmacokinetics: Salicylates are absorbed from stomach and upper small intestine. Particle size, pH of GIT, solubility of preparation and presence of food in stomach influence the absorption. Aspirin is deacetylated in liver, plasma and other tissues to release salicylic acid which is the active form. Plasma t½ of aspirin is 3–5 hours. Elimination follows first order kinetics in small doses and zero order kinetics in higher doses. Salicylates are excreted in urine.

Pharmacological actions (salicylates)

1. **Analgesia:** PGs induce hyperalgesia by affecting the transducing properties of free nerve endings. NSAIDs block the pain sensitizing mechanism induced by bradykinin, TNF-α, interleukins (ILs) and other algesic substances. They are, therefore, more effective against inflammation associated pain.

2. **Antipyresis:** NSAIDs reduce body temperature in fever, but do not cause hypothermia in normo-thermic individuals. Fever during infection is produced by pyrogens including, ILs, TNF-α, interferon's which induce PGE_2 production in hypothalamus, and hence raises its temperature set point. NSAIDs block the action of pyrogens.

3. **Anti-inflammatory:** Most important mechanism of anti-inflammatory action of NSAIDs is by inhibition of PGs synthesis at the site of injury. Certain NSAIDs may act by additional mechanisms including inhibition of expression/activity of some of these molecules and generation of superoxide/ other free radicals. Stabilization of leukocyte lyso-somal membrane and antagonism of certain actions of kinins may be contributing to NSAID action.

4. **Dysmenorrhoea:** NSAIDs lower uterine PG levels, afford excellent relief.

5. **Antiplatelet:** NSAIDs inhibit synthesis of both proaggregatory (TXA_2) and antiaggregatory (PGI_2) prostanoids, but effect on platelet TXA_2 (COX-1 generated) predominates. Therapeutic doses of most NSAIDs inhibit platelet aggregation so bleeding time is prolonged. Aspirin is highly active; it acetylates platelet COX irreversibly in the portal circulation before it is deacetylated by first pass metabolism in liver. Small doses are therefore able to exert antithrombotic effect for several days.

6. **Ductus arteriosus closure:** During fetal circulation ductus arteriosus is kept patent by local elaboration of PGE_2 and PGI_2. This can be closed by small doses of indomethacin or aspirin.

7. **Parturition:** Sudden spurt of PGs synthesis by uterus probably triggers labor and facilitates its progression. Accordingly, NSAIDs have the potential to delay and retard labor.

8. **Gastric mucosal damage:** Gastric pain, mucosal erosion/ulceration and blood loss are produced by all NSAIDs.

9. **Renal effects:** NSAIDs produce renal effects by at least 3 mechanisms:
   - COX-1 dependent impairment of renal blood flow and reduction of GFR which can worsen renal insufficiency.
   - Juxtaglomerular COX-2 dependent Na^+ and water retention.
   - Ability to cause papillary necrosis on habitual intake.

10. **Anaphylactoid reactions:** Aspirin precipitates asthma, angioneurotic swellings, urticaria or rhinitis in certain susceptible individuals.

Therapeutic uses (KUHS, Jan., 2014):

1. As antipyretics and analgesics in the treatment of gout, rheumatic fever, and rheumatoid arthritis. Commonly treated conditions requiring analgesia include headache, arthralgia, and myalgia.

2. Salicylic acid is used topically to treat corns, calluses, and epidermophytosis.

3. Methyl salicylate ("Oil of Wintergreen") is used externally as skin counterirritant in liniments.

4. Salicylates are used to inhibit platelet aggregation.

5. Low doses of aspirin are used prophylactically to decrease the incidence of transient ischemic attack and unstable angina.

6. In patent ductus arteriosus, familial colonic poly-posis, prevention of colon cancer and treatment of Barter's syndrome.

Adverse effects: Gastric (nausea, vomiting, gastritis/ peptic ulcer, occult blood loss); Hemolysis; Rashes, photosensitivity, nephrotoxicity, **Reye's syndrome** (fatal, fulminating hepatitis with cerebral edema in children when aspirin is given during viral infections); **Salicylism** (poisoning with salicylate); Acute salicylate intoxication.

Contraindications (HNBG Uni., July 2015): Bleeding tendencies, children with chickenpox or influenza, chronic liver disease, diabetics, pregnancy, breast feeding mothers, G6PD deficient individuals.

Dose: Analgesic: 300–600 mg q6–8h (q:every; h: hour); Anti-inflammatory: 4–6 g/d; Antiplatelet effects: 75–300 mg/d.

Newer analgesics

1. **Tapentadol immediate-release:** For treatment of moderate to severe pain. Tapentadol is both a μ-opioid agonist and a norepinephrine reuptake inhibitor. Dose: 50–100 mg

2. **Diclofenac potassium soft gelatin capsule (DPSGC):** It is formulated as a liquid-filled capsule using Prosorb technology and a gelatin-containing capsule shell. Drug is indicated for mild to moderate pain only in adults. Dose: 25 mg QID.

3. **Bupivacaine liposome injectable suspension:** Liposomal bupivacaine consists of multivesicular liposomes, which have multiple lipid bilayers that

are arranged like a honeycomb with bupivacaine in the aqueous cores. Bupivacaine concentration is 1.3% (or 13.3 mg/ml). It is indicated for postsurgical analgesia.

Q. 2. Write uses of opioids in dentistry.

(TNMGR, Sept. 2002)

Ans. Opioid analgesia occurs by activation of opioid receptors expressed on neurons in supraspinal sites, spinal sites and in peripheral tissue. Moderate to severe pain can be managed by combination of NSAID with opioids. In acute pain, opioids are not recommended. They are routinely used for chronic, intractable pain. They act as μ-receptor agonist and also mimic the effect of endogenous pain relieving chemicals. Opioids can be prescribed alone if the patient already has a prescription for an NSAID or is taking acetaminophen appropriately. When using these combination analgesics one should still follow the principle of maximizing the nonopioid before adding the opioid. If an opioid is necessary, codeine should be the first to consider. If codeine is insufficient, the next opioid to consider is oxycodone. Meperidine for dental pain should be reserved for the patient who is allergic to morphine and codeine derivatives, but who still requires an opioid. Hydromorphone is most potent, should be used only when all other measure has failed to relieved pain and that only for short duration. If acetaminophen is insufficient, opioids are considered acceptable during pregnancy provided they are given for a short duration. Chronic opioid use can result in fetal dependence, premature delivery and growth retardation. Opioids are considered safe in lactation. In elderly patients, opioid analgesics have an increased likelihood of more profound adverse effects as well as prolonged durations of action. Therefore, it is best not to select an opioid. If it is necessary, reduced doses must be utilized.

Effects of opioids are analgesia, antitussive, sedation, nausea, vomiting, constipation, mood alteration, respiratory depression, tolerance, physical dependence, addiction potential, miosis. Various opioids used are oxycodone (5–10 mg q46h), codeine sulfate (30–60 mg q46h), hydromorphone (2–4 mg q4h), meperidine (50–150 mg), pentazocine (50 mg q4h), tramadol (50–100 mg). Other uses are:

1. As analgesics: Opioids are indicated in severe pain of any type such as fracture of mandible.
2. In preanaesthetic medication: To allay anxiety; to produce pre- and postoperative analgesia; to reduce the dose of anaesthetic required.
3. In acute left ventricular failure.

4. As anxiolytic.
5. As anti-diarrheal.
6. As antitussive agent: Codeine and dextromethorphan are commonly used for dry cough.
7. As a part of conscious sedation: Fentanyl alone or with midazolam.

Contraindications: Severe chronic respiratory disease, inflammatory disease, concurrent use of alcohol.

Q. 3. Discuss the pharmacotherapy of orofacial pain.

(Nagpur Uni., 2002; RGUHS, April, 2006; TNMGR, March 2007)

Ans. Pain is defined as unpleasant sensory and emotional experience associated with actual or potential tissue damage or described in terms of such damage **(International Association for Study of Pain—IASP).** Orofacial pain can be:

1. **Nociceptive:** Because of tissue injury and inflammation, e.g. odontogenic infections, mucosal conditions, musculoskeletal conditions.
2. **Neuropathic:** Because of primary lesion or dysfunction of nervous system, e.g. cranial neuralgias, stomatodynia, phantom tooth pain.

Pharmacotherapy

A. **Nonsteroidal anti-inflammatory drugs:** Ibuprofen, naproxen, celecoxib, diflunisal, ketorolac, meloxicam.

Indication: Mild to moderate nociceptive pain, TMJ disorders.

B. **Opiate analgesics:** Oxycodone, codeine sulfate, tramadol, fentanyl.

Indications: Moderate to severe nociceptive pain.

C. **Adjuvant analgesics:** Carbamazepine, gabapentin, pregablin (anticonvulsants); Amitriptyline, nortriptyline, imipramine (antidepressants); Clonazepam, doxepin (anxiolytic); Baclofen, cyclobenzaprine, tizanidine (muscle relaxants).

Indications: Cranial neuralgia, traumatic neuropathy, neuropathic pain of unknown reason, burning mouth, myofascial pain.

D. **Topical analgesics:** Lidocaine, diphenhydramine, benzocaine, capsaicin.

Indications: Mucosal pain, superficial facial pain, stomatodynia.

Q. 4. Write a note on drugs used in management of trigeminal neuralgia.

(NTR Uni., June 2014)

Ans. Trigeminal neuralgia (TN) is defined as "Unilateral disorder characterized by brief electric shock-like pains, abrupt in onset and termination, and limited to the distribution of one or more divisions of the trigeminal nerve" **(International Headache Society—IHS, 2004).**

Classification: TN has been classified as (IHS):

1. Classic (essential or idiopathic) TN: Absence of a clinically evident neurological deficit.
2. Symptomatic TN: Caused by a demonstrable structural lesion other than vascular compression.

Pharmacological management

1. **First-line therapy:** Carbamazepine (200–1200 mg/day); Oxcarbazepine (600–1800 mg/day).
2. **Second-line treatment:** Lamotrigine (400 mg/day); Baclofen (40–80 mg/day); Pimozide (4–12 mg/day).
3. **Third-line treatment:** Gabapentin (300 mg–1800 mg); Pregablin (150–600 mg); Topiramate (100–400 mg); Levetiracetam (1000–4000 mg); Botulinum toxin A (25–75U).
4. **Others:** Phenytoin and IV phenytoin, fosphenytoin, clonazepam, valproic acid, misoprostol, tocainide (12 mg), topical capsaicin cream, intranasal lidocaine, tizanidine, sumatriptan, and amitriptyline.

Q. 5. Write a short note on surface analgesics.

Ans. Surface analgesics are the drugs used to relieve pain by direct application on the skin or mucous membrane. Surface or topical analgesics are mostly used as gels for application over painful muscles or joints. The drug penetrates the subjacent tissue attaining high concentrations in the affected muscle/joints, while maintaining low blood levels.

Types

1. **Counterirritants:** Topical pain medications that stimulate nerve endings when applied to the skin, and are used to treat musculoskeletal pain. Counterirritants produce hot, cold or tingling sensations. These new sensations are thought to interfere with the sensation of pain.
2. **Topical NSAIDs:** These often contain aspirin, though other forms are available as well. Topical NSAIDs penetrate the tissues beneath the skin with anti-inflammatory medication, reducing swelling at the pain site. They also inhibit pain transmission from sensory nerves. These topical pain medications are used to treat musculoskeletal pain.
3. **Capsaicin creams:** Capsaicin comes from hot peppers, and works to inhibit pain transmissions from sensory nerves in the skin. This topical pain medication can be used for musculoskeletal pain or neuropathic pain.
4. **Local anesthetics:** Patch forms of local anesthetics can be applied to the skin, and may be worn for several hours for pain relief. These topical medications can relieve certain types of neuropathic pain.

Indications: Osteoarthritis, sprains, backache, spondylitis, soft tissue rheumatism.

Advantages: Less gastrointestinal and other systemic adverse effects, bypassing of first pass hepatic metabolism.

Disadvantages: Less efficacious, benefit is difficult to assess, risk of skin/mucosa irritation or swelling, symptoms may worsen if applied in excess or for longer duration.

Q. 6. Write a short note on patient-controlled analgesia. *(NTR Uni., Oct. 2013)*

Ans. Patient-controlled analgesia (PCA) is a method of efficiently delivering pain relief at a patient's preferred dose and schedule by allowing them to administer a predetermined bolus dose of medication on-demand at the press of a button.

Modalities for PCA administration: Intravenous lines, central lines, epidural catheters, peripheral nerve catheters, transdermal delivery systems.

Advantage: More effective pain control with higher patient satisfaction.

Indications: PCA can be an option especially in patients who are unable to tolerate oral medications.

1. PCA can be used to reduce the stress of adhering to a predetermined dosing schedule of analgesics.
2. PCA can be useful in acute pain where there is inadequate pain control from initial opioid administration in emergency.
3. Patients with lower levels of constant chronic pain.
4. Post-surgical patients, especially those with indwelling nerve or epidural catheters.
5. Patients in labor pain.

Contraindications

Absolute

- Systemic infection, burns or trauma at the preferred site of PCA placement.
- Allergic reactions to the selected medication.
- Preexisting neural deficits in the area of a planned indwelling nerve catheter.
- Increased intracranial pressure for epidural catheter placement.

Relative: Chronic renal failure, patient on antithrombotic therapy or with bleeding disorder, OSA.

Medications

1. **Opioid medications:** Pure μ-opioid receptor agonists (morphine, fentanyl, hydromorphone, meperidine,

sufentanil, alfentanil, and remifentanil); µ-opioid receptor agonist-antagonists (butorphanol, nalbuphine, pentazocine); partial µ-opioid receptor agonists (buprenorphine, dezocine). Despite a variety of medication options, morphine remains the gold standard medication for intravenous PCA.

2. **Local anesthetics:** Sodium channel blockers (bupivacaine, levobupivacaine, and ropivacaine).

3. **Other medications:** Ketamine, naloxone, clonidine, magnesium, ketorolac, lidocaine, and droperidol.

7. DENTAL PHARMACOLOGY

Q. 1. Write about uses of antiseptics in dentistry.
(TNMGR, March 2002, HP Uni., May 2018)

Ans. Asepsis is the state of being free from disease causing microorganisms.

Antiseptics (surface disinfectant) are chemicals or products that destroy or inhibit the growth of microorganisms in or on living tissue.

Classification: Refer Microbiology section.

Antiseptics uses

a. As disinfectant of surgical instruments: Formaldehyde, lysol, oxycyanide of mercury, sodium hypochlorite.
b. As antiseptic wash and dressing: Cetrimide (1%), gentian violet (2–5%), methylene blue (1–3%).
c. As cleansing agent for wound: Hydrogen peroxide (10–20%), potassium permanganate (0.5%).
d. As preservative: Phenol or cresol (0.5%), sodium metabisulphite (0.05–0.1%).
e. As parasiticides: Salicylic acid (2%).
f. Insecticides: Pyrethrum.

Q. 2. Discuss the role of fluorides in caries prevention.
(MUHS, June 2017; AIIMS-CDER, May 2019; TNMGR, Oct. 2019)

Ans. The major route of fluoride absorption is through gastrointestinal tract. After absorption, fluoride is carried by blood and distributed to various tissues like teeth and bone; salivary glands; soft tissues. Fluoride level peaks 30 minutes after ingestion. The plasma half life is 4–10 hours. In plasma fluoride exists in two forms: Ionic and nonionic. About 99% of all fluorides in the human body are found in calcified tissues such as bone and teeth. 10–25% of daily intake of fluoride is not absorbed and is excreted in faeces. The elimination of absorbed fluoride occurs almost exclusively via the kidneys. The renal clearance of fluoride in the adult typically is 30–50 ml/min.

Mechanism of action

1. Conversion of hydroxyapatite to fluoridated hydroxyapatite → increase in enamels resistance to acid solubility.
2. Increased rate of post-eruptive maturation.
3. Antibacterial action by inhibiting enzymes required for cell metabolism and growth.
4. Alteration in plaque formation.
5. Alteration of tooth morphology.

Preparations

- Systemic: Fluoridated water, drops, tablets, milk, salt, fruits, vegetable, cereals, seafood, tea leaves.
- Topical: Mouth rinses, gels, foams, rinses saliva, gel, varnish, tablets, fluoride-containing prophylaxis paste, silver diamine fluoride.

Q. 3. Write a short note on anti-plaque agents.
(TNMGR, March 2007; BFUHS, Nov. 2009; NTR Uni., June 2015; May 2019)

Ans. Plaque is defined as a highly specific but variable structural entity formed by sequential colonization of microorganism on the tooth surface, epithelium and restorations **(WHO, 1978).**

Plaque can be controlled by: Mechanical (dentifrices and interdental cleansing aids) or chemical (antiplaque agents).

Antiplaque agents (APA)

Classification

I. First generation: They are capable of reducing plaque scores by about 20–50%. Exhibits poor retention within mouth.

a. **Triclosan:** Triclosan is available in dentifrices and mouth rinses. Triclosan is both a bisphenol and a nonionic germicide with low toxicity. It has broad spectrum of antibacterial activity and lack the staining effects of cationic agents. Triclosan also acts as an anti-inflammatory agent in mouth rinses. It acts on cytoplasmic membrane, induces leakage of cellular constituents leading to bacteriolysis.

b. **Metallic ions:** Zinc and copper, stannous. It reduces the glycolytic activity in bacteria and delays its growth.

c. **Quaternary ammonium compounds:** They are cationic antiseptics and surface active agents. Effective against Gram-positive organisms. The mechanism of action is related to their ability to rupture the cell wall and alter cytoplasmic contents, e.g. cetylpridinium chloride (CPC) of 0.05%. benzathonium chloride, benzalkonium chloride.

d. **Antibiotics:** Vancomycin, erythromycin, nidda-mycin and kanamycin, metronidazole, tetracycline, penicillin.

II. Second generation: Produce an overall plaque reduction of around 70–90% and better retained by the oral tissues.

1. **Bisbiguanide:** Chlorhexidine gluconate (0.2%), alexidine, octenidine.

2. **Enzymes:** Used as active agents, breaks down the formed matrix of plaques and calculus, e.g. mucinase, mutanase, dextranase, etc.

III. Third generation: They block binding of micro-organism to tooth or to each other. Compared to CHX, they do not exhibit good retentive properties.

Various APA agents are

1. **Delmopinol (0.1–0.2%):** It is a morpholinoethanol derivative. It acts by interfering with plaque matrix formation and reduction of bacterial adherence, therefore can be used as pre-brushing mouthrinse. Adverse effects include staining, taste disturbances, mucosal soreness and erosion.

2. **Povidone iodine (PVP-I):** Povidone-iodine is an iodophore and is microbicidal for Gram-positive and Gram-negative bacteria, fungi, Mycobacterium, virus, and protozoas.

3. **Salifluor:** Salifluor is a salicytonide (5n-octanoyl-3-trifeuoromethylsalicylanide), with both antibacterial and anti-inflammatory property.

4. **Natural products**
   a. Sanguinarin chloride: It is an alkaloid extract from blood root plant sanguinaria candensis. It is most effective against Gram-negative organisms, used in mouth rinse.
   b. Propolis or naturally occurring bee product consists of wax and plant extracts and contains flavones, flavanones and flavonls.
   c. Menthol, thymol.

5. **Miscellaneous agents:** Fluorides: Stannous fluo-rides; Alcohol is an ingredient of most mouth rinses with plaque altering abilities. Oxygenating agent: Such as hydrogen peroxide and buffered sodium peroxy-borate and peroxy-carbonate in mouth rinses have a beneficial effect on ANUG. Adverse effects include tissue injury, delayed wound healing, potential carcinogenic effects as well as *Candida albicans* overgrowth.

Q. 4. Write a short note on chlorhexidine.

(TNMGR, April 2003; NTR Uni., June 2014; BBD Uni., May 2019)

Ans. Chlorhexidine (CHX) is a cationic bisbiguanide antiseptic and gold standard in chemical plaque control with bacteriostatic and bactericidal actions. It is active against both Gram-positive and Gram-negative strains, fungi yeasts and viruses.

Available forms: Digluconate, acetate, hydrochloride salts.

Mechanism of action

A. **Antiplaque action**
- Prevents pellicle formation by blocking acidic groups on salivary glycoproteins thereby reducing glycoprotein adsorption on the tooth surface.
- Prevents adsorption of bacterial cell wall to the tooth surface.
- Prevents bonding of mature plaques.

B. **Antibacterial action**

a. **Bacteriostatic (low concentration):** Positively charges CHX molecules react with negatively charged bacterial cell wall, altering the integrity of cell membrane. CHX binds to inner membrane phospholipids and increase permeability (reversible effect). Its long lasting bacteriostatic action is known as "**Sustantivity**".

b. **Bactericidal action:** High concentration of CHX → progressive more damage to membrane → loss of large molecules → coagulation and precipitation of cytoplasm → vital cell activity ceases → cell death.

Dicationic CHX molecule attaches to the pellicle by one cation and to bacteria with other in attempt to colonize the tooth surface (**pin-cushion effect**). This prolongs its action.

Uses

1. As surgical scrub (hand antisepsis)
2. Neonatal bath
3. In obstetrics
4. General skin antiseptic
5. In ocular infections (0.02%)
6. As an adjunct to oral hygiene and professional prophylaxis.

- **For short-term applications**
1. An adjunct to mechanical plaque control
2. Post-oral surgery, periodontal surgery, root planning.
3. As an immediate prophylactic rinse in prevention of post-extraction bacteremia.
4. In recurrent oral ulceration.
5. Treatment of denture stomatitis patient and dry socket.
6. During therapy for oral infections and ANUG.

- **For intermittent term application**
1. For oral hygiene and gingival health in physically and mentally handicapped.

2. Medically compromised individuals predisposed to oral infections.
3. High caries risk patients.
4. Removable and fix orthodontic wearers.
5. Patients with extensive prosthetic reconstruction on abutment teeth with reduced periodontal support.
6. Dental implant patients.

- **For long-term application**
1. Patients who have decreased resistance to bacterial infection due to serious medical problems, e.g. agranulocytosis, leukemia, hemophilia, thrombocytopenia, kidney disease, bone marrow transplant, AIDS.
2. Patient under chemotherapy, radiation therapy, immunosuppressive drugs.
3. Patients with intermaxillary fixation.
4. Patients who are mentally challenged.
5. Patients with physical disability motor-function disturbance.
6. Geriatric patients.

Chlorhexidine is extensively used antiseptic in dentistry. Concentration used is 0.12–0.2%—as mouthwash. 0.5–1% in toothpaste/gel.

Side effects

1. Brown discoloration of teeth or restorations (due to release of pigment melanoidins, free sulphydryl groups)
2. Taste alteration (mainly salty)
3. Oral mucosa erosion.
4. Unilateral or bilateral parotid swelling (due to over vigorous rinsing)
5. Enhanced supragingival calculus formation (due to precipitation of salivary proteins)
6. Hypersensitivity (rare)
7. Idiosyncratic reaction

Dose: 10–15 ml twice daily oral rinse for 30 sec.

CHX Products: Mouthrinses, gels, sprays, toothpastes, varnishes, chewing gums, periodontal dressings.

Q. 5. Write a short note on disclosing agents.
(RGUHS, April 2007; HP, Aug. 2010; NTR Uni., April 2014)

Ans. Disclosing agents are preparations in liquid, tablet or lozenge, which contain dye or other coloring agents, which is used for the identification of bacterial plaque.

Uses

- Diagnosing the dental plaque.
- Personalized patient instruction and motivation.
- Self-evaluation by the patient.

- To evaluate effectiveness of oral hygiene maintenance.
- Preparation of plaque indices.

Ideal properties

1. Its taste should be comfortable to patient.
2. Intensity of colour should contrast to surrounding environment.
3. It should be retentive enough.
4. Non-irritating, non-allergic.
5. Antiseptic property.
6. The dye must be capable of adequately penetrating the plaque.
7. Selective staining efficacy
8. Water-soluble.

Mechanism of action: Dental plaque has ability to retain dyes because of polarity difference between plaque and dye. The dye binds to surface by electrostatic interactions and hydrogen bonds.

Dyes used are:

1. Iodine preparations: Skinner's iodine, diluted tincture of iodine; Plaque turns deep brown or black.
2. Mercurochrome preparations: Mercurochrome solution 5%.
3. Bismark brown (Easlick's disclosing solution).
4. Merbromin.
5. Erythrosine: Most widely used; causes red staining of plaque. Direct rinsing or topical application.
6. Fast green.
7. Fluorescent disclosing agent: 0.75% sodium fluorescein solutions; plaque appears *bright yellow* in normal light, intensive *yellow green* under blue light.
8. Two-tone solution: Multicoloring disclosing agent: Older (thicker) plaque stains blue, Newer (thinner) plaque stains red.
9. Basic fuchsin.

Disclosing agents are available tablet/liquids. The tablet is chewed, swished and spit out. Liquid is applied with the help of cotton applicator.

Q. 6. Write a short note on therapeutic uses of alcohol in dentistry.
(TNMGR, April 1998)

Ans. Alcohol has been both consumed as a beverage and used in medicine since time immemorial.

1. As antiseptic: Ethanol (60–90%).
2. Rubifacient and counter-irritant for sprains, joint pains, etc.
3. Rubbed into the skin to prevent bedsores.
4. Alcoholic sponges to reduce body temperature in fever.

5. Intractable neuralgias like trigeminal neuralgia and others: Injection of alcohol directly into the nerve trunks.
6. Severe cancer pain: Inj. of alcohol is used (50–100%).
7. To ward off cold—may benefit by causing vasodilatation of blanched mucosa.
8. As appetite stimulant and carminative.
9. Reflex stimulation in fainting-1 drop in nose.
10. To treat methanol poisoning.
11. As chemoembolization agent.
12. As sclerosing agent.

Q. 7. Discuss the drugs affecting orthodontic tooth movements. *(TNMGR, Oct. 2012; Sumandeep Uni., June 2017)*

Ans. During orthodontic treatment, drugs are prescribed to manage pain, TMJ problems and some infection throughout the course of treatment. Some of these drugs may have profound effects on short- and long-term outcomes of orthodontic practice.

A. Analgesics
1. NSAIDs like aspirin (COX inhibitor): Slows the tooth movement.
2. Selective NSAIDs (COX-2 inhibitor): No negative effect on tooth movement.
3. Acetaminophen (paracetamol): No effect on tooth movement.
4. Indomethacin: Slows the tooth movement.
5. Flurbiprofen: No significant effect on tooth movement.

B. Vitamin D: Enhances the rate of tooth movement.
C. Fluorides: Delay the tooth movement.
D. Bisphosphonates: Inhibit the tooth movement.

E. Hormones
1. Estrogens: Delay the tooth movement.
2. Thyroid hormones: Enhances the rate of tooth movement.
3. Relaxin: Enhances the rate of tooth movement.
4. Calcitonin: Inhibit the tooth movement.
5. Parathyroid hormone: Enhances the rate of tooth movement.

F. Corticosteroids: Enhances the rate of tooth movement.
G. Prostaglandins: Low concentration enhances tooth movement; whereas high concentration leads to root resorption.
H. Interleukin antagonists: Delay the tooth movement.
I. TNF-α antagonist: Delay the tooth movement.
J. Integrin inhibitors like echistatin: Inhibit tooth movement.
K. Immunomodulators: Delay the tooth movement.
L. Immunosuppressant: Delay the tooth movement.

M. Anticonvulsants: Makes the orthodontic treatment difficult because of gingival overgrowth, gingival bleeding, xerostomia.
N. Anticancer drugs: They damages precursor cell involved in bone remodeling, complicating the tooth movement.
O. Alcohol: Chronic alcoholics develop severe root resorption during orthodontic treatment.

Q. 8. Write a short note on sialogogues and anti-sialogogues. *(TNMGR, March 2007; KUHS, Dec. 2012; NTR Uni., April 2013)*

Ans. Sialogogues are the agents which activate muscarinic cholinergic receptors of the parasympathetic nervous system to increase salivary flow in patients with xerostomia.

A. Sialogogues
I. **Mechanical (masticatory) stimulant:** Xylitol, sorbitol, mannitol, aspartame, acesulfame K (gums and tablets).
II. **Chemical stimulants:** Alcohol-free mucopolysaccharide solution with citric acid, citric acid.
III. **Electrical stimulation:** Intra-oral electronic stimulator of salivary glands.
IV. **Oral moisturizers:** Carboxymethylcellulose, hydroxypropylmethylcellulose (solutions), water glycerin agent and glycerate polymer (gels).
V. **Pharmacologic stimulant:** Cholinergic stimulator:
　1. Pilocarpine: It is FDA approved sialogogue, especially after radiotherapy and in Sjögren's syndrome. It is a parasympathomimetic drug, acting as muscarinic agonist. **Dose:** 5–7.5 mg, TDS.
　2. Cevimeline: It is a parasympathomimetic drug, acting as muscarinic agonist. **Dose:** 30 mg, TDS.
　3. Bromhexine: Mucolytic agent, stimulate the salivary as well as lacrimal secretions.
　4. Anethole trithione: Mucolytic agent, increases salivary secretion by up regulating the muscarinic receptors.

B. Anti-sialogogues *(HP Uni., April 2019)*: These agents are used to decrease salivary secretion by cholinergic antagonist action. They decrease salivary secretion by inhibiting the action of myoepithelial cells in salivary glands.
1. Scopolamine transdermal patch: 0.3–0.6 mg
2. Glycopyrrolate: 1–2 mg q4–6 hr.
3. Atropine: 0.4–1.6 mg q4–6 hr.
4. Hyoscyamine: 0.125–0.75 mg
5. Diphenhydramine hydrochloride.
6. Amisulpride: 400 mg/day.

7. Methantheline: 50–100 mg
8. Propantheline: 15–30 mg
9. Clonidine: 0.2 mg
10. Probanthine: 7.5–15 mg
11. Robinul: 1–2 mg
12. Saltroine: 0.4 mg
13. Antipasbenty: 10–20 mg

Contraindication to antisialogogues: Glaucoma, prostatic hypertrophy, gastrointestinal disorders (ulcerative colitis, obstructive disease, intestinal atony), and myasthenia gravis.

Q. 9. Write a note on antioxidants.

(RGUHS, April 2007; Oct. 2010; TNMGR, Oct. 2011; Sumandeep Vidyapeeth, April 2011; BBD Uni., June 2016)

Ans. Antioxidants are compounds used by aerobic organisms for protection against oxidative stress, induced by free radicals and active oxygen species.

Classification

A. According to their location

1. **Extracellular antioxidants:** β-carotene, ascorbic acid, bilirubin, uric acid, ceruloplasmin, transferrin, superoxide dismutase enzyme-3, selenium glutathione peroxidase, reduced glutathione.
2. **Cell membrane associated:** α-tocopherol.
3. **Intra-cellular antioxidants:** Superoxide dismutase enzymes 1 and 2, catalase, glutathione peroxidase, DNA repair enzymes, reduced glutathione.

B. According to mode of action

1. **Preventative**
   a. **Enzymes:** Superoxide dismutase, catalase, glutathione peroxidase, glutathione reductase, glutathione transferase.
   b. **Metal ion sequestrators:** Albumin, lactoferrin, transferrin, ceruloplasmin, uric acid, polyphenolic flavonoids.
2. **Scavenging:** Ascorbate, carotenoids, uric acid, vit. E, bilirubin, reduced glutathione, other thiols.

C. According to their solubility

1. Water-soluble: Haptoglobin, ceruloplasmin, albumin, ascorbate, uric acid, polyphenolic flavonoids, reduced glutathione and other thiols, cysteine and transferrin.
2. Lipid Soluble: α-tocopherol, carotenoids, bilirubin, quinines.

Commonly used antioxidants are:

1. **Vitamin C:** Vitamin C works synergistically with vitamin E to quench free radicals and also regenerates the reduced form of vitamin E.

2. **Vitamin E:** Its antioxidant function mainly resides in the protection against lipid peroxidation. Vitamin E has been proposed for prevention against colon, prostate and breast cancers, some cardiovascular diseases, ischemia, cataract, arthritis and certain neurological disorders.

3. **β-carotene:** β-carotene is a strong antioxidant and is the best quencher of singlet oxygen.

4. **Selenium:** Selenium forms active site of several antioxidant enzymes including glutathione peroxidase. Similar to selenium, manganese and zinc also form an essential part of various antioxidant enzymes. Selenium is a trace mineral found in soil, water, vegetables (garlic, onion, grains, nuts, soybean), seafood, meat, liver, yeast.

5. **Lycopene:** Lycopene has been hypothesized to prevent carcinogenesis and atherogenesis by protecting critical cellular biomolecules, including lipids, lipoproteins, proteins, and DNA. Lycopene, when given in dose of 4.8 mg/day orally for 3 months leads to the reversal of dysplastic changes in leukoplakia and when given in dosage of 16 mg/day leads to substantial increase in mouth opening in OSMF. Major dietary source of lycopene is tomatoes with lycopene in cooked tomatoes are more bioavailable than that in raw tomatoes.

6. **Flavonoids:** They are polyphenolic compounds which are present in most plants. The main natural sources of flavonoids include green tea, grapes, apple, cocoa, ginkgo biloba, soybean, curcuma, berries, onion, and broccoli. They have been reported to prevent or delay a number of chronic and degenerative ailments such as cancer, cardiovascular diseases, arthritis, aging, cataract, memory loss, stroke, Alzheimer's disease, inflammation, infection. Green tea is a rich source of flavonoids, especially flavonols (catechins) and quercetin. Catechin levels are 4–5 times greater in green tea than in black tea. Many health benefits of green tea reside in its antioxidant, anticariogenic, anti-hypercholesterolemic, antibacterial (dental caries), anti-inflammatory activities.

7. **Omega-3 and omega-6 fatty acids:** They are essential long-chain polyunsaturated fatty acids. Dietary sources of omega-6 fatty acids (linoleic acid) include vegetable oils, nuts, cereals, eggs, and poultry. It is important to maintain an appropriate balance of omega-3 and omega-6 in the diet, as these two substances work together to promote health.

8. **Isoflavones:** These are found chiefly in soy products. Isoflavones are structural isomers of flavonoids and allocate biological properties with

them. They have anti-estrogenic effects, and thus could act as chemopreventive agents in hormone-dependent cancers.

9. **Curcumin:** This is a plant phenol widely used as a spice (curry) and food-coloring agent. *In vivo* and *in vitro* studies have demonstrated that it may prevent initiation of DNA damage and is involved in anti-promotion mechanisms such as apoptosis. A number of studies have shown that curcumin is effective in inhibiting carcinogenesis in the skin, colon, stomach mammary gland and oral cavity.

10. **Retinoid:** Best known retinoid is vitamin A or retinol. They are required for maintenance of normal cell growth and differentiation. In contrast to carotenoid, they act primarily in post-initiation phases of promotion and progression in carcinogenesis. Animal studies have shown that retinoid are potent to suppress or reverse epithelial carcinogenesis at several sites, especially oral carcinogenesis.

11. **Vitamin D:** Vitamin D inhibits proliferation and DNA synthesis, alters expression of several oncogenes, reduces lipid peroxidation and angiogenesis and induces differentiation. Epidemiologic studies support an inverse association among vitamin D intake and colorectal cancer risk.

12. **Folic acid:** It is majorly found in fresh fruits and vegetables. Together with vitamin B_{12}, methionine and choline, it is involved in methyl group metabolism. Much of the basic cancer research has focused on DNA methylation, and hypomethylation has been associated with DNA abnormalities. A converse association involving dietary folate intake and adenomatous polyps or colorectal cancer has been stated in both case-control and cohort studies.

13. **Antioxidant enzymes:** Superoxide dismutase, catalase, and glutathione peroxidase serve as primary line of defense in destroying free radicals.

14. **Polyphenols:** They exert their antioxidant effect by their direct antioxidant properties (e.g. by sparing vitamin E or by regenerating vitamin C) or to their inhibitory effect towards lipoxygenase.

15. **Coenzymes Q10:** It exists in an oxidized form (ubiquinone or CoQ) and a reduced form (ubiquinol or CoQH2) and both of them possess antioxidant activity. CoQ10 is also regarded as a pro-oxidant molecule in response to various pathophysiological events.

16. **Lazaroids:** They are a newly identified family of compounds which are derived from glucocorticoids but lack activity of both glucocorticoids and mineralocorticoids. These compounds scavenge lipid peroxyl radicals and inhibit iron-dependent lipid peroxidation by a mechanism similar to that of vitamin E.

17. **Recent antioxidant:** Phloretin, tetracurcuminoid and ferulic acid, including formulations applied topically, can neutralize cell-damaging free radicals, particularly those caused by UV rays, nicotine, alcohol, and hydrogen peroxide. Certain antioxidants, including phloretin, silymarin, and hesperetin, significantly inhibit the inflammatory response associated with *A. actinomycetem-comitans*. Lutein, dark green vegetables, lignan, oatmeal, barley, rye, grape seed or pine bark extracts can also provide powerful antioxidant protection for the body.

Mechanism of action of antioxidants: Antioxidants neutralize free radicals by donating one of their electrons, which ends the electron stealing reaction. The antioxidant nutrient, however, does not become a free radical by donating an electron because they are stable in either form.

Application in dentistry

I. Periodontology: Reactive oxygen species (ROS) cause periodontal tissue damage by ground substance degradation, collagenolysis either directly or indirectly or as a result of oxidation of proteases, stimulation of excessive pro-inflammatory cytokine release through NF-κβ activation, PG-E2 production via lipid peroxidation and superoxide release, both of them have been linked to bone resorption. Studies suggest that scaling stimulates increase in superoxide dismutase levels, various other antioxidants and total antioxidant capacity of saliva and thus can be considered as prognostic biomarkers of periodontal treatment. It has also been shown that antioxidant therapy can be used as an adjunct to the nonsurgical periodontal therapy.

II. Restorative dentistry: The elevated antioxidant—levels might provide protection against dental caries activity. The oxidative carbohydrate metabolism within the dental plaque might be adversely affected by these antioxidants and thus reducing bacterial activity and growth and consequently dental caries activity.

III. Orthodontics: Application of a topical antioxidant-essential oil gel has been shown to be an effective means of reducing inflammation in orthodontic patients with gingivitis. Bond strength of brackets bonded to bleached human tooth enamel can be increased by pine-bark extract.

IV. Implantology: Antioxidant supplementation with grape seed extract has positive effect on treating peri-implantitis.

V. Oral medicine: Oxidative damage plays a key role in pathogenesis of cancer by causing DNA damage. Antioxidant nutrients act to inhibit the development of cancer cells and destroy them through apoptosis, by stimulation of cytotoxic cytokines, by their action on gene expression, by preventing the development of tumor's necessary blood supply or by cellular differentiation.

- **Therapeutic use of antioxidants for oral lesions**
  1. Prevention of lesions in high-risk individuals with mucosa that clinically appears normal with no history of either premalignant or malignant lesion.
  2. Treatment of premalignant oral lesions.
  3. In patients who have had either premalignant or malignant oral lesions that have been successfully treated, in order to prevent recurrence of the treated initial lesion or to prevent the development of a second or a separate primary.

Q. 10. Drugs and gingival hyperplasia: List the drugs and their mechanism of action.

(TNMGR, Oct. 2012; Sumandeep Uni., April 2015)

Ans. Gingival hyperplasia or hypertrophy is an abnormal overgrowth of gingival tissues. Various drugs inducing gingival hyperplasia are:

I. Anticonvulsants: Phenytoin, sodium valproate, phenobarbitone, vigabatrin, primidone, mephenytoin, ethotoin, ethosuximide, methosuxinimide.

II. Immunosuppressant: Cyclosporine, tacrolimus, sirolimus.

III. Calcium channel blockers: Nifedipine, nitrendipine, felodipine, nicardipine, manidipine, amlodipine, nimodipine, nisoldipine, verapamil, diltiazem.

- **Mechanism of action**
  1. All the drugs induce an increase in epithelial cell proliferation due to overexpression of antigen Ki-67 and slight under expression of the CDK-inhibitors p27KIP1 and p21WAF1.
  2. Disruption of homeostasis of collagen synthesis and degradation in gingival connective tissue, predominantly through the inhibition of collagen phagocytosis of gingival fibroblasts.
  3. Existence of differential proportions of fibroblast subsets in each individual which exhibit a fibrogenic response to these medications.
  4. Synergistic enhancement of collagenous protein synthesis by human gingival fibroblasts.
  5. Negative effects on calcium ion influx across cell membranes, which interfere with the synthesis and function of collagenase.

Q. 11. Justify the importance of ozone therapy during management of pulp diseases. *(BFUHS, May, 2010)*

Ans. Ozone (O_3) is one of the most powerful antimicrobial agents available for use in dentistry.

Mechanism of action

1. **Effect on bacteria:** Ozone acts on bacterial cell membranes, by oxidation of their lipid and lipoprotein components and render the spores defective in germination.
2. **Effect on virus:** Ozone causes damage to polypeptide chains and envelope proteins impairing viral attachment capability, and breakage of viral RNA.
3. **Effect on fungal and protozoa:** Ozone inhibits cell growth at certain stages.
4. **Effect on blood cells:** Ozone reduces or eliminates clumping of RBCs and its flexibility is restored, along with oxygen carrying ability. There is a stimulation of production of glutathione peroxidase, catalase, and superoxide dismutase which act as free radical scavengers.
5. **Effect on leukocytes:** Ozone behaves as a weak cytokine such as TNF-α, IL-2, IL-6, IL-8, TGF-β inducer. Ozone reacts with the unsaturated fatty acids of the lipid layer in cellular membranes, forming H_2O_2, one of the most significant cytokine inducers.
6. **Platelets:** H_2O_2 generated by blood ozonation activate phospholipase C, phospholipase A_2, cyclooxygenases and lipooxygenases, and thromboxane synthetase, allowing a step increase of intracellular calcium, release of prostaglandin E_2, prostaglandin $F_{2\alpha}$, and thromboxane A_2 with irreversible platelet aggregation.

Modes of ozone administration: Ozone gas application with a silicone cup; Ozone aqueous solution; Ozone oil.

Advantages of topical ozone therapy

1. There is no chance of development of resistance oxidative challenges of ozone.
2. In addition, there is evidence that ozone directly inactivates bacterial toxins.

Uses

A. **Uses in endodontics:** The oxidative power of ozone characterizes it as an efficient antimicrobial. *In vitro* studies showed that ozone is effective over most of the bacteria found in cases of pulp necrosis. Ozone works best when there is less organic debris remaining. Therefore, the recommendation is to use either ozonated water or ozone gas at the end of cleaning and shaping process.

B. **Ozone therapy and dental caries:** Ozone therapy is used as an atraumatic treatment modality in dental practice. In small lesions, it showed a greater reduction in number of microorganisms than did larger lesions, and lesions closer to gingival margin. Non-cavitated lesions are more likely to reverse than cavitated lesions. It has been shown that the infusion of ozone into noncarious dentine prevented biofilm formation *in vitro* from *S. mutans* and *L. acidophilus* over a 4-week period. The longer the contact time, the better the microbiological killing rate.

C. **Ozone in management of hypersensitivity:** Ozone removes the smear layer, opens up the dentinal tubules, broadens their diameter and allows the calcium and fluoride ions to flow into the tubules easily, deeply and effectively to plug the dentinal tubules, preventing the fluid exchange through these tubules.

D. **Ozone in dental plaque:** Both caries and periodontal disease are caused primarily by plaque biofilm. Ozone might be useful to control oral infectious microorganisms in dental plaque. Ozonated water is effective in killing Gram-positive, Gram-negative bacteria and oral *C. albicans* causing periodontal disease. Ozonated water had nearly the same antimicrobial activity as 2.5% sodium hypochlorite.

E. **Ozone therapy in oral surgery:** Ozone has a positive influence on bone metabolism and reparative process of bone. Ozone therapy is found to be beneficial for treatment of refractory osteomyelitis in head and neck. Ozone therapy may stimulate cell proliferation and soft tissue healing of bone necrosis or in extraction sites in patients treated with bisphosphonates. Ozone kills the microorganisms causing peri-implantitis and shows a positive wound healing effect due to increase of tissue circulation. Application of ozone after tooth extraction reduced the post-extraction complications.

F. **Antimicrobial efficacy of ozone as denture cleaners:** Application of ozonated water may be useful in reducing the number of *C. albicans* on denture plates.

Contraindications: Pregnancy, severe anaemia, hyperthyroidism, thrombocytopenia, acute alcohol intoxication, recent myocardial infarction, hemorrhage from any organ, G6PD and ozone allergy.

8. HAEMATINICS, COAGULANTS AND ANTICOAGULANTS

Q. 1. Discuss coagulants. *(Sumandeep Vidyapeeth, April 2011; TNMGR, April 2012)*

Q. Mention the role of vitamin K in clotting mechanism. *(TNMGR, March 2007; Sumandeep Uni., April 2015)*

Ans. These are substances which promote coagulation and are indicated in hemorrhagic states. Fresh whole blood or plasma provide all the factors needed for coagulation and are the best therapy for deficiency of any clotting factor; also they act immediately. Other drugs used to restore haemostasis are:

1. **Vitamin K**
- K1 (from plants, fat soluble): Phytonadione (phylloquinone).
- K2 (purified fish): Menaquinone
- K3 (synthetic)
  - Fat-soluble: Menadione, acetomenaphthone.
  - Water-soluble: Menadione sodium bisulfite, menadione sodium diphosphate (K4)

2. **Miscellaneous:** Fibrinogen (human); Antihaemophilic factor; Desmopressin; Adrenochrome monosemicarbazone; Rutin; Ethamsylate.

A. **Vitamin K (clotting vitamin/antihemorrhagic factor):** It is a fat-soluble dietary principle required for synthesis of clotting factors.

Dietary sources: Green leafy vegetables, such as cabbage, spinach; and liver, cheese, nuts, etc.

Daily requirement: 50–100 µg/day.

Action: Vitamin K has an important role in post-translational modification of calcium binding proteins. Vitamin K acts as a cofactor for carboxylase enzyme that catalyzes the carboxylation glutamic acid, resulting in its conversion to gamma-carboxyglutamic acid (Gla).

Role of vitamin K in coagulation: Factors II, VII, IX, and X make up the core of the coagulation cascade. These factors are synthesized in the liver in the inactive form. They undergo post-translational modifications, gamma carboxylation of glutamic acid residues.

Use: Prophylaxis and treatment of bleeding due to deficiency of clotting factors in the following situations: Dietary deficiency of vit K, prolonged antimicrobial therapy, obstructive jaundice or malabsorption syndromes, liver disease, newborns, overdose of oral anticoagulants, hypoprothrombinaemia.

Toxicity: Rapid IV injection of emulsified vit. K produces flushing, breathlessness; constriction in the chest, fall in BP. Menadione and its water-soluble derivatives can cause haemolysis in a dose-dependent manner. In the newborn menadione or its salts can precipitate kernicterus.

B. **Fibrinogen:** To control bleeding in hemophilia, antihaemophilic globulin (AHG) deficiency and acute afibrinogenemic states; 0.5 g IV.

C. **Antihaemophilic factor:** It is indicated (along with human fibrinogen) in hemophilia and AHG deficiency. Dose: 5–10 U/kg IV infusion, repeated 6–12 hourly.

D. **Desmopressin:** It releases factor VIII and von Willebrand's factor from vascular endothelium and checks bleeding in hemophilia and von Willebrand's disease.

E. **Adrenochrome monosemicarbazone:** It is believed to reduce capillary fragility, control oozing from raw surfaces and prevent microvessel bleeding, e.g. epistaxis, haematuria, retinal hemorrhage, secondary hemorrhage from wounds, etc. Dose: 1–5 mg oral/ IM.

F. **Rutin:** It is a plant glycoside claimed to reduce capillary bleeding. It has been used in a dose of 60 mg BD-TDS along with vit. C.

G. **Ethamsylate:** It reduces capillary bleeding when platelets are adequate; probably exerts antihyaluronidase action, improves capillary wall stability, but does not stabilize fibrin (not an antifibrinolytic). Side effects are nausea, rash, headache, and fall in BP (only after IV injection). Dose: 250–500 mg TDS oral/IV.

Q. 2. What are the various haemostatic agents used in dentistry? *(TNMGR, April 1995; Oct. 2019; HP Uni., Aril 2019)*

Ans. Hemostasis is a process which causes bleeding to stop.

Styptics/local haemostatic is the substances used to stop bleeding from a local and approachable site. They are particularly effective on oozing surfaces, e.g. tooth socket, abrasions, etc.

1. **Absorbable materials:** Provide a meshwork which activates the clotting mechanism and checks bleeding. Left *in situ*, these materials are absorbed in 1–4 weeks, e.g. **fibrin (sheet or foam):** Prepared from human plasma; **Gelatin foam, and oxidized cellulose.**

2. **Thrombin:** It is obtained from bovine plasma, may be applied as dry powder or freshly prepared solution to the bleeding surface in hemophiliacs, e.g. bovine thrombin, pooled human plasma thrombin, recombinant thrombin.

3. **Vasoconstrictors:** They act by constricting blood vessels and decreasing their size. **0.1% Adr** solution may be soaked in sterile cotton-gauze and packed in the bleeding tooth socket or nose (in case of epistaxis) to check bleeding.

4. **Astringents:** Tannic acid or metallic salts (alum) are occasionally applied for bleeding gums, bleeding piles, etc. They act by precipitating proteins, hence toughening the surface. Styptics like ferric chloride and $Fe_2(SO_4)_3$ are concentrated forms of astringents, which cause superficial and local coagulation.

5. **Sclerosing agents:** Sodium tetradecyl sulfate, polidocanol. They are injected locally, acts as irritant, which causes inflammation followed by coagulation and fibrosis.

Q. 3. Write a short note on sclerosing agents.

Ans. Sclerotherapy is the use of physical, chemical, and biological properties of an agent used to disrupt target tissue which allows the formation of sclerosed or "hardened" byproducts that following therapy have drastically changed or diminished functions. They are used only for local injection.

1. Ethanol: Its mechanism of action is a combination of cytotoxic damage induced by the denaturation and extraction of surface proteins, hypertonic dehydration of cells, and coagulation and thrombosis when blood products are present. Dose: 1 ml/kg.

2. Sodium tetradecyl sulfate (STS) (3% with benzyl alcohol 2%): 0.5–2 ml at each site.

3. Ethanolamine oleate (5% in 25% glycerine and 2% benzyl alcohol): 1–5 ml inj.

4. Sclerodex: Combination of hypertonic saline (7%) and hypertonic glucose (70%).

5. N-butyl cyanoacrylate (NBCA).

6. Boiling contrast.

7. Sodium morrhuate (5%).

8. Polidocanol (3% inj): 2 ml.

9. Bleomycin.

10. OK 432 (picibanil): It is a natural killer cell activator. Biologic product created from the incubation of group A streptococcus with penicillin.

11. Others: Doxycycline, tetracycline, povidone-iodine, acetic acid, phenol, pantopaque, bismuth, albendazole infusion, and honey.

Q. 4. Write a short note on thrombolytic/anticoagulant drugs. *(TNMGR, March 2002, 2012; KLE Uni. Dec.2008; NTR Uni., April 2014; HP Uni., May 2018)*

Ans. Thrombolytics/fibrinolytics are drugs used to lyse thrombi/clot to recanalize occluded blood vessels. They are curative rather than prophylactic; work by activating the natural fibrinolytic system.

I. Anticoagulants: Used for treatment of arterial and venous thrombosis.

1. **Direct thrombin inhibitors:** Dabigatran, argatroban.

2. **Indirect thrombin inhibitors:** Fondaparinux, heparin (enoxaparin, UFH, LMWH)

3. **Vit. K epoxide reductase inhibitors:** Warfarin.

4. **Direct Xa inhibitors:** Rivaroxiban, apixaban.

II. Antiplatelet: Used for treatment of arterial disease.

1. **COX inhibitors:** Aspirin.

2. **Glycoprotein IIb/IIIa inhibitors:** Abciximab, eptifibatide, tirofiban.

3. **ADP inhibitors:** Clopidogrel, ticlopidine.

4. **Phosphodiesterase inhibitor:** Dipyridamol.

III. Thrombolytic: Used for treatment of arterial and venous thrombosis.

Plasminogen activators

1. **Streptokinase (Stk):** It is obtained from β-hemolytic streptococci group C. It is inactive as such, combines with circulating plasminogen to form an activator complex which then causes limited proteolysis of other plasminogen molecules to plasmin. Its t½ is 30–80 min. Streptokinase is antigenic; can cause hypersensitivity reactions and anaphylaxis.

2. **Urokinase:** It is an enzyme isolated from human urine; now prepared from cultured human kidney cells, which activates plasminogen directly and has a plasma t½ of 10–15 min. It is non-antigenic. Indicated in patients in whom streptokinase has been used for an earlier episode.

3. **Alteplase (recombinant tissue plasminogen activator (rt-PA):** Produced by recombinant DNA technology from human tissue culture, it specifically activates gel phase plasminogen already bound to fibrin, and has little action on circulating plasminogen. It is rapidly cleared by liver and has a plasma t½ of 4–8 min. It is non-antigenic, but nausea, mild hypotension and fever may occur. It is expensive.

4. **Tenecteplase:** It is a mutant variant of rt-PA with higher fibrin selectivity and longer duration of action. A single IV bolus dose (0.5 mg/kg) or split into two doses (30 min apart) is given. The clinical efficacy and risk of bleeding with reteplase and tenecteplase are similar to alteplase.

Uses of fibrinolytic

1. Acute myocardial infarction.

2. Deep vein thrombosis.

3. Pulmonary embolism.

4. Peripheral arterial occlusion.

5. Stroke.

Q. 5. Write about oral and parenteral iron preparations, their indications and toxicity.

(TNMGR, Oct. 1999, April 2012)

Ans. 1. Oral iron preparations

a. Ferrous sulfate (hydrated salt 20% iron, dried salt 32% iron): Cheapest, causes metallic taste in mouth, e.g. tablet Fersolate (200 mg).

b. Ferrous gluconate (12% iron), e.g. tab. Ferronicum (400 mg), Elixer (400 mg/15 ml).

c. Ferrous fumarate (33% iron): Less water-soluble, tasteless. Tab. Nori-A (200 mg).

d. Colloidal ferric hydroxide (50% iron), e.g. tab. Neoferum (200 mg).

e. Ferrous succinate (35% iron).

f. Iron choline citrate.

g. Iron calcium complex (5% iron).

h. Ferric ammonium citrate (scale iron).

i. Ferrous aminoate (10% iron).

j. Ferric glycerophosphate.

k. Iron hydroxyl polymaltose.

2. Parenteral iron preparation

a. Iron-dextran: 50 mg elemental iron/ml, e.g. imferon (2 ml).

b. Iron-sorbitol: Citric acid complex: 50 mg elemental iron/ml, e.g. Jectofer (1.5 ml).

Uses

1. **Iron deficiency anaemia:** It is the most important indication for medicinal iron. A rise in Hb level by 0.5–1 g/dl per week is an optimum response to iron therapy. It is faster in the beginning and when anaemia is severe.

2. **Megaloblastic anaemia:** When brisk haemopoiesis is induced by vit. B_{12} or folate therapy, iron deficiency may be unmasked.

3. **As an astringent:** Ferric chloride is used in throat paint.

Toxicity

Adverse effects of oral iron: Epigastric pain, heartburn, nausea, vomiting, staining of teeth, metallic taste, bloating, colic. Constipation is more common than diarrhea.

Adverse effects of parenteral iron: Local pain at site of IM injection, pigmentation of skin, sterile abscess, fever, headache, joint pains, flushing, palpitation, chest pain, dyspnoea, lymph node enlargement. A metallic taste in mouth lasting few hours occurs with iron-sorbitol injection.

9. ANTI-DIABETICS AND OTHER HORMONES

Q. 1. Write a short note on antidiabetic drugs.

(TNMGR, March 2011; BFUHS, Oct. 2011)

Q. Write a note on oral sulphonylurease.

(TNMGR, Nov. 2001, March 2007)

Ans. Drugs used to treat diabetes are known as Antidiabetic.

Classification of antidiabetic drugs

A. Insulin.

B. Oral hypoglycemic drugs

1. Sulphonylureas

a. **First generation:** Tolbutamide (500 mg), chlorpropamide (250–500 mg).

b. **Second generation:** Glibenclamide (5 mg), glipizide (2.5–10 mg), gliclazide (5–15 mg), glimepiride (1–4 mg).

2. Biguanide:
Reducing hepatic gluconeogenesis and lipogenesis as well as increasing insulin-mediated uptake of glucose in muscles, e.g. metformin (500–1000 mg).

3. Meglitinide analogue:
They enhance insulin release by blocking ATP-sensitive K^+ channels. Repaglinide (0.5–2 mg).

4. D-phenylalanine derivative:
Nateglinide (60–120 mg).

5. Thiazolidinediones:
Increase peripheral uptake of glucose, e.g. rosiglitazone (2–8 mg), pioglitazone (15–45 mg).

6. α-Glucosidase inhibitor:
By inhibiting polysaccharide reabsorption in intestine, e.g. acarbose (25–100 mg), miglitol (25–100 mg).

C. DPP-4 inhibitors:
By prolonging action of glucagon like peptide, e.g. sitagliptin (25–100 mg), saxagliptin (2.5–5 mg), vildagliptin (50 mg), linagliptin (5 mg).

D. SGLT2 inhibitors:
By inhibition of glucose reabsorption in renal glomeruli, e.g. dapagliflozin (500 mg) and canagliflozin (100 mg)

E. Cycloset:
By reversal of insulin resistance, e.g. bromocriptine (0.8 mg).

Mechanism of action of sulfonylureas: Sulfonylureas provoke a brisk release of insulin from pancreas. Sulfonylureas bind to receptors on pancreatic β cells, and block the ATP-sensitive K^+ channels. This reduced K^+ conductance causes depolarization and Ca^{++} influx leading to increased insulin secretion. Thus, some functional β cells are essential for their action.

Pharmacokinetics: All sulfonylureas are well absorbed orally, and are 90% or more bound to plasma proteins. Some are primarily metabolized, may produce active metabolite; others are mainly excreted unchanged in urine.

Interactions: Drugs that enhance sulfonylurea action (may precipitate hypoglycemia) are:

- Displace from protein binding: Phenylbutazone, sulfinpyrazone, salicylates, sulfonamides, PAS.
- Inhibit metabolism/excretion: Cimetidine, sulfonamides, warfarin, chloramphenicol, and acute alcohol intake.

- Synergize with or prolong pharmacodynamic action: Salicylates, propranolol, sympatholytic antihypertensive, lithium, theophylline, alcohol.

Drugs that decrease sulfonylurea action are:

- Induce metabolism: Phenobarbitone, phenytoin, rifampicin, chronic alcoholism.
- Opposite action/suppress insulin release: Corticosteroids, thiazides, furosemide, oral contraceptives.

Adverse effects

1. Hypoglycemia.
2. Nonspecific side effects: Nausea, vomiting, flatulence, diarrhoea or constipation, headache, paresthesias and weight gain.
3. Hypersensitivity: Rashes, photosensitivity, purpura, transient leucopenia, agranulocytosis.

Q. 2. Write a note on types of insulin.
(TNMGR, Oct. 2011)

Ans. In people with type 1 diabetes, the pancreas no longer makes insulin. In type 2 diabetes, insulin secretion is normal, but the body does not respond well to it. Insulin is metabolized in the liver, kidney and muscle.

Mechanism of action: Insulin acts by binding to specific receptors present on almost all cells in the body. This binding stimulates tyrosine kinase activity in the β subunit. This in turn activates a cascade of phosphorylation and dephosphorylation reactions which stimulate or inhibit the enzymes involved in the metabolic actions of insulin.

Insulin can be classified as:

A. Based on source: Bovine insulin; Porcine insulin; Human insulin (regular, lente, NPH).

B. Based on purity: Single peak insulin; Monocomponent insulin.

C. Based on onset and duration of action:

1. Ultra short (rapid) acting insulin: Insulin lispro, insulin aspart, insulin glulinase.
2. Short acting (regular) insulin: Human regular.
3. Intermediate acting insulin: Isophane insulin (NPH), lente.
4. Long acting insulin: Ultralente, protamine zinc insulin.

Use of insulin in diabetes mellitus: Insulin is effective in all types of diabetes mellitus. The dose should be adjusted as per the needs of each patient. **Insulin resistance** is said to be present when the insulin requirement is >200 U/day. It is due to the antibodies to insulin which partly neutralize it.

Side effects: Hypoglycemia, allergy, lipodystrophy, edema.

Q. 3. Write a short note on calcitonin.
(TNMGR, Nov. 2001)

Ans. Calcitonin/thyrocalcitonin is hypocalcemic protein hormone produced by parafollicular 'C' cells of thyroid. Parathyroid, thymus and cells of medullary carcinoma of thyroid also contain calcitonin. Synthesis and secretion of calcitonin is regulated by plasma Ca^{2+}. Plasma t½ of calcitonin is 10 min, but its action lasts for several hours.

Actions: Actions of calcitonin are generally opposite to that of PTH. It inhibits bone resorption by direct action on osteoclasts, decreasing their ruffled surface which forms contact with the resorptive pit. Calcitonin inhibits proximal tubular calcium and phosphate reabsorption by direct action on kidney. However, hypocalcaemia overrides the direct action by decreasing the total calcium filtered at the glomerulus, urinary Ca^{2+} is actually reduced.

Preparation and units: Synthetic salmon calcitonin is used clinically, because it is more potent due to slower metabolism. Human calcitonin has also been produced. 1 IU = 4 µg of standard preparation.

Adverse effects: Nausea, flushing, tingling of fingers, bad taste and allergic reaction.

Uses
1. Hypercalcaemic states: Hyperparathyroidism, hypervitaminosis D, osteolytic bony metastasis and hypercalcemia of malignancy; 4–8 IU/kg IM 6–12 hourly only for 2 days.
2. Postmenopausal osteoporosis: 100 IU SC or IM daily along with calcium and vit. D supplements.
3. Paget's disease: 100 U daily or on alternate days produces improvement for few months.

Q. 4. Write a note on pharmacology of drugs which affects calcium homeostasis.
(TNMGR, Nov. 1995, March 2008)

Q. Write a note on drugs which affect bone resorption.
(NTR Uni., May 2018)

Ans. Normal plasma calcium is 9–11 mg/dl (40% is bound to plasma proteins; 10% is complexed with citrate, phosphate and carbonate in an undissociable form; the remaining (about 50%) is ionized and physiologically important). Plasma calcium level precisely regulated by 3 hormones, viz. PTH, calcitonin and calcitriol (active form of vit D). These regulators control its intestinal absorption, exchange with bone and renal excretion. In addition, several other hormones, metabolites and drugs influence calcium homeostasis.

A. Influences affecting bone turnover: ↑ Bone resorption → ↑ in serum calcium level
- Corticosteroids.
- Parathormone.
- Thyroxine (excess).
- Hypervitaminosis D.
- Prostaglandin E_2.
- Interleukin-1 and interleukin-6.
- Alcoholism.
- Loop diuretics.

B. Influences affecting bone turnover: ↓ Bone resorption → ↓ in serum calcium level
- Androgens/estrogens
- Calcitonin
- Growth hormone
- Bisphosphonates
- Fluoride
- Gallium nitrate
- Mithramycin
- Thiazide diuretics

Preparations
1. Calcium chloride (27% Ca): Freely water-soluble but highly irritating, tissue necrosis occurs if injected IM or extravasation takes place during IV injection. Orally also the solution irritates.
2. Calcium gluconate (9% Ca): It is non-irritating to GIT and vascular endothelium. A sense of warmth is produced on IV injection; extravasation should be guarded. It is the preferred injectable salt.
3. Calcium lactate (13% Ca): Given orally, non-irritating and well tolerated.
4. Calcium dibasic phosphate (23% Ca): Insoluble reacts with HCl to form soluble chloride in the stomach. It is bland; used orally as antacid and to supplement calcium.
5. Calcium carbonate (40% Ca): Insoluble, tasteless and non-irritating. It has been used as antacid.

Side effects: Constipation, bloating and excess gas.

Use
1. **Tetany:** 10–20 ml of calcium gluconate (elemental calcium 90–180 mg) IV over 10 min, followed by slow IV infusion.
2. **As dietary supplement:** In growing children, pregnant, lactating and menopausal women. The dietary allowance recommended by National Institute of Health (1994) is:
- Children (1–10 yr): 0.8–1.2 g

- Young adult (11–24 yr), pregnant and lactating women: 1.2–1.5 g
- Men (25–65 yr), women (25–50 yr) and (51–65) yr if taking HRT: 1.0 g
- Women (51–65 yr) not taking HRT, every one >65 yr: 1.5 g

3. **Osteoporosis:** In the prevention and treatment of osteoporosis with HRT/raloxifene/alendronate.
4. **Empirically,** calcium gluconate IV has been used in dermatoses, paresthesias, weakness and other vague complaints.
5. **As antacid.**

Q. 5. Write a short note on bisphosphonates.

(UHSR, June 2017)

Ans. Bisphosphonates define a class of drugs that are widely indicated since the 1990s to treat osteoporosis both in men and women. Their effectiveness in treating osteoporosis and other conditions is related to their ability to inhibit bone resorption.

Types

1. **Nitrogen-containing bisphosphonates:** They are more potent.
   - **Oral:** Alendronate (35–40 mg), risedronate (35 mg), Ibandronate (150 mg).
   - **Intravenous:** Pamidronate (30–60 mg), zoledronic acid, ibandronate (3 mg).
2. **Non-nitrogen containing bisphosphonates** include etidronate, clodronate, and tiludronate; high potential to inhibit bone mineralization and causes osteomalacia.

Mechanism of action: They inhibit bone resorption by attaching to hydroxyapatite binding sites on the bone, and get released and impair the osteoclast's ability to continue bone resorption.

Indications

- **FDA-approved:** Osteoporosis in postmenopausal women, osteoporosis in men, glucocorticoid-induced osteoporosis, hypercalcemia of malignancy, paget disease of bone, and malignancies with metastasis to bone.
- **Non-FDA-approved:** Osteogenesis imperfecta, prevention of glucocorticoid-induced osteoporosis.

Contraindications: Hypersensitivity to bisphosphonates; Hypocalcaemia; Chronic kidney disease; Esophageal disorders; History of atypical femur fracture; History of bisphosphonate-related osteonecrosis of jaw (BRONJ).

Adverse effects

1. **GIT:** Gastrointestinal reflux, esophagitis, esophageal/gastric ulcers, and gastritis. Abdominal pain, diarrhea, and constipation.
2. **Infusion reaction:** Flu-like symptoms, fevers, myalgias, arthralgias, and headaches.
3. **Hypocalcaemia**
4. **Arthralgia and myalgia**
5. **Ocular:** Uveitis, conjunctivitis, and scleritis.
6. **Atypical femur fractures**
7. **Bisphosphonate-related osteonecrosis of jaw (BRONJ):** Risk factors for BRONJ include: Use of intravenous bisphosphonates, higher dose, prolonged duration of exposure, pre-existing dental disease, dental implants, dental extraction, and poorly fitting dentures, use of glucocorticoids and anticancer therapy, history of diabetes, smoking, and cancer.

Diagnostic criteria of BRONJ

- History of treatment with a bisphosphonate.
- Those who had >8 weeks of exposed bone in maxillofacial region.
- No radiation therapy to jaw.

Stages and management: By American Association of Oral and Maxillofacial Surgeons (AAOMS):

- **Stage 0:** Indicated by no visible bone but nonspecific symptoms. Symptomatic treatment and conservative management of underlying dental issues; antibiotics are recommended if the infection is present.
- **Stage 1:** Indicated by exposed, inflamed necrotic bone without symptoms. Common treatment includes antimicrobial rinses (if the infection is not present).
- **Stage 2:** Indicated by exposed, necrotic bone with local signs or symptoms of infection. Symptomatic treatment, antimicrobial rinses, and systemic antibiotics.
- **Stage 3:** Indicated by exposed, necrotic bone with pain and infection, pathologic fracture, extra-oral fistula, and extensive osteolysis. Symptomatic treatment, systemic antibiotics, and superficial surgical debridement of necrotic bone.

Dental implications and prevention

- Delay the initiation of bisphosphonate therapy for few months to allow healing, if an invasive dental procedure of jaw is planned.
- Stop bisphosphonate 2 months before dental procedure and resume them after jaw healing, in patients who have been on **bisphosphonates** for >4 years.
- When clinically appropriate, consider a drug holiday after 3–5 years of intravenous bisphosphonates and 5–10 years of oral bisphosphonates.

10. CORTICOSTEROIDS

Q. 1. Describe the regulatory mechanism of steroid secretions. Enlist the pharmacological actions of steroids. *(MUHS, May 2010; RGUHS, May 2011; RUHS, May 2018)*

Q. Write about indications for corticosteroid therapy. *(TNMGR, Oct. 1999; NTR Uni., May 2018)*

Ans: Corticosteroids are hormones produced in the cortex of the adrenal gland. Corticosteroids and their biologically active synthetic derivatives differ in their metabolic (glucocorticoid) and electrolyte-regulating (mineralocorticoid) activities.

Classification:

1. **Short-acting (8–12 hr):** Hydrocortisone (20 mg), cortisone (25 mg)
2. **Intermediate-acting (18–36 hr):** Prednisolone (5 mg), methylprednisolone (4 mg), triamcinolone (4 mg), fludrocortisone (2 mg)
3. **Long-acting (36–54 hr):** Paramethasone (2 mg), dexamethasone (0.75 mg), betamethasone (0.6 mg).

Regulatory mechanism of steroid secretions: Following three major mechanisms control ACTH release and the cortisol secretion.

1. **Negative feedback mechanism:** Most important stimulus for secretion of cortisol is the release of ACTH from anterior pituitary. The secretion of ACTH in anterior pituitary is determined by two hypothalamic neurohormones (diurnal release of CRF and AVP) that act synergistically. Circulating cortisol also exerts a direct negative feedback on hypothalamus and anterior pituitary to decrease the release of CRF and ACTH from respective sites.
2. **Diurnal variation:** Cortisol is secreted from adrenal gland in an episodic manner and frequency of pulses follows a circadian rhythm. Levels are highest in morning on waking and lowest in the middle of evening.
3. **Stress:** Stress such as physical; psychological; physiological, can override the negative feedback mechanism and diurnal variation. Cortisol rises immediately (within minutes) and dramatically during stress. Mineralocorticoid release is controlled by the renin-angiotensin system.

Mechanism of action: They have inhibitory effects on B and T cells and phagocytes, having activity on both the innate and acquired immune systems and therefore having efficacy in autoimmune and autoinflammatory diseases. They act on cells by both genomic and non-genomic mechanisms. There is activation of cytosolic GC receptor (cGCR) by a classical genomic mechanism.

This mechanism results in the suppression of proinflammatory molecules called *transrepression* and upregulation of many anti-inflammatory molecules called *transactivation*. Transrepression accounts for many of the desired GC effects, while transactivation is associated with many of undesirable side effects. Genomic effects take hours to days as compared to nongenomic effects that occur rapidly within seconds to minutes. Nongenomic effects include GC signaling through membrane associated receptors and second messengers. The nongenomic effects are far more significant at doses greater than 100 mg/d.

Pharmacokinetics: Most glucocorticoids are well-absorbed orally. Hydrocortisone undergoes high first pass metabolism. It is 95% bound to plasma proteins—corticosteroid binding globulin or transcortin. Glucocorticoids are metabolized in the liver by oxidation and reduction followed by conjugation. Metabolites are excreted by the kidneys. The t½ varies with each agent.

Pharmacological actions: Actions of glucocorticoids are:

1. **Carbohydrate and protein metabolism:** Glucocorticoids promote gluconeogenesis. They also cause protein breakdown.
2. **Fat metabolism:** Promote lipolysis; redistribution of body fat occurs, which is deposited over face, neck and shoulder: 'moon face', 'fish mouth', 'buffalo hump'.
3. **Calcium metabolism:** They inhibit intestinal absorption and enhance renal excretion of Ca^{2+}, also loss of calcium from bone indirectly due to loss of osteoid.
4. **Water excretion:** Effect on water excretion is independent of action on Na^+ transport; hydrocortisone and other glucocorticoids, but not aldosterone, maintain normal GFR.
5. **CVS:** Glucocorticoids restrict capillary permeability; maintain tone of arterioles and myocardial contractility.
6. **Skeletal muscles:** Weakness occurs in both hypo- and hypercorticism.
7. **CNS:** Mild euphoria, increased motor activity, insomnia, and hypomania or depression.
8. **Stomach:** Aggravate peptic ulcer.
9. **Lymphoid tissue and blood cells:** Glucocorticoids enhance the rate of destruction of lymphoid cells (T cells > B cells).
10. **Anti-inflammatory responses:** Glucocorticoids interfere at several steps in the inflammatory response; most important mechanism is limitation of recruitment of inflammatory cells and production

of proinflammatory mediators like PGs, LTs, and PAF through inhibition of phospholipase A_2.

11. **Immunological and allergic responses:** Glucocorticoids impair immunological competence and suppress all types of hyper sensitization and allergic phenomena.

12. **Permissive action:** Action of some hormones is executed only in presence of glucocorticoids, called **permissive action**, e.g. calorigenic effect of glucagon; lipolytic effect of catecholamines.

Indications for corticosteroid therapy

A. Replacement therapy

1. Acute adrenal insufficiency: Hydrocortisone or dexamethasone is given IV
2. Chronic adrenal insufficiency (Addison's disease): Hydrocortisone (orally) along with adequate salt and water.
3. Congenital adrenal hyperplasia (adrenogenital syndrome): Hydrocortisone 0.6 mg/kg/daily in divided doses.

B. Pharmacotherapy: The following general principles must be observed.

- A single dose (even excessive) is not harmful.
- Short courses (even high dose) are not likely to be harmful in the absence of contraindications; starting doses can be high in severe illness.
- Long-term use is potentially hazardous: keep the duration of treatment and dose to minimum.
- Initial dose depends on severity of the disease; start with a high dose in severe illness and reduce gradually as symptoms subside, while in mild cases start with the lowest dose and titrate upwards to find the correct dose.
- No abrupt withdrawal after a corticoid has been given for >2–3 weeks: may precipitate adrenal insufficiency.
- Infection, severe trauma or any stress during corticoid therapy, increase the dose.
- Use local therapy (cutaneous, inhaled, intranasal, etc.) wherever possible.

1. Arthritides

i. Rheumatoid arthritis: Corticosteroids are indicated only in severe cases as adjuvant to NSAIDs.
ii. Osteoarthritis: Intra-articular injection of a steroid may be used to control an acute exacerbation.
iii. Rheumatic fever: Only in severe cases.
iv. Gout: Intra-articular injection of a soluble glucocorticoid.

2. Collagen diseases: Most cases of SLE, polyarteritis nodosa, dermatomyositis, nephrotic syndrome, glomerulonephritis and related diseases need corticoids.

3. **Severe allergic reactions:** Anaphylaxis, angioneurotic edema, urticaria and serum sickness.

4. **Autoimmune diseases:** Autoimmune hemolytic anaemia, ITP, active chronic hepatitis responds to corticoids.

5. **Bronchial asthma:** Inhaled glucocorticoid therapy is recommended.

6. **Other lung diseases:** Aspiration pneumonia and pulmonary edema from drowning.

7. **Infective diseases:** Corticosteroids are indicated only in serious infective diseases to tide over crisis or to prevent complications.

8. **Eye diseases:** Topical instillation as eye drops or ointment is effective in diseases of the anterior chamber: allergic conjunctivitis, iritis, iridocyclitis, keratitis, etc.

9. **Skin diseases:** Topical corticosteroids are widely employed and are highly effective in many eczematous skin diseases. Systemic therapy is needed (may be life-saving) in pemphigus vulgaris, exfoliative dermatitis, Stevens-Johnson syndrome and other severe afflictions.

10. **Intestinal diseases:** Ulcerative colitis, Crohn's disease, celiac disease.

11. **Cerebral edema** due to tumors, tubercular meningitis, etc. responds to corticoids.

A short course of 2–4 weeks oral prednisolone can hasten recovery from Bell's palsy and acute exacerbation of multiple sclerosis. In the latter, methyl prednisolone 1 g IV daily for 2–3 days may be given in the beginning. Neurocysticercosis: Prednisolone 40 mg/day or equivalent is given for 2–4 weeks to suppress the reaction to dying larvae.

12. **Malignancies:** Corticoids are an essential component of combined chemotherapy of acute lymphatic leukemia, Hodgkin's and other lymphomas, because of their marked lympholytic action.

13. **Organ transplantation and skin allograft:** High dose corticoids are given along with other immunosuppressant to prevent rejection reaction.

14. **Septic shock:** Low-dose (hydrocortisone 100 mg TDS IV infusion for 5–7 days) therapy is needed in patients who are adrenal deficient and require vassopressor drug despite adequate fluid replacement.

15. **Thyroid storm:** Corticosteroids reduce peripheral T4 to T3 conversion. Hydrocortisone 100 mg TDS may improve outcome.

16. **To test adrenal-pituitary axis function:** Dexamethasone suppresses adrenal-pituitary axis at doses which do not contribute to steroid metabolites in urine; responsiveness of the axis can be tested by measuring daily urinary steroid metabolite excretion.

Steroids and dentistry: When a patient on long-term steroids requires a dental procedure, adequate precautions are to be taken.

- Antibiotic coverage may be needed depending on the procedure, as these patients are more susceptible to infections.
- Patients on long-term glucocorticoids may require an additional dose of steroid to manage the stress.
- Long-term administration of glucocorticoids may delay wound healing.
- For analgesia, patient should take those ones which do not produce much gastric irritation.

Q. 2. Write a note on adverse effects of corticosteroids/ prednisolone.

(TNMGR, Nov. 2001; RGUHS, April, 2007)

Ans. Adverse effects of glucocorticoids are dependent on dose, duration of therapy and the relative potency.

A. Adverse effects of mineralocorticoids

1. Sodium and water retention.
2. Edema.
3. Hypokalemic alkalosis.
4. Progressive rise in blood pressure.

B. Adverse effects of glucocorticoids

1. Cushing syndrome.
2. Hyperglycemia.
3. Muscular weakness.
4. Susceptibility to infections.
5. Delayed healing.
6. Peptic ulceration.
7. Osteoporosis.
8. Posterior sub-capsular cataract.
9. Glaucoma.
10. Growth retardation.
11. Fetal abnormalities.
12. Psychiatric disturbances.
13. Suppression of hypothalamo-pituitary-adrenal (HPA) axis.
14. Steroid withdrawal syndrome: Rapid withdrawal of steroids may cause a syndrome that could include fatigue, joint pain, muscle stiffness, muscle tenderness, or fever.
    - **Steroid sparing drugs** *(RUHS, June 2018):* Use of non-steroid immune-suppressive drugs that permits partial withdrawal of corticosteroids is known as steroid sparing therapy.

Steroid sparing agents

A. Immunosuppressant

1. Azathioprine.
2. Leflunomide (10–20 mg).

3. Cyclophosphamide: Cyclophosphamide is an alkylating agent that binds to DNA non-specifically during cell cycle and suppresses B cell function > T cell function. Dose: 1 g IV. **Side effects:** Acute myelosuppression, mucosal ulcers, alopecia, nephrotoxicity, cardiotoxicity, hepatotoxicity, carcinogenicity, teratogenicity, and interstitial lung fibrosis.

4. Cyclosporine: Cyclosporine is an immunosuppressive agent with anti-T cell lymphocyte activity. **Side effects:** Electrolyte abnormalities, nephrotoxicity, tremors, hirsutism, hyperlipidaemia, hypertension, gingival hyperplasia.

5. **Dapsone:** It inhibits neutrophil toxicity and chemotaxis by blocking myeloperoxidase activity. **Side effects:** Hemolytic anemia, methemoglobinemia, idiosyncratic peripheral motor neuropathy, psychosis, agranulocytosis, **dapsone hypersensitivity** syndrome (mononucleosis-like reactions, such as fever, erythroderma, hepatitis, eosinophilia, or death).

6. Tacrolimus: Newer immunosuppressant, acts by inhibiting T cell activation and cytokine release. It is available in 0.1 and 0.3% ointment form. **Side effects:** Nephrotoxicity, neurotoxicity, GI complaints, hypertension, hyperkalaemia, hyperglycemia, diabetes, irritation, and burning sensation of applied area.

7. Mycophenolate mofetil: It inhibits *de novo* purine synthesis by non-competitively inhibiting inosine monophosphate dehydrogenase (IMPDH). Dose: 0.5–1.5 g BD; **Side effects:** Gastrointestinal distress, reversible anemia, leucopenia, and thrombocytopenia.

8. Methotrexate.

B. Others: Biological agents: Tocilizumab (8 mg/kg); Anakinra (100 mg); Rituximab (1000 mg); TNF-α blocker.

Q. 3. Write a note on long acting glucocorticoids.

(TNMGR, Aug. 2004)

Ans. Long-acting glucocorticoids have duration of action ~36–54 hr and includes:

1. **Dexamethasone:** Very potent and highly selective glucocorticoid. Long acting, causes marked pituitary-adrenal suppression, but fluid retention and hypertension are not a problem. It is used for inflammatory and allergic conditions (0.5–5 mg/day oral). Shock, cerebral edema (4–20 mg/day IV infusion or IM injection). Also used topically.

2. **Betamethasone:** Similar to dexamethasone, 0.5–5 mg/day oral, 4–20 mg IM, IV injection or infusion, also topical.

Dexamethasone or betamethasone is preferred in cerebral edema and other states in which fluid retention must be avoided.

Q. 4. Discuss the role of corticosteroids in treatment of oral pathologies.
(RGUHS, April, 2008; TNMGR, March 2009; MUHS, May 2010; RGUHS, May 2011; Sumandeep Uni., June 2016)

Q. Write a note on uses of corticosteroids in dentistry.
(Sumandeep Uni., June 2017; HP Uni., April 2019; NTR Uni., May 2019)

Ans. Corticosteroids are one of the most widely used drugs due to their anti-inflammatory, anti-allergic and immunosuppressive effects. Today they are used as systemic, topical, intra-articular and intralesional in the oral and maxillofacial region.

A. Agents used

1. Topical corticosteroids: Beclomethasone (50–100 μg spray), betamethasone (0.1% cream), clobetasol (0.05% cream), fluocinonide (0.05% cream).
2. Injectable corticosteroids: Triamcinolone acetonide (10 mg/ml), dexamethasone (4 mg/ml).
3. Systemic corticosteroids: Prednisolone (1 mg/kg)

B. Therapeutic uses in dentistry and oral lesions

1. **Aphthous stomatitis**
   a. Minor aphthae:
      - Topical: Triamcinolone acetonide (0.1%); Fluocinonide (0.05%), clobetasol (0.05%), 2–3 times a day; Dexamethasone elixir (0.5 mg/5 ml), QID.
   b. Major aphthous:
      - Systemic: Prednisone (1 mg/kg/day), to be tapered after 1–2 weeks.
      - Intralesional steroids can be used to treat large indolent major RAS lesions
2. **Behçet's disease:** Prednisone (40–60 mg/day), used alone or in combination with immunosuppressive agents.
3. **Oral submucous fibrosis (OSMF)**
   - Submucosal injections of dexamethasone (4 mg/ml) and hyaluronidase (1500 IU) diluted in 1 ml of 2 % lidocaine biweekly.
   - Submucosal injection of triamcinolone (10 mg/ml) diluted in 1 ml of lidocaine (2%) biweekly.
4. **Oral lichen planus (OLP)**
   - Topical as ointments, pastes, lozenges, mouthwashes or inhaler, e.g. triamcinolone acetonide (0.1%) ointment, clobetasol propionate gel (0.1–0.05%), betamethasone valerate gel (0.05%), fluocinonide gel (0.05%).
   - In widespread lesions, use triamcinolone acetonide (0.1%) or dexamethasone elixir (0.1 mg/ml).
   - Intralesional inj. triamcinolone acetonide (0.2–0.4 ml, 10 mg/ml) for intractable erosive OLP.
   - Systemic: Prednisone (0.5–1 mg/kg) for acute exacerbation, recalcitrant severe erosive OLP.
5. **Chronic ulcerative stomatitis:** Topical: Fluocinonide (0.05%) gel 4X/d for 3 weeks; Betamethasone dipropionate (0.05%) 4X/d for 2 months
6. **Pyostomatitis vegetans:** Prednisolone 20 mg for 2 days, followed by 15 mg for 1 day and then 10 mg for 1 day and lastly 5 mg for 1 day was used.
7. **Pemphigus**
   - Topical: Clobetasol (0.05%) or fluocinonide acetonide (0.05%)
   - Intralesional: Triamcinolone acetonide (10–20 mg/ml), 0.05–0.1 ml per site every 1–2 week.
   - Systemic: Prednisone (1–2 mg/kg/d) in divided doses for 6–10 weeks or prednisone (40 mg) single daily dose for 2–4 weeks.
   - Pulse therapy: Use of mega doses of steroids, e.g. methylprednisolone 1 g/d IV over 1–3 hr for 3 days.
8. **Pemphigoid**
   - Topical: Clobetasol propionate (0.05%)
   - Intralesional: Triamcinolone acetonide (10–20 mg/ml)
   - Systemic: Prednisone; 0.3 mg/kg/d in mild; 0.6 mg/kg/d in moderate; and 0.75–1 mg/kg/d in severe case.
9. **Erythema multiforme:** Mild: Self-limiting; Prednisone 40 mg/d for 1 week; Moderate to severe: Prednisone 30 mg/d for several weeks.
10. **Lupus erythematosus**
    - Topical: High potency steroids.
    - Intralesional Inj.
    - Systemic: Prednisone 10–20 mg/day or prednisone 20–40 mg alternate day.
11. **Lymphatic malformation:** Intralesional Inj. of triamcinolone acetonide (10 mg)
12. **Orofacial granulomatosis:** Intralesional triamcinolone acetonide (3–10 mL; 10 mg/mL)
13. **Melkerson Rosenthal syndrome:** Systemic: Prednisone (1–1.5 mg/kg/d) tapering over 3–6 weeks; Intralesional inj.
14. **Bell's palsy:** "Fagan Regimen" (for patients presenting within 10 days of onset): Start with 60 mg × 3 days → 40 mg × 3 days → 20 mg × 3 days → 10 mg × 3 days → 5 mg × 3 days.

15. **Ramsay Hunt syndrome:** Prednisone (60 mg for 3–5 days) along with antivirals.

16. **Post-herpetic neuralgia:** Prednisone 40 mg/d for 10 days.

17. **TMJ disorders**
    - Intra articular Inj.: Disodium phosphate ester of betamethasone (3 mg/ml), methylprednisolone acetate, triamcinolone acetonide, 0.5–1 ml.
    - Systemic: Hydrocortisone (20–240 mg/d), prednisone (5–60 mg/d), dexamethasone (0.75–9 mg/d) or betamethasone (0.6–7.2 mg).

18. **Cranial arteritis:** Prednisone 40–60 mg/d; methylprednisolone pulse therapy: 1 g, IV

19. **Mucocele:** Intralesional Inj. of triamcinolone acetonide (10 mg/ml), (0.5–1.5 ml)

20. **Central giant cell granuloma:** Intralesional inj. of triamcinolone acetonide (10–20 mg/ml) with lidocaine (0.5%), per week for 6 weeks.

21. **Localized Langerhans cell histiocytosis (eosinophilic granuloma):** 2 ml of triamcinolone acetonide (25 mg/ml); Methylprednisolone succinate (80–200 mg).

22. **Infectious mononucleosis:** Prednisone (60–80 mg/day)

23. **Adrenal crisis prophylaxis**
    - Primary: Hydrocortisone (20–25 mg) IV
    - Secondary: Hydrocortisone (15–20 mg) IV

24. **Shock:** Hydrocortisone 1.5–3 mg/kg IV or prednisone 1 mg/kg.

25. **Endodontics:** Triamcinolone acetonide application in root canal reduces post-treatment pain. Steroid-antibiotic combinations are used as intracanal medicaments for management of root resorption. Hydrocortisone mixed with zinc oxide eugenol is used as root canal sealers. It has also been used in dentin hyepersentstivity, pulp capping, pulpotomy, topically.

26. **Dentoalveolar surgery (3rd molar extraction, pre-prosthetic surgery, orthognathic surgery, etc.):** Dexamethasone (8 mg), methyl prednisolone (40 mg), prednisone (25 mg), betamethasone (0.5 mg).

27. **Trigeminal nerve injury and chronic facial pain, allergic condition of maxillofacial region.**

28. **Orthodontic tooth movement:** Steroids delay the tooth movement.

Q. 5. Write a short note on methylprednisolone.
(TNMGR, April 2012)

Ans. Methylprednisolone is a corticosteroid medication used to suppress the immune system and decrease inflammation, slightly more potent and more selective than prednisolone. Dose: 4–32 mg/day oral. It has reduced incidence of sodium and water retention.

Pharmacokinetics: It is absorbed from GIT, metabolized mainly in liver and excreted in urine. Methylprednisolone acetate has been used as a retention enema in ulcerative colitis.

Indiactions: In conditions requiring glucocorticocoid activity. **Pulse therapy** with high dose methylprednisolone (1 g infused IV every 6–8 weeks) has been tried in nonresponsive active rheumatoid arthritis, renal transplant, pemphigus, etc. with good results and minimal suppression of pituitary-adrenal axis. Initial effect of methylprednisolone pulse therapy (MPPT) is probably due to its anti-inflammatory action, while long term benefit may be due to temporary switching off of the immune-damaging processes as a consequence of lymphopenia and decreased Ig synthesis.

Q. 6. Classify sympathomimetic drugs based on its therapeutic use.

Ans. Sympathomimetic agents are used to augment the endogenous Catecholamines of the sympathetic nervous system for therapeutic benefit.

1. **Direct sympathomimetic:** They act directly as agonists on ? and/or ? adrenoceptors: Adr, NA, and isoprenaline, Phenylephrine, Methoxamine, Xylometazoline, Salbutamol.

2. **Indirect sympathomimetic:** They act on adrenergic neuron to release NA, which then acts on the adrenoceptors, e.g. Tyramine, Amphetamine.

3. **Mixed action sympathomimetic:** They act directly as well as indirectly, e.g. Ephedrine, Dopamine, and Mephentermine.

FDA approved sympathomimetic indications
- Cardiac: Treatment of hypotension and hypovolemic and neurogenic shock.
- Pulmonary: Treatment of asthma and COPD.
- Sympathomimetic agents are used as nasal decongestants for treatment of allergic rhinitis, and conjunctivitis.
- Ophthalmic: Open-angle glaucoma.
- Neurologic: Local anesthetic effects.
- Psychiatric: Narcolepsy.
- Endocrine: For obesity.
- Genitourinary: For urinary incontinence.

Adverse effects
1. **Direct sympathomimetic:** Hypertensive emergency, reflex bradycardia, piloerection, urinary retention, sedation, respiratory depression, miosis, dry mouth, tachycardia, arrhythmias, acute coronary syndrome,

tremor, insomnia, and diaphoresis, hyperinsulinaemia, hyperglycemia, and hypokalaemia.

2. **Indirect sympathomimetic:** Anorexia, weight loss, insomnia, nausea, vomiting, abdominal cramps, mesenteric ischemia, motor tics, and seizures. Cardiovascular complications of indirect sympathomimetic similar to the direct agents.

Contraindications

1. Hypersensitivity to drug.
2. Phenylephrine (relative) in patients with a history of extreme bradycardia.
3. Hypertrophic obstructive cardiomyopathy relative contraindication for dobutamine.
4. Heart failure or cardiac injury is a relative contraindication for isoproterenol.
5. Asthma or hypersensitivity reactions, hypertension or cardiovascular disease are relative contraindications for cocaine.

11. EMERGENCY DRUGS IN DENTAL PRACTICE

Q. 1. Discuss in detail emergency drugs used in dental practice. *(TNMGR, March 2010; MUHS, May 2010; BBD Uni., April 2014; Sumandeep Uni., June 2016; May 2018)*

Ans. The most essential aspects of patient management when urgencies or emergencies arise consist of a thorough primary assessment of the patient and airway management. Drugs that should be promptly available to the dentist can be divided into two categories. The first category represents those which may be considered **essential**. The second category contains drugs which are also very helpful and should be considered as part of the **emergency kit**.

Essential emergency drugs

1. **Oxygen:** Oxygen is indicated for every emergency except hyper-ventilation. This should be done with a clear full face mask for the spontaneously breathing patient and a bag-valve-mask device for apneic patient. Oxygen should be available in a portable source, ideally in an "E"-size cylinder which holds over 600 liters. If the patient is conscious, or unconscious yet spontaneously breathing, oxygen should be delivered by a full face mask, where a flow rate of 6–10 liters/minute is appropriate for most adults. If the patient is unconscious and apneic, it should be delivered by a bag-valve-mask device where a flow rate of 10–15 liters/minute is appropriate. A positive pressure device may be used in adults, provided that the flow rate does not exceed 35 L/min.

2. **Epinephrine:** Epinephrine is the drug of choice for emergency treatment of anaphylaxis and asthma which does not respond to its drug of first choice, albuterol or salbutamol. Epinephrine is also indicated for management of cardiac arrest. As a drug, epinephrine has a very rapid onset and short duration of action, usually 5–10 minutes when given intravenously. For emergency purposes, epinephrine is available in two formulations. It is prepared as 1:1,000 (1 mg/ml) for IM; 1:10,000, (1 mg/10 ml) for IV injection. These doses should be repeated as necessary until resolution of the event.

3. **Nitroglycerin:** This drug is indicated for acute angina or myocardial infarction. For emergency purpose, it is available as sublingual tablets or sublingual spray. With signs of angina pectoris, one tablet or spray (0.3/0.4 mg) should be administered sublingually. If necessary, this dose can be repeated in 5 minute intervals. Systolic blood pressures below 90 mmHg contraindicate the use of this drug.

4. **Injectable antihistamine:** An antihistamine is indicated for management of allergic reactions. Whereas mild non-life threatening allergic reactions may be managed by oral administration, life-threatening reactions necessitate parenteral administration.

5. **Albuterol (salbutamol):** A selective β_2 agonist such as albuterol (salbutamol inhaler) is the first choice for management of bronchospasm. It has a peak effect in 30–60 minutes, with duration of 4–6 hours. Adult dose is 2 sprays; Pediatric dose is 1 spray, to be repeated as necessary.

6. **Aspirin:** Aspirin (acetylsalicylic acid) reduces overall mortality from acute myocardial infarction. The lowest effective dose of 162 mg should be given immediately.

7. **Oral carbohydrate:** An oral carbohydrate source, such as fruit juice or non-diet soft-drink, should be readily available. Its use is indicated in the management of hypoglycemia in conscious patients.

Additional emergency drugs

1. **Glucagon:** Ideal management of severe hypoglycemia in diabetic emergency is intravenous administration of 50% dextrose. Glucagon is indicated if an intravenous line is not in place and venipuncture is not expected to be accomplished, as in a dental office. Dose for an adult is 1 mg. If patient is <20 kg, recommended dose is 0.5 mg.

2. **Atropine:** This anti-muscarinic, anti-cholinergic drug is indicated for management of hypotension, which is accompanied by bradycardia. The dose recommended is 0.5 mg initially, followed by increments as necessary, up to 3 mg.

3. **Ephedrine:** For the treatment of severe hypotension, it is ideally administered in 5 mg increments intravenously. Intramuscularly it should be given in a dose of 10–25 mg.

4. **Corticosteroid:** Administration of a corticosteroid may be indicated for prevention of recurrent anaphylaxis and in management of an adrenal crisis. Prototype for this group is hydrocortisone, which may be administered in a dose of 100 mg.

5. **Morphine:** Morphine is indicated for management of severe pain which occurs with a myocardial infarction. Advanced cardiac life support recommendations list morphine as the analgesic of choice for this purpose. If an intravenous is not in place, consideration can be given to administering morphine in a dose of approximately 5 mg intramuscularly.

6. **Naloxone:** If either morphine is included in emergency kit, or opioids are used as part of a sedation regimen, then naloxone should also be present for emergency management of inadvertent overdose. Doses should ideally be titrated slowly in 0.1 mg increments to effect.

7. **Nitrous oxide:** Nitrous oxide is a reasonable second choice, if morphine is not available to manage pain from a myocardial infarction. For management of pain associated with a myocardial infarction, it should be administered with oxygen, in a concentration approximating 35%, or titrated to effect.

8. **Injectable benzodiazepine:** Management of status epilepticus may require administration of lorazepam (4 mg) intramuscularly, or midazolam (5 mg) intramuscularly. If an intravenous is in place, these drugs should be slowly titrated to effect.

9. **Flumazenil:** The benzodiazepine antagonist flumazenil should be part of emergency kit. Dose is 0.1–0.2 mg intravenously, incrementally.

In addition to having drugs available, a small amount of basic equipment should be readily available. This includes a stethoscope, blood pressure cuff, an oxygen delivery system, syringes and needles. Dentists should also consider having an automated external defibrillator (AED), as a means to treat cardiac arrest.

Q. 2. Write a note on medical emergencies in dentistry.

Q. Write a note on anaesthetic emergencies.
(RGUHS, October, 2008; NTR Uni., May 2019)

Ans. A medical emergency in the dental office may be an unexpected event that can include accidental or willful bodily injury, central nervous system

Table 11.2: Medical emergencies in dentistry

Emergency condition	Signs and symptoms	Treatment	Drug dosage
Allergic reaction (mild or delayed)	Hives; itching; edema; erythema (skin, mucosa, conjunctiva)	1. Discontinue all sources of allergy causing substances 2. Administer diphenhydramine	Diphenhydramine 1 mg/kg: Oral Child: 10–25 mg QID Adult: 25–50 mg QID
Allergic reaction (sudden onset): Anaphylaxis	Urticaria (itching, flushing, hives); rhinitis; wheezing/difficulty breathing; bronchospasm; laryngeal edema; weak pulse; marked fall in blood pressure; loss of consciousness	This is a true, life-threatening emergency 1. Call for emergency medical services 2. Administer epinephrine 3. Administer oxygen 4. Monitor vital signs 5. Transport to emergency medical facility by advanced medical responders	Epinephrine 1:1000 (0.01 mg/kg) q5 min. until recovery or until help arrives; IM/SC
Acute asthmatic attack	Shortness of breath; wheezing; coughing; tightness in chest; cyanosis; tachycardia	1. Sit patient upright or in a comfortable position 2. Administer oxygen 3. Administer bronchodilator 4. If bronchodilator is ineffective, administer epinephrine 5. Call for emergency medical services with transportation for advanced care if indicated	1. Albuterol inhale 2. Epinephrine 1:1000 (0.01 mg/kg) q15 min as needed; IM/SC

Contd...

Table 11.2: Medical emergencies in dentistry (*Contd...*)

Emergency condition	Signs and symptoms	Treatment	Drug dosage
Local anesthetic toxicity	Light-headedness; changes in vision and/or speech; metallic taste; changes in mental status—confusion; agitation; tinnitis; tremor; seizure; tachypnea; bradycardia; unconsciousness; cardiac arrest	1. Assess and support airway, breathing, and circulation (CPR if warranted) 2. Administer oxygen 3. Monitor vital signs 4. Call for emergency medical services with transportation for advanced care if indicated	Supplemental oxygen-mask
Local anesthetic reaction: vasoconstrictor	Anxiety; tachycardia/palpitations; restlessness; headache; tachypnea; chest pain; cardiac arrest	1. Reassure patient 2. Assess and support airway, breathing, and circulation (CPR if warranted) 3. Administer oxygen 4. Monitor vital signs 5. Call for emergency medical services with transportation for advanced care if indicated	Supplemental oxygen-mask
Overdose: BZDs	Somnolence; confusion; diminished reflexes; respiratory depression; apnea; respiratory arrest; cardiac arrest	1. Assess and support airway, breathing, and circulation (CPR if warranted) 2. Administer oxygen 3. Monitor vital signs 4. If severe respiratory depression, establish IV access and reverse with flumazenil. 5. Monitor recovery (for at least 2 hours after the last dose of flumazenil) and call for emergency medical services with transportation for advanced care if indicated	Flumazenil 0.01–0.02 mg/kg (maximum: 0.2 mg); IV/IM
Overdose: Narcotic	Decreased responsiveness; respiratory depression; respiratory arrest; cardiac arrest	1. Assess and support airway, breathing, and circulation (CPR if warranted) 2. Administer oxygen 3. Monitor vital signs 4. If severe respiratory depression, reverse with naloxone 5. Monitor recovery (for at least 2 hours after the last dose of naloxone) and call for emergency medical services with transportation for advanced care if indicated	Naloxone 0.1 mg/kg up to 2 mg; IV/SC
Seizure	Warning aura—disorientation, blinking, or blank stare; uncontrolled muscle movements; muscle rigidity; unconsciousness; postictal phase—sleepiness, confusion, amnesia, slow recovery	1. Recline and position to prevent injury 2. Ensure open airway and adequate ventilation 3. Monitor vital signs 4. If status is epilepticus, give diazepam and call for emergency medical services with transportation for advanced care if indicated	Diazepam (IV) Child up to 5 years: 0.2–0.5 mg slowly q2–5 min. with max. 5 mg Child 5 years and >1 mg q2–5 min. with max. 10 mg

Contd...

Table 11.2: Medical emergencies in dentistry (*Contd...*)

Emergency condition	Signs and symptoms	Treatment	Drug dosage
Neurogenic or vasovagal syncope (fainting)	Feeling of warmth; skin pale and moist; pulse rapid initially then gets slow and weak; dizziness; hypotension; cold extremities; unconsciousness	1. Recline, feet up 2. Loosen clothing that may be binding 3. Ammonia inhales 4. Administer oxygen 5. Cold towel on back of neck 6. Monitor recovery	Ammonia in vials: Inhale. If bradycardia: Atropine 0.5 mg IM If no bradycardia: Ephedrine 25 mg IM
Chest pain (angina)			Nitroglycerin (0.4 mg) single tablet placed under the tongue and can be continued q5 min
Hypoglycemia	Serum glucose <60 mg/dL: Tachycardia, shakiness, diaphoresis, impaired cognitive and CNS functions		Sweetened beverage, viscous glucose concentrate, should be placed in buccal vestibule. 25–50 ml of 50% dextrose solution (IV). Glucagon 1 mg (IM); 0.5 mg (IV)

stimulation and depression, respiratory and circulatory disturbances, as well as allergic reactions. For all emergencies:

1. Discontinue the dental treatment.
2. Call for assistance/someone to bring oxygen and emergency kit.
3. Position patient: Ensure open and unobstructed airway.
4. Monitor vital signs.
5. Be prepared to support respiration, support circulation, provide CPR and call for emergency medical services (Table 11.2).

Biostatistics, Research Methodology and Ethics

1. BIOSTATISTICS

Q. 1. Discuss role of biostatistics in oral health research. *(TNMGR, March 2010; RGUHS, May 2011; NTR Uni., June 2015)*

Ans. Statistics is a mathematical science pertaining to the collection, analysis, interpretation or explanation, and presentation of data. **Biostatistics** is a branch of statistics that emphasizes the statistical applications in the biomedical and health sciences. It is mainly consists of various steps like generation of hypothesis, collection of data, and application of statistical analysis. The aim of biostatistics is to minimize bias and maximize precision. Steps in scientific investigations are:

1. Formulation of the research problem
2. Identification of key variables
3. Statistical design of an experiment
4. Collection of data
5. Statistical analysis of the data
6. Interpretation of the analytical results

Role of Biostatistics in Health Research

1. In documentation of medical/dental history of disease, their course of progression and variability among patients.
2. In clinical epidemiological studies on etiology of health events, determine the superiority of specific therapies.
3. In planning and conduct of therapeutics and pro-phylactic clinical trials to determine the superiority of specific therapies.
4. In calculation of diagnostic efficacies and likelihood ratio in prognostic studies.
5. In providing methods for the definition of "normal" and indicating at what point of the measure of some bodily characteristic becomes "Abnormal" or "Pathological"

6. In supplying the measurements of accuracy of various laboratory and clinical procedures that are commonly used in medical practice.

Uses of Statistics in Dental Science

1. To find the statistical difference between means of two groups, e.g. mean plaque scores of two groups.
2. To assess the state of oral health in the community and to determine the availability and utilization of dental care facilities.
3. To indicate the basic factors underlying the state of oral health by diagnosing the community and find solutions to such problems.
4. To determine success or failure of specific oral health care programs or to evaluate the program action.
5. To promote oral health legislation and in creating administrative standards for oral health care delivery.

Branches of Biostatistics

- **Descriptive biostatistics:** Methods of producing quantitative summaries of information in biological sciences. Tabulation and graphical presentation.
- **Inferential biostatistics:** Methods of making genera-lizations about a larger group based on information about a sample of that group in biological sciences. Primarily performed in two ways: Estimation; Testing of hypothesis.

Q. 2. Write a short note on mean, mode, median (measures of central tendency). Explain with examples. *(RGUHS, May 2011; NTR Uni., Oct. 2012; BBD Uni., April 2015; HP Uni., April 2019)*

Ans. Central tendency is defined as "the statistical measure that identifies a single value as representative of an entire distribution." It aims to provide an accurate description of the entire data. The measures of central tendency are mean, median and mode. They are summary indices describing the central point or the most characteristic value of a set of measurements.

1. **Mean:** This implies arithmetic average, which is obtained by summing up all the observations and dividing the total by number of observations. Mean is the most commonly used measure of central tendency.

   Types
   - **Arithmetic mean:** Arithmetic mean (or, simply, "mean") is nothing but the average. **Advantages:** Mean uses every value in the data and hence is a good representative of data. It is closely related to SD. **Disadvantages:** It is sensitive to extreme values/outliers, especially when the sample size is small. Therefore, it is not an appropriate measure of central tendency for skewed distribution.
   - **Weighted mean:** It is calculated when certain values in a dataset are more important than the others.
   - **Geometric mean:** It is defined as the arithmetic mean of the values taken on a log scale.
   - **Harmonic mean:** It is the reciprocal of arithmetic mean of the observations.

2. **Median/positional average:** When all the observations of a variable are arranged in either ascending or descending order, the middle observation is known as **median**. It divides the frequency distribution exactly into two halves. **Advantages:** It is easy to compute and comprehend, not distorted by outliers/skewed data and can be determined for ratio, interval, and ordinal scale. **Disadvantages:** It does not take into account the precise value of each observation. It is not amenable to further mathematical calculation.

3. **Mode:** Mode is defined as the value that occurs most frequently in the data. Some datasets do not have a mode because each value occurs only once, whereas others can have >1 mode. It is rarely used as a summary statistic except to describe a bimodal distribution. In a bimodal distribution, taller peak is called **major mode** and shorter one is **minor mode**. **Advantages:** It is the only measure of central tendency that can be used for data measured in a nominal scale. It can be calculated easily. **Disadvantages:** It is not algebraically defined and the fluctuation in the frequency of observation is more when the sample size is small.

Position of measures of central tendency: All three measures are identical in a normal distribution. In skewed distribution, mean is shifted to the tail; Mode lies in the hump; Median lies in between mean and mode.

Q. 3. Write a short note on measures of variability/dispersion.

Ans. Any characteristic that can be observed, measured, or categorized is called a variable. Types of variables are: Nominal (variable has no implied value or order); Ordinal variable (has an order but not at equal intervals); Interval variable (has equal intervals but no meaningful zero); Ratio variable (has equal intervals with a meaningful zero). **Variability** refers to how "spread out" a group of scores is. The terms **Variability, Spread, and Dispersion** are synonyms, refers to how close the data cluster around the measure of central tendency.

Need of Variability

1. It helps to ascertain the measures of deviation.
2. It helps to compare different group.
3. It is useful to supplement the information provided by the measures of central tendency.
4. It is useful to calculate further advance statistics based on the measures of dispersion.

Types of Measures of Variability

1. **Range (R):** It is the difference between the largest (L) and smallest (S) values in a set of values. It defines the normal limits of a biological characteristic.

$$R = L - S.$$

   Advantages: It is easily calculated and readily understood. It provides a quick estimate of the measure of variability. **Disadvantages:** It is not based on all the observations of the series. It only takes the highest and the lowest scores into account. In case of open ended distributions range cannot be used. It is affected greatly by fluctuations in sampling.

2. **Inter-quartile range (IQR):** IQR is a measure of variability, based on dividing a dataset into quartiles. Quartiles divide a rank-ordered dataset into four equal parts. The values that divide each part are called the 1st, 2nd, and 3rd; denoted by Q1, Q2, and Q3, respectively.

$$IQR = Q3 - Q1.$$

3. **Variance:** Variability can also be defined in terms of how close the scores in the distribution are to the middle of the distribution. Using the mean as the measure of the middle of the distribution, the variance is defined as the average squared difference of the scores from the mean.

4. **Standard deviation (SD)** *(NTR Uni., May 2019):* SD is the square root of the variance. It is a measure that summarizes the amount by which every value within a dataset varies from the mean. It is the most robust and widely used measure of dispersion, as it takes into account every variable in the dataset. When the values in a dataset are pretty tightly bunched together, the SD is small. When the values are spread apart, SD will be relatively large. A SD close to 0 indicates that the data points tend to be very close to the mean (also called the **expected value**) of the set. SD is usually presented in conjunction with the mean and is measured in the same units. In many datasets, the values deviate from the mean value due to chance and such datasets are said to display a **normal distribution**. In a dataset with a normal distribution most of the values are clustered around the mean while relatively few values tend to be extremely high or extremely low. For datasets that have a normal distribution, the SD can be used to determine the proportion of values that lie within a particular range of the mean value. For such distributions, it is always the case that 68% of values are <1 SD away from the mean value; 95% of values are <2 SD away from the mean; 99% of values are <3 SD away from the mean. Sample standard deviation formula is:

Where,

$$s = \sqrt{\frac{\Sigma(X - \bar{X})^2}{n - 1}}$$

s = Sample standard deviation
Σ = Sum of ...
$\bar{X}$ = Sample mean
n = Number of scores in sample.

Uses of standard deviation

- It summarises the deviations of a large distribution from mean in one figure used as a unit of variation.
- Indicates whether the variation of difference of an individual form the mean is by chance.
- It helps in finding the standard error.
- It helps in finding the suitable sample size.

5. **Standard error of mean (SEM):** It is calculated by dividing the SD by the square root of n. It is the SD of the error in the sample mean relative to the true mean of total population. With increasing sample size (n), SEM decreases.

Q. 4. Write a short note on normal curve.

[RGUHS, May 2012]

Ans. Normal distribution refers to a family of continuous probability distributions described by the normal equation. **Normal equation** is the probability density function for the normal distribution. If large values are collected for any character, and a frequency table is prepared with small class interval, the frequency curve of this data will give a bell-shaped symmetrical curve, which is known as **gaussian** or **normal curve** (Fig. 1.4). The shape of this curve depends on mean and SD of the data. Mean of the distribution determines the location of center of the graph, and SD determines the height and width of the graph. When SD is large, the curve is short and wide; when SD is small, the curve is tall and narrow. Normal curve is used to find confidence limits of the population parameters. Normal distribution also forms the basis for the tests of significance.

Characteristics

1. It is bell-shaped.
2. It is symmetrical.
3. Mean, median and mode coincide.
4. It has two inflections. The central part is convex while at the points of inflection, the curve changes from convexity to concavity. A perpendicular from the point of inflection will cut the base at a distance of one SD from the mean on either side.

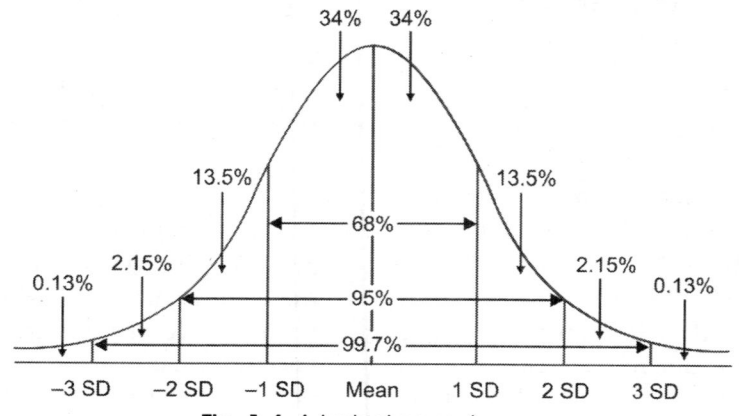

Fig. 1.4: A typical normal curve

5. Shape of the curve tells the probability of occurrence by chance or how often an observation, measured in terms of mean and SD can occur normally in a population.

Probability and the Normal Curve

The normal distribution is a continuous probability distribution. This has several implications for probability.

- Total area under the normal curve is equal to 1.
- Probability that a normal random variable X equals any particular value is 0.
- Probability that X is greater than α equals the area under the normal curve bounded by α and plus infinity.
- Probability that X is less than α equals the area under the normal curve bounded by α and minus infinity.

Additionally, every normal curve conforms to the following "rule".

- About 68% of the area under the curve falls within 1 SD of the mean.
- About 95% of the area under the curve falls within 2 SD of the mean.
- About 99.7% of the area under the curve falls within 3 SD of the mean.

Collectively, these points are known as the **empirical rule** or the **68–95–99.7 rule**. Clearly, given a normal distribution, most outcomes will be within 3 standard deviations of the mean.

Q. 5. What is probability/chance in statistics?
(NTR Uni., April 2014)

Ans. Probability may be defined as the relative frequency or probable chances of occurrence with which an event is expected to occur on an average. An element of uncertainty is associated with every conclusion, which is numerically expressed as probability and is denoted by p (range of 0–1). When p = 0, there is no chance of an event happening or its occurrence is impossible. When p = 1, the chances of an event to occur is 100%.

p = Number of events occurring/total number of trials

Purpose of selecting a representative sample is to know the probability of occurrence of single/group of observations in a normal distribution of any biologic variable. It is important to know whether occurrence of probability is by chance, which can be estimated by using tests of significance. It is estimated based on five laws of probability (Addition law; Multiplication law; Binomial law of probability distribution; Probability from shape of normal curve; Probability of

calculated values from tables), normal curve and tables. **Addition law** is used when one event excludes the possibility of the other (mutually exclusive). **Multiplication law** is applied to two or more events occurring together but they must not be associated. **Binomial law** is formed by the terms of the expansion of the binomial expression (p + q)n, where n = sample size or number of events; p + q = 1.

Q. 6. Write about parametric and non-parametric test.
(RGUHS, Nov. 2011; Sumandeep Uni., June 2016; NTR Uni., Nov. 2017)

Ans. Parametric test/normal distribution statistical tests assume the underlying population to be normally distributed and are based on means and SDs. The samples have the same variance (homogeneity of variances). The samples are randomly drawn from the population, and the observations within a group are independent of each other, e.g. all types of the t-test, F-test, and ANOVA, repeated ANOVA. Numerical data (quantitative variables) that are normally distributed are analyzed with parametric tests.

Nonparametric tests/distribution free tests *(NTR Uni., May 2018):* These tests make no assumption about the population distribution. Non-parametric tests may fail to detect a significant difference when compared with a parametric test. That is, they usually have less power, e.g. Chi-square test, Mann-Whitney U test, Fishers exact probability test, etc. Non-parametric tests are done when:

- Researcher is unaware of the nature of distribution or other required population parameters.
- When the sample may be too small to test the hypothesis.
- When scales of measurements are not numerical.

Advantages of Nonparametric Tests

1. Probability statements obtained from most non-parametric tests are exact probabilities.
2. Can be used for small sample size
3. For treating observations from samples drawn from several different populations.
4. Treat data which are simply classificatory, or the numerical scores having only the strength of ranks.
5. Easier to learn and apply (Table 1.6)
- **Mann-Whitney U test** is a non-parametric test that allows two groups or conditions or treatments to be compared without making the assumption that values are normally distributed. Requirements: Two random, independent samples; The data is continuous. Null hypothesis asserts that the medians of the two samples are identical.

Table 1.6: Uses of parametric and non-parametric tests

Sl. No.	Description	Parametric methods	Non-parametric methods
1.	Descriptive statistics	Mean, SD	Median, IQR
2.	Sample with population (or hypothetical value)	One sample t-test (n<30); one sample Z-test (n≥30)	One sample Wilcoxon signed rank test
3.	Two unpaired groups	Independent sample t-test (unpaired sample t-test)	Mann-Whitney U-test/Wilcoxon rank sum test
4.	Two paired groups	Paired sample t-test	Related sample Wilcoxon rank sum test
5.	≥3 unpaired groups	One-way ANOVA	Kruskal-Wallis H-test
6.	≥3 paired groups	Repeated measures ANOVA	Friedman test
7.	Degree of linear relationship between 2 variables	Pearson's correlation coefficient	Spearman rank correlation coefficient
8.	Predict one outcome variable by at least one independent variable	Linear regression model	Non-linear regression model/log linear regression model or log normal data

Q. 7. Discuss tests of significance.

(AIIMS-CDER, Dec. 1991; HP Uni., July 2013; BBD Uni., April 2014; UHSR; April 2015; AHSUC, May 2017; Sumandeep Uni., May 2018; UOD, June 2019)

Ans. The methods of statistical inference used to support or reject claims based on sample data are known as **tests of significance**. Common tests are Z-test, t-test and χ^2-test.

Stages in performing test of significance:
1. State the research hypothesis
2. State the null hypothesis (H0)
3. Select a probability of error level (α level)
4. Select and compute the test for statistical significance
5. Interpret the results

Z-test: When Z-test is applied, the difference observed between a sample estimate and population is expressed in terms of **standard error (SE)**. The score of value of the ratio between observed difference and SE is called 'Z'. If the distance in terms of SE or Z score falls in the zone of acceptance (95% confidence limit), the null hypothesis (H0) is accepted. The distance from the mean at which H0 is rejected is called **level of significance**. Greater the Z value, lesser will be the P. **In two-tailed** test, the difference is being tested for significance but the direction is not specified. P value of an experiment group includes both sides of extreme results at both ends of scale. In case of 5% level of significance, probability (P) will be 2.5% (0.025 at each end). **In one-tailed test**, one end of the scale is excluded to know specifically whether the results are higher or lower, by specifying the direction on plus or minus side. The significance level or P value will apply to relative end only. The significance level will be half of the P value.

Application
1. To test the significance of difference between a sample mean and a known value of population.
2. To test the significance of difference between two samples mean or between experiment samples mean and control sample mean.

Prerequisite to apply Z-test:
1. Samples must be randomly selected.
2. Data must be quantitative.
3. Variable is assumed to follow normal distribution in the population.
4. Sample size must be >30. If SD of population is known, Z-test can still be applied even if the sample is <30.

Q. 8. Write a short note on chi-square test.

(UHSR, April 2010; NTR Uni., Junr 2015; BBD Uni., April 2018)

Ans. Chi-square test, χ^2 test (or **chi-square test**), is a non-parametric test, not based on any assumption or distribution of any variable. This test follows **Chi-square distribution**. It is most commonly used when data are in frequencies, such as in the number of responses in 2 or more categories. It has very important applications as:

1. **Test of proportions:** To find the significance of difference in 2 or >2 proportions.
    i. To compare the values of two binomial samples even if they are small, <30.
    ii. To compare the frequencies of two multinomial samples.
2. **Test of association:** It measures the probability of association between two discrete attributes. There are two possibilities, they are either independent of

each other or they are dependent on each other. Assumption of independence of each other is made, unless proved otherwise by Chi-square test. This test can be applied to find relationship between two discrete attributes when there are >2 classes/groups.

3. **Test of Goodness of fit:** To determine if actual numbers are similar to the expected or theoretical numbers. Whether or not the observed frequencies of a character differ from the hypothetical or expected ones by chance or due to some factor playing part.

Calculation of χ^2 test: Essential requirements for the calculation are a random sample, qualitative data and lowest expected frequency not <5.

1. Make contingency tables (**2 × 2 Table**). Note the frequencies observed in each class of one event, row wise and then the numbers in each group of the other event, column wise.

2. Determine the expected number in each group of the sample or the cell of table on the assumption of null hypothesis, i.e. no difference in the proportions of the group from that of the universe.

3. Find the difference between the observed (O) and expected (E) frequencies in each cell.

4. Calculate χ^2 values by = $(O-E)^2/E$.

5. Sum up χ^2 values of all the cells.

6. Calculate degrees of freedom; df = (c – 1) (r – 1); c = number of vertical columns, r = number of horizontal rows.

7. Refer to **Fisher's χ^2 table**. If the calculated value of χ^2 is higher or lower than the x^2 value given in the table, it is significant or insignificant at that particular level of significance to which the reference is made for comparison. Exact level can be determined by comparison with the next higher or lower P value in the table.

Limitations

1. It will not give a reliable result with one df, if the expected value in any cell is <5.

2. Interpret χ^2 test with caution if sample total or total of values in all the cells is <40.

3. This test does not measure the strength of association.

4. The statistical finding of relationship does not indicate the cause and effect.

Q. 9. Write a short note on student 't' test.

(RGUHS, May 2011; UHSR, April 2013; HP, May 2013; RUHS, May 2015; BBD Uni., April 2017; UOK, July 2017; DYP Uni., May 2019)

Ans. Student's t-test is a method of testing hypotheses about the mean of a small sample drawn from a normally distributed population when the population SD is unknown. The ratio of observed difference between two means of small samples to the SE of difference in the same is denoted by 't'. This ratio follows the **'t' distribution**. The probability of occurrence of calculated value is determined by reference to **'t' table**. Probability converted into percentage is stated as level of significance. P = 0.05 may be stated as significant at 5% level. If the calculated 't' value exceeds the value given under P = 0.05 in the table, it is said to be significant at 5% level and null hypothesis is rejected and alternate hypothesis is accepted.

Degree of freedom (df): The quantity in the denominator which is 1 < the independent number of observations in a sample is called **degrees of freedom** (df). It is used in preference of sample size. In unpaired 't' test, df = $n_1 + n_2 - 2$; where n_1 and n_2 are the number of observations in each of the two series.

Criteria for applying t-test: Random samples; Quantitative data; Variable normally distributed; Sample size <30.

1. **Unpaired t-test:** This test is applied when comparison is made between two measurements in two different groups/two populations, to test if the difference between the two means is real or it can be attributed to sampling variability. Following steps are taken to test the significance of difference:
   - Find the observed difference between means of two samples.
   - Calculate the standard error between the two means.
   - Calculate the 't' value.
   - Determine the pooled degrees of freedom.
   - Compare calculated value with the table value at particular df to find the level of significance in two-tailed test. In one-tailed test, compare results with values given under P = 0.10 and P = 0.02.

2. **Paired t-test:** It is applied when comparison has to be made between two measurements in the same subjects after two consecutive treatments. This test is used:
   - To study the role of a factor/cause when the observations are made before and after its play.
   - To compare the effect of two drugs, given to same individuals in the sample on two different occasions.
   - To study the comparative accuracy of two different instruments.
   - To compare results of two different laboratory techniques.
   - To compare observations made at two different sites in the same body.

Following steps are taken to test the significance of difference:

1. Find the difference in each set of paired observations before and after.
2. Calculate the mean of the difference.
3. Work out the SD of differences and then the standard error of mean from the same.
4. Determine 't' value.
5. Find the df.
6. Refer 't' table and find the probability of calculated 't' corresponding to n–1 degrees of freedom.
7. If the P is >0.05, the difference observed has no significance. Thus, the factor under study may have no influence on the variable. But if P is <0.05, the difference observed is significant.

Q. 10. Write a short note on ANOVA test.
(HP Uni., May 2017; AIIMS-CDER, Dec. 2017; MUHS, Dec. 2018; Gujarat Uni., April 2019)

Ans. Analysis of variance (**ANOVA**) test or **F-test** is a collection of statistical models used to analyze the differences among group means and their associated procedures, developed by Ronald Fisher. ANOVAs are useful for comparing (testing) three or more means (groups or variables) for statistical significance. ANOVA is used in the analysis of comparative experiments, those in which only the difference in outcomes is of interest. The statistical significance of the experiment is determined by a ratio of two variances. This ratio is independent of several possible alterations to the experimental observations.

Steps

1. Start with null hypothesis.
2. Calculate the sum of squares.
3. Split this into sum of squares between the classes and sum of squares within the classes.
4. Compare the calculated F-ratio with that given in the F-table at df between the classes and at df within the classes at 5% level of significance.
5. If the calculated value is greater than table value, null hypothesis is rejected.

Types of ANOVA

1. **One-way** has one independent variable (with 2 levels). It is an extension of two-sample t-test to three or more samples and deals with statistical test on >2 groups.
2. **Two-way** has two independent variables (it can have multiple levels).
   Assumptions: Population must be close to a normal distribution; Samples must be independent; Popu-

lation variances must be equal; Groups must have equal sample sizes.

3. **MANOVA** *(AIIMS-CDER, May 2014)*: It is just an ANOVA with several dependent variables. MANOVA tests the multiple dependent variables by creating new, artificial, dependent variables that maximize group differences. These new dependent variables are linear combinations of the measured dependent variables.
4. **Factorial ANOVA:** An ANOVA test with >1 independent variable, or "factor". It can also refer to >1 **level of independent variable.** Factorial ANOVA is an efficient way of conducting a test; all the variables can be tested at the same time.
5. **Repeated measures ANOVA:** A repeated measures ANOVA is almost the same as one-way ANOVA, here related groups are tested, not independent ones. It is called *repeated measures* because the same group of participants is being measured over and over again.

   Advantages
   - When you collect data from the same participants over a period of time, individual differences are reduced or eliminated.
   - Testing is more powerful because the sample size is not divided between groups.
   - The test can be economical, same participants are tested.

   Assumptions: There must be one independent variable and one dependent variable; Dependent variable must be continuous, on an interval scale or a ratio scale; Independent variable must be categorical, either on the nominal scale or ordinal scale.
6. **Other methods,** such as planned or post hoc comparisons, are conducted to examine specific comparisons among individual means.
   a. **Planned** comparisons are hypotheses specified before the analysis commences.
   b. **Post hoc** comparisons are for further exploration of the data after a significant effect has been found. This analysis is occurring out of interest after the primary analysis has rejected the null hypothesis.

Q. 11. Write about various methods of data collection.
(RGUHS, May 2007; TNMGR, March 2010; BFUHS, May 2011)

Ans. A collective recording of observations either numerical or otherwise is called data. Data is classified into two broad categories:

A. **Qualitative data:** When the data is collected on the basis of attributes. It can also be descriptions of situations, events, people, interactions and observed behaviors; direct quotations from people and excerpts or entire passages from documents, correspondence, records and case studies. Qualitative data can be best conveyed in the form of words.

B. **Quantitative data:** When the data is collected through the measurements. It can be discrete or continuous. It is feasible to represent such data through ordinal and ratio scales, and are capable of being statistically evaluated.

Data can be calculated through

1. **Primary source:** Data is collected by investigator himself, because no previous records of the data exist. Primary data can be collected using a range of methods like direct personal interview, oral health examination, questionnaire method, surveys, focus groups, etc. Such data is considered to be highly reliable.

2. **Secondary source:** Data already recorded is utilized to serve the purpose of the study. Generally, secondary data includes government reports, census data, departmental records, etc. Using such data is less expensive and faster in comparison to primary data.

Data collection method

1. **Interviews:** An interview is meant to record and analyze people's opinions, experiences, beliefs and ideas on relevant topics. Research interviews can be:
   - **Structured interviews** follow a strict procedure of asking a list of predetermined questions to the participants, and recording the answers using standardized techniques.
   - **Semi-structured interview** is more open as compared to a structured interview, allowing the investigator or respondent to divert, if an idea is to be pursued in more detail.
   - **Unstructured interviews** do not follow a designated set of questions.

2. **Focus groups:** A focus group refers to a group of people who have been purposefully assembled at a place to take part in a discussion on a topic of relevance.

3. **Questionnaire and schedule:** In case of a questionnaire, the respondents comprise heterogeneous and widely scattered groups of people. The **schedule** is a structure of a set of questions on a given topic, which the researcher asks the respondent personally.

4. **Observation:** The researcher observes the behaviour of participants and records the results of these observations.

5. **Case study:** A case study is an in-depth investigation about a person, group, situation or occurrence.

6. **Ethnography:** Ethnography is the study of societies and cultures in a systematic way.

7. **Projective technique:** Projective techniques are methods of eliciting someone's internal ideas, values, attitudes, needs and opinions by responding to stimuli using external objects.

Q. 12. Discuss sampling in detail.
(TNMGR, March 2010; RGUHS, Nov. 2011; MUHS, June 2012;NITTE Uni., April 2016; HP Uni., June 2016; AHSUC, May 2017; Sumandeep Uni., June 2017; RGUHS, Nov.2017; NTR Uni., May 2019)

Ans. Sample means group of individuals who are actually available for the investigations. **Sampling** is an act of extracting a representative part of population for determining characteristics of whole population. The objective of sampling is:

1. Estimation of population parameters from the sample statistics.
2. To test the hypothesis about population from which the samples are drawn.

Stages in Sampling

Advantages of sampling: 1. Reduced cost of the survey; 2. Greater speed; 3. Greater accuracy; 4. More scope; 5. Higher response; 6. Quality information; 7. Allowance of error

Disadvantages: 1. Sampling as well as non-sampling errors; 2. Feeling of discrimination; 3. Requirement of representative sample of optimum size. Characteristics of sample: 1. Representative of population; 2. Optimum sample size.

Sampling methods/techniques *(Gujarat Uni., June 2018):*

A. **Probability/random sampling method** *(NTR Uni., April 2011):* All subjects in the target population have equal chances to be selected in the sample. By this method, samples are more representatives of the target population. **Advantages:** This technique reduces the chance of systematic errors and sampling biases. **Disadvantages:** Time consuming; Exhaustive and expensive.

1. **Simple random sampling:** This method is used when the whole population is accessible and the investigators have a list of all subjects in this target population. The list of all subjects in this population is called the "**Sampling Frame**". From this list, random samples are drawn using **lottery method/computer generated random** list.

2. **Stratified random sampling:** In this method, the whole population is divided into homogeneous strata or subgroups according a demographic

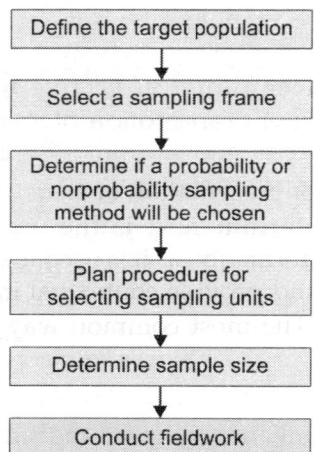

Fig. 1.12: Stages in sampling

factor (e.g. gender, age,) followed by selecting a random sample from the different strata.

Advantages: It allows obtaining samples from minority/under-represented populations.

3. **Systematic random sampling/interval sampling:** In this, systematic sample is formed by selecting one unit at random and then selecting additional units at regular/fixed interval. It is simple and convenient to adopt.

4. **Cluster sampling/multistage:** This method is used when the population forms natural groups/ cluster, such as villages, wards, etc. It is used when creating a sampling frame is nearly impossible due to large size of the population. This method is called **multistage** because the selection passed with two stages: Firstly, the selection of eligible clusters, then, the selection of sample from individuals of these clusters.

Steps in collection of data in cluster sampling:
1. List all cities, towns, villages with their population falling under the area of interest.
2. Calculate cumulative population and divide by 30. This gives the sampling interval.
3. Select a random number less than or equal to sampling interval. This forms the first cluster.
4. The second cluster is n +1st cluster, where n = sampling interval.

    Advantages: Simpler, less time and less cost involved.

    Disadvantages: Cluster sampling gives higher standard error.

5. **Multi-phasic sampling:** In this method, part of the information is collected from whole population and part from sub-samples. This

method may be adopted when the interest is in any specific disease.

6. **Pathfinder surveys** (*NTR Uni., June 2015):* Survey is an investigation in which information is systematically collected, but in which experimental method is not used. In this method, sampling of only a specified proportion of the population is done. In this way statistically significant and clinically relevant information is obtained at minimum expense. It can be **Pilot** or **National pathfinder** survey.

B. **Non-probability sampling method/purposive/ judgment/non-random sampling:** In this, the sample population is selected in a non-systematic process that does not guarantee equal chances for each subject in the target population.

Advantages: The techniques need less effort, less time and less expensive.

Disadvantages: The sampling techniques are prone to encounter with systematic errors and sampling biases. Inferences drawn from sample are not generalisable to the population.

1. **Convenience sampling:** In this method, the investigators enroll subjects according to their availability and accessibility. This method is quick, inexpensive, and convenient.

2. **Judgmental sampling:** In this method, the subjects are selected by the choice of the investigators. This method may be biased by investigator judgment.

3. **Snow-ball/chain sampling:** This method is used when the population cannot be located in a specific place. In this method, the investigator asks each subject to give him access to his colleagues from the same population.

4. **Quota sampling:** In this, the population is divided into quotas according to some specific characteristics (age, sex, religion, etc.) represented to the exact extent that the investigator desires.

• **Estimation of sample size** (*RGUHS, May 2013; Sumandeep Uni., April 2014; NTR Uni., May 2019):* A sample must be of the required size in order to have the required degree of accuracy in the results as well as to be able to identify any significant difference/association that may be present in the study population. Sample size should never be small. Bigger the sample size, higher will be the precision of estimates of samples. The more heterogeneous a population is on a variety of characteristics (e.g. race, age, sexual orientation, religion), then a larger sample is needed to reflect that diversity.

Following factors influence the sample size:

1. Size of the study population (from which the sample is to be selected).
2. The confidence level (generally set at 95% confidence level).
3. An approximate idea of the estimate of the characteristics under study and its variability from unit to unit in the population.
4. Knowledge about the precision of the estimate of the characteristic.
5. The probability level within which the desired precision is to be maintained.
6. The availability of experimental material, resources and other practical considerations.

- **Sampling error** (NTR Uni., May 2019): **Sampling error** is the deviation of selected sample from the true characteristics, traits, behaviours, qualities or figures of the entire population. They are the errors that creep in due to the sampling process and could arise because of faulty sampling design and small sample size. **Non-sampling errors** are:
- **Coverage error:** Due to non-response/non-cooperation of the informant.
- **Observational error:** Due to interviewer's bias or imperfect experimental technique or interaction of both.
- **Processing errors:** Due to errors in statistical analysis.
- **Sampling bias** (RUHS, May 2018; NTR Uni., May 2019): Sampling bias is a tendency to favour a selection of sample unit that possess particular characteristics. It is a systematic error that leads to distortion in the result of study. It may occur in the form of over-representation bias. Bias may be unintentional (accidental), or intentional.

Types of sampling bias (BBD Uni., April 2018):

1. **Self-selection bias/response bias:** This type of bias happens in a situation when the participants in the study have some control over the study to participate or not.
2. **Household bias:** When one type of respondent it over represented because groupings (strata) of different sizes are polled equally.
3. **Exclusion bias/non-response bias:** This type of bias happens when some people of the group are eliminated from the study.
4. **Healthy user bias:** This type of bias occurs when the sample selected has more likelihood to be healthier as compared to general population.

Minimizing sampling bias

1. Large sample size
2. Avoid convenient or judgment sampling.

Q. 13. Write about presentation of statistical data.
(HP, May 2015)

Ans. Methods of presentation of statistical data:

A. **Text presentation:** Text is the main method of conveying information as it is used to explain results and trends, and provide contextual information.

B. **Tabulation:** The most common way of presenting data in the tables is known as **frequency distribution** table. The variable has range from lowest to highest. This range is divided into subgroups called **classes**. The difference between the upper and lower limit of a class is known as **class interval**.

   Rules for making a table

   1. Every table should contain a title as to what is depicted in the table.
   2. Number of the class intervals should not be too many or too less.
   3. Class interval should be at equal width.
   4. Class limit should be clearly defined to avoid ambiguity.
   5. Each row and column should be clearly defined with the headings.
   6. Units of measurements should be specified.
   7. If the data is not original, the source of the data should be mentioned at the bottom of the table.

C. **Graph/diagram:** Diagrams and graphs are extremely useful as they are attractive to eyes, give a bird's eye view, have a lasting impression on mind and facilitate comparison of the data.

Rules for making diagram and graphs

1. Every diagram must be given a title that is self-explanatory.
2. It should be simple and consistent with the data.
3. Values of the variables are presented on horizontal or X-axis and frequency on the vertical line or Y-axis.
4. Diagram should not look clumsy.
5. Scale of presentation should be mentioned at the right hand top corner of the graph.
6. Scale of division of the two axes should be proportional and the division should be marked along with the details of variables and frequencies presented on the axes.

Types of diagrams

1. **Bar diagram:** This is used to represent qualitative data. It represents only one variable. The height (or length) of a bar represents the amount of information

in a category. Bar graphs are flexible, and can be used in a grouped or subdivided bar format in cases of two or more datasets in each category. A **stack vertical bar graph** is used to compare the sum of each category, and analyze parts of a category.

2. **Histogram:** This is used to depict quantitative data of continuous type. It is a bar diagram without gap between the bars.

3. **Multiple bar diagram:** This is used to compare qualitative data with respect to a single variable.

4. **Proportional bar diagram:** This is used to represent qualitative data. It is used to compare only proportion of subgroups between different major groups of observations.

5. **Component bar diagram:** This is used to represent qualitative data. It is used to represent both, the number of cases in major groups as well as the subgroups simultaneously.

6. **Pie diagram:** This shows percentage breakdown of qualitative data. It is generally the most appropriate format for representing information grouped into a small number of categories. It is also used for data that have no other way of being represented aside from a table (i.e. frequency table).

7. **Line diagram:** This is useful to study changes of values in the variable over time.

8. **Frequency polygon:** This is used to represent frequency distribution of quantitative data and is useful to compare two or more frequency distributions.

9. **Cartograms/spot map:** These maps are used to show geographical distribution of frequencies of a characteristic.

Q. 14. Write a short note on correlation and regression.
(AIIMS-CDER, Dec. 2009; RUHS, June 2017; NTR Uni., May 2019)

Q. Discuss statistical tests in assessing the relationship between 2 variables.

Ans. The most commonly used techniques for investigating the relationship between two quantitative variables are correlation and linear regression.

A. Correlation: The relationship between two quantitatively measured variables. The extent of relationship between two sets of figures is called correlation coefficient (r).

Types of correlation

1. Perfect positive correlation: In this, the two variables are directly proportional and fully correlated with each other (r = +1).

2. Perfect negative correlation: The two variables are inversely proportional to each other (r = –1).

3. Moderately positive correlation: In this, the non-zero values of coefficient lie between 0 and +1. ($0 < r < 1$).

4. Moderately negative correlation: In this, the non-zero values of coefficient lie between –1 and 0. ($-1 < r < 0$)

5. Absolutely no correlation: In this, the value of correlation coefficient is zero.

- Calculation of correlation coefficient from ungrouped series: When associated variables are normally distributed, the correlation coefficient is called **Pearson's correlation coefficient.** It is defined as the covariance of two variables divided by the product of their standard deviations.

- Calculation of correlation coefficient from grouped series: When two variables are correlated, but they do not follow the normal distribution, the correlation coefficient used is **Spearman's rank order correlation coefficient** (or Spearman's rho). **Kendall rank correlation coefficient** (or Kendall's tau coefficient) is used to test the association between two measured quantities. The test is nonparametric, since it does not rely on any assumptions on the distribution of X or Y.

Misuse of correlation

- Failure to consider a third variable related to both of the variables being investigated, which is responsible for the apparent correlation.

- A nonlinear relationship may exist between two variables that would be inadequately described, or possibly even undetected, by the correlation coefficient.

- A dataset may sometimes comprise distinct subgroups, resulting in an inflated correlation coefficient.

- When the subjects are not a random sample.

B. Regression is concerned with obtaining a mathematical equation which describes the relationship between two variables. **Independent variable** is the one that is chosen freely or occurs naturally. **Dependent variable** occurs as a consequence of value of the independent variable. It is normally used for estimation purposes.

- Simple linear regression: Analysis of single regressor, one independent variable explains the behavior of dependent variable.

- Multiple regression: Application with more than one regressor. More than one independent variable explains the behavior of dependent variable.

Q. 15. Write about hypothesis. *(NTR Uni., Oct. 2013)*

Ans. Hypothesis is a tentative prediction or explanation of the relationship between two or more variables under study. A hypothesis helps to translate the research problem and objectives into clear explanation or prediction of expected results or outcomes of the research study.

Nature of hypothesis: The hypothesis is a clear statement of what is intended to be investigated. It should be specified before research is conducted and openly stated in reporting the results. This allows to: Identify the research objectives; Identify the key abstract concepts involved in the research; Identify its relationship to both the problem statement and the literature review.

Characteristics of a good hypothesis: Conceptual clarity, empirical referents, objectivity, specificity, relevant, testability, consistency, simplicity, availability of techniques, purposiveness, verifiability, profundity of effect, economical.

Sources of hypothesis: Theoretical/conceptual frameworks, previous research, real life experiences, academic literature.

Types of hypotheses

A. **Null hypothesis** (H0 or HN) (UHSR, May 2016; HP Uni., April 2019): The null hypothesis represents a theory that has been put forward, either because it is believed to be true or because it is to be used as a basis for argument, but has not been proved. It is also known as **statistical hypothesis** and is used for statistical testing and interpretation of statistical outcomes. It states the existence of no relationship between the independent and dependent variables. By starting with the proposition that there is no association, statistical tests can estimate the probability that an observed association could be due to chance.

B. **Alternative hypothesis (H1 or HA)/research hypothesis:** The alternative hypothesis is a statement of what a hypothesis test is set up to establish. It states the existence of relationship between two or more variables. It is opposite of null hypothesis. The alternative hypothesis cannot be tested directly; it is accepted by exclusion if the test of statistical significance rejects the null hypothesis.

Other Types of Hypotheses

- **Simple hypothesis:** It is the statement that reflects the relationship between two variables.
- **Complex hypothesis:** It is the statement that reflects the relationship between more than two variables.
- **Associative hypothesis:** It reflects a relationship between variables that occurs or exists in natural settings without manipulation.

- **Casual hypothesis:** It predicts the cause and effect relationship between two or more dependent and independent variables in experimental/interventional setting, where independent variable is manipulated by research to examine the effect on dependent variable.
- **Directional hypothesis:** It specifies not only existence but also the expected direction of the relationship between the variables.
- **Nondirectional hypothesis:** It reflects the relationship between two or more variables, but it does not specify the anticipated direction.

Q. 16. Write a short note on testing of hypothesis.

Ans. Hypothesis testing (**statistical inference**) is a formal process to determine whether to reject a null hypothesis, based on sample data.

Steps involved in testing of hypothesis are

1. State an appropriate null hypothesis for the problem. Calculate the suitable statistics using the standard error; t, Chi-square, F, etc.
2. Determine the degrees of freedom for the statistic.
3. Find the probability level, P corresponding to the test statistic using the relevant tables.
4. The null hypothesis is rejected if P is less than 0.05; otherwise it is accepted.
5. Formulation of a research question and selection of appropriate research design.
6. Calculation of sample size suitable to the hypothesis to be tested.
7. Apply the test of statistical significance fitting to the hypothesis (stated later in the article).
8. Determine P value from the results.
9. Compare the obtained P value with the critical value of P (either <0.05 or <0.01, as defined in the research protocol)
10. If P value < critical value, reject null hypothesis and accept the alternative hypothesis (difference detected). If P value > critical value, accept null hypothesis (no difference is detected).

Errors in hypothesis testing: In testing of hypothesis, two types of error are possible while accepting or rejecting the null hypothesis:

a. **Type I error (α-error):** A type I error (false-positive) occurs if an investigator rejects a null hypothesis that is actually true in the population. This gives rise to the chances of finding a false-positive result or detecting a difference when no such difference exists. The probability of committing a type I error is called

α/level of statistical significance. Usually, α is taken at 0.05.

b. **Type II error (β-error):** A type II error (false-negative) occurs if the investigator fails to reject a null hypothesis that is actually false in the population. This gives rise to the chances of finding a false-negative result or inability to detect a difference when such a difference exists. The probability of making a type II error is called β. β error should not be >20%.

- **Power of the study:** The probability of detecting a real difference when it does exist is the power of the study. It is denoted by ($1-\beta$). The accepted power of the study is set at 80%.

Ideally α and β would be set at zero, eliminating the possibility of false-positive and false-negative results. Conventional range for α is between 0.01 and 0.10; and for β, between 0.05 and 0.20.

Depending on whether the null hypothesis is true or false in the target population, and assuming that the study is free of bias, 4 situations are possible (Table 1.16).

- **P value:** P denotes the probability of obtaining a result equal to or "more extreme" than what is actually observed, assuming that the null hypothesis is true. Before the test is performed, a threshold value is chosen called the **significance level of the test** (also denoted by α) and this is conventionally taken as 5% or 0.05.
- **P value** <0.05 indicates strong evidence against the null hypothesis, so it is rejected (statistically **"significant"**).
- **P value** <0.01 indicates even stronger evidence against the null hypothesis (statistically **"highly significant"**).
- P value >0.05 indicates weak evidence against the null hypothesis.
- P value $\approx$ 0.05 is considered to be marginal.
- **Confidence interval (CI):** CI is a measure of the precision of the results. The two values that define the interval are called the **"confidence limits"**. A wide CI means that the results are imprecise, whereas a narrow CI indicates the estimate is precise. The upper and lower limits provide the means of assessing whether the results are clinically important.

Table 1.16: Study inference depending on the null hypothesis

Result of experiment	Decision	
	Accept H_0	*Reject* H_0
H_0 (true)	Correct decision	Type I error (α error)
H_0 (false)	Type II error (β error)	Correct decision

The CI of mean is expressed as 95%. CI of mean = mean $\pm$ 1.96 $\times$ standard error of mean. P value must be considered with 95% CI.

2. RESEARCH METHODOLOGY

Q. 1. Define research methodology. Write about principles of research methodology.
(BFUHS, May 2010; BBD Uni., April 2015; RUHS, May 2015, 2018)

Ans. Research is defined as a systematic process of collecting and analyzing data to find an answer to a question or a solution to a problem, to validate or test an existing theory. **Research methods** are all those methods/techniques that are used for conduction of research. **Research methodology** is a way to systematically solve the research problem. It may be understood as a science of studying how research is done scientifically.

All research is different but the following principles are common to all research. The WHO/Ethical Research Committee has developed a series of documents to assist researchers.

a. Clear statement of research aims
b. Information sheet for participants, which sets out clearly what the research, is about, what it will involve and consent is obtained in writing on a consent form prior to research beginning.
c. Appropriate methodology.
d. The research should be carried out in an unbiased fashion.
e. The research should have appropriate and sufficient resources in terms of people, time, transport, money, etc. allocated to it.

The people conducting the research should be trained in research and research methods and this training should provide:

i. Knowledge around appropriate information gathering techniques.
ii. An understanding of research issues.
iii. An understanding of the research area.
iv. An understanding of the issues around dealing with vulnerable social care clients, especially regarding risk, privacy and sensitivity and the possible need for support.

Those involved in designing, conducting, analyzing and supervising the research should have a full understanding of the subject area. If applicable, the information generated from the research will inform the policy-making process. All research should be ethical and not harmful in any way to the participants.

Q. 2. How to prepare a research protocol?

(NTR Uni., May 2008; HP Uni., June 2016)

Ans. A **research proposal** is a detailed description of a proposed study designed to investigate a given problem. Aims of the protocol.

1. To raise the question to be researched and clarify its importance.
2. To collect existing knowledge and discuss the efforts of other researchers who have worked on the related questions (literature review).
3. To formulate a hypothesis and objectives.
4. To clarify ethical considerations.
5. To suggest the methodology required for solving the question and achieving the objectives.
6. To discuss the requirements and limitations in achieving the objectives.

Elements of a research proposal are

1. **Title:** It should be concise and descriptive. It must be informative and catchy.
2. **Abstract:** It is a brief summary, which includes the main research question, the rationale for the study, the hypothesis (if any) and the method.
3. **Introduction:** The introduction provides the background information. It should answer the question of why the research needs to be done and what will be its relevance. It allows the investigator to describe the problem systematically, to reflect on its importance, its priority in the country and region and to point out why the proposed research on the problem should be undertaken..
4. **Objectives:** Research objectives are the goals to be achieved by conducting the research. They may be stated as 'general' and 'specific'. General objective of the research is what is to be accomplished by the research project. Specific objectives relate to the specific research questions the investigator wants to answer through the proposed study and may be presented as primary and secondary objectives.
5. **Variables:** During the planning stage, it is necessary to identify the key variables of the study and their method and units of measurement must be clearly indicated. Four types of variables are important in research: Independent variables, dependent variables, confounding or intervening variables, background variables.
6. **Questions and/or hypotheses:** Hypotheses are not meant to be haphazard guesses, but should reflect the depth of knowledge, imagination and experience of the investigator. In the process of formulating the hypotheses, all variables relevant to the study must be identified.

7. **Methodology:** The method section is very important because it tells how you plan to tackle your research problem. The guiding principle for writing the methods section is that it should contain sufficient information for the reader to determine whether the methodology is sound.

   i. **Research design:** The selection of the research strategy is the core of research design and is probably the single most important decision the investigator has to make. The choice of the strategy, whether descriptive, analytical, experimental, operational or a combination of these depend on a number of considerations but this choice must be explained in relation to the study objectives.

   ii. **Research subjects or participants:** Depending on the type of study:
      a. Inclusion or selection criteria.
      b. Exclusion criteria.
      c. Sampling procedure to ensure representativeness and reliability of the sample and to minimize sampling errors.
      d. Use of controls in study. Some descriptive studies (studies of existing data, surveys) may not require control groups.
      e. Criteria for discontinuation.

   iii. **Sample size:** The proposal should provide information and justification about sample size. A larger sample size than needed to test the research hypothesis increases the cost and duration of the study and will be unethical if it exposes human subjects to any potential unnecessary risk without additional benefit. A smaller sample size than needed can also be unethical as it exposes human subjects to risk with no benefit to scientific knowledge.

   iv. **Interventions:** If an intervention is introduced, a description must be given of the drugs or devices (proprietary names, manufacturer, chemical composition, dose, frequency of administration) if they are already commercially available. If they are in phases of experimentation or are already commercially available but used for other indications, information must be provided on available pre-clinical investigations in animals and/or results of studies already conducted in humans (in such cases, approval of the drug regulatory agency in the country is needed before the study).

   v. **Ethical issues:** Ethical considerations apply to all types of health research. The proposal must describe the measures that will be undertaken to ensure that the proposed research is carried out in accordance with the World Medical Association Declaration of Helsinki on Ethical Principles for Medical Research involving Human Subjects.

vi. **Informed consent form (ICF):** A consent form, where appropriate, must be developed and attached to the proposal. It should be written in the prospective subject's mother tongue and in simple language which can be easily understood by the subject. The approved version of the protocol must have copies of ICF, both in English and the local language in which they are going to be administered.

vii. **Research setting:** It includes all the pertinent facets of the study, such as the population to be studied (sampling frame), place and time of study.

viii. **Study instruments:** Instruments are the tools by which the data are collected. Descriptions of other methods of observations like medical examination, laboratory tests and screening procedures are necessary for established procedures, reference of published work cited but for new or modified procedure, an adequate description is necessary with justification for the same.

8. **Collection of data and analysis:** A short description of the protocol of data collection minimizes the possibility of confusion, delays and errors. The description should include the design of the analysis form, plans for processing and coding the data and the choice of the statistical method to be applied to each data. What will be the procedures for accounting for missing, unused or spurious data?

9. **Monitoring, supervision and quality control:** Detailed statement about the all logistical issues to satisfy the requirements of good clinical practices, protocol procedures, responsibilities of each member of the research team, training of study investigators, steps taken to assure quality control.

10. **Significance of the study:** Indicate how your research will refine, revise or extend existing knowledge in the area under investigation. How will it benefit the concerned stakeholders? What could be the larger implications of your research study? How do you propose to share the findings of your study with professional peers, practitioners, participants and the funding agency?

11. **References:** The proposal should end with relevant references on the subject.

12. **Appendixes** include the appropriate appendixes in the proposal. Regarding original scales or questionnaires, if the instrument is copyrighted then permission in writing to reproduce the instrument from the copyright holder or proof of purchase of the instrument must be submitted.

Q. 3. What are descriptive studies?

Ans. Study design is the set of methods and procedures used to collect and analyze data on variables specified in a particular research question. Study designs are primarily of two types (Fig. 2.3):

A. Observational: i. Descriptive; ii. Analytical.

B. Interventional/experimental.

A. Descriptive study: A descriptive study is one that is designed to describe the distribution of one or more variables, without regard to any causal or other hypothesis. Descriptive studies are useful to assess disease burden and provide information for resource planning.

Advantages: Inexpensive, quick.

Disadvantages: Validity of results is highly dependent on whether the study sample is well representative of studied population.

Types

a. **Case reports and series:** A case report refers to the description of a patient with an unusual disease or with simultaneous occurrence of >1 condition. They may illustrate new or unfamiliar cases or rare manifestations of a common disease, a chance observation using new investigation, uncommon adverse effects of therapies, etc. A case series is similar, except that it is an aggregation of multiple similar cases.

b. **Cross sectional studies.**

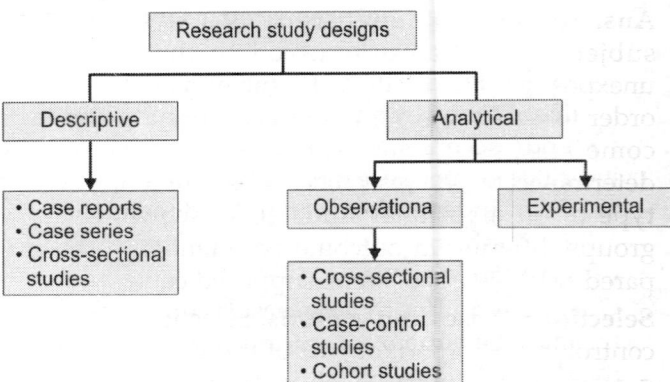

Fig. 2.3: Classification of research study design

c. **Ecological studies:** Ecological (or correlational) study design involves looking for association between an exposure and an outcome across populations rather than in individuals.

Limitations

a. Association between exposure and outcome at the group level may not be true at the individual level (**"Ecological Fallacy"**).

b. The association may be related to a third factor which in turn is related to both the exposure and the outcome (**"Confounding"**).

c. Migration of people between regions with different exposure levels may also introduce an error.

Q. 4. What are qualitative and quantitative researches? *(NTR Uni., May 2019)*

Ans. Qualitative research is primarily exploratory research. It provides insights into the problem or helps to develop ideas or hypotheses for potential quantitative research. Qualitative data collection methods vary using unstructured or semi-structured techniques. Sample size is typically small, and respondents are selected to fulfill a given quota.

Quantitative research is used to quantify the problem by way of generating numerical data or data that can be transformed into usable statistics. It is used to quantify attitudes, opinions, behaviors, and other defined variables and generalize results from a larger sample population. Quantitative data collection methods are much more structured and include various forms of surveys: Online surveys, paper surveys, mobile surveys and kiosk surveys, face-to-face interviews, telephone interviews, longitudinal studies, website interceptors, online polls, and systematic observations.

Q. 5. Write a short note on case control study.

(UOK, July 2017; HP Uni., April 2019)

Ans. An **observational study** is a study in which subjects are not randomized to the exposed or unexposed groups, rather the subjects are observed in order to determine both their exposure and their outcome status and the exposure status is thus not determined by the researcher. Case control study is a type of observational study in which two existing groups differing in outcome are identified and compared on the basis of some supposed causal attribute.

Selection of cases and controls: Selection of cases and controls is an important part of this design.

Selection of case: The investigator should define the cases as specifically as possible. Sometimes, definition of a disease may be based on multiple criteria; thus, all these points should be explicitly stated in case definition.

Selection of a control: An important aspect of selecting a control is that they should be from the same 'study base' as that of the cases. Thus, the pool of population from which the cases and controls will be enrolled should be same.

Types of controls

- **Hospital controls:** An important source of controls is patients attending the hospital for diseases other than the outcome of interest. These controls are easy to recruit and are more likely to have similar quality of medical records.

- **Relative and friend controls:** These controls are easy to recruit and they are also more likely to be similar to the cases in socioeconomic status and other demographic factors.

- **Population controls:** These controls can be easily conducted from the list of all available individuals. However, they can be expensive and time consuming and the response rate may be very low.

- Historic controls: Use of controls from the past (time period when cases did not occur.

Matching in a case-control study: Matching is used in case-control studies to ensure that the cases and controls are similar in certain characteristics. Matching is a useful technique to increase the efficiency of study. 'Individual matching' is one common technique used in case-control study.

Advantages: Efficient sampling of rare disease. Rapid evaluation of chronic disease. Economical: May serve explanatory purpose.

Limitations: Not practical for rare exposures. Sampling is prone to systematic error. Historical information often cannot validate. Relevant cofactors may be difficult to control.

Biases in case control study: Selection bias, bias in investigating controls, confounding bias, problems due to overmatching, analysis bias.

Q. 6. Write a short note on cohort studies.

(AIIMS-CDER, May 1991;
UHSR; May 2016; NTR Uni., May 2019)

Ans. A cohort is a group of people who share a common characteristic or experience within a defined period (e.g. are born, are exposed to a drug or vaccine or pollutant, or undergo a certain medical procedure). The comparison group may be the general population from which the cohort is drawn, or it may be another cohort of persons thought to have had little or no exposure to the substance under investigation, but otherwise similar. A **cohort study** is a form of longitudinal study (a type of observational study), it is an analysis of risk factors and follows a group of people who do not have the disease, and uses correlations to determine the absolute risk of subject contraction. Cohort studies can either be conducted **prospectively or retrospectively** from archived records. In a cohort study, an outcome or disease-free study population is first identified by the exposure or event of interest and followed in time until the disease or outcome of interest occurs. Because exposure is identified before the outcome, cohort studies have a temporal framework to assess causality and thus have the potential to provide the strongest scientific evidence.

Advantages

1. Gather data regarding sequence of events; can assess causality.
2. Examine multiple outcomes for a given exposure.
3. Can calculate rates of disease in exposed and unexposed individuals over time (e.g. incidence, relative risk).
4. Good for investigating rare exposures.

Disadvantages: Large numbers of subjects are required to study rare exposures, susceptible to selection bias.

Disadvantages of prospective cohort study: May be expensive to conduct. May require long durations for follow-up. Maintaining follow-up may be difficult. Susceptible to loss to follow-up or withdrawals.

Disadvantages of retrospective cohort study: Susceptible to recall bias or information bias. Less control over variables.

Q. 7. Write a short note on cross-sectional studies.
(AIIMS-CDER, May 1991)

Ans. Cross-sectional study (non-experimental) is a type of observational study that involves analysis of data collected from a population, or a representative subset, at one specific point in time. Cross-sectional studies differ from case-control studies in that they aim to provide data on the entire population under study. Cross-sectional studies are descriptive studies. They can be used to describe **odds ratio, absolute risks and relative risks** from prevalence. They are often used to assess the prevalence of acute or chronic conditions, or to answer questions about the causes of disease or the results of intervention. Large cross-sectional studies can be made at little or no expense. This is a major advantage over other forms of epidemiological study. A natural progression has been suggested from cheap cross-sectional studies of routinely collected data which suggest hypotheses, to case-control studies testing them more specifically, then to cohort studies and trials which

cost much more and take much longer, but may give stronger evidence.

Q. 8. Write a note on experimental studies.
(AHSUC, May 2018)

Q. Write a short note on randomized controlled trials.
(RGUHS, May 2013;BFUHS, June 2016; Sumandeep Uni., June 2017; BBD Uni., April 2018; RUHS, May 2018; MUHS, Dec. 2018, HP Uni., April 2019)

Q. Goals and types of randomization in randomized control trials.
(AIIMS-CDER, Dec. 2017)

Ans. Experimental studies are ones where researchers introduce an intervention and study the effects. The studies under this category are:

A. Randomised controlled trials (RCTs) *(Gujarat Uni., April 2019):* A study design that randomly assigns participants into an experimental group or a control group. As the study is conducted, the only expected difference between the control and experimental groups in a RCT is the outcome variable being studied. It involves the following steps:

a. Reference population.
b. Protocol.
c. Informed consent.
d. Randomization.
e. Concealment of allocation.
f. Measurement of response variable.
g. Ascertainment of outcome.

Advantages

1. Good randomization will "wash out" any population bias.
2. Easier to blind/mask than observational studies.
3. Results can be analyzed with well-known statistical tools.
4. Populations of participating individuals are clearly identified.

Disadvantages

1. Expensive in terms of time and money.
2. Volunteer biases: The population that participates may not be representative of the whole.
3. Does not reveal causation.
4. Loss to follow-up attributed to treatment.

- **Randomization:** Randomization ensures that each patient has an equal chance of receiving any of the treatments under study, generate comparable intervention groups, which are alike in all the important aspects except for the intervention each group receives.

- **Benefits:** It eliminates the selection bias, balances the groups with respect to many known and unknown confounding or prognostic variables, and forms the basis for statistical tests, a basis for an assumption of free statistical test of the equality of treatments. It can be: Simple randomization, block randomization, stratified randomization, covariate adaptive randomization.
- **Blinding:** Bias is avoided not only by randomization but also by blinding. A study may be double blind, single blind, or open.

B. Field trials

1. Preventive trials: When one has to derive disease-free status in a healthy population using preventive techniques, large scale field trials are required.
2. Risk factor trials: In this, specific risk factors are averted in groups of population and the reduction in disease incidence observed.

C. Community trials: The whole community is taken as the study group. Control communities in the neighbourhood can be selected for comparison.

D. Natural experiments: When natural events lead on to determinants in health.

E. Before and after studies: When no control is available, the past situation can be compared with situation following intervention.

Q. 9. Write a short note on double blind study.
(NTR Uni., April 2014)

Ans. A blind or blinded experiment is an experiment in which information about the test is kept blind from the participant until after the test. Bias may be intentional or unconscious. Blinding is of three types:

a. **Single blind:** When the patient is blind and the investigator is only aware of the drug given.
b. **Double blind:** When the patient and investigator are blind.
c. **Triple blind:** When the patient, investigator and data clean-up people are blind.

Blind testing is used wherever items are to be compared without influences from tester's preferences or expectations.

The main advantage to a double-blind study is that there is more confidence that any differences between the treatment and the placebo are real, since the perceptions of the doctors, patients and data analysts do not factor into the results.

Q. 10. Describe the steps in carrying out the clinical trials. *(NTR Uni., Nov. 2017)*

Ans. According to the National Institutes of Health (NIH), a clinical trial is "a research study in which one or more human subjects are prospectively assigned to one or more interventions to evaluate the effects of those interventions on health-related biomedical or behavioral outcomes."

Types of Clinical Trials

1. Preventive trials
2. Screening trials
3. Diagnostic trials
4. Treatment (intervention) trials
5. Genetic studies
6. Quality of life studies
7. Epidemiological studies.

Phases of clinical trials: The phases of clinical trials are:

1. **Phase 1 trials:** This phase occurs directly after lab testing. Based on the lab testing, researchers have determined that the drug, device or other treatment may provide a benefit to humans. It usually consists of a very small number of participants and is conducted to evaluate the drug's overall safety and determine the safest dose of the drug.
2. **Phase 2 trials:** In this phase, the experimental drug or treatment is tested on a larger group of people (up to several hundred), to see if it is effective and safe. If results from this phase show that the new drug or device may be just as beneficial or more beneficial, then researchers can move to next phase.
3. **Phase 3 trials:** In this phase, the experimental drug or treatment being studied is given to large groups of people. Researchers will use these trials to confirm the drug's efficacy, monitor side effects, compare it to other commonly used treatments or to a placebo, and collect information to ensure safe use of the drug or treatment.
4. **Phase 4 trials:** This phase occurs post-marketing, meaning after a drug has been shown to work and the treatment has received FDA approval. Studies done at this stage are designed to evaluate the long-term risks and benefits of a medication.

Q. 11. Discuss animal model used in dental research.
(NTR Uni., April 2013)

Ans. Animal models are used to test the efficacy and effects of restorative materials on dental pulp; to evaluate the etiopathogenesis, clinical characteristics, and histological and immunologic aspects of periodontal disease; and to test the success of newer surgical techniques prior to its application on humans. They are also used to assess the advanced surgical procedures such as lasers and implant research and to evaluate newer drug efficacy before applying onto clinical trials.

Benefits of animal models in research:

1. Use of animals in research has made a substantial contribution to the understanding of biological processes.
2. It has been responsible for many important bio-medical discoveries.
3. It used in the development of a great number of therapies and preventative treatments, such as antibiotics, insulin, vaccines, and organ transplantation.

Guidelines to use animals in research: Indian National Science Academy developed the updated guidelines to use of animals in scientific research.

1. Depending on the need, one should allow and provide facilities to use animal models for the research purpose.
2. It is recommended to the researchers that one should not use animals unless until it is an unavoidable situation.
3. It should provide adequate care, housing, and make sure that the animal models used for research purpose are physically comfort and in good health
4. Sources of experimental animals for research should be from recognized animal facilities.
5. It should provide training facilities to the scientific researcher and the supporting staff those who take care of the animals during experiment.
6. Alternative animal models should be used to replace experimental animals wherever possible.
7. Forming ethical committees will ensure the minimal usage of animal models.
8. Committee for the Purpose of Control and Supervision of Experiments on Animals (CPCSEA) in India inculcated the credo of **"4 Rs"**—**R**eplacement, **R**eduction, **R**efinement, and **R**ehabilitation of animals used in experimentation.

Commonly used animals in research: Mouse, rat, hamster, guinea pig, rabbit, cat, dog, and monkey.

Alternatives to experimental animal models: Advantages of alternative methods are time efficiency, less manpower, and cost-effectiveness. Examples are: Computer models, cells and tissue cultures, alternative organisms (zebra-fish, fruit fly, eukaryotic nematode), microorganisms (brewing yeast).

Q. 12. What are the measures of disease frequency?

Ans. There are several measures of disease frequency in common use and depending on the research question and the available data, one should choose which measure is appropriate.

a. **Prevalence (P):** It is the number of existing cases (old and new), in a defined population at a specified point of time.

$$P = \frac{\text{Number of people with disease at a specified time}}{\text{Total number of subjects in the population}} \times 10^n$$

Uses of prevalence data:

1. Assess healthcare needs and planning health care services.
2. Study chronic diseases or disease with gradual onset.

b. **Incidence:** It is defined as the number of new cases in a given period in a specified population.

$$I = \frac{\text{Number of people with disease at a specified time}}{\text{Population at risk at the specified time}} \times 10^n$$

Uses of incidence data:

1. Describes trends in diseases; assessment of etiology.
2. Identification of risk factors and evaluates impact of primary prevention program.

Also **Prevalence** = Incidence × Duration.

c. **Risk:** It is the probability that a subject within a population will develop a given disease, or other health outcome, over a specified follow-up period. It can be calculated by:

$$\text{Risk} = \frac{\text{Number of subjects developing the diseases over a time period}}{\text{Total number of subjects followed over that time period}}$$

d. **Incidence rate:** It can be calculated by dividing the number of subjects developing a disease by the total time at risk for all people to get the disease.

$$\text{Incidence rate} = \frac{\text{Number of subjects developing the diseases}}{\text{Total time at risk for the disease for all subjects followed}}$$

Q. 13. Write a note on validity and reliability of diagnostic test. *(NTR Uni. June 2017)*

Ans. Validity of a test refers to ability of a diagnostic test to distinguish between individuals with and without a particular disease.

Evaluation of test with dichotomous variables (positive/negative): Two principal measures of test validity are sensitivity and specificity.

1. **Sensitivity** is defined as the proportion of diseased individuals with a positive test result.

2. **Specificity** is the proportion of disease-free individuals with a negative test result.

3. **Accuracy** is defined as the proportion of all tests results (both positive and negative) that are concordant with true health status.

To properly assess the validity (sensitivity and specificity) of a diagnostic test, the investigator should identify and make use of an existing gold standard. It should be mentioned that an ideal test would have both a sensitivity and specificity of 100%.

4. **Positive predictive value** (PPV) of a test is defined as the proportion of individuals with positive tests that actually have the disease.

5. **Negative predictive value** (NPV) is defined as the proportion of individuals with a negative test result that are actually disease-free.

As the prevalence of disease in the sample being tested increases, PPV of the test increases as well. As the prevalence of a particular disease decreases, NPV increases.

6. **Likelihood ratios (LR)**
   - Positive LR = Probability (+ test) among diseased individuals/probability (+ test) among disease-free individuals.
   - Negative LR = Probability (– test) among disease-free individuals/probability (– test) among diseased individuals.

   In general, LRs >1 indicate that the test result increases the probability that a patient has the disease of interest; LRs <1 decrease the probability of the target disorder. A LR = 1 indicates that the pre-test and post-test probabilities of disease are equivalent.

7. **ROC curve:** ROC curve is a plot of true-positive rate (sensitivity) versus false-positive rate (1-specificity) for a range of diagnostic test thresholds. Accuracy of diagnostic test can be assessed visually by examining the proximity of ROC curve to the upper left-hand corner of the graph. Closer the curve follows the upper left corner of the ROC space, the more accurate the test.

Table 2.13: Evaluation of test with dichotomous variables (positive/negative)

	Disease present	Disease absent
Test positive	a (true positives)	b (false positives)
Test negative	c (false negatives)	d (true negatives)

Sensitivity = a/(a+c); Specificity = d/(b+d);
Accuracy = a+c/(a+b+c+d);
Positive predictive value (PPV) = a/(a+b)
Negative predictive value (NPV) = d/(c+d)

Q. 14. Discuss ethics in dentistry.

Ans. The word 'ethics' is derived from the Greek word *'ethos'* meaning custom or character. Ethics is the philosophy of human conduct, a way of stating and evaluating principles by which problems of behaviour can be solved. Dental ethics means moral duties and obligations of the dentist towards his patients, professional colleagues and to the society.

History: The "Hippocratic Oath" has been regarded as a summing up of a standard of professional ethics. It is widely believed that the oath was written by Hippocrates, the father of medicine, in the 4th century BC.

In India, the Dentist Act was amended via Section 17A empowering the Dental Council of India (DCI) to prescribe standards of professional conducts and etiquette. The code of ethics was framed by DCI in 1975 and later notified by Government of India as "Dentists (code of ethics) Regulations 1976". It is in force from August 1976.

Ethical principles
1. To do no harm (non-maleficence).
2. To do good (beneficence).
3. Respect for persons.
4. Justice.
5. Veracity or truthfulness.
6. Confidentiality.

Ethical Rules for Dentists (Prescribed By DCI)
I. **The duties and obligations of dentist towards the patients**
   1. Every dentist should be courteous, sympathetic, friendly and helpful.
   2. He should observe punctuality in fulfilling his appointments.
   3. He should establish a well merited reputation for professional ability and fidelity.
   4. The welfare of the patient should be conserved to the utmost of the practitioner's ability.
   5. A dentist should not permit considerations of religion, nationality, race, party politics or social standing to intervene between his duties and his patients.
   6. Information of a personal nature which may be learned about or directly from a patient in the course of dental practice should be kept in the utmost confidence.

II. **Duties of dentists towards one another**
   1. Every dentist should cherish a proper pride in his/her colleagues and should not disparage them either by act or word.

2. When the dentist is interested with the care of the patient of other during sickness or absence, mutual arrangements should be made regarding remuneration.
3. A dentist called upon in any emergency to treat the patient of another dentist, should, when the emergency is provided for retire in favour of the regular dentist but shall be entitled to charge the patient for his services.
4. If a dentist is consulted by the patient of another dentist and the former finds that the patient is suffering from previous faulty treatment, it is his duty to institute correct treatment at once with as little comments as possible and in such a manner to avoid reflection on his predecessor.

III. **Duties of dentists to the public:** Dentist has to assume a leadership role in the community on matters related to dental health.
IV. **Some unethical practices**
1. Practice by unregistered persons employed by the dentist.
2. Dentist signed under his name and authority issuing any certificate which is untrue, misleading or improper.
3. Dentist advertising whether directly or indirectly, for the purpose of obtaining patients or promoting his own professional advantage.
4. Use of bogus diplomas, etc.
5. Paying or accepting commissions.
6. Undercutting of charges in order to solicit patients.
7. If the planed treatment is beyond the dentist's skill, the patient is not referred to a consultant.
8. In case of any emergency, consultation during the temporary absence of the patient's dentist, temporary service is provided and the patient is not sent back.
9. If consulted, the dentist accepts charge of the case without request of the referring dentist.

- **Ethics in Research** (*UHSR, May 2012; Gujarat Uni., July 2017; NTR Uni., Nov. 2017*): The Nuremberg code is a set of research ethical principles for human experimentation, set as a result of the Nuremberg trials at the end of 2nd World War. It was the first international instrument on the ethics of medical research, promulgated in 1947. The code, designed to protect the integrity of the research subject, set out conditions for the ethical conduct of research involving human subjects emphasizing their voluntary consent to research.
- **Cardinal Principles of Ethics in Research (By Beauchamp and Childress):** Autonomy, non-maleficence, beneficence, and justice—are fundamental for understanding the current approach to ethical assessment in health care. **Respect for autonomy** stands for acting intentionally after being given sufficient information and time to understand the information. **Beneficence** is directed to promote the well-being of patients and society. **Non-maleficence** implies first do no harm which can be achieved by careful decision-making and having adequate training. **Justice** deals with the equitable distribution of social benefits.
- **Principles of Ethics in Medical Research**
1. **Principles of essentiality:** Refers to whether the research is considered to be absolutely essential after a due consideration of the existing scientific knowledge in the proposed area of research.
2. **Principles of voluntariness, informed consent, and community agreement:** Research participants should be fully apprised of the research and the associated risks and benefits. Where research entails treating any community, the principles of voluntariness and informed consent apply to the community as a whole and to each individual member.
3. **Principles of non-exploitation:** The participants should be fully apprised of all the possible dangers that may arise during the research so that they can appreciate all the physical and psychological risks.
4. **Principles of privacy and confidentiality:** The identity and records of the participants are as far as possible kept confidential (except when required for legal reasons).
5. **Principles of precaution and risk minimization:** Due care and caution should be taken at all stages of the research to ensure that the research participant and those affected by it including the community are put to the minimum risk, suffer from no known irreversible adverse effects, and generally, benefit from the research or experiment.
6. **Principles of professional competence:** Research should be conducted by competent and qualified persons who act with total integrity and impartiality.
7. **Principles of accountability and transparency:** The research or experiment should be conducted in a fair, honest, impartial, and transparent manner after full disclosure is made of each aspect, and any conflict of interest that may exist.
8. **Principles of maximization of public interest and of distributive justice:** The research or

experiment and its subsequent application should be conducted and used to benefit all human kind.

9. **Principles of public domain:** The research findings should be brought into the public domain so that its results are generally made known through scientific and other publications.

10. **Principles of totality of responsibility:** Professional and moral responsibility should be observed, for the due observance of all the principles, guidelines, or prescriptions of those directly or indirectly connected with the medical research.

- **Ethical committee formation** (*NTR Uni., Oct. 2011*): The first appearance of need of ethics committee (EC) was made in Declaration of Helsinki in 1964, while in India, it appeared in 1980 in the ICMR Policy Statement. The establishment of EC requires 5–15 members with at least one basic medical scientist (preferably one pharmacologist), one clinician, a legal expert, a social scientist/representative of NGO/ philosopher or theologian and a lay person from the community. Every institute, where research is going on should have its own EC with its head preferably from outside the institute. Individuals carrying out research can approach to independent ECs. The decisions of EC should be taken only after quorum formation with a minimum of five members having at least one basic medical scientist, one clinician and one legal expert or retired judge. The ECs should have independence from political, institutional, professional, and market influences, in their composition, procedures, and decision-making. ECs are responsible for carrying out the review of proposed research before the commencement of the research. The basic responsibility of EC is to ensure an independent, competent and timely review of all ethical aspects of the project proposals received in order to safeguard the dignity, rights, safety and wellbeing of all actual or potential research participants. The EC should also look into matters like informed consent process, qualifications of principal investigator and supporting staff, adequacy of infrastructure and facilities, risk benefit ratio, plans to maintain confidentiality and plans for post-trial access and compensations. They also need to ensure that there is regular evaluation of the ongoing studies that have received a positive decision. EC is the most important checkpoint for promoting ethical research in the country.

- Informed consent: Informed consent is a process in which a health care provider educates a patient about the risks, benefits, and alternatives of a given procedure or intervention. Informed consent is required for many aspects of health care. These include consent for treatment, dissemination of patient information, discussion of HIPPA laws, specific procedures, surgery, blood transfusions and anesthesia.

Informed consent should include: (1) Describing the proposed intervention, (2) emphasizing the patient's role in decision-making, (3) discussing alternatives to the proposed intervention, (4) discussing the risks of the proposed intervention, and (5) eliciting the patient's preference (usually by signature).

Informed consent is both an ethical and legal obligations of medical practitioners and originates from the patient's right to direct what happens to his/her body.

Informed consent may be waived in emergency situations if there is no time to obtain consent or if the patient is unable to communicate and no surrogate decision maker is available.

Informed consent is also mandatory for participants in research studies. The main purpose of clinical trials is to "study" new medical products in people. It is important for people who are considering participation in a clinical trial to understand their role, as a "subject of research" and not as a patient. Informed consent in case of research studies involves providing a potential participant with:

- Adequate information to allow for an informed decision about participation in the clinical investigation.

- Facilitating the potential participant's understanding of the information.

- An appropriate amount of time to ask questions and to discuss with family and friends the research protocol and whether you should participate.

- Obtaining the potential participant's voluntary agreement to participate.

- Continuing to provide information as the clinical investigation progresses or as the subject or situation requires.

Q. 15. Write a note on applications of evidence-based dentistry. (*NTR Uni., May 2018*)

Ans. The ADA defines evidence-based dentistry (EBD) as "an approach to oral health care that requires the judicious integration of systematic assessments of clinically relevant scientific evidence, relating the patient's oral and medical condition and history, with the dentist's clinical expertise and the patient's treatment needs and preferences."

Applications/uses

1. Evidence-based principles help strengthen professions by identifying knowledge gaps and

encourage formulating clear questions regarding the evidence.

2. It develops questioning attitude in clinicians which lead to more research, better decision and thereby strengthening profession.
3. It helps health professional to decide the best suited treatment for his patient on by weighing benefit to risk ratio.
4. Clinician is able to explain the selection of particular treatment modality and its probable outcome to patient based on best evidence available.
5. EBD practice helps to reduce bias in research and its application in clinical practice.
6. EBD practice helps to curb overzealous and over-confident attitude of clinician about his beliefs on certain traditional procedures and makes him understand need of selection of treatment based on amalgamation of best evidence, his clinical experience and patients' needs and preferences.
7. This ultimately helps to empower the patient by preventing unnecessary treatments and to receive only best suited one.

How to practice EBD: EBD is practiced in following order which is popularly called as 5 'A's.

1. **Ask:** Recognize a need for information and formulate an answerable question. In order to achieve this, the question must be focused and well-articulated for all 4 parts of its "anatomy using '**PICO criteria**' which stand for
   i. **P:** Patient/problem
   ii. **I:** Intervention (or cause/prognosis)
   iii. **C:** Compare (or control)
   iv. **O:** Outcome
2. **Acquire:** Acquire best evidence which can answer that question. Look for scientific literature available to find the evidence. This scientific data can be categorizes based on its framework like: Case report/series, review article, case-control study, cohort study, cross-sectional study, RCTs, systemic reviews, meta-analysis, summaries of evidence, etc. Database is classified as per its level of evidence as follows (Fig. 2.15).
3. **Appraise:** Critically appraise the evidence for its level, validity, reliability, relevance and usefulness. It consists of the process of assessing and interpreting evidence through the systematic consideration of its validity, relevance and results. Grading of Recommendations Assessment, Development and Evaluation (**GRADE**) system is often used to rate the quality of evidence and grading strength of recommendations in systematic reviews and clinical practice guidelines. The GRADE process evaluates the study design, risk of bias, imprecision, inconsistency, indirectness, and magnitude of effect.
4. **Apply:** Apply the evidence with your clinical expertise and your patient's needs.
5. **Access:** Evaluate the overall results and your process. Make any necessary changes.

Resources for EBD: PubMed, The Cochrane Library, EBD at ADA.org, Journal of Evidence Based Dental Practice, database of abstracts of review of effectiveness

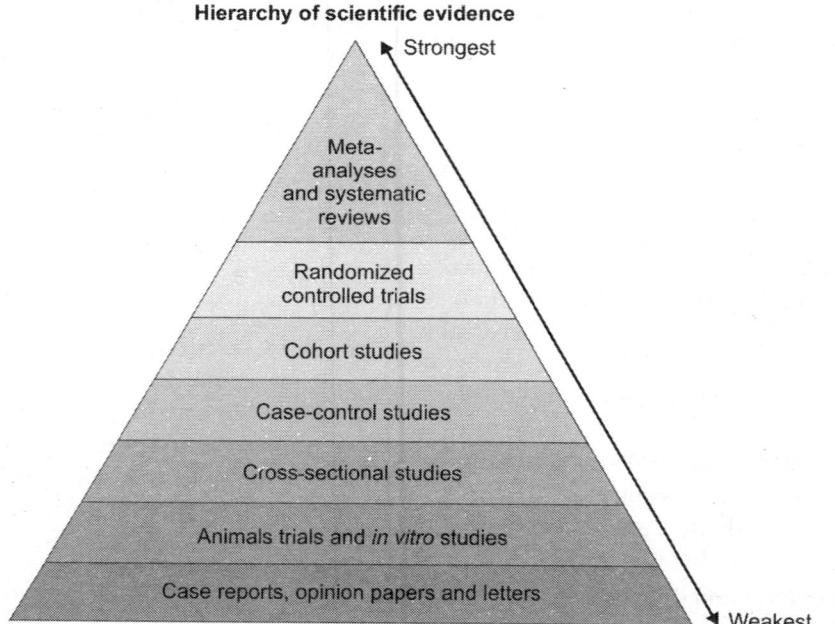

Hierarchy of scientific evidence

Strongest

- Meta-analyses and systematic reviews
- Randomized controlled trials
- Cohort studies
- Case-control studies
- Cross-sectional studies
- Animals trials and *in vitro* studies
- Case reports, opinion papers and letters

Weakest

Fig. 2.15: Pyramid depicting level/quality of evidence

(DARE), Agency for health care research and quality (AHRQ), centre for evidence-based dentistry, ADA evidence-based clinical guidelines, CDC division of oral health.

Hierarchy of evidence/level of evidence pyramid *(BBD Uni., July 2013; UHSR, May 2016):* A fundamental tool for evidence-based practice has been the evidence pyramid, which depicts the hierarchy or levels of evidence from lowest to highest. The levels of evidence were originally described by the Canadian Task Force on the Periodic Health Examination in 1979 to develop recommendations based on evidence in the medical literature. Sackett developed these further into the evidence pyramid. Levels of evidence are arranged in increasing order of internal validity (rigor or freedom from bias) from bottom to top, with *in vitro* and animal studies placed at the lowest level, followed by opinions, case reports, observational studies, RCTs, systematic reviews, and meta-analyses at the tip, representing the highest level of available evidence.

a. **Case reports and case series:** Case studies and case series form the lowest rungs of the evidence ladder, as isolated observations are collected in an uncontrolled, unsystematic manner, and the information gained cannot be generalized to a larger population of patients.

b. **Cross-sectional studies.**

c. **Case-control studies.**

d. **Cohort studies (prospective cohort, concurrent cohort).**

e. **Randomized controlled trials:** RCTs are the gold standard by which all clinical research is judged. This is the strongest type of experimental design.

f. **Systematic reviews and meta-analyses:** Systematic reviews and meta-analyses are considered the gold standard for evidence because of their strict protocols to reduce bias and to synthesize and analyze already

completed studies. A systematic review is a scientific tool that can be used to appraise, summarize, and project results and implications of otherwise unmanageable quantities of research. Systematic reviews appear at the top of the hierarchy of evidence. This reflects the fact that when rigorously conducted, they should give us the best possible estimate of any true effect.

Cochrane Database of Systematic Reviews *(CDSR)* *(AIIMS-CDER, May 2015)* is the leading resource for systematic reviews in health care. CDSR includes all Cochrane reviews (and protocols) prepared by Cochrane Review Groups in the Cochrane Collaboration. Each Cochrane review is a peer-reviewed systematic review that has been prepared and supervised by a Cochrane Review Group (editorial team) in the Cochrane Collaboration according to the Cochrane Handbook for Systematic Reviews of Interventions or Cochrane Handbook for Diagnostic Test Accuracy Reviews.

The Cochrane Library provides reliable and up-to-date information on the effects of interventions in health care.

Includes:

• The Cochrane Database of Systematic Reviews (Cochrane Reviews)

• Database of Abstracts of Reviews of Effects (Other Reviews)

• The Cochrane Central Register of Controlled Trials (Clinical Trials)

• The Cochrane Database of Methodology Reviews (Methods Reviews)

• The Cochrane Methodology Register (Methods Studies)

• Health Technology Assessment Database (Technology Assessments)

• NHS Economic Evaluation Database (Economic Evaluations)

h. **Meta-analysis** *(NTR Uni., June 2017):* Meta-analysis is the statistical pooling of the results of studies that are part of a systematic review. They are statistical procedures that integrate the results of several independent studies considered to be 'combinable'. This means that similar measures from comparable studies are listed systematically and the available effect—measures are combined, where possible. Conducting a systematic review involves proper methodology as described in the Preferred Reporting Items for Systematic Review and Meta-analysis **(PRISMA)**.

Advantages: They increase statistical power of analysis and precision to assess the treatment effects. Well-

Table 2.15: Study designs best suited for the type of study design and objective of the study

Type of question	Suggested best type of study
Therapy	RCT > cohort > case-control > case series
Diagnosis	Prospective, blind comparison to a gold standard
Etiology/harm	RCT > cohort > case-control > case series
Prognosis	Cohort study > case-control > case series
Prevention	RCT > cohort study > case-control > case series
Clinical exam	Prospective, blind comparison to gold standard
Cost	Economic analysis

conducted MAs allow a more objective evaluation of the evidence. MAs produce the highest quality of evidence achievable in medicine.

Limitations: Oversimplified results of research area; Errors in classifying of studies; Errors in estimating effect sizes; Limited number of well conducted studies; Low quality of primary studies; Heterogeneous primary data included in analysis.

Protocol of meta-analysis
- Definitions of the response variables.
- Methods of literature searching for the inclusion of the primary data in the analysis.
- Measures to identify and address publication bias.
- Inclusion and exclusion criteria for the articles to be analyzed.
- Data extraction procedure.
- Statistical analysis of the primary data, including quality and heterogeneity analysis.

Q. 16. Write a short note on IMRAD.
(NTR Uni., May 2018)

Ans. Most scientific papers are prepared according to a format called **IMRAD** (**I**ntroduction, **M**aterials and **M**ethods, **R**esults, **A**nd, **D**iscussion). It indicates a pattern or format rather than a complete list of headings or components of research papers; the missing parts of a paper are: Title, Authors, Keywords, Abstract, Conclusions, and References. Introduction explains the scope and objective of the study in the light of current knowledge on the subject; the materials and methods describe how the study was conducted; the results section reports what was found in the study; and the discussion section explains meaning and significance of the results and provides suggestions for future directions of research.

Q. 17. Write a short note on statistical package for social sciences.
(NTR Uni., May 2018)

Ans. "Statistical Package for Social Sciences" (SPSS) is a package of programs for manipulating, analyzing, and presenting data; the package is widely used in the social and behavioral sciences. SPSS is the set of software programs that are combined together in a single package.

Types of SPSS
1. **SPSS base** *(Manual: SPSS Base 11.0 for Windows User's Guide):* This provides methods for data description, simple inference for continuous and categorical data and linear regression and is, therefore, sufficient to carry out the analyses.

2. **Advanced models module** *(Manual: SPSS 11.0 Advanced Models):* This includes methods for fitting general linear models and linear mixed models and for assessing survival data, and is needed to carry out the analyses.
3. **Regression models module** *(Manual: SPSS 11.0 Regression Models):* This is applicable when fitting nonlinear regression models including logistic regression analysis.
4. **SPSS exact tests module** enables one to use small samples and still feel confident about the results.
5. **SPSS forecasting module** enables analysts to predict trends and develop forecasts quickly and easily, without being an expert statistician.
6. **SPSS missing values module** finds relationships between any missing values in data and other variables.

SPSS for Windows offers a spreadsheet facility for entering and browsing the working data file (Data Editor). Output from statistical procedures is displayed in a separate window (output viewer). It takes the form of tables and graphics that can be manipulated interactively and can be copied directly into other applications. It is its graphical user interface (GUI) that makes SPSS so easy by simply selecting procedures from the many menus available.

One of the **advantages of SPSS** is that data can be imported from other sources, when data is organized as a database, including Excel. Importing an Excel spreadsheet to **SPSS** for the data analysis is a fairly simple process, requiring some preparation and a few basic steps.

3. COMPUTERS, LASERS AND MISCELLANEOUS

Q. 1. Write about applications of computers in dentistry.
(NTR Uni., Nov 2007)

Ans. Computer is a machine capable of receiving, storing, manipulating and yielding information such as numbers, words, pictures. In the field of dentistry, computers are used for a large number of purposes. They can be broadly classified as:
1. **Education/academic applications**
   - Provide a large data bank of information;
   - Aid to time-tabling;
   - Carry out lengthy or complex calculations;
   - Assist teaching and learning processes;
   - Provide students' profiles;
   - Assist in career guidance
2. **Administrative applications:** Computers are used in the administration field. They are aimed for a

smooth running of dental clinics, hospitals and dental institutions. The various activities which are part of administrative applications are mentioned below.

- Patient appointments and recalls.
- Correspondence.
- Billing and accounting.

Inventory controls and supply orders.

- Dental insurance claims.
- Document preparation and word processing.
- Referral information.
- Missed appointments and follow-ups.

3. **Clinical applications:** Computers are also very much useful for the dentist in their professional practice.

- Patient records storage and retrieval.
- Patient evaluation, examination and treatment planning.
- Patient motivation and awareness.
- Appliance designing using CAD, CAM techniques.
- Storage of patient photographs, radiographs and study models.
- Computerized imaging techniques.
- Computerized cephalometrics.
- Growth prediction.
- Radiovisiography (RVG) technique.
- Clinical diagnosis and treatment planning.

4. **In research:** Computers are ideally suited for data analysis concerning large research projects. Software packages are readily available for the various simple and complicated analytical and quantitative techniques of which researchers generally make use of innumerable data can be processed and analyzed with greater ease and speed. Moreover, the results obtained are generally correct and reliable. Not only this, even the design, pictorial graphing and report are being developed with the help of computers. Researchers interested in developing skills in computer data analysis must be aware of the following steps:

  i. Data organization and coding;

  ii. Storing the data in the computer;

  iii. Selection of appropriate statistical measures/techniques;

  iv. Selection of appropriate software package;

  v. Execution of the computer program.

Limitations of computer-based analysis:

1. Computerized analysis requires setting up of an elaborate system of monitoring, collection and feeding of data. All these require time, effort and money.

2. Various items of detail which are not being specifically fed to computer may get lost.

3. The computer does not think; it can only execute the instructions of a thinking person. If poor data or faulty programs are introduced into the computer, the data analysis would not be worthwhile.

4. **Other applications:** Besides administrative purposes and clinical uses the other applications include:

  - Creating a database of **survey** information.
  - Case presentations.
  - Conference presentations.
  - Reviewing of literature.
  - Continuing medical education.

Q. 2. Write a note on health information system.

(NTR Uni., June 2017)

Ans. The health information system provides the underpinnings for decision-making and has four key functions: Data generation, compilation, analysis and synthesis, and communication and use.

Health planners and decision-makers need different kinds of information including:

- Health determinants (socioeconomic, environmental behavioral, genetic factors) and the contextual environments within which the health system operates.

- Inputs to the health system and related processes including policy and organization, health infrastructure, facilities and equipment, costs, human and financial resources, health information systems.

- Performance or outputs of health system responsiveness of the system to user needs, and financial risk protection.

- Health outcomes (mortality, morbidity, disease outbreaks, health status, disability, wellbeing).

  A good health information system brings together all relevant partners to ensure that users of health information have access to reliable, authoritative, useable, understandable, comparative data. Data from different sources are used for multiple purposes at different levels of the health care system.

- Individual level data about the patient's profile, health care needs, and treatment serve as the basis for clinical decision-making.

- Health facility level data, both from aggregated facility-level records and from administrative sources.

- Population level data are essential for public health decision-making and generate information.

- Public health surveillance brings together information from both facilities and communities with a focus mainly on defining problems and providing a timely basis for action. This is especially so when responses need to be urgent, as in the case of epidemic diseases (COVID-19).

Sources
- Indirect sources: Census, Civil Registration System and Sample Registration System.
- Direct sources: Sample surveys and official statistics.

Q. 3. Write a short note on summarization of health data. *(NTR Uni., Nov. 2017)*

Ans. Data summarization strategies can reduce the data burden either directly by limiting the amount of data reported, or indirectly by increasing its interpretability. In order for data summarization to be effective, the analysis plan should be framed according to each of the following:

1. Purpose of analysis: Routine surveillance and monitoring, statewide or community-based needs assessment, quality assurance activities, program evaluation, and special studies each require development of a distinct analysis strategy.
2. Audience for analysis: The degree and type of data summarization must be matched to the needs of each group.
3. Data availability and data quality: Choices about which data to include in an analysis are highly dependent on both the availability of data and on its quality.
4. Variables, methods, and presentation framed by the purpose of the analysis, the audience for which it is intended, and the availability and quality of data, the specifics of analysis planning can proceed.

Data summarization occurs in three successive phases:

Phase I: Selection of variables. This includes selection and definition of primary indicator or indicators that will be the central focus of analysis.

Phase II: Selection of analytic methods. This phase involves decisions about how the indicators and other variables selected will be examined.

Phase III: Selection of presentation format. This phase involves designing a report that effectively communicates the results of the analysis (Table 3.3).

Q. 4. Write a note on third party dental care.

Ans. Oral health is an integral part of general health and, therefore, can be rightly called the gateway of the body. The prohibitive cost of dentistry has been the main hindrance which deprives people of availing the services.

Third party payers (TPP): Any organization, public or private, that pays or contributes for healthcare expenses, on behalf of beneficiaries. such as employers, commercial insurance companies and public health funding mechanisms. These payments, called third-party payments, are distinguished by the separation between the individual receiving the service (first party), the dentist providing the service (second party), and the organization paying for it (third party).

Principles
- TPPs are a source of full or partial payment for dental treatments or dental non-clinical work rendered.
- Their financial involvement should support appropriate oral healthcare for the patient and evidence-based treatment decisions agreed upon by the dentist and the patient.
- TPPs are responsible to provide clarity to patients as to the scope of coverage of their contracts and the terms attached to the provision of treatments covered.
- Patients should receive necessary treatments, and the plans should pay fairly and promptly, to reduce or eliminate patients out of pocket expenses. However, the patient should remain responsible for the payment to the dentist if the TPPs fail to pay.

Table 3.3: Summarizing data: Reducing the data burden

Restricting the amount of data	Increasing interpretability	
Phase I: Variables	*Phase II: Methods*	*Phase III: Presentation*
Limit the number of indicators	Limit the amount of stratification	Text
Limit the number of person, place, time risk variables	Transform variables into:	Tables
	Discrete categories	Charts
	Ranks	Graphs
	Scores	Maps
	Construct indices	
	Use statistical testing	

Q. 5. Write a short note on dental anxiety.

Ans. Anxiety is an emotional state that precedes the actual encounter with the threatening stimuli which sometimes is not even identifiable. Anxiety associated with the thought of visiting the dentist for preventive care and over dental procedures is referred to as **dental anxiety.**

Fear is a reaction to a known or perceived threat or danger. Dental fear is a reaction to threatening stimuli in dental situations. **Phobia** is persistent, unrealistic, and intense fear of a specific stimulus, leading to complete avoidance of the perceived danger. Overwhelming and irrational fear of dentistry associated with devastating feelings of hypertension, terror, trepidation, and unease is termed "**odontophobia**", and has been diagnosed under specific phobias according to the Diagnostic and Statistical Manual (DSM) of mental disorders IV.

Etiology: Dental anxiety can arise due to multiple factors, such as previous negative or traumatic experience (**conditioning experiences**), vicarious learning from anxious family members or peers, individual personality characteristics such as neuroticism and self-consciousness, lack of understanding, exposure to frightening portrayals of dentists in the media. Some common fears giving rise to dental anxiety are fear of pain, blood-injury fears, fear of mercury poisoning, fear of radiation exposure, fear of choking and/or gagging, and lack of control during dental treatment.

Management

1. **Psychotherapeutic interventions** are either behaviorally or cognitively oriented, and recently, the use of cognitive behavior therapy (CBT) has been shown to be highly successful in the management of extremely anxious and phobic individuals.
2. **Ambience of dental operatory:** Receptionists, dental nurses, and dental hygienists should be positive and caring, and elicit information from the patients in a unhurried concerned tone to make the patients comfortable. The office atmosphere can be made calm and unthreatening by the playing of soft music and avoidance of bright lights.
3. **Aromatherapy:** Inhalation of pleasant scents such as essential oils has an anxiolytic effect and improves mood.
4. **Communication, rapport and trust building:** Dentist should first introduce themselves and personally converse with the patient in their office, and listen carefully in a calm, composed, and nonjudgmental way.

A. Psychotherapeutic management

- **Behavior-management techniques:** Behavior modification is based on the principles of learning, both in terms of classical conditioning or operant conditioning and of social learning. It aims to change undesirable behavior in certain situations through learning.
  1. **Relaxation techniques:** A relaxation response is the opposite of a stress response, and when practiced regularly it not only lowers stress and anxiety levels but also enables an individual to cope with the symptoms of anxiety.
  2. **Guided imagery:** Guided imagery has been defined as a directed, deliberate daydream that uses all the senses to create a focused state of relaxation and a sense of physical and emotional well-being.
  3. **Biofeedback:** Biofeedback is also referred to as applied psychophysiological feedback, and is a mind-body technique. Biofeedback therapies use instruments to measure, amplify, and feedback physiological information to the patient being monitored.
  4. **Hypnotherapy:** In this interaction, the hypnotist attempts to influence the subjects' perceptions, feelings, thinking, and behavior by asking them to concentrate on ideas and images that may evoke the intended effects.
  5. **Acupuncture:** It is effective in treating dental problems such as anxiety, temporomandibular dysfunction syndrome, pain, and Sjögren's syndrome.
  6. **Distraction:** It is a useful technique of diverting the patient's attention from what may be perceived as an unpleasant procedure.
  7. **Positive reinforcement:** Positive reinforcement is an effective technique to reward desired behaviors and thus strengthens the recurrence of those behaviors.
  8. **Cognitive behavioural therapy (CBT):** CBT is a combination of behavior therapy and cognitive therapy. It is today the most accepted psychological treatment for anxiety related to particular situations and specific phobias. It involves learning to change negatively distorted thoughts (cognitions) and actions (behaviors).

B. **Pharmacologic management:** Pharmacological control of pain and anxiety can be achieved by the use of sedation and general anesthesia, and should be sought only in situations where the patient is not able to respond and cooperate well with psycho-therapeutic interventions, is not willing to undergo this type of treatment, or is considered dental-phobic.

Q. 2. Write about LASERS in dentistry.

(NTR Uni., June 2014)

Ans. LASER is an acronym for light amplification by stimulated emission of radiation. Lasers are heat pro-ducing devices converting electromagnetic energy into thermal energy. The characteristic of a laser depends on its wavelength (WL), and wavelength affects both the clinical applications and design of laser. The WL used in medicine and dentistry generally range from 193 to 10600 nm, representing a broad spectrum from ultraviolet to the far infra-red range.

Mechanism of action: If radiation energy is absorbed by the tissue, following reactions occurs.

1. **Photochemical interaction:** This type of interaction includes the interaction of beam with the chemical process of the tissue and includes:
   a. Biostimulation: It describes the stimulatory effect of laser light on biochemical and molecular processes that normally occur in tissue like healing and repair.
   b. Photodynamic therapy: It is the therapeutic use of lasers for the treatment of pathological conditions.
   c. Fluorescence: This can be used to detect light reactive substances in the tissues.
2. **Photothermal interaction:** It includes:
   a. Photoablation: This is removal of tissue by vaporization and superheating of tissue fluids, coagulation or hemostasis.
   b. Photopyrolysis: It is burning away of the tissues.
3. **Photomechanical interaction:** It includes:
   a. Photodisruption or photodissociation: It is breaking apart of structure by laser light.
   b. Photoacoustic: This involves removal of tissues with shockwave therapy.
4. **Photoelectrical interaction:** It includes:
   a. Photoplasmolysis: In this, tissue is removed through the formation of electrically charged ions.

Types of Laser: Based on power, lasers can be classified into the following three categories:

1. **High-power lasers (hard, hot):** These lasers increase tissue kinetic energy and produce heat. As a result, they leave their therapeutic effects through thermal interactions. These effects include necrosis, carbonization, vaporization, coagulation and denaturation. These lasers have an output power of >500 mW.

2. **Intermediate-power lasers:** These lasers leave their therapeutic effects without producing significant heat. These lasers have an output power of 250–500 mW.

3. **Low-power lasers (soft, cold):** It is also known as low level laser (LLL). These lasers have no thermal effect on tissues and produce a reaction in cells through light, called **photobiostimulation** or **photo-biochemical reaction.** Output power of these lasers is <250 mW.

Lasers used:

1. **Carbon dioxide laser:** This is most commonly used in soft tissue surgeries. It has a wavelength of 10,600 nm and is readily absorbed by water. Therefore, it does not penetrate too deep into the tissues (0.1–0.23 mm) without repeated or prolonged use. This is used ideally for superficial lesions, resurfacing of the skin and removal of sialoliths.

2. **Nd:YAG laser:** It has a wavelength of 1,064 nm. This is mostly used in soft tissue procedures, in removing tattoos and certain pigmented lesions.

3. **Ho:YAG laser:** This is used for arthroscopic surgery, soft tissue surgery. It has a wavelength of 2,100 nm.

4. **Er:YAG lasers:** These lasers are most commonly used for the treatment of hard tissues and skin resurfacing. They have a wavelength of 2944 nm.

5. **Argon lasers:** With a wavelength of 488,514 nm are readily absorbed by hemoglobin and melanin and are useful in the treatment of pigmented lesions and vascular anomalies.

6. **Diode lasers:** They have a wavelength of 620–900 nm and are used to treat oral soft tissue lesions.

APPLICATIONS OF LASER IN ORAL MEDICINE

A. Oro-mucosal pathologies

1. **Leukoplakia:** The lesions can be removed with laser and encourages regeneration of new, healthy epithelium. Small lesions can be removed with a carbon dioxide laser with a margin of 3–4 mm. Thickened hyper-keratotic lesions have less water content; therefore, vaporization cannot be done. Diffuse lesions cannot be managed by excision. The disadvantage of vaporization is that, a specimen cannot be taken and sent for pathological examination.

2. **Oral lichen planus:** Erosive lichen planus can be controlled by laser treatment. Carbon dioxide laser should be used along with selected local and systemic medications. The contact Nd:YAG laser with round probe can also be used.

3. **Oral submucous fibrosis:** The use of laser to release fibrotic bands leads to healing with minimal scarring, thereby decreasing the probability of procedure induced trismus. Diode laser is a portable device which delivers rays through a fiberoptic cable and, hence, can be delivered to relatively 'difficult to access' areas. Its cutting depth is <0.01 mm, and thus preserves tissues beyond this depth.

4. **Herpes simplex virus infections:** Low level laser therapy (LLLT) can be used in association with conventional therapy. LLLT presents both anti-inflammatory and analgesic effects, contributing to tissue repair and fibroblast proliferation and an increase in the interval between infections.

5. **Recurrent aphthous ulcers:** Recently, LLLT has been used as the treatment modality. It helps in immediate pain relief and accelerates wound healing. Cold lasers (LLLT lasers) accelerate wound healing and reduce pain by perhaps 'stimulating oxidative phosphorylation' in mitochondria and modulating inflammatory responses.

B. Orofacial pain

1. **Trigeminal neuralgic pain:** Low-level laser of 830 nm wavelength is efficient in the treatment of neuralgic pain.

2. **Myofacial pain:** Use of 830 nm wavelength laser in several appointments can reduce or eliminate myofacial pain.

3. **Temporomandibular joint disorder pain:** A potential noninvasive treatment for TMJ pain is LLLT. The efficacy of LLLT to be superior to placebo therapy.

4. **Mucositis pain:** 'Low' or 'low and middle' energy (output power ranged from 5 to 200 mW) irradiation with helium/neon laser (wavelength 632.8 nm) has been reported to be a simple atraumatic technique, useful in the treatment of mucositis of various origins.

C. Salivary gland pathologies

1. **Sialolithiasis:** Various types of lasers have been employed to treat sialolithiasis, including carbon dioxide, diode, Ho:Yag and Nd:YAG lasers. Among these diode laser has been reported to have more advantages. It has a greater absorption by hemoglobin, oxyhemoglobin and melanin, thereby making its penetration depth smaller than Nd:YAG laser.

2. **Mucocele:** CO_2 laser has a high water absorption rate and is well absorbed by all soft tissues with high water content. In addition, its effects on adjacent tissues are minimal. The cut is precise and does not affect the muscle layer, causes minimal hemorrhage and almost no acute inflammatory reaction. The operation time is short (3–5 min.) making it a convenient treatment for children and patients who cannot withstand long treatment.

D. Biopsy: The laser biopsies present some advantages compared those made with the scalpel: Generally these interventions do not require anesthesia or sutures and the healing of the donor site, at least in the initial stages, it is more rapid. The laser most commonly used are: Diode laser, CO_2 laser, Nd:YAG laser, Er:YAG laser.

APPLICATION OF LASERS IN CONSERVATIVE AND ENDODONTICS

1. **Caries detection:** DIAGNOdent is used for caries and calculus detection by emitting a non-ionizing laser beam at a wavelength of 655 nm (at 90° angle) toward a specific darkened groove on the occlusal surface of patient's tooth where bacterial decay is suspected, or along the long axis of a root surface to detect the presence of bacteria-laden calculus. This diagnostic technology, in which the photons of this laser wavelength are absorbed into any existing bacteria in these areas of the patient's tooth, is called **laser-induced fluorescence**.

2. **Cavity preparation:** Er:YAG laser has been successfully used to prepare holes in enamel and dentine with no cracks and low or no charring.

3. **Caries removal:** Carious material contains a higher water content compared with surrounding healthy dental hard tissues. There is a possible selectivity in the removal of carious material using the Er:YAG laser because the ablation threshold of healthy dentine is two times higher than the corresponding threshold of carious dentine. The laser removed infected and softened carious dentine to the same degree as the bur treatment. In addition, a lower degree of vibration is noted with the Er:YAG laser treatment.

4. **Restoration removal:** Er:YAG laser is capable of removing cement, composite resin and glass ionomer. Lasers should not be used to ablate amalgam restorations however, because of potential release of mercury vapour. Er:YAG laser is incapable of removing gold crowns, cast restorations and ceramic materials because of the low absorption of these materials and reflection of the laser light.

5. **Etching:** Er:YAG laser produces micro-explosions during hard tissue ablation that result in microscopic and macroscopic irregularities. These micro-irregularities make the enamel surface micro-retentive and may offer a mechanism of adhesion without acid-etching.

6. **Treatment of dentinal hypersensitivity:** Desensitizing of hypersensitive dentine with an Er:YAG laser

is effective, and maintenance of positive result is more prolonged.

7. **Caries prevention:** Laser irradiation of dental hard tissues modifies the calcium to phosphate ratio, reduces the carbonate to phosphorous ratio, and leads to formation of more stable and less acid soluble compounds, reducing susceptibility to acid attack and caries.

8. **Bleaching:** The objective of laser bleaching is to achieve an effective power bleaching process using the most efficient energy source. The FDA approved standards for tooth whitening has cleared three dental laser wavelengths: Argon, CO_2 and the most recent 980 nm GaAIAs diode.

9. **In Endodontics:** Lasers are being considered to disinfect root canals photothermally. Lasers may be more effective than medications to break up biofilms by denaturing proteins and volatizing the aqueous component. A technique known as **photoactivated disinfection** (PAD) uses tolonium chloride solution to photosensitize bacterial cells such as *E. faecalis*. These cells then selectively absorb laser light at 635 nm and are ablated. Er:YAG laser technology has been used to carry out endodontic therapy from access, to disinfection to root canal preparation without supplemental anesthesia. A further benefit to these lasers when they are preparing the root canal space is that they remove the smear layer.

APPLICATIONS OF LASERS IN PERIODONTOLOGY

1. **Periodontal pocket therapy:** Diodes, Er:YAG, Nd:YAG, and CO_2 devices from various manufacturers have received FDA clearance for sulcular debridement, defined as removal of diseased or inflamed soft tissue in the periodontal pocket to improve clinical indices including gingival index, gingival bleeding index, probe depth, attachment level and tooth mobility. Nd:YAG lasers are useful in periodontal care because of their affinity for pigment allows for selective debridement of diseased sulcular epithelium. Nd:YAG wavelength is also bactericidal, biostimulative, and has the ability to stimulate fibrin formation with the proper parameters. Erbium lasers have been shown to be effective at scaling and root planning, effective pocket decontamination, and can replace scalpels.

2. **Laser biopsy:** All dental laser wavelengths are capable of performing precise biopsies. Smaller lesions can often be removed with a compounded topical anesthetic only. Sutures are rarely needed due to the excellent hemostasis and minimal trauma observed when lasers are used properly. Any lesion removed

needs to be submitted to an oral pathologist for microscopic diagnosis. The dentist should also note what type of laser was used as there is often a tissue effect visible along the incision known as a "**laser artifact**." The artifact varies depending on the thermal effects of the particular laser and settings used.

3. **Gingivectomy:** Gingivectomy is the most common procedure performed with dental lasers. All laser wavelengths can be used to precisely incise gingiva for restorative, cosmetic, and periodontal indications. Rapid healing and reduced pain are commonly seen postoperatively and patients rarely need periodontal packing or sutures.

4. **Frenectomy:** Frenectomies are a very common laser procedure that can be accomplished effectively with any wavelength. Simple ones can often be achieved with topical anesthesia only. Hemostasis is usually excellent, particularly with the more thermal CO_2, Nd:YAG, and diodes.

5. **Crown-lengthening with minimum trauma.**

6. **Implantology:** A diode laser can be used at second stage surgery instead of a scalpel. The laser cuts precisely and effects haemostasis and seems to minimize pain and swelling.

APPLICATIONS IN ORAL SURGERY

CO_2 lasers have been popular in oral surgery due to their precise incisions and excellent hemostasis. Erbium lasers are capable of cutting bone in a less traumatic fashion and can be quite useful for the following procedures:

- Surgical extractions with less traumatic flaps and bone removal
- Alveoloplasty.
- Incision and drainage.
- Operculectomies.
- Treatment of peri-implantitis
- Pre-prosthetic.
  - Ridge preparation/hyperplasic tissue reduction.
  - Tuberosity reductions.
  - Vestibuloplasty.
  - Tori removal

Nd:YAG and diodes have biostimulative properties that can be used to promote healing, osteogenesis, and postoperative comfort. Nd:YAG lasers can also form fibrin rapidly in an extraction site creating a quick and more durable clot. An interesting application of dental lasers is in the treatment of bisphosphonate induce osteonecrosis of jaw. When the necrotic bone is removed with an Er:YAG laser, the remaining bone is so minimally traumatized that osteoclastic needs are minimized. Nd:YAG biostimulation can be used concurrently or separately to promote bone healing as well.

APPLICATIONS IN PEDIATRIC DENTISTRY

Dental lasers offer many advantages when treating children. All procedures previously discussed apply to pediatric treatments as well. The ability to provide care with less use of needles and high-speed handpieces makes for a less traumatic experience. All previously discussed restorative and surgical procedures can be performed safely on children. Dental lasers can also aid in procedures such as pulpotomies and orthodontic surgical needs.

Advantages: Dry surgical field, better visualization, tissue surface sterilization, reduction in bacteremia, pain, swelling/edema, minimal mechanical trauma with faster healing response, widely accepted by patients as operating time is reduced and thus cost-effective.

Disadvantages

1. Relatively high in cost.
2. Lasers require specialized training.
3. No single wavelength will optimally treat all dental disease.
4. They are harmful to eyes and skin.

Dental Material

Q. 1. Write a note on rheological properties of dental materials. *(RGUHS, Oct. 2010)*

Ans. Rheology is the study of flow of matter.

Properties

1. Viscosity: It is the resistance offered by a liquid when placed in motion. It is measured in poise or centipoise.
2. **Creep:** It is defined as time dependant plastic deformation or change of shape that occurs when a metal is subjected to a constant load near its melting point.
   a. Static creep: It is a time dependant deformation produced in a completely set solid subjected to a constant stress.
   b. Dynamic creep: It is produced when the applied stress is fluctuating, such as in fatigue type test.
3. Flow: In dentistry, the term flow is used instead of creep to describe the rheology of amorphous substances, e.g. waxes.
4. Behaviour of liquids:
   a. Newtonian (ideal): Liquids that exhibit a constant viscosity under all the stress conditions.
   b. Pseudoplastic: Exhibit decrease in viscosity, when there is increase in shear rate.
   c. Dilatants: These are liquids that show higher viscosity as shear rate increases, e.g. fluid denture base resins.
5. Thixotropic: These materials exhibit different viscosity, after it is deformed.

Q. 2. Write a short note on hardness tests.
(NTR Uni., May 2019).

Ans. In metallurgy and in most other fields, the resistance to indentation is taken as the measure of hardness. There are many surface hardness tests.

1. **Brinell:** Brinell test utilizes a 10 mm diameter steel ball as an indenter, applying a uniform 3000 kgf (29 kN) force. The load is divided by the area of the surface of indentation and the quotient is referred to as **Brinell hardness number (BHN).**

   Application: Used for measuring hardness of metals and metallic materials.
2. **Rockwell hardness number (RHN):** Like the BH test, a steel ball or a conical diamond point is used. However, instead of measuring the diameter of the impression, the depth is measured directly by a dial gauge on the instrument.

   Application: This has a wider application for materials, even suitable for brittle and plastic materials.
3. **Vickers hardness test (VHN):** This is also similar to the Brinell test, however, instead of a steel ball, a diamond in the shape of a square pyramid is used. The load is divided by the area of indentation.

   Application: Vickers test is used in the ADA for dental casting golds.
4. **Knoop hardness test (KHN):** A diamond indenting tool is used of a different shape from that of Vickers. Knoop hardness value is independent of the ductility of material and values for both exceedingly hard and soft materials can be obtained from this test.

   Knoop and Vickers tests are classified as **microhardness tests**. Brinell and Rockwell tests are classified as **macrohardness tests**.
5. **Shore and the barcol:** A metal indenter that is spring loaded is used. The hardness number is based on depth of penetration and is read directly from a gauge.

   Applications: Used for measuring the hardness of rubber and plastics.

Q. 3. Write a short note on colour and its significance.
(TNMGR, Sept. 2010)

Ans. Colour is formed by the combined intensities of wavelengths present in a beam of light.

Dimensions of colour (TNMGR, Oct. 2017):

1. Hue: It refers to basic colour of an object, e.g. red, green or blue.
2. Value: Colour can be separated into light and a dark shade, this lightness, which is measured independently of the colour hue is called value.
3. Chroma: It represents the degree of saturation of a particular hue.

Measurement of colour: By Munsell system.

Clinical consideration: The ideal restorative material should match the colour of the tooth it restores. In maxillofacial prosthetics, the colour of the gums, external skin and the eyes have to be duplicated. Clinically in the operatory or dental lab, colour selection is usually done by the use of shade guides.

Q. 4. Write about importance of divine proportions.
(NTR Uni., Oct., 2014)

Ans. The golden proportion was described geometrically in the 4th century BC by Euclid as the unique division of a line (AB) into 2 parts (AC and CB) in such a way that AB:AC=AC:CB. A more accurate mathematical approach came from Fibonacci in 12th century, in which the golden proportion was defined as phi, and was found to be equal to 1.618. The apparent widths of the maxillary anterior teeth on smile, and their actual mesio-distal width, differ because of the curvature of the dental arch. For best appearance, the apparent width of the lateral incisor should be 62% of the width of the central incisor, the apparent width of the canine should be 62% of that of the lateral incisor, and the apparent width of the first premolar should be 62% of that of the canine. This ratio of recurring 62% proportions appears in a number of other relationships in human anatomy, and is referred to as the "**Golden Proportion.**"

Divine proportions in human dentition: A rhythm is seen in the natural normal ideal occlusion with the lower incisor phi for the upper central incisors, φ2 for lateral incisor width and φ3 for premolars. A second series of divine proportions was discovered in the teeth. Starting with the widths of all four lower incisors as 1.0 value, a phi relation to the tips of the upper canine widths was found. A φ2 relationship to the four lower incisors was found at the widths of the upper second molars. A third golden proportion was seen from the distal aspect of the lower canines. This measurement as a base revealed the lower first molars at the mesial cusps to be in the phi relationship.

Golden proportion and smile: It has been noticed that there exists another compound golden proportion in which the width of all the 8 anterior teeth together are in the golden proportion to the width of the smiling lips.

Analysis of cephalometric matrix: Eight divine proportions have been established:

- Corpus axis length phi to condyle axis length (to condyle tip).
- Anterior cranial fossa length SN to posterior cranial fossa length S-Ba.
- Basal or cranial anterior base length (cc to N) phi to cranial centre to articulare (Ar).
- Length of the hard palate ANS-PNS phi to depth of nasopharynx and point A to PNS to posterior margin of the condyle neck.
- Anterior length of Frankfort plane (Pt V to orbitale) phi to Pt V to glenoid fossa (GL).
- Vertical height of point A to Pm phi to A to the Frankfort plane.
- Palate at incisive canal to menton phi to canthus of eye.
- Height of the lower incisor tip from Pm phi to distance of incisor tip to point A.

Clinical applications: The findings of the golden relationship can aid the clinician in determining the area most out of harmony and balance and hence determine the best approach to achieve "harmonic unity" in aesthetics. The golden relation of SN and S-Ba may serve as a guide for analysis of the nasopharynx and naso-oro airway and the proportionality of the anterior and posterior cranial base and protrusion of the maxilla. The bony nasal width was also found in a progression through the midface with the lateral dimensions to the lateral articulare and to the maxilla width. In addition, the dental arch width (in the adult) at the first molar was golden to the base of the trihedral eminences, which would be an important determinant for adult treatment planning.

Q. 5. Write a note on tarnish and corrosion.
(TNMGR, March 2008; Oct. 2018; BFUHS, May 2011; UOK, May 2015;AIIMS-CDER, June 2016; RGUHS, July 2017; Gujarat Uni., April 2019)

Ans. Tarnish is a surface discoloration on a metal or even a slight loss or alteration of the surface finish or lustre.

Causes

a. Formation of hard and soft deposits on the surface of the restorations.
b. Pigment producing bacteria, produce strain.
c. Formation of thin films of oxides, sulphides and chlorides.

Corrosion is actual deterioration of a metal by reaction with the environment.

Causes: Water, oxygen, chloride ions, sulphides in the oral cavity.

Classification

1. **Chemical or dry corrosion:** In this the metal reacts to form oxides, sulphides in the absence of electrolytes, e.g. formation of Ag_2S in dental alloys containing silver.
2. **Electrolytic or electrochemical or wet corrosion:** This requires the presence of water or other fluid electrolytes. There is formation of free electrons and electrolyte provides the pathway for the transport of electrons. The surface of anode corrodes due to loss of electrons.
   a. **Galvanic corrosion:** It occurs when dissimilar metals lie in direct physical contact with each other.
   b. **Heterogeneous corrosion (MUHS, June 2018):** It occurs within the structure of the restoration itself. Heterogeneous/mixed compositions can cause the galvanic corrosion. When an alloy containing eutectic is immersed in an electrolyte, the metallic grains with the lower electrode potential are attacked and corrosion results. In a cored structure, differences in the composition within the alloy grains are found. Thus, part of a grain can be anode and part cathode. In metals or alloy, the grain boundaries may act as anodes and the interior of grain as the cathode. Solder joints may also corrode due to the inhomogeneous composition. Impurities in any alloy enhance corrosion.
   c. **Stress corrosion:** A metal which has been stressed by cold working becomes more reactive at the site of maximum stress.
   d. **Concentration cell or crevice corrosion**
      i. **Electrolyte concentration cell:** In a metallic restoration which is partly covered by food debris, the composition of electrolyte under the debris will differ from that of saliva and this can contribute to the corrosion of the restoration.
      ii. **Oxygen concentration cell:** Differences in oxygen tension in between parts of the same restoration causes corrosion of the restoration. Greater corrosion occurs in the part of the restoration having lower concentration of oxygen.

Protection against corrosion

1. **Passivation:** Certain metals readily form strong adherent oxide film on their surface which protects them from corrosion. Such metals are said to be passive, e.g. chromium, titanium, and aluminium.
2. **Increasing noble metal content:** At least 50% of the atoms in a dental alloy should be gold, platinum or palladium to ensure against corrosion.
3. **Polishing:** Polishing metallic restorations like amalgam and cast metal to a high luster minimizes corrosion.
4. **Other methods:** Dissimilar metal restorations should be avoided. Avoid using a high mercury containing amalgam as it is more susceptible to corrosion.

Q. 6. Write a note on biocompatibility of materials.
(TNMGR, March 2009; RGUHS, Nov. 2011; Sumandeep Uni., June 2017; MUHS, June 2018; TNMGR, Oct. 2019)

Q. Discuss tissue response to various dental materials in detail. *(Sumandeep Uni. April 2014)*

Ans. Biocompatibility is defined as the ability of a restorative material to induce an appropriate and advantageous host response during its intended clinical use.

Biocompatibility tests/toxicity evaluation

A. *In vitro* **tests**
   1. Direct cell culture.
   2. Agar diffusion testing.
   3. Filter diffusion testing.
   4. Dentin barrier testing.
   5. Ames test.
   6. Micronucleus test.

B. **Animal tests**
   1. LD_{50} median lethal dose.
   2. Limit test.
   3. Implantation test.
   4. Maximization test.
   5. Buehler test.
   6. Micronucleus test.

C. **Usage tests**
   1. Pulp/dentin test.
   2. Endodontic usage test.
   3. Intraosseous implant test.
   4. Clinical trials: Phase I–Phase IV

Biocompatibility of dental materials

1. Zinc phosphate cement: No reported systemic reaction, allergy, or mutagenic/carcinogenic reaction. Locally, it will provoke a stinging reaction for a short period.
2. Zinc polycarboxylate cement: No reported systemic reaction, allergy, or mutagenic/carcinogenic reaction. Locally, it produces minimal irritation to the pulp.

3. Zinc oxide eugenol cement: No reported systemic reaction, or mutagenic/carcinogenic reaction. It can cause allergic contact dermatitis. Locally, it can produce cytotoxic reaction; eugenol has an obtundant effect when used in deep cavities.

4. Calcium hydroxide: No reported systemic reaction, allergy, or mutagenic/carcinogenic reaction. When used as indirect capping material, it exerts anti-microbial activity and decreases the permeability of dentine. In case of direct pulp capping, it produces superficial coagulation necrosis.

5. Glass ionomer cement: No reported systemic reaction, allergy, or mutagenic/carcinogenic reaction. Unset cement is cytotoxic to pulp.

6. Silver amalgam: No reported mutagenic/carcinogenic reaction. Elemental mercury can lead to systemic toxicity. In deep cavities, it leads to reduced number of odontoblasts, dilated capillaries, and inflammatory cell reaction.

7. Composite resin: No reported systemic reaction, mutagenic/carcinogenic reaction. Some component may produce type IV delayed hypersensitivity reaction. It may cause pulpal inflammation.

8. Ceramics: No reported local, allergy, or mutagenic/carcinogenic reaction. There is risk of silicosis due to inhalation of ceramic dust.

9. Dental casting alloys: No reported systemic reaction. Release of metals may be cytotoxic locally. Lichenoid reactions and allergic reactions have been reported in the oral mucosa. Some components are mutagenic as well as carcinogenic also.

10. Wrought alloys: Release of manganese can lead to nervous and skeletal disorders. Corrosion products may cause local pain and swelling. Lichenoid reaction may be seen in oral mucosa. Nickel is a weak mutagen.

11. Denture base resins: No reported systemic reaction, or mutagenic/carcinogenic reaction. Chemically activated resin is most cytotoxic. Resins may cause severe pulpal reactions.

12. Impression materials: No allergy, or mutagenic/carcinogenic reaction. Some materials are toxic in high concentration. Polyether is highly cytotoxic. Contact dermatitis reaction may also occur.

13. Endodontic materials:
    a. Latex materials: No reported systemic reaction, or mutagenic/carcinogenic reaction. It may result in contact dermatitis and latex allergy.
    b. Obturating material: No reported systemic reaction, or mutagenic/carcinogenic reaction. Gutta-percha is slightly cytotoxic. Allergy to gutta-percha is very rare.

c. Root canal sealers: No reported systemic reaction. Some may cause cytotoxic and allergic reactions.

Q. 7. What are biomimetic substances?
(RGUHS, Nov. 2011; NTR Uni., April 2014)

Ans. Biomimetics can be defined as the study of the structure, formation, and function of biologically produced materials and also biological mechanisms and processes especially for the purpose of synthesizing similar products by artificial mechanisms which mimic natural ones.

Bioactive materials used in dentistry

1. **Synthetic polymer: Biodegradable polymers:** Polylactic acid and Polyglycolic acid copolymers, used as suture materials, bone, skin, and liver substitutes. **Non-biodegradable polymers:** Polyanhydrites, polyphosphazenes, polymethyl methacrylate (PMMA), polytetrafluoroethylene (PTFE), and poly-hydroxyethylmethacrylate. PTFE is used for bone augmentation and guided bone regeneration.

2. **Ceramics:** Alumina, hydroxyapatite, bioceramics.
   - **Biomimetics in restorative dentistry:** Glass ionomer cements (GICs), biodentine.

Biomimetic approaches for regeneration

- **Regeneration of dentin-pulp complex:** Recombinant human BMP2 and BMP4.
- **Stem cell therapy:** SHED, DPSCs, SCAP.
- **Pulp implantation:** Tissue engineering triad of DPSCs, dentin matrix protein I, and a collagen scaffold.
- **Root canal revascularization:** Patient's own blood cells.
- **Injectable scaffold theory:** In this procedure, pulp tissue is obtained by tissue engineering process and then it is administered in a soft three-dimensional scaffold matrix.
- **Gene therapy:** Gene delivery of mineralizing genes into pulp tissue to induce mineralization.
- **Bioengineered tooth:** Whole-tooth regeneration.
- **Biomimetic mineralization:** Guided formation of enamel-like fluoroapatite layer on a mineral substrate.
- **Biomimetic remineralisation:** Biomimetic remineralisation of dentin by ion-containing solutions or ion-leaching silicon-containing materials.
- **Development of artificial salivary gland:** Adult embryonic stem cells are used to develop parenchymal cells and restoration of its secretory functions.
  - **Biomimetic approaches of oral surgery:** Multipotent stem cells (MSCs) have been used in the

tissue engineering of human-shaped temporo-mandibular joints. Mandibular condyles are made up of cartilaginous and bone tissues. MSCs were differentiated into chondrogenic and osteogenic cells and these cells were subsequently encapsulated in a poly (ethylene glycol) diacrylate hydrogel which was then molded into an adult human mandibular condyle in stratified yet integrated layers of cartilage and bone.

Advantages: No toxic reactions, may assist in tissue healing or integration.

Disadvantages

1. They can cause immune reactions.
2. They may contaminated by bacteria and other infectious pathogens.
3. They are difficult to sterilize.
4. They have the tendency to denature at temperature below their melting point.
5. The cost factor is also a limitation.

Q. 8. Write a short note on biodentine.
(RUHS, June 2017; TNMGR, MAY 2018)

Ans. Biodentine (dentine in a capsule) is a bio-compatible and bioactive dentine substitute with dentin like mechanical properties which has beneficial effect on living cells and acts in a biocompatible manner.

Composition of biodentine

- **Powder:** Tri-calcium silicate, di-calcium silicate, calcium carbonate and oxide (filler), Iron oxide (coloring agent), zirconium oxide (radioopacifier).
- **Liquid:** Calcium chloride (accelerator), hydrosoluble polymer (reducing agent).

Mechanism of action: Biodentine induces mineralization after its application. Mineralization occurs in the form of osteodentine by expressing markers of odonto-blasts and increases TGF-β_1 secretion from pulpal cells enabling early mineralization. Biodentine induces apposition of reactionary dentine by odontoblast stimulation and reparative dentin by cell differentiation.

Properties

1. Tissue regeneration and early mineralization.
2. Short setting time.
3. Antibacterial properties.
4. Biocompatibility and is non-genotoxic.
5. Biodentine has significantly higher push-out bond strength than MTA (p <0.5).
6. Good material handling, ease of manipulation, better consistency, safety handling.
7. Elastic modulus, at 22.0 Gpa, is very similar to that of dentine at 18.5; Compressive strength of about 220 MPa is equal to average for dentine of 290 MPa; Micro-hardness of biodentine at 60 HVN is same as that of natural dentin.
8. Good marginal adaptation and sealing ability.

Clinical implications: Pulp capping; Repair of root perforations, Apexification; Root-end filling; As dentine substitute (base) for posterior restorations.

Q. 9. Write a short note on bioceramics.
(NTR Uni., June 2017)

Ans. Bioceramics are biocompatible ceramic materials or metal oxides with the ability to either function as human tissues or to resorbs or encourage the regeneration of natural tissues.

Classification

1. Bioinert: Alumina, zirconia.
2. Bioactive: Bioactive glasses, bioactive glass ceramics, hydroxyapatite, calcium silicates.
3. Biodegradable: Tricalcium phosphate, bioactive glasses.

Advantages

- Excellent biocompatibility properties.
- Intrinsic osteoinductive capacity.
- Function as a regenerative scaffold that is eventually dissolved.
- Ability to achieve excellent hermetic seal, form a chemical bond with the tooth structure and have good radiopacity.
- Antibacterial properties.

Uses

- **Prosthetic uses:** Implants, prosthesis, prosthetic devices, coatings to improve the biocompatibility of metal implants.
- **Surgical uses:** Joint replacements, fill surgical bone defects, alveolar ridge augmentation, sinus obliteration, and correction of orbital floor fracture.
- **Endodontic uses:** Sealers, obturation, perforation repair, retrograde filling, pulpotomy, resorption, apexification, regenerative endodontics.
- **Restorative uses:** Dentin substitute, pulp capping, dentin hypersensitivity, dentin remineralisation.

Q. 10. Write a note one high speeds in dentistry.
(NTR Uni., Oct. 2019)

Ans. Handpieces used in dentistry are generally available low or slow speeds (<6000 rpm), medium or intermediate speeds (6000–1,00,000 rpm), and high or ultra-high speeds (>1,00,000 rpm).

Rationale of increased speeds: The main reason for increasing the speed of rotating instruments is to increases its cutting efficiency. The operator has better control and greater ease of operation. Instruments last longer. Patient is generally less apprehensive because annoying vibrations and operating time are decreased. Several teeth in the same arch must be treated at the same appointment.

Types of high-speed instruments: Low speed: Up to 10,000 rpm; **Intermediate speed**: 25,000–45,000 rpm; **High speeds**-50,000–1,00,000 rpm; and **Ultra-high speeds**: 1,00,000 rpm.

Heat generation: The rotating cutting tools come in contact with the tooth surface, and the heat is generated. It has been found that the temperature rise develops within 10–12s, after the cutting operation is started. The temperatures resorbs by dental burs in cutting human dentin ranges from 125°–275°F. Hence, it is advisable to use some form of coolant.

Coolants: There are three types of coolants usually employed in dental practice such as water, spray of air and water, and air alone.

Cross contamination by ultra-speed cutting tools: The extent of aerosol produced by air turbine may reach hazardous levels of microbial population, with the heaviest concentration being at 2 feet in distances from the patient's mouth. So, standard precautions should be taken like use of double protective face mask, protective eyeglasses with face shield and protective apron.

Biological response to high-speed tools: Pulp changes found are comparable to those produced at lower operating speeds provided that adequate cooling of the cutting instrument is ensured. The enamel showed minute cracks and dentin showed altered staining reactions as a result of localized overheating.

Q. 11. Discuss design and mechanics of cutting of dental burs.

Ans. Dental burs have revolutionized the dentistry field and are used for cutting hard tissues such as bone or tooth. They are normally made of stainless steel, diamond grit or particles, and tungsten carbide and fitted to a dental drill incorporating an air turbine. The dental bur has three parts: Head, neck, and shank. The head contains the blades, which produce cutting action by rotary motion. The blades are positioned at various degree angles in order to change the property of the bur. Dental burs come in many shapes and sizes designed for specific applications and can rotate at speeds of up to 500,000 rpm. Each bur is designed to operate at an optimum speed and intended for use in a specific handpiece motor combination. The optimum speed are also dependent upon the nature of the material being cut. They can be made of steel and then coated with a hard coating, such as tungsten carbide coating, or they can be entirely tungsten carbide. Steel wears rapidly and corrodes easily and thus appears to be a poor choice of material for burs. However, at lower speeds, the wear rate associated with the cutting process is reduced significantly, and steel may be the preferred material.

Generally, geometrical features of the bur are manufactured to have a negative rake angle. However, those with a positive rank angle are designed mainly for cutting soft materials (e.g. acrylics) to remove material during cutting to prevent the tool from clogging with the chips.

Q. 12. Discuss pulp protection materials used.

(NTR Uni., Oct. 2008)

Ans. Pulp capping is a treatment in which a protective agent is applied on the pulp when it is exposed by traumatic injuries, mechanical factors or dental caries, in order to allow pulp healing and to maintain the vitality of the pulp and its functions.

Ideal properties of pulp capping materials

- Stimulate reparative dentin formation and maintain pulpal vitality.
- Release fluoride to prevent secondary caries.
- Bactericidal or bacteriostatic.
- Adhere to dentin and to restorative material.
- Resist forces during restoration placement and during the life of restoration.
- Sterile and radiopaque.
- **Various pulp capping materials used:** Calcium hydroxide ("**Gold standard**"), zinc oxide eugenol (ZnOE) cement, corticosteroids (hydrocortisone, cleocin, cortisone, ledermix-calcium hydroxide + prednisolone), antibiotics (penicillin, neomycin and keflin-cephalothin sodium, vancomycin) with calcium hydroxide, polycarboxylate cement, inert materials (isobutyl cyanoacrylate, tricalcium phosphate ceramic), collagen, bonding agents (4-META-MMA-TBB adhesives, hybridizing dentin bonding agents), calcium phosphate, hydroxyapatite, lasers, glass ionomer/resin modified glass ionomer, MTA, MTYA1-Ca [89.0% microfiller, 10.0% calcium hydroxide and 1.0% benzoyl peroxide + liquid (67.5% triethyleneglycol dimethacrylate, 30.0% glyceryl methacrylate, 1.0% o-methacryloyl tyrosine amide, 1.0% dimethylaminoethylmethacrylate and 0.5% camphorquinone)], growth factors (**BMPs, recombinant insulin-like growth factor I)], other growth factors** (epidermal growth factor, basic

fibroblast growth factor, insulin-like growth factor II, platelet-derived growth factor-BB, TGF-β_1), bone-sialoprotein, biodentin, enzymes (heme-oxygenase 1, simvastatin), stem cells, propolis (Russian penicillin), novel endodontic cement, emdogain, odontogenic ameloblast associated protein, endo sequence root repair material, castor oil bean cement, TheraCal.

Q. 13. Elaborate on materials used in minimum intervention dentistry.   (NTR Uni., May 2019)

Ans. Minimal invasive dentistry (MID) is defined as the maximum preservation of healthy dental tissue.

Principle: MID is dependent on the following factors:
1. Demineralization-remineralization cycle.
2. Adhesion in restorative dentistry.
3. Biomimetic restorative material.

MI preparation techniques: Mechanical rotary high/low-speed bur; non-rotary atraumatic restorative treatment (ART); Air abrasion; Sono abrasion; Air polishing; Chemo-mechanical (Carisolv); Hydro-kinetic laser (CO_2, Er: YAG, Nd:YAG); Ozone technology (O_3).

Q. 14. Write a note on cavity liners and varnishes.   (NTR Uni., Oct. 2012)

Ans. Cavity liner is used to provide a barrier against the passage of irritants from cements or other restorative materials and to reduce the sensitivity of freshly cut dentin.

Composition: Suspension of calcium hydroxide in an organic liquid (methyl ethyl ketone or ethyl alcohol).

Properties: They neither possess mechanical strength nor provide any significant thermal insulation. The calcium hydroxide liners are soluble and should not be applied at the margins of restorations. Fluoride compounds are added to some cavity liners.

Other liners: Type III glass ionomer and ZnOE.

- **Cavity varnish:** Cavity varnish is a solution of one or more resins which when applied onto the cavity walls evaporates leaving a thin resin film that serves as a barrier between the restoration and the dentinal tubules.

Application
1. It reduces micro-leakage around the margins of newly placed restorations, thereby reducing, postoperative sensitivity.
2. It reduces passage of irritants into the dentinal tubules from the overlying restoration or base.

3. Varnish may be used as a surface coating over certain restorations to protect them from dehydration or contact with oral fluids.
4. Varnish may be applied on the surface of metallic restoration as a temporary protection in cases of galvanic shock.

Composition: Natural gum such as copal, resin or synthetic resin dissolved in an organic solvent like alcohol, acetone, or ether. Medicinal agents such as chlorobutanol, thymol and eugenol may be added. Some varnishes also contain fluorides.

Properties: Varnishes neither possess mechanical strength nor provide thermal insulation. The solubility of dental varnishes is low; they are virtually insoluble in water.

Clinical considerations: When placing a silicate restoration, the varnish should be confined to the dentin. Varnish applied on the enamel inhibits the uptake of fluoride by the enamel.

Contraindications
Composite resins: Solvent in the varnish may react with the resin.

Glass ionomer: Varnish eliminates the potential for adhesion, if applied between glass ionomer cement (GIC) and the cavity.

When therapeutic action is expected from the overlying cement, e.g. zinc oxide eugenol and calcium hydroxide.

Q. 15. Write about calcium hydroxide and mineral trioxide.   (BFUHS, Nov. 2006, 2008; TNMGR, June 2017, May 2019)

Ans. Calcium hydroxide is commonly employed for direct or indirect pulp capping agents, as low strength base, in apexification of teeth incomplete root formation.

Mechanism of action: The ionic form of calcium acts on tissue and induces the formation of hard tissue and has antibacterial effects.

Composition
1. **Base paste:** Glycol silicate, calcium sulphate, titanium dioxide, calcium tungstate/barium sulphate.
2. **Catalyst paste:** Calcium hydroxide, zinc oxide, zinc stearate, ethylene toluene, sulphonamide.

Calcium hydroxide reacts with the salicylate ester to form a chelate. Setting time is 2.5–5.5 minutes.

Classification
I. **Based on setting time:** Fast setting; Controlled setting; Low setting; Non setting.

II. **Based on form of availability:** Powder; Single paste (Endocal); Two-paste system (Dycal).

Applications

1. Conservative procedure: Pulp capping (direct/indirect).
2. Endodontics: Pulpotomy, apexification, management of resorption, management of traumatized teeth, intracanal medicament, endodontic sealer.
3. Pediatric dentistry: As obturation material.
   - **Mineral trioxide aggregate (MTA):** It is an excellent alternative to the conventional root canal filling materials.

Composition: Calcium silicate compounds and calcium compounds containing aluminium oxide and bismuth oxide.

Properties

1. Physical state: Solid powder.
2. Specific gravity: 4–4.5
3. pH: 12.5
4. Slightly soluble in water.
5. Setting time: 4 hours.
6. Compressive strength for MTA at 24 hours is 40.0 MPa.
7. MTA has comparable radiodensity as zinc oxide eugenol.
8. MTA has excellent sealing ability.
9. Antibacterial and antifungal action.
10. MTA does not react or interfere with any other restorative material.
11. Tricalcium oxide content of MTA interacts with tissue fluids and form $CaOH_2$, resulting in hard-tissue creation.
12. MTA has the potential to activate the cementoblasts and eventually cementum production. MTA also allows the overgrowth of PDL fiber over its surface.

Types: Gray MTA, white MTA.

Advantages: Excellent biocompatibility; Activates dentinogenesis and cementogenesis; Hydrophilic; Better sealing of setting; Radiopaque.

Disadvantages: Difficult to manipulate, longer setting time.

Clinical applications

1. Vital pulp therapy.
2. Apexification.
3. Perforations.
4. Root resorption.
5. Retrofilling.
6. Obturating material.
7. Barrier for internal bleaching procedures.

Q. 16. Write about root canal filling materials.
(BFUHS, Oct. 2010)

Ans. A root canal filling material should prevent infection/reinfection of treated root canals.

A. Metals: Silver points, titanium wires, stainless steel files.
B. Plastics: Gutta-percha, resilon.
C. Pastes: MTA, ZnOE, calcium hydroxide, iodoform pastes, chlorapercha, eucapercha, biocalex, N_2.
   - **Gutta-percha:** Gutta-percha is a polymeric resin-like material obtained from the coagulation of latex produced by Palaquium gutta tree (Isonandra gutta tree).

Forms of gutta-percha

- α-form: Runny, tacky and sticky, used with the thermo-mechanical and injectable techniques.
- β-form: Solid, compactable and ductile, used with mechanical condensation techniques.
- γ-form: Amorphous and unstable form.

Advantages

1. It is compactable and adapts excellently to the irregularities and contour of the canal.
2. It can be softened and made plastic by heat or by organic solvents.
3. It is inert, dimensional stable; non-allergic.
4. It will not discolor the tooth structure.
5. It is radiopaque.
6. It can be easily removed from the canal when retreatment is indicated.

Disadvantages: Lacks rigidity and adhesive quality; does not bond to any sealers; easily displaced by pressure.

Q. 17. Write a short note on mercury and dental amalgam.
(RGUHS, Nov. 2013; TNMGR, June 2017; NTR Uni., May 2019)

Ans. An amalgam is defined as a special type of alloy in which mercury is one of the components. Mercury is able to react with other metals to form a plastic mass, which is packed into the prepared cavity. Dental amalgam is the most widely used filling material for posterior teeth. The alloys before combining with mercury are known as dental amalgam alloys.

Classification

a. Based on the copper content: Low copper (<6%) and high copper alloys.
b. Based on zinc content: Zinc containing (>0.01%) and zinc-free alloys.
c. Based on the shape of particle: Lathe cut, spherical and spheroidal alloys.

d. Based on number of alloyed metals: Binary, ternary and quaternary alloys.

e. Based on size of alloy: Microcut and macrocut.

Advantages

1. Reasonably easy to insert.
2. Not much technique sensitive.
3. Manifests anatomic form well.
4. Adequate resistance to fracture.
5. Long service life and cheaper.

Disadvantages

1. The colour does not match tooth structure.
2. More brittle.
3. Chances of corrosion, galvanic action and marginal breakdown.
4. Do not bond to tooth structure.
5. Risk of mercury toxicity.

Applications

1. As a permanent filling material in class I, II cavities.
2. In combination with retentive pins to restore a crown.
3. For making dies.
4. In retrograde filling materials.
5. As a core material.

Contraindications

1. Amalgam should not be placed in patients with impaired kidney function.
2. Individuals with allergic hypersensitivity to mercury or components of the alloy.
3. New amalgam fillings should not be placed in contact with non-amalgam restoration.
   - **Technical considerations** (*AIIMS-CDER, April 2016*): The clinical success of amalgam restorations is highly dependent on the correct cavity design and selection and manipulation of the alloy.

Selection of materials

1. **Alloy:** For restorations subjected to occlusal forces, an amalgam with high resistance to marginal fracture is desirable. If strength is needed quickly the best choice is spherical or high copper alloys. A non-zinc alloy is selected in cases where it is difficult to control moisture.
2. **Mercury:** There is only one requisite for dental mercury and that is its purity. High purity mercury is labelled as 'triple distilled'. ADA specification No. 6 for dental mercury requires that the mercury should possess no surface contamination and <0.02% non-volatile residue.
3. **Dispensers:** Tablets, pre-proportioned capsules (400, 600, 800 or 1200 mg of alloy powder with corresponding proportion of mercury).

4. **Mercury:Alloy ratio (proportioning):** Prior to mechanical triturators, when amalgam was triturated manually excess mercury had to be used in order to achieve smooth and plastic amalgam mixes. This excess mercury was removed from the amalgam by: Using a squeeze cloth; increasing dryness technique during condensation of each increment.
   - **Eames' technique:** In 1959 Dr. Wilmer Eames proposed 1:1 ratio of mercury:alloy. This is known as the minimal mercury or Eames' technique.
   - **Trituration:** The objective is to wet all the surfaces of the alloy particles with mercury. Trituration is achieved either by: Manually by hand; Mechanical mixing.
5. **Manual mixing:** A glass mortar and pestle is used. Typically a 25 to 45 second period is sufficient.
6. **Mulling:** It is done to improve the homogeneity of the mass and get a single consistent mix. The mix is enveloped in a dry piece of rubber dam and vigorously rubbed between the first finger and thumb for 2–5 seconds.
7. **Condensation:** The amalgam is placed in the cavity after trituration, and packed (condensed) using suitable instruments.
8. **Shaping and finishing:** Precarve burnishing condenses and smoothes the surface amalgam and reduces the voids and irregularities caused by the serrated condenser.
9. **Carving:** The restoration is carved to reproduce the tooth anatomy.
10. **Burnishing:** After the carving, the restoration is smoothened, by burnishing the surface and margins of the restoration.
11. **Polishing:** Polishing minimizes corrosion and prevents adherence of plaque. The polishing should be delayed for at least 24 hours after condensation, or preferably longer. Wet polishing is advised as dry polishing powders can raise the temperature above 60°C.
    - **Creep (AIIMS-CDER, April 2016):** Creep of dental amalgam is a slow progressive permanent deformation of set amalgam, which occurs under constant stress (static creep) or intermittent stress (dynamic creep).

Significance of creep: Creep is related to *marginal breakdown* of low-copper amalgams. The higher the creep, greater is the degree of marginal deterioration. According to ISO 24234:2015 creep should be <2%.

Creep values: Highest: Lathe-cut low-copper alloys; Lowest: High copper amalgams.

Factors affecting creep

- **Microstructure:** Increased creep rate is shown by larger γ1 volume fractions. Decreased creep rate is shown by larger γ1 grain sizes. γ2 phase is associated with higher creep rates. Single composition high-copper amalgams have very low creep rates. Increased zinc content reduces creep.
- **Effect of manipulative variables:** For increased strength and low creep values: Mercury:alloy ratio should be minimum; Condensation pressure should be maximum for lathe-cut or admixed alloys; Careful attention should be paid to timing of trituration and condensation. Either under- or over-trituration or delayed condensation tend to increase the creep rate.

Recent advances in silver amalgam (*Sumandeep Uni. May 2018*): Resin coated amalgam, fluoridated amalgam, bonded amalgam, and consolidated silver alloy system, gallium—an alternative to amalgam.

Q. 18. Write a short note on mercury hygiene in dental office. (MUHS, May 2012; UHSR, May 2016)

Ans. Mercury is toxic to living creatures. This hazard can arise during trituration, condensation and finishing of the restoration, and also during the removal of old restorations at high speed.

Precautions

1. All the staff involved in handling mercury should be well trained in management and hygiene protocol.
2. The clinic should be well ventilated with fresh air circulation and outside exhaust.
3. All excess mercury and amalgam waste should be stored in well sealed containers.
4. Proper disposal system should be followed to avoid environmental pollution.
5. Amalgam scrap/mercury contaminated material should not be subjected to heat sterilization.
6. Spilled mercury is cleaned as soon as possible as it is extremely difficult to clean it from carpets.
7. Vacuum cleaners are not used as they disperse the mercury through exhaust.
8. Skin contact with mercury should be washed with water and soap.
9. The alloy mercury capsules should have tight fitting cap.
10. While removing old fillings, a water spray, mouth mask and suction should be used.
11. The use of ultrasonic amalgam condenser is not recommended.
12. All scrap amalgam should be salvaged and stored in air tight container.
13. Professional clothing should be removed before leaving the workplace.
14. Annual programme for handling toxic materials should be monitored for actual exposure levels.

Q. 19. Write a short note on direct filling gold. (RGUHS, July 2016)

Ans. Gold in its pure form is very soft (25 BHN). Its malleability and lack of a surface oxide layer permit increments to be welded together.

Applications

1. Pits and small class I restorations.
2. For repair of casting margins.
3. For class II, class V and class VI restorations.
4. Repair of cement vent holes and perforations in gold crowns.

Contraindications

1. Teeth with very large pulp chambers.
2. Periodontally compromised teeth.
3. Handicapped patients.
4. Root canal filled teeth.

Types

1. Foil (fibrous gold): Sheet (cohesive/non-cohesive), ropes, cylinders, laminates, platinized.
2. Electrolytic precipitate (crystalline gold): Mat, mat foil, Gold-calcium alloy.
3. Granulated gold (encapsulated powder)

Gold foil: Gold foil is the oldest of all products described. It is manufactured by beating gold into sheets.

Electrolytic precipitate: Crystalline gold powder is formed by electrolytic precipitation.

Properties

1. **Strength:** Greatest strength is in the most dense area and the weakest part is the porous area, where layers or crystals are not closely compacted.
2. **Hardness:** A reduction in hardness probably indicates the presence of porosity.
3. **Density:** True density of pure gold is 19.3 g/cm^3.
4. **Effect of voids:** Voids on the restoration surface (pits) increase the susceptibility to corrosion and deposition of plaque.
5. **Tarnish and corrosion:** Resistance to tarnish and corrosion is good, if compacted well.
6. **Biocompatibility:** Pulpal response is minimal if compacted well.

Advantages: Esthetic, tarnish and corrosion resistant, good mechanical properties, good biocompatibility.

Disadvantages

1. Non-esthetic because it is not tooth colored.

2. High CTE (coefficient of thermal conductivity).
3. Problems of temperature sensitivity if not insulated with a base.
4. Manipulation is technically challenging.

Q. 20. Write a note on tissue conditioners.
(TNMGR, March 2008; April 2013; AIIMS-CDER, April 2016; AHSUC, July 2016; MUHS, Dec. 2018)

Ans. Tissue conditioners are temporary soft liners, used only for few days to treat irritated mucosa. They are replaced every 3–5 days. Their hardness ranges from 14 to 49 shore. They lose alcohol over time resulting in a weight loss of 5–9%. These materials show both viscous and visco-elastic behaviour which help in both adaptation to tissue and cushioning of masticatory forces.

Uses
1. Poor health conditions, ill-fitting dentures.
2. As functional impression material.
3. As reline materials in surgical obturators.
4. Used to stabilize and enhance retention and comfort of denture base during maxilla-mandibular relation.

Composition
Powder: Poly ethyl methacrylate.
Liquid: Aromatic ester (butyl phthalate, butyl glycolate) in ethanol.

Denture reliner (AIIMS-CDER, April 2016): Reliners may be classified as: Hard or soft (resilient); Heat cured or self cured; Short-term or long-term; Resin based or silicone based.

- **Heat cured acrylic resin (hard liner):** New resin is cured against the old denture by compression molding technique. A low curing temperature is necessary for the relining process to avoid distortion of the denture.

Disadvantages: There is a tendency for it to warp toward the relined side due to: Diffusion of monomer from the reliner before curing, and processing shrinkage of the liner.

- **Chair-side reliners (hard short-term liner):** These materials are used for relining resin dentures directly in the mouth. According to ADA specification No. 17, peak temperature reached during curing should not be >75°C. They have higher porosity and water sorption. They tend to discolor, become foul smelling and may even separate from the denture base.
- **Soft or resilient denture liners:** International Standards Organization describes two categories of soft liners.

1. Short-term soft liners (**tissue conditioners**) (ISO 10139: Part 1).
2. Long-term soft liners (ISO 10139: Part 2).

Long-term soft liners: The purpose of 'permanent' soft liner is to protect the soft tissue by acting as a cushion. They are used when there is irritation of the mucosa, in areas of severe undercut and congenital or acquired defects of palate.

Requirements
1. Good bonding to the denture base.
2. Should be biocompatible, hygienic; maintain its resilience for a long period.
3. Should have good dimensional stability.
4. Low water sorption (max. 20 $\mu g/mm^3$).

Classification (ISO 10139–2:2009)
1. **Based on depth of penetration:** Type A (soft); Type B (extra soft).
2. **Based on their method of processing:** Mouth cured/chairside soft liners; Processed soft liners.

Types
- **Plasticized acrylic resin:** It may be self-cured or heat-cured. **Disadvantages:** They lose plasticizers and harden with use.
- **Vinyl resins:** The plasticized poly (vinyl chloride) and poly (vinyl acetate) resins, like the plasticized acrylic resins, lose plasticizer and harden during use.
- **Silicone rubbers:** These materials retain their elastic properties but may loose adhesion to the denture base.
- **Other polymers:** Polyurethane and polyphosphazine rubber.

Problems associated with soft liners
1. Inadequate bonding to denture.
2. Some silicone liners undergo a high volume change with gain and loss of water.
3. Heat cured soft acrylics bond loose their softness as plasticizer is leached from the liner.
4. It reduces the denture base strength.
5. Trimming, cutting, adjusting and polishing of a soft liner is difficult.

Q. 21. Critically evaluates various types of resins used for provisional restorations. *(BFUHS, Nov. 2009)*

Ans. These materials have more cross-linking agent as compared to denture base resins.

Composition: Polymethylmethacrylate (PMMA), peroxide, oxide particles, methymethacrylate (MMA) liquid, tertiary amines, hydroquinone.

Uses

1. Used as resin facings or veneer on indirect cast restorations.
2. Used in fabrication of provisional crowns and bridges.
3. Acrylic facings of cast partial denture.
4. Immediate acrylic denture.

Types

1. PMMA resins.
2. Polymethyl (isobutyl) methacrylate resins.
3. Epimines.

Q. 22. Write a short note on denture base resins.

(TNMGR, March 2009; AHSUC, July 2016)

Ans. Denture base and other resins used in dentistry are made up of polymers.

Classification

I. **Based on material used**: Metallic (stainless steel), non-metallic (acrylic resin).

II. **Based on duration of use**: Temporary (self cure), permanent (heat cure).

III. **ISO 20795–1:2013 classification**

Type 1: Heat cure polymers: Polymerization at temperature >65°C.

Type 2: Self cure polymers: Polymerization at temperature <65°C.

Type 3: Thermoplastic materials: Moldable polymers.

Type 4: Light cure materials: Polymerization by visible or UV radiation.

Type 5: Microwave materials: Microwave heat polymerization.

Ideal requirements of dental resins: Dental resins should:

1. Be tasteless, odourless, nontoxic and non-irritant to oral tissues.
2. Be esthetically satisfactory and dimensionally stable.
3. Have enough strength, resilience and abrasion resistance.
4. Be insoluble and impermeable to oral fluids.
5. Have a low specific gravity and radiopaque.
6. Be easy to fabricate and repair.
7. Have good thermal conductivity.
8. When used as a filling material it should bond chemically with the tooth.

Composition of heat activated acrylic resin

- **Powder:** PMMA, ethyl/butyl methacrylate (copolymers), benzoyl peroxide (initiator), mercuric/cadmium sulphide (dyes), dibutyl phthalate (plasticizer), zinc/titanium oxide (opacifiers), inorganic fillers like glass fibers, zirconium silicate, alumina, etc. (improves physical properties), dyed synthetic nylon/acrylic fibers (simulate small capillaries).
- **Liquid/Monomer:** MMA, dibutyl phthalate (plasticizer), hydroquinone (inhibitor), glycol dimethacrylate (cross-linking agent).
- **Curing cycle** *(HP Uni., June 2016):* The curing or polymerization cycle is the technical name for the heating process used to initiate, control and complete the polymerization of the resin in the mold. Long curing cycles are recommended for thicker resins to avoid internal porosity. Recommended curing cycles:
  1. **Long cycle:** a. 74°C for 8 hours, b. 74°C for 8 hours, then boil for 1 hour.
  2. **Short cycle:** 74°C for 2 hours, then boil for 1 hour of the thinner portions (short cycle).
    - **Composition of self cure/cold cure/chemically activated acrylic resin**
- **Powder:** PMMA, benzoyl peroxide (initiator), mercuric/cadmium sulphide (dye).
- **Liquid/Monomer:** MMA, tertiary amines (activator), glycol dimethacrylate (cross-linking agent), hydroquinone (inhibitor).
    - **Composition of light activated acrylic resin:** Polyether urethane dimethacrylate (major component), camphoroquinone (photoinitiator), amine (photoactivator), silicone dioxide (inorganic filler), acrylic resin beads (organic fillers), high molecular weight acrylic resin (monomer).

Types of porosity in acrylic resin denture base: Contraction porosity, gaseous porosity, granular porosity.

- **Crazing** *(AIIMS-CDER, April 2016):* Crazing is formation of surface cracks on the denture base resin. In some cases it has a hazy or foggy appearance rather than cracks. Crazing weakens the resin and reduces the esthetic qualities. The cracks formed can cause fracture.

Causes: Mechanical stresses, attack by a solvent, incorporation of water.

Avoided by

1. Using cross-linked acrylics
2. Tin foil separating medium
3. Metal molds

Q. 23. Write a short note on use and abuse of denture adhesives.

(BFUHS, Nov. 2006; TNMGR, Sept. 2010, Oct. 2011)

Ans. These are highly viscous aqueous solutions which are often used to improve the retention of complete dentures.

Composition: Keraya gum, tragacanth, sodium carboxymethyl cellulose, polyethylene oxide, flavouring agent.

They are applied to denture base and inserted. When wet, the polymer portion absorbs water and swells. They improve the retention of the denture base through adhesion. It fills up the spaces between the denture and the tissue.

Disadvantages

1. Unpleasant feel and Difficult to clean.
2. Diluted easily by saliva.
3. In excess may cause gastric irritation.
4. May be allergic to some patient and cause caries because of acidic in nature.

Indications

1. Temporary retention of poorly fitting dentures.
2. Patient with poor neuromuscular control.

Q. 24. Write a short note on bonding primers.

(RGUHS, May 2011)

Ans. Primers contain bifunctional hydrophilic monomers dissolved in solvents such as acetone, ethanol or water. These solvents displace water from the moist collagen network to allow infiltration of monomers through the nanospaces of collagen network. This renders the hydrophilic dentin hydrophobic and spongy for the penetration of the resin into the dentin, e.g. HEMA(hydroxyethyl methacrylate), NMSA (N-methacryloyl 5-amino-salicylic acid), NPG (N-phenylglycine), PMDM (pyromellitic-diethyl methacrylate) and 4-META (methacryloxy ethyl trimellitic anhydride).

Application of primer: Primers should be applied for at least 15 seconds to allow the monomer to diffuse to the complete depth of demineralised dentin. The primer should be air dried with a blow of oil free compressed air to volatilize any remaining excess solvent before the application of adhesive.

- **Bonding agents** *(Sumandeep Uni. May 2018)*: Restorative resins are hydrophobic, therefore, bonding agents should contain both hydrophilic and hydrophobic parts. The hydrophilic part bonds with either calcium in the hydroxyapatite crystals or with collagen. The hydrophobic part bonds with the restorative resin.

Evolution of dentin bond agents *(NTR Uni., Nov. 2007)*:

1. **First generation** (1950–1970): Mineral acids were used to etch enamel. Dentin etching was not recommended. They used glycerophosphoric acid dimethacrylate to provide a bifunctional molecule. These were generally self-cured. The main disadvantage was their low bond strength (2 to 6 MPa).

2. **Second generation** (1970s): Developed as adhesive agents for composite resins which had by then replaced acrylic restorations. One system used NPG-GMA. Other products included phenyl-P, 2-methacryloxy phenyl phosphoric acid. Bond strengths achieved were three times more than the earlier generations, e.g. Prisma, Universal Bond, Clearfil, Scotchbond.

3. **Third generation** (1980s): The third generation bond agents had bond strengths comparable to that of resin to etched enamel. However, their use is more complex and requires two to three application steps. Etching of enamel using 37% phosphoric acid → conditioning of dentin using mild acids → application of separate primer → application of polymerizable monomer → placement of the resin. Examples are tenure, scotch bond 2, prisma, universal bond, mirage bond, etc.

4. **Fourth generation** (early 1990s): Total-etch technique was introduced. Examples are all bond 2, Scotchbond multipurpose, OptiBond, etc. The all bond consists of 2 primers (NPG-GMA and biphenyl dimethacrylate (BPDM) and an unfilled resin adhesive (40% BIS-GMA, 30% UDMA, 30% HEMA). This system bonds composite not only to dentin but to most dental related surfaces like enamel, casting alloys, amalgam, porcelain and composite.

5. **Fifth generation** (mid-1990s): Fifth generation combined the primer and adhesive into one bottle (**self priming adhesive**). Examples: Single bond (3M), one step (BISCO), prime and bond (dentsply). The advantages are: Reduced application steps, less technique sensitive, less volatile liquid, pleasant odor, higher bond strength.

6. **Sixth generation** (mid to late 1990s) *(NTR Uni., May 2019)*: A separate etchant is not required. These are 2 bottle systems. Two varieties are seen—type I and type II.

   - Type I: 2 bottle 2 step systems. Etchant and primer are combined in one bottle (called **self etching primer**). Other bottle contains adhesive. Examples are: Clearfil SE bond, adhese, optibond solo plus, nano bond, etc.

   - Type II: 2 bottle 1 step system. Liquid A contains the primer. Liquid B contains a phosphoric acid modified resin (self etching adhesive). Both liquids are mixed just before application, e.g. Xeno III, Adper prompt L-pop, Tenure Uni-Bond, etc.

7. **Seventh generation** (early 2000): Attempts to combine all three (etchant, primer and adhesive) into

a single product. Thus, seventh generation adhesives may be characterized as 'no mix self-etching adhesives'. Examples include iBond, G bond (GC), Xeno IV (Dentsply) (glass ionomer based), Clearfil S3 (Curare).

8. **Eighth generation**: In 2010, voco America introduced voco Futurabond DC as 8th generation bonding agent, in which the addition of nano-fillers increases the penetration of resin monomers and the hybrid layer thickness, which in turn improves the mechanical properties.

Indications of Bonding Agents

1. For bonding composite to tooth structure.
2. Bonding composite to porcelain and various metals.
3. Desensitization of exposed dentin or root surfaces.
4. Bonding of porcelain veneers.

Contraindication: Bonding should not be done immediately after bleaching a tooth.

- **Universal adhesive systems** (*UHSR, June 2018*): Universal adhesives are in practice since 2011. These new products are known as "**multi-mode**" or "**multi-purpose**" adhesives because they may be used as self-etch (SE) adhesives, etch-and-rinse (ER) adhesives, or as SE adhesives on dentin and ER adhesives on enamel ("selective enamel etching").

Composition: Biphenyl dimethacrylate (BPDM), dipenta-erythritol penta-acrylate phosphoric acid ester (PEN-TA) and polyalkenoic acid copolymer may enhance adhesion to tooth structures. Additionally, the matrix of universal is based on a combination of monomers of hydrophilic (hydroxyethyl methacrylate/HEMA) hydrophobic (decandiol dimethacrylate/D3MA) and intermediate (bis-GMA) nature.

Q. 25. Write a short note on glass ionomers.

[NTR Uni., Nov. 2007; TNMGR, Aug. 2008; RGUHS, Oct. 2010; RUHS, June 2017; UOK, July 2017]

Ans. Glass ionomer cements (GIC) are adhesive tooth coloured anticariogenic restorative materials. Its synonyms are poly (alkenoate) cement, ASPA (aluminosilicate polyacrylic acid).

Applications

1. Anterior esthetic restorative material.
2. For eroded areas.
3. As luting agent.
4. As liners and base.
5. For core build up.

Classification (*BBD Uni., April 2015*):

Type I: Luting and bonding cement.

Type II: For restorations.
Type III: Liners and base.
Type IV: Pit and fissure sealants.

Composition

Powder: Silica, alumina, aluminium fluoride, calcium fluoride, sodium fluoride, aluminium phosphate, zirconium oxide, lanthanum, strontium, barium.

Liquid: Polyacrylic acid (50%), iticonic acid, maleic acid, tricarballylic acid, tartaric acid, water.

Advantages

1. Chemical adhesion to the tooth structure.
2. Anticariogenic potential.
3. Biocompatibility.
4. Tooth coloured restorative material.
5. Good marginal integrity.

Disadvantages

1. Inferior mechanical properties.
2. Poor wear resistance.
3. High moisture sensitivity.
4. Poor aesthetics.

Setting reaction

- When the powder and liquid are mixed together, the acid attacks the glass particles. Thus, calcium, aluminum, sodium and fluoride ions leach out into the aqueous medium.
- The initial set occurs when the calcium ions cross-link (binds) the polyacrylic acid chains. This forms a solid mass.
- In the next phase, the aluminum also begins to cross-link with polyacrylic acid chains.
- Sodium ions combine with fluorine to form sodium fluoride which is uniformly distributed within the cement.
- Water plays a very important role in the cement. Initially it serves as the medium. Later it slowly hydrates the matrix, adding to the strength of the cement (maturation process).
- The unreacted glass (powder) particle is sheathed (covered) by a silica gel. It is formed by the leaching of the ions (Ca^{2+}, Al^{3+}, $Na+$, F^-) from the outer portion of the glass particle.

Properties

1. **Mechanical properties**: Restorative GIC has a compressive strength of 150 MPa. The luting GIC has a compressive strength of 85 MPa.
   - Tensile strength: Luting type: 6.2 MPa; Restorative type: 6.6 MPa hardness (49 KHN).
   - Fracture toughness: Type II GICs are far inferior to composites in this respect.

- Elastic modulus (7.3 GPa): MOE is half that of zinc phosphate cement.
- Wear resistance: They are more susceptible to toothbrush abrasion and occlusal wear when compared to composites.

2. **Solubility and disintegration:** The initial solubility is high due to leaching of intermediate products. Glass ionomer cements are more resistant to attack by organic acids.

3. **Adhesion:** It adheres well to enamel and dentin. Glass ionomer bonds chemically to tooth structure.

4. **Esthetics:** Esthetically they are inferior to silicates and composites.

5. **Biocompatibility:** Pulpal response to GIC is classified as mild.

6. **Anticariogenic properties:** Type II glass ionomer releases fluoride in amounts comparable to silicate cements initially and continue to do so over an extended period of time. In addition, due to its adhesive effect they have the potential for reducing infiltration of oral fluids at the cement-tooth interface, thereby preventing secondary caries.

Q. 26. Write a short note on zinc polycarboxylate cement. *(Gujarat Uni., April 2019)*

Ans. Zinc polycarboxylate cement became the first cement system developed with potential for adhesion to tooth structure.

Applications: Primarily for luting permanent restorations, as bases and liners, for cementation of bands, as root canal fillings in endodontics.

Composition

- **Powder:** Zinc oxide (basic ingredient), magnesium oxide (modifier), oxides of bismuth and aluminum, stannous fluoride (increases strength, modifies setting time and imparts anticariogenic properties).
- **Liquid:** Aqueous solution of polyacrylic acid or copolymer of acrylic acid with other unsaturated carboxylic acids, i.e. itaconic, maleic, or tricarballylic acid.

Setting reaction: When the powder and liquid are mixed, the surface of powder particles are attacked by the acid, releasing zinc, magnesium and tin ions. These ions bind to the polymer chain via the carboxyl groups.

Properties

1. **Mechanical properties:** ISO requires a minimum compressive strength of 50 MPa for this cement. Tensile strength: 6.2 MPa.

2. **Solubility and disintegration:** It tends to absorb water and is slightly more soluble (0.6% wt) than zinc phosphate.

3. **Biocompatibility:** Pulpal response is classified as mild.

4. **Adhesion:** It bonds chemically with the tooth structure.

5. **Optical properties:** They are very opaque.

6. **Anticariogenic properties:** Some manufacturers have attempted to incorporate fluoride within the cement.

7. **Thermal properties:** They are good thermal insulators.

Advantages

1. Comparatively less irritating to the pulp.
2. Chemical bond to tooth structure.

Disadvantages: Limited fluoride release when compared to GIC.

Q. 27. Discuss in detail the various luting agents used in dentistry. *(TNMGR, March 2008; NTR Uni., June 2014; HP Uni., June 2016)*

Ans. Luting/bonding/cementing is the process by which crown, restoration and other devices are attached to tooth structure using an intermediate material called cement.

Types

1. Temporary (short-term) luting cements: Zinc oxide eugenol.
2. Permanent (long-term) luting cementation: Zinc phosphate cement, GIC, resin cement, zinc polycarboxylate cement, reinforced zinc oxide eugenol.

Luting mechanism

1. **Non-adhesive:** Luting cement fills the gap between restoration-tooth, and holds by engaging in small surface irregularities, e.g. all luting cements.
2. **Micromechanical bonding:** Surface irregularities are enhanced through air abrasion/acid etching to provide large irregularities for cement to fill, e.g. resin cements.
3. **Molecular bonding:** This results from van der Waals forces and a chemical bond between the cement and the tooth surface, e.g. zinc polycarboxylate, GIC.

General Requirements of Luting Materials

1. They should be nontoxic and nonirritant to pulp and tissues.
2. They should be insoluble in saliva and liquids taken into the mouth.
3. Mechanical properties: These must meet the requirements for their particular applications, e.g. a cement base should develop sufficient strength rapidly to enable a filling material to be packed on it.

4. **Optical properties:** For cementation of translucent restorations, cement should match the color and translucency of tooth substance.
5. Dental cements should ideally be adhesive to both tooth structure and restorative material, but not to dental instruments.
6. They should be bacteriostatic in a cavity with residual caries.
7. They should have an obtundant effect on the pulp.
8. Luting cement should have sufficiently low viscosity to give a low film thickness.

Recent advances *(MUHS, June 2016)*

- *Resin-modified glass-ionomer cement (NTR Uni., Oct 2014):* Resin-modified glass-ionomer cement (RMGI), developed in 1980s, and is a hybrid material derived from adding polymerizable resins to conventional glass-ionomer cement.

Classification

1. Resin-modified glass ionomer cement (RMGI), e.g. Fuji II LC.
2. Compomers or polyacid-modified composites (PMC), e.g. Dyract Variglass VLC.

Composition

Powder: Ion leachable glasses (silica, alumina), photo-initiators or chemical initiators or both, polymerizable resin, hydroxyethyl methacrylate (HEMA) monomers.

Liquid: Polyacrylic acid, water, methacrylate monomer.

Properties

1. **Strength:** Compressive strength is slightly lower (105 MPa) when compared to conventional GIC. The diametral tensile strength is however greater (20 MPa).
2. **Hardness:** Hardness (40 KHN) is comparable to that of conventional GIC.
3. **Microleakage:** These materials have a greater amount of microleakage when compared to GIC.
4. **Anticariogenicity:** These materials have a significant anticariogenic effect because of the fluoride release.
5. **Pulpal response:** Pulpal response to the cement is mild (similar to conventional GIC).
6. **Esthetics:** They are more translucent and therefore more esthetic than conventional GIC.
   - *Compomers:* The compomers, also known as poly acid-modified composite resins, were described as being a combination of composite resin (comp) and glass-ionomer (omer), offering the advantages of both.
   - *Resins:* Resins are useful for all-ceramic, veneers, metal or metal-ceramic restorations where reten-

tion and resistance form is compromised and for post cementation in endodontically treated teeth.

Q. 28. Write a note on anticariogenic material.
(RGUHS, July 2016; NTR Uni., Oct 2019)

Ans. Fluoride is well documented as an anticariogenic agent. Currently, various restorative materials contain fluorides and they exhibit anticariogenic property. These restorative materials release an adequate amount of fluoride into the oral environment and increase the level of fluoride in saliva, plaque and hard dental tissues.

Fluoride releasing restorative materials

1. **Glass ionomer cements:** Two processes have been proposed to describe the mechanism of fluoride release from glass-ionomers into an aqueous environment. The first process is a short-term reaction in which the outer surfaces of alumino-fluoro-silicate glass particles rapidly dissolves into solution. In second process, there is more gradual dissolution and resulted in the sustained diffusion of ions through the bulk cement.
2. **Modified glass ionomer cements:** Metal reinforced glass ionomers, resin-modified glass-ionomer cements (RMGICs), polyacid modified composite (compomer), polyacid-modified composites containing glass fillers and ytterbium trifluoride,
3. **Composites.**
4. **Amalgam.**

Q. 29. Write a short note on pit and fissure sealants.
(RGUHS, July 2016)

Ans. Deep pits and fissures on posterior teeth are susceptible to decay as they provide shelter for organisms. They are often too narrow making it difficult to clean.

Indications: Deciduous molars and young permanent molars with deep pits and fissures.

Types

1. Based on filler content: Filled and unfilled.
2. Based on curing mechanism: Light cured and chemical cured.

Color: The sealants are available as transparent, tooth colored, opaque, tinted or white materials.

Composition: Bis-GMA, polyurethanes and cyanoacrylates.

Properties

- Sealants must have low viscosity so that they will flow readily into the depths of the pits and fissures and wet the tooth.
- Wettability is also important for proper adaptation and penetration.

- Acid etching with bonding agents is necessary for the retention of the sealant.
- Sealant must have sufficient mechanical properties like strength, stiffness and wear resistance.

Q. 30. Define and classify dental composites. Write in detail about its properties and newer modifications. *(NTR Uni., Oct. 2009; RGUHS, May 2014)*

Ans. Composite is a system composed of a mixture of two or more macromolecules, which are essentially insoluble in each other and differ in form.

Uses

1. Restoration of anterior and posterior teeth.
2. To veneer metal crowns and fixed partial dentures.
3. To build-up cores.
4. Bonding of orthodontic brackets, etched cast restorations, ceramic crowns, posts, inlays, onlays and laminates.
5. Pit and fissure sealant.
6. Esthetic laminates.
7. Repair of chipped porcelain restorations.

Types

I. ISO 4049:2009 Classification:
  1. Type 1: Polymer-based material suitable for restorations involving occlusal surfaces.
  2. Type 2: All other polymer-based materials and luting agents.
II. **Based on curing mechanism (ISO 4049:2009):** Types 1 and 2 are further grouped into 3 classes based on curing mechanism.
  - Class 1: Self-cured materials.
  - Class 2: Light-cured materials: Group 1 (energy applied intraorally), Group 2 (energy applied extraorally).
  - Class 3: Dual-cured materials.
III. Based on filler particle size (Willems 1993)
  1. Fine particle size >3 μm.
  2. Ultrafine particle size <3 μm
  3. Microfine (0.04 μm)
  4. Nano range (5100 nm or 0.0050.01 μm)
IV. **Based on filler particle size:** Macrofillers (10–100 μm); Midifillers (1–10 μm); Minifillers (0.1–1 μm); Microfillers (0.01–0.1 μm)
  a. Homogenous (contains only microfillers)
  b. Heterogenous (microfillers combined with prepolymerized fillers): Splintered prepolymerized particles; Spherical prepolymerized particles.
  c. Agglomerated (microfiller sintered to form larger filler complexes): Nanofillers (0.0050.01 μm); Hybrid.

V. **Based on viscosity:** Conventional, flowable, packable.

Composition

- Resin matrix/binder: Bis-GMA or urethane dimethacrylate
- Filler: Quartz, colloidal silica or heavy metal glasses.
- Coupling agent: Organosilanes.
- Others: A curing system (chemical/light); Inhibitors (0.01%): Prevents premature polymerization, e.g. butylated hydroxytoluene (BHT); UV absorbers to improve color stability; Opacifiers (0.001 to 0.007%) e.g. titanium dioxide and aluminum; Color pigments.
  I. **Resin matrix:** Dental composites use a blend of monomers that are aromatic or aliphatic dimethacrylates of bis-GMA (bisphenol-A-glycidyl methacrylate), urethane dimethacrylate (UDMA) and bis-EMA (bisphenol-A-polyethylene glycol diether dimethacrylate) are most commonly used. Triethylene glycol dimethacrylate (TEGDMA) is added to control the viscosity.
  II. **Filler particles** *(RGUHS, Oct. 2010; MUHS, May 2012):* Composite fillers are classified by material, shape and size. They are broadly classified into 3 groups: Macrofillers, microfillers and nanofillers. A mixture of different particle sizes is referred to as a **hybrid**.
  Functions of fillers: Addition of filler particles into the resin significantly improves its properties.
  1. Improves strength
  2. Reduces shrinkage, wear and water sorption.
  3. Smaller the particle size, the greater the polishability.
  4. Reduces thermal expansion and contraction.
  5. Improves clinical handling and imparts radiopacity.
  Important attributes of fillers: Amount of filler added (filler loading), size of particles and its distribution, shape of fillers, index of refraction, radiopacity, hardness.
  III. **Coupling agent:** Coupling agents bond the filler particles to the resin matrix. Most commonly used coupling agents are organosilanes (i.e. 3-methacryloxypropyltrimethoxysilane).

Functions of coupling agents

1. They improve the properties of the resin through transfer of stresses from more plastic resin matrix to stiffer filler particles.
2. They prevent water from penetrating the filler-resin interface.
3. They bond the fillers to the resin matrix thereby reducing the wear.

- **Polymerization (setting) mechanisms:** They polymerize by the addition mechanism that is initiated by free radicals. The free radicals can be generated by chemical activation or external energy (heat, light or microwave).
- **Polymerization shrinkage and its prevention.** *(TNMGR, Oct. 2016):* During polymerization, reduction in intermolecular distance results in volumetric polymerization shrinkage. At the molecular level, there is a decrease in molecular vibration with increased cross-linking.

Factors Affecting Polymerization Shrinkage

1. **Filler volume fraction:** Filler volume fraction has an inverse relation to volumetric shrinkage.
2. **Degree of conversion of resin matrix:** The volumetric shrinkage is directly proportional to the degree of conversion.
3. **Composition of resin matrix:** The shrinkage is influenced by monomer functionalities, molecular structure, molecular mass, and size.
4. **Configuration factor:** "C factor" or "Configuration factor," is defined as the ratio of bonded to unbonded surfaces of the composite restorations. If the C factor is high, the shrinkage stress is high.
5. **Intensity of curing light:** There exists a linear relationship between polymerization shrinkage and light intensity.
6. **Thickness of composite resin, shade, and opacity of composite:** Incremental curing induces lesser polymerization shrinkage.
7. **Other factors:** Exposure time, mode of curing, compatibility between spectral output of curing light, and photoinitiator system.

Methods to minimize polymerization shrinkage

- **Modification of placement technique:** Incremental technique reduces shrinkage stress. Buccolingual incremental technique induces least strain.
- **Material aspect:** The introduction of ring opening silorane molecules has resulted in low shrinkage composite resins. The rate of polymerization and shrinkage stress is reduced by increasing the concentration of inhibitor.
- **Curing technique:** Pulse delay technique and soft-start polymerization reduce the polymerization shrinkage and stress.
- **Use of stress absorbing liners:** Flowable resin can be used as an intermediate stress absorbing layer as it has a lower elastic modulus which reduces the stress at the tooth-restoration interface, ultimately reducing the cuspal deflection ("**Elastic wall concept**").

- **Preheating:** Preheating resin composites have found to reduce the polymerization shrinkage.

Recent advances

1. **Microfilled/microfine composite:** The microfilled composite is the resin of choice for esthetic restoration of anterior teeth, especially in non-stress bearing situations.
2. **Hybrid composite resins:** Hybrid composites have a surface smoothness and esthetics competitive with microfilled composites for anterior restorations. The hybrids are generally considered as **multipurpose composites** suitable for both anterior and posterior use.
3. **Nano and nanohybrid composite resins:** Nano-composites are similar to the microfilled, comprising of uniformly sized nanofillers. Nanohybrids like the conventional hybrids come in a range of filler sizes including nanofillers. They can be used for both anterior and posterior restorations.

Q. 31. Write a short note on health hazards of photocuring. *(BBD Uni., April 2016)*

Ans. "Blue light hazard": The cumulative exposures to high intensity blue light may cause ocular damage. This blue light hazard to the retina is greatest at 440 nm, which is close to the maximum emission from dental light cure units. Blue light is transmitted through the ocular media and absorbed by the retina. While high levels of blue light cause immediate and irreversible retinal burning, chronic exposure to low levels of blue light is thought to cause accelerated retinal aging and degeneration and can accelerate age-related macular degeneration (ARMD). It should also be noted that the maximum recommended exposure times are for individuals with normal photosensitivity and patients or dental personnel who have had cataract surgery, or who are taking photosensitizing medications, have a greater susceptibility for retinal damage and ocular injury may occur with even shorter exposure times. Blue light filtering glasses ('**Orange blue-blockers**') can reduce the transmission of light below 500 nm to <1%.

Q. 32. Write a short note on titanium.
(TNMGR, Aug. 2008, April 2013)

Ans. Commercially pure titanium has become one of the materials of choice for dental implant material because:

a. It has low density (4.5 g/cm^2) but high strength.
b. It has minimal bio corrosion due to its passivating effect.
c. It is biocompatible.

d. Titanium has good stiffness (5–10 times higher than bone).

Pure titanium has different crystallographic forms at high and low temperatures. At temperature below 885°C the hexagonal close packed or α-lattice is stable, whereas at higher temperature the metal rearranges into a body cantered cubic or β-crystal. α-titanium is not used in orthodontic applications, since they do not have improved springback characteristics. β-titanium can be stabilized down to room temperature by the addition of elements like molybdenum. β-titanium alloy in wrought wire form is used for orthodontic applications.

Properties

1. Modulus of elasticity: 71.7×10^3 MPa.
2. Yield of strength: 860–1170 MPa.
3. The high ratio of yield strength to modulus produces orthodontic appliances that can undergo large elastic activations.
4. Beta titanium can be highly cold worked.
5. Welding: Clinically satisfactory joints can be made by electrical resistance welding of β-titanium.
6. Corrosion resistance: Both forms have excellent corrosion resistance and environmental stability.

Uses

1. Metal-ceramic restorations.
2. Dental implants.
3. Partial denture frames.
4. Complete denture bases.
5. Bar connectors.
6. Titanium mesh membranes (Tiomesh) are used in bone augmentation. (In dentistry, it is especially useful as an alternative alloy to those who are allergic to nickel.)

Disadvantages

1. Poor castability.
2. Highly technique sensitive.
3. Requires expensive machines for casting and machining.
4. Low fusing porcelains (<800°C) required to prevent β-phase transformation.

Q. 33. Write a short note on metal-free ceramics.
(RGUHS, Oct. 2010; HP Uni., June 2016; AHSUC, July 2016)

Q. Write a note on recent advances in ceramics.
(Sumandeep Uni. April 2014)

Ans. Metal-free ceramics/all ceramic restorations without a metallic core or substructure. This makes them esthetically superior to the metal ceramic restorations.

They are:

1. Platinum foil matrix condensed porcelain restorations:
   - Conventional feldspathic porcelain restorations.
   - Porcelain restorations with aluminous core.
   - Ceramic jacket crown with leucite reinforced core (Optec HSP)
2. Castable glass ceramics (Dicor)
3. Pressable glass-ceramics:
   - Leucite reinforced glass-ceramics (IPS Empress).
   - Lithia disilicate reinforced glass-ceramics (IPS Empress 2)
4. Glass infiltrated core porcelains:
   - Glass infiltrated aluminous core (In-Ceram).
   - Glass infiltrated spinel core (In-Ceram Spinell).
   - Glass infiltrated zirconia core (In-Ceram Zirconia)
5. Ceramic restorations from CAD/CAM ceramic blanks:
   - Feldspathic porcelain blanks (Vitablocs Mark II).
   - Lithia disilicate glass ceramic blanks (IPSe max CAD, Kavo).
   - Glass infiltrated blanks (alumina, spinell, zirconia).
   - Partially sintered zirconia blanks (Vita In-Ceram YZ).
   - Sintered zirconia blanks (Everest ZH blanks)
6. Ceramic restorations from copy milled ceramic blanks:
   - Alumina blocks (Celay In-Ceram).
   - $MgAl_2O_4$ blocks (In-Ceram spinell).

Composition: Silica, alumina, calcium oxide, soda, potash, boric oxide, zinc oxide, zirconium oxide.

Q. 34. Write a short note on glazing in ceramics.
(NTR Uni., Oct. 2014)

Ans. The glazing is to obtain a smooth surface that simulates a natural tooth surface. It is done either by:

- **Auto glazing:** Rapid heating up to the fusion temperature for 1–2 minutes to melt the surface particles.
- **Add on glazing:** Applying a glaze to the surface and re-firing. Auto glazing is preferred to an applied glaze.

Significance: The aim of glazing is to seal the open pores in the surface of fired porcelain. Dental glazes are composed of colorless glass powder, applied to the fired crown surface, so as to produce a glossy surface. Unglazed or trimmed porcelain may also lead to inflammation of the soft tissues it contacts.

Q. 35. Write a note on zirconia. *(NTR Uni., May 2019)*
Ans. Zirconia is the oxide of zirconium metal (ZrO_2). Zirconium oxide is a white crystalline oxide ceramic with unique properties.

Indications: It is a material of choice for posterior crowns and short span fixed partial dentures in high stress areas. It is not particularly suited for esthetic zones because of its greater opacity.

Transformation toughening: It has the highest strength among the dental ceramics because of its high degree of crack resistance. This is possible because of a unique property of zirconia to undergo a process known as **transformation toughening**. The stable form of zirconia is the monoclinic form. When zirconia is heated, it changes to its tetragonal high-temperature phase which again reverts back to the monoclinic form on cooling. However, addition of yttrium oxide (3–5%) also known as yttria maintains the zirconia in its high temperature tetragonal form at room temperature. Thus, this form of zirconia is known as **'yttria-stabilized zirconia polycrystal'**. When a stress is applied to the zirconia as in the beginning of a crack formation, it reverts back to its monoclinic form locally with an accompanying increase in volume. The local increase in volume introduces compressive stresses around the crack and slows its growth. This is also known as 'tension expansion'—a phenomenon otherwise known only in the case of steel. For this reason zirconium oxide is also known as **"Ceramic Steel"** *(UHSR, June 2018)*

Composition: Zirconium dioxide (ZrO_2) (90–92%), yttrium oxide (Y_2O_2) (3–5%), hafnium oxide (HfO_2) (<3%), aluminum oxide (Al_2O_3) (<0.25), silicon dioxide (SiO_2) (<1%)

Properties of zirconia
- Dental zirconia is an extremely hard, dense, strong and highly opaque material.
- Density 9 g/cm^3.
- Melting point 2715°C.
- Refractive index 2.13.
- Soluble in hydrofluoric acid and hot sulphuric acid.
- Flexure strength: 900–1200 MPa.
- MOE: 210 GPA.
- CTE: 10.5×10^{-6}/°C.
- Esthetics: Zirconia based restorations are more esthetic because of the elimination of metal display.

Q. 36. Discuss about biomaterials used in implants.
(BFUHS, May 2005; BBD Uni., June 2016)

Ans. A dental implant is a material or device placed in and/or on oral tissues to support an oral prosthesis (GPT-8).

Types of implants: Subperiosteal, transosteal, endosseous.

Materials used
1. **Metals:** Stainless steel, cobalt-chromium-molybdenum based, titanium and its alloys, surface coated titanium.
2. **Ceramics:** Hydroxyapatite, bioglass, aluminum oxide.
3. **Polymers and composites**
4. **Others:** Gold, tantalum, carbon, etc.

1. Titanium and its alloys: Commercially pure titanium (cp Ti) is currently the most widely used material for implants. It has become the material of choice because of its low density (4.5 gm/cm^2) but high strength, minimal bio-corrosion due to its passivating effect, excellent biocompatibility. Titanium also has good stiffness. Its alloyed form contains aluminum (6%) and vanadium (4%).

- **Surface coated titanium:** Newer implant designs use titanium that is coated with a material that bonds and promotes bone growth (**bioactive**). The implant is coated with a thin layer of tricalcium phosphate or hydroxyapatite that has been plasma sprayed.

2. Ceramics: They are primarily used as surface coats on titanium implants.

- **Bioactive,** e.g. hydroxyapatite, bioglass (CaO, NaO, P_2O_5 and SiO_2).
- **Bioinert.** e.g., Aluminum oxide.

3. Stainless steel: 18–8 or austenitic steel.

4. Polymers and composites: For tissue attachment and replacement augmentation and for stress distribution.

5. Other materials: Gold, palladium, tantalum, platinum and alloys, zirconium, tungsten and carbon compounds.

- **Osseointegration** *(MUHS, Dec. 2016):* The term osseointegration was first described by Per Ingvar Branemark. It is defined as an apparent direct connection of an implant surface and host bone without intervening connective tissue **(GPT-8)**. To achieve osseointegration, the bone must be viable, space between the implant and bone should be <10 nm and contain no fibrous tissue.

- **Factors favoring osseointegration:** Atraumatic drilling of bone, selection of proper implant material, implant design, favorable occlusal forces, bone quality, no contraindicating local or systemic factors, nature of the surface coating and surface configuration.

- **Implant surfaces and coatings** *(TNMGR, March 2008):* **Bioactive substances** are coated over the titanium to actively promote a favorable bone response. Examples of bioactive materials are hydroxyapatite, tricalcium phosphate and bioactive glasses.

Commercially available bioactive glasses include Bioglass, Ceravital, Biogran and glass ceramic A-W. In this case the interphase is termed 'Biointegration' because there is no intervening space between the bone and the implant.

Techniques used to modify implant surfaces

1. **Ablative procedures**: Ablation is removal of material from the surface of an object by blasting, vaporization, chipping, or other erosive processes, e.g. grit blasting, acid etching, anodizing, shot/laser peening.
2. **Additive procedures**: It is a process of creating a layer by addition of material, e.g. plasma spraying, electrophoretic deposition, sputter deposition, soluble gel coating, soluble blast media, pulsed laser deposition, biomimetic precipitation.

Dental implant surface should stimulate bone growth around them upon placement. Surface characteristics are classified based on the following:
1. Roughness: Smooth: <0.5 µm; Rough: 0.5–3 µm.
    i. Minimally rough: 0.5–1 µm
    ii. Intermediately rough: 1–2 µm
    iii. Rough: 2–3 µm
2. Texture:
    a. Concave: By additive treatment.
    b. Convex: By subtractive treatment.

Q. 37. Write a short note on gypsum material.
(RGUHS, May 2011)

Ans. Gypsum products are derived from the mineral gypsum, chemically known as calcium sulphate dehydrate.

Applications
1. Study models for oral and maxillofacial structures.
2. Cast and die material.
3. Impression material.
4. Investing material in flasking procedure.
5. Investment material for casting of metallic restorations.
6. For mounting stone models onto articulators.

Types: ISO 6873:2013 classification
- Type I: Impression plaster (water/powder ratio = 0.40–0.75)
- Type II: Model plaster, plaster of Paris (water/powder ratio = 0.40–0.55). Class 1: For mounting; Class 2: For models.
- Type III: Dental stone (water/powder ratio = 0.28–0.33).
- Type IV: Die stone (high strength and low expansion) (water/powder ratio = 0.22–0.26).
- Type V: Dental stone (high strength and high expansion) (water/powder ratio = 0.18–0.22).

Advantages
1. Good reproducibility.
2. Dimensionally accurate and stable.
3. Inexpensive and easy to use.
4. Good colour contrast.

Disadvantages
1. Poor mechanical properties cause fracture of teeth from stone cast.
2. Poor abrasive resistance.
3. Poor compatibility with hydrocolloid impression materials.
4. Poor wetting of rubber impression materials.

Specialized gypsum products: Dental casting investment, divestment, synthetic gypsum, orthodontic stone, resin modified stones, mounting plaster, fast setting stone.

- **Setting expansion of plaster of Paris** *(AIIMS-CDER, April 2016)*: Setting expansion is measured using an extensometer. Setting expansion is of two types:

1. Normal setting expansion (0.05 to 0.5%): All gypsum products show a linear expansion during setting, due to the outward thrust of the growing crystals during setting.

Significance: Setting expansion is undesirable in impression plaster, dental plaster and stone as it will result in an inaccurate cast or changes in the occlusal relation if used for mounting. Increased setting expansion is desired in case of investment materials as it helps to compensate the shrinkage of metal during casting. This can be reduced by: Mechanical mixing; Increase in W/P ratio; Using modifiers; Potassium sulphate (4%), sodium chloride and borax.

2. Hygroscopic setting expansion: When a gypsum product is placed under water before the initial set stage, a greater expansion is seen. This is due to hygroscopic expansion. When expansion begins, externally available water is drawn into pores forming in the setting mass and this maintains a continuous aqueous phase in which crystal growth takes place freely. It is greater in magnitude than normal setting expansion.

Importance: Used to expand some gypsum bonded investments.

- **Improved dental stone or die stone** *(RGUHS, May 2014)*: The most commonly used die materials are alpha hemihydrate type IV and type V gypsum products. The setting expansion has been increased from 0.01–0.3%. This higher setting expansion is required in the stone used for the die to aid in compensation for the base metal alloy solidification shrinkage.

Advantages

1. Good strength with minimal shrinkage.
2. Easy manipulation, good working time and sets quickly.
3. Compatible with impression materials.
4. Has smooth, hard surface.
5. Can be easily trimmed.
6. Has good color contrast and is economical.

Disadvantages: Brittle. Not as abrasion resistant as the epoxy and electroformed dies. Edges and occlusal surface may be rubbed off.

Q. 38. Enumerate and explain various die materials in dentistry. *(BFUHS, May 2005; Sumandeep Uni., April 2014; MUHS, June; Dec. 2017; AHSUC, May 2018)*

Ans. Models are used primarily for observation, diagnosis and patient education, e.g. orthodontic study models. A working model or master **cast** is the positive replica on which restorations or appliances are fabricated, e.g. complete denture. **Dies** is/are a positive replica of a prepared tooth or teeth in a suitable hard substance on which inlays, crowns and other restorations are made.

Types of die materials

1. **Gypsum:** Type IV, type V
2. **Metal and metal-coated dies:** Electroformed, sprayed metals, amalgam.
3. **Polymers:** Metal or inorganic filled resins, Polyurethane, epoxy.
4. **Cements:** Silicophosphate or polyacrylic acid bonded cement.
5. **Refractory materials:** Investments and divestments. Investment casts are used to make patterns for RPD frames. Divestment dies are used in direct baking of porcelain crowns or preparation of wax patterns.

Ideal requirement of die materials: An ideal die material should:

1. Be dimensionally accurate.
2. Have good abrasion resistance, strength and toughness to allow burnishing of foil and resist breakage.
3. Have a smooth surface and able to reproduce all fine details in the impression.
4. Be compatible with all impression materials.
5. Have a color contrast with wax, porcelain and alloys.
6. Be easy to manipulate and quick to fabricate.
7. Be non-injurious to health by touch or inhalation.

Q. 39. Write a note on investment material. *(MUHS, June 2016; AIIMS-CDER, April 2017)*

Ans. An **investment** can be described as a ceramic material which is suitable for forming a mold into which molten metal or alloy is cast. The procedure for forming the mold is described as '**investing**'.

Requirements of an Investment Material

1. Investment mold must expand to compensate for the alloy shrinkage.
2. Powder should have a fine particle size to give a smooth surface to the casting.
3. The manipulation should be easy with suitable setting time.
4. The material should have a smooth consistency when mixed.
5. The set material should be porous enough to permit air in the mold cavity to escape easily during casting.
6. At higher temperatures, the investment must not decompose to give off gases.
7. It must have adequate strength at room temperature to permit handling.
8. Casting temperatures should not be critical.
9. After casting, it should break away readily from the surface of metal.
10. The material should be economical.

Classification of Refractory Materials

A. Classification based on application (ISO 15912:2006)

- Type 1: For construction of inlays, crowns and other fixed restorations.
- Type 2: For construction of complete or partial dentures or other removable appliances.
- Type 3: For construction of casts used in brazing procedures.
- Type 4: For construction of refractory dies.

B. Sub-classification based on method of burnout (ISO 15912:2006)

- Class 1: For burn-out by a slow- or step-heating method.
- Class 2: For burn-out by a quick-heating method.

C. Classification based on type of binder used: They all contain silica as refractory material.

1. Gypsum bonded investments: They are used for casting gold alloys. They can withstand temperature up to 700°C.
2. Phosphate bonded investments: For metal ceramic and cobalt-chromium alloys. They can withstand higher temperatures.
3. Ethyl silica bonded investments: They are an alternative to phosphate bonded investments, for high

temperature casting. They are principally used in the casting of base metal alloy partial dentures.

General composition of investments: All investment materials contain a refractory, a binder and modifiers.

1. Refractory: A refractory is a material that will withstand high temperatures without decomposing or disintegrating, e.g. silica. Allotropic forms: Quartz, tridymite, cristobalite, fused quartz.

Significance *(NTR Uni., Oct. 2019)*: They can withstand high temperatures and regulate thermal expansion.

2. Binder: A material which will set and bind together the particles of refractory substance, e.g. gypsum, phosphate and silicate. The common binder used for gold alloys is dental stone (alpha-hemihydrate). The investments for casting cobalt chromium alloys use ethyl silicate, ammonium sulphate or sodium phosphate.

3. Chemical modifiers: Chemicals such as sodium chloride, boric acid, potassium sulfate, graphite, copper powder or magnesium oxide are added in small quantities to modify properties.

Phosphate bonded investment *(NTR Uni., Nov. 2007; TNMGR, March 2008)*: Phosphate bonded investments are perhaps the most widely utilized investment in dentistry. This is because a substantial amount of cast dental structures today use high fusing noble or base metal alloys.

Uses: For casting high fusing alloys, e.g. high fusing noble metal alloys, metal ceramic alloys and base metal alloys like nickel-chromium and cobalt-chromium.

Composition

a. **Powder**: Ammonium diacid phosphate (binder), silica (refractory material), magnesium oxide, carbon (modifier).

b. **Liquid**: Silica solution in water.

Setting reaction: Ammonium diacid phosphate reacts with magnesium oxide to give the investment room temperature strength. At higher temperature, ammonium diacid phosphate reacts with silica to form silicophosphate, which increases the strength at higher temperature.

Manipulation: Powder/liquid ratio: 16–23 ml/100 gm.

Factors affecting setting time

1. Warmer temperatures accelerate the setting. Cooling the liquid prolongs the working time.
2. Increasing the mixing time accelerates the set.
3. An increased L/P ratio delays setting and gives more working time.

Properties

1. Phosphate investments have wax pattern expansion, setting expansion and thermal expansion.
2. Regular investments are generally materials of low strength.
3. Phosphate bonded investments undergo thermo chemical reactions when heated to high temperatures.
4. Investments appear to have low flow when mixed. However, they flow readily and envelope the pattern when poured into the mold under vibration.
5. Early phosphate investments produced rough castings when compared to gypsum based investments.

Q. 40. Discuss casting defects in detail. How to avoid various casting defects? *(NTR Uni., Nov. 2007; BFUHS, May 2007, 2008; TNMGR, Sept. 2010; HP Uni., May 2012; HP Uni., June 2016; May 2018; AHSUC, May 2018)*

Ans. A casting defect is an irregularity in the metal casting process that is very undesired.

1. Distortion: Usually due to distortion of wax pattern. This can be minimized by manipulating wax at high temperature, investing pattern within one hour after finishing.

2. Surface roughness: Surface irregularities can range from surface roughness to larger nodules and fins. It can be because of:

a. Air bubbles on wax pattern.
b. Too rapid heating of investment.
c. Higher water/powder ratio.
d. Prolonged heating.
e. Too high or too low casting pressure.
f. Foreign body inclusion.

- **Nodules** on the inner surface of a casting can are caused by air or gas bubbles trapped on the wax pattern. Minimized by: Proper mixing of investment, vibration of mix, vacuum investing, application of wetting agent.

- **Fins** are narrow raised areas on a casting usually corresponding to a crack in the investment. Molten alloy fills and solidifies in these cracks resulting in fins. Cracks are usually caused by weak investment or too rapid a heating of the investment. Minimized by: Proper water/powder ratio, avoid prolonged and rapid heating of mold, heat the ring gradually to 700°C, proper spruing, avoid premature use.

3. Porosity: External porosity causes discolouration, whereas internal porosity weakens the restoration.

a. **Shrink spot/localized shrinkage porosity** *(May 2015):* Large irregular voids usually found near the sprue-casting junction, occurs due to incorrect cooling sequence, and the sprue freezes before the rest of the casting. This allows more molten metal to flow into the mold to compensate for the shrinkage of the casting as it solidifies. If the sprue solidifies before the rest of the casting no more molten metal can be supplied from the sprue. It is avoided by: Using sprue of correct thickness, attach sprue to thickest portion of wax pattern, flaring the sprue at the point of attachment or placing a reservoir close to the wax pattern.

b. **Suck back porosity** *(MUHS, June 2012; Sharda Uni., July 2017):* This is an external void usually seen in the inside of a crown opposite the sprue. A hot spot is created by the hot metal impinging on the mould wall near the sprue, which causes this region to freeze last. Since the sprue has already solidified, no more molten material is available and the resulting shrinkage causes a type of shrinkage called suck back porosity. It is avoided by reducing the temperature difference between the mold and the molten alloy.

c. **Microporosity:** Fine irregular voids within the casting, occurs when the casting freezes too rapidly.

d. **Pinhole porosity:** Tiny voids due to release of incorporated gases during solidification.

e. **Gas inclusion porosity**: Large voids, due to dissolved gases.

f. **Back pressure porosity:** Porous casting with rounded short margins. It occurs due to inadequate venting of the mould. It can be avoided by using adequate casting force, using investment of adequate porosity, by placing pattern not more than 6–8 mm away from the end of the ring and providing vents in large castings.

g. **Casting with gas blow hole:** This occurs due to wax residue in the mould, which yields large volumes of gases.

4. Incomplete casting: It may occur due to insufficient use of alloy, when mould is not heated to casting temperature, premature solidification of alloy, blocked sprue, back pressure due to gases and low casting pressure.

5. Too bright/shiny casting with short and rounded margins: It occurs due to incomplete elimination of wax.

6. Small casting: It occurs when the compensation for shrinkage of alloy has not been done by adequate expansion of mould cavity.

7. Contamination: It occurs due to oxidation by overheating, using oxidizing zone of flame, failure to use flux.

8. Black casting: It occurs due to release of sulphur when the investment is overheated due to incomplete elimination of wax pattern.

Q. 41. Write a short note on sprue former.

(MUHS, June 2018)

Ans. A sprue former is made of wax, plastic or metal. The thickness is in proportion to the wax pattern. A reservoir is attached to the sprue or the attachment of the sprue to the wax pattern is flared. The length of the sprue is adjusted so that the wax pattern is approximately 1/4" from the other end of the ring.

Functions

1. To form a mount for the wax pattern.
2. To create a channel for the elimination of wax during burnout.
3. Forms a channel for entry of molten alloy during casting.
4. Provides a reservoir of molten metal which compensates for alloy shrinkage during solidification.

Q. 42. Write a note on dental waxes.

(Sumandeep Uni. May 2018)

Ans. Waxes are used to prepare patterns for alloy castings.

Components: Dental waxes contain natural waxes, synthetic waxes and additives.

Chemical nature: Natural waxes are long chain, complex combinations of organic compounds of reasonably high molecular weight.

- Hydrocarbons, e.g. saturated alkanes.
- Esters, e.g. myricyl palmitate (beeswax).

Various types of waxes are

1. **Mineral waxes:** Paraffin and microcrystalline waxes.
2. **Plant waxes:** Carnauba/Brazil wax/Palm wax, Ouricury wax, Candelilla, Japan wax and cocoa butter.
3. **Insect wax:** Beeswax, shellac wax.
4. **Animal wax:** Spermaceti, lanolin.
5. **Synthetic waxes:** Ozokerite, montan wax, ceresin, barnsdall.

Wax additives: Gums (gum arabic and tragacanth), fats (beef tallow and butter); Oils (hydrocarbon oils, silicone oils), resins, synthetic resins.

Classification

I. According to origin: Mineral, plant, insect, animal.

II. According to use

1. **Pattern waxes**: Inlay casting, RPD casting, and base plate.
2. **Processing waxes**: Boxing, utility, sticky, carding, shellac.
3. **Impression waxes**: Corrective, bite registration.

III. ISO classification (ISO 15854: 2005) for casting inlay and baseplate wax:

1. Type I (casting wax): For cast metal restorations. Class 1: Soft; Class-2: Hard.
2. Type II (baseplate wax) For denture bases and occlusion rims. Class 1: Soft; Class 2: Hard; Class 3: Extra hard.

General properties

1. **Melting range**: Waxes have melting ranges rather than melting points.
2. **Thermal expansion**: Waxes expand when subjected to a rise in temperature and contract as the temperature is decreased.
3. **Mechanical properties**: The elastic modulus, proportional limit and compressive strength of waxes are low compared to other dental materials.
4. **Flow**: Flow increases as the melting point of the wax is approached.
5. **Residual stress**: Regardless of the method used, residual stresses will exist in the completed pattern.
6. **Ductility**: It increases as the temperature of wax is increased.
   - **Inlay wax** (RGUHS, Nov. 2011; TNMGR, Oct. 2019): Inlay wax is a specialized dental wax that can be applied onto the prepared cavity or to the dies to form direct or indirect pattern.

Uses: Pattern for inlays, crown and bridges.

Ideal requirements

1. When softened, it should be uniform, without graininess.
2. The colour should contrast with the die.
3. The wax should not pull or chip.
4. On burnout, it should completely vaporize.
5. The wax pattern should be rigid and dimensionally stable.

Classification: According to ISO 15854:2005, inlay casting waxes are classified as:

1. Class 1: Soft—extra oral or laboratory use
2. Class 2: Hard—intraoral use (direct)

Composition: Paraffin wax (base), ceresin, gum dammar, carnauba (modifiers), candellila, and colouring agents.

Properties

1. Flow: Requirements according to ISO 15854:2005

- At 45°C: Both class 1 and class 2 should have a flow between 70 and 90%.
- At 37°C: Class 2 should not flow >1%.
- At 30°C: Class 1 should not flow >1%.

2. Thermal properties: Thermal conductivity of inlay wax is low. Inlay wax has a high coefficient of thermal expansion (CTE). It has a linear expansion of 0.7% with increase in temperature of 20°C.

3. Wax distortion: Wax distortion is due to release of stresses in the pattern caused due to: 1. Contraction on cooling, 2. Occluded gas bubbles, 3. Change of shape of the wax during molding, 4. From manipulation.

4. Residue on ignition: Waxes vaporize during burnout. ISO 15854:2005 limits the non-vaporizable residue to a maximum of 0.1%.

Q. 43. Write a note on polishing agents used in dentistry. *(BFUHS, May 2009;NTR Uni., Oct. 2011)*

Ans. Abrasion is wearing away of a substance or structure through a mechanical process, such as grinding, rubbing or scraping (**GPT-8**). **Finishing abrasives** are hard, coarse abrasives which are used initially to develop contour and remove gross irregularities, e.g. coarse stones. **Polishing abrasives** have finer particle size and are less hard than abrasives used for finishing. They are used for smoothening surfaces that have been roughened by finishing abrasives, e.g. polishing cakes, pumice, etc. **Cleansing abrasives** are soft materials with small particle sizes and are intended to remove soft deposits that adhere to enamel or a restorative material.

Examples

1. Pure alumina	7. Rouge
2. Polishing cakes	8. Tin oxide
3. Pumice	9. Chalk
4. Garnet	10. Chromic oxide
5. Kieselgurh	11. Zirconium silicate
6. Tripoli	12. Zinc oxide

Q. 44. Write a note on orthodontic wires.
(AIIMS-CDER, Dec. 2017)

Ans. Various types of wires are used in fixed and removable orthodontics for tooth movement and stabilization.

Classification (ISO 15841:2014)

1. Type 1 wires: Wires displaying linear elastic behaviour during unloading at temperatures up to 50°C.
2. Type 2 wires: Wires displaying nonlinear elastic behaviour during unloading at temperatures up to 50°C.

General properties of orthodontic wires

1. Force generated: For a given design, the force generated is proportional to the wire's stiffness.
2. Elastic deflection and working range: Biologically, low constant forces are less damaging. This is best achieved by a large elastic deflection.

Maximum elastic deflection = Proportional limit (PL)/Modulus of elasticity (MOE)

Load deflection rate (LDR) is defined as the external loading needed for the unit deformation and, signifies the force generated by the unit length deformation. Orthodontic arch wires with high LDR not only apply excessive force on teeth, but their strength decreases quickly with tooth movement. Wires with low LDR generate light and continuous force.

3. Springiness: It is a measure of how far a wire can be deflected without causing permanent deformation.
4. Stiffness: Amount of force required to produce a specific deformation. Stiffness = 1/springiness.
5. Resilience: It is the energy storage capacity of the wires which is a combination of strength and springiness.
6. Formability: It represents the amount of permanent bending; the wire will tolerate before it breaks.
7. Ductility of the wire.
8. Ease of joining: Most wires can be soldered or welded together.
9. Corrosion resistance and stability in the oral environment is important for the appliance durability.
10. Most orthodontic wires are biocompatible.
11. Titanium alloy wires are more expensive than the stainless steel or cobalt chromium nickel wires.

Types: Wrought gold alloys, wrought base-metal alloys, stainless steel, cobalt-chromium-nickel, nickel-titanium, β-titanium (TMA).

- Stainless steel (TNMGR, April 2012): It is an iron based alloy which contains <1.2% carbon. When chromium (12–30%) is added to steel, the alloy is called stainless steel. These are resistant to tarnish and corrosion, because of the passivating effect of the chromium.

Types: Based upon the lattice arrangement of iron:
1. Ferritic stainless steel: Body centred cubic structure.
2. Martenistic stainless steel: Body cantered tetragonal structure.
3. Austenitic stainless steel (18-8 stainless steel): Face cantered cubic.
4. Duplex.
5. Precipitation hardening.

Properties

1. Sensitization: It is loss resistance to corrosion of stainless steel if it is heated between 400 and 900°C. It occurs because of precipitation of chromium carbide at the grain boundaries at high temperatures.
2. Stabilization: This is used to minimize the sensitization. In this method, some metal is introduced that precipitates as carbide in preference to chromium, e.g. titanium.
3. Annealed and partially annealed wires: When stainless steel wires are fully annealed, they become soft and highly formable. When it is partially annealed, the yield strength is increased and formability decreased.
4. Mechanical properties: In orthodontic wires, strength and hardness may increase with a decrease in the diameter. Tensile strength: 2100MPa; Yield strength: 1400 MPa; Hardness: 600 KHN.
   - Nickel-titanium alloys (Ni-Ti) (BFUHS, May 2011; TNMGR, Oct. 2017): These nickel-titanium alloy (NITINOL) wires have large elastic deflections or working range and limited formability. They are used extensively as arch wires in fixed orthodontic treatment and to manufacture endodontic instruments.

Composition: Nickel: 54%, titanium: 44%, cobalt: 2%. Other additions made to alter the phase transformation temperature are elements such as iron and chromium which lower the temperature.

Properties

- Shape memory and superelasticity: It refers to the ability of the material to remember its original shape after being plastically deformed while in the martensitic form. At high temperature, a stable body centered cubic lattice (austenitic phase) exists. On appropriate cooling or an application of stress, this transforms to a close-packed hexagonal martensitic lattice with associated volumetric change. The 'memory' effect is achieved by first establishing a shape at temperatures near 482°C. The appliance, e.g. archwire is then cooled and formed into a second shape. Subsequent heating through a lower transition temperature (37°C mouth temperature) causes the wire to return to its original shape. Superelasticity/Pseudoelasticity is stress-induced change in the form from austenitic to martensitic form, which gets reversed on the removal of the stress. Stressing an alloy initially results in standard proportional stress-strain behavior. However, at the stress where it induces the phase transformation, there is an increase in strain, referred to as **superelasticity**. At the completion of the phase, it reverts to standard proportional stress strain behavior. Unloading results in the reverse transition and recovery. This characteristic is useful in some orthodontic situations because it results in low forces and a very large working range or springback.

Types of Ni-Ti alloys
1. Martensitic stabilized alloys.
2. Austenite active alloy.
3. Martensite active alloy.

Advantages
1. Excellent resiliency.
2. Good springback property.
3. Low load deflection rate.
4. Exert very low forces.

Disadvantages
1. Lack of formability.
2. Loops for closing spaces or bends for opening bites cannot be placed.
3. Wires can easily move in the mouth and can cause trauma to mucosa.
4. Brittleness.
5. High cost.

Clinical uses
1. Ideal for use in initial alignment stage.
2. They can be used as an early levelling and alignment wires.
3. They can be used to make NiTi palatal expanders, coil springs and separators.
4. As actuators.
5. As robotics.
   - **Titanium alloys (TMA wires)** *(NTR Uni., Oct. 2012, June 2015):* Pure titanium has different crystallographic forms at high and low temperatures. At temperatures below 885°C the hexagonal close packed (HCP) or alpha lattice is stable, whereas at higher temperatures the metal rearranges into a body-centered cubic (BCC) form called β-titanium. α-titanium is not used in orthodontic applications. The β-form is more useful in orthodontics. However, to retain the β-form as it cools to room temperature elements like molybdenum are added. This stabilizes the β-form and prevents its transformation to the α-form.

Composition: Ti (79%), Mo (11%), Zr (6%), Sn (4%).

Mechanical properties of titanium-molybdenum
1. Modulus of elasticity: 70 GPa.
2. Yield strength: 860–1200 MPa.

3. The high ratio of yield strength to modulus produces orthodontic appliances that can undergo large elastic activations.
4. β-titanium can be highly cold-worked.
5. Clinically satisfactory joints can be made by electrical resistance welding of β-titanium.
6. Both forms have excellent corrosion resistance and environmental stability.
7. Heat treatment can alter its properties, therefore, heat treatment of these wires is not recommended.

Q. 45. Write a short note on elgiloy.
(BBD Uni., June 2016; HP Uni., May 2017)

Ans. Elgiloy is a non-magnetic cobalt-chromium-nickel-molybdenum alloy having a unique combination of very high strength while maintaining excellent formability, excellent corrosion resistance, and high fatigue strength. Cobalt chromium alloy was marketed as Elgiloy by Rocky Mountain Orthodontics.

Composition: Cobalt (40%), molybdenum (7%), chromium (20%), manganese (2%), nickel (15%), iron (15.8%), carbon (0.15%), beryllium (0.04%).

Types of elgiloy
1. **Blue elgiloy:** Softest of the four wire tempers. Used when considerable bending, soldering and welding is required.
2. **Yellow elgiloy:** It is relatively ductile and more resilient than blue.
3. **Green elgiloy:** More resilient than yellow elgiloy, can be shaped with pliers before heat treatment.
4. **Red elgiloy:** Most resilient and provides high spring qualities. Heat treatment makes it extremely resilient.

Properties
1. **Springiback:** With exception of red temper elgiloy, non-heat treated Co-Cr wires have smaller springback.
2. **Stiffness:** High modulus of elasticity.
3. **Formability:** Good formability. Modified by heat treatment.
4. **Joinability:** It can be soldered and welded.
5. **Good biocompatibility and environmental stability.**
6. **Friction:** Resistance to tooth movement along stainless steel and cobalt chromium wires may be comparable.
7. **Heat treatment:** 900°F (482°C) for 7–12 min in a dental furnace. Temp >1200°F (749°C) results in partial annealing—↓ in resistance to deformation.

Clinical applications
- Elgiloy is easier to bend than SS, NiTi and β-Ti in its "as received state".

- It is preferred in techniques in which loops are used.
- Along with SS considered most ideal and economical finishing wire.

Advantages: Greater resistance to fatigue and distortion. Longer function as a resilient spring. Excellent corrosion resistance.

Drawbacks: High elastic force delivery. Lower spring back than stainless steel.

Q. 46. Write a short note on esthetic brackets.
(NTR Uni., April 2014; HP Uni., May 2017)

Ans. Aesthetic orthodontic brackets can be broadly classified into two categories:

1. **Plastic brackets:** Plastic brackets having better esthetics, composed of unfilled polycarbonate, but they lack strength and stiffness resulting in tie-wing fracture and slot distortion. These brackets also have increased slot roughness and get stained due to intraoral fluid adsorption.

2. **Ceramic brackets:** Ceramic brackets are made of aluminium oxide in two different forms that are polycrystalline and monocrytalline depending on method of manufacturing. Monocrystalline brackets are more translucent than polycrystalline brackets. Both types are resistant to staining and discoloration in oral cavity. Ceramic brackets are nine times harder than stainless steel brackets and can cause enamel abrasion if there is contact between bracket and tooth. Polycrystalline zirconia brackets, an alternative to alumina ceramic brackets have greatest toughness. These have good sliding properties, less plaque accumulation, and clinically acceptable bond strength.

Esthetic arch wires: Optiflex wires, organic polymer wire, Teflon coated wires, Epoxy coated wires, Nitanium tooth tone plastic coated wires, Bioforce wires, Invisalign wires.

Q. 47. Write a short note on base metal alloy.
(Sumandeep Uni. June 2016)

Ans. Alloys which contain little or no noble metals are known as **base metal alloys (BMA)**. These include:

1. Nickel-chromium alloys
2. Cobalt-chromium alloys
3. Pure titanium
4. Titanium-aluminum-vanadium alloys

I. Nickel-chromium alloys
Composition
- **Basic elements:** Nickel (61–81%), chromium (11–27%), molybdenum (2–9%).
- **Minor additions:** Beryllium, aluminum, iron, silicon, copper, manganese, cobalt, tin.

Properties
1. They are the cheapest of the casting alloys.
2. They are white in color.
3. **Melting range:** 1155–1304°C.
4. **Density:** 7.8–8.4 g/cm^3.
5. **Castability:** They are extremely technique sensitive.
6. **Hardness and workability:** 175–360 VHN.
7. **Yield strength:** 310–828 MPa.
8. **Modulus of elasticity:** 150–218 GPa.
9. **Percent elongation:** 10–28%.
10. **Porcelain bonding:** These alloys form an adequate oxide layer which is essential for successful porcelain bonding.
11. **Sag resistance:** They have a higher sag resistance.
12. **Tarnish and corrosion resistance:** These alloys are highly resistant to tarnish and corrosion, due to passivation.
13. **Casting shrinkage:** These alloys have a higher casting shrinkage than the gold alloys.
14. **Etching:** Etching of base metal alloys is done in a electrolytic etching bath.
15. **Biological considerations:** Nickel may produce allergic reactions in some individuals. It is also a potential carcinogen.

II. Cobalt-chromium alloys: These alloys are also known as 'Stellite' because of their shiny, star-like appearance.

Applications: Denture base, cast removable partial denture framework, crowns and fixed partial dentures, bar connectors.

Composition: Cobalt (35–65%), chromium (23–30%), nickel (0–20%), molybdenum (0–7%), iron (0–5%), carbon up to 0.4%, tungsten, manganese, silicon and platinum traces.

According to ADA specification No. 14, a minimum of 85% by weight of chromium, cobalt, and nickel is required.

Properties
1. **Density:** The density is half that of gold alloys (8 to 9 g/cm^3).
2. **Fusion temperature:** ADA specification No. 14 divides it into two types, based on fusion temperature (liquidus temperature). Type I (high fusing): Liquidus temperature >1300°C; Type II (low fusing): Liquidus temperature <1300°C.
3. **Yield strength:** It is higher than that of gold alloys (710 MPa).
4. **Elongation:** The elongation value is 1–12%.
5. **Modulus of elasticity:** They are twice as stiff as gold alloys (225 × 10^3 MPa).

6. **Hardness:** These alloys are 50% harder than gold alloys (432 VHN).
7. **Tarnish and corrosion resistance (passivation):** Formation of a layer of chromium oxide on the surface of these alloys prevents tarnish and corrosion in the oral cavity.
8. **Casting shrinkage:** Casting shrinkage is much greater (2.3%) than that of gold alloys.
9. **Porosity:** Porosity is due to shrinkage of the alloy and release of dissolved gases.

Advantages of base metal alloys

1. Lighter in weight.
2. Better mechanical properties (exceptions are present).
3. As corrosion resistant as gold alloys (due to passivating effect).
4. Less expensive than gold alloys.

Disadvantages

1. More technique sensitive.
2. Complexity in production of dental appliance.
3. High fusing temperatures.
4. Extremely hard, so requires special tools for finishing.
5. The high hardness can cause excessive wear of restorations and natural teeth contacting the restorations.

Q. 48. Write a short note on allergy due to nickel alloy.   *(RGUHS, May 2011; NTR Uni., May 2019)*

Ans. Nickel is known allergen, more so in females than males. It results in contact dermatitis and hypersensitivity. OSHA regulations allow 15 μg/m^3 of nickel in air.

Immune response: Type IV cell-mediated delayed hypersensitivity/allergic contact dermatitis.

Diagnosis: A diagnosis can be confirmed by conducting a cutaneous sensitivity test called a patch test using 5% nickel sulphate in petroleum jelly. Oral clinical signs and symptoms of nickel allergy can include: Burning sensation, gingival hyperplasia, labial desquamation, angular chelitis, erythema multiforme, periodontitis, stomatitis with mild to severe erythema, papular perioral rash, loss of taste or metallic taste, numbness, soreness at the side of tongue.

Treatment

1. Nickel titanium arch wire should be removed and replaced with a stainless steel arch wire or preferably a titanium molybdenum alloy (TMA).
2. Resin coated Ni-Ti wires are also an option. These resin-coated wires have had their surface treated with nitrogen ions, which form an amorphous surface layer.
3. If any severe allergic reaction develops, the patient should be referred to a physician to be treated with antihistamines, anesthetics or topical corticosteroids.

Q. 49. Write a short note on biomaterials used for alveolar ridge augmentation.   *(TNMGR, April 2013)*

Ans. A. Bone replacement grafts

1. **Autogenous bone grafts/autografts:** From same individual. Intraoral from mandibular symphysis, maxillary tuberosity, ramus, exostosis. Extra oral from iliac crest, tibial plateau.
2. **Allograft:** From a genetically dissimilar member of the same species, e.g. mineralized or demineralized freeze dried bone allograft.
3. **Xenograft/heterograft:** From donor of another species, e.g. bovine.
4. **Isograft:** It refers to a graft between genetically identical individuals.
5. **Alloplasts:** Natural or synthetic materials, e.g. ceramic materials, synthetic calcium phosphate ceramics, calcium carbonate, HTR polymers, bioactive glass ceramics.

B. Membranes used in guided tissue and bone regeneration

1. **Non-resorbable membranes:** Cellulose filters, expanded polytetrafluoroethylene membrane (e-PTFE), dental rubber dam, titanium membranes.
2. **Resorbable membrane:** Collagen membranes, PLA/PGA, synthetic liquid polymer, polyglactin, calcium sufate.

Q. 50. Write a short note on CAD/CAM.
    (RGUHS, July 2016; MUHS, Dec. 2017)

Ans. Dental copings, crowns and FDP frameworks also can be machined from metal blanks via computer-aided designing and computer-aided machining (CAD/CAM).

Advantages

1. Improved fit.
2. Possibility of one visit restorations like inlays and crowns.
3. Complex castings can be fabricated with greater ease and accuracy.
4. Structures are homogenous with minimum porosity and defects.

Commercially available CAD/CAM systems: Cerec (Sirona), Sirona InLab, Everest (Kavo), Cercon (Dentsply), Lava (3M ESPE), Zeno (Weiland), 5-tec (Zirkonzahn), etc.

Essentials of CAD/CAM system

1. Scanner or digitizer-virtual impression
2. Computer-virtual design (CAD)
3. Milling station: Produces the restoration or framework
4. Ceramic blanks: Raw material for the restoration
5. Furnace:For post-sintering, ceramming etc.

CAD process: CAD process aids in designing either the restoration, coping or the FPD substructure. The computer can automatically detect the finish line. Some use a library of tooth shapes that is stored on the computer to suggest the shape of the proposed restoration. A recording of the bite registration is also added to the data. The combined information together with the 3D optical impression of the prepared tooth establishes the approximate zone in which the new restoration can exist. The proposed restoration can then be morphed to fit into this zone in an anatomically and functionally correct position. The dentist can make corrections or modify the design if required and then send it to the milling unit for completion.

Classification of machinable ceramic blanks

1. Feldspathic porcelain blanks [Vitablocs Mark II].
2. Glass ceramic blanks: Tetrasilicic fluormica based glass ceramic [Dicor MGC], leucite based [ProCad, Everest G], lithia disilicate glass ceramic [IPS e max CAD].
3. Glass infiltrated blanks: Alumina (Vita In-Ceram Alumina); Spinell (Vita In-Ceram Spinell); Zirconia (Vita In-Ceram Zirconia).
4. Presintered blanks: Alumina (Vita In-Ceram AL), ytrria stabilized zirconia (Vita In-Ceram YZ).
5. Sintered blanks: Ytrria stabilized zirconia (Everest ZH blanks).

Copy Milled (CAM) system: In copy milling, a wax pattern of the restoration is scanned and a replica is milled out of the ceramic blank.

Commercial systems available

1. Celay (Mikrona AG).
2. Cercon (Degudent). Cercon has both CAD/CAM and copy-milling systems.
3. Ceramill system.

Fabrication of a copy-milled restoration substructure: A stone die is prepared from the impression of the preparation. A pattern of the restoration is created using wax. The pattern is fixed on the left side of the milling machine (Cercon brain). A pre-sintered zirconia blank is attached to the right side (milling section) of the machine. The machine reads the bar code on the blank which contains the enlargement information. On activation the pattern on the left side is scanned while the milling tool on the right side mills out the enlarged replica (30% larger) of the pattern from the attached ceramic blank. The milled structure is removed from the machine and sectioned off from the frame. The zirconia structure is then placed in a sintering furnace (Cercon heat) and fired for 6 hours at 1350°C to complete the sintering process. The restoration is completed using compatible veneering porcelains.

Q. 51. Write a short note on 3D stereolithographic model. *(UHSR, May 2016)*

Ans. Stereolithography is a rapid prototyping systems (RPS) designed to create solid and detailed, three-dimensional (3D) physical models that can accurately replicate complex anatomical structures directly from computer data. Combining the scanned information of reconstructed computed tomography (CT) images with an ultraviolet (UV) laser beam sequentially passed over a photosensitive resin, it is possible to produce, from a two-dimensional (2D) image, a dimensionally accurate 3D anatomical model, as a complete replica of the external surface and internal structures (including soft tissues) in a layer-by-layer fashion. **Color stereolithography,** allows for the selective coloring of determined anatomical structures in solid 3D models.

Technique: The stereolithographic apparatus consists of a container or bath with a liquid photosensitive resin, a model-building platform, and a curing ultraviolet laser. The laser beam moves in sequential cross-sectional increments of 1 mm or less. The model is initially designed through CAD (computer assisted design) software; the CAD data file is converted into slices of known dimensions and transferred to the stereolithographic apparatus for building. The laser beam is computer controlled and directed to the resin and, on contact, polymerizes the surface layer; when this layer is completed, a mechanical platform moves down 1 mm (or less) into the resin bath, carrying and exposing a new layer of resin, and this second layer is then cured and bonded on the previous one, in a sequential fashion. This process is repeated, layer-by-layer, as necessary, until completing the stereolithographic model of the anatomical structures-of-interest. About 80% of the total polymerization takes place in the device's container and the remaining 20% is completed by means of a conventional UV curing unit.

Advantages: Great surface finish and accuracy.

Applications

- Stereolithography has become a well-known technique in the processes of diagnosis, preoperative planning, and surgery simulation, primarily in cases of reconstructive and orthognathic surgery.

- By coloring tumors with stereolithography, it is possible to visually establish their extension and clarify their relationship to alveolar nerve in mandible and hard surrounding structures; thus, the surgical team may estimate the extent of the tumor resection in complex areas.

- In orthognathic surgical field, 3D physical models are accurate and predicative anatomical replicas for documentation, analysis, treatment planning, and long-term follow up; furthermore, these models are useful for developing and teaching surgical and orthodontics protocols; additionally, the following different purposes may be achieved primarily: Guiding the treatment to the desired result, giving the patient a reasonable preview of the outcome, serving as a communication tool among the orthodontist, surgeon, pediatric dentist, and other specialists, and the patient.

- **Implant planning:** Computer-aided designing and fabrication techniques provide a preoperative view of anatomical structures and restorative information for achieving the ideal implant position. Subsequently, this clinical evidence can be accurately transferred to the patient and guide the pre-prosthetic surgical procedure.

Q. 52. Write a short note on impression materials.
(RGUHS; Nov. 2017)

Ans. Dental impression is the negative replica of hard and soft tissues of the mouth.

Purpose of impression: To study alignment of teeth. Construction of special (custom) tray. Treatment planning. Fabrication of indirect restorations.

Desirable properties of an impression *(BBD Uni., April 2015):*

1. A pleasant odour, taste, and acceptable color.
2. Absence of toxic or irritant constituents.
3. Adequate shelf life for requirements of storage and distribution.
4. Not expensive and easy to use with the minimum of equipment.
5. Setting characteristics that meet clinical requirements.
6. Readily wets oral tissues.
7. Elastic properties that allow easy removal of the set material from the mouth and good elastic recovery.
8. Adequate strength to avoid breaking or tearing upon removal from the mouth.

9. Dimensional stability over temperature and humidity ranges normally found in clinical and laboratory procedures for a period long enough.
10. Compatibility with cast and die materials.
11. Readily disinfected without loss of accuracy.

Classification of impression materials
I. According to mode of setting and elasticity
1. Thermoset (chemical/irreversible): Impression plaster, ZnOE, alginate, elastomeric impression material.
2. Thermoplastic (temperature/reversible): Compound, waxes, agar.
3. Rigid: Impression plaster, ZnOE impression paste, compound, waxes.
4. Elastic: Alginate, elastomeric impression material, agar.

II. According to tissue displacement
1. Mucostatic, e.g. plaster, ZnOE, low viscosity alginates, low viscosity elastomeric materials, etc.
2. Mucocompressive: Compound, high viscosity alginates, high viscosity elastomers, etc.

III. According to use
1. **Impression materials used for complete denture prosthesis:** Impression plaster, impression compound and impression paste.
2. **Impression materials used for dentulous mouths:** Alginates and rubber base impressions.

   ♦ **Impression compound fusion and glass transition temperature** *(AIIMS-CDER, April 2016):*

   - **Fusion temperature:** When impression compound is heated in a hot water bath, the material starts to soften at 39°C. However, at this stage, it is still not plastic or soft enough for making an impression. This temperature at which the material looses its hardness on heating or forms a rigid mass upon cooling is referred to as **fusion temperature.** Impression compound exhibits a fusion temperature range rather than a fixed point. On continued heating above 43.5°C, the material continues to soften and flow to a plastic mass that can be manipulated.

   - **Glass transition temperature** (Tg) is the temperature at which an amorphous solid becomes soft upon heating or brittle upon cooling. The glass transition temperature is always lower than the melting temperature (Tm) of the crystalline state of the material, if one exists. The glass transition temperature is more important in plastic applications than is the melting point, because it tells a lot about how the polymer behaves under ambient conditions. If a polymer's glass transition temperature is well above ambient room temperature, the material behaves like a brittle glassy polymer; if the Tg is well below room temperature, the material is what is commonly termed a rubber or elastomers. Those materials whose Tg is reasonably close to the ambient temperature exhibit plastic material behavior. Plasticizers are used to decrease the glass transition temperature.

♦ **ZnOE impression paste** (*AIIMS-CDER, April 2016*):

Uses

1. Cementing and insulating medium.
2. Temporary filling material.
3. Root canal filling material.
4. Surgical pack in periodontal surgical procedures.
5. Bite registration paste.
6. Temporary relining material for dentures.
7. Impressions for edentulous patients.

Zinc oxide eugenol is popular as an impression material for making impressions of edentulous arches for the construction of complete dentures.

Classification: ADA specification No. 16.: Type I (hard) and Type II (soft).

Composition

- **Base paste**: Zinc oxide (87%), vegetable or mineral oil (13%).
- **Accelerator paste**: Oil of cloves/eugenol (12%), gum/polymerized rosin (50%), filler (silica type) 20%, lanolin (3%), resinous balsam (0%), calcium chloride and color (5%).

Setting reaction: The setting reaction is a typical acid-base reaction to form a chelate (zinc eugenolate).

Initial setting time (final setting time): Type I: 3–6 minutes (10 minutes); Type II: 3–6 minutes (15 minutes).

Properties

1. **Consistency and flow:** A paste of thick consistency can compress the tissues. Clinically, these materials have a very good flow.
2. **Detail reproduction:** It registers surface details quite accurately.
3. **Rigidity and strength:** The compressive strength of hardened ZOE is approximately 7 MPa two hours after mixing.
4. **Dimensional stability:** Dimensional stability is quite satisfactory with negligible shrinkage (<0.1%).
5. **Biological considerations:** Some patients experience a burning sensation in the mouth due to eugenol.

Advantages

1. It has enough working time to complete border molding.
2. It can be checked in the mouth repeatedly without deforming.
3. It registers accurate surface details.
4. It is dimensionally stable.
5. Does not require separating media since it does not stick to the cast material.

Disadvantages

1. It requires a special tray for impression making.
2. It is sticky in nature and adheres to tissues.
3. Eugenol can cause burning sensation and tissue irritation.
4. It cannot be used for making impression of teeth and undercut areas.

Q. 53. Write a short note on elastomers. *(TNMGR, Aug. 2008; NTR Uni., Nov. 2017; HP Uni., May 2018)*

Ans. These are basically synthetic rubber base materials which are also known as non-aqueous elastomeric impression materials.

Types

a. According to chemistry:
   1. Polysulfide.
   2. Condensation polymerizing silicones.
   3. Addition polymerizing silicones.
   4. Polyether.
b. According to viscosity:
   1. Light body/syringe consistency.
   2. Medium/regular body.
   3. Heavy body/tray consistency.
   4. Very heavy body/putty consistency.

Uses

1. In fixed partial dentures for impressions of prepared teeth.
2. Impressions of dentulous mouths for removable partial dentures.
3. Impressions of edentulous mouths for complete dentures.
4. Polyether is used for border molding of edentulous custom trays.
5. For bite registration.
6. Silicone duplicating material is used for making refractory casts during cast partial denture construction.

I. Polysulfide *(TNMGR, Oct. 2017):* This was the first elastomeric impression material to be introduced (1950). It is also known as **mercaptan or thiokol.**

Composition

- Base paste: Liquid polysulfide polymer = 80–85%; Inert fillers (titanium dioxide, zinc sulfate, copper carbonate or silica) = 16–18%.
- Reactor paste: Lead dioxide (60–68%); Dibutyl phthalate (30–35%); Sulfur (3%); other substances like magnesium, stearate (retarder) and deodorants (2%)
- **Properties**
  1. Unpleasant odor and color. It stains linen and is messy to work with.
  2. These materials are extremely viscous and sticky. Mixing is difficult.
  3. It has a long setting time of 12.5 minutes (at 37°C).
  4. Excellent reproduction of surface detail.
  5. The curing shrinkage is high (0.45%). It has the highest permanent deformation (3–5%).
  6. It has high tear strength (4000 g/cm^2)
  7. It has good flexibility (7%) and low hardness.
  8. It is hydrophobic.
  9. It can be electroplated.
  10. The shelf life is good (2 years).

II. Condensation polymerizing silicones/conventional silicones

Composition

- Base: Polydimethyl siloxane (hydroxyl-terminated) (80–85%); Colloidal silica or microsized metal oxide filler (35–75%); Color pigments (16–18%).
- Reactor paste/accelerator: Orthoethyl silicate (crosslinking agent); Stannous octoate (catalyst).

Properties

1. Pleasant colour and odour.
2. Setting time is 6–9 minutes. Mixing time is 45 seconds.
3. Excellent reproduction of surface details.
4. High curing shrinkage (0.4–0.6%), and permanent deformation is also high (1–3%).
5. Tear strength (3000 g/cm^2) is lower than the polysulfides.
6. It is stiffer and harder than polysulfide.
7. It is hydrophobic.

III. Addition polymerizing silicones (polyvinyl siloxanes) (HP Uni., April 2019): Currently, the addition silicones are most widely used elastomeric impression material worldwide.

Composition

- **Base paste:** Poly (methyl hydrogen siloxane), other siloxane prepolymers, fillers (amorphous silica or fluorocarbons), palladium-hydrogen absorber fillers, retarders, coloring agents.

- **Reactor paste:** Divinyl polysiloxane, other siloxane prepolymers, fillers, platinum salt-catalyst (chloroplatinic acid).

Properties

1. Pleasant odor and color.
2. May also cause allergic reaction.
3. Excellent reproduction of surface details.
4. Setting time ranges from 5 to 9 minutes. Mixing time is 45 seconds.
5. It has a low curing shrinkage (0.17%) and the lowest permanent deformation (0.05–0.3%).
6. It has good tear strength (3000 g/cm).
7. It is extremely hydrophobic.
8. It can be electroplated with silver or copper.
9. It has low flexibility and is harder than polysulfides.
10. Shelf-life is 1–2 years.

IV. Polyether (HP Uni., April 2019):

Composition

Base: Polyether polymer (80–85%), colloidal silica filler, glycolether or phthalate plasticizer.

Reactor/accelerator paste: Aromatic sulfonate ester (crosslinking agent), colloidal silica (filler), phthalate/glycolether (plasticizer).

Properties

1. Pleasant odor and taste.
2. Sulfonic ester can cause skin reactions.
3. Setting time is around 6–8 minutes. Mixing should be done quickly that is 30 seconds.
4. Curing shrinkage is low (0.24%). The permanent deformation is also low (0.8–1.5%).
5. It is extremely stiff (flexibility 3%). It is harder than polysulfides.
6. Tear strength is good (3000 g/cm).
7. It is hydrophilic.
8. It can be electroplated with silver or copper.
9. The shelf life is excellent >2 years.
10. It has excellent detail reproduction (20 μm).

Q. 54. Write a note on recent advances in maxillofacial impression materials.

(Sumandeep Uni. April 2015)

Ans. Maxillofacial prosthetics are the branch of prosthodontics concerned with the restoration and/or replacement of the stomatognathic and craniofacial structures with the prosthesis that may or may not be removed on a regular or elective basis.

Classification of maxillofacial materials

1. Surgical reconstruction (alloplastic implantable material).
2. Prosthetic reconstruction.

Ideal Requisites for Maxillofacial Materials

1. Materials used should be biocompatible.
2. Should be flexible at temperatures from 4.4° to 60°C.
3. Color should blend with the adjacent skin as close as possible.
4. Chemical and environmental stability.
5. Poor thermal conductivity.
6. Ease of processing and ease of duplication.
7. Light weight and easily retained in position and be comfortable to the patient.

Materials: Acrylic resins (polymethyl methacrylate), plasticized methylmethacrylate, vinyl polymers and copolymers (realistic—polyvinyl chloride; Mediplas—polyvinyl acetate chloride), chlorinated polyethylene, polyurethane, silicones (room temperature vulcanizing—silastic 382, 386, 399; High temperature vulcanized silicones—PDM siloxane, MDX 4-4210; Silastic 891).

Recent advancements: Silicone block copolymers, polyphosphazenes fluoroelastomer, newer version SM4, A-2186 (factor II).

Genetics

Q. 1 Write a short note on genes.

(NTR Uni., April 2009)

Ans. Genes represent the smallest physical and functional units of inheritance that resides in specific sites called loci or locus for a single location. The term gene was coined by Wilhelm Johannsen in 1909. A gene can be defined as the entire DNA sequence necessary for the synthesis of a functional polypeptide molecule or RNA molecule (tRNA and rRNA).

Functions of genes: Genes accomplish their function:

1. Through replication that result in more units like themselves.
2. Through transcription and translation, whereby proteins that function as determiners in metabolism of cell are synthesize.

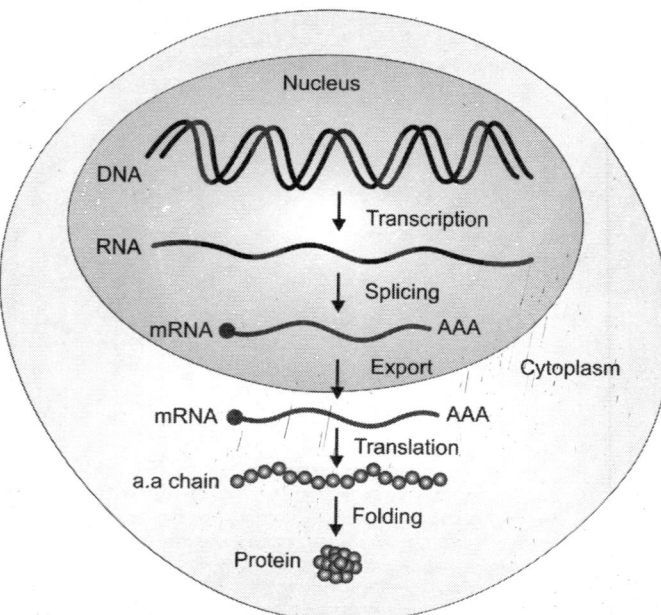

Fig. 1.1: Mechanism of gene expression/regulation

3. By determining the structure of proteins, which are responsible for directing cell metabolism through their activity as enzymes.

Regulation of gene expression *(UOK, June 2019):* Expression of genes can be controlled with the help of regulatory proteins at numerous levels. These regulatory proteins bind to DNA and send signals that indirectly control the rate of gene expression.

Mechanism: Sequence of events:

1. **Chromatin structure:** Eukaryotic DNA is compacted into chromatin structures which can be altered by histone modifications. Such modifications can result in the up- or down-regulation of a gene.
2. **Initiation of transcription:** Several factors such as promoters and enhancers alter the ability of RNA polymerase to transcribe the mRNA, thus modulating the expression of the gene.
3. **Post-transcriptional processing:** Modifications such as polyadenylation, splicing, and capping of the pre-mRNA transcript can lead to different levels and patterns of gene expression.
4. **RNA transport:** After post-transcriptional processing, the mature mRNA must be transported from the nucleus to the cytosol so that it can be translated into a protein.
5. **Stability of mRNAs:** Eukaryotic mRNAs differ in their stability and some unstable transcripts usually have sequences that bind to mRNAs, reducing their stability, resulting in downregulation of the corresponding proteins.
6. **Initiation of translation:** At this stage, the ability of ribosome in recognizing the start codon can be modulated, thus affecting the expression of the gene.
7. **Post-translational processing:** Common modifications in polypeptide chains include glycosylation, fatty acylation, and acetylation, these can help in

regulating expression of the gene and offering vast functional diversity.

8. **Protein transport and stability:** Following translation and processing, proteins must be carried to their site of action in order to be biologically active.

♦ **Gene mutations** (*TNMGR, March 2010*): A mutation is a sudden, permanent inheritable change in the genetic material. The mutation may be due to the insertion or deletion of a nucleotide, the substitution of one nucleotide with another or inversion of two nucleotides. A 'nonsense' mutation changes an amino acid specifying codon into a chain terminating codon. 'Frame shift' is a mutation arising from the insertion or deletion of one or more nucleotides that causes gene to be misread during translation into the polypeptide.

Causes of mutation

1. Spontaneous mutations: Result from errors in replication of DNA, due to enzyme defect.
2. Induces mutations: Changes in the DNA caused by the effects of mutagens, e.g.:
   i. Ionizing radiation: X-rays, cosmic rays, etc.
   ii. Non-ionizing radiations: UV rays.
   iii. Chemicals: Mustard gas.

Q. 2. Write a short note on structure of chromosomes.
(NTR Uni., June 2014)

Ans. Chromosome is made up of DNA tightly coiled many times around proteins called histones that support its structure. Chromosomes were first described by Strasburger (1815), and the term 'chromosome' was first used by Waldeyer in 1888. They appear as rod-shaped dark stained bodies during the metaphase stage of mitosis when cells are viewed under a light microscope.

Structure: Each chromosome typically has one centromere and one or two arms that project from the centromere. Structurally, each chromosome is differentiated into three parts:

• **Pellicle:** It is the outer envelope around the substance of chromosome. It is very thin and is formed of achromatic substances.
• **Matrix:** It is the ground substance of chromosome which contains the chromonemata. It is also formed of non-genic materials.
• **Chromonemata:** Embedded in the matrix of each chromosome are two identical, spirally coiled threads, the chromonemata. Each chromonemata consists of about 8 microfibrils, each of which is formed of a double helix of DNA.
• **Centromere:** A small structure in the chromonema, marked by a constriction which is recognised as

permanent structure in the chromosome is termed as the **centromere**, also known as **kinetochore** or **primary constriction**. It divides the chromosome into two sections, or "arms"; short arm ("**p arm**") and long arm ("**q arm**").

• **Secondary constriction or nucleolar organizer:** The chromosome also possesses secondary constriction at any point of the chromosome. The chromosome region distal to the secondary constriction, i.e. the region between the secondary constriction and the nearest telomere is known as satellite. Therefore, chromosomes having secondary constrictions are called **satellite chromosomes** or **sat-chromosomes**. Nucleolus is always associated with the secondary constriction of sat-chromosomes. Therefore, secondary constrictions are also called **nucleolus organizer region** (NOR) and sat-chromosomes are often referred to as **nucleolus organizer chromosomes**.

• **Telomeres:** These are specialized ends of a chromosome which exhibits physiological differentiation and polarity.

Types of chromosomes

A. Autosomes and sex chromosomes: Humans have 23 pairs of chromosomes in their cells, of which 22 pairs are autosomes and one pair of sex chromosomes, making a total of 46 chromosomes in each cell.

B. On the basis of number of centromeres
• **Monocentric** with one centromere.
• **Dicentric** with two centromeres.
• **Polycentric** with more than two centromeres.
• **Acentric** without centromere.
• **Diffused or non-located** with indistinct centromere diffused throughout the length of chromosome.

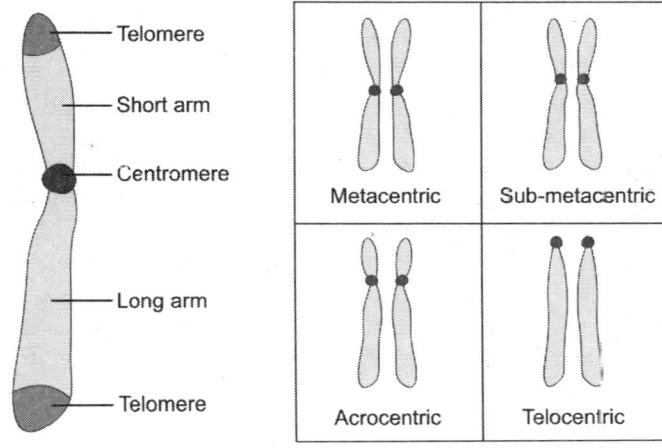

Fig. 1.2: Structure of a chromosome

C. On the basis of location of centromere

- **Telocentric** chromosomes are rod-shaped chromosomes with centromere occupying the terminal position, so that the chromosome has just one arm.
- **Acrocentric** chromosomes are rod-shaped chromosomes with centromere occupying a sub-terminal position. One arm is very long and the other is very short.
- **Sub-metacentric** chromosomes are with centromere slightly away from the mid-point so that the two arms are unequal.
- **Metacentric** chromosomes are V-shaped chromosomes in which centromere lies in the middle of chromosome so that the two arms are almost equal.

Functions and significance

- As the number of the chromosomes is constant for a particular species, they are useful in determination of phylogeny and taxonomy of the species.
- **Genetic code storage**: Chromosome contains the genetic material that is required by the organism to develop and grow.
- **Sex determination**: If X chromosome is passed out of XY chromosome, the child will be a female and if a Y chromosome is passed, a male child develops.
- **Control of cell division**: The chromosomes of the parent cells insure that the correct information is passed on to the daughter cells required by the cell to grow and develop correctly.
- **Formation of proteins and storage**: The chromosomes direct the sequences of proteins formed in the body and also maintain the order of DNA. The proteins are also stored in the coiled structure of the chromosomes.

Q. 3. Write a note on chromosomal aberrations.

(NTR Uni., Oct. 2012; UHSR, April 2015)

Ans. Chromosomal aberrations are classified based upon following criterions:

A. Structural abnormalities

1. Deletion: Breaking away or loss of a portion of chromosome, e.g. Turner's syndrome.
2. Translocation: Two chromosomes break and exchange their broken segments in reciprocal translocation, e.g. Philadelphia chromosome.
3. Inversion: The broken fragment reattaches itself in reverse orientation to the same chromosome, e.g. increase in miscarriages.
4. Duplication: An over representation of specific chromosomal region.
5. Transverse centromeric division: Instead of dividing longitudinally, centromere divides in transverse plane forming an isochromosome, thereby resulting in duplication of one arm and deletion of another arm of the involved chromosome.
6. Ring chromosome.

B. Numerical abnormalities

1. Involving chromosomes sets: Monoploidy, euploidy, polyploidy.
2. Involving individual chromosomes: Autosomal derivatives: Monosomy; Trisomy (Down's syndrome/Trisomy 21, Edward syndrome/Trisomy 18, Patau syndrome/Trisomy 13); Sex-linked derivatives: Turner's syndrome, superfemale, Klinefelter's syndrome.
3. Type of chromosomal abnormality: Gross chromosomal aberrations; Single gene disorders; Polygenic disorders.

The genetic factors cause variations in following features of dental relation. They include:

- Variations in size, shape of jaws
- Variations in size, number, shape, form of teeth.
- Malocclusion.
- Periodontal conditions.
- Incidence of facial clefts.
- Growth and development.

Q. 4. Discuss pedigree and its importance.

(NTR Uni., June 2015)

Ans. A pedigree is a pictorial representation of a family history, essentially a family tree that outlines the inheritance of one or more characteristics. The person from whom the pedigree is initiated is called the **proband** and is usually designated by an arrow. Pedigree analysis is useful when studying any population when progeny data from several generations is limited. Pedigree analysis is also useful when studying species with a long generation time. A series of symbols are used to represent different aspects of a pedigree (Fig. 1.4a).

Once phenotypic data is collected from several generations and the pedigree is drawn, careful analysis will allow determining whether the trait is dominant or recessive.

A. For traits exhibiting dominant gene action

(Fig. 1.4b):

- Affected individuals have at least one affected parent.
- The phenotype generally appears every generation.
- Two unaffected parents only have unaffected offspring.

B. For traits exhibiting recessive gene action (Fig. 1.4c):

- Unaffected parents can have affected offspring.
- Affected progeny are both male and female.

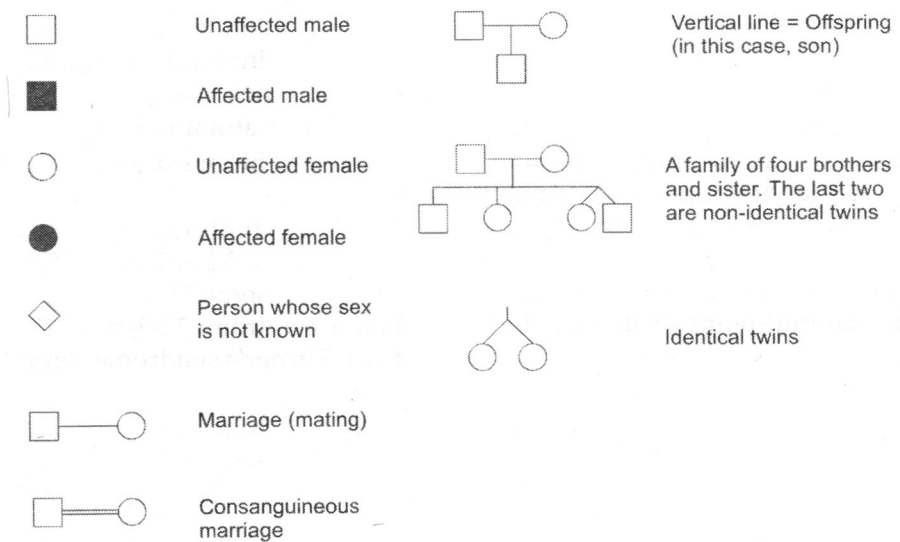

Fig. 1.4a: Symbols used for pedigree analysis

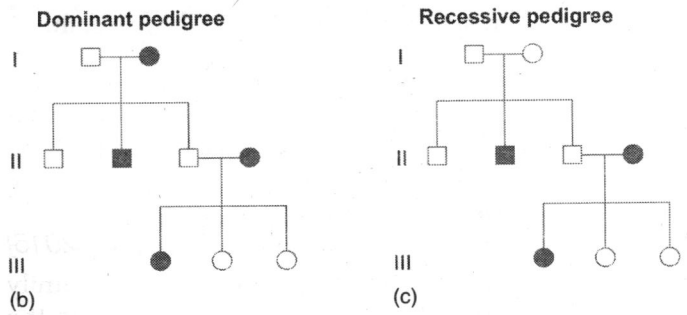

Fig. 1.4: (b) Pedigree of a trait controlled by dominant gene; (c) Pedigree of a trait controlled by recessive gene

Q. 5. Write about principle of orofacial genetics.

(NTR Uni., April 2013; NTR Uni., May 2018)

Ans. Genetics is concerned with the inheritance of traits (normal or abnormal), and interaction of genes and the environment. **Genotype** is genetic constitution of an individual. **Phenotype** is observable characteristic of the individual. The proportion of phenotypic variance attributable to the genotype is known as **heritability**.

1. In specific traits, individual genotypes are readily identified and differences are qualitative, e.g. ABO blood.
2. In continuous traits, difference is characterized quantitatively between individuals, e.g. height, weight, tooth size.
3. The quantitative traits are modified by environmental factors.
4. The genetic variation may be dependent on segregation of multiple genes, polygenes.
5. The genetic difference caused by polygene is known as polygenic variation.

6. Different types of genetic product are being considered as different distances from the fundamental level of gene activity, e.g. enzymes and its genetic variants.
7. Morphological characters are the end result of vast complexity of interacting, hierarchical, biochemical and developmental process.
8. Each gene influences many morphological characters (pleiotropic), so that a deleterious mutation results in a syndrome.
9. Each morphological character may be dependent on many different genes.

Modes/pattern of inheritance: *(KUHS, June 2013; RUHS, May 2015; HP Uni., April 2019)*

The different ways in which genes are handed down from parents to offspring's and expresses them.

1. **Autosomal dominant** *(RUHS, May 2018)*: When one member of the allelic pair is able to express itself irrespective of the presence of other member, e.g. dentinogenesis imperfecta, amelogenesis imperfecta, achodroplasia.
2. **Autosomal recessive** *(RUHS, May 2018)*: Inheritance depends on the expression of both the members of the allelic pair, e.g. cystic fibrosis, hypophosphatasia.
3. **Sex-linked:** These traits carried by genes present on sex chromosomes X and Y, e.g. ectodermal dysplasia, hemophilia.
4. **Co-dominant:** When both members of the chromosomes pair are able to express themselves fully in the phenotype, e.g. ABO blood group.
5. **Intermediate:** When a trait is expressed as a result of partial expression of both chromosomes of a pair, e.g. sickle cell trait.

6. **Monogenic:** These traits are produced and regulated by a single gene locus, e.g. albinism, neurofibromatosis.

7. **Polygenic inheritance** *(NTR Uni., May 2018):* Multiple genes control the trait. e.g. height of an individual.

8. **Multifactorial inheritance** *(Gujarat Uni., July 2017):* These traits are determined by the interaction of multiple genes and environmental factors, e.g. cleft lip and palate (CLP).

Q. 6. Write a short note on twin studies.

(RGUHS, May 2013; UOK, July 2017; Gujarat Uni., April 2019)

Ans. Twin studies have been a valuable source of information about the genetic basis of complex traits. To maximize the potential of twin studies, large, worldwide registers of data on twins and their relatives have been established. Twin studies can be used to obtain insights into the genetic epidemiology of complex traits and diseases, to study the interaction of genotype with sex, age and lifestyle factors, and to study the causes of co-morbidity between traits and diseases. By facilitating comparisons between monozygotic (MZ) and dizygotic (DZ) twins, twin registers represent some of the best resources for evaluating the importance of genetic variation in susceptibility to disease.

Classification

1. **Classical MZ-DZ comparison:** These studies estimate the contributions of genetic and environmental effects to phenotypic variance, and test, e.g. age, cohort and sex differences in gene expression.

2. **Multivariate analyses (simultaneous analysis of correlated traits):** This involves direction of phenotypic causality, causes of co-morbidity of two or more traits, multivariate modeling of environmental and genetic correlations between traits.

3. **Co-twin control study:** Case control studies of MZ twins who are perfectly matched for genes and family background; also used to study gene expression in discordant twins.

4. **Extended twin study (studies of twins and their families):** In this study, parents can be included to study cultural transmission, to determine genetic and environmental stability; Social interactions and special twin effects. Also maternal effects and imprinting can be studied if offspring of MZ twins are included.

5. **Genotyping at candidate loci:** These include genotyping of MZ twins to detect variability genes and penetrance; genotyping of DZ twins to estimate associations within and between families.

6. **Genotyping at marker loci:** These include genotyping of DZ twins to detect linkage with quantitative trait loci; selecting informative families from large twin registers.

Methods used in twin studies: Twin studies intend to measure the heritability of a trait, which can be determined by concordance rates. Concordance rate (CR) for a disease or trait among identical and fraternal twin pairs is actually a statistical measure of probability. Historically, CRs are computed separately for monozygotic (MZ) and dizygotic (DZ) pairs. When MZ concordances are greater than DZ concordances, genetic influences are indicated.

Advantages

- Twin studies allow disentanglement of the shared genetic and environmental factors for the trait of interest.
- Researchers can estimate the proportion of variance in a trait attributable to genetic variation versus the proportion that is due to shared environment or unshared environment.
- The use of twins can improve the statistical power of a genetic study by reducing the amount of genetic and/or environmental variability.

Limitations

- Results from twin studies cannot be directly generalized to the general population, due to lack of randomization.
- Some researchers suggest that genetic factors may lead to a higher incidence of twin births in some women.
- Findings from twin studies are often misunderstood, misinterpreted, and blown out of proportion.
- Many twin registries depend on the voluntary participation of twins, leading to volunteer bias or recruitment bias.
- Use of twins does not allow the researcher to consider the effects of both shared—environment and gene/environment interaction simultaneously.

Q. 7. Write a short note on single gene disorders.

(KUHS, Jan., 2014)

Ans. Single gene inheritance is also known as Mendelian inheritance. Single gene diseases are usually inherited in one of several patterns depending on the location of the gene and whether one or two normal copies of the gene are needed for the disease phenotype to manifest. There are five basic modes of inheritance for single-gene diseases: Autosomal dominant, auto-somal recessive, X-linked dominant, X-linked recessive, and mitochondrial.

Classification/Mendelian pattern of inheritance *(NTR Uni., Nov. 2017):*

A. Autosomal disorders

1. **Autosomal dominant disorders**: Arise due to defect in at least one gene out of pair of genes on autosomes.

   Features:

   a. Disease appears in each generation.

   b. Delayed age of onset.

   c. Vertically transmitted.

   d. Affected individual has an affected parent.

   e. Male and female are equally affected.

   f. Capability of transmission is same in both the parents.

   g. Each child is at 50% risk of inheriting the abnormal gene.

   Examples: Osteogenesis imperfecta, mesiodens, dentinogenesis imperfecta, dentin dysplasia, Apert's syndrome.

2. **Autosomal recessive disorders**: They occur when both the genes on autosome are affected. Since two abnormal genes are required for obtaining a given clinical phenotype, their incidence is low as com-pared to autosomal dominant disorders.

   Features

   a. Sudden onset of illness.

   b. Male and female are equally affected.

   c. Early age of onset.

   d. Consanguinity increases the incidence.

   e. Most of the offspring are normal.

   f. Affected individual may or may not have affected parent.

   Examples: Dentin dysplasia (coronal type), amelo-genesis imperfecta (hypocalcified II), hypophos-phatasia, Hurler's syndrome.

B. X-linked disorders

1. **X-linked dominant disorders**: They arise from an affected heterozygote female.

   Features

   a. Both sexes are affected, female > male.

   b. Absence of father to son transmission.

   c. All the female of affected father are affected.

   d. Affected females have deficiency of live born sons.

   Examples: Vitamin D resistant rickets, orofacial digital syndrome.

2. **X-linked recessive disorders**: They arise in female recessive homozygotes or less commonly male hemizygotes.

Features

   a. Males are mostly affected.

   b. Complete absence of male to male transmission.

   c. Female carrier has a 25% chance of having affected son.

   d. Each child of affected parents is at 50% risk of transmission.

   Examples: Hemophilia, Fabry disease.

C. Mitochondrial: This can affect both males and females, but only passed on by females, can appear in every generation, e.g. Leber's hereditary optic neuro-pathy, Kearns-Sayre syndrome.

Q. 8. Write a short note genetic polymorphism.
(TNMGR, Sept. 2009)

Ans. Genetic diseases have been broadly classified into two groups:

1. **Simple Mendelian diseases (monogenic disorders).**

2. **Complex genetic diseases (polygenic disorders):** They are a result of the interaction of multiple diffe-rent gene loci, environmental, and behavioral factors. Many of the diagnostic features of these complex diseases also called quantitative trait disorders are regulated by several genes. Complex diseases are associated with variations in multiple genes, each having a small overall contribution and relative risk for the disease process. When a specific allele occurs, in at least 1% of the population, it is said to be genetic polymorphism. In contrast to mutations that have been casually linked with Mendelian diseases, genetic polymorphisms are often not directly casually linked, but rather specific alleles are reported to be found more frequently in diseased individuals than in non-affected controls. Examples: Cytokine gene polymorphisms, receptor gene poly-morphisms, antigen-antibody gene polymorphisms, polymorphisms in genes encoding enzymes.

Q. 9. Write about craniofacial anomalies.
(AIIMS-CDER, May 2014)

Ans. Craniofacial anomalies are a diverse group of deformities in the growth of head and facial bones. These are congenital and may vary in severity.

1. Cleft lip and/or palate: Most common congenital craniofacial anomalies seen at birth.

2. Cleft lip.

3. Cleft palate.

4. Craniosynostosis: Crouzan syndrome, Apert syn-drome.

5. Hemifacial microsomia (Goldenhar syndrome, brachial arch syndrome, facio-auriculo-vertebral syndrome, oculo-auriculo-vertebral spectrum, or lateral facial dysplasia).

6. Vascular malformation: Hemangioma, lymphangioma.
7. Deformational or positional plagiocephaly: Holoprosencephaly, Stickler syndrome.

Q. 10. Write a short note on homebox gene.
[Sumandeep Uni., June 2017;UHSR, Gujarat Uni., June 2018; MUHS Dec. 2018; AIIMS-CDER, Dec. 2018]

Ans. A homeobox (HOX) is a DNA sequence of about 180 base pairs long, found within genes that are involved in the regulation of development (morphogenesis) of animals, fungi, and plants. Genes that have a homeobox are called **homeobox genes** and form a homeobox gene family. HOX genes are a particular cluster of homeobox genes which function in patterning the body axis thereby providing the identity of particular body region and they determine where body segments grow in a developing fetus. Mutations in any one of these genes can lead to the growth of extra, typically non-functional body parts. Humans generally contain homeobox genes in four clusters, called HOXA (or HOXI), HOXB, HOXC, or HOXD, on chromosomes 2, 7, 12, and 17, respectively. HOX gene network appears to be active in human tooth germs between 18–24 weeks of development. Examples:

1. **PAX-9 gene**: PAX-9 is widely expressed in the neural crest derived mesenchyme involved in craniofacial and tooth development. PAX-9 gene is mapped onto 14q12-q13 and mutations in this gene can lead to non-syndromic tooth agenesis.
2. **MSX-1 gene**: At present, two human MSX genes—MSX-1 and MSX-2, have been isolated. MSX-1 gene is mapped onto 4p16.1. They are expressed in undifferentiated multipotential cells that are proliferating or dying and they provide positional information, and regulate epithelial–mesenchymal signaling in craniofacial development.
3. **DLX gene**: DLX (distal less) family of homeobox genes consists of six members (DLX 1–6) and is expressed in the epithelium and mesenchyme of branchial arches, tooth bud mesenchyme, dental lamina, cranial neural crest, dorsal neural tube, and frontonasal process. Mutation in these genes results in abnormalities affecting first four branchial arch derivatives including mandible and calvaria.
4. **LHX gene**: Lim homeodomain transcription factors (LHX-1 and LMX 1b) are expressed in neural crest derived ectomesenchyme of first branchial arch. Improper expression of this gene leads to tooth agenesis and cleft palate.
5. **BARX gene:** Improper expression of this gene results in failure of nervous system to develop and cleft palate formation. BARX-1 is expressed in the mesenchyme of the mandibular and maxillary process and in the tooth primordial, while BARX-2 is expressed in the oral epithelium prior to the tooth development.
6. **RUNX gene:** RUNX-2 (runt related protein) is a transcription factor and a key regulator of osteoblast differentiation and bone formation. Also, analysis of RUNX-2 showed that it is restricted to dental mesenchyme between the bud and early bell stages of tooth development.

Q. 11. Write about genetic basis of dental caries.
[RGUHS, May 2011]

Ans.

1. Variation in caries risk and protection has a strong genetic component.
2. Traits such as tooth morphology, immune response saliva, and diet contribute the genetic determination of dental caries.
3. Only a few specific genes are associated with caries risk, e.g. amelogenin, ameloblastin and tuftelin.
4. Variation in genetics also influences the difference in dietary habits that influence the caries risk.
5. The genes associated with enamel formation, taste, saliva contribute to caries risk and/protection.
6. Fluoride and other environmental factors can override this genetic influence.
7. An association has been found between caries experience and the proline rich protein in saliva.
8. The inheritance of proline rich proteins follows an autosomal dominant mode.

Q. 12. Write about genetic basis of malocclusion.
[TNMGR, March 2010; NTR Uni., May 2019]

Ans. Genetics and environmental factors play important role in etiology of malocclusion.

1. Class II division 1: Studies have shown a higher correlation between the patients and his immediate family and data from random pairings of unrelated siblings, thus supporting the concept of polygenic inheritance for class II division 1 malocclusion.
2. Class II division 2: Family occurrence has been reported in twin and triplet studies and in family pedigrees.
3. Class III malocclusion: Family studies of mandibular prognathism are suggestive of heredity in the etiology of this condition.
4. Population differences: Growth records of aborigines have shown that a fairly large percentage of variations observed in tooth size are due to genetic factors. Certain teeth show more variability in size, shape and eruption, e.g. third molars.

Q. 13. Describe in detail the various congenital anomalies causing malocclusion.

(TNMGR, Oct. 2013)

Ans. Many congenital malformations involve malocclusion of the teeth.

1. Clefts of the lip and palate.
2. Hemifacial microsomia.
3. Mandibulofacial dysostosis.
4. Robin complex.
5. Nager acrofacial dysostosis.
6. Wildervanck Smith syndrome.
7. Hallermann-Streiff syndrome.
8. Basal cell nevus syndrome (Gorlin-Goltz syndrome).
9. Klinefelter syndrome.
10. Marfan syndrome.
11. Crouzan's syndrome

Q. 14. Write a short note on gingival lesion of genetic origin.

(TNMGR, Oct. 2012)

Ans. These are following diseases of genetic origin, which manifest as gingival lesion:

1. Ehlers-Danlos syndrome.
2. Familial fibromatoses.
3. Neurofibromatosis 1.
4. Acatalasia.
5. Hypophosphatasia.
6. Papillon-Lefèvre syndrome.
7. Down's syndrome.
8. Leukocyte adhesion defect.
9. Cyclic neutropenia.
10. Chédiak-Higashi syndrome.

Q. 15. Discuss significance of development of genetic control of cleft lip and palate.

(AIIMS-CDER, May 2018)

Ans. Orofacial clefts, notably cleft lip (CL) and cleft palate (CP), are the most common craniofacial birth defects in humans and represent a substantial personal and societal burden. Clefts affect approximately 1 in 700 individuals.

1. Syndromic forms of CL/P: Simple Mendelian inheritance patterns, more suitable for conventional genetic mapping strategies, e.g.

- Van der Woude syndrome is an autosomal dominant form of orofacial clefting. Mutation in the interferon regulatory factor 6 (IRF6) gene causes clefting as IRF6 is expressed in medial edge epithelia of palatal shelves.
- CL/P in ectodermal dysplasia syndrome, autosomal recessive trait, mutations identified in the poliovirus receptor-like 1 (PVRL1) gene. PVRL1 is expressed in the epithelia of the palatal shelves, nose and skin, as well as the dental ectoderm.
- X-linked cleft palate and ankyloglossia: An X-linked recessive pattern on the long arm of chromosome X. Gene was identified as TBX22 which is expressed in the palatal shelves and tongue during development. If a male inherits a mutated TBX22, it is highly likely that he will have the disease.

2. Genetics of non-syndromic CL/P: CL/P is a genetic trait; 40-fold risk for CL/P among 1st degree relatives of an affected individual, greater concordance in MZ compared with DZ twins, concordance rate in MZ is only 40–60%, suggesting the influence of environmental factors is also important. High association between IRF6 variants, MSX1 and CL/P.

- Genetic variation in IRF6 contributes to 12% of CL/P and triples the recurrence risk in some families.
- MSX1 is involved in both primary and secondary palatogenesis.
- MSX1 inactivation results in cleft palate and tooth agenesis.
- Mutations in MSX1 in 2% of patients with non-syndromic clefting.

Q. 16. Write a short note on genetic engineering.

(BFUHS, Oct. 2010)

Ans. Genetic engineering/genetic modification is the direct manipulation of an organism's genome using biotechnology, to change the genetic makeup of cells, including the transfer of genes within and across species boundaries to produce improved or novel organisms. New DNA may be inserted in the host genome by first isolating and copying the genetic material of interest using molecular cloning methods to generate a DNA sequence, or by synthesizing the DNA, and then inserting this construct into the host organism. Genes may be removed, or "knocked out", using a nuclease. **Gene targeting** is a different technique that uses homologous recombination to change an endogenous gene, and can be used to delete a gene, remove exons, add a gene, or introduce point mutations. An organism that is generated through genetic engineering is considered to be a **genetically modified organism** (GMO). If genetic material from another species is added to the host, the resulting organism is called **transgenic**. If genetic material from the same species or a species that can naturally breed with the host is used the resulting organism is called **cisgenic**.

Genome editing: Genome editing is a type of genetic engineering in which DNA is inserted, replaced, or removed from a genome using artificially engineered nucleases, or "molecular scissors." There are currently four families of engineered nucleases: Meganucleases, zinc finger nucleases (ZFNs), transcription activator-like effector nucleases (TALENs), and Cas9-guide RNA system.

Applications: Genetic engineering has applications in medicine, research, industry and agriculture and can be used on a wide range of plants, animals and microorganisms.

1. Medicine: In medicine, genetic engineering has been used in manufacturing drugs, to create model animals and do laboratory research, and in gene therapy.
2. Manufacturing: Genetic engineering is used to mass-produce insulin, human growth hormones, human albumin, monoclonal antibodies, anti-hemophilic factors, vaccines and many other drugs. Genetically engineered viruses are being developed that can still confer immunity, but lack the infectious sequences.
3. Research: Genetic engineering is used to create animal models of human diseases. Genetically modified mice are the most common genetically engineered animal model. They have been used to study and model cancer, obesity, heart disease, diabetes, arthritis, substance abuse, anxiety, aging and Parkinson disease.
4. Gene therapy: Gene therapy is the genetic engineering of humans, generally by replacing defective genes with effective ones. This can occur in somatic tissue or germ-line tissue.

Q. 17. Write a short note on gene therapy.

Ans. Gene therapy is the replacement of person's faulty genetic material with normal genetic material to treat or cure a disease or abnormal medical condition (US Food and Drug Administration). The procedure involved in gene therapy includes:

1. Pinpoint gene of interest.
2. Acquiring a normal copy of gene (therapeutic gene) by restrictive endonuclease enzyme (cutting and splicing).
3. Finally cloning of therapeutic gene into a vector, which is a vehicle to deliver the gene of interest.

Faulty genes can be corrected by several methods:
1. Regulation of particular gene can be changed.
2. Faulty gene can be replaced for a normal gene through homologous recombination.
3. Normal gene is inserted into non-specific location within the genome to replace a non-functional gene.

4. Abnormal gene is repaired through selective reverse mutation which returns the gene to its normal functional status.

General principles of gene transfer: The concept of gene therapy involves the introduction of exogenous genes into somatic cells that form the organs of the body to produce a desired therapeutic effect. The selected DNA fragment is first cleaved using restriction endonucleases. Then vector or vehicle is prepared to transfer the genetic material. The vector is isolated, purified and cleaved to allow insertion of the DNA fragment. The DNA fragments then must be joined to the cleaved ends of the vector, effectively closing the molecule. This successful insertion of an exogenous DNA molecule into a vector results in a **DNA chimera**. These vector constructs are the basis of **recombinant DNA techniques**. Next step involves introduction of the construct into a cell, allowing the production of a line of genetically identical cells containing the DNA sequence introduced by the vector. This allows mass production of cells with a specifically designed genetic make-up. Vector delivers the therapeutic gene into patient's target. The target cells become infective with therapeutic gene through vector. Functional proteins are created from the therapeutic gene causing the cell to return to a normal stage.

Requirements for vector: Ideal requirements for vectors are:

1. It should not be identified by immune system (non-immunologic).
2. Should be stable and easy to reproduce.
3. Should have longevity of expression.
4. Should have high efficiency (100% cells transfected).
5. High specificity and low toxicity.
6. It should be able to protect and deliver DNA across the cell membrane into the nucleus.
7. It should be able to target gene delivery to specific cells.
8. It should be easy to be produced in large amounts and be inexpensive.

Types of vector for gene therapy:

A. Viral vectors: Adenovirus; Adeno associated virus (AAV), retro virus and herpes simplex virus.

B. Non-viral vectors: Gene transfer mediated by non-viral vectors is referred to as **transfection.**

1. **Physical vectors:** Electrophoration, microinjection, use of ballistic particles.
2. **Chemical vectors:** Calcium vectors, lipids and protein complexes.

Non-viral methods present certain advantages over viral methods, with simple large scale production and low host immunogenicity.

Types of gene therapy

1. **Germline gene therapy**: Repair or replace defective gene in germ line cell. Modified gene would be inherited.
2. **Somatic gene therapy**: Repair or replace defective gene in some or all body cells of an individual. But the change is not passed to next generation.

Types of delivery

1. *In vivo:* During *in vivo* gene transfer, the foreign gene is injected into the patient by viral and non-viral methods.
2. *Ex vivo:* Ex vivo gene transfer involves a foreign gene transduced into tissue cells cultivated in the laboratory, and then resulting genetically modified cells are transplanted back into the patient.

Difficulties in gene therapy include

1. Difficulty to deliver genes in some sites like lung cells.
2. Genes might integrate at sites where it can affect the functioning of another gene.
3. Vectors may be recognized as foreign by immune system triggering immune response.
4. Viral vector may cause toxicity, inflammatory response and might recover their ability to cause disease.
5. Multigene disorders are difficult to treat by gene therapy.
6. Gene therapy is expensive.

Applications in dentistry

1. **Bone repair**: Bone defects in the oral and maxillofacial region can be repaired by transferring genes encoding BMPs. The advantage of an *ex vivo* gene transfer approach is that specific cells like bone marrow cells or stem cells can be selected as the cellular delivery vehicle for specific clinical problems.
2. **Pain**: The use of gene transfer in place of drug delivery to achieve the continuous release of short-lived bioactive peptides in or near the spinal dorsal horn underlies the most common strategies for gene therapy of pain. Also direct gene delivery to the articular surface of the temporomandibular joint has been found to be feasible.
3. **DNA vaccination**: Immunization of salivary gland using plasmid DNA encoding the *P. gingivalis* fimbrial gene leads to the production of fimbrial protein locally in the salivary gland tissue with consequent production of specific salivary IgA, and IgG, antibodies and serum IgG antibodies.

4. **Keratinocyte**: Cultured oral keratinocytes have been grafted to oral surgical defects. They persist at these sites and exhibit normal epithelial morphology. Human growth hormone, apolipoprotein E and coagulation factor IX are successfully delivered by genetically modified keratinocytes. Gene therapy can be used to treat keratinocytes disorders and dermatologic disorders like ichthyosis and epidermolysis bullosa.

5. **Salivary glands**: Salivary glands produce large amount of proteins and are sites easily accessible for gene transfer with minimum invasiveness through intraductal cannulation. The opening of the main duct in the oral cavity is cannulated and gene delivery vectors are infused by a retrograde injection that increases salivary secretions by transferring genes that encode secretory proteins into salivary glands.

6. **Oral cancer**: The general strategy in cancer treatment is to express a gene product that will result in cancer cell death. It can be achieved by:
   a. Addition of a tumor suppressor gene (**gene addition therapy**).
   b. Deletion of a defective tumor gene (**gene excision therapy**).
   c. Downregulation of expression of genes that stimulate tumor growth.
   d. Enhancement of immune surveillance (**immunotherapy**).
   e. Activation of prodrugs that have a chemotherapeutic effect and cause toxicity only to tumor cells ("**Suicide**" **gene therapy**).
   f. Introduction of genes to inhibit tumor angiogenesis.
   g. "Cancer vaccination" with genes for tumor antigens.

   The goal of gene therapy in cancer is to introduce new genetic material into cancer cells that will selectively kill the cancerous cells, causing no toxicity to surrounding normal cells. Vectors such as adenoviruses are useful for gene therapy of head and neck cancers. Replacing a mutated p53 gene with a wild-type (normal) p53 gene is a potential approach to head and neck cancer treatment. The tumor suppressor genes p16, p21, p27, and Rb are frequently mutated in head and neck cancer, and therefore are potential gene therapy targets. In gene-directed enzyme–prodrug therapy, a recombinant virus is generated which encodes a prodrug-activating enzyme such as nitroreductase, thymidine kinase or cytosine deaminase. The activated drug is able to leech out of the virus-infected cell to kill surrounding non-infected cells, creating a bystander effect in cancer.

7. **Orthodontic tooth movement**: Gene therapy with osteoprotegerin (OPG) and RANKL has been used to inhibit and accelerate orthodontic tooth movement in a rat model. Local RANKL gene transfer to the periodontal tissue accelerated orthodontic tooth movement by approximately 150% after 21 days, without eliciting any systemic effects. Local OPG gene transfer inhibited tooth movement by about 50% after 21 days of forced application.

8. **Gene therapy to grow new teeth**: This approach is generally presented in terms of adding molecules to induce *de novo* tooth initiation in the mouth. It might be combined with gene-manipulated tooth regeneration.

Q. 18. Write a short note on gene mapping.
(NTR Uni., April 2013)

Ans. Gene mapping refers to the mapping of genes to specific locations on chromosomes. It is a critical step in the understanding of genetic diseases. There are two types of gene mapping:

1. **Genetic mapping**: Using linkage analysis to determine the relative position between two genes on a chromosome. It is best if measured between "close" markers. Unit of distance in genetic maps = centiMorgans (cM). 1 cM =1% chance of recombination between markers.

2. **Physical mapping**: Using all available techniques or information to determine the absolute position of a gene on a chromosome. Physical mapping relies upon observable experimental outcomes: Hybridization and amplification. It may or may not have a distance measure.

The ultimate goal of gene mapping is to clone genes, especially disease genes. Once a gene is cloned, we can determine its DNA sequence and study its protein product.

Gene maps: Genetic map; Physical map; Transcription map; Sequence map.

Techniques of gene mapping:

1. **Gene mapping by *in situ* hybridization (ISH)**: It is a molecular hybridization technique which allows localization of nucleic acid sequence directly in the intact cell (i.e. *in situ*) without DNA extraction. ISH involves specific hybridization of a single strand of a labelled nucleic acid probe to a single strand of complementary target DNA or RNA in the tissue. The end-product of hybridisation is visualized by radioactive labelled probe (32P, 125I), or non-radioactive-labelled probe (e.g. biotin, digoxigenin).

Applications: ISH is used for the following:
  i. In viral infections, e.g. HPV, EBV, HIV, CMV, HCV, etc.
  ii. In human tumours for detection of gene expression and oncogenes.
  iii. In chromosomal disorders, particularly by use of fluorescent *in situ* hybridisation (FISH).

2. **Gene mapping by somatic cell hybridization**: In this, cells from two different species (e.g. humans and rodents) are artificially fused together in the presence of the Sendai virus. The virus facilitates the fusing of the two cell types to form a hybrid cell.

3. **Gene mapping by gene dosage using patient cells**: The method used to detect dosage differences in either gene products or gene sequences themselves between patient's cell lines containing different numbers of copies of a particular gene.

4. **Gene mapping by chromosomal aberration**: It is done to detect directly chromosomal aberration involving genes leading to particular disease.

5. **Gene mapping by linkage analysis**: Linkage analysis is a method of mapping genes that uses family studies to determine whether two genes show linkage when passed on from one generation to the next.

Q. 19. Write a short note on genetic markers.
(RGUHS, Sept. 2006 BBD Uni., April 2014)

Ans. A genetic marker is a DNA sequence that is readily detected and whose inheritance can easily be monitored. They are used to flag the position of a particular characteristic.

Types

1. **Non-PCR based**: RFLP (restriction fragment length polymorphism).

2. **PCR based**
   a. RAPD (random amplification of polymorphic DNA)
   b. AFLP (amplified fragment length polymorphism)
   c. SCAR (sequence characterize amplified region)
   d. STS (sequence tagged sites)
   e. EST (express sequence tags)
   f. SNP (single nucleotide polymorphism)
   g. SSR (simple sequence repeats)
   h. CAPS (cleaved amplified polymorphic sequence)
   i. SSLP (simple sequence length polymorphism)
   j. VNTR (variable number tandem repeat)
   k. STR (short tandem repeat)
   l. SFP (single feature polymorphism)
   m. DArT (diversity arrays technology)
   n. RAD markers (restriction site associated DNA markers)

Genetic markers can exhibit two modes of inheritance, i.e. dominant/recessive or co-dominant. Generally co-dominant markers are more informative than the dominant markers. Out of above mentioned markers, SNPs have been identified as one of the most common types of polymorphism. It has been incorporated into studies referred to as **genome-wide association studies (GWAS).**

Methods of detection: Southern blotting (a nuclear acid hybridization technique) and PCR.

In **Southern blot**, prior DNA-size fractionation is done by gel electrophoresis. Extracted target DNA is then immobilised on nitrocellulose filter or nylon. Hybridization of the target DNA is then done with labelled probe. **In PCR**, a single strand of DNA generates another by DNA polymerase using a short complementary DNA fragment; this is done using a primer which acts as an initiating template. A cycle of PCR consists of three steps:

i. Heat denaturation of DNA (at 94°C for 60–90 seconds).

ii. Annealing of the primers to their complementary sequences (at 55°C for 30–120 seconds).

iii. Extension of the annealed primers with DNA polymerase (at 72°C for 60–180 seconds).

Classification of genetic markers

- **Type I:** They are associated with genes of known function. They serve as a bridge for comparison and transfer of genomic information from a map rich species into a relatively map-poor species, e.g. RFLP, allozyme, EST.

- **Type II:** They are associated with anonymous genomic segments. They have found widespread use in population genetic studies, e.g. RAPD, AFLP, microsatellites, most of SNP.

Molecular genetic markers can be divided into two classes:

1. **Biochemical markers:** They detect variation at the gene product level such as changes in proteins and amino acids.

2. **Molecular markers:** They detect variation at the DNA level such as nucleotide changes: Deletion, duplication, inversion and/or insertion.

Properties of ideal genetic marker

1. It must be polymorphic.
2. Co-dominant inheritance.
3. It should be evenly and frequently distributed throughout the genome.
4. It should be easy, fast and cheap to detect.
5. It should be reproducible.
6. It has high exchange of data between laboratories.

Applications

1. Measure of genetic diversity.
2. Finger printing.
3. Genotypic selection.
4. Genotyping, pyramiding and introgression.
5. Indirect selection using quantitative traits loci.
6. Marker assisted selection.
7. Identification of genotype.
8. In genetic maps.

Genetic markers and oral diseases

- **Dental caries:** Genes consistently associated with caries experience in recent studies are as follows: Ameloblastin (AMBN), amelogenin (AMELX), aquaporin 5 (AQP5), carbonic anhydrase VI (CA6), enamelin (ENAM), estrogen related receptor beta (ESRRB), kallikrein 4 (KLK4), matrix metallo-proteinase 16 (MMP16), MMP-20, mucin 5 (MUC5B), polycystin-2 (PKD2), tuftelin 1 (TUFT1).

- **Periodontal diseases:** Genetics plays a role in the etiology of periodontal disease by controlling periodontal structural integrity as well as affecting the host response to subgingival microbiota. Out of various responsible genes identified, vitamin D receptor gene, VDR, interleukin-10 (IL-10), and the immunoglobulin platelet receptor gene Fc-γRIIA are the strongest candidates. Other genes identified are: IL-1α, IL-1β, IL-6, MMP-2, MMP-3, MMP-8, MMP-9.

- **Oral cancer:** Alterations in the EGFR gene copy number or alterations in miR-7, miR-21, mRNA-KIFGA, OPN, DEPDC1B, EZH2, deltaNp63, and DNMT3B are significant for early evaluation and correlation with oral cancer. Increase in the levels of Bcl-2 and Bcl-X expression is observed in dysplastic oral lesions and in oral cancer. A high expression of p53 was observed in 40–67% of cases of carcinoma of the head and neck, indicating an important role of p53 in the carcinogenesis process, as an early event of malignant transformation, and of the histological progression of the tumor.

Q. 20. Write a note on genetic counseling.
(TNMGR, Sept. 2010; RUHS, June 2017; UHSR, June 2018; NTR Uni., May 2019)

Ans. Genetic counseling is a communication process in which individuals seeking advice are provided with all the scientific information to enable them in making a decision about current or future pregnancies.

- **Procedures for prenatal diagnosis:**

1. Visualization of fetus:

- **Ultrasonography:** With this technique it is now possible to visualize the embryo as early as 5½–6 weeks of pregnancy and cardiac activity is detectable at 7–8 weeks. Ultrasonography has now become a routine procedure for verification of viable embryo, determination of gestational age, diagnosis of multiple gestation, determination placental and fetal position, diagnosis of fetal anomalies, detection of uterine malformation and guide for passage of instrument for invasive procedures.

- **Radiography**: Although mineralization of fetal skeleton at 11 weeks of gestation is adequate to permit radiographic examination, this procedure has been discarded due to safety reasons.
- **Fetoscopy**: It has been employed for cannulation of umbilical vessels and for blood sampling transfusion and fetal tissue biopsies.

2. Analysis of fetal tissue:

- **Amniocentesis:** (optimum time: 16–18 weeks of gestation): Under strict aseptic conditions and local anesthesia, 20–30 ml of fluid is aspirated. The fibroblast-like cells obtained at amniocentesis can be cultured in a variety of tissue culture media enriched with fetal bovine serum for 1–3 weeks permitting accumulation of sufficient dividing cells for karyotyping. Sex determination of fetus is 99% accurate by this method.
- **Chorionic villus sampling (CVS):** The chorion contains the mitotically active villus cells and is therefore, the area to be biopsied. At 9–12 weeks of gestational age villi float freely within the inter-villous space and are attached only loosely to the underlying structure. In CVS sampling 10–25 mg of chorionic villi is collected. Because the Langer-hans cells of the cytotrophoblast are in dividing phase, it is possible to perform a "direct" chromo-some analysis, immediately after sampling, or alternately after 24 hours of incubation in a tissue culture medium.
- **Fetal and maternal blood analysis:** Isolation and analysis of fetal cells in maternal blood is an attractive method of non-invasive prenatal diag-nosis. Flow cytometric test of maternal blood with anti-gamma globin MAb (monoclonal antibody to gamma chain of hemoglobin molecule) is highly specific for examining fetal cells with respective of its gender because the amount of gamma hemoglobin chain produce per cell is significantly higher in fetus in comparison to that of adults.
- **Fetal liver biopsy:** A variety of enzymes inter-mediary metabolism is expressed only in the liver. The prenatal diagnosis of disorders associated with abnormalities of this enzyme is made by fetal liver biopsy, like in glycogen storage diseases, etc.

- **Fetal skin biopsy:** This approach is used only in those disorders where skin is involved, e.g. epidermolytic hyperkeratosis.
- **Preimplantation diagnosis:** In this procedure one or two cells are removed from cleavage stage embryos from the patients. The embryos are identified by using molecular technique. Subsequently, healthy embryo is reimplanted in the uterine cavity enabling further development till full term. A number of strategies deve-loped to design optimal procedures for the preimplan-tation diagnosis of genetic defects are:

- **Polar body biopsy:** The chromatin polar body is virtually "mirror image" of the chromatin of the oocyte.
- **Multicell biopsy:** Prior to the late 8-cell stage, 1–3 blastomeres of the pre-embryo are dissociated with pipetting after boring a small hole in zona pellucida, that heals rapidly afterwards.
- **Blastocyst biopsy:** From trophoblast (which later forms placenta) of the blastocyst a number of cells can be safely removed for analysis without adversely affecting the fetus.

Basic information required for genetic counseling

A genetic counseling must have:
1. Precise and fully confirmed diagnosis of the diseases.
2. Accurate pedigree of the family.
3. Knowledge of the mode of the inheritance of the condition.

Indications for Prenatal Diagnosis

1. Advanced maternal age (e.g. Down syndrome).
2. Previous child with chromosome aberration.
3. Intrauterine growth delay.
4. Biochemical disorder.
5. Congenital anomaly.
6. Previous history of neural tube defect in the family.
7. Structural anomalies found on ultrasonography.
8. Person with mental retardation or developmental delay (e.g. fragile X syndrome).
9. Couples with a history of recurrent miscarriages.

How to Identify Genetic Diseases?

Step1

1. Buildup the pedigree tree "bottom-up", starting with the index case and ending up with grandparents, cousins, uncles, aunts, etc.
2. Ask the mother of the patient about her siblings, children, parents and all the immediate blood relatives that she can remember from her side or from her groom's side.
3. Fill in the appropriate pedigree symbols to indicate normal, carrier, affected individuals, stillbirths,

spontaneous abortions, twins, consanguinity, unknown gender, etc.

Step 2

1. Analyze the pedigree chart and determine the mode of inheritance.
2. The negative family history should not be considered conclusive evidence against the presence of heritable condition. The presence of consanguinity does not prove recessive inheritance.

Step 3

Calculate risk of recurrence. The perception of what constitutes "high or low" depends on the investigator. In the risk, figure has two components:

1. The probability of occurrence of the disease.
2. The burden of the diseases.

Step 4

The decision making:

1. Allow the patient or his family members to decide on continuation and termination of pregnancy.
2. Counseling should be supportive.
3. Conditions with Mendelian inheritance usually have high risk of recurrence.
4. Support your conclusion with chromosomal and molecular data wherever possible.
5. Autosomal dominant condition: 50% risk to offspring of affected parents.
6. Autosomal recessive condition: 25% risk to offspring of carrier parents.
7. X-linked recessive condition: 50% risk to siblings.
8. On observing a structural chromosomal anomaly in the patient, check the parent chromosome.
9. Duplication or deletion of chromosome can result in congenital malformation or mental retardation.

Q. 21. Write a note on human races.

(NTR Uni., Oct 2012)

Ans. Races are defined as a distinct evolutionary lineage within a species. An evolutionary lineage is a population of organisms characterized by a continuous line of descent such that the individuals in the population at any given time are connected by ancestor/descendent relationships. Race refers to classification of humans into relatively large and distinct population groups based on appearance through heritable phenotypic characteristics, often influenced by and correlated with culture, ethnicity and socioeconomic status.

Race formation is a complex process where several factors are involved. These may be summarized as:

1. **Mutation:** The basic mechanism by which genetic variability is introduced through mutation. As soon as a new mutant gene appears, it multiplies from one generation to another and becomes a distinctive characteristic of the particular population, provided other conditions are favorable.

2. **Natural selection:** Natural selection moulds the genotypes of an organism such that they produce phenotypes fitting to the environment in which organism lives. Advantageous genes are multiplied more rapidly and disadvantageous gene will be eliminated by nature.

3. **Genetic drift:** Chance fluctuations of gene frequencies may lead to appreciable genetic differences between completely isolated sub-populations. This effect becomes stronger, if the effective breeding size of population is small. In this process, increase or decrease of the frequency of a gene in a certain population happens merely as an accident or chance.

Table 1.21: Classification of human race by Ashley Montagu (1951)

Sl. no.	Characters	Caucasoid	Negroid	Mongoloid
1.	Skin colour	Light reddish white to olive brown. Some are brown	Brown to brown black. Some are yellow-brown	Light yellow to yellow brown. Some are reddish brown.
2.	Head hair	Light blond to dark brown in colour, colour, fine to medium in texture, straight to wavy in form	Brown-black in colour. Coarse in texture, curly to frizzly or woolly in form	Brown to brown blac in colour, coarse in texture, straight in form
3.	Head form	Dolichocephalic to brachycephalic, height is medium to very high	Predominantly dolicho-cephalic, height is low to medium	Predominantly brachycephalic height is medium
4.	Body hair quantity	Moderate to profuse	Slight	Sparsely distributed
5.	Face	Narrow to medium broad	Medium broad to narrow. Prognathism is very often present	Medium broad to very broad. Check bones are high and flat

4. **Migration:** Migration plays an important role in racial differentiation. It helps in isolation, hybridization and mixing of different populations with the migrants.

5. **Isolation:** Isolation may be geographical or social and is considered to be a great race maker. The natural selection and genetic drift, will act effectively only when a particular population is isolated from the neighbouring populations.

6. **Hybridization:** Hybridization is a process by which genes within a species are introduced into other populations resulting in genetic combinations which are entirely new. Through hybridization, genetic variation is introduced in a population called gene flow that leads to the formation of new race.

7. **Sexual selection:** It is a process of selecting mates on the basis of some preferred qualities, as a result of which the sexually preferred type would become the dominant variety of the individuals.

8. **Social selection:** In social selection, breeding is regulated by artificially instituted barriers between socially approved individual and groups within a population, so that mating occurs between individuals preferred by such social standards rather than at random.

I. Boyd's Classification (1958):

1. **European Group:** Early European; Lapps; Northwest Europeans; Eastern and Central Europeans; Mediterranean.

2. **African Group:** The African races, excluding inhabitants of North Africa, which belong to European group.

3. **Asian Group:** The Asian races; Indo-Dravidian.

4. **American Group:** American Indians 60 biological diversity.

5. Pacific; Indonesian race; Melanesian race; Polynesian race.

6. **Australian Group:** Australian aborigines.

II. Ashley Montagu Classification (1951): He used skin colour, hair form and head form. He classified mankind into three main groups, viz. 1. Negroid, 2. Mongoloid, and 3. Caucasoid.

Q. 22. Write about stem cells in dentistry.
(NTR Uni., April 2007; May 2018; RUHS, June 2017)

Ans. Stem cells are primitive cells found in all multicellular organisms that are characterized by self-renewal and the capacity to differentiate into any mature cell type. There are 2 main types of stem cells: Embryonic stem cells and adult stem cells.

Stem cells have the following capabilities:

1. They are able to continuously produce daughter cells having the same characteristics as themselves (**self-renewal**).

2. They can generate daughter cells that have different, more restricted properties.

3. They can re-populate a host *in vivo* (**differentiation**).

Sources of stem cells: There are many potential sources for stem cells:

1. Embryonic stem (ES) cells are derived from the inner cell mass of a blastocyst from a 4/5 days old embryo.

2. Embryonic germ (EG) cells are collected from fetal tissue at a somewhat later stage of development (from gonadal ridge).

3. Adult stem cells that are derived from mature tissues and are found in adult tissues. They act as a repair system for the body, replenishing specialized cells, but also maintain the normal turnover of regenerative organs, such as blood, skin, or intestinal tissues.

Generic criteria for pluripotent embryonic stem or embryonic germ cells:

1. Originate from a pluripotent cell population.

2. Maintain normal karyotype.

3. Immortal and can be propagated indefinitely in the embryonic state.

4. Clonally-derived cultures capable of spontaneous differentiation into extra-embryonic tissue and somatic cells representative of all 3 embryonic germ layers in teratoma or *in vitro*.

Characteristics of mesenchymal stem cells (MSCs): MSCs are described as multipotent because of their ability, even as clonally isolated cells, to exhibit the potential for differentiation into a variety of different cells/tissue lineages.

1. **Bone marrow mesenchymal stem cell (BMSCs) from orofacial bones:** Human BMSCs can also be isolated from orofacial (maxilla and mandible) bone marrow aspirates obtained during dental surgical procedures such as dental implant treatment, wisdom tooth extraction, extirpation of cysts and orthodontic osteotomy.

2. **Dental tissue-derived stem cells**

a. **Dental pulp stem cells (DPSCs)** are cells that had phenotypic characteristics similar to those of BMSCs. DPSCs are putative candidate for dental tissue engineering due to: Easy surgical access to the collection site and very low morbidity after extraction of dental pulp. DPSCs can generate much more typical dentin tissues within a short period and can be safely cryopreserved and recombined with many scaffolds. They possess immunoprivilege and anti-inflammatory abilities favorable for the allotransplantation experiments.

b. **Stem cells from human exfoliated deciduous teeth; SHED** (UHSR, May 2016): Dr Songtao Shi discovered SHED in 2003. The main task of these cells seems to be the formation of mineralized tissue, which can be used to enhance orofacial bone regeneration. Types of stem cells present in human exfoliated deciduous teeth are:

- Adipocytes: They can be used to treat various spine and orthopedic conditions, Crohn's disease, cardiovascular diseases and may also be useful in plastic surgery.
- Chondrocytes and osteoblasts: They have been used to grow intact teeth in animals.
- Mesenchymal stem cells (MSCs): They have successfully been used to repair spinal cord injury, to treat neuronal degenerative disorders such as Parkinson's disease, cerebral palsy, Alzheimer's disease, and other such disorders. MSCs have better curative potential than other type of adult stem cells.

    Advantages of SHED: It is a simple painless technique to isolate them and being an autologous transplant they do not possess any risk of immune reaction or tissue rejection. SHED is also be useful for close relatives of the donor such as grandparents, parents and siblings. SHED banking is more economical and may be complementary to cord cell banking. These cells are not subjected to same ethical concerns as embryonic stem cells.

c. **Periodontal ligament** is another adult MSC source in dental tissues, and periodontal ligament stem cells (PDLSCs) can even be isolated from extracted teeth. PDLSCs have demonstrated the ability to regenerate periodontal tissues (cementum, PDL and alveolar bone) in experimental animal models.

d. **SCAP:** MSCs residing in the apical papilla of permanent teeth with immature roots are known as SCAP. SCAP are capable of forming odontoblast-like cells, producing dentin in vivo, and are likely cell source of primary odontoblasts for the formation of root dentin. SCAP supports apexogenesis, which can occur in infected immature permanent teeth with periradicular periodontitis or abscess. SCAP residing in the apical papilla survive such pulp necrosis because of their proximity to the periapical tissue vasculature.

3. **Oral mucosa-derived stem cells:**

a. **Oral epithelial progenitor/stem cells,** which are a subpopulation of small oral keratinocytes. Although these cells seem to be unipotential stem cells, i.e. they can only develop into epithelial cells. They may be useful for intra-oral grafting.

b. **In the lamina propria of the gingiva,** which attaches directly to the periosteum of underlying bone with no intervening submucosa.

4. **Periosteum-derived stem/progenitor cells:** Cultured periosteum-derived cells have been used for alveolar ridge or maxillary sinus floor augmentation in clinical research that successfully demonstrated enhanced bone remodeling and lamellar bone formation with subsequent reliable implant insertion and reduced postoperative waiting time after implant placement.

5. **Salivary gland-derived stem cells:** Stem cells in the adult salivary gland are expected to be useful for autologous transplantation therapy in the context of tissue engineered—salivary glands or direct cell therapy.

Applications of Stem Cell Research in Dentistry

1. **Alveolar bone augmentation:** Alveolar bone regeneration by stem cells helps to regenerate the tissue. Stem cell based therapies carry the drawbacks of high cost and labor.

2. **Tooth/root regeneration:** The ultimate goal of tooth regeneration is to develop fully functioning bioengineered teeth that can replace lost teeth. Tooth engineering to form dental structures in vivo has been established using many different types of stem cells from mice, rats, and pigs.

3. **Mandible condyle regeneration:** Damage to TMJ disc or condyle arising from trauma or arthritis can result in lifelong pain and disturbed masticatory function for patients. Tissue regeneration strategy on these defects can hold promise to affect the quality of life (QOL) of these patients.

4. **Tongue regeneration:** Loss of tongue tissue from surgical resection can profoundly affect the quality of life. Advances in stem cell biology and tissue engineering may enable the reconstruction of the damaged or resected tongue with normal physiological function.

Aging of mesenchymal stem cell: A number of changes occurred in physiological, functional, and molecular parameters of stem cells during long-term cultures. These changes included:

a. Typical hay flick phenomenon of cellular aging.

b. Gradual decreasing proliferation potential.

c. Telomere shortening.

d Impairment of functions.

The proliferative potential of MSC decreases faster after 120 days of *in vitro* expansion.

♦ **Tooth stem cell banking** (*BBD Uni., April 2014*): Although tooth banking is currently not very popular the trend is gaining acceptance mainly in the developed countries. BioEden (Austin, Texas, USA), has International Laboratories in UK (serving Europe) and Thailand (serving South East Asia) with global expansion plans. Stem cell banking companies like Store–A–Tooth (Provia Laboratories, Littleton, Massachusetts, USA) and StemSave (StemSave Inc, New York, USA) are also expanding their horizon internationally. In Japan, the first tooth bank was established in Hiroshima University and the company was named "Three Brackets" (Suri Buraketto) in 2005. Nagoya University (Kyodo, Japan) also came up with a tooth bank in 2007. Taipei Medical University in collaboration with Hiroshima University opened the nation's first tooth bank in September, 2008. The Norwegian Tooth Bank (a collaborative project between the Norwegian Institute of Public Health and the University of Bergen) set up in 2008 is collecting exfoliated primary teeth from 1,00,000 children in Norway. Not last but the least, Stemade introduced the concept of dental stem cells banking in India recently by launching its operations in Mumbai and Delhi.

Q. 23. Discuss nanotechnology in dentistry.

(RGUHS, July 2016; Gujarat Uni., June 2018)

Ans. Nanotechnology is the manipulation of matter on the molecular and atomic levels. (Greek: "dwarf"). The concept of nanotechnology was first elaborated in 1959 by Richard Feynman.

♦ **Nanomaterials:** Nanomaterials are those materials with components <100 nm in at least one dimension. Nanomaterials in one dimension are termed sheets, in two dimensions as nanowires and nanotubes, and as quantum dots in three dimensions. Nanomaterial properties vary majorly from other materials due to two reasons: The increase in surface area and quantum effects. Quantum effects become more dominant at the nanoscale.

Nanotechnology has applications in many fields like:

• Medicine: Diagnostics, drug delivery, tissue engineering.

• Chemistry and environment: Catalysis, filtration.

• Energy: Reduction of energy consumption, increasing the efficiency of energy production.

♦ **Nanodentistry:** Approaches to nanodentistry.

• **Bottom-up approaches:** Assembly of small components into compound structures.

• **Top-down approaches:** Creation of small structures by using bigger ones in guiding their assembly

A. Dental nanorobotics: Bottom-up approach

1. **Local nano-anaesthesia:** A colloidal suspension containing millions of anesthetic dental nanorobots would be used to induce local anesthesia. Deposited on the gingival tissue, the nanorobots would reach the dentin and move toward the pulp via the dentinal tubules.

2. **Hypersensitivity cure:** Nanorobots, using local organic materials, could result in effective occlusion of particular tubules, resulting in rapid and stable treatment.

3. **Tooth repositioning:** All the periodontal tissues may be directed by orthodontic nano-robots leading to swift and pain-free corrective movements.

4. **Nano-robotic dentifrice (dentifrobots):** Toothpastes or mouthwashes could contain the dentifrobots which would then survey all gingival surfaces regularly. They would also break down harmful materials into harmless substances and undertake constant calculus removal.

5. **Dental durability and cosmetics:** Changing the superficial enamel layer with materials like sapphire 12 or diamond may enhance the toughness and appearance of teeth as these materials have 20–100 times the hardness of enamel.

6. **Nanodiagnostics (photosensitizers and carriers):** Quantum dots may also play the role of a photosenstizer and carrier. They attach the antibody to the target cell and on stimulation by UV light, result in the formation of reactive oxygen species which destroy the target cells. Another role of nanotechnology may lie in overcoming some drawbacks of biochip technology.

7. **Therapeutic aid in oral diseases**

• **Nanotherapeutics/drug delivery:** Nanotechnology will eliminate the solubility problems, lead to a reduction in the dosage of drug and reduce the adverse effects. It may also lead to increased bioavailability.

• **Diagnosis of oral cancer**

• Nanoscale cantilevers: Elastic beams used to attach with cancer-linked molecules.

• Nanopores: Small holes that enable DNA pass one strand at a time, thus making DNA sequencing highly efficient.

- **Nanotubes:** Carbon rods that can detect affected genes and also localize their location.
- **Quantum dots:** They attach to proteins associated with cancer cells, thus localizing tumors.
- **Treatment of oral cancer:** Options include the following:
  - Nano-materials for brachytherapy: BrachySil™
  - Nanovectors for gene therapy.
  - Nonviral gene delivery systems.
  - Drug delivery across the blood–brain barrier.

B. Dental nano-materials: Nano-dentistry as top-down approach

1. **Nanocomposites:** Nanocomposites, defined by filler-particle sizes of $\leq$100 nm, can broadly be divided into nano-hybrid and nano-filled resin-based composites. Nanocomposites have comparable or better finishing, polishing ability, shade matching, flexural strength and hardness than conventional composites.
2. **Nano-solution (nano-adhesives):** Nano-solutions are constituted by dispersible nanoparticles, which are used as a component in bonding agents.
- **Advantages:** Higher dentine and enamel bond strength, high stress absorption, longer shelf life, durable marginal seal, no separate etching required, fluoride release.
3. **Nano light-curing glass ionomer restorative:** This blends nanotechnology initially developed for Filtek™ supreme universal restorative with fluoro-aluminosilicate technology. **Advantages:** Excellent polish, superb esthetics, enhanced wear resistance.
   - **Clinical indications:** Primary teeth restoration, transitional restoration, small class I restoration, sandwich restoration, class III and V restoration, core build-up.
4. **Impression materials:** Traditional vinyl poly siloxanes have incorporated nanofillers, which produce a distinctive material with improved flow, enhanced hydrophilic properties and superior detail precision.
5. **Nano-composite denture teeth:** These are made of polymethylmethacrylate (PMMA) and homogeneously distributed nano-fillers.
   - **Advantages:** Excellent polishing ability and stain-resistant, superb esthetics, enhanced wear resistance and surface hardness.
6. **Nano-encapsulation:** Specifically targeted release systems have been developed by South West Research Institute (SWRI). These include nano-capsules in the form of new vaccines, antibiotics, and delivery of drugs with fewer adverse effects.

7. **Dentifrices:** These are mainly made up of nano-sized hydroxyapatite molecules. They will result in protective shell on tooth surface and may even repair damaged areas.
8. **Laser plasma application for periodontia:** Application of nano-sized titania particle emulsion on human skin followed by laser irradiation, leads to the disintegration of the particles along with other results like: Shock waves, micro-abrasion of hard tissues, stimulus to produce collagen. **Applications:** Periodontal therapy, melanin removal, Soft tissue incision (without anesthesia), cavity preparation—enamel and dentin cutting.
9. **Bone replacement materials:** Bone is a natural nano-composite made up of organic compounds (mainly collagen) toughened with inorganic compounds like hydroxyapatite. This rule has been utilized by Nano-Bone®. Characteristics of bone graft materials are: Osteoinductive, completely synthetic, non-sintered, extremely porous, nano-structured, degradation by osteoclasts, excellent processability, no products in ionic solution.
10. **Materials for induction of osseous growth:** A new calcium sulphate based composite has been developed (bone gen-TR), which breaks down more slowly and regenerates bone more effectively.
11. **Prosthetic implants:** Nanotechnology has aid in the development of surfaces with definite topography and chemical composition leading to predictable tissue integration.
12. **Radiopacity:** Nanoparticles may be incorporated in materials and instruments to achieve radiopacity.
13. **Orthodontic wires:** Orthodontic wires may be drawn from a novel stainless steel material, with very high strength along with excellent deformability, corrosion resistance and fine surface finish.
14. **Nano-needles:** Nano-structured stainless steel crystals have been used to manufacture suture needles.
15. **Nano-sterilizing solution:** A new sterilizing solution following nano-emulsion concept has been developed. **Advantages:** Broad spectrum, hypoallergic, non-coroding, does not stain fabric; Require no protective clothing, environment friendly, compatible with various impression materials.

C. Regenerative nanotechnology: Bio-mimicry

1. **Dentition renaturalization:** This technique may revolutionarise cosmetic dentistry. Initially, the old restorations are removed followed by complete coronal renaturalization—all the teeth remanufactured to become identical to natural teeth.

2. Dentition replacement therapy (major tooth repair): Nanotechnology may utilize genetic engineering, tissue engineering and tissue regeneration initially, followed by growing whole new teeth *in vitro* and their installation.

Challenges faced by nanotechnology

- Precise positioning and manufacture of nanoscale parts.
- Cost-effective nano-robot mass manufacturing methods.
- Synchronization of numerous independent nano-robots.
- Biocompatibility concern.
- Financing and tactical concerns.
- Inadequate assimilation of clinical research.
- Social issues of public acceptance, ethics, regulation and human safety.

Supplementary Questions 2020

HUMAN ANATOMY, EMBRYOLOGY AND HISTOLOGY

Q. 1. Discuss the anatomy and functioning of muscles of mastication. Add a note on the role in maintaining temporomandibular joint. *(UHSR, RUHS, Yenepoya Uni., June 2020; MUHS, KLE Uni., BFUHS, July 2020; People's Uni., Aug. 2020)*

Q. 2. Write in detail about the development, anatomy and physiology of salivary glands. *(CDER-AIIMS, UHSR, June 2020; KLE Uni., July 2020)*

Q. 3. Describe the anatomy of the parotid gland and add a note on applied anatomy. *(NTR Uni., Sept. 2020)*

Q. 4. Development of mandible, age changes and its anomalies. *(RUHS, UHSR, June 2020; RGUHS, July 2020; UOK, Aug. 2020)*

Q. 5. Describe the development of TMJ. Discuss the common disorders of TMJ. *(RUHS, June 2020; MUHS, KLE Uni., July 2020)*

Q. 6. Anatomy of the TMJ and its applied aspects. *(UHSR, June 2020; UOK, NTR Uni., Aug. 2020)*

Q. Elaborate the temporomandibular disorder criteria in detail. *(UOK, Aug. 2020)*

Q. Discuss its age-related adaptive changes. *(BFUHS, July 2020)*

Q. 7. Enumerate the paranasal sinuses. Describe in detail the applied anatomy of maxillary air sinus. *(UHSR, June 2020; RGUHS, MUHS, July 2020)*

Q. 8. Draw a neat labeled diagram of taste buds and write about distribution in oral cavity. *(RGUHS, July 2020; People Uni. Aug. 2020)*

Q. 9. Lymphatic drainage of the head and neck region. *(RUHS, June 2020)*

Q. 10. Danger areas of the face and their significance. *(NTR Uni., Aug. 2020)*

Q. 11. Describe in detail the anatomy, development and nerve supply of tongue. Add a note on developmental disorders of the tongue and their pathogenesis. *(UHSR, June 2020; MUHS, KUHS, July 2020)*

Q. 12. Embryological development of palate. *(People Uni., Aug.2020)*

Q. 13. Describe briefly development of face. *(MUHS, July 2020)*

Q. 14. Pharyngeal arches. *(NTR Uni., Sept. 2020)*

Q. 15. Muscles of facial expressions. *(RUHS. June 2020)*

Q. 16. Describe mandibular nerve and discuss in detail its importance in dentistry. *(NTR Uni., Sept. 2020)*

Q. 17. Explain the course of inferior alveolar nerve. Add a note on applied anatomy. *(NTR Uni., Sept. 2020)*

Q. 18. Lingual nerve. *(RUHS, June 2020)*

Q. 19. Describe in detail the extracranial and intracranial course of facial nerve. Add a note on its applied aspect. *(RUHS, KNRUHS, June 2020; MUHS, July 2020; UOK, Aug. 2020)*

Q. 20. Anterior triangle of the neck. *(RUHS, June 2020)*

Q. 21. Discuss fifth cranial nerve. *(RUHS, June 2020; PAHER, MUHS, July 2020)*

Q. 22. Describe in detail the course of external carotid artery. *(MUHS, BFUHS, July 2020)*

Q. 23. Layers of SCALP. *(UOK, Aug. 2020)*

Q. 24. Histology of bone. *(NTR Uni., Sept. 2020)*

DENTAL ANATOMY AND DENTAL HISTOLOGY

Q. 1. Discuss the development of teeth and write about the developmental defects of teeth. *(Manipal Uni., KLE Uni., July 2020)*

Q. 2. Development of a tooth and stages of eruption. *(NTR Uni., Aug.2020)*

Q. 3. Describe the various theories of eruption.
(UHSR, June 2020)

Q. 4. Write in detail development, composition, physical characteristics and structure of enamel.
(MUHS, July 2020; NTR Uni., Sept. 2020)

Q. 5. Discuss the composition and function of gingival crevicular fluid. *(RUHS, June 2020)*

Q. 6. Describe the anatomical, histological and clinical aspects of cementum. *(RUHS, June 2020)*

Q. 7. Discuss the ultrastructure and biological importance of dentogingival unit. *(People's Uni., Aug.2020)*

Q. 8. Discuss in detail the age changes in enamel, dentin and pulp with their clinical significance.
(UHSR, June 2020; NTR Uni., Sept. 2020)

Q. 9. Discuss the anatomy of maxillary first molar.
(NTR Uni., Sept. 2020)

Q. 10. List structural components of pulp. Explain the functions of pulp. *(UHSR, June 2020)*

Q. 11. Gingival pigmentation. *(RUHS, June 2020)*

Q. 12. Development of attachment apparatus.
(RUHS, June 2020)

Q. 13. Nerve supply of periodontal ligament.
(People's Uni., Aug. 2020)

Q. 14. Management of dentinal hypersensitivity.
(People's Uni., Aug.2020)

Q. 15. Apical third anatomy and its clinical significance. *(UHSR, June 2020)*

Q. 16. Bone morphogenic protein. *(MUHS, July 2020)*

Q. 17. Salivary immunoglobulins. *(UOK, Aug. 2020)*

Q. 18. Describe the macroscopic and microscopic features of gingiva. *(UOK, Aug. 2020)*

Q. 19. Nerve supply of peridontium.
(UOK, Aug. 2020)

Q. 20. Structure of cementum. *(UOK, Aug. 2020)*

Q. 21. Structure of periodontal ligament.
(NTR Uni., Sept. 2020)

Q. 22. Growth prediction methods.
(NTR Uni., Sept. 2020)

Q. 23. Postnatal growth of maxilla and its clinical significance. *(NTR Uni., Sept. 2020)*

PHYSIOLOGY

Q. 1. Calcium metabolism in the body.
(UHSR, RUHS, Yenepoya Uni., June 2020; MUHS, July 2020; People Uni., Aug 2020)

Q. 2. Discuss the clotting factors and mechanism. Add a note on clotting disorders. *(RUHS, June 2020; KLE Uni , MUHS, July 2020)*

Q. 3. Saliva and its importance in oral health.
(UHSR, June 2020; KUHS, Manipal Uni., July 2020; UOK, Aug. 2020)

Q. 4. Biological role of saliva. *(PAHER, July 2020; People Uni., Aug. 2020)*

Q. 5. Describe the composition and function of saliva.
(BFUHS, July 2020; NTR Uni., Sept. 2020)

Q. 6. Factors controlling the secretion and regulation of saliva. *(NTR Uni., Sept. 2020)*

Q. 7. Describe the pharyngeal phase of deglutition.
(NTR Uni., Sept. 2020)

Q. 8. Stages of deglutition. *(UHSR, June 2020)*

Q. 9. Discuss pain and mechanism of pain in detail. How will you differentiate the pulpal pain from periodontal pain? *(KNRUHS, RUHS, UHSR, June 2020)*

Q. 10. Neuromuscular junction.
(Yenepoya Uni., June 2020)

Q. 11. Neuromuscular transmission.
(UOK, Aug. 2020)

Q. 12. Write a note on the physiology of nerve conduction. *(BFUHS, July 2020)*

Q. 13. Pulpal pain. *(MUHS, July 2020)*

Q. 14. Theories of pain pathways. *(MUHS, July 2020)*

Q. 15. Define blood pressure. Regulation of blood pressure. *(KNRUHS, RUHS, June 2020; BFUHS, July 2020; UOK, Aug. 2020)*

Q. 16. List the composition of blood. Explain the stages of erythropoiesis. *(UHSR, June 2020)*

Q. 17. Discuss the components and functions of blood. *(UOK, Aug. 2020)*

Q. 18. Blood groups.   *(UOK, Aug. 2020)*

Q. 19. Blood sugar regulation.
                              (Yenepoya Uni., June 2020)

Q. 20. Regulation of parathyroid hormone. Add a note on tetany.   *(NTR Uni., Sept. 2020)*

Q. 21. Glycosylated form of hemoglobin.
                              (NTR Uni., Sept. 2020)

Q. 22. Secondary hypertension.   *(BFUHS, July 2020)*

Q. 23. Role of sodium in homeostasis.
                              (BFUHS, July 2020)

BIOCHEMISTRY

Q. 1. Role of laboratory investigations in oral surgery.
                              (RUHS, June 2020)

Q. 2. Vitamins.   *(NTR Uni., Aug 2020)*

Q. 3. Explain the metabolism of carbohydrates.
                              (UHSR, June 2020)

Q. 4. Gluconeogenesis.   *(UHSR, June 2020)*

Q. 5. Nutrition in edentulous geriatric patient.
                       (AIIMS-CDER, RUHS, June 2020)

Q. 6. Role of vitamins in oral health.   *(Manipal Uni., July 2020; NTR Uni., Sept. 2020)*

Q. 7. Discuss Krebs cycle.   *(KLE Uni., July 2020)*

Q. 8. Protein energy malnutrition. *(RUHS, June 2020)*

Q. 9. Basal metabolic rate.   *(RUHS, June 2020)*

Q. 10. Balanced diet.   *(RUHS, June 2020)*

Q. 11. Explain the impact of nutrition on oral health.
                              (RUHS, June 2020)

Q. 12. Renal function tests.   *(UOK, Aug. 2020)*

Q. 13. Discuss role of diet in dental caries.
                              (NTR Uni., Sept. 2020)

Q. 14. Vitamin D.   *(NTR Uni., Sept. 2020)*

MICROBIOLOGY

Q. 1. Discuss about bio waste management.
                              (RUHS, June 2020)

Q. 2. How to achieve adequate mercury hygiene in dental clinic?   *(RUHS, June 2020)*

Q. 3. Sterilization and disinfection in dentistry.
                  (RUHS, June 2020; MUHS, July 2020; UOK, Aug. 2020)

Q. 4. Disinfection protocol in prosthodontics.
                          (CDER-AIIMS, June 2020)

Q. 5. Infection control.   *(UHSR, June 2020)*

Q. 6. Asepsis in dental clinic.   *(RUHS, June 2020)*

Q. 7. Autoclaving.   *(RUHS, June 2020)*

Q. 8. Plaque microflora.   *(RUHS, June 2020)*

Q. 9. Describe about the structure of *Streptococcus mutans.*   *(UHSR, June 2020; NTR Uni., Sept. 2020)*

Q. 10. Pathogenesis of dental caries.
                              (UHSR, June 2020)

Q. 11. Caries vaccine.   *(RUHS, June 2020)*

Q. 12. Immunoglobulins.   *(UHSR, June 2020; UOK, NTR Uni., Aug., 2020)*

Q. 13. Role of immunoglobulins in dental caries.
                              (NTR Uni., Sept. 2020)

Q. 14. Antigen–antibody system. *(PAHER, July 2020)*

Q. 15. Cell-mediated immunity. *(RGUHS, July 2020)*

Q. 16. Acquired immunity.   *(NTR Uni., Sept. 2020)*

Q. 17. Differentiate T cells from B cells.
                              (UHSR, June 2020)

Q. 18. Anaphylaxis.
                  (UHSR, June 2020; NTR Uni., Sept. 2020)

Q. 19. Culture media.   *(UOK, Aug. 2020)*

Q. 20. Oral microbial flora.   *(UOK, Aug. 2020)*

Q. 21. Hypersensitivity.   *(RUHS, June 2020, BFUHS, KUHS, July 2020; NTR Uni., Sept. 2020)*

Q. 22. Delayed hypersensitivity.
                              (NTR Uni., Sept. 2020)

Q. 23. Discuss in brief the various theories of antibody formation.   *(BFUHS, July 2020)*

Q. 24. Write a note on the microbiology of primary and secondary endodontic infections.
                              (BFUHS, July 2020)

PATHOLOGY

Q. 1. Differential diagnosis of periapical swelling.
(RUHS, June 2020)

Q. 2. Vitamin C and its role in maintaining the health of oral mucosa. *(RUHS, June 2020)*

Q. 3. Compare and contrast benign and malignant tumors. *(Yenepoya Uni., June 2020)*

Q. 4. Define oral cancer. Discuss the role of various risk factors of oral cancer in its causation.
(KLE Uni., July 2020)

Q. 5. Viral carcinogenesis. *(KUHS, July 2020)*

Q. 6. Spread of tumors. *(UHSR, June 2020)*

Q. 7. Metastasis. *(RUHS, June 2020)*

Q. 8. Define acute inflammation. Describe the vascular changes occurring due to acute inflammation. *(UHSR, June 2020; NTR Uni., Sept. 2020)*

Q. 9. Chemical mediators of inflammation.
(RUHS, June 2020)

Q. 10. Process of inflammation and its mediators.
(Manipal Uni., July 2020)

Q. 11. Role of leukocytes in inflammation.
(RUHS, June 2020)

Q. 12. Hemorrhage and shock.
(Manipal Uni., July 2020)

Q. 13. Explain stages of shock and its etiopathogenesis. *(KNRUHS, June 2020)*

Q. 14. Pathophysiology and management of hypovolaemic shock. *(MUHS, July 2020)*

Q. 15. Anaphylactic shock. *(RUHS, June 2020)*

Q. 16. Discuss in detail about wound healing. Add a note on healing of an extraction wound.
(KLE Uni., BFUHS, July 2020)

Q. 17. Factors that determine wound healing.
(MUHS, July 2020; UOK, Aug. 2020)

Q. 18. Define repair. Describe the process of healing of surgical wound. *(RUHS, June 2020)*

Q. 19. Complications of wound healing in orofacial area. *(UOK, Aug. 2020)*

Q. 20. Healing of oral tissues after radiation injury.
(UHSR, June 2020)

Q. 21. "Mouth is the mirror of health," discuss.
(UHSR, June 2020)

Q. 22. Osteoradionecrosis. *(CDER-AIIMS, June 2020)*

Q. 23. Oral manifestations of HIV. *(PAHER, July 2020)*

Q. 24. AIDS in children. *(RUHS, June 2020)*

Q. 25. Autoimmune disease. *(PAHER, July 2020)*

Q. 26. Significance of viral diseases in dentistry.
(PAHER, July 2020)

Q. 27. Blood disorders. *(PAHER, July 2020)*

Q. 28. Dry socket. *(KNRUHS, June 2020)*

Q. 29. Lower lip parasthesia. *(KNRUHS, June 2020)*

Q. 30. Trigeminal neuralgia. *(RUHS, June 2020)*

Q. 31. Periapical cyst. *(MUHS, July 2020)*

Q. 32. Add a note on xerostomia and its pharmacological management. *(KUHS, July 2020)*

Q. 33. Aphthous ulcers. *(UHSR, June 2020)*

Q. 34. Anaemia. *(RUHS, June 2020).*
Q. Management of anaemia. *(MUHS, July 2020)*

Q. 35. Denture stomatitis and its management.
(MUHS, July 2020)

Q. 36. Xerostomia and its effects on prosthodontics treatment. *(MUHS, July 2020)*

Q. 37. Write about pathophysiology of residual ridge.
(MUHS, July 2020)

Q. 38. Wallerian degeneration. *(UOK, Aug. 2020)*

Q. 39. Osteomyelitis of jaw. *(BFUHS, July 2020)*

Q. 40. Hyperglycemia and its significance in medical history. *(BFUHS, July 2020)*

Q. 41. Write a note on gingival enlargement of and its management. *(BFUHS, July 2020)*

Q. 42. Primary herpetic gingivostomatitis.
(BFUHS, July 2020)

PHARMACOLOGY

Q. 1. Classify anti-inflammatory agents. Write a note on merits and demerits of each. *(RUHS, June 2020)*

Q. 2. NSAIDs. *(PAHER Uni., July 2020)*

Q. 3. Analgesics and anti-inflammatory drugs used in dentistry. *(Manipal Uni., July 2020)*

Q. 4. Management of dental pain during endodontic treatment. *(MUHS, July 2020)*

Q. 5. Selective COX-2 inhibitors and their mechanism of action. *(RGUHS, July 2020)*

Q. 6. Analgesics for pediatric dental patients. *(NTR Uni., Sept. 2020)*

Q. 7. Emergency drugs used in dentistry. *(KNRUHS, June 2020)*

Q. 8. Antioxidants. *(RGUHS, July 2020)*

Q. 9. Discuss drugs affecting orthodontic treatment. *(RUHS, June 2020)*

Q. 10. Adverse drug reactions. *(RUHS, June 2020)*

Q. 11. Describe the principles of antibiotic therapy. Add a note on factors influencing the selection of antibiotics. *(RUHS, June 2020; MUHS, July 2020; UOK, Aug. 2020)*

Q. 12. Role of broad spectrum antibiotics in orofacial infections. *(MUHS, July; NTR Uni., Aug. 2020)*

Q. 13. Discuss the antibiotics used in dentistry. *(UHSR, June 2020)*

Q. 14. Antibiotic resistance. *(KUHS, July 2020)*

Q. 15. Hemostatics used in dentistry. *(UHSR, June 2020)*

Q. 16. Local anesthetics. *(RUHS, Yenepoya Uni., June 2020)*

Q. 17. Side effects of long-term corticosteroid therapy. *(RGUHS, July 2020)*

Q. 18. Corticosteroids. *(RUHS, June 2020; BFUHS, July 2020)*

Q. 19. Dental implications of immune suppressive therapy. *(RUHS, June 2020)*

Q. 20. Antiviral drugs. *(NTR Uni., Aug. 2020)*

Q. 21. Antifungal drugs. *(UHSR, June 2020; NTR Uni., Sept. 2020)*

Q. 22. Antisialogogues. *(MUHS, July 2020)*

Q. 23. Mention factors modifying drug action. *(BFUHS, July 2020; NTR Uni., Sept. 2020)*

Q. 24. Chlorhexidine and its uses in dentistry. *(NTR Uni.. Sept. 2020)*

Q. 25. Management of patient suffering from hepatitis B for oral surgical procedure. *(BFUHS, July 2020)*

BIOSTATISTICS AND RESEARCH METHODOLOGY

Q. 1. Define biostatistics. Discuss various methods of summarization of data. *(KLE Uni., July 2020)*

Q. 2. Discuss various types of research and explain research protocol in detail. *(Manipal Uni., July 2020)*

Q. 3. What is sample? Discuss in detail about various sampling techniques used in research. *(RUHS, June 2020)*

Q. 4. Write on sampling and sampling designs in scientific research. *(MUHS, July 2020; NTR Uni., Sept. 2020)*

Q. 5. General principles of research methodology. *(People's Uni., Aug. 2020)*

Q. 6. Ethical considerations of research. *(UHSR, June 2020)*

Q. 7. Parametric and nonparametric tests. *(PAHER, July 2020)*

Q. 8. Qualitative research. *(PAHER, July 2020)*

Q. 9. What is H-index, i-10 index and G-index? *(Manipal Uni., July 2020)*

Q. 10. Tests of significance. *(RUHS, UHSR, June 2020)*

Q. 11. What is chi-square test? *(RUHS, June 2020)*

Q. 12. Case control studies. *(UHSR, June 2020)*

Q. 13. Data collection. *(MUHS, July 2020)*

Q. 14. Statistics. *(UOK, Aug 2020)*

Q. 15. Randomized controlled trials. *(NTR Uni., Sept. 2020)*

Q. 16. Write a note on research tools and data collection methods. *(BFJHS, July 2020)*

Q. 17. Describe in brief the concept of evidence based dentistry. *(BFUHS, July 2020)*

DENTAL MATERIALS

Q. 1. Recent advances in dental ceramics.
(RUHS, June 2020; MUHS, July 2020)

Q. 2. Methods for testing biocompatibility of dental materials. *(RUHS, June 2020)*

Q. 3. Discuss about the biomaterials used in dental implants. *(RUHS, June 2020)*

Q. 4. Write a note on polymerization shrinkage and its management. *(RUHS, June 2020)*

Q. 5. Discuss current orthodontic bonding materials.
(RUHS, June 2020)

Q. 6. Describe the evolution and recent trends in dental ceramics. *(People's Uni., Aug. 2020)*

Q. 7. Colour science applied to prosthodontics.
(UOK, People's Uni., Aug.2020)

Q. 8. Casting machines. *(People's Uni., Aug.2020)*

Q. 9. Inlay waxes. *(MUHS, July 2020)*

Q. 10. Tarnish and corrosion.
(BFUHS, MUHS, July 2020)

Q. 11. Colour changing composite.
(UHSR, June 2020)

Q. 12. Coefficient of correlation. *(UHSR, June 2020)*

Q. 13. Von Mise's stress. *(UHSR, June 2020)*

Q. 14. Annealing. *(UHSR, June 2020)*

Q. 15. Ceramic steel. *(UHSR, June 2020)*

Q. 16. Chairside reliners. *(UHSR, June 2020)*

Q. 17. Glass ionomer cement. *(MUHS, July 2020)*

Q. 18. Discuss various suture materials used in oral surgery. *(MUHS, July 2020)*

Q. 19. Die materials and die systems.
(MUHS, July 2020)

Q. 20. Denture adhesives. *(UOK, Aug. 2020)*

Q. 21. Discuss anticariogenic materials.
(NTR Uni., Sept. 2020)

Q. 22. Biocompatibility tests for dental materials.
(NTR Uni., Sept. 2020)

Q. 23. Castable ceramics. *(BFUHS, July 2020)*

GENETICS AND MISCELLANEOUS

Q. 1. Recent advances in genetics.

Q. 2. Stem cells.

Q. 3. Discuss epidemiology of dentofacial traits.
(RUHS, June 2020)

Q. 4. Discuss importance of genetics in orthodontics.
(RUHS, June 2020)

Q. 5. Regulation of gene function. *(KUHS, July 2020)*

Q. 6. Syncope. *(KUHS, July 2020)*

Q. 7. Evolution of face. *(NTR Uni., Sept. 2020)*

Q. 8. Twin studies. *(NTR Uni., Sept. 2020)*

Q. 9. Gene mapping. *(NTR Uni., Sept. 2020)*

Suggested Reading

Anatomy, Embryology and Histology

1. Lipski M, Tomaszewska IM, Lipska W, Lis GJ, Tomaszewski KA. The mandible and its foramen: Anatomy, anthropology, embryology and resulting clinical implications. Folia Morphol (Warsz). 2013; 72(4):285–92.
2. Owusu JA, Stewart CM, Boahene K. Facial Nerve Paralysis. Med Clin North Am. 2018;102(6):1135–1143.
3. Smith KK. The evolution of mammalian development. Bull Mus Comp Zool 2001;156:119–35.
4. Alomar X, Medrano J, Cabratosa J, Clavero JA, Lorente M, Serra I, Monill JM, Salvador A. Anatomy of the temporomandibular joint. Semin. Ultrasound CT MR. 2007;28(3):70–83.
5. House JW, Brackmann DE. Facial nerve grading system. Otolaryngol Head Neck Surg. 1985;93(2):146–7.
6. Patel VN, Hoffman MP. Salivary gland development: a template for regeneration. Semin. Cell Dev. Biol. 2014;26:52–60.
7. Singh TP, Bala S, Kalsey G, Singla RK. Applied anatomy of Fascial spaces in Head and neck. J Anat Soc India. 2000; 49(1):78–88.
8. Grégoire V, Ang K, Budach W, Grau C, Hamoir M, Langendijk JA, Lee A, Le QT, Maingon P, Nutting C, O'Sullivan B, Porceddu SV, Lengele B. Delineation of the neck node levels for head and neck tumors: a 2013 update. DAHANCA, EORTC, HKNPCSG, NCIC CTG, NCRI, RTOG, TROG consensus guidelines. Radiother Oncol. 2014; 110(1):172–81.
9. BD Chaurasia's Human Anatomy, Vol-3 (Head-Neck and Brain). 6th Edition.
10. Inderbir Singh's Human Embryology. 10th Edition.
11. Inderbir Singh's Textbook of Human Histology. 7th Edition.
12. K.Sembulingam, Prema Sembulingam. Essentials of Medical Physiology, 6th Edition.
13. Harvey B. Sarnat, Laura Flores Sarnat. Embryology of the neural crest: Its inductive role in neurocutaneous syndrome. J Clin Neurology. 2005;20:637.

Dental Anatomy and Dental Histology

1. Almonnaitiene R, Balciuniene I, Tutkuviene J. Factor's influencing permanent teeth eruption. Stomatologija, Baltic Dental and Maxillofacial Journal. 2010;12: 67–72.
2. Santosh AB, Jones TJ. The epithelial-mesenchymal interactions: Insights into physiological and pathological aspects of oral tissues. Oncol Rev. 2014;8(1):239.
3. Presland RB, Dale BA. Epithelial structural proteins of the skin and oral cavity: Function in health and disease. Crit Rev Oral Biol Med 2000;11(4):383–408
4. Avila Rodríguez MI, Rodríguez Barroso LG, Sánchez ML. Collagen: A review on its sources and potential cosmetic applications. J Cosmet Dermatol 2018;17:20–6.
5. GS Kumar. Orban's Oral Histology and Embryology. 2nd Edition. 2019. Elsevier India.
6. Wheeler's Dental Anatomy, Physiology and Occlusion. Stanley J. Nelson. 1st Edition. 2015. Elsevier India.
7. Ten Cate's Oral Histology-Development, structure and function-Antonio Nanci. 8th Edition. Mosby
8. Newman and Carranza's Clinical Periodontology. 13th Edition. Saunder 2019.
9. Clinical Outline of Oral Pathology. Lewis R. Eversole. 4th Edition.2012. CBS Publishers and Distributors. New Delhi.
10. Contemporary Orthodontics by Proffit. 6th Edition. 2018. Mosby

Physiology

1. O'Grady NP, Barie PS, Bartlett JG, et al. Guidelines for evaluation of new fever in critically ill adult patients: 2008 update from the American College of Critical Care Medicine and the Infectious Diseases Society of America. Crit Care Med. 2008; 36:1330–49.
2. Yaddanapudi S, Yaddanapudi L. Indications for blood and blood product transfusion. Indian J Anaesth. 2014;58(5):538–42. doi:10.4103/0019-5049.144648.
3. Melissa Chudow, Michelle Carter, Mark Rumbak. Pharmacological Treatments for Acute Respiratory Distress Syndrome. American Association of Critical-Care Nurses. 2015;26(3);185–191.
4. Vila T, Rizk AM, Sultan AS, Jabra-Rizk MA. The power of saliva: Antimicrobial and beyond. PLoS Pathog. 2019;15(11):e1008058.
5. Herenia P, Lawrence Salivary markers of systemic disease: noninvasive diagnosis of disease and

monitoring of general health J Can Dent Assoc 2002; 68(3):170–4.

6. Review of Medical Physiology: Ganong. 26th Edition. 2019.

7. Gyton and Hall Textbook of Medical Physiology. 2nd South Asia Edition. 2016.

8. Das S. Concise textbook of Surgery. 10th Edition. 2008.

9. Harrison's Principle of Internal Medicine. 19th Edition. 2015.

10. Bell's orofacial pain: Guidelines for Assessment, Diagnosis and Management. 7th Edition

11. K. Sembulingam, Prema Sembulingam. Essentials of Medical Physiology, 6th Edition.

12. Burket's Oral medicine. 12th Edition.

13. Neelima A. Malik. Textbook of Oral and Maxillofacial Surgery. 3rd Edition.

Biochemistry

1. Muenzer J. Overview of the mucopolysaccharidoses. Rheumatology. 2011;50:v4–v12.

2. Bhattacharya PT, Misra SR, Hussain M. Nutritional Aspects of Essential Trace Elements in Oral Health and Disease: An Extensive Review. Scientifica (Cairo). 2016;2016:5464373. doi:10.1155/2016/5464373

3. Palmer CA. Gerodontic nutrition and dietary counseling for prosthodontic patients. Dent Clin N Am 2003;47:355–71.

4. American Diabetes Association. Classification and diagnosis of diabetes: Standards of Medical Care in Diabetes-2019. Diabetes Care. 2019;42(Suppl. 1):S13–S28.https://doi.org/10.2337/dc19-S002

5. World Health Organization: Definition, Diagnosis and Classification of Diabetes Mellitus and its Complications: Report of a WHO Consultation. Part 1: Diagnosis and Classification of Diabetes Mellitus. Geneva, World Health Org., 1999.

6. Vasudevan DM, Sreekumari S, Vaidyanathan K. Textbook of biochemistry for dental students. JP Medical Ltd., 2011.

7. Badwal RS, Bennett J. Nutritional considerations in the surgical patient. Dent Clin North Am. 2003; 47:373–93.

8. Satyanarayana U, Chakrapani U. Fundamentals of Biochemistry. Books and Allied Ltd. 2008. Kolkata, India, 2nd Edition, 2008.

9. Soben Peter. Essentials of Public Health Community Dentistry. 5th Edition.

Microbiology

1. Walker DM. Oral mucosal immunology: An Overview. Ann Acad Med 2004;33:27S–30S

2. Upendran A, Geiger Z. Dental Infection Control. [Updated 2020 Feb 17]. In: StatPearls [Internet].

Treasure Island (FL): StatPearls Publishing; 2020 Jan. Available from: https://www.ncbi.nlm.nih.gov/books/NBK470356/

3. Yoo JH. Review of Disinfection and Sterilization-Back to the Basics. Infect Chemother. 2018;50(2): 101–109.

4. Lehner T. Immunology of dental caries. Immunology of oral diseases. 3rd Edition. Blackwell scientific publications; 1992.

5. CDC. Immunization of Health-Care Personnel: Recommendations of the Advisory Committee on Immunization Practices (ACIP). MMWR, 2011; 60 (RR-7).

6. Silindir M, Ozer AY. Sterilization methods and the comparison of E-Beam sterilization with Gamma Radiation sterilization. FABAD J Pharm Sci. 2009; 34:43–53.

7. Wilson AP, Treasure T, Sturridge MF, Gruneberg RN. A scoring method (ASEPSIS) for postoperative wound infections for use in clinical trials of antibiotic prophylaxis. Lancet 1986;1(8476): 311–3.

8. Rao S.www.microrao.com

9. Dey NC, Dey TK, Sinha D. Medical Bacteriology Including Medical Mycology and AIDS. 17th Edition. Kolkata, India: New Central Book Agency; 2004.

10. Ananthanarayan and Paniker's Textbook of Microbiology. 9th Edition.

11. Richard G Topazian, Morton H Goldberg, James R. Hupp. Oral and Maxillofacial Infections. 4th Edition.

12. Surinder Kumar. Textbook of Microbiology. 1st Edition.

13. Grossman's Endodontic Practice. 13th Edition.

Pathology

1. Harshmohan's Textbook of Pathology, 7th Edition.

2. Shafer's Textbook of Oral Pathology, 7th Edition.

3. Burket's Oral medicine, 12th Edition.

4. Norman K. Wood, Paul W. Goaz. Differential Diagnosis of Oral and Maxillofacial Lesions, 5th Edition.

5. Neelima A. Malik. Textbook of Oral and Maxillofacial Surgery, 3rd Edition.

6. K. Sembulingam, Prema Sembulingam. Essentials of Medical Physiology, 6th Edition.

7. Davidson's Principles and Practice of Medicine, 22nd Edition.

8. Promod John. Textbook of Oral medicine, 3rd Edition.

9. Oliver RJ, Sloan P, Pemberton MN. Oral biopsies: methods and applications. British Dental Journal 2004;196:329.

10. Hazar Shekarchizadeh, Mohammed R Khami, Simin Z. Mohebbi, Hamed Ekhtiari, Jorma I Virtanen.

Oral Health of Drug Abusers: A Review of Health Effects and Care. Iranian Journal of Public Health 2013;42(9):929–940.

11. Joel B Epstein. The Mouth: A Window on Systemic Disease. Canadian Family Physician 1980;26:953–957.

12. Jayanthi P, Priya Thomas, Bindhu PR, Rekha Krishnapillai. Prion Diseases in Humans: Oral and Dental Implications. North American Journal of Medical Sciences 2013;5(7):399–403.

13. Stephen R Porter. Prions and Dentistry. Journal of Royal Society of Medicine. 2002;95(4):178–181.

14. Ryungsa Kim, Manabu Emi, Kazuaki Tanabe. Cancer immune-editing from immune surveillance to immune escape 2007;121:1–14.

15. Amin MB, Edge SB, Greene FL, et al. (Eds). AJCC Cancer Staging Manual. 8th edn. New York: Springer; 2017.

Pharmacology

1. Paderni C, Compilato D, Giannola LI, Campisi G. Oral local drug delivery and new perspectives in oral drug formulation. Oral Surg Oral Med Oral Pathol Oral Radiol. 2012;114:e25–e34.

2. Craig DC. Royal College of Anaesthetists, Royal College of Surgeons of England. Conscious sedation for dentistry: An update. Br Dent J. 2007;203: 629–31.

3. Surbhi Leekha, MBBS; Christine L. Terrell, MD; and Randall S. Edson. General Principles of Antimicrobial Therapy. Mayo Clin Proc. 2011;86(2):156–167.

4. Flynn TR, Halpern LR. Antibiotic selection in head and neck infections. Oral and Maxillo Facial Surg Clinics of North America 2003;15(1):17–38.

5. Golub LM, Suomalainen K, Sorsa T. Host modulation with tetracyclines and their chemically modified analogues. Curr Opin Dent 1992;2:8090.

6. Wilson W, Taubert KA, Gewitz M, et al. Prevention of infective endocarditis: Guidelines from the American Heart Association: A guideline from the American Heart Association Rheumatic Fever, Endocarditis, and Kawasaki Disease Committee, Council on Cardiovascular Disease in the Young, and the Council on Clinical Cardiology, Council on Cardiovascular Surgery and Anesthesia, and the Quality of Care and Outcomes Research Inter-disciplinary Working Group. Circulation 2007; 116(15):1736–54.

7. Zhanel GG, Sniezek G, Schweizer F, Zelenitsky S, Lagacé-Wiens PR, Rubinstein E, Gin AS, Hoban DJ, Karlowsky JA. Ceftaroline: A novel broad-spectrum cephalosporin with activity against meticillin-resistant Staphylococcus aureus. Drugs. 2009;69(7):809–31.

8. Romero-Reyes M, Uyanik JM. Orofacial pain management: Current perspectives. J Pain Res. 2014;7:99115. Published 2014 Feb 21. doi:10.2147/JPR.S37593

9. Tyrovola JB, Spyropoulos MN. Effects of drugs and systemic factors on orthodontic treatment. Quintessence Int, 2001;32(5):365–71.

10. Alok Sharma, et al. "Antioxidants in Dentistry: A Review". EC Dental Science. 2016;34:580–584.

11. Daniel E Becker. Emergency Drug Kits: Pharmacological and Technical Considerations. Anesth Prog. 2014;61(4):171–179.

12. Stamatova I, Meurman JH. Probiotics: Health benefits in the mouth. Am J Dent. 2009;22:329–38.

13. Pastino A, Lakra A. Patient Controlled Analgesia (PCA) [Updated 2019 Dec 8]. In: StatPearls [Internet]. Treasure Island (FL): StatPearls Publishing; 2020 Jan. Available from: https://www.ncbi.nlm.nih.gov/books/NBK551610/

14. Nogales CG, Ferrari PH, Kantorovich EO, Lage-Marques JL. Ozone therapy in medicine and dentistry. J Contemporary Dental Practice. 2008; 9(4):75.

15. Padmaja Udaykumar. Textbook of Pharmacology for Dental and Allied Health Sciences. 2nd Edition 2007.

16. K.D. Tripathi's Essential of Medical Pharmacology. 7th Edition.

17. Tara Shanbhag, Smita Shenoy, Veena Nayak. Pharmacology for Dentistry. 2nd Edition.

18. Davidson's Principles and Practice of Medicine. 22nd Edition.

Biostatistics, Research Methodology and Ethics

1. Elfil M, Negida A. Sampling methods in Clinical Research; an Educational Review. Emerg (Tehran). 2017;5(1):e52.

2. In J Lee S. Statistical data presentation. Korean J Anesthesiol. 2017;70(3):267276.

3. Thomas MV, Straus SE. Evidence-Based Dentistry and the Concept of Harm. Dent Clin N Am. 2009;53: 23–32.

4. Pandey A, Roy N, Bhawsar R, Mishra RM. Health Information System in India: Issues of Data Availability and Quality. Demography India 2010;39(1): 111–128.

5. Struillou X, Boutigny H, Soueidan A, Layrolle P. Experimental animal models in periodontology: A review. Open Dent J. 2010;4:37–47.

6. Martin Schittek, Nikos Mattheos, HC Lyon, Rolf Attström. Computer assisted learning. A Review. European Journal of Dental Education. 2001;5:93–100.

7. Walsh LJ. The current status of low level laser therapy in dentistry. Part 1 Soft tissue applications. Australian Dental Journal. 1997;42(4):247–254.

8. Walsh LJ. The current status of low level laser therapy in dentistry. Part 2 Hard tissue applications. Australian Dental Journal. 1997;42(5):302–306.
9. Mahajan BK. Methods in Biostatistics. 7th Edition.
10. Soben Peter. Essentials of Public Health Community Dentistry. 5th Edition.
11. Kothari CL. Research Methodology: Methods and Techniques. 2nd Edition. 2004.

Dental Material

1. Yeli M, Kidiyoor KH, Nain B, Kumar P. Recent advances in composite resins-A review. J Oral Res Rev 2010;2:8–14.
2. Zinelis S, Eliades T, Eliades G, Makou M, Silikas N. Comparative assessment of the roughness, hardness and wear resistance of aesthetic brackets materials. Dental Materials 2005;21:890–94.
3. Slavkin HC. Biomimetics: replacing body parts is no longer science fiction, J Am Dent Assoc, 1996; 127:1254–1257.
4. Malkondu O, Kazandag MK, Kazazoglu E. A review on Biodentine, a contemporary Dentine Replacement and repair material. Biomed Res Int 2014;1–10.
5. Hepdarcan SS, Yýlmaz RBN, Nalbantgil D. Which Orthodontic Wire and Working Sequence Should be Preferred for Alignment Phase? A Review. Turk J Orthod. 2016;29(2):4750. doi:10.5152/TurkJ Orthod. 2016.160009
6. Raghavendra SS, Jadhav GR, Gathani KM, Kotadia P. Bioceramics in endodontics-a review. J Istanb Univ Fac Dent. 2017;51(3 Suppl 1):S128–S137.
7. Qureshi A, ES Nandakumar, Pratapkumar, Sambashivarao. Recent advances in pulp capping materials: an overview. J Clin Diagn Res. 2014;8(1): 316321. doi:10.7860/JCDR/2014/7719.3980
8. Ma. del Socorro Islas Ruiz; Miguel Ángel Noyola Frías DDS; Ricardo Martínez Rider; Amaury PozosGuillén, Arturo Garrocho Rangel. Fundamentals of Stereolithography, an Useful Tool for Diagnosis in Dentistry. http://dx.doi.org/10.15517/ijds.v0i0.20730
9. Mannappalli JJ. Basic Dental Materials. 4th Edition. 2016.
10. Mahalaxmi S. Materials Used in Dentistry. 2nd Edition. 2018. Wolters Kluwer India Private Limited.
11. Anusavice KJ. Philips' Science of Dental Materials. 11th Edition. Elsevier, India. 2010;471–486.

Genetics and Miscellaneous

1. Ghergie M, Cocîrla E, Lupan I, Kelemen BS, Popescu O. Genes and dental disorders. Clujul Med. 2013;86(3): 196–199.
2. Griffiths AJF, Gelbart WM, Miller JH, et al. Modern Genetic Analysis. New York: W. H. Freeman; 1999. Human Pedigree Analysis. Available from: https://www.ncbi.nlm.nih.gov/books/NBK21257/
3. Leslie EJ, Marazita ML. Genetics of Cleft Lip and Cleft Palate. Am J Med Genet C Semin Med Genet. 2013 November; 163(4):246–258. doi:10.1002/ajmg.c.31381.
4. Ivens A, Flavin N, Williamson R. Dixon M, Bates G, Buckingham M, et al. The human homeobox gene HOX7 maps to chromosome 4p16.1 and may be implicated in Wolf-Hirschhorn syndrome. Hum Genet 1990; 84:473–76.
5. Siddique N, Raza H, Ahmed S, Khurshid Z, Zafar MS. Gene Therapy: A Paradigm Shift in Dentistry. Genes 2016;7:98; doi:10.3390/genes7110098.
6. Campanella V. Dental Stem Cells: Current research and future applications. Eur J Paediatr Dent. 2018 Dec; 19(4):257.
7. Ensanya Ali Abou Neel, Laurent Bozec, Roman A Perez, Hae-Won Kim, Jonathan C Knowles. Nano-technology in dentistry: prevention, diagnosis, and therapy. International Journal of Nanomedicine 2015;10:6371–6394.
8. Harold C. Slavkin, Mahvash Navazesh, Pragna Patel. Basic Principles of Human Genetics: A Primer for Oral Medicine. In Michael Glick, editor. Burket's Oral Medicine. People's Medical Publishing House-USA 2015. 12th Ed. P. 625–651.
9. Proffit WR. Contemporary orthodontics. 4th Edition. St Louis: Mosby, 2007.
10. Gangane SD. Human Genetics. 4th Edition. 2012. Elsevier.
11. Shobha Tandon. Textbook of Pedodontics. 2nd Edition. 2008
12. Damle SG. Textbook of Pediatric Dentistry. 4th Edition.